ESSENTIALS OF CLINICAL
RADIATION ONCOLOGY

ESSENTIALS OF CLINICAL RADIATION ONCOLOGY

Third Edition

Editors

Jenna E. Kocsis, MD
Chief Resident
Department of Radiation Oncology
Cleveland Clinic Foundation
Cleveland, Ohio

Sarah M. C. Sittenfeld, MD
Assistant Professor
Department of Radiation Oncology
University of Cincinnati
Cincinnati, Ohio

Matthew C. Ward, MD
Adjunct Assistant Professor
Department of Radiation Oncology
Levine Cancer Institute
Atrium Health
Charlotte, North Carolina

Rahul D. Tendulkar, MD, FASTRO
Professor
Cleveland Clinic Lerner College of Medicine
Staff Physician
Department of Radiation Oncology
Cleveland Clinic Foundation
Cleveland, Ohio

Gregory M. M. Videtic, MD, CM, FRCPC, FACR, FASTRO
Professor of Medicine
Cleveland Clinic Lerner College of Medicine
Staff Physician
Department of Radiation Oncology
Cleveland Clinic Foundation
Cleveland, Ohio

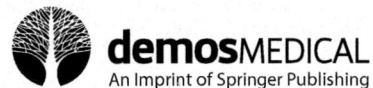

demosMEDICAL
An Imprint of Springer Publishing

Springer Publishing Company, LLC
902 Carnegie Center/Suite 140, Princeton, NJ 08540
www.springerpub.com
connect.springerpub.com

Acquisitions Editor: David D'Addona
Production Editor: Joe Stubenrauch
Compositor: Exeter Premedia Services Private Limited.

ISBN: 978-0-8261-5456-9
e-book ISBN: 978-0-8261-9199-1
DOI: 10.1891/9780826191991

25 26 27 28 / 5 4 3 2 1

Medicine is an ever-changing science. Research and clinical experience are continually expanding our knowledge, in particular our understanding of proper treatment and drug therapy. The authors, editors, and publisher have made every effort to ensure that all information in this book is in accordance with the state of knowledge at the time of production of the book. Nevertheless, the authors, editors, and publisher are not responsible for any errors or omissions or for any consequence from application of the information in this book and make no warranty, expressed or implied, with respect to the content of this publication. Every reader should examine carefully the package inserts accompanying each drug and should carefully check whether the dosage schedules therein or the contraindications stated by the manufacturer differ from the statements made in this book. Such examination is particularly important with drugs that are either rarely used or have been newly released on the market.

The work is provided, "as is," and the publisher disclaims any and all warranties, express or implied, including any warranties as to accuracy, comprehensiveness, or currency of the content of this work or any information that can be accessed through the work via a hyperlink or otherwise, the persistence and accuracy of which is hereby disclaimed. Neither the publisher nor its licensors shall be liable to you or anyone else for any inaccuracy, error or omission, regardless of cause, in the work or for any damages resulting therefrom.

Library of Congress Control Number: 2025023804

Publisher's Note: **New and used products purchased from third-party sellers are not guaranteed for quality, authenticity, or access to any included digital components.**

Printed in the United States of America by Gasch Printing.

To the enduring commitment of past, present, and future residents in the pursuit of knowledge, without whom this work would not have been possible.

CONTENTS

XIII. BENIGN DISEASES

CONTRIBUTORS

Salem Alfaifi, MD, FRCPC, Staff Physician, Department of Radiation Oncology, Taussig Cancer Center, Cleveland Clinic Foundation, Cleveland, Ohio

Katherine R. Amarell, MD, Resident Physician, Department of Radiation Oncology, Taussig Cancer Center, Cleveland Clinic Foundation, Cleveland, Ohio

Sudha R. Amarnath, MD, Assistant Professor of Medicine, Department of Radiation Oncology, Taussig Cancer Center, Cleveland Clinic Foundation, Cleveland, Ohio

Carryn M. Anderson, MD, FASTRO, Clinical Professor, Department of Radiation Oncology, University of Iowa Health Care, Iowa City, Iowa

Ehsan H. Balagamwala, MD, Assistant Professor, Cleveland Clinic, Cleveland, Ohio

Cole Billena, MD, Resident Physician, Department of Radiation Oncology, Cleveland Clinic Foundation, Cleveland, Ohio

Anirudh Bommireddy, MD, Resident Physician, Department of Radiation Oncology, Taussig Cancer Center, Cleveland Clinic Foundation, Cleveland, Ohio

James R. Broughman, MD, Resident Physician, Department of Radiation Oncology, Taussig Cancer Center, Cleveland Clinic Foundation, Cleveland, Ohio

David S. Buchberger, MD, MSc, Resident Physician, Department of Radiation Oncology, Taussig Cancer Center, Cleveland Clinic Foundation, Cleveland, Ohio

Shauna R. Campbell, DO, Assistant Professor, Department of Radiation Oncology, Taussig Cancer Center, Cleveland Clinic Foundation, Cleveland, Ohio

Samuel T. Chao, MD, Professor at CCLCM at Case Western Reserve University, Department of Radiation Oncology, Rose Ella Burkhardt Brain Tumor and Neuro-Oncology Center, Taussig Cancer Institute, Cleveland Clinic Foundation, Cleveland, Ohio

Sheen Cherian, MD, Assistant Professor, Cleveland Clinic Foundation, Cleveland, Ohio

Erik M. Davies, MD, MEd, Resident Physician, Department of Radiation Oncology, Taussig Cancer Center, Cleveland Clinic Foundation, Cleveland, Ohio

Christopher W. Fleming, MD, Associate Staff, Department of Radiation Oncology, Maroone Cancer Center, Cleveland Clinic Florida, Weston, Florida

Ahmed Halima, MD, Resident Physician, Department of Radiation Oncology, Taussig Cancer Center, Cleveland Clinic Foundation, Cleveland, Ohio

Jason W. D. Hearn, MD, Associate Professor, Department of Radiation Oncology, University of Michigan, Ann Arbor, Michigan

Nikhil P. Joshi, MD, Associate Professor, Department of Radiation Oncology, Rush University Medical Center, Chicago, Illinois

Aditya Juloori, MD, Assistant Professor, Department of Cellular and Radiation Oncology, University of Chicago, Chicago, Illinois

Sarah S. Kilic, MD, Radiation Oncologist, Arizona Oncology, Tucson, Arizona

Jeffrey A. Kittel, MD, Radiation Oncologist, Radiation Oncology Associates, Ltd.; Department of Radiation Oncology, Aurora St. Luke's Medical Center, Milwaukee, Wisconsin

Jana M. Kobeissi, MD, Resident Physician, Cleveland Clinic, Cleveland, Ohio

Jenna E. Kocsis, MD, Chief Resident, Department of Radiation Oncology, Cleveland Clinic Foundation, Cleveland, Ohio

Shlomo A. Koyfman, MD, Associate Professor, Director of Head and Neck and Skin Cancer Radiation, Cleveland Clinic, Cleveland, Ohio

Aryavarta M. S. Kumar, MD, PhD, Assistant Professor, Department of Radiation Oncology, Louis Stokes Cleveland VA Medical Center, Cleveland, Ohio

Gaurav Marwaha, MD, Associate Professor and Interim Chairperson, Department of Radiation Oncology, Rush University Medical Center, Chicago, Illinois

Zachary S. Mayo, MD, Resident Physician, Department of Radiation Oncology, Taussig Cancer Center, Cleveland Clinic Foundation, Cleveland, Ohio

Omar Y. Mian, MD, PhD, Associate Professor, Cleveland Clinic and Case Western Reserve University, Cleveland, Ohio

Jacob A. Miller, MD, Assistant Professor, Department of Radiation Oncology, Taussig Cancer Center, Cleveland Clinic Foundation, Cleveland, Ohio

Erin S. Murphy, MD, Associate Professor, Department of Radiation Oncology, Taussig Cancer Center, Cleveland Clinic Foundation, Cleveland, Ohio

Bryn M. Myers, MD, Resident Physician, Department of Radiation Oncology, Taussig Cancer Center, Cleveland Clinic Foundation, Cleveland, Ohio

Elizabeth E. Obi, MD, Resident Physician, Department of Radiation Oncology, Taussig Cancer Center, Cleveland Clinic Foundation, Cleveland, Ohio

Sean M. Parker, MD, Resident Physician, Cleveland Clinic, Cleveland, Ohio

Shireen Parsai, MD, Radiation Oncologist, Department of Radiation Oncology, Riverside Methodist Hospital, Columbus, Ohio

Praveen Pendyala, MD, Staff Physician, Department of Radiation Oncology, Taussig Cancer Center, Cleveland Clinic Foundation, Cleveland, Ohio

Yvonne D. Pham, MD, Radiation Oncologist, Department of Radiation Oncology, Saint Luke's Hospital, Kansas City, Missouri

Bindu V. Rusia, MD, Assistant Professor, Department of Radiation Oncology, Allegheny Health Network Cancer Institute, Pittsburgh, Pennsylvania

Jacob G. Scott, MD, DPhil, Staff Physician-Scientist, Department of Radiation Oncology, Taussig Cancer Center, Cleveland Clinic Foundation; Professor, Department of Molecular Medicine, Cleveland Clinic Lerner College of Medicine, Cleveland, Ohio

Chirag Shah, MD, Chair, Department of Radiation Oncology, Allegheny Health Network, Pittsburgh, Pennsylvania

Monica E. Shukla, MD, Associate Professor, Department of Radiation Oncology, Medical College of Wisconsin, Milwaukee, Wisconsin

Arun D. Singh, MD, Professor of Ophthalmology, Director of Department of Ophthalmic Oncology, Cole Eye Institute, Cleveland Clinic Foundation, Cleveland, Ohio

Sarah M. C. Sittenfeld, MD, Assistant Professor, Department of Radiation Oncology, University of Cincinnati, Cincinnati, Ohio

Timothy D. Smile, MD, Radiation Oncologist, Department of Radiation Oncology, OSF HealthCare Cancer Institute, Saint Francis Medical Center, Peoria, Illinois

Kevin L. Stephans, MD, Associate Professor, Department of Radiation Oncology, Taussig Cancer Center, Cleveland Clinic Foundation, Cleveland, Ohio

Abigail L. Stockham, MD, Consultant and Assistant Professor, Department of Radiation Oncology, Mayo Clinic, Rochester, Minnesota

John H. Suh, MD, Professor and Enterprise Chair, Department of Radiation Oncology, Taussig Cancer Center, Cleveland Clinic Foundation, Cleveland, Ohio

Rahul D. Tendulkar, MD, FASTRO, Professor, Cleveland Clinic Lerner College of Medicine; Staff Physician, Department of Radiation Oncology, Cleveland Clinic Foundation, Cleveland, Ohio

Martin C. Tom, MD, Assistant Professor, Department of Radiation Oncology, The University of Texas MD Anderson Cancer Center, Houston, Texas

Adannia N. Ufondu, MD, Resident Physician, Cleveland Clinic Radiation Oncology, Cleveland, Ohio

Andrew D. Vassil, MD, Staff Physician, Department of Radiation Oncology, Taussig Cancer Center, Cleveland Clinic Foundation, Cleveland, Ohio

Gregory M. M. Videtic, MD, CM, FRCPC, FACR, FASTRO, Professor of Medicine, Cleveland Clinic Lerner College of Medicine; Staff Physician, Department of Radiation Oncology, Cleveland Clinic Foundation, Cleveland, Ohio

Winston Vuong, MD, Resident Physician, Department of Radiation Oncology, Taussig Cancer Center, Cleveland Clinic Foundation, Cleveland, Ohio

Matthew C. Ward, MD, Adjunct Assistant Professor, Department of Radiation Oncology, Levine Cancer Institute, Atrium Health, Charlotte, North Carolina

Ian W. Winter, MD, Radiation Oncologist, Radiation Oncology Consultants, Ltd.; Department of Radiation Oncology, Advocate Lutheran General Hospital, Park Ridge, Illinois

Neil M. Woody, MD, MS, Assistant Professor, Department of Radiation Oncology, Taussig Cancer Institute, Cleveland Clinic Foundation, Cleveland, Ohio

Kailin Yang, MD, PhD, Resident Physician, Department of Radiation Oncology, Taussig Cancer Center, Cleveland Clinic Foundation, Cleveland, Ohio

Jennifer S. Yu, MD, PhD, Staff, Department of Radiation Oncology, Department of Cancer Biology, Burkhardt Brain Tumor and Neuro-Oncology Center, Cleveland Clinic Foundation; Associate Professor, Program Leader, Developmental Therapeutics Program, Co-Leader, Cancer Stem Cell Working Group, Case Comprehensive Cancer Center, Cleveland, Ohio

PREFACE

Essentials of Clinical Radiation Oncology was born out of the long-standing tradition in the Cleveland Clinic Radiation Oncology Residency program of preparing yearly "handouts" summarizing the most recent and high-yield data to complement the formal teaching curriculum. As recent graduates of the Cleveland Clinic residency program, we attest to their value not only in learning the basics of radiation oncology, but in our continued education as independent clinicians. It was with great pride that we shared the hard work of decades of residents with the broader radiation oncology community in the publication of our first and second editions, and we were pleased to receive validation of its worth from a diverse group of readers.

The field of radiation oncology is continually evolving, as developing data inform new treatment paradigms or updates established ones. With the third edition of *Essentials of Clinical Radiation Oncology*, we aim to keep pace with the changing clinical environment by providing readers with the most up-to-date studies and treatment approaches. We have included two new chapters to comprehensively cover the broadest range of clinical topics and added over 230 studies to the Evidence-Based Q&A sections.

While much has changed in the field over the past several years, the outstanding dedication of current Cleveland Clinic Radiation Oncology residents, recent graduates, and current faculty to education has remained strong. Without them, this update would not have been possible. It is with deep gratitude to these many coauthors and on their behalf that we now offer this present edition to the radiation oncology community. As with the prior editions, we appreciate readers' suggestions and welcome any feedback. We trust this resource will prove valuable to all practitioners in their continued efforts to provide excellent patient care.

Jenna E. Kocsis, MD
Sarah M.C. Sittenfeld, MD
Matthew C. Ward, MD
Rahul D. Tendulkar, MD, FASTRO
Gregory M. M. Videtic, MD, CM, FRCPC, FACR, FASTRO

ABOUT THE FORMAT OF THIS BOOK

The intention of this book is to serve as a resource for all levels of practitioners, from medical students to practicing physicians. Therefore, the reader will find clinically pertinent details starting from basic epidemiology and culminating in an evidence-based approach to important and up-to-date clinical questions. The front matter of each chapter contains information about the disease and its natural history. This includes a summary of the American Joint Committee on Cancer staging system (and other relevant risk stratification systems), printed in an abbreviated format intended for physician understanding. Next, general Treatment Paradigms are included in the midpart of each chapter to give the reader an overview of the role of each anticancer modality in the multidisciplinary care of the patient. Finally, the highlight of this resource is the Evidence-Based Q&A format of clinical studies presented to guide the reader through the most pertinent literature. Each study is block-quoted from the source with a quick-access citation to the original reference in combination with a condensed summary intended to highlight the pertinent findings. It should be noted that our intention with this book is to provide a manual of information useful to the clinician, rather than to be "prescriptive" in terms of staging, radiation delivery, or chemotherapy dosing. Our hope is that this format provides an efficient yet thorough method for practitioners to develop a deeper understanding of a disease and the current state of its treatment.

PART I: Central Nervous System

1 GLIOBLASTOMA, IDH-WILD-TYPE

Salem Alfaifi, Martin C. Tom, Jennifer S. Yu, and Samuel T. Chao

QUICK HIT In the 2021 WHO classification system, glioblastoma (GBM) is grade 4 and defined by IDH-wild-type gene status with presence of any one or more of the following: microvascular proliferation, necrosis, EGFR amplification, TERT promoter mutation, and/or chr 7 gain/chr 10 loss. GBM is the most common primary malignant brain tumor in adults and has a poor prognosis, with a median survival of ~14 months. Treatment is maximal safe resection with neurologic preservation followed by adjuvant RT + TMZ, followed by TMZ with or without tumor treating fields (TTF). The standard RT dose is 60 Gy/30 fx. The most common site of treatment failure is within or adjacent to the RT field. For older or frail patients, options include short-course RT ± TMZ, TMZ alone (particularly for MGMT promoter hypermethylated tumors), or best supportive care.

EPIDEMIOLOGY: Most common (50%) primary malignant brain tumor in adults.[1] Incidence: 3 to 4 cases per 100,000 or ~13,000 cases per year in the United States. Median age at diagnosis is 65, and the M:F ratio is ~1.5:1.[2,3]

ANATOMY: Diffusely infiltrative tumor that invades along white matter tracts. Location is dependent on the amount of white matter: 75% are supratentorial (31% temporal, 24% parietal, 23% frontal, 16% occipital), <20% multifocal (enhancing foci encompassed by FLAIR hyperintensity), 2% to 7% multicentric (enhancing foci with intervening FLAIR nonhyperintense normal brain).[4,5]

PATHOLOGY

Origin: Cell of origin is not clear but presumed to arise from neural stem cells and neural progenitor cells in subventricular zone.[6]

Grading and WHO Classification[2,7-11]: Historically, glioma type was based primarily on histopathologic appearance (e.g., oligodendroglioma with "fried egg appearance" and "chicken-wire vasculature" vs. astrocytoma with pleomorphic giant cells and prominent cytoplasmic processes). Grade was based on the presence or extent of anaplasia, mitotic activity, microvascular proliferation, and necrosis. Presence of microvascular proliferation and/or necrosis was typically enough to classify a glioma as grade 4. However, with advances in our understanding of the molecular basis of gliomas, major restructuring began with the WHO 2016 classification, and subsequently the WHO 2021 classification (Figure 1.1), which uses an integrated diagnosis based on both histopathologic appearance and molecular characteristics. To qualify as GBM, the tumor must lack an IDH mutation (i.e., IDH-wild-type) AND have any one or more of the following: microvascular proliferation, necrosis, EGFR amplification, TERT promoter mutation, and/or chr 7 gain/chr 10 loss. By definition, GBM is grade 4. The WHO 2016 classification previously had an entity termed "GBM, IDH-mutant"; however, in the WHO 2021 classification, this has been replaced with "astrocytoma, IDH-mutant, grade 4."

GENETICS

IDH1/2: IDH genes encode essential enzymes that participate in metabolic processes. Mutations in IDH1 and less commonly IDH2 are prevalent in different malignancies including gliomas (see Chapters 2 and 3). In the 2021 WHO classification, the diagnosis of GBM was restricted only to tumors that are IDH-wild-type and thus eliminated the term "Glioblastoma, IDH-mutant" from the 2016 classification.[11] However, it is worth noting that prior to molecular classification, IDH mutations were present in ~10% of GBMs and associated with increased age and secondary tumors that developed from previous low-grade gliomas.[9,13] Thus, many GBM clinical trials prior to molecular classification included patients with IDH mutations. IDH1 mutation is an independent positive prognostic factor in grade 4 gliomas (MS 27.4 months for IDH1-mutant vs. 14 months for IDH1-wildtype).[14,15]

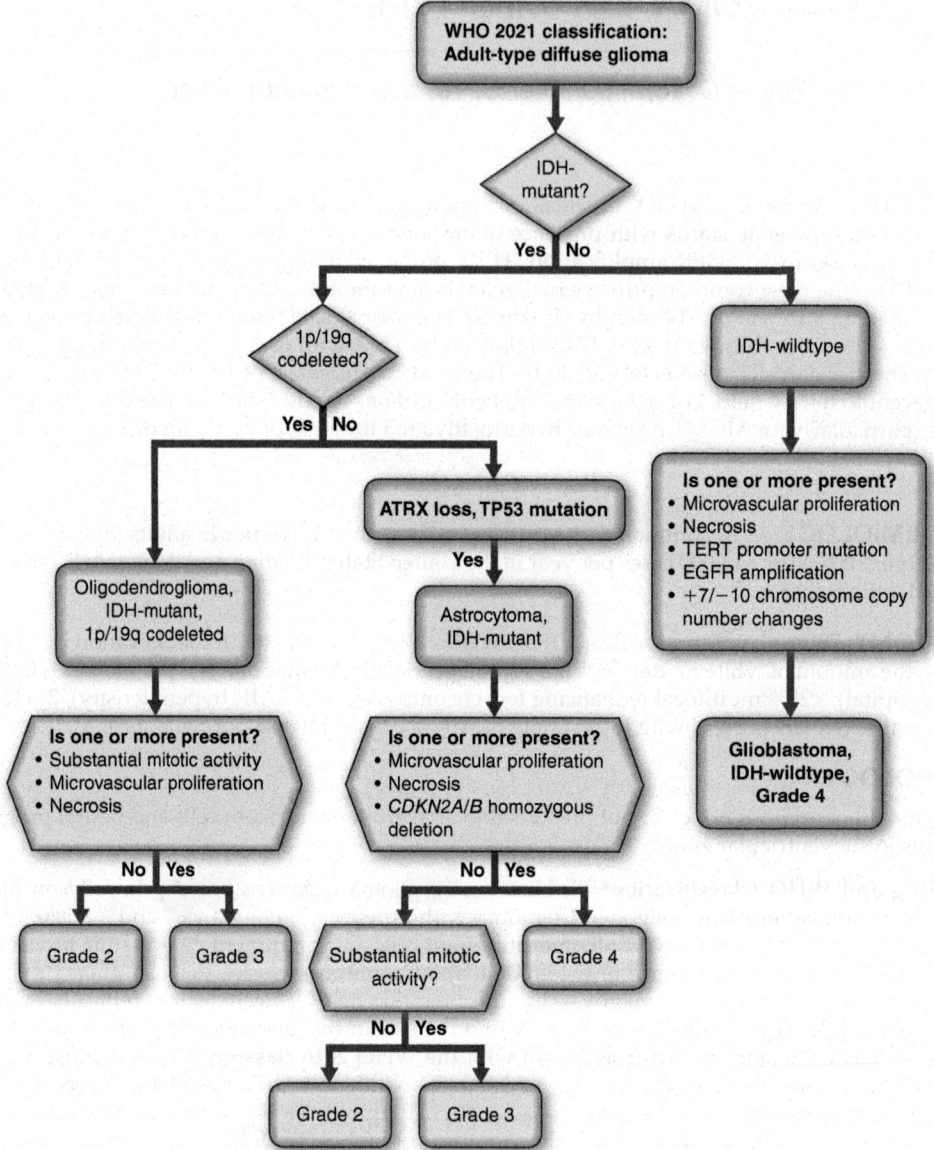

Figure 1.1 WHO 2021 CNS classification of adult diffuse gliomas.

Source: Adapted and modified from Halasz LM, Attia A, Bradfield L, et al. Radiation therapy for IDH-mutant grade 2 and grade 3 diffuse glioma: an ASTRO clinical practice guideline. *Pract Radiat Oncol.* 2022;12(5):370–386. doi:10.1016/j.prro.2022 .05.004.

EGFR/EGFRvIII: EGFR plays a central role in cell division, migration, adhesion, differentiation, and apoptosis. Amplification of EGFR and its active mutant EGFRvIII variant occurs frequently in GBM. EGFRvIII is an in-frame deletion of exons 2 to 7 of the EGFR gene affecting 801 base pairs and is an independent predictor of worse prognosis with standard CRT. Novel strategies to target EGFR/EGFRvIII-amplified GBM are evolving.[15–18] EGFR amplification is now one of the molecular defining features of GBM, IDH-wild-type.[11]

TERT Promoter Mutation: TERT encodes the catalytic subunit of the telomerase complex. TERT promoter mutation facilitates reactivation of telomerase, thereby maintaining telomere length that overcomes replicative senescence. TERT promoter mutation is a negative prognostic factor and is now one of the molecular defining features of GBM, IDH-wild-type.[11,15,19,20]

Chr 7 Gain and Chr 10 Loss: This chromosomal change is a negative prognostic factor and is also now one of the molecular defining features of GBM, IDH-wild-type.[11,15]

MGMT Promoter Methylation: O^6-methylguanine-DNA methyltransferase is located on chr 10q26. Its purpose is to repair alkylation of guanine at the O^6 position. When the promoter undergoes epigenetic silencing by methylation, the gene is downregulated, allowing greater efficacy of alkylating agents. MGMT promoter hypermethylation in GBM is predictive of response to alkylating agents. The Hegi study (see Evidence-Based Q&A) demonstrated that MGMT promoter hypermethylation is both a favorable prognostic and predictive factor. MGMT promoter hypermethylation is present in ~1/2 of patients (45% in the Hegi study, varies drastically).[15,21] MGMT promoter methylation status is not part of the WHO 2021 classification.

See Chapters 2 and 3 for a discussion of 1p19q codeletion, ATRX mutation, TP53 mutation, BRAF mutation, and CDKN2A/B homozygous deletion.

CLINICAL PRESENTATION: Headache (~70%), cognitive changes, seizure (good prognostic factor[22]), motor weakness, nausea/vomiting, visual loss, sensory loss, language disturbance, dysphagia, papilledema, gait disturbance, intracranial bleed (~5%) depending on tumor location.

WORKUP: H&P with neurologic exam. Fundoscopic exam (if suspicious of increased ICP).

Labs: CBC to establish baseline for CHT.

Imaging: MRI brain with and without gadolinium. GBMs are typically hypointense on T1 with heterogeneous contrast enhancement, central necrosis, and surrounding edema; T2/FLAIR hyperintense. Following surgical resection, obtain a postoperative MRI within 72 hours (ideally 24–48 hours) to determine the extent of resection and residual disease.

Pathology: Stereotactic or open biopsy with histopathologic and molecular assessment can be performed for unresectable tumors or an uncertain clinical diagnosis. Typically, if clinical findings are consistent with glioma, maximum safe resection is performed for both treatment and to establish the pathologic diagnosis without the need for biopsy.

PROGNOSTIC FACTORS: Clinical factors as established by Li et al.[23]: KPS, age, extent of resection, and neurologic function. MGMT promoter methylation status as well as other molecular markers discussed above. See Table 1.1 for RTOG RPA.

Table 1.1 RTOG RPA Classification for Glioblastoma			
RPA Class	**Defining Variables**	**MS (mos)**	**OS at 1, 3, and 5 Yrs**
III	<50 y/o and KPS ≥90	17.1	70%, 20%, 14%
IV	<50 y/o and KPS <90 ≥50 y/o, KPS ≥70, resection, and working	11.2	46%, 7%, 4%
V + VI	≥50 y/o, KPS ≥70, resection, and not working ≥50 y/o, KPS ≥70, biopsy only ≥50 y/o, KPS <70	7.5	28%, 1%, 0%

Source: From Li J, Wang M, Won M, et al. Validation and simplification of the radiation therapy oncology group recursive partitioning analysis classification for glioblastoma. *Int J Radiat Oncol Biol Phys.* 2011;81(3):623–630. doi:10.1016/j.ijrobp.2010 .06.012.

NATURAL HISTORY: GBMs, like other gliomas, are locally aggressive and frequently cause symptoms related to local progression, mass effect, and edema of surrounding tissue by alterations in permeability of blood–brain barrier.[24]

TREATMENT PARADIGM

Surgery: Primary treatment is surgical resection with the aim of maximal safe resection with neurologic preservation. For technically unresectable tumors, a biopsy is warranted to obtain tissue. Various tools may be applied to improve the safety of resection, such as intraoperative ultrasound/MRI, functional mapping (phase reversal, direct brain stimulation, awake anesthesia). To evaluate the extent of resection, obtain a contrast-enhanced MRI within 72 hours of surgery (ideally 24–48 hours) to avoid confounding with subacute blood products. Contraindications to GTR include eloquent/inaccessible areas involved (brainstem, motor cortex, language centers, etc.), significant infiltration past midline, periventricular or very diffuse lesions, and medical comorbidities.

Chemotherapy: As established in the Stupp trial,[25] TMZ 75 mg/m^2 daily with RT including weekends, followed by 150 to 200 mg/m^2 daily on days 1 to 5 of 28-day cycles, with the first cycle beginning 28 days after the completion of RT. Major side effects of TMZ are constipation, thrombocytopenia, and neutropenia. Patients treated with TMZ are sometimes given prophylaxis against pneumocystis pneumonia and can be given daily DS trimethoprim/sulfamethoxazole, or alternatively two pentamidine inhalation treatments during the RT course. TMZ is a prodrug converted to MTIC, which alkylates DNA. Numerous systemic therapies are under investigation, but only TMZ has demonstrated a clear survival benefit and remains the standard of care.

Radiation

Indications: Adjuvant RT after surgery improves OS vs. observation or CHT alone and is indicated in all patients with sufficient functional status to tolerate treatment.

Dose: 60 Gy/30 fx is standard. For older or frail individuals, various hypofractionated schemes have been investigated, including 40 Gy/15 fx, 34 Gy/10 fx, and 25 Gy/5 fx. In the palliative setting, RT is superior to best supportive care in terms of OS.

Toxicity: Common acute side effects may include fatigue, headache, exacerbation of presenting neurologic deficits, alopecia, skin erythema, nausea, memory changes, or cerebral edema. Late effects are dependent on tumor location but may include radiation necrosis, memory/cognitive changes, hearing loss, optic neuritis, cataracts, and hypopituitarism.

Procedure: See *Handbook of Treatment Planning in Radiation Oncology*, Chapter 3.[26]

EVIDENCE-BASED Q&A

What is considered optimal surgery for GBM?

Lacroix, MDACC (*J Neurosurg* 2001, PMID 11780887): RR showing improved OS with ≥98% resection in better prognostic patients (young, good KPS, no MRI evidence of necrosis). GTR also limits risk of cerebral edema during RT. **Conclusion: GTR with ≥98% resection improves OS, especially when other predictive variables are favorable.**

Karschnia, RANO Resect Group (*Neuro-Oncology* 2023, PMID 35961053): RR of 1,008 patients with newly diagnosed GBM assessing the impact of the extent of surgical resection on outcomes. The extent of resection was categorized according to RANO categories (Table 1.2). Lower absolute residual tumor volumes (in cm^3) were favorably associated with outcomes: Patients who underwent "maximal contrast-enhancement (CE) resection" (class 2) had better outcomes compared with those with "submaximal CE resection" (class 3) or "biopsy" (class 4). Extensive resection of non-CE tumor (≤5 cm^3 residual non-CE tumor) was associated with better survival among patients with complete CE resection, thus defining class 1 ("supramaximal CE resection"). The prognostic value of the resection classes was maintained on MVA when adjusting for molecular and clinical markers. **Conclusion: In newly diagnosed GBM, lower residual tumor volumes following surgical resection were favorably associated with outcomes.**

Table 1.2 RANO Categories for Extent of Resection in GBM[27]					
1: Supramaximal CE Resection	**2: Maximal CE Resection**			**3: Submaximal CE Resection**		**4: Biopsy**
	2A: Complete CE Resection	**2B: Near Total CE Resection**	**3A: Subtotal CE Resection**	**3B: Partial CE Resection**	
0 cm^3 CE + ≤5 cm^3 non-CE	0 cm^3 CE + >5 cm^3 non-CE	≤1 cm^3 CE	≤5 cm^3 CE	>5 cm^3 CE	No reduction of tumor volume
mPFS 11 months	mPFS 9 months		mPFS 8 months		mPFS 5 months
MS 24 months	MS 19 months		MS 15 months		MS 10 months

Source: Adapted from Karschnia P, Young JS, Dono A, et al. Prognostic validation of a new classification system for extent of resection in glioblastoma: a report of the RANO resect group. *Neuro Oncol.* 2023;25(5):940–954. doi:10.1093/neuonc/noac193.

How did we arrive at the current standard RT dose?

The BTCG 69-01[28] and 1981 SGSG[29] studies demonstrated a doubling of survival with adjuvant RT over best supportive care. Dose escalation was beneficial to 60 Gy/30 fx, but there was no benefit to escalating to 70 Gy. A subsequent University of Michigan experience[30] showed that escalating to 90 Gy still resulted in 90% in-field failures with an increase in toxicity. Thus, 60 Gy/30 fx is considered the standard dose for GBM. However, a single-arm phase I study from the University of Michigan has shown a promising median OS of 20.1 months with safe dose escalation to 75 Gy/30 fx along with concurrent and adjuvant TMZ.[31] This has raised the question again about the potential benefit of dose escalation in the TMZ era and has in part led to the ongoing NRG BN001 trial.

What chemotherapies have been used after surgery?

Historically, nitrosoureas were utilized until a meta-analysis of PRTs of RT vs. RT + nitrosoureas showed only modest 1-year OS benefit.[32] BCNU was the RTOG standard of care for many years. BCNU wafers (Gliadel) were investigated in a phase III trial of RT ± BCNU wafers: MS improved to 13.9 months vs. 11.8 months.[33] However, the survival advantage was possibly driven by grade 3 patients, and a subsequent 2007 meta-analysis suggested BCNU wafers are not effective or cost-effective in GBM.[34]

What trial defines the current standard of care in GBM management?

RT + concurrent and adjuvant TMZ is the standard of care based on the Stupp trial. TTF is discussed below as a separate Q&A.

Stupp, EORTC 26899/NCIC (*NEJM* 2005, PMID 15758009; Update *Lancet Oncol* 2009, PMID 19269895): PRT of 573 patients with GBM, ages 18 to 70 with ECOG PS 0 to 2. All patients received EBRT 60 Gy/30 fx and were randomized to RT alone or CRT with concurrent TMZ 75 mg/m^2 7 days per week and then adjuvant TMZ 150 to 200 mg/m^2 d1–5 q4 weeks × 6 cycles. Eighty-five percent completed CRT, and 47% of patients completed six cycles of adjuvant TMZ. OS and PFS were significantly improved (see Table 1.3) with the benefit holding across all subgroups. MGMT promoter hypermethylation was the strongest prognostic and predictive factor. **Conclusion: Concurrent CRT and adjuvant TMZ established as standard of care for GBM.**

Table 1.3 Stupp Trial Results, Including 2009 Update (All Differences Statistically Significant)				
	MS (mos)	**2-Yr PFS**	**2-Yr OS**	**5-Yr OS**
RT	12.1	2%	11%	2%
RT + TMZ	14.6	11%	27%	10%

What is the impact of MGMT promoter methylation status on the prognosis for GBM and their response to TMZ?

MGMT promoter hypermethylation is both prognostic (better outcome regardless of treatment) and predictive (better response to a specific treatment—TMZ in this case) for GBM.

Hegi (*NEJM* 2005, PMID 15758010): Subset analysis of 206 GBM patients in the Stupp trial, 45% of whom had epigenetic silencing of MGMT promoter by hypermethylation. Regardless of TMZ use, MGMT promoter hypermethylation was associated with improved OS (MS 15.3 vs. 11.8 months). Survival in hypermethylated tumors treated with RT + TMZ vs. RT alone was 21.7 vs. 15.3 months (*p* = .007) and 2-year OS was 46% vs. 23% (*p* = .007). In patients with nonhypermethylated MGMT promoter, MS difference between the groups was NS (12.7 vs. 11.8 months); however, 2-year OS was significant (13% vs. 2%). **Conclusion: MGMT promoter hypermethylation is both prognostic and predictive of response to TMZ.** *Comment: The use of TMZ for patients with nonhypermethylated MGMT promoter is controversial; some feel the subset was underpowered and patients may still benefit.*

Is there any benefit to increasing the dose density of TMZ?

The RTOG 0525[35] investigated the use of adjuvant TMZ 75 to 100 mg/m^2 × 21 days q4 weeks × 6–12 cycles vs. adjuvant Stupp regimen. This approach did not show benefit.

Is there any role for hyperfractionation in GBM?

RTOG 8302[36] and RTOG 9006[37] examined this question and showed no benefit to hyperfractionated RT compared with standard fractionation in patients with malignant glioma.

Does a radiosurgery boost improve disease control for GBM patients?

Souhami, RTOG 9305 (*IJROP* 2004, PMID 15465203): PRT of GBM patients with KPS ≥70 and unifocal, enhancing, well-demarcated, ≤4 cm lesion randomized to RT + BCNU ± upfront SRS (15–24 Gy, depending on size). MS was 13.5 months in SRS arm vs. 13.6 months in standard arm. **Conclusion: There is no role for an upfront SRS boost in GBM.**

Is there a role for a brachytherapy boost in malignant gliomas?

Two trials[38,39] showed no improvement in OS with brachytherapy boost including using I-125 implant prior to EBRT or after EBRT in malignant gliomas.

What is the role of WBRT in GBM?

WBRT can be considered for multifocal disease/subependymal spread/gliomatosis cerebri or poor performance patients (KPS <60) with comparable outcomes (MS ~7 months) to limited volume RT.[39,40]

What is the basis for the treatment volumes used during standard CRT?

After standard treatment, over 80% of recurrences occur within a 2-cm margin of the contrast-enhancing lesion seen on CT or MRI at original diagnosis.[41] Thus, the high-dose treatment volume typically includes a 2-cm CTV expansion of the resection cavity and any residual enhancing tumor, as used in RTOG protocols. Although peritumoral edema seen on T2 and FLAIR MRI sequences is typically targeted in the low-dose PTV, retrospective single-institution reviews have suggested that there are no increased rates of LR when peritumoral edema is not specifically targeted during RT treatment.[42] In fact, EORTC protocols for GBM do not include targeting edema volumes.[41] A more recent phase I/II study treated 27 patients with 5-fx SRS in escalated doses from 25 to 40 Gy with a 5-mm CTV expansion and showed that only one patient may have dosimetrically benefitted from conventional 2-cm margins.[43]

Is there a benefit to the addition of bevacizumab to TMZ?

Two phase III randomized trials[44,45] showed only improvement of PFS without OS benefit when adding bevacizumab to standard CRT.

What are TTF and is there a benefit in GBM?

Electric fields can be used to disrupt the polarization within a cell that normally occurs during the spindle formation process in mitosis, thus inhibiting cell division. The FDA-approved NovoTTF-100A (Optune) is a device that a patient wears on their head along with an attached portable battery pack that emits alternating electric fields.

Stupp, EF-14 (*JAMA* 2017, PMID 29260225): PRT of 695 patients with GBM treated with CRT (Stupp regimen), without early progression, and then randomized to either conventional adjuvant TMZ ± TTF. MFU 40 months, minimum follow-up 24 months. TTF significantly improved OS (20.9 vs. 16.0 months, $p < .001$) and PFS (6.7 vs. 4.0 months, $p < .001$). Mild to moderate skin toxicity underneath the transducer arrays occurred in 52% of patients who received TTF vs. no patients who received TMZ alone. **Conclusion: NovoTTF + adjuvant TMZ as part of the Stupp protocol is associated with a 5-month OS benefit. Comment: Criticism of this study focuses on the lack of a sham device in the control arm.**

Taphoorn (*JAMA Oncol* 2018, PMID 29392280): Secondary analysis of patients in the Stupp TTF study (above). Of the patients, 639 completed HR-QOL questionnaires. Deterioration-free survival (deterioration = 10-point drop in scores) was significantly longer with TTF for global health, physical and emotional functioning, and leg weakness. Time to deterioration was worse only for itchy skin (8.2 vs. 14.4 months). **Conclusion: NovoTTF + adjuvant TMZ as part of the Stupp protocol is associated with improved survival without a negative influence on HR-QOL, except for more itchy skin.**

What is the role of proton therapy (PBT) in GBM?

Brown (*Neuro-Oncology 2021*, PMID 33647972): PRT of 67 patients with newly diagnosed GBM randomized to receive either PBT (28 patients) or IMRT (39 patients). After MFU of 49 months, there was no significant difference in time to cognitive failure between treatment arms ($p = .74$). PBT was associated with a lower rate of fatigue (24% vs. 58%, $p = .05$), but otherwise there were no significant differences in patient-reported outcomes at 6 months. There were no differences in PFS ($p = .24$) or OS ($p = .60$). Grade 2+ toxicities were significantly higher in patients who received IMRT ($p = .02$). **Conclusion: PBT was not associated with a neurocognitive benefit in comparison to IMRT.**

MANAGEMENT OF OLDER/FRAIL PATIENTS WITH GLIOBLASTOMA

What is the role of RT over best supportive care?

RT improves OS over best supportive care in older patients with good KPS.

Keime-Guibert, France (*NEJM* 2007, PMID 17429084): PRT of 81 patients age ≥70 (all KPS ≥70) with newly diagnosed anaplastic astrocytoma or GBM randomized to RT 50.4 Gy/28 fx vs. best supportive care after biopsy/resection. MS improved with RT (29.1 vs. 16.9 weeks, $p = .002$). No difference between the arms in terms of QOL or cognition. Trial closed early after interim analysis demonstrated improved OS with use of RT. **Conclusion: RT plays an important role in improving OS in GBM patients, even in the older population, without a decline in QOL or measured cognitive function.**

Is hypofractionation comparable to standard fractionation for older adults/poor performance status GBM patients?

Multiple trials have demonstrated the efficacy of hypofractionated, shortened regimens for select patients who are not receiving systemic therapy. An important caveat is that these trials generally have not taken into account molecular markers, and thus the durability of control is unknown when compared with standard therapy for those with favorable molecular profiles. Prospectively validated regimens include 40 Gy/15 fx, 34 Gy/10 fx, and 25 Gy/5 fx.

Roa, Canadian (*JCO* 2004, PMID 15051755): PRT of 100 patients age ≥60 randomized to 60 Gy/30 fx vs. 40 Gy/15 fx, both without CHT. MS was 5.1 months for standard vs. 5.6 for shorter course RT (NS). The shorter course arm required less steroid use at the end of treatment (49% vs. 23%); 26% of patients stopped long-course RT vs. 10% in short-course arm. **Conclusion: In patients older than 60 who are not receiving CHT, there is no difference in OS between 40 Gy/15 fx and standard fractionation.**

Roa, IAEA (*JCO* 2015, PMID 26392096): PRT of 98 older/frail patients (age ≥50 and KPS 50–70 or age ≥65 with KPS ≥50) with GBM randomized to 25 Gy/5 fx vs. 40 Gy/15 fx. No CHT given. Patients receiving 25 Gy/5 fx had noninferior OS compared with those receiving 40 Gy/15 fx, and no difference in PFS or QOL. **Conclusion: Short-course RT delivered in 1 week (25 Gy/5 fx) is a treatment option for older and/or frail patients with newly diagnosed GBM.**

Can TMZ be substituted for RT in elderly patients?

TMZ alone is a noninferior option compared with standard RT in older patients and may be preferred over RT alone in patients with MGMT promoter hypermethylation.

Wick, NOA-08 (*Lancet Oncol* 2012, PMID 22578793): PRT of 373 patients with anaplastic astrocytoma (11%) or GBM (89%), age >65, and with KPS ≥60 randomized to TMZ alone (100 mg/m^2 for 7 days, alternating with 7 days off, for as long as tolerated) vs. standard RT alone (60 Gy/30 fx). OS for patients receiving TMZ alone was noninferior to those receiving standard RT (8.6 vs. 9.6 months). Patients with MGMT promoter hypermethylation had improved OS compared with unmethylated patients. Patients with MGMT promoter hypermethylation had significantly improved EFS with receipt of TMZ compared with RT. Patients without MGMT promoter hypermethylation had significantly improved EFS when receiving RT compared with TMZ. **Conclusion: TMZ alone is noninferior to standard RT alone in this older patient population. MGMT promoter hypermethylation is an important prognostic factor and may be predictive of appropriate treatment regimens.**

Malmström, Nordic Trial (*Lancet* 2012, PMID 22877848): PRT of 342 patients with GBM and age >60 randomized to CHT alone (TMZ 200 mg/m^2 d1–5 of 28-day cycle for up to 6 cycles) vs. 60 Gy/30 fx vs. 34 Gy/10 fx. Median OS significantly improved for patients receiving TMZ alone (8.3 months) vs. standard RT (6 months) but not vs. hypofractionated RT (7.5 months). For patients >70 years, survival was improved in both the TMZ and hypofractionated arms compared with standard fractionation. **Conclusion: Older patients had a detriment in OS when receiving standard RT compared with TMZ alone. Use of TMZ alone or hypofractionated RT should be considered in the elderly population, especially if over age 70. Comment: See following Perry trial.**

Should TMZ be added to short-course RT?

Perry, EORTC 26062 (*NEJM* 2017, PMID 28296618): PRT of patients age ≥60 with newly diagnosed GBM treated with 40 Gy/15 fx and randomized to no systemic therapy vs. 3 weeks concurrent TMZ and monthly adjuvant TMZ up to 12 cycles. RT + TMZ significantly improved OS compared with RT alone (9.3 vs. 7.6 months, $p = .0001$). PFS was also improved (5.3 vs. 3.9 months, $p < .0001$). OS improved in patients with MGMT promoter hypermethylation who received RT + TMZ vs. TMZ alone (13.5 vs. 7.7 months, $p = .0001$) but not statistically significant in patients with unmethylated MGMT status (10 vs. 7.9 months, $p = .055$). **Conclusion: There is an OS benefit to the addition of TMZ to RT even for those receiving a hypofractionated regimen among elderly patients. Patients with MGMT promoter hypermethylation benefit most from RT + TMZ with a ~6-month improvement in OS.**

RECURRENT/PROGRESSIVE GLIOBLASTOMA

What are the options when there is disease recurrence?

Recurrence is common, with 80% of recurrences occurring within 2 cm of primary.[41] Options include re-resection, bevacizumab, CCNU, re-RT, and TTF.

Is re-resection an option for recurrence?

Karschnia, RANO Resect Group (*Neuro Oncol* 2023, PMID 37253096): RR of 681 patients with first recurrence of GBM, including 310 patients who underwent re-resection. Patients were stratified based on the residual tumor volumes following re-resection according to RANO classification system: "supramaximal CE resection" (class 1): 0 cm^3 CE tumor + ≤5 cm^3 non-CE tumor; "maximal CE resection" (class 2): 0–1 cm^3 CE tumor ± >5 cm^3 non-CE tumor; or "submaximal CE resection" (class 3): >1 cm^3 CE tumor. Patients designated as RANO class 1 or 2 (per definition had a residual CE tumor of ≤1 cm^3) had superior survival compared with RANO class 3 (MS 12 vs. 9 months, $p = .001$). The outcomes for patients in RANO class 3 were comparable to patients without re-resection (MS 9 vs. 7 months, $p = .73$). No difference in survival between patients with RANO class 1 vs. 2 (MS 12 months in both), but the rate of postoperative neurologic deficits was higher among patients with RANO class 1. **Conclusion: Re-resection is associated with favorable outcomes when a postoperative volume of <1 cm^3 residual CE tumor can be surgically achieved.**

Is re-irradiation an option for progression?

Fokas (*Strahlenther Onkol* 2009, PMID 19370426): RR of 53 patients with recurrent GBM. Demonstrated MS of 9 months after re-RT with a median dose of 30 Gy in 3 Gy/fx; only KPS <70 predicted for poor survival. Well-tolerated, no >G2 acute or late toxicity. **Conclusion: Hypofractionated RT is safe and feasible for re-RT of GBM. Comment: See RTOG 1205 below.**

What is the role of pulsed-reduced dose-rate (PRDR) re-irradiation to minimize toxicity?

The inverse dose-rate effect may allow for reassortment of tumor cells while the treatment is delivered, perhaps leading to increased tumor kill with decreased toxicity due to normal tissue repair.

Adkison, Wisconsin (*IJROBP* 2011, PMID 20472350): RR of 103 patients (86 with GBM) treated with PRDR re-RT. RT was delivered slowly at 0.0667 Gy/min to a median dose of 50 Gy. Four of 15 patients had significant RT necrosis on autopsy. MS for GBM patients after PRDR was 5.1 months. **Conclusion: PRDR appears safe in the re-RT setting in order to treat larger volumes to a higher dose.**

Is bevacizumab effective for recurrent GBM?

Bevacizumab is beneficial in improving PFS as a second-line therapy with or without re-RT. Prospective and observational studies showed safety and efficacy when added to re-RT.[41,46]

Wong (*JNCCN* 2011, PMID 21464145): Meta-analysis of 15 trials (mainly phase II data) with a total of 548 patients treated with bevacizumab at recurrence. MS was 9.3 months; 6% CR, 49% PR, and 29% stable disease.

Tsien, RTOG 1205 (*JCO* 2022, PMID 36260832): PRT of 170 patients with recurrent GBM randomized to hypofractionated re-RT (35 Gy/10 fx) with concurrent bevacizumab 10 mg/kg q2 weeks vs. bevacizumab alone. Primary endpoint was median survival time (MST). No difference in MST between re-RT with concurrent bevacizumab vs. bevacizumab alone (10.1 vs. 9.7 months, p = .5). However, re-RT with concurrent bevacizumab improved 6-month PFS vs. bevacizumab alone (54% vs. 29%, p = .001). There was 5% acute grade 3 toxicity with no late high-grade toxicity. **Conclusion: Re-RT with concurrent bevacizumab is safe and effective with improvement in PFS but not OS.**

REFERENCES

1. Ostrom QT, Price M, Neff C, et al. CBTRUS statistical report: primary brain and other central nervous system tumors diagnosed in the United States in 2015–2019. *Neuro Oncol.* 2022;24(suppl 5):v1–v95. doi:10.1093/neuonc/noac202
2. Berger TR, Wen PY, Lang-Orsini M, Chukwueke UN. World Health Organization 2021 classification of central nervous system tumors and implications for therapy for adult-type gliomas. *JAMA Oncol.* 2022;8(10):1493–1501. doi:10.1001/jamaoncol.2022.2844
3. Melhem JM, Detsky J, Lim-Fat MJ, Perry JR. Updates in IDH-wildtype glioblastoma. *Neurotherapeutics.* 2022;19(6):1705–1723. doi:10.1007/s13311-022-01251-6
4. Grochans S, Cybulska AM, Simińska D, et al. Epidemiology of glioblastoma multiforme–literature review. *Cancers.* 2022;14(10):2412. doi:10.3390/cancers14102412
5. Li Y, Zhang ZX, Huang GH, et al. A systematic review of multifocal and multicentric glioblastoma. *J Clin Neurosci.* 2021;83:71–76. doi:10.1016/j.jocn.2020.11.025
6. Matarredona ER, Pastor AM. Neural stem cells of the subventricular zone as the origin of human glioblastoma stem cells. therapeutic implications. *Front Oncol.* 2019;9:779. doi:10.3389/fonc.2019.00779
7. Marquet G, Dameron O, Saikali S, Mosser J, Burgun A. Grading glioma tumors using OWL-DL and NCI thesaurus. *AMIA Annu Symp Proc.* 2007;2007:508–512. PMID:18693888
8. Halperin EC, Wazer DE, Perez CA, Brady LW. *Perez & Brady's Principles and Practice of Radiation Oncology.* 7th ed. Wolters Kluwer; 2019.
9. Louis DN, Perry A, Reifenberger G, et al. The 2016 World Health Organization classification of tumors of the central nervous system: a summary. *Acta Neuropathol.* 2016;131(6):803–820. doi:10.1007/s00401-016-1545-1
10. Gritsch S, Batchelor TT, Gonzalez Castro LN. Diagnostic, therapeutic, and prognostic implications of the 2021 World Health Organization classification of tumors of the central nervous system. *Cancer.* 2022;128(1):47–58. doi:10.1002/cncr.33918
11. Louis DN, Perry A, Wesseling P, et al. The 2021 WHO classification of tumors of the central nervous system: a summary. *Neuro Oncol.* 2021;23(8):1231–1251. doi:10.1093/neuonc/noab106
12. Halasz LM, Attia A, Bradfield L, et al. Radiation therapy for IDH-mutant grade 2 and grade 3 diffuse glioma: an ASTRO clinical practice guideline. *Pract Radiat Oncol.* 2022;12(5):370–386. doi:10.1016/j.prro.2022.05.004
13. Han S, Liu Y, Cai SJ, et al. IDH mutation in glioma: molecular mechanisms and potential therapeutic targets. *Br J Cancer.* 2020;122(11):1580–1589. doi:10.1038/s41416-020-0814-x
14. Sanson M, Marie Y, Paris S, et al. Isocitrate dehydrogenase 1 codon 132 mutation is an important prognostic biomarker in gliomas. *J Clin Oncol.* 2009;27(25):4150–4154. doi:10.1200/jco.2009.21.9832
15. Śledzińska P, Bebyn MG, Furtak J, Kowalewski J, Lewandowska MA. Prognostic and predictive biomarkers in gliomas. *Int J Mol Sci.* 2021;22(19):10373. doi:10.3390/ijms221910373
16. An Z, Aksoy O, Zheng T, Fan Q-W, Weiss WA. Epidermal growth factor receptor and EGFRvIII in glioblastoma: signaling pathways and targeted therapies. *Oncogene.* 2018;37(12):1561–1575. doi:10.1038/s41388-017-0045-7
17. Pelloski CE, Ballman KV, Furth AF, et al. Epidermal growth factor receptor variant III status defines clinically distinct subtypes of glioblastoma. *J Clin Oncol.* 2007;25(16):2288–2294. doi:10.1200/jco.2006.08.0705
18. Lassman AB, Pugh SL, Wang TJC, et al. Depatuxizumab mafodotin in EGFR-amplified newly diagnosed glioblastoma: a phase III randomized clinical trial. *Neuro Oncol.* 2023;25(2):339–350. doi:10.1093/neuonc/noac173
19. Olympios N, Gilard V, Marguet F, Clatot F, Di Fiore F, Fontanilles M. *TERT* promoter alterations in glioblastoma: a systematic review. *Cancers.* 2021;13(5):1147. doi:10.3390/cancers13051147

20. Stichel D, Ebrahimi A, Reuss D, et al. Distribution of EGFR amplification, combined chromosome 7 gain and chromosome 10 loss, and TERT promoter mutation in brain tumors and their potential for the reclassification of IDHwt astrocytoma to glioblastoma. *Acta Neuropathol.* 2018;136(5):793–803. doi:10.1007/s00401-018-1905-0

21. Hegi ME, Diserens AC, Gorlia T, et al. MGMT gene silencing and benefit from temozolomide in glioblastoma. *N Eng J Med.* 2005;352(10):997–1003. doi:10.1056/nejmoa043331

22. Berendsen S, Varkila M, Kroonen J, et al. Prognostic relevance of epilepsy at presentation in glioblastoma patients. *Neuro Oncol.* 2016;18(5):700–706. doi:10.1093/neuonc/nov238

23. Li J, Wang M, Won M, et al. Validation and simplification of the radiation therapy oncology group recursive partitioning analysis classification for glioblastoma. *Int J Radiat Oncol Biol Phys.* 2011;81(3):623–630. doi:10.1016/j.ijrobp.2010.06.012

24. Zoccarato M, Nardetto L, Basile AM, Giometto B, Zagonel V, Lombardi G. Seizures, edema, thrombosis, and hemorrhages: an update review on the medical management of gliomas. *Front Oncol.* 2021;11:617966. doi:10.3389/fonc.2021.617966

25. Stupp R, Mason WP, Van Den Bent MJ, et al. Radiotherapy plus concomitant and adjuvant temozolomide for glioblastoma. *N Eng J Med.* 2005;352(10):987–996. doi:10.1056/nejmoa043330

26. Vassil AD, Mossolly LM, Woody NM, et al, eds. *Handbook of Treatment Planning in Radiation Oncology.* 3 ed. Springer Publishing Company; 2020.

27. Karschnia P, Young JS, Dono A, et al. Prognostic validation of a new classification system for extent of resection in glioblastoma: a report of the RANO resect group. *Neuro Oncol.* 2023;25(5):940–954. doi:10.1093/neuonc/noac193

28. Walker MD, Alexander E, Hunt WE, et al. Evaluation of BCNU and/or radiotherapy in the treatment of anaplastic gliomas. A cooperative clinical trial. *J Neurosurg.* 1978;49(3):333–343. doi:10.3171/jns.1978.49.3.0333

29. Kristiansen K, Hagen S, Kollevold T, et al. Combined modality therapy of operated astrocytomas grade III and IV. Confirmation of the value of postoperative irradiation and lack of potentiation of bleomycin on survival time: a prospective multicenter trial of the scandinavian glioblastoma study group. *Cancer.* 1981;47(4):649–652. doi:10.1002/1097-0142(19810215)47:4<649::aid-cncr2820470405>3.0.co;2-w

30. Chan JL, Lee SW, Fraass BA, et al. Survival and failure patterns of high-grade gliomas after three-dimensional conformal radiotherapy. *J Clin Oncol.* 2002;20(6):1635–1642. doi:10.1200/jco.2002.20.6.1635

31. Tsien CI, Brown D, Normolle D, et al. Concurrent temozolomide and dose-escalated intensity-modulated radiation therapy in newly diagnosed glioblastoma. *Clin Cancer Res.* 2012;18(1):273–279. doi:10.1158/1078-0432.ccr-11-2073

32. Fine HA, Dear KBG, Loeffler JS, Mc Black PL, Canellos GP. Meta-analysis of radiation therapy with and without adjuvant chemotherapy for malignant gliomas in adults. *Cancer.* 1993;71(8):2585–2597. doi:10.1002/1097-0142(19930415)71:8<2585::aid-cncr2820710825>3.0.co;2-s

33. Westphal M, Hilt DC, Bortey E, et al. A phase 3 trial of local chemotherapy with biodegradable carmustine (BCNU) wafers (Gliadel wafers) in patients with primary malignant glioma. *Neuro Oncol.* 2003;5(2):79–88. doi:10.1093/neuonc/5.2.79

34. Garside R, Pitt M, Anderson R, et al. The effectiveness and cost-effectiveness of carmustine implants and temozolomide for the treatment of newly diagnosed high-grade glioma: a systematic review and economic evaluation. *Health Technol Assess.* 2007;11(45):iii–iv, ix–221. doi:10.3310/hta11450

35. Gilbert MR, Wang M, Aldape KD, et al. Dose-dense temozolomide for newly diagnosed glioblastoma: a randomized phase III clinical trial. *J Clin Oncol.* 2013;31(32):4085–4091. doi:10.1200/jco.2013.49.6968

36. Werner-Wasik M, Scott CB, Nelson DF, et al. Final report of a phase I/II trial of hyperfractionated and accelerated hyperfractionated radiation therapy with carmustine for adults with supratentorial malignant gliomas: radiation therapy oncology group study 83-02. *Cancer.* 1996;77(8):1535–1543. doi:10.1002/(sici)1097-0142(19960415)77:8<1535::aid-cncr17>3.0.co;2-0

37. Ali AN, Zhang P, Yung WKA, et al. NRG oncology RTOG 9006: a phase III randomized trial of hyperfractionated radiotherapy (RT) and BCNU versus standard RT and BCNU for malignant glioma patients. *J Neurooncol.* 2018;137(1):39–47. doi:10.1007/s11060-017-2558-x

38. Laperriere NJ, Leung PM, McKenzie S, et al. Randomized study of brachytherapy in the initial management of patients with malignant astrocytoma. *Int J Radiat Oncol Biol Phys.* 1998;41(5):1005–1011. doi:10.1016/S0360-3016(98)00159-X

39. Selker RG, Shapiro WR, Burger P, et al. The Brain Tumor Cooperative Group NIH Trial 87-01: a randomized comparison of surgery, external radiotherapy, and carmustine versus surgery, interstitial radiotherapy boost, external radiation therapy, and carmustine. *Neurosurgery.* 2002;51(2):343–355. PMID:12182772

40. Shapiro WR, Green SB, Burger PC, et al. Randomized trial of three chemotherapy regimens and two radiotherapy regimens in postoperative treatment of malignant glioma. *J Neurosurg.* 1989;71(1):1–9. doi:10.3171/jns.1989.71.1.0001

41. Niyazi M, Brada M, Chalmers AJ, et al. ESTRO-ACROP guideline "target delineation of glioblastomas". *Radiother Oncol.* 2016;118(1):35–42. doi:10.1016/j.radonc.2015.12.003

42. Chang EL, Akyurek S, Avalos T, et al. Evaluation of peritumoral edema in the delineation of radiotherapy clinical target volumes for glioblastoma. *Int J Radiat Oncol Biol Phys*. 2007;68(1):144–150. doi:10.1016/j.ijrobp.2006.12.009

43. Mendoza MG, Azoulay M, Chang SD, et al. Patterns of progression in patients with newly diagnosed glioblastoma treated with 5-mm margins in a phase 1/2 trial of 5-fraction stereotactic radiosurgery with concurrent and adjuvant temozolomide. *Pract Radiat Oncol*. 2023;13(3):e239–e245. doi:10.1016/j.prro.2023.01.008

44. Gilbert MR, Dignam JJ, Armstrong TS, et al. A randomized trial of bevacizumab for newly diagnosed glioblastoma. *N Engl J Med*. 2014;370(8):699–708. doi:10.1056/NEJMoa1308573

45. Chinot OL, Wick W, Mason W, et al. Bevacizumab plus radiotherapy-temozolomide for newly diagnosed glioblastoma. *N Engl J Med*. 2014;370(8):709–722. doi:10.1056/NEJMoa1308345

46. Tsien CI, Pugh SL, Dicker AP, et al. NRG Oncology/RTOG1205: a randomized phase II trial of concurrent bevacizumab and reirradiation versus bevacizumab alone as treatment for recurrent glioblastoma. *J Clin Oncol*. 2023;41(6):1285–1295. doi:10.1200/JCO.22.00164

2 IDH-MUTANT GLIOMAS: GRADE 3

Salem Alfaifi, Shireen Parsai, Jennifer S. Yu, Samuel T. Chao, and Martin C. Tom

QUICK HIT In the 2021 WHO classification, IDH-mutant gliomas are further subdivided into astrocytomas and oligodendrogliomas based on molecular features. Oligodendroglioma is defined by presence of IDH mutation and 1p/19q codeletion, whereas astrocytoma is defined by presence of IDH mutation and absence of 1p/19q codeletion or by presence of *ATRX* loss and/or *TP53* mutations. Grade 3 gliomas were previously referred to as "anaplastic gliomas," but this term no longer appears in the updated classification. Grade 3 oligodendroglioma (formerly anaplastic oligodendroglioma) has an MS of ~14 years, whereas grade 3 astrocytoma (formerly anaplastic astrocytoma) has an MS of ~10 years. The general treatment paradigm includes maximal safe surgical resection followed by adjuvant RT and CHT. For oligodendrogliomas, PCV improves OS compared with no CHT, and trials are ongoing comparing PCV with TMZ. For astrocytoma, RT followed by TMZ improves OS compared with no TMZ.

EPIDEMIOLOGY: The average annual incidence of grade 3 astrocytoma and oligodendroglioma in the United States is ~1,409 and 374, respectively.[1]

RISK FACTORS: Previous ionizing radiation exposure.[2] Genetic syndromes (<5% of gliomas) associated with gliomas include NF1 (17q, café au lait spots, Lisch nodules, neurofibroma, optic glioma, astrocytoma), NF2 (22q, bilateral acoustic neuroma, glioma, meningioma, ependymoma), tuberous sclerosis (ash-leaf macules, subependymal giant cell astrocytoma, gliomas), Li–Fraumeni syndrome, and VHL (hemangioblastoma).[3]

ANATOMY: Most arise in the cerebral hemispheres. The frontal lobe is more common than parietal/temporal, which is more common than occipital. Cerebellar tumors are uncommon.[1,3]

PATHOLOGY

Grading and WHO Classification[2,4,5]**:** Historically, glioma type was based primarily on histopathologic appearance (e.g., oligodendroglioma with "fried egg appearance" and "chicken-wire vasculature" vs. astrocytoma with pleomorphic giant cells and prominent cytoplasmic processes). Grade was based on the presence or extent of anaplasia, mitotic activity, microvascular proliferation, and necrosis. Grade 3 gliomas were historically termed "anaplastic gliomas," which is no longer used in the classification. Mixed tumors with both oligodendroglial and astrocytic components were historically called "oligoastrocytomas" and were included on many trials of oligodendrogliomas. However, they are no longer part of the classification as molecular characteristics can group them into either oligodendroglioma or astrocytoma. With advances in our understanding of the molecular basis of gliomas, major restructuring began with the WHO 2016 classification, and subsequently the WHO 2021 classification, which uses an integrated diagnosis based on both histopathologic appearance and molecular characteristics.

- Oligodendroglioma, IDH-mutant (grades 2–3): Defined by IDH mutation and presence of 1p/19q codeletion. Grade 3 oligodendrogliomas have features of anaplasia, increased mitotic activity, microvascular proliferation, and/or necrosis. Grade 2 oligodendrogliomas lack these characteristics. The distinction between grades 2 and 3 can be subjective. There is no grade 4 oligodendroglioma.
- Astrocytoma, IDH-mutant (grades 2–3): Defined by IDH mutation and the absence of 1p/19q codeletion (i.e., 1p19q intact) or by presence of *ATRX* loss and/or *TP53* mutations. Grade 3 astrocytomas have features of anaplasia and/or increased mitotic activity. Grade 2 astrocytomas lack these characteristics. The distinction between grades 2 and 3 can be subjective. Grades 2 and 3 astrocytomas lack grade 4 characteristics (see below).
- Astrocytoma, IDH-mutant, grade 4: Defined by IDH mutation and the absence of 1p/19q codeletion or by presence of *ATRX* loss and/or *TP53* mutations; and the presence of one or more of the following grade 4 features: necrosis, microvascular proliferation, and/or CDKN2A/B

homozygous deletion. Given their aggressive behavior and that many were likely included in prior GBM trials based on older classification, they are typically treated similar to GBMs (see Chapter 1).

See Figure 1.1 *WHO 2021 CNS Classification of Adult Diffuse Gliomas.*

See Chapter 3 for other updates on IDH-mutant low-grade gliomas.

GENETICS

IDH Mutation: See Chapter 1 for overview. IDH-mutant diffuse gliomas, encompassing astrocytomas and oligodendrogliomas, are characterized by a class defining IDH1 or (less commonly) IDH2 gene mutation.[6,7] IDH1 R132H is the most common IDH mutation and should be tested on all gliomas. If absent, noncanonical IDH mutations (i.e., other less common IDH1 and IDH2 mutations) should be tested in patients who are <55 years old.[8]

1p19q Codeletion: Codeletion of the short arm of chr 1 and the long arm of chr 19 (1p19q) is a defining feature of oligodendroglioma, and it has a favorable prognosis.[9]

TP53 Mutation and/or ATRX Loss: ATRX is a gene that is involved in chromatin regulation. *ATRX* loss and/or *TP53* mutation are characteristic of astrocytoma and are mutually exclusive with 1p19q codeletion.[7,10]

CDKN2A/B Homozygous Deletion: Associated with poor prognosis in IDH-mutant astrocytomas and, if present, automatically upgrades it to grade 4, even in the absence of microvascular proliferation or necrosis. This should be tested in IDH-mutant astrocytomas that otherwise lack grade 4 characteristics (microvascular proliferation or necrosis).[11,12]

CLINICAL PRESENTATION: Headache and seizures are the most common symptoms. Other symptoms may include memory loss, motor weakness, visual symptoms, language deficit, cognitive changes, and personality changes. In general, size and location dictate presenting symptoms.[3]

WORKUP: H&P with neurologic exam. Fundoscopic exam (if suspicious of increased ICP).

Labs: CBC and other basic labs prior to CHT. Pregnancy test in women of childbearing age.

Imaging: MRI brain with and without gadolinium. Grade 3 gliomas are typically hypointense on T1 with heterogeneous contrast enhancement, central necrosis, and surrounding edema; T2/FLAIR hyperintense. However, some grade 3 gliomas are nonenhancing with only T2/FLAIR hyperintensity. Following surgical resection, obtain a postoperative MRI within 48 to 72 hours (ideally 24–48 hours) to determine the extent of resection and residual disease without confounding by blood products.

Pathology: Stereotactic or open biopsy with histopathologic and molecular assessment can be performed for unresectable tumors or an uncertain clinical diagnosis. Typically, if clinical findings are consistent with glioma, maximum safe resection is performed for both treatment and to establish the pathologic diagnosis, without the need for biopsy.

PROGNOSTIC FACTORS

Patient-Related: Historically, an RPA by the RTOG classified patients based on factors such as age (<50 vs. ≥50 years), KPS (<90 vs. 90–100), mental status changes, and duration of symptoms (<3 vs. ≥3 months).[13–15]

Tumor-Related: Oligodendroglioma has a better prognosis compared with astrocytoma. 1p19q codeletion and MGMT promoter hypermethylation are positive molecular genetic alterations.[9,12,16,17] CDKN2A/B homozygous deletion is a poor prognostic factor within IDH-mutant astrocytomas and thus automatically upgrades it to grade 4.[11,12] The role of CDKN2A/B homozygous deletion in IDH-mutant oligodendrogliomas is less clear, but has been associated with worse prognosis.[18]

Treatment-Related: Extent of surgical resection.[15]

NATURAL HISTORY: IDH-mutant gliomas typically occur in younger patients (fourth and fifth decades) and have better prognosis than IDH-wild-type gliomas. IDH-mutant grade 3 oligodendroglioma has better prognosis (MS ~14 years) than grade 3 astrocytoma (MS ~10 years). Astrocytoma,

IDH-mutant, grade 4 (formerly IDH-mutant GBM) has better prognosis (MS ~32 months) than IDH-wild-type GBM (MS ~14 months). Despite this better prognosis, this new subgroup has not been tested in clinical trials; they were included in prior GBM trials and are typically managed according to GBM protocols (see Chapter 1).[7,10]

TREATMENT PARADIGM

Surgery: Primary treatment is surgical resection with the aim of maximal safe surgical resection with neurologic preservation.

Chemotherapy: Randomized trials including RTOG 9402 and EORTC 26951 have established a survival benefit with the addition of PCV CHT to RT for IDH-mutant grade 3 gliomas (PCV: procarbazine, lomustine, and vincristine). The addition of sequential TMZ following RT improves OS for IDH-mutant grade 3 astrocytoma per the CATNON study. To date, there is no survival benefit from the use of concurrent TMZ, although further maturation of the CATNON trial is pending. TMZ vs. PCV is currently being compared on the CODEL trial for grade 3 oligodendroglioma. Some institutions favor TMZ over PCV given that it is better tolerated. TMZ is given 75 mg/m^2 daily with RT including weekends, followed by 150 to 200 mg/m^2 daily on days 1 to 5 of 28-day cycles, with the first cycle beginning 28 days after the completion of RT. Up to 12 cycles of adjuvant TMZ are administered.

Radiation

Indications: Adjuvant RT improves OS vs. observation or CHT alone after surgery (see the following studies) and is indicated in most patients of sufficient functional status to tolerate treatment.

Dose: The most common dose used in clinical trials is 59.4 Gy/33 fx.

Toxicity: See Chapter 1.

Procedure: See *Handbook of Treatment Planning in Radiation Oncology*, Chapter 3.[19]

EVIDENCE-BASED Q&A

Most of the randomized studies on grade 3 gliomas were designed prior to molecular classification. Prior terminology used "anaplastic" synonymously with "grade 3." Thus, using historical terminology, anaplastic astrocytomas (AA) were often included in GBM trials. Anaplastic oligodendroglioma (AO) and mixed anaplastic oligoastrocytoma (AOA; no longer existent with molecular classification) were both included in grade 3 trials. Many trials subsequently underwent post-hoc analysis using molecular classification.

What is the role of RT in the management of grade 3 gliomas?

The role of RT was initially established in the 1970s and 1980s due to a survival benefit.

Walker (*J Neurosurg* 1978, PMID 355604): 303 patients with anaplastic gliomas s/p surgical resection randomized to one of four arms: (a) best supportive care, (b) BCNU alone, (c) RT alone, (d) RT + BCNU. RT was delivered as 50 to 60 Gy to the whole brain. MS was 14 weeks, 18.5 weeks, 35 weeks, and 34.5 weeks, respectively. **Conclusion: Adjuvant treatment with RT is associated with a survival benefit.**

What is the role of CHT in addition to RT?

Two landmark studies from RTOG and EORTC established the utility of adding CHT (PCV) to RT in grade 3 gliomas. It is important to note that RTOG 9402 and EORTC 26951 included histologic AO and AOA but did not include histologic AA. However, in the current era of integrated histologic and molecular diagnosis, and when stratifying results by IDH status and 1p19q status, these studies are likely applicable as well to grade 3 IDH-mutant astrocytoma.

Cairncross, RTOG 9402 (*JCO* 2006, PMID 16782910; Update *JCO* 2013, PMID 23071247; Subset *JCO* 2014, PMID 24516018): PRT of 291 patients newly diagnosed with AO/AOA randomized after surgery to four cycles of intensified PCV *prior* to RT vs. RT alone. RT dose 59.4 Gy/33 fx. Seventy-nine percent of RT-alone patients eventually received CHT (PCV or TMZ); only 46% of PCV + RT patients received all four cycles of CHT. Original analyses in 2006 did not demonstrate a survival benefit with PCV + RT as compared with RT alone for the entire cohort (4.7 vs. 4.6 years, respectively).

However, on subset analysis in 2014, patients with IDH-mutated tumors lived longer after PCV + RT as compared with those with RT alone. Within the IDH-mutant subgroup, patients with 1p19q codeletion lived the longest. For IDH-wild-type patients, PCV + RT did not increase survival compared with RT alone (see Table 2.1). **Conclusion: No survival benefit in AO/AOA cohort as a whole with PCV + RT vs. RT alone. OS benefit was demonstrated for IDH-mutant tumors with PCV + RT, and within this group those who also had 1p/19q codeletion lived the longest (14.7 vs. 6.8 years).**

Table 2.1 Results of Cairncross RTOG 9402, 2014 Subset Analysis			
	RT + PCV (MS, Yrs)	RT Alone (MS, Yrs)	*p* value
All patients	4.6	4.7	NS
IDH-mutated, 1p19q codeleted	14.7	6.8	.01
IDH-mutated, 1p19q intact	5.5	3.3	.05
IDH-wild-type	1.8	1.3	NS

van den Bent, EORTC 26951 (*JCO* 2006, PMID 16782911; Update *JCO* 2013, PMID 23071237): PRT of 368 patients newly diagnosed with AO/AOA randomized after surgery to RT followed by PCV × 6 cycles vs. RT alone. RT 59.4 Gy/33 fx. Thirty-eight percent of PCV patients discontinued CHT prematurely. On post-hoc pathology review, one-third of the patients were found to have GBM. MFU 11.7 years. OS significantly improved among the entire group with PCV: 3.5 vs. 2.6 years (see Table 2.2). Significant improvements in PFS were noted in both 1p19q codeleted (13 vs. 4.2 years) and 1p19q intact (15 vs. 9 months). No long-term difference in QOL reported after PCV. IDH mutation and 1p19q codeletion were independently significant on multivariate prognostic model. MGMT promoter hypermethylation status was not an independent prognostic factor of survival. **Conclusion: RT + PCV improved both OS and PFS compared with RT alone, with significant improvement in PFS in both the 1p/19q codeleted and intact groups. 1p/19q codeleted tumors derive more benefit compared with 1p/19q intact tumors.**

Table 2.2 2013 Results of EORTC 26951 for Anaplastic Gliomas			
	RT + PCV (MS, Yrs)	RT Alone (MS, Yrs)	*p* value
All patients	3.5	2.6	.018
1p19q codeleted	Not reached (14.2 on longer follow-up[20])	9.3	.059
1p19q intact	2.1	1.8	.185

What is the management of grade 3 astrocytoma?

As mentioned earlier, the contemporary definition of grade 3 astrocytoma uses molecular markers, and post-hoc subset analyses of RTOG 9402 or EORTC 26951 showed only a modest benefit to PCV for IDH-mutant astrocytoma (1p19q intact). It is worth mentioning that prior to this molecular classification, the standard of care of CRT for this group was derived from historical GBM trials, of which grade 3 astrocytoma constituted a minority of patients. They also made up a small minority of the patients on the Stupp trial (see Chapter 1).

What is the role of TMZ for grade 3 gliomas?

Despite the survival advantage demonstrated with PCV in patients with grade 3 gliomas, many substitute TMZ as it is easier to administer and generally better tolerated. Furthermore, astrocytomas (1p19q intact) derived less of a benefit with PCV than oligodendrogliomas (1p19q codeleted). RTOG 0131, NOA-04, and the early results of CATNON support TMZ, particularly for grade 3 astrocytomas. Whether PCV is superior to TMZ for oligodendrogliomas is under evaluation on the CODEL trial.

Vogelbaum, RTOG 0131 (*J Neuroncol* 2015, PMID 26088460): Phase II, single-arm trial including 48 patients with AO/AOA undergoing pre-RT TMZ × 6 cycles followed by concurrent RT + TMZ (for those without complete radiographic response). RT 59.4 Gy/33 fx. MFU 8.7 years, mPFS 5.8 years, MS not reached. 1p19q status available in 37 cases. OS and PFS not reached for codeleted patients. Codeleted patients show a trend toward improved 6-year survival when compared with similar population in the PCV + RT arm in RTOG 9402 (67%; 95% CI 55%–79%). **Conclusion: Pre-RT TMZ followed by concurrent RT + TMZ is indirectly comparable to PCV followed by RT.**

Wick, NOA-04 (*JCO* 2009, PMID 19901110; Update *Neuro Oncol* 2016, PMID 27370396): PRT of 318 patients with anaplastic glioma randomly assigned 2:1:1 (A:B1:B2) to receive (A) RT 54 to 60 Gy, (B1) PCV, or (B2) TMZ. In Arm A, patients received CHT after progression, and in Arm B1 or B2 patients received RT after progression. The primary endpoint was time-to-treatment failure (TTF), defined as progression after RT and one CHT in either sequence. The initial results reported in 2009 did not identify any difference in TTF, PFS, or OS between primary CHT and RT. This was confirmed with the report of long-term results in 2016. The study also identified IDH1 mutation as a positive prognostic factor with a stronger impact as compared with 1p19q codeletion or MGMT promoter hypermethylation. Subset analysis demonstrated that AO (IDH-mutant, 1p19q codeleted) had improved PFS with PCV vs. TMZ, suggesting PCV may be more effective for oligodendrogliomas than astrocytomas. **Conclusion: No difference in TTF between RT alone vs. PCV vs. TMZ. IDH mutation was shown to have a stronger impact on prognosis compared with 1p/19q codeletion or MGMT promoter hypermethylation.**

van den Bent, EORTC CATNON (*Lancet* 2017, PMID 28801186; Update *Lancet* 2021, PMID 34000245): Phase III PRT of 748 patients with newly diagnosed AA (specifically patients had to be *1p19q intact; IDH mutation was not required at initial trial design*) randomized to one of four arms: (a) RT alone, (b) RT + concurrent TMZ, (c) RT + adjuvant TMZ, or (d) RT + concurrent and adjuvant TMZ. RT 59.4 Gy/33 fx. Stratified based on MGMT promoter methylation status, age, 1p loss of heterozygosity, presence of oligodendroglial elements, and performance status. At second interim analysis with MFU of 4.6 years, futility of concurrent TMZ was declared among the entire cohort (MS 5.6 years with concurrent TMZ vs. 5 years without, $p = .76$). Adjuvant TMZ improved OS vs. no adjuvant TMZ (MS 6.9 vs. 3.9 years, $p < .01$). Of patients with IDH mutation, MS with concurrent TMZ vs. no concurrent TMZ was 9.7 vs. 7.7 years ($p = .17$); MS with adjuvant TMZ vs. no adjuvant TMZ was 9.7 vs. 6.5 years ($p < .01$). **Conclusion: Adjuvant TMZ, but not concurrent TMZ, improved PFS and OS for 1p19q intact anaplastic gliomas. Pending data maturation to determine if there is a benefit to concurrent TMZ in patients with IDH mutation.**

Jaeckle, CODEL (*Neuro Oncol* 2020, PMID 32678879): PRT of the initial design of the CODEL trial (prior to changing randomization to RT + PCV vs. RT + TMZ) including 36 patients with 1p19q codeleted grade 3 oligodendrogliomas randomized to RT alone, RT with concurrent and adjuvant TMZ, or TMZ alone. RT 59.4 Gy/33 fx. With 7.5-year follow-up, PFS was shorter with TMZ alone compared with the RT arms (HR 3.12, 95% CI 1.26–7.69). The comparison was underpowered to determine OS differences. No differences were observed in neurocognitive decline. **Conclusion: Patients with 1p19q codeleted grade 3 oligodendrogliomas had significantly shorter PFS when treated with TMZ alone compared with RT arms. The CODEL trial is now redesigned to compare RT + PCV vs. RT + TMZ and is ongoing.**

REFERENCES

1. Ostrom QT, Price M, Neff C, et al. CBTRUS statistical report: primary brain and other central nervous system tumors diagnosed in the United States in 2015–2019. *Neuro Oncol.* 2022;24(suppl 5):v1–v95. doi:10.1093/neuonc/noac202
2. Braganza MZ, Kitahara CM, Berrington De Gonzalez A, Inskip PD, Johnson KJ, Rajaraman P. Ionizing radiation and the risk of brain and central nervous system tumors: a systematic review. *Neuro Oncol.* 2012;14(11):1316–1324. doi:10.1093/neuonc/nos208
3. Halperin EC, Wazer DE, Perez CA, Brady LW. *Perez & Brady's Principles and Practice of Radiation Oncology.* 7th ed. Wolters Kluwer; 2019.
4. Marquet G, Dameron O, Saikali S, Mosser J, Burgun A. Grading glioma tumors using OWL-DL and NCI Thesaurus. *AMIA Annu Symp Proc.* 2007;2007:508–512. PMID:18693888
5. Louis DN, Perry A, Wesseling P, et al. The 2021 WHO classification of tumors of the central nervous system: a summary. *Neuro Oncol.* 2021;23(8):1231–1251. doi:10.1093/neuonc/noab106
6. Sanson M, Marie Y, Paris S, et al. Isocitrate dehydrogenase 1 codon 132 mutation is an important prognostic biomarker in gliomas. *J Clin Oncol.* 2009;27(25):4150–4154. doi:10.1200/jco.2009.21.9832
7. Gritsch S, Batchelor TT, Gonzalez Castro LN. Diagnostic, therapeutic, and prognostic implications of the 2021 World Health Organization classification of tumors of the central nervous system. *Cancer.* 2022;128(1):47–58. doi:10.1002/cncr.33918
8. Dewitt JC, Jordan JT, Frosch MP, et al. Cost-effectiveness of IDH testing in diffuse gliomas according to the 2016 WHO classification of tumors of the central nervous system recommendations. *Neuro Oncol.* 2017;19(12):1640–1650. doi:10.1093/neuonc/nox120

9.   Cairncross JG, Wang M, Jenkins RB, et al. Benefit from procarbazine, lomustine, and vincristine in oligodendroglial tumors is associated with mutation of IDH. *J Clin Oncol.* 2014;32(8):783–790. doi:10.1200/jco.2013.49.3726

10. Berger TR, Wen PY, Lang-Orsini M, Chukwueke UN. World Health Organization 2021 classification of central nervous system tumors and implications for therapy for adult-type gliomas. *JAMA Oncol.* 2022;8(10):1493–1501. doi:10.1001/jamaoncol.2022.2844

11. Fortin Ensign SP, Jenkins RB, Giannini C, Sarkaria JN, Galanis E, Kizilbash SH. Translational significance of CDKN2A/B homozygous deletion in isocitrate dehydrogenase-mutant astrocytoma. *Neuro Oncol.* 2023;25(1):28–36. doi:10.1093/neuonc/noac205

12. Śledzińska P, Bebyn MG, Furtak J, Kowalewski J, Lewandowska MA. Prognostic and predictive biomarkers in gliomas. *Int J Mol Sci.* 2021;22(19):10373. doi:10.3390/ijms221910373

13. Curran WJ Jr, Scott CB, Horton J, et al. Recursive partitioning analysis of prognostic factors in three Radiation Therapy Oncology Group malignant glioma trials. *J Natl Cancer Inst.* 1993;85(9):704–710. doi:10.1093/jnci/85.9.704

14. Lamborn KR, Chang SM, Prados MD. Prognostic factors for survival of patients with glioblastoma: recursive partitioning analysis. *Neuro Oncol.* 2004;6(3):227–235. doi:10.1215/s1152851703000620

15. Gorlia T, Delattre JY, Brandes AA, et al. New clinical, pathological and molecular prognostic models and calculators in patients with locally diagnosed anaplastic oligodendroglioma or oligoastrocytoma. A prognostic factor analysis of European Organisation for Research and Treatment of Cancer Brain Tumour Group Study 26951. *Eur J Cancer.* 2013;49(16):3477–3485. doi:10.1016/j.ejca.2013.06.039

16. Wick W, Hartmann C, Engel C, et al. NOA-04 randomized phase III trial of sequential radiochemotherapy of anaplastic glioma with procarbazine, lomustine, and vincristine or temozolomide. *J Clinical Oncology.* 2009;27(35):5874–5880. doi:10.1200/jco.2009.23.6497

17. Van Den Bent MJ, Carpentier AF, Brandes AA, et al. Adjuvant procarbazine, lomustine, and vincristine improves progression-free survival but not overall survival in newly diagnosed anaplastic oligodendrogliomas and oligoastrocytomas: a randomized European Organisation for Research and Treatment of Cancer Phase III trial. *J Clin Oncol.* 2006;24(18):2715–2722. doi:10.1200/jco.2005.04.6078

18. Appay R, Dehais C, Maurage CA, et al. CDKN2A homozygous deletion is a strong adverse prognosis factor in diffuse malignant IDH-mutant gliomas. *Neuro Oncol.* 2019;21(12):1519–1528. doi:10.1093/neuonc/noz124

19. Vassil AD, Mossolly LM, Woody NM, et al. *Handbook of Treatment Planning in Radiation Oncology.* 3 ed. Springer Publishing Company.

20. Lassman AB, Hoang-Xuan K, Polley MC, et al. Joint final report of EORTC 26951 and RTOG 9402: phase III trials with procarbazine, lomustine, and vincristine chemotherapy for anaplastic oligodendroglial tumors. *J Clin Oncol.* 2022;40(23):2539–2545. doi:10.1200/jco.21.02543

3 LOW-GRADE GLIOMAS

Adannia N. Ufondu, Erik M. Davies, Martin C. Tom, and Erin S. Murphy

QUICK HIT WHO grades 1 to 2 gliomas are commonly referred to as low-grade gliomas (LGGs), which are an uncommon and heterogeneous group of primary brain tumors presenting primarily in younger adults or children. Molecular and genomic factors have improved prognostic and predictive stratification and improved our understanding of LGGs. Grade 2 adult diffuse gliomas are now defined by the presence of an IDH mutation and the lack of aggressive histologic features. Ongoing studies seek to define management based on molecular classification, but established treatment paradigms remain largely based on clinical factors and require patient-specific decision-making (Table 3.1). Following maximal safe surgical resection, options include observation, RT, CHT, or combined CRT. RT dose is typically 45 to 54 Gy. CHT consists of either temozolomide (TMZ) or PCV (procarbazine, lomustine/CCNU, and vincristine).

Table 3.1 General Postoperative Treatment Paradigm for LGGs		
Classification	Risk Factors	Postoperative Management
Grade 1 gliomas	GTR	• Observation
	STR	• Observation • RT
Grade 2; oligodendroglioma, IDH-mutant and 1p19q codeleted OR Grade 2; diffuse astrocytoma, IDH-mutant	Low risk*	Observation
	High risk†	• RT → PCV • RT → TMZ • RT + TMZ → TMZ • Observation in select patients • Vorasidenib (IDH inhibitor) in select patients

Note: RT dose is 45–54 Gy at 1.8 Gy/fx; treatment paradigms defined based on clinical and molecular characteristics.
*Low risk per RTOG 9802 defined as age <40 and GTR.
†High risk per RTOG 9802 defined as age ≥40 and/or STR; per RTOG 0424 defined as ≥3 risk factors (age ≥40, tumor ≥6 cm, tumor crossing midline, preoperative NFS >1, astrocytoma histology).

EPIDEMIOLOGY: Between 2018 and 2020, there were ~1,238 total cases of IDH-mutant grade 2 astrocytomas and ~1,411 cases of grade 2 IDH-mutant 1p/19q-codeleted oligodendrogliomas diagnosed in the United States. Between 2016 and 2020, there were ~5,417 total cases of pilocytic astrocytoma (grade 1) diagnosed in the United States.[1]

RISK FACTORS: Ionizing radiation, genetic syndromes including NF-1 (AD mutation on chr 17q, café au lait spots, Lisch nodules, neurofibromas, optic gliomas, astrocytomas), NF-2 (AD mutation on chr 22q, bilateral acoustic neuromas, meningiomas, ependymomas, gliomas), tuberous sclerosis (ash-leaf macules, shagreen patches, hamartomas, angiofibromas, periungual fibromas, subependymal giant cell astrocytomas, gliomas), and Li–Fraumeni syndrome (AD mutation, TP53 mutation, gliomas, sarcomas, breast cancer, leukemia, adrenocortical carcinomas).

ANATOMY: Typically, LGGs arise from the supratentorial cortex. Brainstem gliomas and optic pathway gliomas, when biopsied, are often classified as low-grade and are discussed elsewhere.

PATHOLOGY: Gliomas represent a group of tumors with characteristics of neuroglial cells (astrocytes or oligodendrocytes). LGGs represent a heterogeneous group of WHO grade 1 (noninfiltrative) and grade 2 (infiltrative/diffuse) glial neoplasms.

WHO GRADING[2–4]**:** Historically, glioma type was based primarily on histopathologic appearance (i.e., oligodendroglioma with "fried egg appearance" and "chicken-wire vasculature" vs.

astrocytoma with pleomorphic giant cells and prominent cytoplasmic processes). Grade was based on the presence or extent of anaplasia, mitotic activity, microvascular proliferation, and necrosis. Grade 3 gliomas were historically termed "anaplastic gliomas," which is no longer used in the classification. Mixed tumors with both oligodendroglial and astrocytic components were historically called "oligoastrocytomas" and were included on many trials of oligodendrogliomas. However, they are no longer part of the classification as molecular characteristics can group them into either oligodendroglioma or astrocytoma. With advances in our understanding of the molecular basis of gliomas, major restructuring began with the WHO 2016 classification, and subsequently the WHO 2021 classification, which uses an integrated diagnosis based on both histopathologic appearance and molecular characteristics.

Grades 2–3 Tumors

- Oligodendroglioma, IDH-mutant (grades 2–3): Defined by IDH mutation and presence of 1p/19q codeletion. Grade 3 oligodendrogliomas have features of anaplasia, increased mitotic activity, microvascular proliferation, and/or necrosis. Grade 2 oligodendrogliomas lack these characteristics. The distinction between grades 2 and 3 can be subjective. There is no grade 4 oligodendroglioma.
- Astrocytoma, IDH-mutant (grades 2–3): Defined by IDH mutation and the absence of 1p/19q codeletion (i.e., 1p19q intact) or by presence of *ATRX* loss and/or *TP53* mutations. Grade 3 astrocytomas have features of anaplasia and/or increased mitotic activity. Grade 2 astrocytomas lack these characteristics. The distinction between grades 2 and 3 can be subjective. Grades 2 and 3 astrocytomas lack grade 4 characteristics (see Chapter 2).

See Figure 1.1 *WHO 2021 CNS Classification of Adult Diffuse Gliomas.*

Grade 1 Tumors

- Pilocytic astrocytoma: Slow-growing, posterior fossa, often cystic tumor in children and young adults demonstrating Rosenthal fibers. BRAF is a driver mutation. Enhances on MRI due to degenerative hyalinization of blood vessels. Malignant transformation is rare.
- Pleomorphic xanthoastrocytoma: Large, peripheral tumor frequently with leptomeningeal involvement. Often benign despite aggressive histologic appearance.
- Subependymal giant cell astrocytoma: Well-defined tumor typically along lateral ventricles.
- Ganglioglioma: Composed of both neoplastic neurons and astrocytes, commonly in temporal lobe, indolent course.

GENETIC MARKERS

IDH1 and IDH2 Mutations: See Chapter 1 for overview. Favorable prognosis compared with IDH-wild-type (wt).[5] IDH-mutant (mut) diffuse gliomas, encompassing astrocytomas and oligodendrogliomas, are characterized by a class defining IDH1 or (less commonly) IDH2 gene mutation.[6,7] IDH1 R132H is the most common IDH mutation and should tested on all gliomas. If absent and patient <55 years, noncanonical IDH mutations (i.e., other less common IDH1 and IDH2 mutations [R132C, R132S, R132G, R132L, R172K, R172M, R172W]) should be tested.[8]

1p19q Codeletion: Codeletion of the short arm of chr 1 and the long arm of chr 19 (1p19q) is a defining feature of oligodendroglioma, and it has a favorable prognosis.[5,9]

TP53 Mutation and/or ATRX Loss: ATRX is a gene that is involved in chromatin regulation. *ATRX* loss and/or *TP53* mutation are characteristic of astrocytoma and are mutually exclusive with 1p19q codeletion.[7,10] Less favorable prognosis than 1p19q codeletion.

MGMT Methylation: Associated with improved OS among high-risk grade 2 glioma treated with RT + TMZ.[11,12] MGMT works by removing alkyl adducts from the O6 position of guanine at DNA level, thus antagonizing the effects of alkylating agents. Methylation of MGMT silences the gene, thus leading to inadequate repair and improved response to alkylating agents.

BRAF: Mutations present in ganglioglioma, pilocytic astrocytoma, and pleomorphic xanthoastrocytoma.[13] KIAA1549-BRAF fusion is observed in the majority of pilocytic astrocytomas.

CLINICAL PRESENTATION: Depends on location, but most commonly presents as a transient neurologic disturbance or seizure (seizure in >80% of grade 2 glioma compared with 50% GBM[14]). Seizure activity associated with increased production of 2-hydroxyglutarate in IDH mutants.

WORKUP: H&P with complete neurologic exam.

Imaging: MRI with and without contrast (functional if in critical region). Grade 2 gliomas are most commonly seen as a nonenhancing hemispheric lesion (~20% do enhance[15]), rarely with mass effect. Best seen as T2/FLAIR hyperintensity (hypointense on T1, nonenhancing with gadolinium). Calcifications may be present, most classically in oligodendrogliomas. Of note, pilocytic astrocytomas enhance via a different mechanism than anaplastic astrocytomas and GBM (degenerative hyalinization of blood vessels).

Procedures: Establish preoperative neurocognitive baseline with formal testing if possible. EEG if seizures.

Pathology: Obtain tissue via a maximal safe resection, with biopsy only if a resection is not possible or diagnosis is unclear. Send for molecular profile as detailed above. Obtain a postoperative MRI within 72 hours of surgery (ideally 24–48 hours) to determine the extent of surgical resection/residual disease and avoid confounding by blood products.

PROGNOSTIC FACTORS: There is no agreed-upon definition of low-risk and high-risk patients. Various cooperative groups have defined risk factors differently. Pignatti et al. combined EORTC trials and established five poor prognostic factors: age ≥40, astrocytoma histology, tumors ≥6 cm, tumor crossing midline, and preoperative neurologic deficits.[16] RTOG 9802 stratified patients based on age and resection status, with those <40 years old s/p GTR composing the low-risk group. Seizure at presentation is a positive prognostic factor.[17] An update combined EORTC/RTOG/NCCTG analysis with pathologic grade 2 confirmation by Gorlia et al. identified four externally validated factors that predict worse PFS and OS: neurologic deficit at presentation, <30 weeks since first symptoms, astrocytic histology, and tumor >5 cm.[18] Note that age was not prognostic in this analysis. Molecular markers have since been found to be more important predictors of outcome, but it is likely that both molecular and clinical characteristics contribute to outcomes (see section on Genetic Markers).

NATURAL HISTORY: Varies widely depending on histology, prognostic factors, and molecular markers. Grade 2 gliomas have a long natural history but typically recur. At recurrence, up to 70% of tumors will have undergone malignant transformation (i.e., WHO grade 3/4).[19] Grade 1 gliomas can be cured with GTR alone.

TREATMENT PARADIGM: For grade 2 adult diffuse glioma, upfront maximal safe resection is recommended followed by postoperative MRI to evaluate extent of resection within 48 to 72 hours. Low-risk patients may be observed, whereas adjuvant CRT is recommended for high-risk patients (see Prognostic Factors for definition of low and high risk).

Surgery: Surgery is generally required to establish a diagnosis and debulk the tumor for those with extensive neurologic symptoms. There are no trials directly assessing extent of resection in LGG; however, the degree of resection is a strong prognostic factor.[20] The low-risk arm of RTOG 9802 showed significant correlation between the amount of residual tumor on imaging and recurrence.[21]

Observation: Following surgery, observation is an option for low-risk patients. This was supported by the "Non-Believers Trial" (below) and the phase II portion of RTOG 9802, which defined low-risk as those <40 years old s/p GTR. However, close follow-up is crucial, as RTOG 9802 showed a 50% risk of progression at 5 years in low-risk patients observed postoperatively.

Chemotherapy: The use of adjuvant CHT (and RT) in grade 2 glioma continues to evolve. RTOG 9802 (phase III) found that adjuvant RT followed by six cycles of PCV improves OS compared with RT alone. RTOG 0424 (phase II) supports RT with concurrent and adjuvant TMZ as it was associated with improved OS compared with a historical control. Both regimens have activity in grade 2 gliomas, but level I evidence (RTOG 9802) exists only for PCV. However, many institutions favor TMZ over PCV given better tolerance and ease of administration. EORTC 22033-26033 showed no difference in PFS if patients were treated with dose-dense TMZ alone vs. RT alone; however, further data maturation is necessary. TMZ monotherapy is not favored, and TMZ is typically used in conjunction with RT. Concurrent TMZ is 75 mg/m² taken daily (even on weekends). Adjuvant TMZ schedule: 150 to 200 mg/m² daily on days 1 to 5 q28 days, with cycle 1 beginning 28 days post-RT for a total of 12 cycles. Side effects of TMZ: constipation, thrombocytopenia, opportunistic infection. Prophylaxis against *Pneumocystis jirovecii* can be considered while on TMZ.

The IDH inhibitor, vorasidenib, is a new FDA-approved treatment option for select patients with residual/recurrent grade 2 glioma not having received prior RT. See the INDIGO trial in the Evidence-Based Q&A section.

Radiation

Indications: High-risk patients should undergo adjuvant CRT as established by RTOG 9802 (defined as age ≥40, or <40 years old s/p STR).

Dose: Doses of 45 to 54 Gy are acceptable.[22] There is no benefit to escalating dose from 45–50.4 Gy to 59.4–64.8 Gy per EORTC 22844 "Believers Trial" and RTOG 9110 discussed below. RTOG 9802 and RTOG 0424 used 54 Gy/30 fx, and the European trial E3F05 used 50.4 Gy/28 fx.

Toxicity: Acute: fatigue, headache, exacerbation of presenting neurologic deficits, alopecia, nausea, cerebral edema, side effects related to TMZ. Late: cognitive changes, radiation necrosis (2% on the standard arm of RTOG 9110), hypopituitarism (2 years post-RT), cataracts, vision loss (rare and location-dependent), secondary malignancy (<0.1%/yr).

Procedure: See *Handbook of Treatment Planning in Radiation Oncology*, Chapter 3.[23]

PEDIATRIC LOW-GRADE GLIOMA

LGGs are the most common type of brain tumor in children, which tend to be indolent with rare malignant transformation. Major histologic groups are pilocytic astrocytoma (grade 1) and diffuse fibrillary astrocytoma (grade 2). At the molecular level, the vast majority of tumors are mediated by a single genetic hit (mostly in MAPK pathway), while IDH mutation is less frequent. Common alterations include NF1 (hypothalamic/optic tract low-grade glioma), BRAF fusion, BRAF-V600E, NTRK (neurotrophic tyrosine receptor kinase) fusion, and FGFR fusion. Surgical resection or biopsy (except for children with NF1) should be attempted before adjuvant therapy. Complete surgical resection is the most prognostic factor, with >90% OS/PFS (GTR) and 45% to 65% PFS (STR) at 5 to 10 years. For tumors arising within the cerebellar and superficial cerebral hemispheres, GTR alone is considered definitive. For tumors in supratentorial midline structures, biopsy followed with focal RT (45–54 Gy) was considered first-line historically. Given risk of radiation-related neurocognitive impairment (age <12 years), there is an increasing role for adjuvant CHT, with common regimens including carboplatin/vincristine and TPCV (thioguanine, procarbazine, lomustine/CCNU, vincristine [VCR]). COG-A9952 (prospective RCT) compared carboplatin/VCR with TPCV and showed a trend of improved 5-year PFS for TPCV (52% vs. 39%, *p* = .10). Subsequent COG-ACNS0223 found that the addition of TMZ to carboplatin/VCR led to a 5-year PFS of 46% and OS of 87%. The LGG 14C03 trial is currently evaluating carboplatin alone vs. carboplatin/VCR for previously untreated pediatric/AYA LGG. TPCV should be avoided in NF1 patients (commonly with hypothalamic/optic tract low-grade glioma) due to increased risk of secondary malignancy from procarbazine/CCNU. A phase III RCT is underway to evaluate selumetinib (MEK1/2 inhibitor) vs. carboplatin/VCR for NF1-associated LGG (COG-ACNS1831). Studies employing BRAF and mTOR inhibitors are ongoing.

EVIDENCE-BASED Q&A

Does early surgical resection improve outcomes compared with watchful waiting?

No prospective trials are available to answer this question in grade 2 glioma, but retrospective studies favor upfront maximal safe resection.

Jakola, Norwegian University Hospitals (*JAMA* 2012, PMID 23099483): Population-based study of surgical resection (and extent) compared with observation. Chosen based on patients' residential address. In hospital A, patients were biopsied and observed (50% ultimately underwent resection), and in hospital B an early resection was performed. MFU 7 years. OS was significantly better with early surgical resection (5-year OS 60% vs. 74%, *p* = .01). Fewer patients underwent any resection if delayed (89% vs. 50%). **Conclusion: Early resection is warranted if safe and feasible.**

Is it safe to observe patients after surgery and reserve RT for progression?

Yes, but the ideal population to observe is unclear in the genomic era, and routine observation is associated with reduced PFS and increased seizure rates.

van den Bent, EORTC 22845 "Non-Believers Trial" (*Lancet* 2005, PMID 16168780): PRT of 311 patients (WHO PS 0–2) with LGG (astrocytoma [50%], oligodendroglioma [13%], mixed [13%], and incompletely resected pilocytic astrocytomas [1%]) s/p surgery randomized to immediate RT (54 Gy/30 fx) vs. observation with RT at progression. Resection >90% noted in 42%, 50% to 89% resection in 20%, and <50% resection or biopsy in 38%. Sixty-five percent of patients in observation arm eventually received RT. Rates of pathology-confirmed malignant transformation (70%) equal between groups. Primary endpoints OS and PFS; results are summarized in Table 3.2. **Conclusion: Immediate (vs. delayed) RT improved PFS and decreased seizure rate, but it did not improve OS.**

Table 3.2 Results of EORTC "Non-Believers Trial"					
	MS	5-Yr OS	mPFS	5-Yr PFS	Seizures at 1 Yr
Observation	7.4 yrs	66%	3.4 yrs	35%	41%
Postop 54 Gy/30 fx	7.2 yrs	69%	5.3 yrs	55%	25%
p value	.872		<.0001		.0329

Shaw, RTOG 9802 Phase II (*J Neurosurg* 2008, PMID 18976072): Phase II portion of RTOG 9802 observing 111 patients <40 years old s/p surgeon-defined GTR. 5-year OS 93% and 5-year PFS 48%. Review of postop MRI revealed that 59% of patients had <1 cm residual disease (subsequent 26% recurrence rate), 32% had 1 to 2 cm residual disease (68% recurrence), and 9% had >2 cm residual disease (89% recurrence). Poor prognostic factors included large tumor size (≥4 cm), astrocytoma or mixed oligoastrocytoma histology, and residual disease ≥1 cm by MRI. **Conclusion: Patients <40 years old s/p surgeon-determined GTR of a grade 2 glioma have a >50% risk of progression at 5 years and should be closely followed with consideration of adjuvant treatment.**

Does RT dose escalation improve outcomes?

Despite early retrospective data supporting dose escalation, two PRTs have failed to confirm a benefit.[24]

Karim, EORTC 22844 "Believers Trial" (*IJROBP* 1996, PMID 8948338): PRT of 379 patients with supratentorial low-grade astrocytomas, oligodendrogliomas, and mixed oligoastrocytoma, ages 16 to 65, KPS ≥60, randomized to 45 Gy/25 fx vs. 59.4 Gy/33 fx after surgery (any degree of resection). There was no difference in 5-year OS (59% vs. 58%) or PFS (50% vs. 47%). Radionecrosis 2.5% vs. 4% at 2 years. **Conclusion: Dose-escalated RT for grade 2 gliomas does not improve OS or PFS.**

Shaw, RTOG 9110 (*JCO* 2002, PMID 11980997; Update *Neuro Oncol* 2020, PMID 32002556): PRT of 203 patients with supratentorial grades 1 to 2 astrocytoma, oligodendroglioma, or mixed oligoastrocytoma randomized to 50.4 Gy/28 fx vs. 64.8 Gy/36 fx, following surgery (any degree of resection). No difference in 5-year OS (64% vs. 72%, *p* = .48) with higher rate of grade 3+ radiation necrosis seen in high-dose arm (2% vs. 5%). Ninety-two percent of failures were in-field. 15-year update showed no improvement in OS (22% vs. 25%, *p* = .98). PFS was improved in patients with oligodendroglioma compared with astrocytoma. MMSE was stable after RT. **Conclusion: No difference in 5-year or 15-year OS between high-dose and low-dose RT for adult low-grade gliomas.**

Does adjuvant CRT improve outcomes compared with adjuvant RT alone?

The addition of PCV to RT substantially improves survival in high-risk patients.

Shaw, RTOG 9802 Phase III (*JCO* 2012, PMID 22851558; Update Buckner *NEJM* 2016, PMID 27050206): Phase III component of RTOG 9802, which randomized 251 high-risk patients (age >40 or <40 years s/p STR) with grade 2 glioma (astrocytoma, oligodendroglioma, and mixed oligoastrocytoma in 26%, 42%, and 32%) to RT alone vs. RT followed by six cycles of PCV. RT dose was 54 Gy/30 fx. Addition of PCV led to higher grade 3 and 4 hematologic toxicities (51% vs. 8% grade 3 and 15% vs. 3% grade 4 toxicities). The addition of PCV improved OS and PFS (see Table 3.3). Favorable prognostic variables for both OS and PFS included receipt of PCV and oligodendroglioma histology. Exploratory analysis of patients with IDH1-mut demonstrated significantly longer OS (13.1 vs. 5.1 years). Power insufficient to investigate IDH1-wt. **Conclusion: The addition of PCV to RT significantly improves OS in high-risk patients.**

Table 3.3 Final Results of RTOG 9802 Phase III Component				
	MS	**10-Yr OS**	**mPFS**	**10-Yr PFS**
RT alone	7.8 yrs	41%	4 yrs	21%
RT followed by PCV	13.3 yrs	62%	10.4 yrs	51%
p value	.003		<.001	

Bell, RTOG 9802 Genomic Analysis (*JCO* 2020, PMID 32706640): Post-hoc genomic analysis of RTOG 9802 that grouped patients (106 of the initial 251) with available tissue into the following categories based on WHO 2016 molecular classifications: IDHmut/1p19q-codel, IDHmut/1p19q-noncodel, and IDHwt. MFU 9 years. OS and PFS were analyzed for each respective group and for some individual mutations; see Table 3.4 for the results. IDH1/2mut, 1p/19q codel, and TERT promoter mutations were significantly associated with improved OS and PFS. TERT promoter mutations were not significantly associated with improved PFS. **Conclusion: Significant OS and PFS benefit with the addition of PCV to RT for IDHmut/codel and IDHmut/noncodel, but not IDHwt patients.**

Table 3.4 Genomic Analysis of RTOG 9802 Phase III Component						
	IDH-Mut, 1p19q-Codel		**IDH-Mut, 1p19q-Noncodel**		**IDH-Wild-Type**	
	mOS	**mPFS**	**mOS**	**mPFS**	**mOS**	**mPFS**
RT alone	13.9 yrs	5.8 yrs	4.3 yrs	3.3 yrs	1.9 yrs	0.7 yrs
RT followed by PCV	NR	NR	11.4 yrs	10.4 yrs	1.9 yrs	0.7 yrs
p value	.029	<.001	.013	.003	.94	.41

Are outcomes similar if TMZ is substituted for PCV?

Level I data suggest that PCV improves survival, but it is toxic and difficult to administer. Many clinicians therefore give TMZ, extrapolating from high-grade glioma data. This question is being further addressed in the ongoing CODEL study, a phase III trial randomizing grades 2 to 3 glioma patients with 1p19q codeletion to adjuvant RT followed by PCV vs. RT + TMZ followed by TMZ.

Fisher, RTOG 0424 (*IJROBP* 2015, PMID 25680596; Update *IJROBP* 2020, PMID 32251755): Single-arm phase II trial of 129 high-risk WHO grade 2 glioma patients (astrocytomas, oligodendrogliomas, and mixed oligoastrocytoma) treated with RT (54 Gy/30 fx) with concurrent daily TMZ followed by 12 cycles of monthly adjuvant TMZ. Patients must have three or more of the following risk factors: age ≥40, tumor ≥6 cm, tumor crossing midline, astrocytoma histology, preoperative NFS >1. The 3-year OS was 74% comparing favorably to historical rate of 54% (*p* < .001) and higher than the hypothesized rate of 65%. The 3-year PFS was 59%. Grade 3/4 toxicity in 44%/10% and one patient with grade 5 infection attributed to TMZ/steroids. Notably, rates of hematologic toxicities were 24% for grade 3 events and 8% for grade 4. Favorable factors for OS and PFS included MGMT methylation and female sex. **Conclusion: Long-term results with concurrent and adjuvant TMZ are favorable.**

Bell, RTOG 0424-MGMT (*JAMA Oncol* 2018, PMID 29955793): Subsequent analysis of RTOG 0424 examining 75 (of the total 129) patients with MGMT status available, 76% methylated vs. 24% unmethylated. In MVA (including IDH1/2 status), unmethylated MGMT was associated with worse OS (HR 2.70, 95% CI 1.02–7.14) and PFS (HR 2.74, 1.19–6.33). **Conclusion: MGMT promoter methylation was an independent prognostic biomarker of high-risk grade 2 glioma treated with TMZ-RT.**

Are there subsets of patients who can be treated initially with CHT alone?

Given the long and variable natural history of grade 2 gliomas and relatively younger patient population, studies have evaluated whether RT can be deferred to avoid toxicity. EORTC 22033-26033 compared high-risk grade 2 glioma treated with RT alone vs. dose-dense TMZ alone and found no difference in PFS, HR-QOL, or impaired cognitive dysfunction. It is important to note that the median PFS of 39 months (TMZ alone) and 46 months (RT alone) in the EORTC study was far less than the median PFS of 10.4 years (RT + PCV) seen on RTOG 9802.

Baumert, EORTC 22033-26033 (*Lancet Oncol* 2016, PMID 27686946): PRT of 477 patients with grade 2 glioma, age ≥18, and with ≥1 high-risk feature (age >40, size >5 cm, progressive disease, tumor crossing midline, neurologic symptoms) randomized to RT alone (50.4 Gy/28 fx) vs. dose-dense TMZ alone (75 mg/m^2 days 1–21 of a 28-day cycle, max 12 cycles). Stratified by 1p deletion, contrast enhancement, age ≥40, and ECOG ≥1. Primary endpoint PFS. At MFU of 48 months, mPFS was 46 months for RT alone vs. 39 months for TMZ alone (*p* = .22). OS not reached. Exploratory analysis showed IDH-mut/1p19q noncodel had longer PFS if treated with RT alone vs. TMZ alone (*p* = .0043), but no difference for IDH-mut/1p19q codeleted or IDH-wt. Grades 3 to 4 hematologic toxicity <1% RT vs. 14% TMZ, moderate/severe fatigue 3% RT vs. 7% TMZ, grades 3 to 4 infections 1% RT vs. 3% TMZ. Furthermore, TMZ monotherapy did not improve QOL, MMSE, or cognition, compared with RT. **Conclusion: TMZ monotherapy did not improve PFS, QOL, or neurocognition compared with RT alone in grade 2 glioma.**

Klein, EORTC 22033-26033 Correlative Analysis (*Neuro Oncol* 2021, PMID 33130890): Neuropsychological assessment completed in 98 patients (53 RT, 46 TMZ) using the Visual Verbal Learning Test (VVLT) revealed baseline similar memory functioning between the arms. Both arms, over time, showed improvement in immediate recall and total number of words recalled, although patients in the RT group showed delayed improvement. There was no correlation between memory functioning and RT GTV, CTV, or PTV. **Conclusion: No evidence that RT significantly affects memory function compared with TMZ monotherapy in the first year after treatment for patients with high-risk low-grade glioma.**

Reijneveld, EORTC 22033-26033 HR-QOL Analysis (*Lancet Oncol* 2016, PMID 27686943): Secondary endpoint reporting on HR-QOL and global cognitive functioning (using the MMSE) from EORTC 22033-26033. The difference in HR-QOL was not significantly different during the 36 months of follow-up between the RT alone and TMZ alone arms. No significant difference recorded between the groups for change in MMSE scores during follow-up from baseline. **Conclusion: The effects of TMZ or RT on HR-QOL or MMSE scores do not differ in patients with grade 2 gliomas.**

What is the role of IDH inhibitors for grade 2 gliomas?

Vorasidenib is an oral CNS-penetrant inhibitor of mutant IDH1 and IDH2 enzymes and is newly FDA-approved for select patients with residual/recurrent grade 2 glioma not having received prior RT. Per NCCN, it can be considered in those in whom upfront treatment with RT and CHT is "not preferred."[22]

Mellighoff, INDIGO Trial (*NEJM* 2023, PMID 37272516): Double-blind, phase III trial of 331 patients with residual or recurrent grade 2 IDH-mut glioma with no previous treatment other than surgery (1–5 years from surgery; not sooner, not later) randomized to either oral vorasidenib (40 mg once daily) vs. placebo in 28-day cycles. Over 80% of patients had ≥2 cm of residual tumor. MFU 14.2 months. PFS significantly improved with vorasidenib (mPFS 27.7 vs. 11.1 months). Time to next intervention was significantly improved in vorasidenib group vs. placebo; at 24 months, 73% of placebo patients required treatment compared with 17% on vorasidenib. Grade 3+ AEs: 23% in vorasidenib vs. 14% in placebo. The most frequent grade 3+ toxicity was rise in ALT in 10% of patients. **Conclusion: Vorasidenib in residual/recurrent grade 2 IDH-mut gliomas treated with surgery alone improves PFS by 16.6 months compared with placebo and can delay time to further treatment.** *Comment: The study is controversial given that it did not compare outcomes or toxicity with the standard of care, which is adjuvant CRT. MFU was just 14.2 months and OS has yet to be reported, so long-term outcomes are unclear.*

How do tumor progression and RT affect cognition?

One reason to delay RT is to avoid the initial neurocognitive effects of treatment, but this is associated with reduced PFS ("Non-Believers Trial" above), which may also affect cognition. Analysis of RTOG 9110 showed stable MMSE scores for most patients after RT and improvement in MMSE for those with lower baseline scores.[25] Analysis of RTOG 9802 showed improved MMSE scores with the addition of CHT to RT.[26] However, MMSE may not be as reliable in evaluating neurocognitive function as more formal testing. A more extensive analysis of 20 patients in RTOG 9110 used formal cognitive testing and showed stable neurocognitive function up to 5 years out from RT.[27] RT dose escalation may worsen QOL, as shown in the "Believers Trial."[28] Several secondary analyses of EORTC 22033-26033 demonstrate that there are no differences in HR-QOL or cognitive function when comparing RT with TMZ. Brain target volumes were also not found to be associated with HR-QOL, but tumor progression was associated with short-term decline.[29,30]

REFERENCES

1. Ostrom QT, Price M, Neff C, et al. CBTRUS statistical report: primary brain and other central nervous system tumors diagnosed in the United States in 2016–2020. *Neuro Oncol.* 2023;25(12 suppl 2):iv1–iv99. doi:10.1093/neuonc/noad149

2. Braganza MZ, Kitahara CM, Berrington De Gonzalez A, Inskip PD, Johnson KJ, Rajaraman P. Ionizing radiation and the risk of brain and central nervous system tumors: a systematic review. *Neuro Oncol.* 2012;14(11):1316–1324. doi:10.1093/neuonc/nos208

3. Marquet G, Dameron O, Saikali S, Mosser J, Burgun A. Grading glioma tumors using OWL-DL and NCI thesaurus. *AMIA Annu Symp Proc.* 2007;2007:508–512. PMID:18693888

4. Louis DN, Perry A, Wesseling P, et al. The 2021 WHO classification of tumors of the central nervous system: a summary. *Neuro Oncol.* 2021;23(8):1231–1251. doi:10.1093/neuonc/noab106

5. Brat DJ, Verhaak RG, Aldape KD, et al. Comprehensive, integrative genomic analysis of diffuse lower-grade gliomas. *N Engl J Med.* 2015;372(26):2481–2498. doi:10.1056/NEJMoa1402121

6. Sanson M, Marie Y, Paris S, et al. Isocitrate dehydrogenase 1 codon 132 mutation is an important prognostic biomarker in gliomas. *J Clin Oncol.* 2009;27(25):4150–4154. doi:10.1200/jco.2009.21.9832

7. Gritsch S, Batchelor TT, Gonzalez Castro LN. Diagnostic, therapeutic, and prognostic implications of the 2021 World Health Organization classification of tumors of the central nervous system. *Cancer.* 2022;128(1):47–58. doi:10.1002/cncr.33918

8. DeWitt JC, Jordan JT, Frosch MP, et al. Cost-effectiveness of IDH testing in diffuse gliomas according to the 2016 WHO classification of tumors of the central nervous system recommendations. *Neuro Oncol.* 2017;19(12):1640–1650. doi:10.1093/neuonc/nox120

9. Cairncross JG, Wang M, Jenkins RB, et al. Benefit from procarbazine, lomustine, and vincristine in oligodendroglial tumors is associated with mutation of IDH. *J Clin Oncol.* 2014;32(8):783–790. doi:10.1200/JCO.2013.49.3726

10. Berger TR, Wen PY, Lang-Orsini M, Chukwueke UN. World Health Organization 2021 classification of central nervous system tumors and implications for therapy for adult-type gliomas. *JAMA Oncol.* 2022;8(10):1493–1501. doi:10.1001/jamaoncol.2022.2844

11. Thon N, Eigenbrod S, Kreth S, et al. IDH1 mutations in grade II astrocytomas are associated with unfavorable progression-free survival and prolonged postrecurrence survival. *Cancer.* 2012;118(2):452–460. doi:10.1002/cncr.26298

12. Watanabe T, Katayama Y, Yoshino A, et al. Aberrant hypermethylation of p14ARF and O6-methylguanine-DNA methyltransferase genes in astrocytoma progression. *Brain Pathol.* 2007;17(1):5–10. doi:10.1111/j.1750-3639.2006.00030.x

13. Olar A, Sulman EP. Molecular markers in low-grade glioma-toward tumor reclassification. *Semin Radiat Oncol.* 2015;25(3):155–163. doi:10.1016/j.semradonc.2015.02.006

14. Gunderson LL, Tepper JE. *Clinical Radiation Oncology,* 4th ed. Elsevier; 2015:1648.

15. Lote K, Egeland T, Hager B, Skullerud K, Hirschberg H. Prognostic significance of CT contrast enhancement within histological subgroups of intracranial glioma. *J Neurooncol.* 1998;40(2):161–170. doi:10.1023/a:1006106708606

16. Pignatti F, van den Bent M, Curran D, et al. Prognostic factors for survival in adult patients with cerebral low-grade glioma. *J Clin Oncol.* 2002;20(8):2076–2084. doi:10.1200/JCO.2002.08.121

17. Reichenthal E, Feldman Z, Cohen ML, Loven D, Zucker G. Hemispheric supratentorial low-grade astrocytoma. *Neurochirurgia.* 1992;35(1):18–22. doi:10.1055/s-2008-1052239

18. Gorlia T, Wu W, Wang M, et al. New validated prognostic models and prognostic calculators in patients with low-grade gliomas diagnosed by central pathology review: a pooled analysis of EORTC/RTOG/NCCTG phase III clinical trials. *Neuro Oncol.* 2013;15(11):1568–1579. doi:10.1093/neuonc/not117

19. van den Bent MJ, Afra D, de Witte O, et al. Long-term efficacy of early versus delayed radiotherapy for low-grade astrocytoma and oligodendroglioma in adults: the EORTC 22845 randomised trial. *Lancet.* 2005;366(9490):985–990. doi:10.1016/s0140-6736(05)67070-5

20. Aghi MK, Nahed BV, Sloan AE, Ryken TC, Kalkanis SN, Olson JJ. The role of surgery in the management of patients with diffuse low grade glioma: a systematic review and evidence-based clinical practice guideline. *J Neurooncol.* 2015;125(3):503–530. doi:10.1007/s11060-015-1867-1

21. Shaw EG, Berkey B, Coons SW, et al. Recurrence following neurosurgeon-determined gross-total resection of adult supratentorial low-grade glioma: results of a prospective clinical trial. *J Neurosurg.* 2008;109(5):835–841. doi:10.3171/jns/2008/109/11/0835

22. NCCN Clinical Practice Guidelines in Oncology: Central Nervous System Cancers. Accessed September 24, 2016. https://www.nccn.org/professionals/physician_gls/pdf/cns.pdf

23. Gregory M. M. Videtic MDCMF, Vassil AD, Woody NM. *Handbook of Treatment Planning in Radiation Oncology.* Springer Publishing Company; 2020.

24. Shaw EG, Daumas-Duport C, Scheithauer BW, et al. Radiation therapy in the management of low-grade supratentorial astrocytomas. *J Neurosurg.* 1989;70(6):853–861. doi:10.3171/jns.1989.70.6.0853

25. Brown PD, Buckner JC, O'Fallon JR, et al. Effects of radiotherapy on cognitive function in patients with low-grade glioma measured by the folstein mini-mental state examination. *J Clin Oncol*. 2003;21(13):2519–2524. doi:10.1200/jco.2003.04.172

26. Prabhu RS, Won M, Shaw EG, et al. Effect of the addition of chemotherapy to radiotherapy on cognitive function in patients with low-grade glioma: secondary analysis of RTOG 98-02. *J Clin Oncol*. 2014;32(6): 535–541. doi:10.1200/jco.2013.53.1830

27. Laack NN, Brown PD, Ivnik RJ, et al. Cognitive function after radiotherapy for supratentorial low-grade glioma: a North Central Cancer Treatment Group prospective study. *Int J Radiat Oncol Biol Phys*. 2005;63(4):1175–1183. doi:10.1016/j.ijrobp.2005.04.016

28. Kiebert GM, Curran D, Aaronson NK, et al. Quality of life after radiation therapy of cerebral low-grade gliomas of the adult: results of a randomised phase III trial on dose response (EORTC trial 22844). EORTC Radiotherapy Co-operative Group. *Eur J Cancer*. 1998;34(12):1902–1909. doi:10.1016/s0959-8049(98)00268-8

29. Dirven L, Reijneveld JC, Taphoorn MJB, et al. Impact of radiation target volume on health-related quality of life in patients with low-grade glioma in the 2-year period post treatment: a secondary analysis of the EORTC 22033-26033. *Int J Radiat Oncol Biol Phys*. 2019;104(1):90–100. doi:10.1016/j.ijrobp.2019.01.003

30. Reijneveld JC, Taphoorn MJB, Coens C, et al. Health-related quality of life in patients with high-risk low-grade glioma (EORTC 22033-26033): a randomised, open-label, phase 3 intergroup study. *Lancet Oncol*. 2016;17(11):1533–1542. doi:10.1016/s1470-2045(16)30305-9

4 MENINGIOMA

Anirudh Bommireddy, Abigail L. Stockham, Martin C. Tom, and Jennifer S. Yu

QUICK HIT Meningiomas are the most common primary brain tumor in adults, representing ~40% of all primary brain tumors with ~37,000 cases per year in the United States, 80% of which are WHO grade 1. Asymptomatic grade 1 meningiomas can be observed, whereas maximal safe resection is otherwise the standard of care for lesions that are surgically accessible. The extent of surgical resection and the grade of meningioma determine the initial postsurgical approach (see Table 4.1). In combination with MRI, DOTATATE PET/CT can aid in determining the extent of resection and RT target volumes. Recurrent meningiomas are generally managed with re-resection followed by RT when no previous RT has been administered. Unresectable meningiomas are managed with fractionated RT or SRS, depending on grade, size, and location. Similar strategies are employed in the setting of spinal meningiomas (~10% of cases). While the vast majority of meningiomas are benign, they may ultimately cause significant morbidity and mortality. Particularly in young patients, the likelihood and morbidity of recurrence must be weighed against the potential long-term sequelae of RT to the brain. Grade 2 meningiomas have an intermediate prognosis, while grade 3 meningiomas have high rates of recurrence and mortality. Several molecular classifiers have been developed to better understand prognosis and predict response to treatment beyond the WHO 2021 classification.

Table 4.1 RT Dose Guidelines for Meningioma			
Extent of Resection	**WHO Grade 1**	**WHO Grade 2**	**WHO Grade 3**
GTR	Observe	EBRT 54–59.4 Gy/30–33 fx (preferred) OR observe in well-selected patients	60–66 Gy/30–33 fx
STR	Observe OR EBRT 54 Gy/30 fx OR SRS 12–14 Gy	59.4–66 Gy/30–33 fx	60–66 Gy/30–33 fx
Recurrent disease	Consider further resection + EBRT 54 Gy/30 fx OR SRS 12–14 Gy	Consider further resection + 59.4–66 Gy/30–33 fx (preferred) OR SRS 16 Gy	Consider further resection 60–66 Gy/30–33 fx (preferred) OR SRS 18–24 Gy (based on size)
	Consider targeted therapy or radionuclide treatment for multiple recurrent and/or previously irradiated disease.		
Unresectable disease	EBRT 54 Gy/30 fx OR SRS 12–14 Gy	59.4–66 Gy/30–33 fx (preferred) OR SRS 16 Gy	60–66 Gy/30–33 fx (preferred) OR SRS 18–24 Gy (based on size)

EPIDEMIOLOGY: 37,000 cases per year in the United States; approximate 1-, 5-, and 10-year survival rates are 80%, 65%, and 58%, respectively (decreased survival rates with increasing age). Incidence increases with age (especially >65).[1,2] There is ~2–3:1 female predominance, although males are slightly more likely to have atypical or malignant meningiomas.[1,3,4]

RISK FACTORS: Older age, ionizing radiation, NF2, MEN1, exogenous/endogenous hormones, elevated BMI, decreased physical activity, increased height (women), uterine fibroids, and breast cancer.[2,5–11] The degree to which estrogen exposure is an independent risk factor from BMI, decreased physical activity, increased height, uterine fibroids, and breast cancer is unclear.

ANATOMY: Arises from the arachnoid layer of the meninges between the dura mater and pia mater, commonly at sites of high density of arachnoid villi and associated arachnoid cap cells. Most frequently noted at supratentorial sites of dural reflection, such as at the cerebral convexity (~20%) and parafalcine/parasagittal (~25%), along the sphenoid wing (~20%) and skull base (resulting in decreased surgical accessibility), intraventricular and suprasellar region, and olfactory groove (~10%) and in the posterior fossa most commonly along the petrous bone (~10%).

PATHOLOGY: Classified by the WHO into three grades (Table 4.2): WHO grade 1 (benign), WHO grade 2 (atypical, yet still benign), and WHO grade 3 (malignant). Choroid and clear cell meningiomas have a higher risk of recurrence and are assigned WHO grade 2, as are brain-invasive meningiomas. While rhabdoid and papillary meningiomas have more aggressive behaviors, the presence of these subtypes alone is not sufficient to designate them as grade 3.[12] Several molecular classifiers have been developed to better understand prognosis and predict response to treatment beyond the WHO 2021 classification.[13–15]

Table 4.2 Summary of WHO Grading for Meningiomas				
WHO Grade	Frequency	Subtypes	Characteristics	Recurrence After GTR
Grade 1	80%–85%	Meningothelial Fibroblastic Transitional Psammomatous Angiomatous Microcystic Secretory Metaplastic Lymphoplasmacyte-rich	Psammoma bodies Cellular whorls Calcifications	7%–25%
Grade 2	15%–18%	Chordoid Clear cell Atypical	≥4 mitoses/10 HPF, brain invasion, OR ≥3 features below: • Hypercellularity • Small cells with high nuclear:cytoplasm ratio • Prominent nucleoli • Patternless/sheet-like growth • Foci of spontaneous necrosis	30%–50%
Grade 3	1%–3%	Anaplastic	≥20 mitoses/10 HPF and/or • Carcinomatous features • Sarcomatous features • Melanomatous features • Loss of usual growth pattern • Abundant mitoses with atypia • Multifocal necrotic foci • *TERT* promoter mutation • Homozygous *CDKNA2A/B* loss	50%–94%

GENETICS: Genetic mutations are common, but the clinical impact of mutations is evolving. DNA methylation profiling and other molecular signatures are promising to better risk-stratify meningiomas.[11] Relevant molecular alterations include *NF2* mutation, *TRAF7* mutation, *TERT* promotor mutation, *SMARCE1* mutation, *BAP1* mutation, *CDKNA2A/B* loss, *H3K27me3* loss, and DNA methylation profiling.[12,16]

CLINICAL PRESENTATION: May be asymptomatic. If symptomatic, presents with headaches, seizure, altered cognition, focal neurologic deficit—these are further detailed in Table 4.3 (data modified from Raizer).[17]

Table 4.3 Common Presenting Symptoms of Meningioma Based on Location
Parasagittal: motor and/or sensory changes
Frontal: personality change, avolition, executive dysfunction, disinhibition, urinary incontinence, Broca aphasia
Temporal: memory changes, Wernicke aphasia (left), aprosody (right), olfactory symptoms including seizures

(continued)

Table 4.3 Common Presenting Symptoms of Meningioma Based on Location (*continued*)
Cavernous sinus: CN symptoms (CN III, IV, V1–V2, VI pass through the cavernous sinus), decreased visual acuity, impaired extraocular motion with resultant diplopia, numbness
Occipital lobe: visual field deficit
Cerebellopontine angle: unilateral deafness/decreased hearing, facial numbness, facial weakness
Optic nerve sheath: ipsilateral decreased visual acuity/blindness, exophthalmos, ipsilateral pupillary dilation nonreactive to direct light but with retained consensual contraction
Sphenoid wing: cranial neuropathy, seizures
Tentorium: extra-axial compression with associated occipital/parietal/cerebellar symptoms
Foramen magnum: paraparesis, urinary/anal sphincter dysfunction, tongue atrophy ± fasciculation
Spinal canal: back pain, Brown-Séquard (hemispinal cord) syndrome

WORKUP: H&P with neurologic exam, head CT, MRI brain. Classically presents with a well-circumscribed, homogeneously enhancing extra-axial mass with a dural tail (present in more than half of meningiomas—may also be present in patients with chloroma, lymphoma, and sarcoidosis). Meningiomas are T1 isointense and CT isodense with normal brain parenchyma unless contrast is administered, underscoring the importance of IV contrast when possible. DOTATATE-PET scans are more sensitive and specific than MRI for meningioma identification, and may be helpful when diagnostic uncertainty exists and to augment target delineation in RT treatment planning in addition to traditional MRI co-registration.[18] Evaluate for bone invasion and/or reactive hyperostosis. Modest perilesional edema may be present; this is more frequently encountered with rapidly enlarging atypical and/or malignant meningiomas as well as convexity or parasagittal meningiomas. Extensive perilesional edema is a relative contraindication to SRS as patients may have considerable posttreatment edema (especially convexity meningiomas).

PROGNOSTIC FACTORS: Worse prognosis with increasing grade, decreasing extent of resection, proliferative index (Ki-67) >1%, brain invasion, age <45, chromosomal abnormalities involving 14 and 22, aggressive clinical behavior, p53 overexpression.[19–25]

NATURAL HISTORY: Grade 1 meningiomas grow ~1 to 2 mm annually. Most failures occur locally, and local progression can further aggravate associated neurologic symptoms. Marginal failure around the meninges is possible, particularly with high-grade meningioma.

TREATMENT PARADIGM

Observation: Observation may be appropriate for incidentally discovered small, asymptomatic meningiomas. Observation is also appropriate for WHO grade 1 tumors following GTR and may be considered following STR as well. Observation following GTR for grade 2 meningiomas is under investigation. Surveillance with MRI is recommended annually for patients with WHO grade 1 meningiomas undergoing observation to assess need for treatment.

Surgery: Standard is maximal safe surgical resection. Often requires craniotomy, but for sphenoid wing/skull base lesions endoscopic surgery may be indicated. Simpson grade correlates with LF (Table 4.4). Postoperative brain MRI should be obtained within 48 hours of surgery.

Table 4.4 Simpson Grading System for Meningioma Resection		
Grade	Extent of Resection	5-Yr LR (%)
0	GTR, including dural attachment and bone plus stripping of 2–4 cm dura	0
1	GTR, including dural attachment and any abnormal bone	9
2	GTR, with coagulation instead of resection of dural attachment	19
3	GTR of meningioma without resection or coagulation of dural attachment	29
4	Subtotal resection	44
5	Tumor debulking or decompression only	N/A

Systemic Therapy: No primary role for CHT. Despite the use of appropriate surgery ± RT, there is a subset of patients who continue to do poorly. Targeted agents that are being studied, particularly in the recurrent setting, include somatostatin analogues, interferons, tyrosine kinase inhibitors, and VEGF inhibitors. The role of radionuclide treatment, such as Lutathera (177Lu-DOTATATE), is also continuing to develop.

Radiation

Adjuvant: Following surgery, adjuvant RT is typically indicated for WHO grades 2 and 3 meningiomas, with consideration of RT for WHO grade 1 following STR. WHO grade 1 meningiomas are generally treated to 50.4 Gy/28 fx or 54 Gy/30 fx. WHO grade 2 meningiomas following GTR are generally treated to 54–59.4 Gy/30–33 fx. WHO grade 2 meningiomas following STR and WHO grade 3 meningiomas are treated to 60–66 Gy/30–33 fx. See RTOG 0539 for common dosing strategy and target delineation. Recent data suggest that dose escalation ≥66 Gy for grade 2 or 3 meningioma is associated with improved LC and PFS with an acceptable risk of radiation necrosis.[26]

Unresectable/Medically Inoperable: SRS dose, when feasible, is 12 to 14 Gy for grade 1 tumors. Fractionated stereotactic RT (FSRT) 25 Gy/5 fx is an option for large-volume or critically located grade 1 meningiomas.[27] When surrounding tissues allow, 16 Gy for grade 2 tumors may be considered. RTOG 9005 dosing (18–24 Gy) is commonly used for grade 3 tumors.

Brachytherapy is utilized at select institutions for multiply recurrent meningiomas.

Following treatment, prior NCCN guidelines suggested that surveillance imaging with contrast-enhanced MRI should be performed at 3, 6, and 12 months, then q6–12 months for 5 years, then q1–3 years thereafter for WHO grade 1/2. For WHO grade 3 meningiomas, contrast-enhanced MRI should be performed q2–4 months for 3 years, then q3–6 months thereafter; however 2025 NCCN guidelines no longer make such recommendations.[28]

Procedure: See *Handbook of Treatment Planning in Radiation Oncology*, Chapter 3.[29]

EVIDENCE-BASED Q&A

Do incidentally discovered meningiomas require aggressive intervention?

Incidentally appreciated meningiomas may not require additional intervention. In at least one study, more than half demonstrated no growth at 5 years. These patients may be followed with imaging at 3 to 6 months and then annually thereafter if no growth is appreciated.[30]

What is the optimal first-line management in the treatment of meningiomas?

Maximal safe surgical resection provides the greatest opportunity for minimizing recurrence rates. The extent of resection is graded according to the Simpson grading system, which was the foundational study in meningioma.[31] A Mayo Clinic study showed a 5- and 10-year PFS of 88% and 75% for GTR, but only 61% and 39% for STR.[21] SRS is commonly employed for grade 1 meningiomas, with LC rates similar to that of GTR.[32]

What is the role of RT in the management of WHO grade 1 meningiomas?

GTR (Simpson 1–3) is generally considered definitive, and patients may be followed with surveillance imaging. However, with longer follow-up, recurrence rates as high as 20%, 40%, and 60% have been reported at 5, 10, and 15 years, likely reflecting modern imaging capabilities.[21,33,34] RT is typically reserved for salvage in these patients. For those with STR (Simpson 4–5), LR rates of 40% at 5 years and 60% at 10 years can be reduced to those of GTR (approximately halved) with adjuvant RT using doses >50.4 Gy.[35,36]

What is the role of RT in the management of WHO grade 2 meningiomas?

Adjuvant RT is generally recommended after GTR and strongly recommended after STR. Adjuvant RT dose after GTR of a WHO grade 2 meningioma was 54 Gy on RTOG 0539 and 59.4 Gy on BN003. After STR of a WHO grade 2, adjuvant RT to 59.4 Gy/33 fx, 60 Gy/30 fx, or 66 Gy/33 fx is recommended to minimize risk of LR based on multiple retrospective series.[37–39] Without RT, LR rates of up to 60% at 5 years and CSS of only 70% at 10 years have been observed. Following GTR (Simpson 1–2), 5-year PFS is roughly doubled, from ~40% to 80% with adjuvant RT. Following STR, adjuvant RT is strongly recommended due to high recurrence rates.[33,40]

Can RT margins be reduced in patients with WHO grade 2 meningioma treated with IMRT?

Although RTOG 0539 used at least a 1-cm CTV expansion for WHO grade 2 meningiomas, retrospective data suggest a 5-mm CTV and a 3-mm PTV may be used without undue risk of LR.[41]

What is the role of RT in the management of WHO grade 3 meningiomas?

Adjuvant RT is necessary regardless of resection extent. WHO grade 3 meningiomas are rare, with <300 cases per year in the United States.[1] Grade 3 tumors are significantly more aggressive, with OS rates of 50% to 60% at 5 years (compared with >90% for low-grade meningiomas). A systematic review showed a median 5-year PFS and OS of 48% and 56%, respectively, in patients with grade 3 meningioma. Incomplete resection and RT dose <50 Gy had significantly poorer 5-year PFS. A minimum dose of 60 Gy is recommended.[37–39,42,43]

Are there prospective data to guide the treatment of meningiomas in the modern era?

Rogers, RTOG 0539 (Low Risk, *Neuro Oncol*, PMID 35657335; Intermediate Risk, *J Neurosurg* 2018, PMID 28984517; High Risk, *IJROBP* 2020, PMID 31786276): RTOG 0539 was the first prospective trial guiding the use of RT for meningiomas. Three risk groups were defined: low, intermediate, and high; and the results are summarized in Table 4.5. **Conclusion: This trial supports observation for low-risk patients and 54 Gy for intermediate-risk patients. WHO grade 1 s/p STR may warrant adjuvant RT (crude failure rate 40%).**

Table 4.5 RTOG 0539 Summary				
Risk Group	**Definition**	**EBRT Dose**	**Target Volume**	**Outcomes**
Low (*n* = 63)	WHO grade 1 meningioma s/p GTR or STR	Observation	N/A	5-yr PFS: 89% 5-yr LF: 9% 5-yr OS: 98%
Intermediate (*n* = 48)	WHO grade 2 meningioma s/p GTR Recurrent WHO grade 1 meningioma	54 Gy/30 fx	Tumor bed + 1 cm CTV, reduced to 5 mm around barriers	3-yr PFS: 94% 3-yr LF: 4%
High (*n* = 51)	WHO grade 3 meningioma (any resection) WHO grade 2 meningioma s/p STR Recurrent WHO grade 2 meningioma	60 Gy/30 fx (high-dose PTV) with simultaneous low-dose PTV 54 Gy	HD PTV: gross tumor + resection bed + 1 cm	3-yr PFS: 59% 3-yr LF: 31% 3-yr OS: 79%
			LD PTV: gross tumor + resection bed + 2 cm	

Weber, EORTC 22042-26042 (*Radiother Oncol* 2018, PMID 29960684): Single-arm phase II study of 56 patients with grade 2 meningioma s/p GTR and RT 60 Gy/30 fx designed to show 3-year PFS >70%. With MFU of 5.1 years, the 3-year PFS was 89% and OS was 98%. Late grade ≥3 toxicity was 14%. **Conclusion: Grade 2 meningioma s/p GTR and 60 Gy/30 fx result in PFS of 89%.** *Note: Observational cohorts of grade 2 meningiomas s/p STR and grade 3 meningiomas s/p any extent of resection have not yet been reported.*

Is there a role for dose-escalated RT?

Zeng, Toronto (*IJROBP* 2024, PMID 37793575): Single-institution cohort study of 118 patients with grades 2 and 3 meningiomas s/p surgery treated with adjuvant or salvage RT. Dose-escalation cohort was ≥66 Gy, while standard-dose cohort was <66 Gy. Residual disease was present in 100% of dose-escalated patients and 66% of standard-dose patients ($p < .001$). The 5-year PFS in the dose-escalated and standard-dose cohorts was 65% and 41%, respectively ($p = .030$). On MVA, dose escalation was associated with improved PFS and less LF. No difference in rate of symptomatic radiation necrosis (6%) between the cohorts. **Conclusion: Dose escalation ≥66 Gy for grade 2 or 3 meningiomas, particularly after STR, is associated with improved LC and PFS with acceptable rates of radiation necrosis.**

Should patients previously treated with RT be screened for meningioma?

No. The incidence of clinically relevant meningioma in patients with a history of cranial RT is ~3% at 30 years from the time of RT.[44] The incidence of any meningioma in patients with no history of cranial RT may be as high as ~13% at 10 years.[45] The incidence may reach 20% in patients with previous cranial RT who undergo screening with MRI at 20 years following RT.[46] The estimated risk of neoplastic transformation from modern, highly conformal or SRS techniques is low at ~1 in 1,000.[47] Therefore, a multidisciplinary working group in the UK has advised against screening as the risks of anxiety from serial MRI examinations and potential knowledge of an asymptomatic (and sometimes unresectable) tumors outweigh the benefits.[48]

What dose of SRS should be used to treat meningioma and what are the outcomes?

Similar to brain metastases, SRS dose depends on the volume being treated and the dose to adjacent critical structures. For grade 1 meningiomas, common doses generally have ranged from 12 to 14 Gy for single-fraction SRS and 25 Gy/5 fx for fractionated SRS. Marginal doses of 10 Gy or less have shown lower LC rates compared with 12 Gy or higher, while higher doses are associated with increased toxicity, including cranial neuropathies.[32,49–53] Higher doses are used for grade 2 (e.g., 16 Gy) and grade 3 meningiomas (e.g., 18–24 Gy). Fractionated SRS with BED >50 Gy may decrease toxicity rates for patients in whom critical structures limit SRS dose.[54] Most SRS series report excellent LC, with 10-year rates ranging from >90% for WHO grade 1 to >60% for WHO grades 2 and 3.[49,51–53] In general, SRS is an accepted treatment option for grade 1 meningiomas over fractionated RT. For grades 2 to 3 meningiomas, fractionated RT is often preferred over SRS.

How should large meningiomas and those located near critical structures be managed?

Pinzi, Italy (*IJROBP* 2023, PMID 36075299): Phase II trial of hypofractionated SRS given in 5 fx for 178 patients with WHO grade 1 large tumors >3 cm and those located <3 mm from critical structures. MFU 53 months. 87% had skull base tumors and 70% with neurologic dysfunction. GTV included enhancing tumor with no CTV/PTV margin. The majority (89%) received 25 Gy/5 fx. LC was 95%, with 50% PR and 45% stable disease. Baseline oculomotor dysfunction improved in 55%, visual deficits remained stable in 87%, and trigeminal pain and numbness improved in 91% and 13% of the affected patients. Treatment-related toxicity was seen in 13%, with visual acuity changes (5%) and trigeminal sensory loss (4%) most common. **Conclusion: Hypofractionated SRS for WHO grade 1 meningioma provides excellent LC with reasonable toxicity profile.**

How does peritumoral edema impact SRS decision-making?

Peritumoral edema is a common complication of SRS for meningioma, occurring in up to 40% of patients, and may require initiation of steroids. The mechanism is unclear, but is likely mediated by VEGF, HIF-1, and MMP-9.[55,56] Risk factors for peritumoral edema include parasagittal location, presence of pretreatment edema, sagittal sinus occlusion, high treatment dose, large tumor volume, high-grade histology, and most significantly tumor–brain contact interface area.[57,58] Although parasagittal location is not an absolute contraindication to SRS, if there is significant edema present, consider other options or preprocedure steroids.

What is meningiomatosis and how should it be managed?

Meningiomatosis is commonly associated with NF or MEN syndromes. Treatment should be coordinated in a multidisciplinary fashion, with surgery given primary consideration due to concerns of secondary malignancy induction. RT is indicated for surgically unresectable or recurrent lesions.[59]

REFERENCES

1. Ostrom QT, Price M, Neff C, et al. CBTRUS statistical report: primary brain and other central nervous system tumors diagnosed in the United States in 2016–2020. *Neuro Oncol.* 2023;25(12 suppl 2):iv1–iv99. doi:10.1093/neuonc/noad149
2. Wiemels J, Wrensch M, Claus EB. Epidemiology and etiology of meningioma. *J Neurooncol.* 2010;99(3):307–314. doi:10.1007/s11060-010-0386-3
3. Claus EB, Bondy ML, Schildkraut JM, Wiemels JL, Wrensch M, Black PM. Epidemiology of intracranial meningioma. *Neurosurgery.* 2005;57(6):1088–1095. doi:10.1227/01.neu.0000188281.91351.b9

4. Cao J, Yan W, Li G, Zhan Z, Hong X, Yan H. Incidence and survival of benign, borderline, and malignant meningioma patients in the United States from 2004 to 2018. *Int J Cancer*. 2022;151(11):1874–1888. doi:10.1002/ijc.34198

5. Asgharian B, Chen YJ, Patronas NJ, et al. Meningiomas may be a component tumor of multiple endocrine neoplasia type 1. *Clin Cancer Res*. 2004;10(3):869–880. doi:10.1158/1078-0432.ccr-0938-3

6. Jhawar BS, Fuchs CS, Colditz GA, Stampfer MJ. Sex steroid hormone exposures and risk for meningioma. *J Neurosurg*. 2003;99(5):848–853. doi:10.3171/jns.2003.99.5.0848

7. Benson VS, Pirie K, Green J, Casabonne D, Beral V, Million Women Study Collaborators. Lifestyle factors and primary glioma and meningioma tumours in the Million Women Study cohort. *Br J Cancer*. 2008;99(1):185–190. doi:10.1038/sj.bjc.6604445

8. Johnson DR, Olson JE, Vierkant RA, et al. Risk factors for meningioma in postmenopausal women: results from the Iowa Women's Health Study. *Neuro Oncol*. 2011;13(9):1011–1019. doi:10.1093/neuonc/nor081

9. Wiedmann M, Brunborg C, Lindemann K, et al. Body mass index and the risk of meningioma, glioma and schwannoma in a large prospective cohort study (The HUNT Study). *Br J Cancer*. 2013;109(1):289–294. doi:10.1038/bjc.2013.304

10. Niedermaier T, Behrens G, Schmid D, Schlecht I, Fischer B, Leitzmann MF. Body mass index, physical activity, and risk of adult meningioma and glioma: a meta-analysis. *Neurology*. 2015;85(15):1342–1350. doi:10.1212/WNL.0000000000002020

11. Custer BS, Koepsell TD, Mueller BA. The association between breast carcinoma and meningioma in women. *Cancer*. 2002;94(6):1626–1635. doi:10.1002/cncr.10410

12. Torp SH, Solheim O, Skjulsvik AJ. The WHO 2021 classification of central nervous system tumours: a practical update on what neurosurgeons need to know-a minireview. *Acta Neurochir (Wien)*. 2022;164(9):2453–2464. doi:10.1007/s00701-022-05301-y

13. Chen WC, Choudhury A, Youngblood MW, et al. Targeted gene expression profiling predicts meningioma outcomes and radiotherapy responses. *Nat Med*. 2023;29(12):3067–3076. doi:10.1038/s41591-023-02586-z

14. Landry AP, Wang JZ, Liu J, et al. Development and validation of a molecular classifier of meningiomas. *Neuro Oncol*. 2025;noae242 . doi:10.1093/neuonc/noae242

15. Maas SLN, Stichel D, Hielscher T, et al. Integrated molecular-morphologic meningioma classification: a multicenter retrospective analysis, retrospectively and prospectively validated. *J Clin Oncol*. 2021;39(34):3839–3852. doi:10.1200/JCO.21.00784

16. Suppiah S, Nassiri F, Bi WL, et al. Molecular and translational advances in meningiomas. *Neuro Oncol*. 2019;21(Suppl 1):i4–i17. doi:10.1093/neuonc/noy178

17. Raizer J. Meningiomas. *Curr Treat Options Neurol*. 2010;12(4):360–368. doi:10.1007/s11940-010-0081-x

18. Perlow HK, Siedow M, Gokun Y, et al. ^{68}Ga-DOTATATE PET-based radiation contouring creates more precise radiation volumes for patients with meningioma. *Int J Radiat Oncol Biol Phys*. 2022;113(4):859–865. doi:10.1016/j.ijrobp.2022.04.009

19. Anvari K, Hosseini S, Rahighi S, Toussi MS, Roshani N, Torabi-Nami M. Intracranial meningiomas: prognostic factors and treatment outcome in patients undergoing postoperative radiation therapy. *Adv Biomed Res*. 2016;5:83. doi:10.4103/2277-9175.182214

20. Durand A, Labrousse F, Jouvet A, et al. WHO grade II and III meningiomas: a study of prognostic factors. *J Neurooncol*. 2009;95(3):367–375. doi:10.1007/s11060-009-9934-0

21. Stafford SL, Perry A, Suman VJ, et al. Primarily resected meningiomas: outcome and prognostic factors in 581 Mayo Clinic patients, 1978 through 1988. *Mayo Clin Proc*. 1998;73(10):936–942. doi:10.4065/73.10.936

22. Pasquier D, Bijmolt S, Veninga T, et al. Atypical and malignant meningioma: outcome and prognostic factors in 119 irradiated patients. A multicenter, retrospective study of the rare cancer network. *Int J Radiat Oncol Biol Phys*. 2008;71(5):1388–1393. doi:10.1016/j.ijrobp.2007.12.020

23. Yang SY, Park CK, Park SH, Kim DG, Chung YS, Jung HW. Atypical and anaplastic meningiomas: prognostic implications of clinicopathological features. *J Neurol Neurosurg Psychiatry*. 2008;79(5):574–580. doi:10.1136/jnnp.2007.121582

24. Cai DX, Banerjee R, Scheithauer BW, Lohse CM, Kleinschmidt-Demasters BK, Perry A. Chromosome 1p and 14q FISH analysis in clinicopathologic subsets of meningioma: diagnostic and prognostic implications. *J Neuropathol Exp Neurol*. 2001;60(6):628–636. doi:10.1093/jnen/60.6.628

25. Vranic A, Popovic M, Cor A, Prestor B, Pizem J. Mitotic count, brain invasion, and location are independent predictors of recurrence-free survival in primary atypical and malignant meningiomas: a study of 86 patients. *Neurosurgery*. 2010;67(4):1124–1132. doi:10.1227/NEU.0b013e3181eb95b7

26. Zeng KL, Soliman H, Myrehaug S, et al. Dose-escalated radiation therapy is associated with improved outcomes for high-grade meningioma. *Int J Radiat Oncol Biol Phys*. 2024;118(3):662–671. doi:10.1016/j.ijrobp.2023.09.026

27. Pinzi V, Marchetti M, Viola A, et al. Hypofractionated radiosurgery for large or in critical-site intracranial meningioma: results of a phase 2 prospective study. *Int J Radiat Oncol Biol Phys*. 2023;115(1):153–163. doi:10.1016/j.ijrobp.2022.08.064

28. National Comprehensive Cancer Network. NCCN Clinical Practice Guidelines in Oncology: Central Nervous System Cancers 4.2024; 2025. Accessed January 27, 2025. https://www.nccn.org/professionals/physician_gls/pdf/cns.pdf

29. Videtic GMM. *Handbook of Treatment Planning in Radiation Oncology*. 3rd ed. Demos Medical; 2020. doi:10.1891/9780826168429

30. Yano S, Kuratsu J, Kumamoto Brain Tumor Research Group. Indications for surgery in patients with asymptomatic meningiomas based on an extensive experience. *J Neurosurg*. 2006;105(4):538–543. doi:10.3171/jns.2006.105.4.538

31. Simpson D. The recurrence of intracranial meningiomas after surgical treatment. *J Neurol Neurosurg Psychiatry*. 1957;20(1):22–39. doi:10.1136/jnnp.20.1.22

32. Bloch O, Kaur G, Jian BJ, Parsa AT, Barani IJ. Stereotactic radiosurgery for benign meningiomas. *J Neurooncol*. 2012;107(1):13–20. doi:10.1007/s11060-011-0720-4

33. Komotar RJ, Iorgulescu JB, Raper DM, et al. The role of radiotherapy following gross-total resection of atypical meningiomas. *J Neurosurg*. 2012;117(4):679–686. doi:10.3171/2012.7.JNS112113

34. Perry A, Scheithauer BW, Stafford SL, Lohse CM, Wollan PC. "Malignancy" in meningiomas: a clinicopathologic study of 116 patients, with grading implications. *Cancer*. 1999;85(9):2046–2056. doi:10.1002/(sici)1097-0142(19990501)85:9<2046::aid-cncr23>3.0.co;2-m

35. Miralbell R, Linggood RM, de la Monte S, Convery K, Munzenrider JE, Mirimanoff RO. The role of radiotherapy in the treatment of subtotally resected benign meningiomas. *J Neurooncol*. 1992;13(2):157–164. doi:10.1007/BF00172765

36. Rogers L, Barani I, Chamberlain M, et al. Meningiomas: knowledge base, treatment outcomes, and uncertainties. A RANO review. *J Neurosurg*. 2015;122(1):4–23. doi:10.3171/2014.7.JNS131644

37. Sughrue ME, Sanai N, Shangari G, Parsa AT, Berger MS, McDermott MW. Outcome and survival following primary and repeat surgery for World Health Organization grade III meningiomas. *J Neurosurg*. 2010;113(2):202–209. doi:10.3171/2010.1.JNS091114

38. Boskos C, Feuvret L, Noel G, et al. Combined proton and photon conformal radiotherapy for intracranial atypical and malignant meningioma. *Int J Radiat Oncol Biol Phys*. 2009;75(2):399–406. doi:10.1016/j.ijrobp.2008.10.053

39. Hug EB, Devries A, Thornton AF, et al. Management of atypical and malignant meningiomas: role of high-dose, 3D-conformal radiation therapy. *J Neurooncol*. 2000;48(2):151–160. doi:10.1023/a:1006434124794

40. Aghi MK, Carter BS, Cosgrove GR, et al. Long-term recurrence rates of atypical meningiomas after gross total resection with or without postoperative adjuvant radiation. *Neurosurgery*. 2009;64(1):56–60. doi:10.1227/01.NEU.0000330399.55586.63

41. Press RH, Prabhu RS, Appin CL, et al. Outcomes and patterns of failure for grade 2 meningioma treated with reduced-margin intensity modulated radiation therapy. *Int J Radiat Oncol Biol Phys*. 2014;88(5):1004–1010. doi:10.1016/j.ijrobp.2013.12.037

42. Dziuk TW, Woo S, Butler EB, et al. Malignant meningioma: an indication for initial aggressive surgery and adjuvant radiotherapy. *J Neurooncol*. 1998;37(2):177–188. doi:10.1023/a:1005853720926

43. Kaur G, Sayegh ET, Larson A, et al. Adjuvant radiotherapy for atypical and malignant meningiomas: a systematic review. *Neuro Oncol*. 2014;16(5):628–636. doi:10.1093/neuonc/nou025

44. Friedman DL, Whitton J, Leisenring W, et al. Subsequent neoplasms in 5-year survivors of childhood cancer: the Childhood Cancer Survivor Study. *J Natl Cancer Inst*. 2010;102(14):1083–1095. doi:10.1093/jnci/djq238

45. Muller HL, Gebhardt U, Warmuth-Metz M, et al. Meningioma as second malignant neoplasm after oncological treatment during childhood. *Strahlenther Onkol*. 2012;188(5):438–441. doi:10.1007/s00066-012-0082-7

46. Banerjee J, Paakko E, Harila M, et al. Radiation-induced meningiomas: a shadow in the success story of childhood leukemia. *Neuro Oncol*. 2009;11(5):543–549. doi:10.1215/15228517-2008-122

47. Niranjan A, Kondziolka D, Lunsford LD. Neoplastic transformation after radiosurgery or radiotherapy: risk and realities. *Otolaryngol Clin North Am*. 2009;42(4):717–729. doi:10.1016/j.otc.2009.04.005

48. Sugden E, Taylor A, Pretorius P, Kennedy C, Bhangoo R. Meningiomas occurring during long-term survival after treatment for childhood cancer. *JRSM Open*. 2014;5(4):2054270414524567. doi:10.1177/2054270414524567

49. Kano H, Takahashi JA, Katsuki T, et al. Stereotactic radiosurgery for atypical and anaplastic meningiomas. *J Neurooncol*. 2007;84(1):41–47. doi:10.1007/s11060-007-9338-y

50. Choi CY, Soltys SG, Gibbs IC, et al. Cyberknife stereotactic radiosurgery for treatment of atypical (WHO grade II) cranial meningiomas. *Neurosurgery*. 2010;67(5):1180–1188. doi:10.1227/NEU.0b013e3181f2f427

51. Lee JY, Niranjan A, McInerney J, Kondziolka D, Flickinger JC, Lunsford LD. Stereotactic radiosurgery providing long-term tumor control of cavernous sinus meningiomas. *J Neurosurg*. 2002;97(1):65–72. doi:10.3171/jns.2002.97.1.0065

52. Spiegelmann R, Cohen ZR, Nissim O, Alezra D, Pfeffer R. Cavernous sinus meningiomas: a large LINAC radiosurgery series. *J Neurooncol*. 2010;98(2):195–202. doi:10.1007/s11060-010-0173-1

53. Skeie BS, Enger PO, Skeie GO, Thorsen F, Pedersen PH. Gamma knife surgery of meningiomas involving the cavernous sinus: long-term follow-up of 100 patients. *Neurosurgery.* 2010;66(4):661–669. doi:10.1227/01. NEU.0000366112.04015.E2

54. Arvold ND, Lessell S, Bussiere M, et al. Visual outcome and tumor control after conformal radiotherapy for patients with optic nerve sheath meningioma. *Int J Radiat Oncol Biol Phys.* 2009;75(4):1166–1172. doi:10.1016/j.ijrobp.2008.12.056

55. Iwado E, Ichikawa T, Kosaka H, et al. Role of VEGF and matrix metalloproteinase-9 in peritumoral brain edema associated with supratentorial benign meningiomas. *Neuropathology.* 2012;32(6):638–646. doi:10.1111/j.1440-1789.2012.01312.x

56. Kan P, Liu JK, Wendland MM, Shrieve D, Jensen RL. Peritumoral edema after stereotactic radiosurgery for intracranial meningiomas and molecular factors that predict its development. *J Neurooncol.* 2007;83(1):33–38. doi:10.1007/s11060-006-9294-y

57. Unger KR, Lominska CE, Chanyasulkit J, et al. Risk factors for posttreatment edema in patients treated with stereotactic radiosurgery for meningiomas. *Neurosurgery.* 2012;70(3):639–645. doi:10.1227/NEU.0b013e3182351ae7

58. Cai R, Barnett GH, Novak E, Chao ST, Suh JH. Principal risk of peritumoral edema after stereotactic radiosurgery for intracranial meningioma is tumor-brain contact interface area. *Neurosurgery.* 2010;66(3):513–522. doi:10.1227/01.NEU.0000365366.53337.88

59. Wentworth S, Pinn M, Bourland JD, et al. Clinical experience with radiation therapy in the management of neurofibromatosis-associated central nervous system tumors. *Int J Radiat Oncol Biol Phys.* 2009;73(1):208–213. doi:10.1016/j.ijrobp.2008.03.073

5 PRIMARY CENTRAL NERVOUS SYSTEM LYMPHOMA

Sean M. Parker, Erin S. Murphy, and Samuel T. Chao

QUICK HIT Primary CNS lymphoma (PCNSL) accounts for ~2% of primary brain tumors, with increased incidence among the immunosuppressed population. Treatment options include methotrexate-based CHT ± WBRT for consolidation, cytarabine (Ara-C) ± etoposide, or high-dose CHT followed by autologous stem cell transplant (ASCT). Careful patient selection and clinical trial availability often determine therapy (Table 5.1).

Table 5.1 General Treatment Paradigm for Primary CNS Lymphoma	
Induction Phase	**Consolidation Phase After Complete Response**
MTX-based CHT	WBRT 23.4 Gy/13 fx (higher dose/boost if incomplete response)
	Ara-C ± etoposide
	High-dose CHT + ASCT

EPIDEMIOLOGY: PCNSL accounts for ~2% of primary brain tumors, with a yearly estimated incidence of 4.5 per million.[1] In the mid-1990s, the incidence rose significantly but has since declined due to improvements in the management and incidence of HIV/AIDS. However, the incidence among immunocompetent older adults has gradually risen.[2] Peak incidence occurs in adults aged 70 to 79.[3] It is considered an AIDS-defining illness, and those with an HIV infection have a 3,600-fold increased risk of developing PCNSL.[2] In this population, EBV infection is associated with PCNSL development.

RISK FACTORS: Congenital or acquired immunodeficiency: HIV infection, iatrogenic immunosuppression, severe combined immunodeficiency, Wiskott–Aldrich syndrome, ataxia–telangiectasia, common variable immunodeficiency, or organ transplant recipients. Autoimmune disease may be an independent risk factor, although likely secondary to use of immunosuppressant medications.[4] In immunocompetent patients, the risk factors are less established.

ANATOMY: Presentations include intracranial, leptomeningeal, periventricular, vitreous, and/or spinal lesions. Location in order of decreasing frequency: frontal lobe, parietal lobe, temporal lobe, basal ganglia, corpus callosum, cerebellum, brainstem, insula, occipital lobe, and fornix.[5] Twenty percent of cases involve the eyes (commonly bilateral) and ~1% have isolated spinal cord involvement, typically involving the lower cervical or upper thoracic regions.[6]

PATHOLOGY: The large majority (90%–95%) of PCNSL are diffuse large B-cell lymphomas, with the other 5% to 10% composed of Burkitt, lymphoblastic, marginal zone, or T-cell lymphoma. Neoplastic B lymphocytes are classically described by "perivascular cuffing" with expression of CD20, CD19, CD22, BCL-6, and IRF4/MUM1, markers of B-cells, germinal center B-cells, and late germinal center B-cells, respectively.[6]

CLINICAL PRESENTATION: The clinical presentation is highly variable depending on location of disease (see Table 5.2). Most patients present with a single lesion (66%). Nonspecific symptoms include confusion, lethargy, headaches, focal neurologic deficits, neuropsychiatric symptoms, increased intracranial pressure, or seizures.[6] In a small percentage of patients (10%–15%), gastrointestinal symptoms or respiratory illness may be seen before manifestation of neurologic symptoms.[5]

Table 5.2 Presentation of Primary CNS Lymphoma by Location	
Primary cerebral lymphoma	Focal deficits (70%), neuropsychiatric symptoms (43%), increased intracranial pressure (33%), seizures (14%)[5]
Primary leptomeningeal lymphoma	Cranial neuropathies (58%), spinal symptoms (48%), headache (44%), leg weakness (35%), ataxia (25%), encephalopathy (25%), bowel and bladder dysfunction (21%)[7]
Primary intraocular lymphoma	Ocular complaints (62%), behavioral/cognitive changes (27%), hemiparesis (14%), headache (14%), seizures (5%), ataxia (4%), visual field deficit (2%)[8]
Primary spinal lymphoma	Myelopathies[9]
Neurolymphomatosis	Painful neuropathies including sensorimotor or pure sensory neuropathy, and pure motor neuropathy[10]

WORKUP: H&P with complete neurologic and lymphatic exam including peripheral LNs and testicular exam. Mini-Mental State Exam. Document KPS. Ophthalmologic and slit-lamp exam.

Labs: LDH, liver function tests, renal function tests, HIV status. Lumbar puncture (at least 1 week after surgery) with assessment of CSF cytology, total protein, cell count, glucose, beta-2 microglobulin, immunoglobulin heavy gene rearrangement, MYD88 mutation, IL-10 levels, and flow cytometry.[7,11]

Imaging: Contrast-enhanced MRI brain; if spinal symptoms are present, MRI spine. CT chest, abdomen, pelvis with IV contrast or whole-body PET/CT scan. Consider testicular ultrasound in men over age 60 or patients who have positive findings on physical exam.

Biopsy: Stereotactic needle biopsy is standard. Needle biopsy is preferred over surgical resection due to less risk and lack of clinical benefit with surgical resection. An ocular biopsy or CSF cytology can also be used for diagnosis.[8] Bone marrow biopsy is also indicated. If biopsy is nondiagnostic in the context of steroids, discontinue steroids and rebiopsy or repeat CSF evaluation at progression.[12]

PROGNOSTIC FACTORS: No formal staging system exists for PCNSL, but multiple prognostic systems have been described (Tables 5.3 and 5.4).

Table 5.3 IELSG Score for Primary CNS Lymphoma[13]			
Number of Risk Factors	2-Yr OS: All Patients	2-Yr OS (With High-Dose MTX)	Risk factors: age >60, ECOG PS >1, elevated LDH, elevated CSF protein concentration (45 mg/dL in patients ≤60 years old; 60 mg/dL if >60 years old), and involvement of deep structures of the brain (e.g., periventricular regions, basal ganglia, corpus callosum, brainstem, cerebellum)
0–1	80% ± 8%	85% ± 8%	
2–3	48% ± 7%	57% ± 8%	
4–5	15% ± 7%	24% ± 11%	

Source: Data from Ferreri AJM, Blay JY, Reni M, et al. Prognostic scoring system for primary CNS lymphomas: the international extranodal lymphoma study group experience. *J Clin Oncol.* 2003;21(2):266–272. doi:10.1200/jco.2003.09.139.

Table 5.4 MSKCC Prognostic Classification[14]		
	MS	FFS
Class 1: ≤50 years	8.5 yrs	2 yrs
Class 2: >50 years, KPS ≥70	3.2 yrs	1.8 yrs
Class 3: >50 years, KPS <70	1.1 yrs	0.6 yrs

Source: Data from Abrey LE, Ben-Porat L, Panageas KS, et al. Primary central nervous system lymphoma: the memorial sloan-kettering cancer center prognostic model. *J Clin Oncol.* 2006;24(36):5711–5715. doi:10.1200/jco.2006.08.2941.

TREATMENT PARADIGM

Surgery: Biopsy alone is sufficient for diagnosis, and surgical resection is not indicated. PCNSL involvement is classically widespread and involves deep brain structures. Therefore, resection is potentially risky and has not prospectively improved OS, although a post-hoc analysis suggests a potential advantage.[6,15]

Chemotherapy: CHT is considered the mainstay of treatment. High-dose MTX (3.5–8 g/m^2) is standard and can be administered as monotherapy (older adults) or more commonly as part of multidrug therapy. The ideal combination regimen has yet to be defined but may include MTX, rituximab, and various combinations of temozolomide (TMZ), cytarabine (Ara-C), ifosfamide, procarbazine, and vincristine (VCR). After a CR, consolidation therapy with Ara-C ± etoposide and ASCT are options.

Radiation

Indications: Whole brain radiation therapy (WBRT) is used for consolidation after MTX-based CHT or for palliation. Historically, high-dose WBRT alone was the mainstay of treatment but is no longer considered the best long-term option for disease control. The utility of low-dose WBRT to 23.4 Gy/13 fx as consolidation approximately 3 to 5 weeks after CR remains controversial.[16] In patients >60 years old, WBRT in combination with MTX is associated with increased neurotoxicity. It has yet to be determined if RT should be withheld in this patient population. Ocular RT can be considered for ocular involvement not responding to CHT. Consider WBRT for palliation in patients ineligible for CHT. Substitution of consolidative SRS for WBRT remains under investigation.

Dose: If WBRT is delivered after CR to CHT, standard is 23.4 Gy/13 fx. If PR, consider WBRT 30 to 36 Gy with boost to 45 Gy/25 fx.[12]

Toxicity: Acute: fatigue, headache, nausea, alopecia, skin erythema, high-frequency hearing loss, changes to hearing and taste, dry mouth. For ocular RT: dry eyes, less commonly retinal injury and cataracts. Late: neurotoxicity changes such as short-term memory loss, verbal fluency/recall, gait changes, ataxia, Parkinson-like features, behavioral changes, and leukoencephalopathy.

Procedure: See *Handbook of Treatment Planning in Radiation Oncology,* Chapter 3.[17]

Medical: Traditionally, corticosteroids are held prior to biopsy unless medically necessary.[18] After biopsy, steroids can be used for quick alleviation of neurologic symptoms. Radiologic regression can be transiently seen with steroids in ~40%, which is suggestive but not diagnostic of PCNSL.

EVIDENCE-BASED Q&A

What is the role of RT alone for PCNSL?

Historically, RT alone was the initial treatment for PCNSL. However, WBRT alone has shown little success in long-term disease control with high rates of LR. On RTOG 8315, 61% of patients treated with RT alone recurred in the brain and the median OS was 11.6 months from start of RT.[19]

Can combination CHT with WBRT improve outcomes when compared with WBRT alone?

DeAngelis, RTOG 9310 (*JCO* 2002, PMID 12488408): Multicenter, single-arm, phase II prospective study evaluating upfront MPV (MTX, procarbazine, VCR) CHT with RT; 102 immunocompetent patients were enrolled; five cycles of MTX 2.5 g/m^2, VCR, intra-Ommaya MTX, procarbazine, and consolidation WBRT followed by Ara-C. WBRT was 45 Gy (1.8 Gy/fx) in 63 patients, but due to late neurotoxicity seen with this dose 16 patients who achieved CR after induction received 36 Gy (1.2 Gy/fx BID) for 15 days instead; 34% relapsed during follow-up period. Median PFS 24 months, MS 37 months. Between 45 Gy WBRT and 36 Gy hyperfractionated RT, there was no difference noted in PFS (25 vs. 23 months, $p = .81$) and OS (37 vs. 48 months, $p = .65$). Side effects of RT included the following: myelosuppression (63%) and delayed neurologic toxicities classified mostly as leukoencephalopathy (15%); eight cases of neurologic toxicities progressed to fatalities. **Conclusion: HD-MTX in combination with other agents improved survival compared with historical rates of RT alone. This CHT combination provides a high response rate, but in conjunction with WBRT there is a significant late risk of neurotoxicity.**

Is consolidation WBRT superior to CHT alone?

Thiel, G-PCNSL-SG1 (*Lancet Oncol* 2010, PMID 20970380): Phase III PRT to compare HD-MTX vs. HD-MTX + WBRT; 551 patients received six cycles of HD-MTX and HD-MTX + ifosfamide and were randomly assigned to immediate WBRT (45 Gy/30 fx) or delayed WBRT. For patients with PR after CHT, they received high-dose Ara-C or WBRT; 13% died during initial CHT. In addition, there was a high dropout rate, leaving 318 patients to be analyzed. No significant difference in MS and PFS; in HD-MTX + WBRT patients, MS was 32 months and mPFS was 18 months. In patients who received CHT alone, the MS was 37 months and mPFS was 12 months. Neurotoxicity was higher in the WBRT group vs. the non-WBRT group in both clinical (49% vs. 26%) and neuroradiology (71% vs. 46%) assessment. **Conclusion: No statistically significant difference was found in OS or PFS between the WBRT + CHT and CHT alone, but the noninferiority endpoint of 0.9 was not met. Therefore, the study was unable to conclude if WBRT has an impact on OS when added to CHT. In addition, the neurotoxicity rates were greater in the WBRT cohort.** *Comment: A small percentage of patients were treated per protocol.*

Can the dose of WBRT be reduced to avoid neurotoxicity but still maintain benefit?

Most trials comparing WBRT with other consolidative therapies have used higher RT dose regimens, which have often been associated with increased neurotoxicity. The below MSKCC trial demonstrates that reduced-dose WBRT is feasible. A retrospective direct comparison similarly found comparable PFS and OS with reduced-dose WBRT.[20]

Morris, MSKCC (*JCO* 2013, PMID 24101038): Single-arm, phase II, multicenter trial assessing consolidation with reduced-dose (rd)-WBRT 23.4 Gy and addition of rituximab to MPV (R-MPV); 45 Gy was delivered for those with PR. Of 52 patients, 31 achieved CR postinduction. Both CR and PR received Ara-C as consolidation after RT. MFU 5.9 years. In the rd-WBRT group, mPFS was 7.7 years, 5-year OS was 80%, and MS was not reached. For the entire cohort, mPFS was 3.3 years and MS was 6.6 years. No evidence of cognitive decline was observed, with the exception of motor speed. **Conclusion: rd-WBRT and Ara-C following R-MPV demonstrated good control with minimal neurotoxicity.**

What is the role of temozolomide?

Glass, RTOG 0227 (*JCO* 2016, PMID 27022122): Single-arm phase I/II trial of induction CHT (rituximab, TMZ, and MTX) followed by WBRT (36 Gy/30 fx at 1.2 Gy BID), followed by adjuvant TMZ. Fifty-three patients treated in phase II portion. Primary endpoint 2-year OS. The 2-year OS was 81% and PFS was 64%, significantly improved from historical controls; 66% of patients experienced grade 3 to 4 toxicities prior to WBRT, and 45% experienced grade 3 to 4 toxicities attributable to post-WBRT CHT. **Conclusion: Induction with rituximab, TMZ, and MTX followed by hyperfractionated WBRT and adjuvant TMZ is safe with 2-year OS superior to that of historical controls.**

What is the role of rituximab?

Rituximab has been frequently studied in combination CHT regimens with mixed results. Of note, the addition of rituximab to MTX and Ara-C alone improved OS and CR in the IELSG-32 trial.[21] However, direct evaluation of rituximab on the phase III HOVON 105 trial demonstrated no benefit.

Bromberg, HOVON 105 (*Lancet Onc* 2019, PMID 30630772; *Neuro Oncol* 2024, PMID 38037691): Phase III RCT of 200 patients randomized to induction CHT (MTX/carmustine/teniposide) ± rituximab. Patients with response after induction received high-dose cytarabine and those <60 years also received reduced-dose WBRT. MFU 60 months. EFS was not significantly different with the addition of rituximab (*p* = .33). **Conclusion: Addition of rituximab to MTX-based induction CHT did not improve EFS.**

Does low-dose WBRT improve PFS as compared with CHT alone?

Omuro, RTOG 1114 (ASCO Abstract 2020): Phase II study of 91 PCNSL patients who underwent R-MPV-A induction CHT ± consolidative low-dose (LD)-WBRT (23.4 Gy/13 fx). MFU 55 months. PFS was improved with the addition of WBRT (25 months vs. NR): 2-year PFS 54% (CHT alone) vs. 78% (CRT; *p* = .015). Moderate to severe neurotoxicity was similar between groups (11% vs. 14%, *p* = .75). **Conclusion: Preliminary results suggest worse PFS with omission of WBRT following induction CHT.**

Is there a role for stem cell transplant with high-dose CHT?

High-dose CHT plus ASCT has a role in both initial and salvage therapy for patients with PCNSL.[22,23] *CALGB 51101 demonstrated myeloablative CHT with ASCT improved PFS over nonmyeloablative CHT alone.*

Batchelor, CALGB 51101 (*Blood Adv* 2024, PMID 38598710): Phase II randomized trial of 113 patients with PCNSL treated with induction CHT (MTX, TMZ, rituximab, cytarabine) then randomized to either myeloablative CHT with ASCT or nonmyeloablative consolidation CHT (etoposide + cytarabine). The 2-year PFS was higher in the ASCT arm (73% vs. 51%, $p = .02$) with less progressive disease or death (28% vs. 11%, $p = .05$). **Conclusion: ASCT offers improved PFS over nonmyeloablative consolidation therapy.** *Comment: WBRT was omitted from both regimens.*

Does consolidation with ASCT improve outcomes compared with WBRT?

Two phase II trials demonstrate mixed results. IELSG-32 suggests both WBRT and ASCT are effective consolidation options, whereas PRECIS suggests more durable response and less neurotoxicity with ASCT over high-dose WBRT.

Ferreri, IELSG-32 (*Lancet Haematol* 2016, PMID 27132696; *Lancet Haematol* 2017, PMID 29054815; *Leukemia* 2022, PMID 35562406): International phase II study with double randomization investigating both MTX-based initial CHT + WBRT vs. high-dose CHT (HDT) + ASCT as consolidation. For the first randomization, 227 HIV-negative patients with newly diagnosed PCNSL were randomized to three different induction regimens, with MTX + cytarabine + rituximab + thiotepa (MATRix) demonstrating the best 7-year OS of 56% at the cost of increased hematologic toxicity. For the second randomization, 118 patients with responsive or stable disease were randomized to WBRT 36 Gy (with a 9-Gy boost in patients with PR) or carmustine–thiotepa followed by ASCT. At long-term analysis, 7-year PFS (55% vs. 50%, $p = .46$) and OS (63% vs. 57%, $p = .26$) were similar between WBRT and ASCT arms, respectively. **Conclusion: WBRT and ASCT are both feasible and effective consolidation therapies following high-dose MTX-based induction therapy.**

Houillier, PRECIS (*JCO* 2019, PMID 30785830; *JCO* 2022, PMID 35834762): Phase II RCT of 140 PCNSL patients randomized after induction CHT with R-MBVP + R-AraC to either WBRT (40 Gy/20 fx) or ASCT (thiotepa, busulfan, CYC). At MFU of 8 years, ASCT demonstrated better EFS (67% vs. 39%, $p = .03$) than WBRT but no difference in OS (69% vs. 65%, $p = $ NS). Of note, neurocognition (64% vs. 13%, $p < .001$) and balance (52% vs. 10%, $p \leq .001$) were worse in WBRT arm. **Conclusion: Compared with high-dose WBRT, ASCT provided more durable EFS and reduced long-term neurocognitive toxicity compared with WBRT.**

How is response assessed in PCNSL?

According to the International PCNSL Collaborative Group guidelines,[24] *MRI must be completed within 2 months of finishing treatment in order to assess response. LP and/or ophthalmologic exam must be completed if initially positive (Table 5.5).*

Table 5.5 Response Criteria in PCNSL per International PCNSL Collaborative Guidelines				
Response	**Steroid Use**	**Eye Exam**	**CSF**	**MRI**
CR	None	Normal	Negative	No enhancement
Unconfirmed CR	Any	Normal or minor abnormality	Negative	No enhancement or minor abnormality
PR	N/A	Decrease in vitreous cells/retinal infiltrate	Persistent or suspicious	≥50% decrease in enhancement
PD	N/A	New ocular disease	Recurrent or positive	≥25% increase or new lesion/site

Source: Adapted from Abrey LE, Batchelor TT, Ferreri AJM, et al. Report of an international workshop to standardize baseline evaluation and response criteria for primary CNS lymphoma. *J Clin Oncol.* 2005;23(22):5034–5043. doi:10.1200/jco.2005.13.524.

What is the role of WBRT as salvage therapy?

WBRT provides an adequate option as salvage therapy for recurrent or refractory PCNSL. Other options include additional CHT or HDT + ASCT.

Nguyen (*JCO* 2005, PMID 15735126): Evaluation of 27 patients with tumor relapse or progression of a refractory tumor after primary CHT with HD-MTX. Salvage WBRT ± boost was delivered, with the majority (67%) of patients remaining on steroids. Median WBRT dose was 36 Gy (1.5 Gy/fx was most prevalent); five patients received a boost to a median dose of 10 Gy and two patients received an SRS boost of 12 or 16 Gy; 74% had either a CR ($n = 10$) or a PR ($n = 10$) to WBRT; eight patients later progressed or recurred at a median of 19 months post-WBRT. Delayed neurotoxicity was diagnosed in three patients, at a median of 25 months, with none resulting in death. **Conclusion: WBRT is an effective option in the salvage setting. For older patients, withholding WBRT until the time of progression may decrease neurotoxicity rates.**

REFERENCES

1.   Ostrom QT, Price M, Neff C, et al. CBTRUS statistical report: primary brain and other central nervous system tumors diagnosed in the United States in 2016–2020. *Neuro Oncol.* 2023;25(suppl 4):iv1–iv99. doi:10.1093/neuonc/noad149

2.   Villano JL, Koshy M, Shaikh H, Dolecek TA, McCarthy BJ. Age, gender, and racial differences in incidence and survival in primary CNS lymphoma. *Br J Cancer.* 2011;105(9):1414–1418. doi:10.1038/bjc.2011.357

3.   Mendez JS, Ostrom QT, Gittleman H, et al. The elderly left behind—changes in survival trends of primary central nervous system lymphoma over the past 4 decades. *Neuro Oncol.* 2018;20(5):687–694. doi:10.1093/neuonc/nox187

4.   Mahale P, Herr MM, Engels EA, Pfeiffer RM, Shiels MS. Autoimmune conditions and primary central nervous system lymphoma risk among older adults. *Br J Haematol.* 2020;188(4):516–521. doi:10.1111/bjh.16222

5.   Bataille B, Delwail V, Menet E, et al. Primary intracerebral malignant lymphoma: report of 248 cases. *J Neurosurg.* 2000;92(2):261–266. doi:10.3171/jns.2000.92.2.0261

6.   Ferreri AJM, Marturano E. Primary CNS lymphoma. *Best Pr Res Clin Haematol.* 2012;25(1):119–130. doi:10.1016/j.beha.2011.12.001

7.   Taylor JW, Flanagan EP, O'Neill BP, et al. Primary leptomeningeal lymphoma. *Neurology.* 2013;81(19):1690–1696. doi:10.1212/01.wnl.0000435302.02895.f3

8.   Grimm SA, McCannel CA, Omuro AMP, et al. Primary CNS lymphoma with intraocular involvement. *Neurology.* 2008;71(17):1355–1360. doi:10.1212/01.wnl.0000327672.04729.8c

9.   Flanagan EP, O'Neill BP, Porter AB, Lanzino G, Haberman TM, Keegan BM. Primary intramedullary spinal cord lymphoma. *Neurology.* 2011;77(8):784–791. doi:10.1212/wnl.0b013e31822b00b9

10. Grisariu S, Avni B, Batchelor TT, et al. Neurolymphomatosis: an international primary CNS lymphoma collaborative group report. *Blood.* 2010;115(24):5005–5011. doi:10.1182/blood-2009-12-258210

11. Ferreri AJM, Calimeri T, Lopedote P, et al. MYD88 L265P mutation and interleukin-10 detection in cerebrospinal fluid are highly specific discriminating markers in patients with primary central nervous system lymphoma: results from a prospective study. *Br J Haematol.* 2021;193(3):497–505. doi:10.1111/bjh.17357

12. Nabors LB, Portnow J, Ahluwalia M, et al. Central nervous system cancers, version 3.2020, NCCN clinical practice guidelines in oncology. *J Natl Compr Cancer Netw.* 2020;18(11):1537–1570. doi:10.6004/jnccn.2020.0052

13. Ferreri AJM, Blay JY, Reni M, et al. Prognostic scoring system for primary CNS lymphomas: the international extranodal lymphoma study group experience. *J Clin Oncol.* 2003;21(2):266–272. doi:10.1200/jco.2003.09.139

14. Abrey LE, Ben-Porat L, Panageas KS, et al. Primary central nervous system lymphoma: the memorial sloan-kettering cancer center prognostic model. *J Clin Oncol.* 2006;24(36):5711–5715. doi:10.1200/jco.2006.08.2941

15. Weller M, Martus P, Roth P, Thiel E, Korfel A, German PCNSL Study Group. Surgery for primary CNS lymphoma? Challenging a paradigm. *Neuro Oncol.* 2012;14(12):1481–1484. doi:10.1093/neuonc/nos159

16. Shah GD, Yahalom J, Correa DD, et al. Combined immunochemotherapy with reduced whole-brain radiotherapy for newly diagnosed primary CNS lymphoma. *J Clin Oncol.* 2007;25(30):4730–4735. doi:10.1200/jco.2007.12.5062

17. Videtic GM, Woody NM, Vassil AD. *Handbook of Treatment Planning in Radiation Oncology.* 3rd ed. Demos Medical; 2020.

18. Ferreri AJM. How I treat primary CNS lymphoma. *Blood.* 2011;118(3):510–522. doi:10.1182/blood-2011-03-321349

19. Levinson K, Beavis AL, Purdy C, et al. Beyond sedlis-a novel histology-specific nomogram for predicting cervical cancer recurrence risk: an NRG/GOG ancillary analysis. *Gynecol Oncol.* 2021;162(3):532–538. doi:10.1016/j.ygyno.2021.06.017

20. Lesueur P, Damaj G, Hoang-Xuan K, et al. Reduced-dose WBRT as consolidation treatment for patients with primary CNS lymphoma: an LOC network study. *Blood Adv.* 2022;6(16):4807–4815. doi:10.1182/bloodadvances.2022007011

21. Ferreri AJM, Cwynarski K, Pulczynski E, et al. Long-term efficacy, safety and neurotolerability of MATRix regimen followed by autologous transplant in primary CNS lymphoma: 7-year results of the IELSG32 randomized trial. *Leukemia.* 2022;36(7):1870–1878. doi:10.1038/s41375-022-01582-5

22. Illerhaus G, Marks R, Ihorst G, et al. High-dose chemotherapy with autologous stem-cell transplantation and hyperfractionated radiotherapy as first-line treatment of primary CNS Lymphoma. *J Clin Oncol.* 2006;24(24):3865–3870. doi:10.1200/jco.2006.06.2117

23. Soussain C, Hoang-Xuan K, Taillandier L, et al. Intensive chemotherapy followed by hematopoietic stem-cell rescue for refractory and recurrent primary CNS and intraocular lymphoma: Société Française de Greffe de Moëlle Osseuse-Thérapie Cellulaire. *J Clin Oncol.* 2008;26(15):2512–2518. doi:10.1200/jco.2007.13.5533

24. Abrey LE, Batchelor TT, Ferreri AJM, et al. Report of an international workshop to standardize baseline evaluation and response criteria for primary CNS lymphoma. *J Clin Oncol.* 2005;23(22):5034–5043. doi:10.1200/jco.2005.13.524

6 PITUITARY NEUROENDOCRINE TUMOR

Bryn M. Myers, John H. Suh, and Praveen Pendyala

QUICK HIT Pituitary neuroendocrine tumor (PitNET), formally known as pituitary adenoma, can be observed in up to 17% of the population but is often asymptomatic and found incidentally by MRI or autopsy.[1,2] For those who present with symptoms, visual impairment, headache, or symptoms related to hormonal aberrations are most frequent. Treatment options include observation, surgery, medication, or SRS/fractionated RT (Figure 6.1). When defining response to treatment in the literature, LC refers to radiographic response (size criteria), whereas remission/response refers to normalization of hormone secretion (complete or partial).

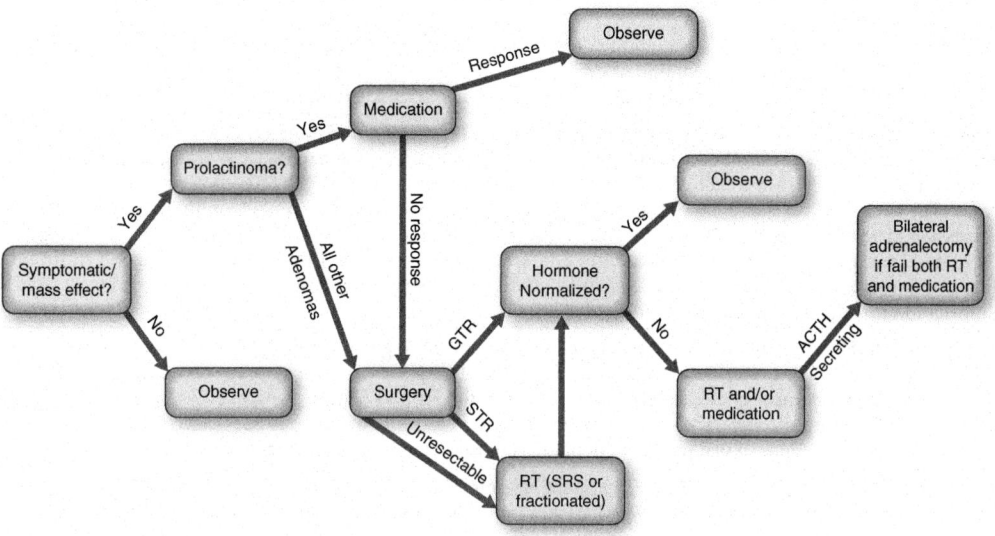

Figure 6.1 General treatment paradigm for PitNET.

EPIDEMIOLOGY: Accounts for 10% to 15% of CNS neoplasms, and ~14,000 cases are diagnosed in the United States each year.[3] Typically diagnosed between 30 and 50 years of age. Male-to-female ratio 1:1, but females are more frequently symptomatic and have higher incidence rates until age 30, when pattern reverses; 70% are secretory.

RISK FACTORS: Personal or family history of colorectal cancer, surgically induced menopause.[4,5] Associated syndromes: MEN1 (mnemonic: 3 Ps; pituitary [25%], parathyroid, and pancreatic islet cell tumors), isolated familial somatotropinoma, Carney complex (spotty skin pigmentation, myxomas, endocrine overactivity, schwannomas).

ANATOMY: The pituitary gland lies within the concave sella turcica of the sphenoid bone. The anterior–posterior clinoid processes make up the anterior–posterior sella borders, respectively. The diaphragma sellae is a dural fold comprising the superior border, and the cavernous sinus (contains internal carotid arteries and CN III, IV, V1, V2, and VI) lies laterally. Embryologically, the anterior lobe (adenohypophysis) develops from Rathke's pouch and the posterior lobe (neurohypophysis) from the third ventricle. PitNETs arise in the anterior lobe, which secretes FSH, LH, ACTH, TSH, PRL, and GH (mnemonic: FLAT PiG). The posterior lobe secretes oxytocin and ADH.

PATHOLOGY: Pituitary tissue has been classically stained with PRL, ACTH, GH, TSH, LH, and FSH to characterize functional status. In the modern era, IHC for pituitary transcription factors is also utilized for defining PitNET lineage. Somatotrophs, lactotrophs, mammosomatotrophs, and thyrotrophs are of PIT1 lineage, corticotrophs are of TPIT lineage, and gonadotrophs are of SF1 lineage. Crooke cell tumors are an aggressive subtype of corticotroph PitNET. Of clinically nonfunctioning PitNETs, 70% to 75% are gonadotroph tumors, with corticotroph tumors being the second most common. Null cell tumors are nonfunctioning PitNETs with no biomarker of lineage determination.

CLINICAL PRESENTATION: Often an asymptomatic, incidental finding. Symptoms can manifest as endocrinopathies (see Table 6.1 for specific tumors) due to hormonal deficiency/hypersecretion, visual field deficits due to optic chiasm compression/involvement (bitemporal hemianopsia, homonymous hemianopsia, temporal quadrantanopia), or apoplexy (acute hemorrhage/infarction). Cavernous sinus invasion can cause CN palsies.

Table 6.1 Overview of PitNET Subtypes
Prolactinoma: Most common PitNET. First-line treatment is medical management with dopamine agonists (e.g., bromocriptine, cabergoline). Most patients have >50% reduction in PRL level with medication. Prolactin levels fall within the first 2 to 3 weeks; 80% show >25% reduction in volume, with decrease in size beginning within 6 weeks. Surgery should be considered if dopamine agonist is unsuccessful, in women wishing to become pregnant, or in patients with pituitary apoplexy. Lower RT remission rate when RT is given alone without medical management compared with other adenoma subtypes. SRS CR rate is 15% to 50% alone, but with medical management increases to 40% to 80% at 2 to 8 years. Fractionated RT alone CR rate is 25% to 50% and with addition of medical therapy increases to 80% to 100% at 1 to 10 years.[6]
Cushing disease (ACTH): First-line treatment is surgery. Remission rate after surgery: 89% for microadenomas, 63% for macroadenomas, and 81% for macroadenomas where GTR anticipated.[7] Tumor extension beyond sella is predictive of nonremission and late recurrence. RT is the preferred second-line treatment over medical management. Fractionated RT remission rate is 50% to 80% with median time to remission of 18 to 42 months. SRS with medical therapy leads to LC rates of 85% to 100% with median time of 7.5 to 33 months for ACTH normalization.[6] Bilateral adrenalectomy, which can lead to Nelson syndrome (rapid enlargement of PitNET, muscle weakness, and skin hyperpigmentation due to melanocyte stimulating hormone), is a final salvage approach.
Acromegaly (GH): First-line treatment is surgery. For patients failing surgery, 50% to 60% show reduced GH/IGF-1 levels with somatostatin analogues (side effects: malabsorptive diarrhea, nausea/vomiting, gallbladder sludge, abdominal cramping). Remission rates of fractionated RT and SRS are similar: 50% to 60% at 5 to 10 years and 65% to 87% at 15 years.[6] GH receptor antagonist, pegvisomant, reduces IGF-1 levels (not GH) if other treatments fail. Side effects of pegvisomant: nausea/vomiting, flu syndrome, diarrhea, and abnormal LFTs.
Hyperthyroidism (TSHoma): First-line treatment is surgery. Consider postoperative RT to a higher dose of 54 Gy as TSHomas are locally aggressive. Medical therapy with somatostatin analogues or methimazole/propylthiouracil, which inhibits thyroperoxidase (converts T3 to T4). Can also consider thyroid ablation.
Metastatic PitNET (formerly known as pituitary carcinoma): Extremely rare (0.2% of pituitary tumors). Frequently metastatic (CSF or systemic), with a mean survival of 1.9 years.[1] First-line treatment is temozolomide, which is also used to treat *aggressive pituitary tumors*—not defined by histology but rather as locally aggressive and not controlled by surgery, RT, or medication. Low MGMT on IHC (not promoter methylation) may be a predictive marker for treatment response.[8,9]
Nonsecretory/functioning: Incidental/asymptomatic, stable microadenomas can be safely observed. Indications for surgery include size >1 cm, mass effect including compression of optic structures, or tumor growth on serial imaging. RT recommended for STR or recurrence.[10] At least partial reduction in size expected in two-thirds of cases. The 10-year LC is >90% with RT. Cabergoline may be used for treating residual nonfunctioning pituitary adenoma.[11]

WORKUP: H&P with focus on CN exam and visual field testing.

Labs: CBC, CMP, baseline endocrine function. Examine respective secretory status with TSH, T3/T4, ACTH, 24-hour urinary free cortisol, PRL, IGF-1, LH, and FSH. Additionally, AFP, beta-hCG, and LDH to investigate other possible etiologies such as germ cell tumors.

Imaging: T1-weighted MRI with gadolinium; high spatial resolution images are required with slice thickness 3 mm or less. Best seen on coronal views. Sellar masses, including pituitary adenomas, meningiomas, and craniopharyngiomas, are less vascular than normal pituitary and take up gadolinium to a lesser degree; they appear hypointense in early phase of DCE MRI.[1] Picoadenoma

<0.3 cm, microadenoma <1 cm diameter, macroadenoma ≥1 cm, giant adenoma >4 cm. Skeletal survey if acromegaly is present.

Differential for Pituitary Mass

Neoplasms: Pituitary tumor, craniopharyngioma, meningioma, germ cell tumor, metastatic tumor, glioma, lymphoma, chordoma.

Benign: Pituitary hyperplasia (pregnancy, long-standing hypothyroidism/hypogonadism), Rathke's cleft cyst, arachnoid cyst, aneurysm, empty sella syndrome, inflammatory lesions (granuloma), abscess.

PROGNOSTIC FACTORS: Immature PIT1-lineage tumors tend to be aggressive. Macroadenomas are more likely to enlarge than microadenomas.[12] Better prognosis with GTR. Significantly higher risk of recurrence with extrasellar invasion such as cavernous sinus invasion and extrasellar post-operative residual disease.[13] There is no formal staging for PitNET. Higher risk of recurrence after surgery with prolactinomas than other pituitary adenomas. The extrasellar and lateral extension of sellar lesions can be characterized using the Hardy–Wilson and Knosp classifications. The Hardy–Wilson classification characterizes pituitary adenomas based on the extent of suprasellar/extrasellar extension, and the Knosp classification characterizes the presence of cavernous sinus invasion.[14] *Hardy grading:* 0: intrapituitary microadenoma with normal sella appearance; I: normal sella size with asymmetric floor; II: enlarged sella with intact floor; III: localized erosion of sella floor; IV: diffusely eroded sella floor.[15]

TREATMENT PARADIGM

Observation: Most asymptomatic PitNETs without lab abnormalities can be safely observed. Intervention is required in <50% of patients.[16]

Surgery: Surgery is first-line treatment for all except prolactinoma and metastatic PitNET.

Surgical Technique: (a) **Transsphenoidal surgery** (**TSS**) performed in >95% cases. TSS has two approaches: sublabial (older technique) and transnasal (microscopic or endoscopic endonasal). Endoscopic is minimally invasive and improves surgical visualization, which may allow for more complete resection and reduced complications.[15] Complications include death (1%), meningitis, CSF leak, diabetes insipidus (6%), hemorrhage, stroke, and visual deficit. (b) **Transcranial approach** for large tumors. LC ~95%, hormone normalization 70% to 80% short term and 40% long term. Postoperatively, new endocrine deficiencies occur in 5% to 15% of patients. Diabetes insipidus occurs in 18% to 30% of patients but resolves in 90% of people within several weeks. Evolution of surgical technique from transcranial to microscopic TSS to endoscopic TSS has improved the outcomes (lower incidence of revision surgery, postoperative hemorrhage, diabetes insipidus, and panhypopituitarism).[17,18] Intraoperative MRI can improve the extent of surgical resection for both microscopic and endoscopic TSS.[19]

Medical Management

Medical management plays a key role in the treatment of secretory PitNETs, particularly when hormone hypersecretion persists after local therapy. The choice of pharmacologic therapy is guided by the specific hormone being secreted and the clinical manifestations of hormone excess or deficiency. Table 6.2 summarizes common secretory PitNET subtypes, associated hormonal disturbances, clinical features, and recommended medical therapies.

Table 6.2 Medical Management of Secretory PitNETs			
Hormone (Frequency)	Hormone Levels	Signs and Symptoms	Medical Therapy
Prolactin (30%)	High	Female: amenorrhea, oligomenorrhea, or infertility. Male: low libido or erectile dysfunction, galactorrhea, osteoporosis	Cabergoline, bromocriptine, quinagolide (not available in the United States)
	Low	Inability to lactate after delivery	No treatment currently available

(continued)

Table 6.2 Medical Management of Secretory PitNETs (*continued*)			
Hormone (Frequency)	Hormone Levels	Signs and Symptoms	Medical Therapy
Growth hormone (25%)	High	Gigantism (before puberty) Acromegaly (after puberty): thickening of bones in the jaw, fingers, and toes; frontal bossing; macroglossia, hyperhidrosis, muscle weakness, glucose intolerance (50%), hypogonadism, cardiomegaly, fatigue, paresthesias, arthralgias, hypothyroidism	Octreotide, lanreotide, pegvisomant injection (expensive but more effective)
	Low	Infancy and childhood: growth failure Adults: loss of strength, stamina, bone density, and musculature, poor memory, depression	Recombinant human GH preparations (i.e., somatropin)
ACTH (15%)	High	Cushing disease (not syndrome): central obesity, hypertension, glucose intolerance, hirsutism, easy bruising, striae, osteoporosis, psychological changes, hypogonadism	Ketoconazole, mitotane, metyrapone
	Low	Hypoglycemia, dehydration, weight loss, weakness, tiredness, dizziness, low blood pressure, nausea/vomiting, diarrhea	Hydrocortisone
TSH (1%)	High	Hyperthyroidism, weight loss, anxiety, heat intolerance, palpitations, diaphoresis, irritability, muscle weakness, Graves ophthalmopathy	Somatostatin analogue (octreotide, lanreotide), methimazole, propylthiouracil
	Low	Cold intolerance, constipation, weight gain, fatigue, anhidrosis, dry skin, brittle hair/fingernails, infertility, hyperprolactinemia, goiter	Levothyroxine

Radiation

Indications: RT indicated if STR s/p surgery, unresectable/inoperable, recurrence after surgery, and/or refractory to medical management. Discontinue medical management 1 month prior to RT and resume after RT completed. Improved response when RT delivered off medical therapy (may alter cell cycle and radiosensitivity) as well as reduce the risk of hypopituitarism.[20-23] Goal is to stabilize or reduce mass effect and normalize hormone levels (takes many years). Excellent LC of 90% to 100% in most studies regardless of RT technique and adenoma subtype. Smaller tumors have improved response and lower risk of hypopituitarism.

SRS vs. Fractionated RT: SRS preferred due to faster time to hormone normalization and patient convenience. Fractionated RT if tumor >3 cm or <3 to 5 mm from chiasm due to risk of visual deficits.[6] Given the potential for 1 to 2 mm of head movement with mask-based immobilization and recommendation for a 1-mm PRV around optic structures, consider conventionally fractionated RT over hypofractionated RT if <2 mm gap between optic structures and tumor. Risk of hypopituitarism is high for both modalities (20% at 5 years; 80% at 10–15 years).[24] Panhypopituitarism occurs in 5% to 10% of patients at 5 years.[6]

Dose: SRS: 14 to 20 Gy for nonsecretory tumors; 20 Gy or higher for secretory tumors.

Fractionated RT: 45–50.4 Gy/25–28 fx for nonsecretory; 50.4–54 Gy/28–30 fx for secretory.

Fractionated SRS: 17–21 Gy/3 fx, 22–25 Gy/5 fx for nonsecretory; 17.4–26.8 Gy/3 fx, 30–32 Gy/5 fx for secretory tumors.[25,26]

Re-RT: 35 to 49.6 Gy, median dose 42 Gy at 1.8 to 2 Gy/fx.[27,28]

(Note: Fractionated SRS and re-RT doses require further validation.)

Constraints: Optic pathway: maximum: 8 to 10 Gy (1 fx), 17.4 Gy (3 fx), 25 Gy (5 fx), 54 Gy (conventional fractionation).

Toxicity: Acute: fatigue, headache, infection, alopecia, otitis. Late: hypopituitarism, radionecrosis, vision impairment, hearing loss, stroke (relative risk 2–4),[29-31] second malignancy (2% at 10–20 years).[32]

EVIDENCE-BASED Q&A

What are the expected outcomes with SRS?

Multiple RRs show excellent 5-year LC for secretory and nonsecretory PitNETs treated with SRS. Hypopituitarism was seen in 20% to 25% at 5 years, and CN dysfunction ranged from 2% to 9%.[33–36]

Kotecha, ISRS Guidelines (*Neuro Oncol* 2020, PMID 31790121): Meta-analysis of 35 retrospective studies of nonfunctioning PitNETs treated with SRS (median 15 Gy, range: 5–35 Gy) or hypofractionated RT (median 21 Gy, range: 12–25 Gy in 3–5 fx). After SRS, 5- and 10-year LC was 94% and 83%, respectively. After hypofractionated RT, 5-year LC was 97%. The most common toxicity was hypopituitarism, ~21%. **Conclusion: Both SRS and hypofractionated RT provide excellent LC for nonfunctioning PitNETs.**

Mathieu, ISRS Review (*J Neurosurg* 2022, PMID 34479203): A systematic review of 45 studies on the use of single-fraction SRS (range: 13.2–35 Gy) for hormone-producing PitNETs. Crude tumor control rate was estimated as 97% for acromegaly, 92% for Cushing disease, and 93% for prolactinomas. Crude endocrine remission rate was 44%, 48%, and 28% for acromegaly, Cushing, and prolactinomas, respectively. **Conclusion: SRS provides effective tumor control for hormone-producing PitNETs but with a lower rate of endocrine remission.**

Is there a difference between time to endocrine response when comparing fractionated RT vs. SRS?

Hormone normalization appears to occur faster after SRS in some series. Important to note that SRS cases usually have smaller volume tumors compared with fractionated RT cases, which may influence outcomes.

Kong, Korea (*Cancer* 2007, PMID 17599761): Compared outcomes of fractionated RT vs. SRS in 125 patients. Hormone complete remission rate was 26% at 2 years and 76% at 4 years; median time to complete remission was 63 months for fractionated RT vs. 26 months for SRS ($p = .007$). **Conclusion: Both fractionated RT and SRS are effective in controlling tumor growth, but SRS may have a quicker effect on hormone normalization.**

What are the expected outcomes with proton therapy for PitNET?

Wattson, Harvard (*IJROBP* 2014, PMID 25194666): RR of 144 patients treated with 3D-conformal passive scattered proton therapy using 2 to 5 beams. Median dose to tumor margin: 20 CGE. LC 98% at MFU of 43 months. New hypopituitarism developed at a median time of 40 months, with larger target volume predictive of hypopituitarism (HR 1.3, $p = .004$); 3-year hypopituitarism rate 45%, 5-year rate 62%; four patients developed temporal lobe seizures. No CVA or secondary malignancies at MFU of 4.3 years. See Table 6.3 for biochemical CR results. **Conclusion: Proton RT is an effective treatment, but the risk of hypopituitarism remains.**

Table 6.3 Biochemical Outcomes After Proton Therapy for Secretory PitNET				
Syndrome	N	3-Yr CR (%)	5-Yr CR (%)	Median Time to CR (mos)
Cushing	74	54	67	32
Nelson	8	63	75	27
Acromegaly	50	26	49	62
Prolactinoma	9	22	38	60
TSHoma	3	0	33	51

What is the risk of secondary malignancy with RT for PitNET?

Pollock, Mayo Clinic (*IJROBP* 2017, PMID 28333013): RR of 188 patients treated with GKRS. Median dose was 18 Gy to tumor margin. No secondary malignancy or malignant transformation reported at MFU of 8.5 years (5–22.3). **Conclusion: Risk of RT-induced tumors after SRS is very low.**

Minniti, Royal Marsden (*J Clin Endocrinol Metab* 2005, PMID 15562021): RR of 462 patients who received fractionated RT; 76% received conventional three-field RT to 45 Gy/25 fx. At MFU of 12 years, 11 patients developed secondary brain tumors (5 meningiomas, 4 high-grade astrocytomas, 1 meningeal sarcoma, 1 PitNET). Cumulative risk 2% at 10 years and 2.4% at 20 years. Relative risk 10.5 compared with normal population. **Conclusion: There is a low risk of second malignancy after fractionated RT, and it should not preclude the use of RT as an effective treatment option.**

REFERENCES

1. Suh JH, Chao ST, Murphy SM, Recinos PF. Pituitary tumors and craniopharyngiomas. In: Tepper JE, Foote RL, Michalski JM. *Gunderson & Tepper's Clinical Radiation Oncology.* 5th ed. Elsevier 2021:528–549.

2. Ezzat S, Asa SL, Couldwell WT, et al. The prevalence of pituitary adenomas: a systematic review. *Cancer.* 2004;101(3):613–619. doi:10.1002/cncr.20412

3. Ostrom QT, Cioffi G, Gittleman H, et al. CBTRUS statistical report: primary brain and other central nervous system tumors diagnosed in the United States in 2012–2016. *Neuro Oncol.* 2019;21(suppl 5):v1–v100. doi:10.1093/neuonc/noz150

4. Hemminki K, Forsti A, Ji J. Incidence and familial risks in pituitary adenoma and associated tumors. *Endocr Relat Cancer.* 2007;14(1):103–109. doi:10.1677/ERC-06-0008

5. Schoemaker MJ, Swerdlow AJ. Risk factors for pituitary tumors: a case-control study. *Cancer Epidemiol Biomarkers Prev.* 2009;18(5):1492–1500. doi:10.1158/1055-9965.EPI-08-0657

6. Loeffler JS, Shih HA. Radiation therapy in the management of pituitary adenomas. *J Clin Endocrinol Metab.* 2011;96(7):1992–2003. doi:10.1210/jc.2011-0251

7. Johnston PC, Kennedy L, Hamrahian AH, et al. Surgical outcomes in patients with Cushing's disease: the Cleveland clinic experience. *Pituitary.* 2017;20(4):430–440. doi:10.1007/s11102-017-0802-1

8. Bengtsson D, Schroder HD, Andersen M, et al. Long-term outcome and MGMT as a predictive marker in 24 patients with atypical pituitary adenomas and pituitary carcinomas given treatment with temozolomide. *J Clin Endocrinol Metab.* 2015;100(4):1689–1698. doi:10.1210/jc.2014-4350

9. McCormack AI, Wass JA, Grossman AB. Aggressive pituitary tumours: the role of temozolomide and the assessment of MGMT status. *Eur J Clin Invest.* 2011;41(10):1133–1148. doi:10.1111/j.1365-2362.2011.02520.x

10. Sheehan J, Lee CC, Bodach ME, et al. Congress of neurological surgeons systematic review and evidence-based guideline for the management of patients with residual or recurrent nonfunctioning pituitary adenomas. *Neurosurgery.* 2016;79(4):E539–E540. doi:10.1227/NEU.0000000000001385

11. Batista RL, Musolino NRC, Cescato VAS, et al. Cabergoline in the management of residual nonfunctioning pituitary adenoma: a single-center, open-label, 2-year randomized clinical trial. *Am J Clin Oncol.* 2019;42(2):221–227. doi:10.1097/COC.0000000000000505

12. Tritos NA, Miller KK. Diagnosis and management of pituitary adenomas: a review. *JAMA.* 2023;329(16):1386–1398. doi:10.1001/jama.2023.5444

13. O'Sullivan EP, Woods C, Glynn N, et al. The natural history of surgically treated but radiotherapy-naive nonfunctioning pituitary adenomas. *Clin Endocrinol (Oxf).* 2009;71(5):709–714. doi:10.1111/j.1365-2265.2009.03583.x

14. Lu L, Wan X, Xu Y, Chen J, Shu K, Lei T. Prognostic factors for recurrence in pituitary adenomas: recent progress and future directions. *Diagnostics (Basel).* 2022;12(4):977. doi:10.3390/diagnostics12040977

15. Roelfsema F, Biermasz NR, Pereira AM. Clinical factors involved in the recurrence of pituitary adenomas after surgical remission: a structured review and meta-analysis. *Pituitary.* 2012;15(1):71–83. doi:10.1007/s11102-011-0347-7

16. Ho KKY, Kaiser UB, Chanson P, et al. Pituitary adenoma or neuroendocrine tumour: the need for an integrated prognostic classification. *Nat Rev Endocrinol.* 2023;19(11):671–678. doi:10.1038/s41574-023-00883-8

17. Linsler S, Quack F, Schwerdtfeger K, Oertel J. Prognosis of pituitary adenomas in the early 1970s and today-Is there a benefit of modern surgical techniques and treatment modalities? *Clin Neurol Neurosurg.* 2017;156:4–10. doi:10.1016/j.clineuro.2017.03.002

18. Molitch ME. Nonfunctioning pituitary tumors and pituitary incidentalomas. *Endocrinol Metab Clin North Am.* 2008;37(1):151–171. doi:10.1016/j.ecl.2007.10.011

19. Pala A, Brand C, Kapapa T, et al. The value of intraoperative and early postoperative magnetic resonance imaging in low-grade glioma surgery: a retrospective study. *World Neurosurg.* 2016;93:191–197. doi:10.1016/j.wneu.2016.04.120

20. Sheehan JP, Pouratian N, Steiner L, Laws ER, Vance ML. Gamma Knife surgery for pituitary adenomas: factors related to radiological and endocrine outcomes. *J Neurosurg.* 2011;114(2):303–309. doi:10.3171/2010.5.JNS091635

21. Castinetti F, Nagai M, Dufour H, et al. Gamma knife radiosurgery is a successful adjunctive treatment in Cushing's disease. *Eur J Endocrinol.* 2007;156(1):91–98. doi:10.1530/eje.1.02323

22. Pollock BE, Jacob JT, Brown PD, Nippoldt TB. Radiosurgery of growth hormone-producing pituitary adenomas: factors associated with biochemical remission. *J Neurosurg.* 2007;106(5):833–838. doi:10.3171/jns.2007.106.5.833

23. Pouratian N, Sheehan J, Jagannathan J, Laws ER Jr, Steiner L, Vance ML. Gamma knife radiosurgery for medically and surgically refractory prolactinomas. *Neurosurgery.* 2006;59(2):255–266. doi:10.1227/01.NEU.0000223445.22938.BD

24. Molitch ME. Diagnosis and treatment of pituitary adenomas: a review. *JAMA.* 2017;317(5):516–524. doi:10.1001/jama.2016.19699

25. Iwata H, Sato K, Nomura R, et al. Long-term results of hypofractionated stereotactic radiotherapy with CyberKnife for growth hormone-secreting pituitary adenoma: evaluation by the Cortina consensus. *J Neurooncol.* 2016;128(2):267–275. doi:10.1007/s11060-016-2105-1

26. Iwata H, Sato K, Tatewaki K, et al. Hypofractionated stereotactic radiotherapy with CyberKnife for nonfunctioning pituitary adenoma: high local control with low toxicity. *Neuro Oncol.* 2011;13(8):916–922. doi:10.1093/neuonc/nor055

27. Schoenthaler R, Albright NW, Wara WM, Phillips TL, Wilson CB, Larson DA. Re-irradiation of pituitary adenoma. *Int J Radiat Oncol Biol Phys.* 1992;24(2):307–314. doi:10.1016/0360-3016(92)90686-c

28. Flickinger JC, Deutsch M, Lunsford LD. Repeat megavoltage irradiation of pituitary and suprasellar tumors. *Int J Radiat Oncol Biol Phys.* 1989;17(1):171–175. doi:10.1016/0360-3016(89)90385-4

29. Brada M, Burchell L, Ashley S, Traish D. The incidence of cerebrovascular accidents in patients with pituitary adenoma. *Int J Radiat Oncol Biol Phys.* 1999;45(3):693–698. doi:10.1016/s0360-3016(99)00159-5

30. Erridge SC, Conkey DS, Stockton D, et al. Radiotherapy for pituitary adenomas: long-term efficacy and toxicity. *Radiother Oncol.* 2009;93(3):597–601. doi:10.1016/j.radonc.2009.09.011

31. Sattler MG, Vroomen PC, Sluiter WJ, et al. Incidence, causative mechanisms, and anatomic localization of stroke in pituitary adenoma patients treated with postoperative radiation therapy versus surgery alone. *Int J Radiat Oncol Biol Phys.* 2013;87(1):53–59. doi:10.1016/j.ijrobp.2013.05.006

32. Minniti G, Traish D, Ashley S, Gonsalves A, Brada M. Risk of second brain tumor after conservative surgery and radiotherapy for pituitary adenoma: update after an additional 10 years. *J Clin Endocrinol Metab.* 2005;90(2):800–804. doi:10.1210/jc.2004-1152

33. Sheehan JP, Starke RM, Mathieu D, et al. Gamma Knife radiosurgery for the management of nonfunctioning pituitary adenomas: a multicenter study. *J Neurosurg.* 2013;119(2):446–456. doi:10.3171/2013.3.JNS12766

34. Minniti G, Osti MF, Niyazi M. Target delineation and optimal radiosurgical dose for pituitary tumors. *Radiat Oncol.* 2016;11(1):135. doi:10.1186/s13014-016-0710-y

35. Hung YC, Lee CC, Yang HC, et al. The benefit and risk of stereotactic radiosurgery for prolactinomas: an international multicenter cohort study. *J Neurosurg.* 2019;133(3):717–726. doi:10.3171/2019.4.JNS183443

36. Ding D, Mehta GU, Patibandla MR, et al. Stereotactic radiosurgery for acromegaly: an international multicenter retrospective cohort study. *Neurosurgery.* 2019;84(3):717–725. doi:10.1093/neuros/nyy178

7 TRIGEMINAL NEURALGIA

Jana M. Kobeissi and Samuel T. Chao

QUICK HIT Trigeminal neuralgia, also referred to as "tic douloureux," is a rare condition characterized by episodic, debilitating pain of the face. It is typically unilateral and described as an electric or shock-like sensation.[1] First-line therapy is antiepileptic medication, such as carbamazepine or oxcarbazepine.[2] Second-line therapy options include microvascular decompression (gold standard, best pain control rate), percutaneous balloon microcompression, radiofrequency rhizotomy, and SRS.[3] Long-term follow-up demonstrates good outcomes of pain relief with SRS.[2]

EPIDEMIOLOGY: Trigeminal neuralgia (TGN) is the most common facial pain syndrome, with an annual incidence of 5.9 cases per 100,000 women and 3.4 cases per 100,000 men in the United States.[4] Male-to-female ratio is 1:1.5.[5] It usually presents in the fifth through the seventh decades of life.[6]

RISK FACTORS: TGN is more common in women, and patients with multiple sclerosis are at higher risk. Hypertension is a suggested risk factor due to the precipitation of tortuous vasculature, although this association is uncertain.[7]

ANATOMY: The trigeminal nerve (CN V) emerges from the midlateral surface of the pons, providing the sensory supply to the face and the motor supply to the muscles of mastication. The semilunar or Gasserian ganglion of the trigeminal nerve is located in Meckel's cave near the apex of the petrous part of the temporal bone. The trigeminal nerve has three branches: **ophthalmic nerve (V1)**, which exits the superior orbital fissure and supplies the cornea, ciliary body, iris, lacrimal glands, conjunctiva, and skin of the upper face; **maxillary nerve (V2)**, which exits through the foramen rotundum and supplies the pterygopalatine fossa, infraorbital canal, and the skin of the external nasal/superior labial face; and **mandibular nerve (V3)**, which exits through the foramen ovale and supplies the teeth and gums of the mandible, skin of the temporal region, lower lip, muscles of mastication, and sensation of the two-thirds of the tongue.

ETIOLOGY: Etiologies include vascular compression of the trigeminal root (most common), benign tumors, malignancy, and multiple sclerosis.[1] Compression due to an ectatic loop of artery or vein is the etiology in 80% to 90% of cases. The compression usually occurs within a few millimeters of emergence from the pons (also called the "root entry zone" [REZ]).[8]

CLINICAL PRESENTATION: The ICHD-3 defines the diagnostic criteria of classic TGN as at least three attacks of unilateral facial pain occurring in one or more divisions of the trigeminal nerve without radiation beyond the trigeminal distribution and at least three of the following characteristics: (a) recurring paroxysmal attacks lasting from a fraction of a second to 2 minutes; (b) severe intensity; (c) electric shock-like shooting, stabbing, or sharp in quality; and (d) at least three attacks precipitated by innocuous stimuli to the affected side of the face (some attacks may be, or may appear to be, spontaneous). There must not be clinical evidence of neurologic deficit and the condition should not be accounted for by another ICHD-3 diagnosis.[1] Of note, pain is typically within the V2 and/or V3 distribution, with V1 the least common distribution. Unlike other facial pain syndromes, TGN does not usually wake patients from sleep. Involvement of the V1 distribution can also be associated with autonomic symptoms of lacrimation, conjunctival injection, and rhinorrhea.

WORKUP: TGN can be diagnosed based on the classic clinical features described. A careful dental exam should be performed. An MRI is indicated to rule out other etiologies, such as demyelinating lesions, a mass in the cerebellopontine angle, or an ectatic blood vessel. The CISS sequence is especially helpful in identifying aberrant vessels. If the patient is unable to get an MRI, a CT cisternogram can be obtained.

TREATMENT PARADIGM

Observation: Observation is appropriate for patients whose symptoms are tolerable and infrequent.

Medical: Antiepileptic drugs are first-line therapy.[9] More than 25% do not respond to medical therapy or have poor tolerance secondary to the associated toxicities of dose escalation necessary for adequate pain control. Carbamazepine (600–800 mg daily) is the first-line agent and has been shown to be effective in four RCTs.[10-13] The most common side effects include drowsiness, dizziness, nausea, and vomiting.[9] Leukopenia and aplastic anemia are rare but more serious complications. Second-line agents include clonazepam, gabapentin, lamotrigine, oxcarbazepine, and topiramate.[9]

Surgery: Typically used if patients have symptoms refractory to medical therapy.[3]

- Microvascular decompression (gold standard): Removal or separation of various vascular structures, usually an ectatic superior cerebellar artery, away from the trigeminal nerve.[14] About 70% of patients are pain-free at 10 years.[15] Risk of complications include 0.2% perioperative mortality, 0.1% brainstem infarction, and 1% ipsilateral hearing loss.[2]
- Radiofrequency rhizotomy: Application of heat to the Gasserian ganglion, thought to selectively destroy pain impulses carried by unmyelinated or thinly myelinated fibers.[16] A heat probe is inserted through foramen ovale in cycles of 45 to 90 seconds at 60°C to 90°C.[17] About 75% are pain-free at 14 years.[18]
- Glycerol rhizolysis: Injection of 0.1 to 0.4 mL of glycerol into the trigeminal cistern.[19] Provides instant pain relief, with a 92% success rate at a follow-up of 1 to 4 years.[20]
- Balloon compression: Use of a Fogarty catheter to compress the Gasserian ganglion by inflating with 0.5 to 1.0 mL of contrast dye for 1 to 6 minutes.[21]

Radiation

Indications: SRS is a minimally invasive option that is preferred for patients with medically refractory disease who are not good candidates for surgery. Pooled observational data suggest SRS may be associated with lower rates of pain control compared with microvascular decompression (MVD) or percutaneous rhizotomy for recurrent/refractory TGN.[22,23] Target is the proximal trigeminal root.

Dose: Typical SRS dose is 70 to 90 Gy in a single fx prescribed to the 100% IDL via a 4-mm shot directed at the REZ of the trigeminal nerve into the pons. RT causes axonal degeneration and necrosis.

Toxicity: Risks of complications include <10% facial numbness/paresthesia and <1% anesthesia dolorosa.[24] A nomogram developed by Lucas et al. quantifies the durability of pain relief and demonstrated that Burchiel pain type prior to treatment (type 1: >50% of symptoms are episodic; type 2: >50% of symptoms are constant), the BNI pain score after SRS, and post-SRS facial numbness were predictive of outcomes. Patients with type 1 Burchiel pain, low BNI pain score after SRS, and absence of post-SRS facial numbness tend to have more durable pain relief.[25]

EVIDENCE-BASED Q&A

MEDICAL THERAPY

What are the outcomes with carbamazepine?

Wiffen (*Cochrane Database Syst Rev* 2011, PMID 21249671): Meta-analysis of 15 PRTs and 629 patients with chronic neuropathic pain of different etiologies (TGN, postherpetic neuralgia, etc.) treated with carbamazepine. Seventy percent of patients reported some degree of improvement in pain, with an NNT of 1.7. Sixty-six percent of patients who received carbamazepine experienced at least one adverse event compared with 27% with placebo, although serious adverse events were not reported. **Conclusion: Carbamazepine is effective in the treatment of chronic neuropathic pain but is associated with higher rate of adverse events.**

STEREOTACTIC RADIOSURGERY

What is the appropriate target volume for SRS, and does increasing the treatment volume improve outcomes?

Flickinger, Pittsburgh/Mayo Clinic (*IJROBP* 2001, PMID 11567820): PRT of 87 patients treated with SRS randomized to a one-isocenter (n = 44) or two-isocenter (n = 43) technique; 75 Gy was prescribed to the maximum point. At MFU of 26 months, complete pain relief (with or without medication) was 66%. Pain relief was identical between one- and two-isocenter SRS treatments. Improved pain relief was associated with younger age (p = .025) and fewer prior procedures (p = .039). Complications (numbness or paresthesias) were correlated with the nerve length irradiated (p = .018). **Conclusion: Increasing the treatment volume to include longer nerve length does not significantly improve pain relief but may increase complications.**

Does Gamma Knife SRS dose escalation improve outcomes?

Kotecha, Cleveland Clinic/Mid-Michigan (*IJROBP* 2016, PMID 27325473): RR of 870 patients from two institutions, divided into three groups based on treatment dose using GKRS and prescribed to the 100% IDL: ≤82 Gy (352 patients), 83 to 86 Gy (85 patients), and ≥90 Gy (433 patients). The 4-year rates of pain response were 79%, 82%, and 92% in patients treated to ≤82 Gy, 83 to 86 Gy, and ≥90 Gy, respectively. Patients who received ≤82 Gy had an increased risk of treatment failure compared with those who received ≥90 Gy (HR 2.0, p = .0007). Treatment-related facial numbness was similar among those receiving ≥83 Gy. The rate of anesthesia dolorosa was 1%. **Conclusion: Dose escalation >82 Gy prescribed to the 100% IDL may be associated with increased pain relief and duration of pain relief but at the expense of increased treatment-related facial numbness.**

What are the outcomes with LINAC-based radiosurgery for trigeminal neuralgia, and does increasing the dose improve outcomes?

Smith, UCLA (*IJROBP* 2011, PMID 21236592): RR of 179 patients treated with LINAC-based radiosurgery for TGN. Significant pain relief was noted at a mean duration of 28.8 months in 79% of the patients, with average time to pain relief of 1.92 months; 19% had recurrent pain at 13.5 months. Of the 28 patients treated with 70 Gy with the 30% IDL touching the brainstem, 64% had significant pain relief and 36% had numbness. Of the 82 patients treated with 90 Gy with the 30% IDL touching the brainstem, 79% had significant pain relief and 49% had numbness. Of the 59 patients treated with 90 Gy with the 50% IDL touching the brainstem, 88% had significant pain relief and 50% experienced numbness. **Conclusion: Increased RT dose and greater volume of brainstem irradiation may improve patient-reported outcomes but may increase numbness and trigeminal dysfunction.**

How do the different radiosurgery modalities compare in terms of outcomes?

Tuleasca (*J Neurosurg* 2018, PMID 29701555): Systematic review of 65 eligible studies, including 6,461 patients, receiving either Gamma Knife, LINAC-based, or CyberKnife SRS. Target was most commonly the REZ. The average rates of initial freedom from pain with or without medication were similar among the three modalities: 85%, 87%, and 79% for Gamma Knife, LINAC-based, and CyberKnife SRS, respectively, with average recurrence rates of 25%, 32%, and 26%. The available studies do not report long-term outcomes for LINAC-based or CyberKnife SRS, with the longest report being 60% pain relief at 3 years. In contrast, long-term evidence exists for GKRS, with 30% to 45% pain relief at 10 years. Overall hypesthesia rates were similar among the three modalities, but slightly higher average rates of bothersome or very bothersome hypesthesia were noted with CyberKnife compared with GKRS (9% vs. 3%, p = .05). Of note, all studies were retrospective, except for one. **Conclusion: Available studies, which are limited in level of evidence, suggest similar outcomes for the different radiosurgery modalities.**

How does SRS for trigeminal neuralgia affect quality of life?

Kotecha, Cleveland Clinic (*IJROBP* 2017, PMID 28721891): Prospective observational study of 50 patients who underwent SRS for TGN. At 12 months, 92% of patients were pain-free and 89% were free from facial numbness. QOL outcomes were collected before and after SRS, demonstrating significant improvement at 12 months, with scores improving by 55% and 59% for EQ-5D (p < .01) and PHQ-9 questionnaires (p = .03), respectively. This was driven by freedom from pain, enhanced ability to care for self, and lower rates of depression. Receiving a higher prescription dose (i.e., 86 Gy vs. ≤82 Gy) was correlated with an improved EQ-5D. **Conclusion: SRS not only provides relief from pain and facial numbness but also improves QOL and depression from TGN.**

Can SRS be repeated for recurrent trigeminal neuralgia?

Limited, retrospective data exist, with success rates varying from 68% to 95%. Success is more likely in those who had a positive pain response to the first procedure.[26–29] *A large RR of 152 patients at Wake Forest who underwent repeat GKRS for TGN (median initial dose 90 Gy, median second treatment dose 80 Gy) found that 84% of patients had at least a BNI IIIb pain relief, with 46% achieving BNI I.*[26]

How do SRS, microvascular decompression, and percutaneous rhizotomy compare?

Lu (*Br J Neurosurg* 2018, PMID 29745268): Systemic review and meta-analysis of 13 eligible studies, with patients treated with SRS (n = 683) or MVD (n = 670) for a first treatment or retreatment. SRS was associated with lower rates of pain freedom in both the short term (OR 0.16, 95% CI 0.11–0.22) and long term (OR 0.31, 0.22–0.44). It was also associated with lower rates of postoperative complications (OR 0.06, 0.02–0.16), higher rates of facial numbness (OR 1.64, 1.08–2.49), and higher rates of pain recurrence (OR 2.28, 1.32–3.93). Of note, all included studies were observational. **Conclusion: Pooled observational data suggest SRS may be associated with lower rates of pain control compared with MVD.**

Rheaume (*World Neurosurg* 2024, PMID 38403014): Systematic review and meta-analysis of 61 eligible studies, including 2,165 patients undergoing repeat MVD, percutaneous rhizotomy, or SRS, for recurrent/refractory TGN pain. Overall, 69% of all patients had complete pain relief after repeat treatment, with 50% maintaining CR at around 3 years postop. SRS had lower rates of pain relief (estimated proportion of complete pain response 0.35) compared with MVD (0.57) and percutaneous rhizotomy (0.60). Of note, all included studies were observational. **Conclusion: Pooled observational data suggest repeat SRS may be associated with lower rates of pain control compared with repeat MVD or percutaneous rhizotomy for recurrent/refractory TGN.**

REFERENCES

1. The international classification of headache disorders, 3rd edition (beta version). *Cephalalgia*. 2013;33(9): 629–808. doi:10.1177/0333102413485658
2. Gronseth G, Cruccu G, Alksne J, et al. Practice parameter: the diagnostic evaluation and treatment of trigeminal neuralgia (an evidence-based review): report of the quality standards subcommittee of the American Academy of Neurology and the European Federation of Neurological Societies. *Neurology*. 2008;71(15):1183–1190. doi:10.1212/01.wnl.0000326598.83183.04
3. Bennetto L, Patel NK, Fuller G. Trigeminal neuralgia and its management. *BMJ*. 2007;334(7586):201–205. doi:10.1136/bmj.39085.614792.BE
4. Zakrzewska JM, Linskey ME. Trigeminal neuralgia. *Am Fam Physician*. 2016;94(2):133–135. PMID:27419329
5. Maarbjerg S, Gozalov A, Olesen J, Bendtsen L. Trigeminal neuralgia–a prospective systematic study of clinical characteristics in 158 patients. *Headache*. 2014;54(10):1574–1582. doi:10.1111/head.12441
6. Ritter PM, Friedman WA, Bhasin RR. The surgical treatment of trigeminal neuralgia: overview and experience at the University of Florida. *J Neurosci Nurs*. 2009;41(4):211–214. PMID:19678507
7. Lin KH, Chen YT, Fuh JL, Wang SJ. Increased risk of trigeminal neuralgia in patients with migraine: a nationwide population-based study. *Cephalalgia*. 2016;36(13):1218–1227. doi:10.1177/0333102415623069
8. Love S, Coakham HB. Trigeminal neuralgia: pathology and pathogenesis. *Brain*. 2001;124(Pt 12):2347–2360. doi:10.1093/brain/124.12.2347
9. Attal N, Cruccu G, Haanpää M, et al. EFNS guidelines on pharmacological treatment of neuropathic pain. *Eur J Neurol*. 2006;13(11):1153–1169. doi:10.1111/j.1468-1331.2006.01511.x
10. Campbell FG, Graham JG, Zilkha KJ. Clinical trial of carbazepine (tegretol) in trigeminal neuralgia. *J Neurol Neurosurg Psychiatry*. 1966;29(3):265–267. doi:10.1136/jnnp.29.3.265
11. Killian JM, Fromm GH. Carbamazepine in the treatment of neuralgia. Use of side effects. *Arch Neurol*. 1968;19(2):129–136. doi:10.1001/archneur.1968.00480020015001
12. Nicol CF. A four year double-blind study of tegretol in facial pain. *Headache*. 1969;9(1):54–57. doi:10.1111/j.1526-4610.1969.hed0901054.x
13. Rockliff BW, Davis EH. Controlled sequential trials of carbamazepine in trigeminal neuralgia. *Arch Neurol*. 1966;15(2):129–136. doi:10.1001/archneur.1966.00470140019003
14. Jannetta PJ. Microsurgical management of trigeminal neuralgia. *Arch Neurol*. 1985;42(8):800. doi:10.1001/archneur.1985.04210090068018
15. Barker FG 2nd, Jannetta PJ, Bissonette DJ, Larkins MV, Jho HD. The long-term outcome of microvascular decompression for trigeminal neuralgia. *N Engl J Med*. 1996;334(17):1077–1083. doi:10.1056/nejm19960 4253341701

16. Attassi M, Seegenschmiedt MH, Körner M. Trigeminal neuralgia. In: Seegenschmiedt MH, Makoski HB, Trott KR, Brady LW, eds. *Radiotherapy for Non-Malignant Disorders*. Springer; 2008:665–677.

17. Tang YZ, Yang LQ, Yue JN, Wang XP, He LL, Ni JX. The optimal radiofrequency temperature in radiofrequency thermocoagulation for idiopathic trigeminal neuralgia: a cohort study. *Medicine (Baltimore)*. 2016;95(28):e4103. doi:10.1097/md.0000000000004103

18. Taha JM, Tew JM Jr, Buncher CR. A prospective 15-year follow up of 154 consecutive patients with trigeminal neuralgia treated by percutaneous stereotactic radiofrequency thermal rhizotomy. *J Neurosurg*. 1995;83(6):989–993. doi:10.3171/jns.1995.83.6.0989

19. Lopez BC, Hamlyn PJ, Zakrzewska JM. Systematic review of ablative neurosurgical techniques for the treatment of trigeminal neuralgia. *Neurosurgery*. 2004;54(4):973–983. doi:10.1227/01.neu.0000114867.98896.f0

20. Mintzer B, Devarajan J. Peripheral neurolysis. In: Deer TR, Leong MS, Buvanendran A, et al, eds. *Comprehensive Treatment of Chronic Pain by Medical, Interventional, and Integrative Approaches: The AMERICAN ACADEMY OF PAIN MEDICINE Textbook on Patient Management*. Springer; 2013:441–452.

21. de Siqueira SR, da Nóbrega JC, de Siqueira JT, Teixeira MJ. Frequency of postoperative complications after balloon compression for idiopathic trigeminal neuralgia: prospective study. *Oral Surg Oral Med Oral Pathol Oral Radiol Endod*. 2006;102(5):e39–e45. doi:10.1016/j.tripleo.2006.03.028

22. Lu VM, Duvall JB, Phan K, Jonker BP. First treatment and retreatment of medically refractive trigeminal neuralgia by stereotactic radiosurgery versus microvascular decompression: a systematic review and Meta-analysis. *Br J Neurosurg*. 2018;32(4):355–364. doi:10.1080/02688697.2018.1472213

23. Rheaume AR, Pietrosanu M, Ostertag C, Sankar T. Repeat surgery for recurrent or refractory trigeminal neuralgia: a systematic review and meta-analysis. *World Neurosurg*. 2024;185:370–380. doi:10.1016/j.wneu.2024.02.097

24. Nurmikko TJ, Eldridge PR. Trigeminal neuralgia–pathophysiology, diagnosis and current treatment. *Br J Anaesth*. 2001;87(1):117–132. doi:10.1093/bja/87.1.117

25. Lucas JT Jr, Nida AM, Isom S, et al. Predictive nomogram for the durability of pain relief from gamma knife radiation surgery in the treatment of trigeminal neuralgia. *Int J Radiat Oncol Biol Phys*. 2014;89(1):120–126. doi:10.1016/j.ijrobp.2014.01.023

26. Helis CA, Lucas JT Jr, Bourland JD, Chan MD, Tatter SB, Laxton AW. Repeat radiosurgery for trigeminal neuralgia. *Neurosurgery*. 2015;77(5):755–761. doi:10.1227/NEU.0000000000000915

27. Herman JM, Petit JH, Amin P, Kwok Y, Dutta PR, Chin LS. Repeat gamma knife radiosurgery for refractory or recurrent trigeminal neuralgia: treatment outcomes and quality-of-life assessment. *Int J Radiat Oncol Biol Phys*. 2004;59(1):112–116. doi:10.1016/j.ijrobp.2003.10.041

28. Gellner V, Kurschel S, Kreil W, Holl EM, Ofner-Kopeinig P, Unger F. Recurrent trigeminal neuralgia: long term outcome of repeat gamma knife radiosurgery. *J Neurol Neurosurg Psychiatry*. 2008;79(12):1405–1407. doi:10.1136/jnnp.2007.142794

29. Park KJ, Kondziolka D, Berkowitz O, et al. Repeat gamma knife radiosurgery for trigeminal neuralgia. *Neurosurgery*. 2012;70(2):295–305. doi:10.1227/NEU.0b013e318230218e

8 VESTIBULAR SCHWANNOMA

Elizabeth E. Obi, Jeffrey A. Kittel, John H. Suh, and Praveen Pendyala

QUICK HIT Vestibular schwannoma (VS), previously called "acoustic neuroma," is a slow-growing, benign nerve sheath tumor of the cerebellopontine angle (CPA) that typically presents with unilateral hearing loss and tinnitus. Treatment options include observation, microsurgical resection, and RT (SRS or fractionated). SRS is generally prescribed up to 13 Gy and conventional fractionation to 45 to 54 Gy. Tumor control outcomes appear equivalent between surgery and RT, but RT may minimize impact on QOL.

EPIDEMIOLOGY: Incidence is approximately 3 to 5 per 100,000 person-years, making up 8% of intracranial tumors and 85% of tumors arising from the CPA.[1,2] Incidence is increasing given utilization of diagnostic imaging.[3,4] Median age at diagnosis is 50 to 55, and incidence increases with age.[3,5] The incidence for those over 70 years of age may be as high as 20 per 100,000 person-years.[2]

RISK FACTORS: Increasing age, NF2 (96% of patients with NF2, often bilateral), NF1 (5% of patients with NF1, unilateral), childhood exposure to RT (relative risk 1.14 per Gy).[6]

ANATOMY: VS typically arises from the vestibular portion of CN VIII and is unilateral in 90% of cases. CN VIII arises from the junction of the pons and medulla, enters the internal auditory foramen along with the facial nerve (CN VII), and then divides into the vestibular and cochlear nerves. The cochlear nerve runs to the spiral ganglion and innervates the spiral organ of Corti and the cochlea. The vestibular nerve runs to the vestibular ganglion and splits into three branches. The superior branch innervates the utricle and the superior and lateral semicircular ducts. The inferior branch innervates the saccule, and the posterior branch innervates the posterior semicircular duct. VS arises with equal frequency in the superior and inferior branches and rarely arises in the cochlear nerve. It tends to occur in the vestibular region of the foramen where the nerve acquires a Schwann cell sheath, although it can sometimes arise from or grow into the CPA.

PATHOLOGY: VS is composed of atypical proliferations of Schwann cells, which are found lining the peripheral nerves. Histopathologically, they are similar to other peripheral schwannomas and are composed of alternating zones of dense and sparse cellularity, termed "Antoni A" and "Antoni B," respectively. Antoni A pattern is arranged in fascicles of elongated cells with cytoplasmic processes with little stromal matrix. Atoni B demonstrates loose, less dense meshwork of cells with microcyst and myxoid changes.[7] IHC demonstrates S100 positivity.[8] Malignant degeneration is extremely rare. There are no known markers that predict aggressive or recurrent behaviors.[9]

GENETICS: Biallelic inactivation of NF2 on chr 22, which produces the tumor suppressor merlin (schwannomin), is common in sporadic VS and is the cause of bilateral VS in NF2.[10] This inactivation leads to the dysregulation of receptor tyrosine kinases and other intracellular signaling pathways, including Pac1, RAS, PAK1, and mTORC1. Other tumor suppressors linked to the development of VS include LZTR1, SMARCB1, and COQ6.[11,12] There are studies suggesting that NF2-associated VS has a polyclonal mutation pattern, which may account for the differences seen in treatment outcomes when compared with sporadic VS.[13,14]

CLINICAL PRESENTATION: Hearing loss, which is typically of high frequency range (95%; only two-thirds are aware of it; average duration ~4 years, although 16% develop sudden hearing loss), tinnitus (63%; average duration ~3 years), vestibular symptoms (61%; typically imbalance and vertigo, often mild to moderate, nonspecific, and fluctuating; average duration ~2 years), headache (12%; most often occipital), trigeminal symptoms (17%; typically facial numbness/hyperesthesia/pain; average duration ~1 year), and facial nerve symptoms (6%; typically facial weakness, less commonly taste disturbance; average duration ~2 years); other symptoms from brainstem compression (ataxia, hydrocephalus, dysarthria, dysphagia, hoarseness) are uncommon.[15] The House–Brackmann and Gardner–Robertson scales are common metrics of facial paralysis and hearing loss, respectively (Tables 8.1 and 8.2).

Table 8.1 House–Brackmann Facial Paralysis Scale[16]	
Grade I	Normal
Grade II	Mild dysfunction (slight weakness, normal symmetry at rest)
Grade III	Moderate dysfunction (obvious but not disfiguring weakness, synkinesis) with normal symmetry at rest Complete eye closure with maximal effort Good forehead movement
Grade IV	Moderately severe dysfunction (obvious and disfiguring asymmetry, significant synkinesis) Incomplete eye closure Moderate forehead movement
Grade V	Severe dysfunction (barely perceptive motion)
Grade VI	Total paralysis

Source: House JW, Brackmann DE. Facial nerve grading system. *Otolaryngol Head Neck Surg.* 1985;93(2):146–147. doi:10.1177/019459988509300202.

Table 8.2 Gardner–Robertson Hearing Loss Scale[17]	
Grade I	Good–excellent (70%–100% speech discrimination)
Grade II	Serviceable (50%–69%)
Grade III	Nonserviceable (5%–49%)
Grade IV	Poor (1%–4%)
Grade V	None

Source: Adapted from Gardner G, Robertson JH. Hearing preservation in unilateral acoustic neuroma surgery. *Ann Otol Rhinol Laryngol.* 1988;97(1):55–66. doi:10.1177/000348948809700110.

WORKUP: H&P including Weber and Rinne tests to assess asymmetric sensorineural hearing loss, CN exam, and audiometry. Consider BAER testing to assess cochlear nerve damage (BAER/ABR; 60%–90% sensitive with lower sensitivity for small tumors; 60%–90% specific).[18]

Imaging: MRI of the brain with contrast is the gold standard for diagnosis. High-resolution CT with IV contrast if unable to obtain MRI. MRI shows isointense or slightly hypointense signal on T1, typically with homogeneous contrast enhancement, although occasional cystic degeneration (more commonly in larger tumors) and hemorrhagic areas can be seen.[19] Classic finding is "ice-cream cone" shape with widening of the porus acusticus.[20] Erosion and widening of the internal acoustic canal may be seen on CT.[21] Differential includes meningioma, glomus tumor, ependymoma, facial or trigeminal schwannoma, epidermoid cyst, and metastasis.

PROGNOSTIC FACTORS: Baseline level of hearing loss, growth rate >2.5 mm/yr, and delay in diagnosis.[22–25] Initial tumor size is not prognostic.[24] Patients with growth rate >2.5 mm/yr have decreased rates of hearing preservation (32% vs. 75%, $p < .0001$) and decreased median time to total hearing loss (7.0 vs. 14.8 years, $p < .0001$).[24,25] Malignant transformation is rare and typically seen with NF2-associated VS.[26]

STAGING: VS are not staged but can be graded on the Koos grading scale (Table 8.3).[27]

Table 8.3 Koos Grading Scale for VS[27]	
Grade I	Intracanalicular
Grade II	Tumor extending into the posterior fossa (PF), with or without an intracanalicular component, without touching the brainstem
Grade III	Tumor extending into the PF, compressing the brainstem, but not shifting it from the midline
Grade IV	Tumor extending into the PF, compressing the brainstem, and shifting it from the midline

Source: Data from Koos WT, Day JD, Matula C, Levy DI. Neurotopographic considerations in the microsurgical treatment of small acoustic neurinomas. *J Neurosurg.* 1998;88(3):506–512. doi:10.3171/jns.1998.88.3.0506.

TREATMENT PARADIGM

Optimal candidates for observation include patients with small- to medium-sized sporadic VS with good–excellent speech discrimination (Gardner–Robinson grade I).

Observation: Consider observation with MRI every 6 to 12 months in patients without baseline hearing loss and stability or slow growth rate. Observation is especially favored in older patients with significant comorbidities. Indications for treatment vary but can include >2.5 mm growth/yr and new onset or worsening of symptoms. Only one-third of VS grow in the first 3 years, and up to 50% grow in the first 5 years. Patients undergoing observation should be counseled that they have a risk of hearing loss without treatment (see Table 8.4). Current consensus guidelines suggest annual imaging at least up to 5 years, with possible longer duration up to 10 years.[28–30]

Table 8.4 General Probability of Hearing Preservation in Favorably Selected Patients[28]			
	2 Yrs	**5 Yrs**	**10 Yrs**
Observation	>75%–100%	>50%–5%	Insufficient data
SRS	>75%–100%	>50%–75%	>25%–50%
Surgery	>25%–50%	>25%–50%	>25%–50%

Source: Data from Olson JJ, Kalkanis SN, Ryken TC. Congress of neurological surgeons systematic review and evidence-based guidelines on the treatment of adults with vestibular schwannomas: executive summary. *Neurosurgery.* 2018;82(2):129–134. doi:10.1093/neuros/nyx586.

Surgery: In general, surgery has excellent results for resection of the entire tumor but can have poor rates of hearing preservation. Hearing preservation is most likely when the tumor is <1.5 to 2 cm in size.[31] Other major morbidities include CSF leaks, tinnitus, headaches, and facial paralysis.[32] Surgery is still the most common treatment for VS and is especially considered for younger patients, larger tumors (Koos grade IV), tumors causing mass effect or dizziness, cystic tumors, and small anatomically favorable tumors with good hearing.[33] There are three main surgical approaches for resection (see Table 8.5).[32–34] The goal of resection is to maximize tumor removal while minimizing morbidity. There is no difference between tumor recurrence or mortality rates between these approaches.[35]

Table 8.5 Surgical Techniques for VS		
Approach	**Advantages**	**Disadvantages**
Retrosigmoid/suboccipital	Possible hearing conservation and facial nerve sparing	Associated with increased risk of CSF leaks and headaches
Translabyrinthine	Possible preservation of facial function	No hearing preservation, a fat graft is required, and the sigmoid sinus is more prone to injury
Middle fossa	Possible hearing conservation for small tumors (≤1.5 cm)	Facial nerve more vulnerable to injury, dural lacerations likely in older patients, may cause trismus from temporalis muscle injury

Chemotherapy: There is generally no role for systemic therapy, although bevacizumab has shown response in rare progressive situations associated with NF2.[36]

Radiation: RT is appropriate when the tumor is <3 to 4 cm in size or when surgery is refused or is not an option.[37] Following an STR, salvage RT can be given upfront (within 12 months of surgery) or later at the time of progression as waiting does not offer inferior tumor control.[38] Follow-up after RT typically consists of exams, audiometry, and MRIs annually for 5 years. Follow-up frequency can be increased to every 6 months during year 1 and for larger tumors.[29,39] Nearly half of VS may demonstrate pseudo-progression, defined as temporary tumor expansion after RT followed by subsequent regression, and it may be necessary to wait at least 3 years following RT to distinguish between pseudo-progression and treatment failure.[40,41]

SRS: Current guidelines recommend doses ≤13 Gy for single-fraction SRS, with most common dose ranging from 12 to 13 Gy, typically prescribed to the 50% isodose line (IDL) with GKRS and the 80%

IDL with LINAC-based radiosurgery. Long-term results show >95% control with minimal morbidity or impact on QOL. Doses >13 Gy are associated with increased morbidity with regard to facial paralysis, trigeminal neuralgia, and hearing loss.[42–44] Impact on hearing preservation and relative differences between treatment modalities appears to vary with time.[45,46] In a series of 440 patients with long-term follow-up, 1 patient (0.3%) developed malignant transformation.[47]

FSRT: The most commonly used hypofractionated SRS (HFSRT) regimens include 21 Gy/3 fx, 22 Gy/5 fx, and 25 Gy/5 fx. Typical conventionally fractionated RT doses range from 45 to 54 Gy in 1.8 to 2 Gy/fx and were historically used for larger tumors prior to the advent of HFSRT.[41] Controversy exists whether fractionation is superior to single-fraction SRS, but fractionation is recommended with larger tumors (>3–4 cm) in an effort to spare adjacent normal structures such as the brainstem and cochlea.[48]

Proton Therapy: Can be used to deliver SRS or fractionated RT when dose constraints cannot be met with other techniques. At 4 years, LC >90% with serviceable hearing ~30%.[49,50]

Important Max Dose Constraints[26,51–54]:

Single-fraction SRS: Brainstem: D0.03cc <15 Gy; cochlea mean: <4 Gy.

Hypofractionated FSRT:

- 3 fx: Brainstem: D0.03cc <18–23.1 Gy; cochlea mean <17 Gy.
- 5 fx: Brainstem: D0.03cc <23–31 Gy; cochlea mean <25 Gy.

Conventionally fractionated: Brainstem D0.03cc <54 Gy; cochlea mean <45 Gy.

Procedure: See *Handbook of Treatment Planning in Radiation Oncology*, Chapter 3.[44]

EVIDENCE-BASED Q&A

What are the outcomes of treatment with surgical resection for patients with VS?

Surgical resection is achievable with high rates of control and low risks of significant complications.[31,32] Can consider maximal safe resection rather than GTR in order to reduce complications[32]; however, patients who undergo STR are at a higher risk of recurrence than patients who undergo GTR/NTR.[55]

Carlson, Mayo Clinic (*Laryngoscope* 2012, PMID 22252688): RR of 203 patients treated at a single institution. Of the patients, 144 underwent GTR, 32 NTR, and 27 STR. Twelve patients (6%) had a recurrence at a mean of 3.0 years after surgery; 5-year RFS ~91%. Patients who received STR were 9× more likely to fail than patients undergoing NTR/GTR. No significant difference between patients with NTR and GTR was noted. Patients with nodular enhancement on initial postop MRI had a 16× higher risk of recurrence compared with patients with linear patterns. **Conclusion: STR increases risk of recurrence compared with GTR/NTR.**

How does SRS compare with observation? What percentage of patients who undergo observation will ultimately experience progression and require treatment?

In a Norwegian cohort study from 2013, patients who underwent GKRS compared with observation had similar rates of hearing loss, symptoms, and QOL. In the V-REX RCT, immediate SRS at the time of initial diagnosis was associated with significantly greater tumor volume reduction at 4 years when compared with a "wait and scan" approach in which SRS was delayed until radiographic tumor growth. Forty-four percent of patients on the wait and scan protocol received SRS due to tumor progression at 4 years.

Breivik, Norway (*Neurosurgery* 2013, PMID 23615094): Prospective cohort study of patients who underwent GKRS (113) or observation (124). Patients underwent GKRS with small tumors (<20 mm) after growth was observed by referring physician (*n* = 31), by patient choice (*n* = 26), or with tumors >20 mm who refused surgery. GKRS dose was 12 Gy to the tumor periphery. Serviceable hearing was lost in 76% of patients on observation and 64% with GKRS (NS). Patients treated with GKRS had significantly less need for future treatment. Symptoms and QOL did not differ between groups. **Conclusion: GKRS appears to prevent the need for further treatment and appears not to significantly impact rates of hearing loss, symptoms, or QOL compared with observation.**

Dhayalan, V-REX (*JAMA*, 2023, PMID 37526718): PRT of 100 patients with newly diagnosed unilateral vestibular schwannoma (<6 months) and a maximal tumor diameter <2 cm randomized to receive either upfront SRS vs. a "wait and scan" protocol for which treatment was given upon tumor growth. Participants assigned to upfront SRS received treatment within 2 months of randomization. Primary endpoint: ratio between tumor volume at 4 years and baseline (V4:V0). Six percent of patients in the upfront SRS group needed additional treatment at 3 years due to progression. In the "wait and scan" group, 44% received SRS. The V4:V0 was significantly lower among those who received upfront SRS than those who underwent "wait and scan" approach. **Conclusion: Among patients with VS <2 cm, upfront SRS at diagnosis results in superior tumor volume reduction compared with an observational wait and scan approach.**

How does RT compare with microsurgical resection?

Studies have shown equivalent tumor control with SRS compared with microsurgical resection with generally better functional outcomes and less impact on QOL with SRS.[45,56–58] *However, there is no consensus on the optimal management. The ideal population of patients for each modality overlaps (small tumors with preserved hearing), but surgery may be preferred in larger tumors, especially in patients with mass effect.*

Pollock, Mayo Clinic (*Neurosurgery* 2006, PMID 16823303): Prospective cohort study of 82 patients with unilateral <3 cm VS undergoing surgical resection ($n = 36$) or GKRS ($n = 46$). No difference in tumor control (100% vs. 96%, $p = .50$). At 1 year, GKRS patients had better facial nerve preservation (100% vs. 69%, $p < .001$), better hearing preservation (63% vs. 5%, $p < .001$), and better physical functioning, energy, and pain. **Conclusion: Similar tumor control with GKRS or surgery, but less morbidity with GKRS.**

Maniakas, Montreal (*Otol Neurotol* 2012, PMID 22996165): Meta-analysis of 16 studies comparing microsurgical resection and SRS. Overall, SRS showed significantly better long-term hearing preservation rates than microsurgery (70% vs. 50%, $p < .001$). Crude rates of long-term tumor progression were not significantly different between SRS and microsurgery (4% vs. 1%). **Conclusion: SRS and microsurgery offer similar control rates, with SRS having less long-term hearing effects.**

What are the long-term results of SRS?

Long-term results for SRS show excellent LC. However, it appears that rates of hearing preservation may continue to decline.[46,47,59]

Hasegawa, Japan (*J Neurosurg* 2013, PMID 23140152): RR of 440 patients treated with GKRS between 1991 and 2000. MFU 12.5 years. Actuarial 5- and 10-year PFS was 93% and 92%, respectively. No patient failed >10 years after treatment. On MVA, significant brainstem compression, marginal dose ≤13 Gy, prior treatment, and female sex correlated with decreased PFS. Patients treated with ≤13 Gy had an increased rate of facial nerve preservation (100% vs. 97%); 10 patients (2%) developed delayed cyst formation. One patient developed malignant transformation. **Conclusion: GKRS is a safe and effective treatment for VS with >10 years of follow-up.**

Carlson, Mayo Clinic (*J Neurosurg* 2013, PMID 23101446): RR of 44 patients with long-term audiometric follow-up after SRS. SRS was given with 12 to 13 Gy to the periphery of the tumor. MFU 9.3 years; 36 patients developed nonserviceable hearing at a mean of 4.2 years after SRS. Kaplan–Meier estimated rates of serviceable hearing at 1, 5, and 10 years following SRS were 80%, 48%, and 23%, respectively. MVA revealed that pretreatment ipsilateral pure tone average ($p < .001$) and tumor size ($p = .009$) were associated with time to nonserviceable hearing. **Conclusion: The percent of patients with serviceable hearing after SRS decreases over time.**

Can SRS be used for larger tumors (>3 cm)?

Yang, Pittsburgh (*J Neurosurg* 2011, PMID 20799863): RR of 65 patients with VS between 3 and 4 cm in one extracanalicular maximum diameter (median tumor volume 9 mL) who underwent GKRS; 17 patients (26%) had previously undergone resection. At 2 years, seven tumors (11%) had grown; 18 (82%) of 22 patients with serviceable hearing before SRS still had serviceable hearing after SRS more than 2 years later. Patients who had a previous resection ($p = .010$), those with tumor volume >10 mL ($p = .05$), and those with Koos grade 4 tumors ($p = .02$) had less likelihood of tumor control after SRS. **Conclusion: GKRS can be used in larger tumors; however, previous resection, volume >10 mL, and Koos grade 4 tumors are associated with worse control.**

How does fractionated RT compare with SRS?

Fractionation offers a theoretical radiobiologic advantage compared with single-fx treatment, which should allow for improved sparing of normal structures. However, evidence for differences in outcome between SRS and 5-fx or longer treatment courses is limited to retrospective data and may only improve hearing preservation.[43,60,61]

Coombs, Heidelberg (*IJROBP* 2010, PMID 19604653): Prospective study of 200 patients with 202 VS treated with either LINAC-based SRS (*n* = 30) or fractionated stereotactic RT (FSRT; *n* = 172). Median SRS dose was 13 Gy to 80% IDL, and median FSRT dose was 57.6 Gy/32 fx. MFU 75 months. No difference in 5-year LC (96% overall). FSRT and SRS (dose ≤13 Gy) showed equivalent hearing preservation (76% at 5 years). For SRS dose >13 Gy (*n* = 11), hearing preservation was significantly worse than FSRT. Both patients who developed trigeminal neuralgia in the SRS group were treated with >13 Gy. Rate of facial nerve weakness was 17% in the SRS group and 2% in the FSRT group. Only one patient treated with SRS to ≤13 Gy developed facial weakness. **Conclusion: SRS with doses ≤13 Gy is a safe and effective alternative to FSRT. FSRT should be reserved for larger lesions.**

Meijer, Netherlands (*IJROBP* 2003, PMID 12873685): RR of 129 patients treated with either single-fx or 5-fx RT using LINAC-based SRS techniques. Patients were prospectively selected for single fx if edentate and 5 fx if dentate due to the immobilization device used. Single-fx arm treated with 10 to 12.5 Gy and 5-fx arm treated with 20 to 25 Gy. No significant differences in 5-year LC (100% vs. 94%), facial nerve preservation (93% vs. 97%), or hearing preservation (75% vs. 61%); 5-year trigeminal nerve preservation was significantly different (92% vs. 98%, *p* = .048), favoring the fractionated group. **Conclusion: Single-fx SRS has similar outcomes to FSRT with a small detriment to trigeminal nerve preservation.**

Is there an emerging role for antiangiogenic agents in the treatment of VS?

Multiple small studies have demonstrated that bevacizumab can decrease tumor growth rates, cause tumor regression, and improve hearing in patients with NF2.[36,62–64] *A phase II study from Johns Hopkins suggested that bevacizumab q3 weeks for 46 weeks demonstrated durable hearing response for ≥3 months in five (36%) patients and suggested that imaging responses are associated with higher blood levels of VEG-F and stromal cell-derived factor 1α.*[63] *Larger studies with long-term follow-up are required.*

REFERENCES

1. Singh K, Singh MP, Thukral C, Rao K, Singh K, Singh A. Role of magnetic resonance imaging in evaluation of cerebellopontine angle schwannomas. *Indian J Otolaryngol Head Neck Surg*. 2015;67(1):21–27. doi:10.1007/s12070-014-0736-0

2. Marinelli JP, Beeler CJ, Carlson ML, Caye-Thomasen P, Spear SA, Erbele ID. Global incidence of sporadic vestibular schwannoma: a systematic review. *Otolaryngol Head Neck Surg*. 2022;167(2):209–214. doi:10.1177/01945998211042006

3. Babu R, Sharma R, Bagley JH, Hatef J, Friedman AH, Adamson C. Vestibular schwannomas in the modern era: epidemiology, treatment trends, and disparities in management. *J Neurosurg*. 2013;119(1):121–130. doi:10.3171/2013.1.JNS121370

4. Cioffi G, Yeboa DN, Kelly M, et al. Epidemiology of vestibular schwannoma in the United States, 2004–2016. *Neurooncol Adv*. 2020;2(1):vdaa135. doi:10.1093/noajnl/vdaa135

5. Propp JM, McCarthy BJ, Davis FG, Preston-Martin S. Descriptive epidemiology of vestibular schwannomas. *Neuro Oncol*. 2006;8(1):1–11. doi:10.1215/S1522851704001097

6. Shore-Freedman E, Abrahams C, Recant W, Schneider AB. Neurilemomas and salivary gland tumors of the head and neck following childhood irradiation. *Cancer*. 1983;51(12):2159–2163. doi:10.1002/1097-0142(19830615)51:12<2159::aid-cncr2820511202>3.0.co;2-l

7. Kumar V, Abbas AK, Fausto N, Robbins SL. *Robbins and Cotran Pathologic Basis of Disease*. Elsevier Saunders; 2005.

8. Sobel RA. Vestibular (acoustic) schwannomas: histologic features in neurofibromatosis 2 and in unilateral cases. *J Neuropathol Exp Neurol*. 1993;52(2):106–113. doi:10.1097/00005072-199303000-00002

9. Sughrue ME, Fung KM, Van Gompel JJ, Peterson JEG, Olson JJ. Congress of neurological surgeons systematic review and evidence-based guidelines on pathological methods and prognostic factors in vestibular schwannomas. *Neurosurgery*. 2018;82(2):E47–E48. doi:10.1093/neuros/nyx514

10. Sughrue ME, Yeung AH, Rutkowski MJ, Cheung SW, Parsa AT. Molecular biology of familial and sporadic vestibular schwannomas: implications for novel therapeutics. *J Neurosurg*. 2011;114(2):359–366. doi:10.3171/2009.10.JNS091135

11. Brodhun M, Stahn V, Harder A. Pathogenesis and molecular pathology of vestibular schwannoma. *HNO*. 2017;65(5):362–372. doi:10.1007/s00106-016-0201-3

12. Mehta GU, Feldman MJ, Wang H, Ding D, Chittiboina P. Unilateral vestibular schwannoma in a patient with schwannomatosis in the absence of LZTR1 mutation. *J Neurosurg*. 2016;125(6):1469–1471. doi:10.3171/2015.11.JNS151766

13. Havik AL, Bruland O, Myrseth E, et al. Genetic landscape of sporadic vestibular schwannoma. *J Neurosurg*. 2018;128(3):911–922. doi:10.3171/2016.10.JNS161384

14. Dewan R, Pemov A, Kim HJ, et al. Evidence of polyclonality in neurofibromatosis type 2-associated multilobulated vestibular schwannomas. *Neuro Oncol*. 2015;17(4):566–573. doi:10.1093/neuonc/nou317

15. Matthies C, Samii M. Management of 1000 vestibular schwannomas (acoustic neuromas): clinical presentation. *Neurosurgery*. 1997;40(1):1–10. doi:10.1097/00006123-199701000-00001

16. House JW, Brackmann DE. Facial nerve grading system. *Otolaryngol Head Neck Surg*. 1985;93(2):146–147. doi:10.1177/019459988509300202

17. Gardner G, Robertson JH. Hearing preservation in unilateral acoustic neuroma surgery. *Ann Otol Rhinol Laryngol*. 1988;97(1):55–66. doi:10.1177/000348948809700110

18. Doyle KJ. Is there still a role for auditory brainstem response audiometry in the diagnosis of acoustic neuroma? *Arch Otolaryngol Head Neck Surg*. 1999;125(2):232–234. doi:10.1001/archotol.125.2.232

19. Schmalbrock P, Chakeres DW, Monroe JW, Saraswat A, Miles BA, Welling DB. Assessment of internal auditory canal tumors: a comparison of contrast-enhanced T1-weighted and steady-state T2-weighted gradient-echo MR imaging. *AJNR Am J Neuroradiol*. 1999;20(7):1207–1213. PMID:10472973

20. DeLong M, Kaylie, D, Kranz, PG, Adamson, CD. Vestibular Schwannomas: lessons for the neurosurgeonpart idiagnosis, neuroimaging, and audiology. *Contemp Neurosurg*. 2011;33(20):1–5. doi:10.1097/01.CNE.0000408560.95604.48

21. Gaillard F MQ, Bell D, et al. Vestibular schwannoma. Accessed August 18, 2024. https://radiopaedia.org/articles/vestibular-schwannoma.

22. Bakkouri WE, Kania RE, Guichard JP, Lot G, Herman P, Huy PT. Conservative management of 386 cases of unilateral vestibular schwannoma: tumor growth and consequences for treatment. *J Neurosurg*. 2009;110(4):662–669. doi:10.3171/2007.5.16836

23. Stangerup SE, Tos M, Thomsen J, Caye-Thomasen P. Hearing outcomes of vestibular schwannoma patients managed with 'wait and scan': predictive value of hearing level at diagnosis. *J Laryngol Otol*. 2010;124(5):490–494. doi:10.1017/S0022215109992611

24. Sughrue ME, Kane AJ, Kaur R, et al. A prospective study of hearing preservation in untreated vestibular schwannomas. *J Neurosurg*. 2011;114(2):381–385. doi:10.3171/2010.4.JNS091962

25. Sughrue ME, Yang I, Aranda D, et al. The natural history of untreated sporadic vestibular schwannomas: a comprehensive review of hearing outcomes. *J Neurosurg*. 2010;112(1):163–167. doi:10.3171/2009.4.JNS08895

26. Kano H, Kondziolka D, Khan A, Flickinger JC, Lunsford LD. Predictors of hearing preservation after stereotactic radiosurgery for acoustic neuroma. *J Neurosurg*. 2009;111(4):863–873. doi:10.3171/2008.12.JNS08611

27. Koos WT, Day JD, Matula C, Levy DI. Neurotopographic considerations in the microsurgical treatment of small acoustic neurinomas. *J Neurosurg*. 1998;88(3):506–512. doi:10.3171/jns.1998.88.3.0506

28. Olson JJ, Kalkanis SN, Ryken TC. Congress of neurological surgeons systematic review and evidence-based guidelines on the treatment of adults with vestibular schwannomas: executive summary. *Neurosurgery*. 2018;82(2):129–134. doi:10.1093/neuros/nyx586

29. Goldbrunner R, Weller M, Regis J, et al. EANO guideline on the diagnosis and treatment of vestibular schwannoma. *Neuro Oncol*. 2020;22(1):31–45. doi:10.1093/neuonc/noz153

30. Paldor I, Chen AS, Kaye AH. Growth rate of vestibular schwannoma. *J Clin Neurosci*. 2016;32:1–8. doi:10.1016/j.jocn.2016.05.003

31. Gormley WB, Sekhar LN, Wright DC, Kamerer D, Schessel D. Acoustic neuromas: results of current surgical management. *Neurosurgery*. 1997;41(1):50–60. doi:10.1097/00006123-199707000-00012

32. Samii M, Matthies C. Management of 1000 vestibular schwannomas (acoustic neuromas): surgical management and results with an emphasis on complications and how to avoid them. *Neurosurgery*. 1997;40(1):11–23. doi:10.1097/00006123-199701000-00002

33. Carlson ML, Link MJ, Wanna GB, Driscoll CL. Management of sporadic vestibular schwannoma. *Otolaryngol Clin North Am*. 2015;48(3):407–422. doi:10.1016/j.otc.2015.02.003

34. Lanman TH, Brackmann DE, Hitselberger WE, Subin B. Report of 190 consecutive cases of large acoustic tumors (vestibular schwannoma) removed via the translabyrinthine approach. *J Neurosurg.* 1999;90(4): 617–623. doi:10.3171/jns.1999.90.4.0617

35. Sughrue ME, Yang I, Aranda D, et al. Beyond audiofacial morbidity after vestibular schwannoma surgery. *J Neurosurg.* 2011;114(2):367–374. doi:10.3171/2009.10.JNS091203

36. Plotkin SR, Duda DG, Muzikansky A, et al. Multicenter, prospective, phase ii and biomarker study of high-dose bevacizumab as induction therapy in patients with neurofibromatosis type 2 and progressive vestibular schwannoma. *J Clin Oncol.* 2019;37(35):3446–3454. doi:10.1200/JCO.19.01367

37. Yang HC, Kano H, Awan NR, et al. Gamma Knife radiosurgery for larger-volume vestibular schwannomas. Clinical article. *J Neurosurg.* 2011;114(3):801–807. doi:10.3171/2010.8.JNS10674

38. Dhayalan D, Perry A, Graffeo CS, et al. Salvage radiosurgery following subtotal resection of vestibular schwannomas: does timing influence tumor control? *J Neurosurg.* 2023;138(2):420–429. doi:10.3171/2022.5.JNS22249

39. Heller RS, Joud H, Flores-Milan G, et al. Changing enhancement pattern and tumor volume of vestibular schwannomas after subtotal resection. *World Neurosurg.* 2021;151:e466–e471. doi:10.1016/j.wneu.2021.04.059

40. Woodson E. Radiation for sporadic vestibular schwannoma: an update on modalities, emphasizing hearing loss, side effects, and tumor control. *Otolaryngol Clin North Am.* 2023;56(3):521–531. doi:10.1016/j.otc.2023.02.011

41. Brun L, Mom T, Guillemin F, Puechmaille M, Khalil T, Biau J. The recent management of vestibular schwannoma radiotherapy: a narrative review of the literature. *J Clin Med.* 2024;13(6):1611. doi:10.3390/jcm13061611

42. Mendenhall WM, Friedman WA, Buatti JM, Bova FJ. Preliminary results of linear accelerator radiosurgery for acoustic schwannomas. *J Neurosurg.* 1996;85(6):1013–1019. doi:10.3171/jns.1996.85.6.1013

43. Combs SE, Welzel T, Schulz-Ertner D, Huber PE, Debus J. Differences in clinical results after LINAC-based single-dose radiosurgery versus fractionated stereotactic radiotherapy for patients with vestibular schwannomas. *Int J Radiat Oncol Biol Phys.* 2010;76(1):193–200. doi:10.1016/j.ijrobp.2009.01.064

44. Videtic GMM, Vassil AD, Woody NM. *Handbook of Treatment Planning in Radiation Oncology.* 3rd ed. Demos Medical; 2020.

45. Carlson ML, Tveiten OV, Driscoll CL, et al. Long-term quality of life in patients with vestibular schwannoma: an international multicenter cross-sectional study comparing microsurgery, stereotactic radiosurgery, observation, and nontumor controls. *J Neurosurg.* 2015;122(4):833–842. doi:10.3171/2014.11.JNS14594

46. Carlson ML, Jacob JT, Pollock BE, et al. Long-term hearing outcomes following stereotactic radiosurgery for vestibular schwannoma: patterns of hearing loss and variables influencing audiometric decline. *J Neurosurg.* 2013;118(3):579–587. doi:10.3171/2012.9.JNS12919

47. Hasegawa T, Kida Y, Kato T, Iizuka H, Kuramitsu S, Yamamoto T. Long-term safety and efficacy of stereotactic radiosurgery for vestibular schwannomas: evaluation of 440 patients more than 10 years after treatment with Gamma Knife surgery. *J Neurosurg.* 2013;118(3):557–565. doi:10.3171/2012.10.JNS12523

48. Sheikh MM. Vestibular Schwannoma. In: De Jesus O, ed. *StatPearls.* StatPearls Publishing; 2023.

49. Weber DC, Chan AW, Bussiere MR, et al. Proton beam radiosurgery for vestibular schwannoma: tumor control and cranial nerve toxicity. *Neurosurgery.* 2003;53(3):577–588. doi:10.1227/01.neu.0000079369.59219.c0

50. Bush DA, McAllister CJ, Loredo LN, Johnson WD, Slater JM, Slater JD. Fractionated proton beam radiotherapy for acoustic neuroma. *Neurosurgery.* 2002;50(2):270–275. doi:10.1097/00006123-200202000-00007

51. Mayo C, Yorke E, Merchant TE. Radiation associated brainstem injury. *Int J Radiat Oncol Biol Phys.* 2010;76(3 suppl):S36–S41. doi:10.1016/j.ijrobp.2009.08.078

52. Bentzen SM, Constine LS, Deasy JO, et al. Quantitative analyses of normal tissue effects in the clinic (QUANTEC): an introduction to the scientific issues. *Int J Radiat Oncol Biol Phys.* 2010;76(3 suppl):S3–S9. doi:10.1016/j.ijrobp.2009.09.040

53. Bhandare N, Jackson A, Eisbruch A, et al. Radiation therapy and hearing loss. *Int J Radiat Oncol Biol Phys.* 2010;76(3 suppl):S50–S57. doi:10.1016/j.ijrobp.2009.04.096

54. Diez P, Hanna GG, Aitken KL, et al. UK 2022 Consensus on normal tissue dose-volume constraints for oligometastatic, primary lung and hepatocellular carcinoma stereotactic ablative radiotherapy. *Clin Oncol (R Coll Radiol).* 2022;34(5):288–300. doi:10.1016/j.clon.2022.02.010

55. Carlson ML, Van Abel KM, Driscoll CL, et al. Magnetic resonance imaging surveillance following vestibular schwannoma resection. *Laryngoscope.* 2012;122(2):378–388. doi:10.1002/lary.22411

56. Regis J, Pellet W, Delsanti C, et al. Functional outcome after gamma knife surgery or microsurgery for vestibular schwannomas. *J Neurosurg.* 2002;97(5):1091–1100. doi:10.3171/jns.2002.97.5.1091

57. Pollock BE, Driscoll CL, Foote RL, et al. Patient outcomes after vestibular schwannoma management: a prospective comparison of microsurgical resection and stereotactic radiosurgery. *Neurosurgery.* 2006;59(1): 77–85. doi:10.1227/01.NEU.0000219217.14930.14

58. Maniakas A, Saliba I. Microsurgery versus stereotactic radiation for small vestibular schwannomas: a meta-analysis of patients with more than 5 years' follow-up. *Otol Neurotol.* 2012;33(9):1611–1620. doi:10.1097/MAO.0b013e31826dbd02

59. Lunsford LD, Niranjan A, Flickinger JC, Maitz A, Kondziolka D. Radiosurgery of vestibular schwannomas: summary of experience in 829 cases. *J Neurosurg.* 2005;102 Suppl:195–199. PMID:15662809

60. Andrews DW, Suarez O, Goldman HW, et al. Stereotactic radiosurgery and fractionated stereotactic radiotherapy for the treatment of acoustic schwannomas: comparative observations of 125 patients treated at one institution. *Int J Radiat Oncol Biol Phys.* 2001;50(5):1265–1278. doi:10.1016/s0360-3016(01)01559-0

61. Meijer OW, Vandertop WP, Baayen JC, Slotman BJ. Single-fraction vs. fractionated linac-based stereotactic radiosurgery for vestibular schwannoma: a single-institution study. *Int J Radiat Oncol Biol Phys.* 2003;56(5):1390–1396. doi:10.1016/s0360-3016(03)00444-9

62. Plotkin SR, Stemmer-Rachamimov AO, Barker FG 2nd, et al. Hearing improvement after bevacizumab in patients with neurofibromatosis type 2. *N Engl J Med.* 2009;361(4):358–367. doi:10.1056/NEJMoa0902579

63. Blakeley JO, Ye X, Duda DG, et al. Efficacy and biomarker study of bevacizumab for hearing loss resulting from neurofibromatosis type 2-associated vestibular schwannomas. *J Clin Oncol.* 2016;34(14):1669–1675. doi:10.1200/JCO.2015.64.3817

64. Morris KA, Golding JF, Axon PR, et al. Bevacizumab in neurofibromatosis type 2 (NF2) related vestibular schwannomas: a nationally coordinated approach to delivery and prospective evaluation. *Neurooncol Pract.* 2016;3(4):281–289. doi:10.1093/nop/npv065

9 UVEAL MELANOMA

Bryn M. Myers, Gaurav Marwaha, John H. Suh, and Arun D. Singh

QUICK HIT   Uveal melanoma (UM) is the most common form of ocular melanoma, with the uvea consisting of the iris, ciliary body, and choroid. It is unrelated to cutaneous melanoma. Historically, management was enucleation. Now, the standard of care for small- to medium-sized tumors is definitive RT with either episcleral plaque brachytherapy or charged particle RT, which offers >90% tumor control and is vision-sparing (Table 9.1). Larger tumors have less favorable tumor control and are managed with either charged particle RT or enucleation. Diagnosis is often made without biopsy by a well-trained ophthalmic oncologist with ultrasound assistance. It is imperative to rule out distant metastases, particularly liver metastases, with dedicated CT/MRI at the time of diagnosis.

Table 9.1 Treatment Paradigm of Uveal Melanoma[1]		
Classification (COMS)	Size	Management
Small	Diameter 5–16 mm and thickness ≤2.5 mm	Low suspicion for melanoma (<3 risk factors*): Monitor High suspicion for melanoma: Plaque brachytherapy[†] Particle beam RT[‡]
Medium	Diameter 5–16 mm and thickness 2.5–10.0 mm	Plaque brachytherapy[†] Particle beam RT[‡] Enucleation
Large[§]	Diameter >16 mm and thickness >10.0 mm	Enucleation Plaque brachytherapy[†] Particle beam RT[‡]

*Risk factors: symptomatic, diameter >12 mm, thickness >2 mm, subretinal fluid or orange pigment, tumor within 3 mm of optic disc, ultrasound hollowness.
[†]Plaque brachytherapy: ^{106}Ru or ^{125}I to 85 Gy is commonly used.
[‡]Particle beam RT: 56–60 GyE in 4 daily fxs or up to 70 GyE in 5 fxs.
[§]Consider neoadjuvant trial.
Source: From Melanoma: Uveal. NCCN Clinical Practice Guidelines in Oncology;1.2024. May 23, 2024.

EPIDEMIOLOGY: Uncommon, with 1,500 to 2,000 cases per year. Most common primary eye tumor in adults, median age 62 years. Often affects fair-skinned individuals (98%). The most common locations are choroid (85%–90%), ciliary body (5%–8%), and iris (3%–5%).[2]

RISK FACTORS: The vast majority of cases are sporadic. However, the following factors may increase risk: fair iris/skin color; propensity to sunburn; strong personal or family history of cancer; occupational history of welding; choroidal nevi; oculodermal melanocytosis[3–5]; germline BAP1, PALB-2, or MBD4 mutation; dysplastic nevus syndrome; and NF-1. Presence of sporadic cutaneous melanoma does not increase the risk of uveal melanoma.

ANATOMY: The posterior uvea is composed of the choroid (the retina's vascular support layer), which is where light-protective melanocytes reside. The anterior uvea includes the iris and ciliary body and controls accommodation and lens movement. The entire uveal tract lies beneath the sclera (the white fibrous protective layer of the eye).

PATHOLOGY: Uveal melanocytes arise from neural crest cells. The degree of pigmentation determines iris color. Pathologic types: spindle cell (best prognosis), mixed (majority of cases), and epithelioid (worst prognosis).

GENETICS: Unlike cutaneous melanoma, UM is not typically associated with BRAF or NRAS gene mutations. Rather, GNAQ and GNA11 mutations are evident early in the tumorigenesis process.

There is increasing evidence of association with germline BAP1 mutations as well as somatic mutations in BAP1, EIF1AX, and SF3B1.[6] Combination of monosomy 3 and 8q gain is associated with metastasis. A 15-gene expression profile (GEP) is an accurate prognostic marker, and GEP class 2 is associated with a higher rate of metastasis.[7]

CLINICAL PRESENTATION: Visual symptoms (blurred vision, photopsia, metamorphopsia, visual field loss), retinal detachment (larger tumors), and rarely pain/eye inflammation. A third of patients are asymptomatic.

WORKUP: Ophthalmologists can make a clinical diagnosis 95% of the time.[2] Diagnostic techniques should include the following: slit-lamp examination, indirect ophthalmoscopy, fundus photography, transillumination, fluorescein angiography, and ocular US (for tumor height/diameter). Tumor distance from the optic disc and fovea, ciliary body involvement, presence of subretinal fluid (SRF), and presence of orange pigment should be reported. Typical UMs are subretinal, brown, raised, and dome-shaped. Internal extension of the tumor results in a mushroom-shaped mass apparent on ultrasonography. Consider MRI of the orbit for large tumors, tumors close to the optic nerve, or suspicion of extraocular involvement. Biopsy is indicated in clinically atypical tumors and is also helpful for prognostication.[3] Risk of seeding due to biopsy is rare.[8] Differential diagnosis includes metastases, benign nevus, hemangioma, and retinal detachment. Metastatic evaluation includes CT abdomen (MRI if highly concerned about liver metastases).

PROGNOSTIC FACTORS: Poor prognostic factors include symptomatic tumors, epithelioid cell, large tumor (>10.0 mm thick, >16 mm diameter), involvement of ciliary body, older age, monosomy 3 and 8q gain, and GEP class 2.

NATURAL HISTORY: The uvea lacks lymphatic channels; thus, metastases from the uvea spread hematogenously to the liver (90% of metastases), lungs, skin, bones, and soft tissues. In small-, medium-, and large-sized tumors, about 1%, 10%, and 25% will develop metastatic disease, respectively. After RT, tumors tend to regress slowly over a few years. Useful vision (>20/200) is preserved in 50% of patients, with tumor size and location being the main drivers for visual outcomes (i.e., >6 mm tumors and proximity to optic nerve/fovea predict for worse visual outcomes).

STAGING: See Tables 9.2 and 9.3.

Table 9.2 AJCC 8th Edition Staging (2017) and COMS Staging for uveal melanoma*				
Choroidal and Ciliary Body Melanoma		**Iris Melanoma**		
T1	a Size category 1 without ciliary body involvement and extracellular extension	T1	a Limited to the iris, ≤3 clock hours in size	
	b Size category 1 with ciliary body involvement		b Limited to the iris, >3 clock hours in size	
	c Size category 1 without ciliary body involvement but with extraocular extension ≤5 mm		c Limited to the iris with secondary glaucoma	
	d Size category 1 with ciliary body involvement and extraocular extension ≤5 mm	T2	a Confluent with or extending into ciliary body without secondary glaucoma	
T2	a Size category 2 without ciliary body involvement or extraocular extension		b Confluent with or extending into ciliary body and choroid, without secondary glaucoma	
	b Size category 2 with ciliary body involvement		c Confluent with or extending into the ciliary body, choroid, or both with secondary glaucoma	

(continued)

Table 9.2 AJCC 8th Edition Staging (2017) and COMS Staging for uveal melanoma* *(continued)*			
Choroidal and ciliary body melanoma		**Iris Melanoma**	
	c Size category 2 without ciliary body involvement, with extraocular extension ≤5 mm	**T3**	Confluent with or extending into the ciliary body, choroid, or both with scleral extension
	d Size category 2 with ciliary body involvement and extraocular extension ≤5 mm	**T4**	**a** Episcleral extension ≤5 mm in largest diameter
T3	**a** Size category 3 without ciliary body involvement and extraocular extension		**b** Episcleral extension >5 mm in largest diameter
	b Size category 3 with ciliary body involvement		
	c Size category 3 without ciliary body involvement, with extraocular extension ≤5 mm	**N1**	**a** Metastasis in ≥1 regional LN
	d Size category 3 with ciliary body involvement and extraocular extension ≤5 mm		**b** No regional LNs, but discrete tumor deposits in orbit that are not contiguous to the eye (choroidal and ciliary body)
T4	**a** Size category 4 without ciliary body involvement and extraocular extension		
	b Size category 4 with ciliary body involvement	**M1**	**a** Distant metastasis, all ≤3.0 cm
	c Size category 4 without ciliary body involvement but with extraocular extension ≤5 mm		**b** Distant metastasis, largest 3.1-8 cm
	d Size category 4 with ciliary body involvement and extraocular extension ≤5 mm		**c** Distant metastasis, largest ≥8.1 cm
	e Any size category with extraocular extension >5 mm		
AJCC Group Staging		**COMS Staging**	
I	T1aN0M0	**Small**	*1–3 mm in apical height and 5-16 mm basal diameter*
IIA	T1b-dN0M0, T2aN0M0	**Medium**	*3.1–8 mm in apical height and <16 mm basal diameter*
IIB	T2bN0M0, T3aN0M0	**Large**	*>8 mm in apical height or >16 mm basal diameter*
IIIA	T2c-dN0M0, T3b-cN0M0, T4aN0M0		
IIIB	T3dN0M0, T4b-cN0		
IIIC	T4d-eN0M0		
IV	Any T, N1M0 or any T, any N, M1a-c		

Because of the intricacy of the AJCC staging, in practice and in most studies, the COMS staging system is utilized. It is broken into three groups: small (5-yr OS >90%), medium (5-yr OS 80%–85%), and large (5-yr OS 60%).

Table 9.3 Size Categories (Ciliary Body and Choroidal UM)							
Thickness (mm)							
>15					4	4	4
12.1–15.0				3	3	4	4
9.1–12.0		3	3	3	3	3	4
6.1–9.0	2	2	2	2	3	3	4
3.1–6.0	1	1	1	2	2	3	4
≤3.0	1	1	1	1	2	2	4
	≤3.0	3.1–6.0	6.1–9.0	9.1–12.0	12.1–15.0	15.1–18.0	>18.0
	Largest Basal Diameter (mm)						

TREATMENT PARADIGM

Observation: Close ophthalmic surveillance q3–6 months is a reasonable option for asymptomatic T1a lesions (treat for any growth or symptoms). NCCN guidelines recommend surveillance if less than three of the following risk factors are present: symptomatic, diameter >5 mm, thickness >2 mm, SRF or orange pigment, tumor within 3 mm of optic disc, ultrasound hollowness, and absence of halo.[1]

Surgery: Enucleation was the historical standard of care, but in the 2000s episcleral brachytherapy became the first-line treatment for small- to medium-sized (<10 mm in apical height) tumors and offered equivalent survival with vision-sparing capability. *Enucleation* under general anesthesia with orbital implant continues to be used when brachytherapy or particle beam RT is not feasible (i.e., for tumor replacing >50% of the globe, blind or painful eyes, extensive extraocular involvement, or neovascular glaucoma). For select larger tumors, in an effort to avoid RT side effects, fragmentation and vitreous cutter *endoresection* can be performed a few weeks postbrachytherapy.[3] Definitive, local resection (*exoresection*) may be feasible as well, in select anterior or large tumors. *Orbital exenteration* is utilized in the setting of massive orbital extension causing pain/blindness.

Chemotherapy/Immunotherapy: In stage IV disease, cytotoxic agents are of limited benefit, whereas dual checkpoint inhibition (nivolumab + ipilimumab) provides modest benefit.[9] For isolated liver metastases, locally ablative therapies are employed (e.g., chemoembolization, metastatectomy, RFA, internal/external RT), although recurrence is frequent. Tebentafusp, a first-in-class immune-mobilizing monoclonal T-cell receptor against cancer (ImmTAC), demonstrated significant improvement in OS in an open-label, phase III trial for patients with stage IV disease. Patients were randomized 2:1 to tebentafusp or investigator's choice of pembrolizumab, ipilimumab, or dacarbazine (82% received pembrolizumab), and the median OS was 21.7 months for tebentafusp vs. 16.0 months for the investigator's choice of therapy.[10]

Radiation

- *Episcleral brachytherapy* typically with ^{125}I or [106]Ru (more common in Europe and better for smaller tumors due to more rapid dose falloff). The half-lives of ^{125}I and [106]Ru are 60 days and 374 days, respectively. Plaques come in a variety of shapes/sizes and are generally gold-plated, with grooves in which radiation sources are glued or molded. Procedure occurs under general anesthesia; the plaque is sutured onto the episcleral surface overlying the tumor with a 2-mm margin of safety. The ophthalmologist makes a conjunctival peritomy, the globe is transilluminated, and the tumor is outlined. Next, a dummy plaque is used to verify the proper position, and the radioactive plaque is placed. Dose is 85 Gy (at a dose rate of 0.6–1.05 Gy/hr) prescribed to tumor apex from inner scleral surface.[11,12] The plaque remains in place for 3 to 7 days, during which time the patient wears a lead eye shield. The plaque is removed by the ophthalmologist, and the patient returns home with bandages and pain medications.
- *Charged particle beam RT* is most commonly delivered with protons (56–60 GyE in 4 daily fx or up to 70 GyE in 5 fx). Tantalum marker rings are surgically placed at the tumor borders for tumor delineation and to serve as fiducials, and multiple additional planning inputs are used for target delineation, including US, surgeon mapping, and CT/MRI. The optimal gaze direction to minimize dose to the cornea, lens, macula, and optic nerve is used.

Side Effects: Acute: pain (brachytherapy), dry eye (rare). Late: vasculopathy (driven by disc/fovea proximity), cataract formation (especially anterior tumors), maculopathy, retinopathy (most common side effect with brachytherapy), optic neuropathy.

Other Modalities: Transpupillary thermotherapy alone is associated with high-risk LR but can easily be combined with brachytherapy as an adjunct. For RT failures, transpupillary thermotherapy or repeat brachytherapy can be employed.[13]

EVIDENCE-BASED Q&A

SMALL TUMORS

Is it necessary to treat all small UMs?

No, the risk of death is low, provided patients are serially monitored with ophthalmologic exams. Significant growth on follow-up exams is an indication for treatment.

COMS Report No. 5, "Small" Choroidal Melanoma Series (*Arch Ophthalmol* 1997, PMID 9400787): Nonrandomized prospective study of 204 patients with **small** choroidal melanomas (i.e., 1–3 mm height and ≥5 mm in basal diameter). MFU 92 months. Eight percent of patients were treated at study enrollment and 33% treated during follow-up. Tumor growth noted in 21% at 2 years and 31% at 5 years. Twenty-seven percent died, six from DM. The 5-year OS was 94% and the 8-year OS was 85%. **Conclusion: Many patients with "small" choroidal melanomas (66%) may represent choroidal nevus and therefore can be closely monitored. Observation of small tumors may be appropriate until progression is noted.**

Singh, Small Choroidal Melanoma Surveillance vs. Treatment (*Am J Opthalmol* 2022, PMID 35358487): Retrospective cohort study of 167 patients that compared the outcomes of surveillance vs. immediate treatment for small choroidal melanoma. Patients in the immediately treated cohort were then classified as low- or high-risk melanoma based on a prediction model. The low-risk, immediate-treatment group was compared with the surveillance group with respect to visual and survival outcomes. MFU 34.6 months. There was no difference in visual acuity at 12, 24, and 36 months. The Kaplan–Meier estimates of MFS at 3 years for the surveillance group and the low-risk immediate-treatment group were 100% and 96%, respectively. **Conclusion: Low-risk choroidal melanoma, as identified by a prediction model, may be managed by surveillance with treatment after documented growth without detriment to visual or systemic outcomes at 3 years.**

What factors determine the use of each isotope (^{125}I vs. ^{106}Ru)?

In the management of smaller tumors (<5 mm), ^{106}Ru offers a more rapid dose falloff than ^{125}I, which may aid in sparing critical vision structures without compromising oncologic outcomes.

Takiar, MD Anderson (*PRO* 2015, PMID 25423888): RR of 107 patients treated with ^{125}I (*n* = 67) or ^{106}Ru (*n* = 40). ^{106}Ru: 5-year LC, PFS, and OS: 97%, 94%, and 92%, respectively. ^{125}I: 5-year LC, PFS, and OS: 83%, 65%, and 80%, respectively. In patients with apical tumor height ≤5 mm, PFS was slightly better for ^{106}Ru (*p* = .02). Enucleation-free survival was better in ^{106}Ru patients (*p* = .02), as was RT retinopathy (*p* = .03) and cataracts (*p* < .01). **Conclusion: Both isotopes offer excellent LC for small UMs, although ^{106}Ru does so with reduced toxicity but is limited to tumors with height ≤5.0 mm.**

MEDIUM TUMORS

How does the historical standard of enucleation compare with episcleral plaque brachytherapy?

No difference in OS, but brachytherapy offers eye- and vision-sparing. In the rare event of RT failure, patients can be salvaged effectively with enucleation.

COMS Report No. 28, "I-125 vs. Enucleation" (*Arch Ophthalmol* 2006, PMID 17159027): PRT of 1,317 patients with medium-sized choroidal melanomas (≥2.5–10 mm height and <16 mm in largest basal diameter)—enucleation vs. episcleral plaque brachytherapy with ^{125}I (85 Gy Rx dose). Exclusions: fovea/optic disc/ciliary body involvement. Thirteen percent of episcleral plaque patients were salvaged (due to tumor progression or RT complications) with enucleation by 5 years. **Conclusion: Episcleral plaque brachytherapy offers equivalent OS compared with enucleation. This PRT set the precedent for plaque brachytherapy as the standard of care in this patient population (see Table 9.4).**

Table 9.4 Results of COMS 28 Trial of I-125 vs. Enucleation for Choroidal Melanoma						
	5- and 12-Yr OS	12-Yr DM	I-125 Arm	Median Visual Acuity	20/40 or Better	20/200 or Worse
Enucleation	81%/59%	17%	Baseline	20/32	70%	10%
I-125 plaque 85 Gy	82%/57%	21%	3 yrs after I-125	20/125	34%	45%
p value	NS	NS				

LARGE TUMORS

What are the management options for large tumors that are not amenable to plaque brachytherapy?

Plaque brachytherapy is limited by suboptimal dosimetry for large tumors and by technical challenges for those near the optic disc. Historically, enucleation was the standard. Neoadjuvant EBRT was assessed on COMS 15, but it did not result in improved outcomes compared with enucleation alone. Charged particle RT does not have the same limitations of plaque brachytherapy for large tumors, and it is used as globe-sparing treatment with favorable outcomes.

COMS Report No. 15, "Large Tumors" (*Arch Ophthalmol* **2001, PMID 11346394**): PRT of 1,003 patients with large choroidal melanomas (>16 mm in largest basal diameter regardless of height, or >10 mm in height regardless of diameter, or >8 mm in height if <2 mm from optic disc)—enucleation vs. preoperative 20 Gy/5 fx EBRT + enucleation. See Table 9.5 for the results. Preoperative EBRT did not increase complication rate, but did have fewer LRs (0 vs. 5). DM was most commonly seen in the liver (93%), lung (24%), and bone (16%). **Conclusion: No role for preoperative EBRT.**

Table 9.5 Results of COMS 15 Trial of Neoadjuvant EBRT for Large UMs		
	5-Yr OS	5-Yr DSS
Enucleation alone	57%	72%
Preop EBRT 20 Gy + enucleation	62%	74%
p value	.32	.64

Papakostas, Harvard (*JAMA Ophthalmol* **2017, PMID 29049518**): RR of 336 patients with large tumors (as defined by COMS 15) treated with proton RT 70 CGE in 5 fx. The 10-year outcomes included tumor control: 88%; eye retention: 70%; melanoma-related mortality: 49%; OS: 61%; visual acuity retention >20/200: 9%; ability to count fingers: 22%. A 1-mm increase in diameter was associated with 20% increased risk of melanoma-related mortality. **Conclusion: Eye conservation is possible in the treatment of large choroidal melanomas.**

CHARGED PARTICLE RT

How does plaque brachytherapy compare with charged particle RT?

Charged particle RT, most commonly protons, is the second most common treatment modality after plaque brachytherapy and has been used to treat UM for decades; 5-year estimates with proton RT treatment include LC >90%, OS 70% to 85%, DMFS 75% to 90%, and DSS 75% to 90%.[14] Advantages of using charged particle RT include the ability to treat larger tumors or those encircling the optic disc where plaque brachytherapy is limited and enucleation is the alternative. Data from a meta-analysis and a single RCT using helium ions suggest charged particle RT is associated with improved LC rates compared with plaque brachytherapy but at the expense of increased anterior eye complications.

Char, UCSF (*Ophthalmology* 1993, PMID 8414414): PRT of 184 patients randomized to helium ion 70 Gy/5 fx vs. episcleral plaque brachytherapy (^{125}I) for tumors <10 mm height and <15 mm diameter. Helium ion therapy had greater LC (100% vs. 83%), comparable survival, and fewer salvage enucleations (9% vs. 17%), however with more anterior eye complications (dry eye, neovascular glaucoma, epiphora). **Conclusion: Compared with brachytherapy, helium ion therapy was associated with better LC and less salvage enucleation but more anterior segment toxicity.**

Chang, Meta-Analysis (*Br J Ophthalmol* 2013, PMID 23645818): Analysis of 49 studies reporting LF after globe-conserving therapy. Surgery included endoresection or transscleral resection, and laser included transpupillary thermotherapy. Results in Table 9.6. **Conclusion: LF rates vary by treatment modality.**

Table 9.6 Results of Meta-Analysis of Globe-Conserving Therapy for UM			
Modality	Weighted Mean LF (%)	Weighted Mean Tumor Diameter (mm)	Weighted Mean Tumor Height (mm)
Brachytherapy (*n* = 3,868)	9	11.00	4.48
Charged particle RT (*n* = 7,043)	4	13.93	5.54
Photon RT (*n* = 542)	8	11.40	6.15
Surgery (*n* = 537)	19	12.96	7.98
Laser (*n* = 552)	21	7.00	2.50

What is the optimal dose to treat UM with charged particle RT?

Only one RCT compared proton RT (PBT) 50 CGE/5 fx vs. 70 CGE/5 fx and reported similar outcomes. A recent survey demonstrated the most commonly used dose was 60 GyE in 4 fx.[15]

Gragoudas, Proton Dose (*Arch Ophthalmol* 2000, PMID 10865313): PRT of 188 patients with UM <15 mm diameter and <5 mm height randomized to PBT 50 CGE vs. 70 CGE both in 5 fx over a 7-day period. At 5 years, there were no differences in LR or metastatic deaths; ~10% of patients in each arm had an LR or DM. The proportion of patients with visual acuity of at least 20/200 was ~55% in both groups. RT maculopathy rates were also similar. Patients treated with 50 CGE had significantly less visual field loss. **Conclusion: Lower dose PBT was not associated with improved visual acuity but had less visual field loss. LF and DM rates were similar.**

Thariat, France (*Int J Radiat Oncol Biol Phys* 2023, PMID 37257661): Single-masked phase II trial of 32 patients randomized to either standard 52 Gy in 4 fxs or moderately hypofractionated 52 Gy in 8 fxs PBT. Mean tumor diameter and thickness were 16.5 mm and 9.1 mm, respectively. MFU 56.7 months. The 2-year LR-free survival rate without enucleation was 79%, similar in both arms. The 2-year OS was 82% and 67% for the standard and experimental arms, respectively (*p* = .56). Grade 3 to 4 ocular toxicity was noted in 72% of the standard arm and 61% of the experimental arm patients. **Conclusion: Both 52 Gy/4 fx and 52 Gy/8 fx yield similar tumor control and enucleation rates.**

OTHER OCULAR TUMORS

A number of other ocular tumors are treated with RT, although given the relative rarity limited data are available. Conjunctival melanoma is distinct from UM and is primarily treated with wide local excision and adjuvant CHT, RT (brachytherapy or charged particle RT), and/or cryotherapy.[16] Other rare conjunctival tumors, such as squamous cell carcinoma, are managed similarly. Choroidal metastases are typically treated with palliative EBRT but have been treated with brachytherapy and charged particle RT in select cases. Angiomas and retinal hemangiomas can be treated with surgery, laser therapy, cryotherapy, plaque brachytherapy, or charged particle RT.[17,18] Retinoblastoma is the most common malignant primary intraocular tumor of childhood. EBRT was previously used as a globe-sparing treatment, but alternatives such as CHT (systemic and local) and other focal therapies (e.g., laser therapy, cryotherapy) with less secondary malignancy risk are now preferred. Plaque brachytherapy has been used for smaller tumors, but its use has similarly been replaced with other focal therapies with less side effects.[19] Currently, EBRT is typically not prescribed due to the risk of second malignant neoplasms.[20]

REFERENCES

1. National Comprehensive Cancer Network. Melanoma: Uveal. NCCN Clinical Practice Guidelines in Oncology;1.2024. May 23, 2024. https://www.nccn.org/guidelines/category_1

2. Aronow ME, Topham AK, Singh AD. Uveal melanoma: 5-year update on incidence, treatment, and survival (SEER 1973-2013). *Ocul Oncol Pathol*. 2018;4(3):145–151. doi:10.1159/000480640

3. Seregard S, Pelayes DE, Singh AD. Radiation therapy: uveal tumors. *Dev Ophthalmol*. 2013;52:36–57. doi:10.1159/000351055

4. Singh AD, Rennie IG, Seregard S, Giblin M, McKenzie J. Sunlight exposure and pathogenesis of uveal melanoma. *Surv Ophthalmol*. 2004;49(4):419–428. doi:10.1016/j.survophthal.2004.04.009

5. Weis E, Shah CP, Lajous M, Shields JA, Shields CL. The association between host susceptibility factors and uveal melanoma: a meta-analysis. *Arch Ophthalmol*. 2006;124(1):54–60. doi:10.1001/archopht.124.1.54

6. Field MG, Harbour JW. Recent developments in prognostic and predictive testing in uveal melanoma. *Curr Opin Ophthalmol*. 2014;25(3):234–239. doi:10.1097/ICU.0000000000000051

7. Onken MD, Worley LA, Char DH, et al. Collaborative ocular oncology group report number 1: prospective validation of a multi-gene prognostic assay in uveal melanoma. *Ophthalmology*. 2012;119(8):1596–1603. doi:10.1016/j.ophtha.2012.02.017

8. Singh AD, Medina CA, Singh N, Aronow ME, Biscotti CV, Triozzi PL. Fine-needle aspiration biopsy of uveal melanoma: outcomes and complications. *Br J Ophthalmol*. 2016;100(4):456–462. doi:10.1136/bjophthalmol-2015-306921

9. Nathan P, Ascierto PA, Haanen J, et al. Safety and efficacy of nivolumab in patients with rare melanoma subtypes who progressed on or after ipilimumab treatment: a single-arm, open-label, phase II study (CheckMate 172). *Eur J Cancer*. 2019;119:168–178. doi:10.1016/j.ejca.2019.07.010

10. Nathan P, Hassel JC, Rutkowski P, et al. Overall survival benefit with tebentafusp in metastatic uveal melanoma. *N Engl J Med*. 2021;385(13):1196–1206. doi:10.1056/NEJMoa2103485

11. Marwaha G, Macklis R, Singh AD, Wilkinson A. Brachytherapy. *Dev Ophthalmol*. 2013;52:29–35. doi:10.1159/000351053

12. Meidenbauer K, Richards Z, Yupari RJ, et al. Outcomes for posterior uveal melanoma: Validation of American brachytherapy society guidelines. *Brachytherapy*. 2021;20(6):1226–1234. doi:10.1016/j.brachy.2021.05.165

13. Bellerive C, Aziz HA, Bena J, et al. Local failure after episcleral brachytherapy for posterior uveal melanoma: patterns, risk factors, and management. *Am J Ophthalmol*. 2017;177:9–16. doi:10.1016/j.ajo.2017.01.024

14. Verma V, Mehta MP. Clinical outcomes of proton radiotherapy for uveal melanoma. *Clin Oncol (R Coll Radiol)*. 2016;28(8):e17–e27. doi:10.1016/j.clon.2016.01.034

15. Hrbacek J, Mishra KK, Kacperek A, et al. Practice patterns analysis of ocular proton therapy centers: the international OPTIC survey. *Int J Radiat Oncol Biol Phys*. 2016;95(1):336–343. doi:10.1016/j.ijrobp.2016.01.040

16. Wong JR, Nanji AA, Galor A, Karp CL. Management of conjunctival malignant melanoma: a review and update. *Expert Rev Ophthalmol*. 2014;9(3):185–204. doi:10.1586/17469899.2014.921119

17. Singh AD, Nouri M, Shields CL, Shields JA, Perez N. Treatment of retinal capillary hemangioma. *Ophthalmology*. 2002;109(10):1799–1806. doi:10.1016/s0161-6420(02)01177-6

18. Mishra KK, Daftari IK. Proton therapy for the management of uveal melanoma and other ocular tumors. *Chin Clin Oncol*. 2016;5(4):50. doi:10.21037/cco.2016.07.06

19. Ortiz MV, Dunkel IJ. Retinoblastoma. *J Child Neurol*. 2016;31(2):227–236. doi:10.1177/0883073815587943

20. American Brachytherapy Society - Ophthalmic Oncology Task Force. Electronic address pec, Committee AO. The American brachytherapy society consensus guidelines for plaque brachytherapy of uveal melanoma and retinoblastoma. *Brachytherapy*. 2014;13(1):1–14. doi:10.1016/j.brachy.2013.11.008

10 SPINE TUMORS

Elizabeth E. Obi, Sarah S. Kilic, Ehsan H. Balagamwala, and Samuel T. Chao

QUICK HIT Chondrosarcomas and chordomas are rare spine and skull base tumors. Chondrosarcomas are usually low-grade, indolent cartilage-producing tumors that rarely metastasize; however, high-grade or rare histologies can behave more aggressively. Surgery is the preferred management and is usually curative. Most tumors are chemo- and radioresistant, with no major role for CHT, and RT is reserved for the incompletely resected or unresectable setting. Chordomas are locally destructive tumors that arise from remnants of the embryonic notochord. They most commonly occur in the skull base, spine, and sacrum. Optimal management of resectable lesions includes en bloc resection with adjuvant RT (Table 10.1). Treatment of skull base chordomas is challenging due to the delicate anatomic location, which mandates maximally safe resection followed by adjuvant RT, often using advanced techniques (protons, heavy ions) if available.

Table 10.1 General Treatment Paradigm for Chondrosarcomas and Chordomas	
Chordoma, resectable	GTR + adjuvant RT to ≥70 Gy if incomplete resection
Chondrosarcoma, low grade	GTR; no role for CHT or RT
Chondrosarcoma, high grade or unconventional histology	GTR; consider preoperative RT to 50.4 Gy if positive margins likely; consider postop RT to 70 Gy for R1 resection, up to 78 Gy for R2 resection
Chordoma or chondrosarcoma, unresectable or incompletely resectable	Maximal safe resection + RT to >70 Gy; strongly consider protons, heavy ions, or SRS if skull base location
Chordoma or chondrosarcoma, oligometastatic	Resection of all lesions or SRS/SBRT to unresectable sites; trial enrollment
Chordoma or chondrosarcoma, widely metastatic	Surgery or RT for symptomatic sites; systemic therapy for select histologies; trial enrollment

EPIDEMIOLOGY: Chondrosarcoma is the third most common primary bone tumor (after myeloma and osteosarcoma).[1] It is the most common primary bone tumor in older populations; most patients are >50 years at diagnosis.[2] Incidence is 0.5 in 100,000 per year, with slight male predominance.[2,3] Chordomas are exceedingly rare, with an incidence of 0.08 in 100,000 per year.[4] Similarly to chondrosarcoma, chordoma is more common in older populations, with most arising between 40 and 60 years of age, with male predominance.[5,6]

RISK FACTORS: There are no known environmental risk factors for chordoma or chondrosarcoma and no known predisposing conditions for chordoma. Most chondrosarcomas are sporadic and de novo. However, some can arise from the malignant transformation of osteochondromas and enchondromas, the latter of which can be solitary or multiple in the context of enchondromatosis. Osteochondromas are cartilage-capped projections from bony surfaces, of which 5% transform to chondrosarcoma. Solitary enchondromas are benign cartilaginous tumors within the bone marrow, in which transformation is extremely rare. Enchondromatosis is associated with Ollier disease, Maffucci syndrome, or multiple hereditary exostoses; 25% to 30% transform to chondrosarcoma.[1,7]

ANATOMY: *Chondrosarcomas:* Can arise in any bone with equal incidence in axial and appendicular skeleton. The proximal femur is the most common site, followed by the proximal humerus, distal femur, and ribs.[3] They can also involve the spine, scapula, and sternum, and rarely involve the facial bones, neck, forearm, clavicle, and small tubular bones.[3] They are further subdivided into conventional and rare types based on a combination of anatomic location within the bone and pathologic features.

Conventional chondrosarcomas include the following:

- Central (75%): Arise within the medullary cavity of any bone; up to 40% arise from enchondroma; typically present in an older male patient.[8]

- Peripheral (10%): Arise within the cartilage cap of preexisting osteochondroma.[9]
- Periosteal (<1%): Arise on the surface of bone; patients typically younger (20–30s).[3]

Rare chondrosarcoma subtypes are based on histology rather than anatomy, and include dedifferentiated, mesenchymal, clear cell, and myxoid. See Pathology section.

Chordomas: As these malignancies arise from remnants of the notochord, they are most commonly found in the midline, although they can also arise in the clinoid process or temporal bone because the notochord projects into these areas. Historically, chordomas were thought to occur most commonly in the sacrum, but newer series demonstrate an approximately equal incidence in the skull base, mobile spine, and sacrum.[10]

PATHOLOGY: *Chondrosarcomas:* Conventional chondrosarcomas are classified as grade 1, 2, or 3 based on cellularity, abundance of hyaline matrix, nuclear size, and frequency of mitoses. Grade 1 chondrosarcomas, or atypical cartilaginous tumor (ACT), are often difficult to distinguish from benign enchondroma. Compared with enchondromas, they demonstrate higher degrees of cellularity and have irregularly distributed, occasionally binucleated cells. Grades 2 and 3 tumors demonstrate increasing degrees of cellularity, nuclear and cellular pleomorphism, myxoid changes, and mitoses. Rare, "nonconventional" subtypes represent <15% of chondrosarcomas and include dedifferentiated, mesenchymal (the only radiosensitive histology), clear cell, and myxoid.[11–14]

Chordomas: Arise from remnants of the embryonic notochord. Three histologic subtypes: conventional, dedifferentiated, and poorly differentiated.[6] Conventional chordomas appear as soft, gray–white, lobulated tumors composed of groups of cells separated by fibrous septa. These cells have round nuclei and an abundant vacuolated cytoplasm, termed *physaliferous* cells. Chondroid chordoma, a subtype of conventional, has a better prognosis and has a predilection for skull base location. Dedifferentiated chordomas are biphasic with an abrupt transition between conventional chordoma and high-grade sarcoma components.[6] Poorly differentiated chordomas have a poor prognosis and demonstrate cohesive sheets of epithelioid cells with eosinophilic cytoplasm.[6] Chordomas stain positive for S100, cytokeratins, and brachyury; expression of brachyury is helpful in differentiating chordoma from chondrosarcoma.[10,11]

GENETICS: *Chondrosarcoma:* ~90% of patients with multiple osteochondromas have an inherited germline mutation in tumor suppressors EXT1 or EXT2; however, presence or absence of the mutation is not associated with malignant transformation. Ollier disease and Maffucci syndrome are both caused by somatic mosaic mutations in IDH1 or IDH26. However, there are no known genes associated with sporadic chondrosarcoma.[12,13]

Chordoma: The vast majority are sporadic, and there are no known syndromes associated with chordoma. However, the transcription factor brachyury, which is involved in notochord development, is overexpressed in >95% of chordomas. Brachyury is not expressed in chondrosarcomas.[14,15]

CLINICAL PRESENTATION: Dependent on site and histology. Patients with chondrosarcomas usually have a long, indolent course; 80% present with bony pain, which is often insidious, slowly progressive, and worse at night.[3] Approximately 27% present with an associated pathologic fracture.[3] Soft tissue swelling is also common. Symptoms may persist for months or years before diagnosis. Similarly, chordomas are often indolent and slow-growing, and patients are often asymptomatic or endorse nonspecific symptoms until late stages. Chordoma of the mobile spine and sacrum can present with pain and neurologic deficits at the corresponding spinal nerve root level. Skull base chordoma presentation varies with location (see Table 10.2).[16]

Table 10.2 Skull Base Tumor Locations and Their Associated Presentations	
Middle fossa	Sensory deficits in the first, second, or third branches of CN V; masseter weakness; diplopia; dysarthria and dysphagia; headache
Jugular foramen	Occipital headache that worsens with movement; CN IX–XII dysfunction (dysarthria, dysphagia, reduced tongue/palate sensation, sternocleidomastoid and shrug weakness, deviation of the tongue on protrusion); glossopharyngeal neuralgia (shooting pain in the throat)

(continued)

Table 10.2 Skull Base Tumor Locations and Their Associated Presentations (*continued*)	
Clivus	Headache most severe at the vertex that worsens with neck flexion; possible dysfunction of CN IV–XII
Orbital or parasellar	Frontal or orbital headache, diplopia, visual deficits, restricted extraocular movements, proptosis
Sphenoid sinus	Frontal headache with or without orbital pain, nasal congestion, diplopia, restricted extraocular movements (especially abduction)
Occipital condyle	Occipital headache and deviation of the tongue on protrusion due to CN XII dysfunction

WORKUP: H&P including complete musculoskeletal and neurologic exam.

Labs: For skull base tumors, consider endocrine and ophthalmologic evaluation.

Imaging: Plain radiograph of affected bone, CT, MRI. Chondrosarcomas have high water content, which leads to low attenuation on CT and high signal intensity on T2 MRI. Classic descriptions of central chondrosarcomas on XR: fusiform expansion in metaphysis or diaphysis, mixed radiolucent and sclerotic appearance, punctate or ring-and-arc pattern of calcifications. Periosteal chondrosarcomas appear as a round soft tissue mass on the bone surface. For grades 2 to 3 chondrosarcomas, obtain CT chest to evaluate for lung metastases.[17–19] Chordomas often originate in bone and demonstrate an extensive and destructive adjacent soft tissue component; calcifications and expansion of the involved bone are common. They are typically iso- or hypointense on T1 MRI, hyperintense on T2 MRI, and heterogeneously enhancing with gadolinium contrast due to intratumoral necrosis, which leads to a "honeycomb" appearance.[20] For newly diagnosed chordomas, NCCN guidelines recommend complete imaging (screening MRI) of the spinal axis.[21]

Biopsy: For nonskull base locations, core biopsy is preferred to establish the diagnosis. May start with a percutaneous approach, but the grade may not be accurately reflected due to lesion heterogeneity; biopsy should be aimed at the most aggressive-looking part of the lesion (soft tissue or enhancing components).[22] For skull base lesions, open, endoscopic, or fine needle biopsy is appropriate as anatomically feasible. For chordomas, there is a risk of seeding with biopsy, and the biopsy tract should be included in the future resection.[23]

PROGNOSTIC FACTORS: Extent of resection is the most important treatment-related prognostic factor for both chondrosarcoma and chordoma. Grade is the most important tumor-related prognostic factor for chondrosarcomas, as demonstrated by worsening OS with increasing grade: grade 1, 10-year OS 83% to 95%; grade 2, 10-year OS 64% to 86%; grade 3, 10-year OS 29% to 55%. Risk of DM is 1% in grade 1 chondrosarcoma, 10% to 15% in grade 2, and up to 70% in grade 3.[17,24–26] Dedifferentiated and poorly differentiated chordomas are associated with worse prognosis. Overall, SEER data suggest MS of ~7.5 years for chordoma.[27]

STAGING: The Musculoskeletal Tumor Society (MSTS) staging system is most commonly used for chondrosarcoma (Table 10.3). AJCC 8th edition staging also exists for bone tumors of appendicular skeleton/trunk/skull/facial bones, spine, and pelvis and can be used to stage chondrosarcoma and chordoma; however, no AJCC prognostic stage groupings exist for the spine and pelvis (Table 10.4). In MSTS, "extracompartmental" is defined as extension of the tumor through the cortex of the involved bone.[28,29]

Table 10.3 MSTS Staging for Sarcomas	
Stage IA	Low grade, intracompartmental
Stage IB	Low grade, extracompartmental
Stage IIA	High grade, intracompartmental
Stage IIB	High grade, extracompartmental
Stage III	Systemic or regional metastases

Table 10.4 AJCC 8th Edition (2017): Staging for Bony Tumors of Appendicular Skeleton, Trunk, Skull, and Facial Bones

Tumor*		Node		Distant Metastasis		Grade	
T1	≤8 cm	N0	No regional LNs	M0	No distant metastasis	G1	Well-differentiated, low grade
T2	>8 cm	N1	Regional LNs	M1a	Distant metastasis to lung	G2	Moderately differentiated, high grade
T3	Discontinuous tumors in primary bone site			M1b	Distant metastasis to nonlung site	G3	Poorly differentiated, high grade

There is no T4 designation for these sites.

TNM	Grade	Group Stage
T1N0M0	G1	IA
T2–3N0M0	G1	IB
T1N0M0	G2–G3	IIA
T2N0M0	G2–G3	IIB
T3N0M0	G2–G3	III
Any T, N0, M1a	Any G	IVA
Any T, N1, any M	Any G	IVB

TREATMENT PARADIGM

Surgery

Chondrosarcoma: Complete resection is considered the only curative option. The surgical approach depends on stage, grade, and location. For grade 1 lesions, the goal is to minimize functional disability. For small grade 1 lesions in the extremity, manage with intralesional curettage followed by phenolization or cryotherapy and then cementation or bone grafting of cavity; this approach has fewer complications than wide local excision (WLE) and offers excellent outcomes, with LC and OS >90% at 10 years.[30–34] For a large grade 1 lesion in an extremity or any-size lesion in the axial/pelvis location, WLE is recommended due to the difficulty of complete curettage and therefore higher LR rate, with LC and OS >90% at 5 years.[35] For grade 2 to 3 disease, wide en bloc local excision is required for all nonmetastatic cases and may entail an extensive reconstruction; the 10-year OS is 70%.[36] For peripheral chondrosarcomas, cartilage cap with its pseudocapsule must be completely resected; the 10-year LC is 82% and the 10-year OS is 95%.[9] For recurrent disease, the preferred management is repeat resection based on grade, as in the preceding discussion.

Chordoma: Similarly to chondrosarcoma, surgery is the mainstay of treatment.[37–39] However, complete resection is often impossible due to anatomic location; in these cases, postoperative RT (PORT) is recommended. Local debulking can provide symptom relief and result in a smaller target for PORT. The surgical approach and technique are dependent on anatomic location. For sacral lesions below S3, en bloc resection is often feasible with a posterior or transperineal approach and is associated with low morbidity. Sacral lesions above S3 often require both an anterior and a posterior approach, with open laparotomy and dissection of the tumor away from viscera, therefore significantly increasing morbidity.[23,40] All approaches are associated with a significant risk of bowel and bladder incontinence. For skull base lesions, a variety of approaches can be employed depending on specific patient and tumor anatomy, including open transsphenoidal, transmaxillary, transnasal, transoral, or endoscopic approaches.

Chemotherapy

Essentially no role for CHT in most cases of chondrosarcoma and chordoma. Chondrosarcomas have poor vascularity, large amounts of extracellular matrix, and expression of the efflux pump MDR1, rendering them particularly chemoresistant; CHT response rates are as low as 0%.[41–45] Per NCCN guidelines, dasatinib can be attempted for widely metastatic chondrosarcoma, with an 18%

response rate in one phase II study.[46] Traditional CHT agents are similarly ineffective in chordomas. Very small series have suggested some efficacy of imatinib or sunitinib.[5,47]

Radiation

Chondrosarcoma: Indications: Generally, radioresistant due to the low proportion of actively dividing cells and therefore no major role for RT, with the following few specific indications: definitive management of unresectable lesions, locally recurrent disease, and postoperative after incomplete resection of high-grade, dedifferentiated, or mesenchymal tumor. RT may also be employed in the palliative setting for symptomatic metastatic lesions.[18,48,49] No guidelines exist for target delineation. Dose: Postoperative doses of ≥60 Gy are commonly used. Cases of true definitive RT (i.e., without any degree of preceding resection) are rare in the literature, and the optimal dose is unknown, but recommend >60 to 70 Gy.

Chordoma: Indications: Similarly to chondrosarcoma, chordoma is a radioresistant histology. Doses <70 Gy are associated with dismal LC. Treating to >70 Gy with photons to certain anatomic sites, particularly the skull base or sacrococcygeal region, may not be feasible and may require consideration of proton or carbon ion therapy.[50,51]

Toxicity: Skull base: hearing loss, trismus, osteoradionecrosis, brain necrosis, cranial nerve dysfunction. Spine: pain flare, vertebral compression fracture, nausea/vomiting/diarrhea, radiation myelopathy.

EVIDENCE-BASED Q&A

Is there a role for PORT in chondrosarcoma and chordoma?

For completely resected lesions, no OS or LC benefit has been seen with adjuvant RT. Evidence is mixed regarding the utility of PORT in patients with less than completely resected disease.

York et al. (*J Neurosurg* 1999, PMID 10413129): Single-institution RR of 28 patients with chondrosarcoma of the spine treated with surgery ± PORT over 43 years. Eighteen patients underwent 28 surgeries; 75% STR. Ten patients had PORT; doses ranged from 40 to 70 Gy. mDFS was not significantly different between surgery alone and surgery + RT (16 months vs. 44 months, *p* = .16). However, STR was associated with a statistically significant lower DFS compared with GTR. **Conclusion: No clear benefit to PORT for spine chondrosarcomas. Complete resection is associated with better DFS.**

Sahgal (*Neuro Oncol* 2015, PMID 25543126): RR of 18 patients with skull base chondrosarcoma and 24 with skull base chordoma treated with surgery and postop IMRT. Thirty-six percent had GTR. Chondrosarcomas treated to a median dose of 70 Gy; 5-year LC 88%, 5-year OS 87%. Chordomas treated to a median dose of 76 Gy; 5-year LC 86%, 5-year OS 65%. GTR and age were the only predictors of LC. **Conclusion: Good LC and OS with surgery + PORT compared with other series. Complete resection is associated with better LC and OS.**

Goda (*Cancer* 2011, PMID 21246520): RR of 60 patients with extracranial chondrosarcoma who had surgery with preop (40%) or postop (60%) RT; 50% had R0 resection. RT dose ranged from 40 to 70 Gy; 10-year LC for R0, R1, and R2 resection was 100%, 94%, and 42%, respectively. Only grade and younger age were associated with poorer outcomes. **Conclusion: In a population with a significant proportion of patients with incomplete resection, surgery with preop or postop RT offers good long-term LC.**

Is there a role for SRS in chondrosarcoma and chordoma?

SRS offers good outcomes in the skull base and spine, as demonstrated by the following studies. For a discussion of the role of SRS in the management of spine metastases, see Chapter 69.

Kano, North American Gamma Knife Consortium (*J Neurosurg* 2011, PMID 21135744): RR of 71 patients who underwent definitive, postoperative, or salvage SRS for skull base chordomas. Median dose 15 Gy (range 9–25 Gy). The 5-year LC was 66% and the 5-year OS was 80% for the cohort. On subset analysis based on receipt of prior RT, LC was similar, but OS was significantly higher for patients who did not receive prior RT (93% vs. 43%). On MVA, older age, prior RT, and larger tumor size were associated with worse LC. **Conclusion: SRS offers modest LC for skull base chordomas. Poor prognostic factors include age, prior RT, and larger tumor size.**

Kano, North American Gamma Knife Consortium (*J Neurosurg* 2015, PMID 26115468): RR of 46 patients who underwent definitive or postoperative SRS for skull base chondrosarcoma. Median dose 15 Gy (range 10.5–20 Gy). The 5-year PFS was 85%, 10-year PFS 70%, 5-year OS 86%, and 10-year OS 76%. Thirteen percent of patients had cranial nerve toxicities attributable to RT. **Conclusion: SRS offers excellent LC with modest toxicity outcomes.**

What are the roles of proton and heavy particle therapy in the treatment of chordoma and chondrosarcoma?

Given that many of these lesions occur in anatomically critical locations (skull base, sacrococcygeus), there has been interest in particle therapy given the potential ability to dose-escalate while relatively sparing OARs. Institutional series and a meta-analysis suggest that particle therapy may offer good LC outcomes with acceptable toxicity.

Imai, Japan (*IJROBP* 2016, PMID 27084649): RR of 188 patients with unresectable sacral chordoma treated with definitive carbon ion RT. All but one patient treated to 67.2 GyE or higher (maximum 73.6 GyE). The 5-year LC was 77% and the 5-year OS was 81%. Ninety-seven percent of patients retained ability to walk; worst toxicities were grade 3 neuropathy in six patients and grade 4 skin toxicity in two patients. **Conclusion: Carbon ion RT offers good LC outcomes with acceptable toxicity and has the ability to preserve ambulation.**

Guan, China (*Radiat Oncol* 2019, PMID 31752953): RR of 91 patients with skull base or C-spine chordoma or chondrosarcoma treated with protons (PBT), carbon ions, or both; 50% definitive, 50% re-RT. Proton-only therapy was 70 GyE/35 fx; combination or carbon ion therapy was to a total dose of 63 to 71 GyE in 2 to 3 Gy/fx. The 2-year LC was 86%, 2-year PFS 77%, and 2-year OS 87%. Twenty-one percent of patients had late grade 1 to 2 toxicities (most commonly hearing loss); no grade 3+ late toxicities. On MVA, tumor volume >60 mL was associated with inferior PFS and OS. Re-RT was also associated with inferior OS. **Conclusion: For chordomas and chondrosarcomas of the skull base and cervical spine, particle therapy offers good LC outcomes with acceptable toxicity.**

Zhou, Meta-Analysis (*World Neurosurg* 2018, PMID 29879512): Meta-analysis of 25 studies with a total of 996 patients with chordoma s/p resection who underwent PORT via conventionally fractionated photons, SRS, PBT, or carbon ions. The 3-year OS was comparable for SRS, PBT, and carbon ions (92%, 89%, and 93%, respectively; NS), which were all superior to conventional RT (70%). Similarly, the 5-year OS was favorable for SRS, PBT, and carbon ions (81%, 79%, and 87%, respectively) compared with conventional RT (46%). Long-term data were limited, but at 10 years PBT appeared to be associated with the most favorable OS (60%) compared with conventional RT (21%), SRS (40%), and carbon ions (45%). **Conclusion: For patients s/p surgery who receive PORT, SRS and particle therapy may offer more favorable survival outcomes compared with conventionally fractionated RT.**

Ioakeim-Ioannidou, MGH (*IJROBP* 2024, PMID 39303998): Single-institution RR of 84 chondrosarcoma patients, with a median age of 19 years, treated with PBT between 1981 and 2023. Of the patients, 9 underwent GTR (11%), 64 STR (76%), and 11 biopsy (13%). Median dose 70 Gy (range 50–79.7 Gy). MFU 18 years. The 10-year OS, chondrosarcoma-specific survival (CSS), and PFS rates were 93%, 95%, and 88%. The 20-year OS, CSS, and PFS were 93%, 97%, and 89%. Eight patients (10%) with late grade 3+ toxicity. **Conclusion: Following resection, high-dose PBT achieves excellent disease control with minimal toxicity.**

Are there any society guidelines regarding the management of recurrent chordoma?

In 2017, the Chordoma Global Consensus Group (CGCG) defined consensus recommendations for the management of recurrent chordoma.

Stacchiotti, CGCG Position Paper (*Ann Oncol* 2017, PMID 28184416): Defined recommendations for the management of recurrent chordoma. For skull base recurrence, high-dose (re)RT preferred over resection. For mobile spine/sacrum recurrence, high-dose (re)RT preferred in most cases, except those with surgically accessible tumor without history of prior piecemeal resection or surgical rupture, in which case maximal safe resection preferred. For any site, if neither high-dose RT nor GTR is feasible, palliative management (which may include palliative RT or surgical debulking) is recommended. **Conclusion: Re-RT to high doses is generally preferred for recurrent chordoma when feasible.**

REFERENCES

1. Gelderblom H, Hogendoorn PC, Dijkstra SD, et al. The clinical approach towards chondrosarcoma. *Oncologist*. 2008;13(3):320–329. doi:10.1634/theoncologist.2007-0237
2. van Praag Veroniek VM, Rueten-Budde AJ, Ho V, et al. Incidence, outcomes and prognostic factors during 25 years of treatment of chondrosarcomas. *Surg Oncol*. 2018;27(3):402–408. doi:10.1016/j.suronc.2018.05.009
3. Kim MJ, Cho KJ, Ayala AG, Ro JY. Chondrosarcoma: with updates on molecular genetics. *Sarcoma*. 2011; 2011:405437. doi:10.1155/2011/405437
4. Frezza AM, Botta L, Trama A, Dei Tos AP, Stacchiotti S. Chordoma: update on disease, epidemiology, biology and medical therapies. *Curr Opin Oncol*. 2019;31(2):114–120. doi:10.1097/CCO.0000000000000502
5. Alan O, Akin Telli T, Ercelep O, et al. Chordoma: a case series and review of the literature. *J Med Case Rep*. 2018;12(1):239. doi:10.1186/s13256-018-1784-y
6. Ulici V, Hart J. Chordoma. *Arch Pathol Lab Med*. 2022;146(3):386–395. doi:10.5858/arpa.2020-0258-RA
7. Silve C, Juppner H. Ollier disease. *Orphanet J Rare Dis*. 2006;1:37. doi:10.1186/1750-1172-1-37
8. Brien EW, Mirra JM, Kerr R. Benign and malignant cartilage tumors of bone and joint: their anatomic and theoretical basis with an emphasis on radiology, pathology and clinical biology. I. The intramedullary cartilage tumors. *Skeletal Radiol*. 1997;26(6):325–353. doi:10.1007/s002560050246
9. Ahmed AR, Tan TS, Unni KK, Collins MS, Wenger DE, Sim FH. Secondary chondrosarcoma in osteochondroma: report of 107 patients. *Clin Orthop Relat Res*. 2003;(411):193–206. doi:10.1097/01.blo.0000069888 .31220.2b
10. George B, Bresson D, Herman P, Froelich S. Chordomas: a review. *Neurosurg Clin N Am*. 2015;26(3):437–452. doi:10.1016/j.nec.2015.03.012
11. Shen J, Shi Q, Lu J, et al. Histological study of chordoma origin from fetal notochordal cell rests. *Spine (Phila Pa 1976)*. 2013;38(25):2165–2170. doi:10.1097/BRS.0000000000000010
12. Pedrini E, Jennes I, Tremosini M, et al. Genotype-phenotype correlation study in 529 patients with multiple hereditary exostoses: identification of "protective" and "risk" factors. *J Bone Joint Surg Am*. 2011;93(24): 2294–2302. doi:10.2106/JBJS.J.00949
13. Pansuriya TC, van Eijk R, d'Adamo P, et al. Somatic mosaic IDH1 and IDH2 mutations are associated with enchondroma and spindle cell hemangioma in Ollier disease and Maffucci syndrome. *Nat Genet*. 2011;43(12):1256–1261. doi:10.1038/ng.1004
14. Vujovic S, Henderson S, Presneau N, et al. Brachyury, a crucial regulator of notochordal development, is a novel biomarker for chordomas. *J Pathol*. 2006;209(2):157–165. doi:10.1002/path.1969
15. Kitamura Y, Sasaki H, Yoshida K. Genetic aberrations and molecular biology of skull base chordoma and chondrosarcoma. *Brain Tumor Pathol*. 2017;34(2):78–90. doi:10.1007/s10014-017-0283-y
16. Jacox A, Carr DB, Payne R, et al. *Management of Cancer Plan. Clinical Practice Guideline No. 9* (AHCPR Pub. No. 94–0592). Rockville, MD: Agency for Health Care Policy and Research, U.S. Department of Health and Human Services, Public Health Service; 1994:31–32.
17. Evans HL, Ayala AG, Romsdahl MM. Prognostic factors in chondrosarcoma of bone: a clinicopathologic analysis with emphasis on histologic grading. *Cancer*. 1977;40(2):818–831. doi:10.1002/1097-0142(197708)40 :2<818::aid-cncr2820400234>3.0.co;2-b
18. Gelderblom A, Bovée, J VMG. Chondrosarcoma. *UpToDate*. Accessed April 27, 2023. https://www .uptodate.com/contents/chondrosarcoma.
19. Murphey MD, Walker EA, Wilson AJ, Kransdorf MJ, Temple HT, Gannon FH. From the archives of the AFIP: imaging of primary chondrosarcoma: radiologic-pathologic correlation. *Radiographics*. 2003;23(5): 1245–1278. doi:10.1148/rg.235035134
20. Youssef C, Aoun SG, Moreno JR, Bagley CA. Recent advances in understanding and managing chordomas. *F1000Res*. 2016;5:2902. doi:10.12688/f1000research.9499.1
21. National Comprehensive Cancer Network (NCCN). NCCN clinical practice guidelines in oncology (NCCN Guidelines). Bone Cancer. Version 2.2025. Accessed May 6, 2025. https://www.nccn.org/professionals/ physician_gls/pdf/bone.pdf
22. Normand AN, Cannon CP, Lewis VO, Lin PP, Yasko AW. Curettage of biopsy-diagnosed grade 1 periacetabular chondrosarcoma. *Clin Orthop Relat Res*. 2007;459:146–149. doi:10.1097/BLO.0b013e3180619554
23. Tenny S. Chordoma. In: Varacallo MA, ed. *StatPearls*. StatPearls Publishing; 2024.
24. Angelini A, Guerra G, Mavrogenis AF, Pala E, Picci P, Ruggieri P. Clinical outcome of central conventional chondrosarcoma. *J Surg Oncol*. 2012;106(8):929–937. doi:10.1002/jso.23173
25. Bjornsson J, McLeod RA, Unni KK, Ilstrup DM, Pritchard DJ. Primary chondrosarcoma of long bones and limb girdles. *Cancer*. 1998;83(10):2105–2119. PMID:9827715
26. WHO. *Soft Tissue and Bone Tumours*. 5th ed. IARC Press; 2020.
27. Smoll NR, Gautschi OP, Radovanovic I, Schaller K, Weber DC. Incidence and relative survival of chordomas: the standardized mortality ratio and the impact of chordomas on a population. *Cancer*. 2013;119(11):2029–2037. doi:10.1002/cncr.28032

28.   Enneking WF. A system of staging musculoskeletal neoplasms. *Clin Orthop Relat Res.* 1986;(204):9–24. PMID:3456859

29.   Wolf RE, Enneking WF. The staging and surgery of musculoskeletal neoplasms. *Orthop Clin North Am.* 1996;27(3):473–481. PMID:8649730

30.   Bauer HC, Brosjo O, Kreicbergs A, Lindholm J. Low risk of recurrence of enchondroma and low-grade chondrosarcoma in extremities. 80 patients followed for 2–25 years. *Acta Orthop Scand.* 1995;66(3):283–288. doi:10.3109/17453679508995543

31.   Donati D, Colangeli S, Colangeli M, Di Bella C, Bertoni F. Surgical treatment of grade I central chondrosarcoma. *Clin Orthop Relat Res.* 2010;468(2):581–589. doi:10.1007/s11999-009-1056-7

32.   Hickey M, Farrokhyar F, Deheshi B, Turcotte R, Ghert M. A systematic review and meta-analysis of intralesional versus wide resection for intramedullary grade I chondrosarcoma of the extremities. *Ann Surg Oncol.* 2011;18(6):1705–1709. doi:10.1245/s10434-010-1532-z

33.   van der Geest IC, de Valk MH, de Rooy JW, Pruszczynski M, Veth RP, Schreuder HW. Oncological and functional results of cryosurgical therapy of enchondromas and chondrosarcomas grade 1. *J Surg Oncol.* 2008;98(6):421–426. doi:10.1002/jso.21122

34.   Leerapun T, Hugate RR, Inwards CY, Scully SP, Sim FH. Surgical management of conventional grade I chondrosarcoma of long bones. *Clin Orthop Relat Res.* 2007;463:166–172. doi:10.1097/BLO.0b013e318146830f

35.   Streitburger A, Ahrens H, Balke M, et al. Grade I chondrosarcoma of bone: the Munster experience. *J Cancer Res Clin Oncol.* 2009;135(4):543–550. doi:10.1007/s00432-008-0486-z

36.   Fiorenza F, Abudu A, Grimer RJ, et al. Risk factors for survival and local control in chondrosarcoma of bone. *J Bone Joint Surg Br.* 2002;84(1):93–99. doi:10.1302/0301-620x.84b1.11942

37.   Stacchiotti S, Casali PG, Lo Vullo S, et al. Chordoma of the mobile spine and sacrum: a retrospective analysis of a series of patients surgically treated at two referral centers. *Ann Surg Oncol.* 2010;17(1):211–219. doi:10.1245/s10434-009-0740-x

38.   Osaka S, Kodoh O, Sugita H, Osaka E, Yoshida Y, Ryu J. Clinical significance of a wide excision policy for sacrococcygeal chordoma. *J Cancer Res Clin Oncol.* 2006;132(4):213–218. doi:10.1007/s00432-005-0067-3

39.   York JE, Kaczaraj A, Abi-Said D, et al. Sacral chordoma: 40-year experience at a major cancer center. *Neurosurgery.* 1999;44(1):74–79. doi:10.1097/00006123-199901000-00041

40.   Yin X, Fan WL, Liu F, Zhu J, Liu P, Zhao JH. Technique and surgical outcome of total resection of lower sacral tumor. *Int J Clin Exp Med.* 2015;8(2):2284–2288. PMID:25932164

41.   Wyman JJ, Hornstein AM, Meitner PA, et al. Multidrug resistance-1 and p-glycoprotein in human chondrosarcoma cell lines: expression correlates with decreased intracellular doxorubicin and in vitro chemoresistance. *J Orthop Res.* 1999;17(6):935–940. doi:10.1002/jor.1100170619

42.   van Oosterwijk JG, Herpers B, Meijer D, et al. Restoration of chemosensitivity for doxorubicin and cisplatin in chondrosarcoma in vitro: BCL-2 family members cause chemoresistance. *Ann Oncol.* 2012;23(6):1617–1626. doi:10.1093/annonc/mdr512

43.   van Oosterwijk JG, Meijer D, van Ruler MA, et al. Screening for potential targets for therapy in mesenchymal, clear cell, and dedifferentiated chondrosarcoma reveals Bcl-2 family members and TGFbeta as potential targets. *Am J Pathol.* 2013;182(4):1347–1356. doi:10.1016/j.ajpath.2012.12.036

44.   Terek RM, Schwartz GK, Devaney K, et al. Chemotherapy and P-glycoprotein expression in chondrosarcoma. *J Orthop Res.* 1998;16(5):585–590. doi:10.1002/jor.1100160510

45.   Italiano A, Mir O, Cioffi A, et al. Advanced chondrosarcomas: role of chemotherapy and survival. *Ann Oncol.* 2013;24(11):2916–2922. doi:10.1093/annonc/mdt374

46.   Schuetze SM, Bolejack V, Choy E, et al. Phase 2 study of dasatinib in patients with alveolar soft part sarcoma, chondrosarcoma, chordoma, epithelioid sarcoma, or solitary fibrous tumor. *Cancer.* 2017;123(1):90–97. doi:10.1002/cncr.30379

47.   Casali PG, Messina A, Stacchiotti S, et al. Imatinib mesylate in chordoma. *Cancer.* 2004;101(9):2086–2097. doi:10.1002/cncr.20618

48.   Le A, Ball D, Pitman A, Fox R, King K. Chondrosarcoma of bone complicating Ollier's disease: report of a favourable response to radiotherapy. *Australas Radiol.* 2003;47(3):322–324. doi:10.1046/j.1440-1673.2003.01187.x

49.   van Maldegem AM, Gelderblom H, Palmerini E, et al. Outcome of advanced, unresectable conventional central chondrosarcoma. *Cancer.* 2014;120(20):3159–3164. doi:10.1002/cncr.28845

50.   Imai R, Kamada T, Araki N, Working Group for Bone and Soft Tissue Sarcomas. Carbon ion radiation therapy for unresectable sacral chordoma: an analysis of 188 cases. *Int J Radiat Oncol Biol Phys.* 2016;95(1):322–327. doi:10.1016/j.ijrobp.2016.02.012

51.   Nishida Y, Kamada T, Imai R, et al. Clinical outcome of sacral chordoma with carbon ion radiotherapy compared with surgery. *Int J Radiat Oncol Biol Phys.* 2011;79(1):110–116. doi:10.1016/j.ijrobp.2009.10.051

PART II: Head and Neck

11 OROPHARYNX CANCER

Zachary S. Mayo, Shireen Parsai, Aditya Juloori, and Jacob A. Miller

QUICK HIT Squamous cell carcinoma (SCC) of the oropharynx is the second most common H&N cancer in the United States.[1] The majority of oropharyngeal carcinomas (OPC) in the United States are associated with the human papillomavirus (HPV), and the incidence of this disease is increasing.[2-4] There are two distinct etiologies: those associated with tobacco and alcohol, which are typically HPV-negative (HPV−), and those associated with HPV infection (HPV+). These are classified as two distinct diseases per the AJCC 8th edition staging system. Treatment of HPV+ and HPV− OPC has historically been similar, but treatment paradigms are increasingly divergent owing to differences in natural history and cure rate (Table 11.1).

Table 11.1 General Treatment Paradigm for Oropharynx Cancer	
	Treatment Options
T1–2N0–1*	Definitive IMRT OR TORS (or other function-preserving surgery), neck dissection, and risk-adapted adjuvant therapy (Chapter 17)
T3–4 and/or N2–3*	Definitive CRT OR Surgery (select patients) with risk-adapted postoperative RT ± CHT

*Based on AJCC 7th edition.

EPIDEMIOLOGY: Estimated 20,441 OPC cases in 2017 with ~5,648 deaths.[5] M:F ratio is approximately 4:1.[6] In the United States, the incidence of HPV+ OPC increased by 225% from 1988 to 2004, and HPV− cancer declined by 50% in the same time frame.[7] Prevalence of HPV was 40% on RTOG 9003, which increased to 64% on RTOG 0129 and further to 73% on RTOG 0522.[8-10] Peak prevalence of oral HPV DNA is bimodal: 7% for ages 30 to 34 and 11% for ages 60 to 64.[8]

RISK FACTORS: Age, number of oral sexual partners (HPV+), tobacco and alcohol abuse (HPV−).[8,11,12]

ANATOMY: The oropharynx consists of the base of tongue (BOT; lingual tonsil), vallecula, palatine tonsils, soft palate, and posterior oropharyngeal wall. The superior border is the soft palate, and the inferior border is the hyoid/lingual surface of the epiglottis. The BOT is the posterior third of the tongue and is separated from the oral tongue by the circumvallate papillae. The surface of the BOT is composed of lymphoid tissue. The palatine tonsils are located between an arch formed by the anterior and posterior tonsillar pillars (Table 11.2).

Table 11.2 Borders of the Oropharynx	
Site	**Boundaries**
Base of tongue (BOT)	Anteriorly by the circumvallate papillae, laterally by the glossopalatine sulci, and inferiorly by the vallecula. Includes the pharyngoepiglottic and glossoepiglottic folds.
Tonsillar complex	Composed of the anterior and posterior tonsillar pillars, true palatine tonsil, and tonsillar fossa. Tonsillar pillars are mucosal folds over the glossopalatine and pharyngopalatine muscles. The tonsillar fossa is a triangular region bounded by the pillars, inferiorly by the glossotonsillar sulcus and pharyngoepiglottic fold, and laterally by the pharyngeal constrictor muscles.

(continued)

Table 11.2 Borders of the Oropharynx (*continued*)	
Site	Boundaries
Soft palate	Anteriorly by the hard palate, laterally by the palatopharyngeal and superior pharyngeal constrictor muscles, and posteriorly by the palatopharyngeal arch/uvula. Forms roof of the oropharynx and floor of the nasopharynx.
Posterior pharyngeal wall (PPW)	Continuous structure spanning the nasopharynx, oropharynx, and hypopharynx. The oropharyngeal PPW begins superiorly at the soft palate and ends inferiorly at the epiglottis.

PATHOLOGY: Approximately 95% of OPC are SCC.[13] The remaining 5% are lymphomas, minor salivary gland cancers (e.g., mucoepidermoid, adenoid cystic; see Chapter 15), and sarcomas. HPV+ and HPV− cancers appear different pathologically. HPV+ tumors originate from the lymphoid tissue of the tonsil or BOT and are more likely to be poorly differentiated/nonkeratinizing and basaloid in appearance. HPV− tumors have no predilection for location and are often keratinizing. Positive IHC staining for p16 is a surrogate for HPV+ tumors, requiring diffuse positive staining in ≥70% of cells.[14] Confirmatory HPV testing with RNA in situ hybridization or PCR is often performed. Patients with p16+ and HPV+ tumors have improved prognosis compared with p16+ and HPV− tumors. Both have a better prognosis than p16− and HPV− (Table 11.3).[15]

HPV 16 serotype accounts for ~85% of HPV-associated cases.[4,16] HPV viral proteins E6 and E7 bind p53 and Rb, respectively, with functional loss of tumor suppression. When E7 binds to Rb, transcription factor E2F is released and allows cyclin to bypass G1/S checkpoint. Reflexive expression of p16 protein inhibits cyclin D-CDK4 complex to prevent uncontrolled cell cycling. Overexpression of p16 protein serves as surrogate marker of HPV-associated oncogenesis. EGFR is more commonly amplified in HPV− tumors and is associated with poor prognosis.[6,17]

Table 11.3 Factors Associated With HPV Status in OPC	
HPV+	HPV−
– Younger – Absent or limited smoking history – Caucasian – Multiple oral sexual partners – More likely palatine tonsil/base of tongue – Poorly differentiated – Nonkeratinizing – Basaloid – p16 upregulated	– Older – Tobacco/alcohol abuse – Non-Caucasian – Unrelated to sexual behavior – No tissue preference – Keratinizing – p53 mutation – EGFR amplified

CLINICAL PRESENTATION: The most common presentation of OPC is a painless neck mass. Other symptoms related to primary tumors include dysphagia, odynophagia, or otalgia referred from CN IX via the tympanic nerve of Jacobson. Impaired oral tongue mobility suggests deep musculature involvement. Trismus suggests medial pterygoid invasion.

WORKUP: H&P with careful attention to the H&N including palpation of the oropharynx, dental exam, neurologic exam, mirror exam, and/or flexible laryngoscopy.

Labs: CBC and CMP with attention to renal function. Plasma circulating tumor HPV DNA may be measured before and after treatment as an emerging biomarker for posttreatment surveillance.[18]

Imaging: PET/CT and CT neck with contrast are necessary for staging and delineation of the primary tumor and involved LN. Consider MRI to evaluate for perineural spread or invasion of the skull base, oral tongue, or pterygoid muscles.[6,19] After CRT, it is more cost-effective to perform PET/CT at 12 weeks and proceed to neck dissection for incomplete response than to perform a planned neck dissection.[20]

Procedures: FNA of lymphadenopathy may be performed but consider direct laryngoscopy/examination under anesthesia with confirmatory tonsillectomy or biopsy of the primary tumor. Tumor HPV testing is recommended per NCCN.[19]

Other: Dental clearance, nutrition consultation, speech and swallowing evaluation/therapy, and audiogram as clinically indicated. Smoking cessation should be advised.

PROGNOSTIC FACTORS: Age, p16 and HPV status, smoking history (both 10 and 20 pack-year cutoffs have been proposed, which may be less relevant than current/former smoking status),[21,22] stage, pathologic or radiographic extranodal extension, comorbidities, performance status, and PET SUV.[22–24] Staging and prognostic stratification of HPV+ patients are evolving (Tables 11.4 and 11.5). On RTOG 0129, the 3-year OS was 82% for HPV+ patients compared with 57% for HPV– patients.[22]

NATURAL HISTORY: Nodal involvement is common, and the initial site of drainage from the oropharynx is to neck level II and subsequently down the jugular chain to levels III and IV. Levels IB and V and retropharyngeal nodes can be involved but are less common.[13] Historically, LRR was responsible for the majority of cancer-related morbidity and mortality.[25] While this remains true for HPV– disease, LRR of HPV+ disease is less common. DM, however, develops in both subgroups at similar rates. The most common sites of DM are lung and bone.[22,26]

Table 11.4 AJCC 8th Ed. (2017) Staging for Oropharynx (p16–)		cN0	cN1	cN2a	cN2b	cN2c	cN3a	cN3b
T1	• ≤2 cm	I						
T2	• >2–4 cm	II	III		IVA			
T3	• >4 cm • Extension to lingual surface of epiglottis							
T4a	• Invasion[1]							
T4b	• Invasion[2]				IVB			
M1	• Distant metastasis				IVC			

Note: Invasion[1] = invasion into larynx, extrinsic musculature of tongue, medial pterygoid muscle, hard palate, or mandible. Invasion[2] = invasion into lateral pterygoid, pterygoid plates, lateral nasopharynx, skull base, or encases carotid artery.
cN1, single ipsilateral LN (≤3 cm) without extranodal extension (–ENE); cN2a, single ipsilateral LN (3–6 cm) and –ENE; cN2b, multiple ipsilateral LN (≤6 cm) and –ENE; cN2c, bilateral or contralateral LN (≤6 cm) and –ENE; cN3a, LN (>6 cm) and –ENE; cN3b, clinically overt ENE.
pN1, single LN (≤3 cm) and –ENE; pN2a, single ipsilateral LN (≤3 cm) and +ENE or single ipsilateral LN (3–6 cm) and –ENE; pN2b, multiple ipsilateral LN (≤6 cm) and –ENE; pN2c, bilateral or contralateral LN (≤6 cm) and –ENE; pN3a, LN (>6 cm) and –ENE; pN3b, LN (>3 cm) and +ENE or multiple LN with any +ENE.

Table 11.5 AJCC 8th Ed. (2017) Staging for HPV-Mediated (p16+) Oropharyngeal Cancer		cN0	cN1	cN2	cN3
T1	• ≤2 cm	I		II	III
T2	• >2–4 cm				
T3	• >4 cm • Extension to lingual surface of epiglottis				
T4	• Invasion into larynx, extrinsic muscles of tongue, medial pterygoid, hard palate, mandible, or beyond				
M1	• Distant metastases			IV	

cN1, one or more ipsilateral LN (≤6 cm); cN2, contralateral or bilateral LN (≤6 cm); cN3, LN (>6 cm).
pN1, ≤4 LNs; pN2 >4 LNs.

TREATMENT PARADIGM

Surgery

Classic oncologic surgery for OPC consisted of radical tonsillectomy (simple tonsillectomy performed for biopsy is generally not sufficient for oncologic control), glossectomy (often requiring mandibulotomy), palatectomy, or pharyngectomy with an ipsilateral or bilateral neck dissection depending on nodal status and laterality of primary tumor. Because of the functional deficits left by these procedures, nonoperative approaches became standard in the 1970s after trials such as RTOG 7303 found similar survival.[27] Over the past decade, however, minimally invasive procedures such as transoral laser microsurgery (TLM) and transoral robotic surgery (TORS) have reduced the morbidity of surgery and are now standard options for T1–2 and select T3 lesions (see Evidence-Based Q&A).[19] Patient selection is critical and generally TORS should be avoided in patients who will require multimodal therapy (e.g., positive LN with ENE) or in tumors that will result in significant functional deficits following surgery (tumors involving the soft palate or epiglottis, deep endophytic tumors of the BOT). This is the same with the modern ORATOR trial.[28]

Radical neck dissection: levels IB to V with sacrifice of internal and external jugular veins, sternocleidomastoid (SCM), omohyoid, CN XI, and submandibular gland. Modified radical neck dissection: levels IB to V but leaves one or more of jugular veins, SCM, omohyoid, or CN XI. Selective neck dissection: modified radical but leaves one or more of levels IB to V. Supraomohyoid neck dissection: resection of levels I to III. SLNB, followed by neck dissection if positive, is an emerging option for cT1–T2N0 OPC cancer.[29]

Chemotherapy

Standard: For patients with indications for systemic therapy (definitive: Table 11.1, postoperative: Chapter 17), concurrent cisplatin is standard for fit patients. Cisplatin can be given concurrently with RT as 100 mg/m^2 weeks 1, 4, and 7 (NCCN Category 1) or 40 mg/m^2 weekly (NCCN Category 2B).[19] *Platinum-ineligible alternatives:* Cetuximab given concurrent with RT is an inferior option without a reduction in toxicity.[19,30,31] Cetuximab starts 1 week prior to RT as a loading dose of 400 mg/m^2 followed by 250 mg/m^2 weekly during RT.[32] Other less common concurrent regimens include carboplatin/paclitaxel, cisplatin/5-FU, and 5-FU/hydroxyurea.

Induction: Cisplatin-based induction CHT has not been proven to increase OS as compared with proceeding directly to concurrent CRT.[33] Typically, docetaxel, cisplatin, and 5-FU (TPF) is given every 3 weeks for 4C and is typically completed 4 to 7 weeks prior to RT alone or concurrent CRT.[19,34]

Immunotherapy: There is no established role for immunotherapy in the initial definitive treatment of HNSCC. HN004 (durvalumab + RT vs. cetuximab + RT), GORTEC 2015-01 PembroRad (pembrolizumab + RT vs. cetuximab + RT), JAVELIN HN100 (CRT +/− avelumab), and KEYNOTE-412 (CRT +/− pembrolizumab) all failed to show a benefit with the addition of immunotherapy to standard CRT.[35-38]

Radiation

Indications: RT is indicated for definitive treatment of OPC or in the postoperative setting (see Chapter 17).

Dose: In the definitive setting, standard dose is 70 Gy/35 fx. Various elective nodal doses have been used, including 56 Gy/35 fx (simultaneous boost) and 50 Gy/25 fx (sequential boost to 70 Gy). RTOG 1016 used a third lower dose to "low-risk" neck to 50 to 52.5 Gy/35 fx. For cT1–2N0–1 OPC, 66 Gy/30 fx RT alone with elective dose of 54 Gy/30 fx (simultaneous) is reasonable based on RTOG 0022 (see Evidence-Based Q&A).[39,40] Dose reduction for HPV+ tumors is the subject of active investigation (see Evidence-Based Q&A). In the postoperative setting, deintensified RT with 50 Gy/25 fx can be considered for patients with intermediate-risk disease (PNI, LVI, close margin, <1 mm ENE, and/or 2–4 LN [pN1]) based on phase II ECOG 3311.[41]

Toxicity: Acute: fatigue, mucositis, dysphagia, odynophagia, xerostomia, dermatitis, aspiration. Chronic: dysphagia, neck fibrosis, xerostomia, trismus, osteoradionecrosis, hypothyroidism, brachial plexopathy, secondary malignancies.

Procedure: See *Handbook of Treatment Planning in Radiation Oncology*, Chapter 4.[42]

EVIDENCE-BASED Q&A

Can definitive RT lead to similar control and survival compared with radical surgeries?

This was a key question in the 1970s when surgery was the definitive therapy of choice, often requiring a mandibulotomy for BOT access leading to subsequent functional deficits. RTOG 7303 is a historical prospective randomized trial addressing this question and found similar 4-year OS and LRC; definitive RT subsequently became a standard option to preserve functional outcomes.

Kramer, RTOG 7303 (*Head Neck Surg* 1987, PMID 3449477): Advanced SCC of the oropharynx or oral cavity randomly assigned to preoperative RT, PORT, or definitive RT (65–70 Gy). Larynx or hypopharynx cancers were randomized to either preoperative (50 Gy) or PORT (60 Gy). For oral cavity or OPC patients, the 4-year OS was similar between all groups: 30% preoperative, 36% postoperative, 33% definitive. The 4-year LRC was 43% preoperative, 52% postoperative, and 38% definitive. **Conclusion: Definitive RT is a justified alternative compared with radical surgery given similar 4-year OS and LRC rates.**

Can the efficacy of RT be improved by altering fractionation?

SCC is known to undergo accelerated repopulation and is sensitive to reoxygenation, so fractionation was thought to play an important role on outcomes with definitive RT. Multiple trials and a meta-analysis demonstrated improved LRC and OS with altered fractionation (AF) for treating locoregionally advanced patients.

Fu, RTOG 9003 (*IJROBP* 2000, PMID 10924966; Update Beitler, *IJROBP* 2014, PMID 24613816): PRT of 1,073 patients with stage III to IV SCC of the oral cavity, oropharynx, and supraglottic larynx or stage II to IV of BOT or hypopharynx randomized to one of four arms: (1) standard fractionation to 70 Gy/35 fx, (2) hyperfractionation to 81.6 Gy/68 fx at 1.2 Gy/fx BID with 6-hour interfraction interval, (3) split-course accelerated hyperfractionation to 67.2 Gy/42 fx given 1.6 Gy/fx BID with 6-hour interfraction interval and 2-week rest after 38.4 Gy, or (4) accelerated hyperfractionation with concomitant boost to 72 Gy/42 fx given at 1.8 Gy/fx 5 days a week with 1.5 Gy/fraction to boost field as second daily treatment given 6 hours apart for the last 12 treatment days. Primary endpoint was 2-year LRC. Results at initial report (Table 11.6): At MFU of 23 months, both hyperfractionation (Arm 2) and concomitant boost (Arm 4) showed improved LRC but no significant difference in OS. All three AF arms showed increased acute toxicity but only concomitant boost arm showed increased late effects. In the final update, hyperfractionation (Arm 2) and concomitant boost (Arm 4) decreased the 5-year LRR compared with standard fractionation, but hyperfractionation did not increase late effects. When using only 5-year follow-up, hyperfractionation improved OS (HR 0.81, *p* = .05) but not when all follow-up data were included. **Conclusion: AF improves disease control in locoregionally advanced SCC of H&N.**

Table 11.6 Results of RTOG 9003			
	Regimen	2-Yr LRC	2-Yr OS
1. Standard	70 Gy/35 fx daily	46%	46%
2. Hyperfractionation	81.6 Gy/68 fx BID	54%*	55%†
3. Split course	67.2 Gy/42 fx BID with 2-week break	48%	46%
4. Concomitant boost	72 Gy/42 fx (BID final 12 days)	55%‡	51%

*Statistically significant difference in the original and final reports.
†Statistically significant difference (only when limited to 5-year follow-up).
‡Statistically significant difference compared with standard arm in the original report.

Overgaard, DAHANCA 6 and 7 Combined Analysis (*Lancet* 2003, PMID 14511925): Combined analysis of two trials performed from 1992 to 1999 including 1,485 patients with stage I to IV SCC: DAHANCA 6 of glottis carcinoma testing fractionation and DAHANCA 7 of supraglottic, pharynx, and oral cavity cancers testing fractionation and the radiosensitizer nimorazole. RT given to 62 to 68 Gy at 2 Gy/fx and randomized to either five or six fractions per week. Overall, 5-year LRC was improved with acceleration (70% vs. 60%, *p* = .0005). Disease-specific but not OS improved by acceleration. **Conclusion: Six fractions weekly became standard in Denmark. This result was independent of p16 status.**[43]

Bourhis, MARCH Meta-Analysis (*Lancet* 2006, PMID 16950362; Update Lacas, *Lancet Oncol* 2017, PMID 28757375): Meta-analysis of 11,969 patients from 34 trials with MFU of 6 years, 75% oropharynx and larynx cancers and 75% stage III to IV. AF was associated with a significant OS benefit of 3% at 5 years ($p = .003$). The significant survival benefit was attributed to hyperfractionation alone, which had the most OS benefit (8%). OS was significantly worse (6% decrement at 5 years) with AF RT alone compared with concurrent CRT (HR 1.22, $p = .01$). **Conclusion: AF, specifically hyperfractionation, improves OS in H&N cancer. The comparison between hyperfractionated RT and concurrent CRT remains to be specifically tested.**

Does CHT add benefit to conventionally fractionated RT?

Adelstein, Head and Neck Intergroup (*JCO* 2003, PMID 12506176): PRT of 271 of planned 362 patients between 1992 and 1999 with stage III to IV unresectable SCC (all sites except sinus, nasopharynx, or salivary) randomized to either (A) RT alone (70 Gy/35 fx), (B) cisplatin with RT (100 mg/m² weeks 1, 4, and 7), or (C) split-course CRT (cisplatin 75 mg/m² with 5-FU 1,000 mg/m² every 4 weeks with 30 Gy/15 fx first course followed by surgical evaluation, and if CR or unresectable another 30–40 Gy given with third cycle of CHT). Trial closed early due to slow accrual. See Table 11.7 for results. The 3-year OS for CRT (Arm B) was superior to Arm A or C. Eighty-nine percent of patients in Arm B experienced grades 3 to 5 toxicities. **Conclusion: High-dose cisplatin when added to conventionally fractionated RT improves OS.**

Table 11.7 Results of H&N Intergroup			
	CR	3-Yr OS	Grades 3–5 toxicities
Arm A: RT	27.4%	23%	52%
Arm B: CRT	40.2%	37%*	89%*
Arm C: Split-course CRT	49.4%*	27%	77%*

*Statistically significant relative to Arm A.

Pignon, MACH-NC Meta-Analysis (*Lancet* 2000 PMID 10768432; Update Pignon, *Radiother Oncol* 2009, PMID 19446902; By Disease Site: Blanchard, *Radiother Oncol* 2011, PMID 21684027; Update Lacas, *Radiother Oncol* 2021, PMID 33515668): Meta-analysis of ~17,000 patients from 93 trials demonstrated OS benefit to addition of CHT of 4.5% at 5 years. Concurrent CRT showed absolute benefit of 6.5% at 5 years (SS); induction 2.4% at 5 years (NS). No OS benefit in patients above 70 years. Both concurrent and induction CHT improved distant control (HR 0.73 and 0.88, $p = .0001$ and .04, but not different when compared with each other). The 2021 update included 18,951 patients from 101 trials and the benefit of concurrent CRT remained with a 5-year absolute benefit of 6.5% and 10-year benefit of 3.6% (SS). **Conclusion: There is a survival benefit to CHT in addition to RT for HNSCC; the effect of concurrent CHT is greater than that of induction CHT.**

Does CHT add benefit to hyperfractionated RT?

Although hyperfractionated RT alone is superior to conventional RT alone, concurrent CHT remains beneficial for both conventional and hyperfractionated RT.

Brizel, Duke (*NEJM* 1998, PMID 9632446): PRT of 116 patients with T3–4 N0–3 HNSCC (and T2N0 BOT) treated to 75 Gy/60 fx BID and randomized to either no concurrent therapy or concurrent cisplatin (60 mg/m²) and 5-FU (600 mg/m²) weeks 1 and 6. At MFU of 41 months, the 3-year OS was 55% in CHT arm vs. 34% in hyperfractionated group ($p = .07$). LRC was also improved (44% vs. 70%, $p = .01$). Toxicity was comparable. **Conclusion: Concurrent CHT adds benefit to hyperfractionated RT with similar toxicity.**

Bourhis, GORTEC 99-02 (*Lancet Oncol* 2012, PMID 22261362): PRT of stage III to IV HNSCC randomized to standard CRT (70 Gy/35 fx with carboplatin/5-FU), accelerated CRT (70 Gy in 6 weeks with carboplatin/5-FU), or very accelerated RT alone (64.8 Gy/36 fx BID in 3.5 weeks). Standard CRT and accelerated CRT with similar PFS ($p = .88$). Conventional CRT improved PFS compared with very accelerated RT ($p = .04$). **Conclusion: Acceleration alone cannot completely compensate for lack of CHT.**

Does hyperfractionated RT add benefit to CRT?

This question is the inverse of the previous question and was partially addressed by GORTEC 99-02 but was also addressed by RTOG 0129. RTOG 0129 is noteworthy particularly because secondary retrospective analysis defined the importance of HPV status in OPC prognosis (see HPV section later).[22]

Nguyen-Tan, RTOG 0129 (*JCO* 2014, PMID 25366680): PRT of 721 patients with SCC of the oral cavity, oropharynx, larynx, or hypopharynx to either 70 Gy/35 fx or 72 Gy/42 fx over 6 weeks with concomitant boost schedule (see RTOG 9003 earlier). Both arms received cisplatin 100 mg/m^2 every 3 weeks (two cycles for accelerated arm, three for standard arm). After MFU of 7.9 years, no differences were observed in any endpoint (OS, PFS, LRC, or DM). **Conclusion: No benefit to acceleration in the presence of concurrent CHT.**

Is cetuximab of benefit compared with RT alone?

An EGFR inhibitor, cetuximab, is active against H&N cancer and improved OS compared with RT alone.

Bonner (*NEJM* 2006, PMID 16467544; Update *Lancet Oncol* 2010, PMID 19897418): PRT of 424 patients from 1999 to 2002 with stage III to IV SCC of the oropharynx, hypopharynx, or larynx randomized to either RT alone (three regimens permitted: daily, BID, and concomitant boost) or RT with cetuximab given 400 mg/m^2 loading dose 1 week before RT and 250 mg/m^2 weekly during RT. Primary endpoint was LRC. Cetuximab improved LRC and OS (MS 29 vs. 49 months, p = .03). Toxicity was not different, with the exception of infusion reactions and acneiform rash. Subsequent analyses did not show interaction with HPV status.[44] Survival was improved among patients receiving cetuximab who developed grade 2+ acneiform rash compared with those without rash. **Conclusion: Cetuximab improves OS compared with RT alone.**

Does cetuximab improve survival when added to cisplatin?

Ang, RTOG 0522 (*JCO* 2014, PMID 25154822; Update *IJROBP* 2023, PMID 36549347): PRT of 891 patients with stage III to IV H&N cancer randomized to RT with cisplatin ± cetuximab. The addition of cetuximab did not improve OS, DFS, LRC, or DM but did increase toxicity. There was no benefit to cetuximab when stratifying by p16 status. EGFR expression did not predict outcome. **Conclusion: There is no benefit to the addition of concurrent cetuximab to cisplatin.**

Is concurrent cetuximab directly comparable and less toxic than concurrent cisplatin?

It was hypothesized that concurrent cetuximab may provide similar oncologic outcomes to cisplatin but with reduced toxicity. Multiple RCTs directly compared RT with concurrent cetuximab vs. concurrent cisplatin among HPV+ OPC and each demonstrated reduced survival with cetuximab without dramatic reductions in toxicity.[30,31,45,46]

Gillison, RTOG 1016 (*Lancet* 2019, PMID 30449625): PRT of HPV+ OPC (AJCC 7th T1–2, N2a–N3 or T3–4, N0–3) treated with accelerated IMRT (70 Gy/35 fx, 6 fx/wk) with either concurrent cisplatin (100 mg/m^2 days 1 and 22) or concurrent cetuximab. Primary endpoint OS. Of 805 patients with 4.5-year MFU, OS with cetuximab was not noninferior to cisplatin (HR 1.45, p = .5). Furthermore, cetuximab was associated with significantly inferior OS, PFS, and LRF, but not DM (Table 11.8). Moderate to severe acute and late toxicities were similar. **Conclusion: For HPV+ OPC, concurrent cetuximab has inferior OS compared with concurrent cisplatin without a dramatic reduction in toxicity.**

Table 11.8 Results of RTOG 1016						
	5-Yr OS	5-Yr PFS	5-Yr DM	5-Yr LRF	Acute G3–4 Toxicity	Late G3–4 Toxicity
Cisplatin	85%	78%	9%	10%	82%	20%
Cetuximab	78%	67%	12%	17%	77%	17%
p value	.016	.0002	.09	.0005	.16	.19

Mehanna, De-ESCALATE (*Lancet Oncol* 2019, PMID 30449623): PRT of 334 patients with HPV+ low-risk (p16+ and <10 smoking pack-years) OPC treated with RT (70 Gy/35 fx) with either concurrent cisplatin (100 mg/m^2 days 1, 22, and 43) or concurrent cetuximab. Primary endpoint of overall G3–5 toxicity at 2 years was not significantly different (p = .98). The 2-year OS was worse with cetuximab vs. cisplatin (89% vs. 98%, p = .001), as was the 2-year any-recurrence (16% vs. 6%, p = .0007). Giving cetuximab instead of cisplatin was estimated to lead to one extra death at 2 years for every 12 patients treated. **Conclusion: For low-risk HPV+ OPC, concurrent cetuximab showed no benefit in terms of reduced toxicity, but instead showed inferior OS and disease control compared with cisplatin.**

Can hypofractionated RT be utilized in patients with locally advanced HNSCC?

Hypofractionated RT is not standardly used in the management of HNSCC except for early-stage laryngeal cancer. The HYPNO trial, presented at ASTRO 2023 (results not yet published), found that in low- to middle-income countries, LRC, PFS, and OS were noninferior with hypofractionated RT (55 Gy/20 fx; 5 fx per week) compared with accelerated RT (66 Gy/33 fx; 6 fx per week).[47]

Can induction CHT improve survival by reducing rate of distant metastases?

This has been extensively studied and is controversial. In summary, TPF is the preferred induction regimen, but superiority of induction CHT to concurrent CRT has not yet been established. TAX 323 randomized patients to induction cisplatin/5-FU (PF) +/– docetaxel (TPF) followed by RT alone and found an OS benefit to TPF.[34] Similarly, TAX 324 randomized patients to induction PF vs. TPF followed by CRT with concurrent carboplatin and found a survival benefit to TPF.[48,49] The PARADIGM and DeCIDE trials randomized patients to induction CHT followed by CRT vs. CRT alone and found no benefit to induction CHT.[33,50]

What is the role of concurrent immunotherapy in definitive treatment of HNSCC?

At this time, there is no established role for immunotherapy in the upfront definitive treatment of HNSCC. HN004[69] compared RT with concurrent durvalumab to RT with concurrent cetuximab in cisplatin-ineligible patients and showed a PFS (51% vs. 66%) and LRF (32% vs. 15%) detriment to durvalumab. JAVELIN Head and Neck 100 was a phase III PRT investigating CRT +/– concurrent and maintenance avelumab and found no benefit to the addition of immunotherapy.[35] Similarly, KEYNOTE-412 compared CRT (6 fx/wk over 6 weeks with concurrent cisplatin) +/– concurrent and maintenance pembrolizumab for an unselected population of locally advanced HNSCC and found no statistically significant EFS benefit with the addition of immunotherapy (63% with pembrolizumab vs. 56% without).[36] HN005 is a phase II/III PRT for HPV+ OPC and included a concurrent nivolumab arm. Interim analysis reported at ASTRO 2024 noted inferior PFS for both experimental arms (60 Gy over 5 weeks + nivolumab and 60 Gy over 6 weeks + cisplatin), and a phase III trial will not proceed.[51]

Which tonsil tumors can be treated with unilateral neck RT?

O'Sullivan published the classic series defining unilateral RT safe for T1–2N0 lateralized tonsil tumors with ≤1 cm of soft palate or superficial BOT invasion. Subsequent series have expanded indications to well-lateralized N+ patients, although more controversial.[52–55] Modern trials (NRG HN002) recommend unilateral RT for cT1–3 tonsil tumors, well-lateralized (<1 cm soft palate or BOT invasion, no PPW involvement) with minimal nodal disease (N0–2a, no ECE) and unilateral RT optional for N2b patients confined to level II without ECE. A recent meta-analysis found that contralateral neck failure is strongly associated with T stage (1.3% for T1; 3% T2; 11% T3; 16% T4).[56] Guidelines exist on this topic for clarity.[57]

O'Sullivan, PMH (*IJROBP* 2001, PMID 11567806): RR of 228 patients with carcinoma of the tonsillar region treated with unilateral RT between 1970 and 1991. Eighty-four percent were T1–2, 58% N0. Crude rate of contralateral failure was 3.5%: T1 0% (0/67), T2 1.5% (2/118), T3 10% (3/30), T4 0% (0/7). Risk was >10% if involving the medial one-third of the soft palate or BOT involved. **Conclusion: Unilateral RT is safe in select tonsil cancers with <1 cm of medial extension.**

Huang, PMH (*IJROBP* 2017, PMID 28258895): RR of 379 patients treated with unilateral RT. T1–T2N0–N2b tonsil cancer treated between 1999 and 2014 stratified by HPV status. MFU 5 years. Regional control was not statistically different between HPV+ or HPV– patients. Overall, the 5-year contralateral neck failures were 2%. **Conclusion: Ipsilateral RT to selected T1–T2N0–N2b tonsil patients results in equally excellent outcomes regardless of tumor HPV status. When considering ipsilateral RT, ≤1 cm superficial involvement of soft palate or BOT is safe, but suspicion of deeper invasion should be approached cautiously.**

Taku, MDACC (*IJROBP* 2022, PMID 35504500): RR of 403 patients with well-lateralized AJCC 7th edition T1–2/N0–2b tonsillar cancer treated with unilateral RT. Eligible patients included those with tumors confined to the tonsillar fossa without >1 cm extension to the soft palate, no evidence of BOT involvement, tumor size ≤4 cm after diagnostic tonsillectomy, and clinical N0–2b disease. MFU 5.8 years. Eighty-five percent had ipsilateral cervical nodal disease and 45% had multiple involved LNs. Disease recurrence was uncommon, with 9 patients (2%) developing primary site recurrence and 13 (3%) developing neck recurrence. Among those with neck recurrence, four were ipsilateral and nine were contralateral. The 5- and 10-year OS were 94% and 89%, respectively. **Conclusion: Ipsilateral RT for well-lateralized tonsillar tumors offers favorable outcomes with low rates of contralateral neck failure.**

When is it necessary to irradiate levels IB, V, or contralateral retropharyngeal (RP) nodes?

With modern imaging, it is likely safe to spare levels IB and V for T1–2 OPC if not involved on imaging. Contralateral RP nodes were not routinely spared historically, but the following study from a prospective institutional database identified minimal risk of failure in a clinically uninvolved neck and significantly improved QOL. Contemporary retrospective data also suggest it is safe to spare contralateral RP nodes for T1–2N1 disease.[58]

Sanguineti, Johns Hopkins (*IJROBP* 2009, PMID 19131181): RR of 103 patients with T1–2, clinically N+ OPC staged with CT imaging who underwent initial neck dissection. Overall, if CT was negative, levels IB, IV, and V were involved in 3%, 6%, and 1%. Levels IB and V were <4% regardless of pathologic involvement of II to IV. Level IV was 5% if level III was not involved, but 11% if level III was involved. **Conclusion: Levels IB and V are low risk (<5%) and can be spared in cT1–2N+ OPC.**

Sanguineti, Johns Hopkins (*Acta Oncol* 2014, PMID 24274389): RR of 91 patients with HPV+ OPC and cN+ who underwent ipsilateral neck dissection between 1998 and 2010. Pathology reviewed to determine risk of subclinical disease at each neck level (not evident on CT). Risk of subclinical disease in both IB and V is <5%, while it is 6.5% (95% CI 3.1%–9.9%) for level IV. Level IB subclinical involvement is >5% when 2+ ipsilateral levels besides IB are involved. Risk of occult disease in level IV is <5% when level III is not involved. Low number of events in level V did not allow analysis of predictors. **Conclusion: Consider electively covering level IB if ≥2 other levels are involved. Level IV may be spared when level III is negative.**

Spencer (*Cancer* 2014, PMID 25143048): 748 patients from a single-institution prospective database with primary oral cavity, oropharynx, hypopharynx, larynx, and unknown primary treated with RT to comprehensive LNs (Group 1), elimination of contralateral high level II (Group 2), and elimination of contralateral RP LNs in patients with cN0 neck (Group 3). There were 488 patients in Groups 2 and 3 and there were no failures in the contralateral high level II or RP. QOL was significantly better in all domains (*p* < .0007) for patients with contralateral RP sparing. **Conclusion: In cN0 patients, sparing the contralateral RP LN is safe and results in improved QOL.**

What prospective data guided the adoption of IMRT for OPC in the United States?

RTOG 0022 is one of the few prospective trials that investigated the safety and efficacy of IMRT in the cooperative group setting. It also demonstrated good outcomes for T1–2N0–1 OPC treated with RT alone.

Eisbruch, RTOG 0022 (*IJROBP* 2010, PMID 19540060; Update *IJROBP* 2023, PMID 36925074): Initial RTOG multi-institutional trial demonstrating the safety and efficacy of IMRT. Prospective phase II trial of 69 T1–2N0–1 OPC patients treated with RT alone to 66 Gy/30 fx with IMRT. The 2-year LRF was 9%. LRF was increased in those with major deviations: 2/4 patients with deviations (50%) vs. 3/49 without (6%; *p* = .04). At an MFU of 12 years on the 2023 update, 5- and 10-year LRF rates were 14% and 15%, 5- and 10-year DFS rates were 66% and 50%, and 5- and 10-year OS rates were 84% and 67%, respectively. Acute grades 3 to 4 toxicities occurred in 39% of patients, while late grades 3 and 4 toxicities were seen in 13% and 9% of patients, respectively. **Conclusion: IMRT is feasible with encouraging acute and late toxicity. Quality of IMRT is important to avoid LRF.**

Does prognosis differ between HPV+ and HPV− tumors when treated uniformly?

HPV+ OPC is now classified as a distinct disease given outcomes differ vastly from HPV− OPC.

Ang, RTOG 0129 (*NEJM* 2010, PMID 20530316): Secondary analysis of RTOG 0129 (see Nguyen-Tan [2014] in the preceding) investigating the prognostic role of HPV. HPV status was determined by both FISH for HPV DNA and IHC for p16. Sixty-four percent of patients had HPV+ tumors and the 3-year OS was markedly improved for these patients (82% vs. 57%, $p < .001$). The 3-year rate of local–regional disease relapse was lower for patients with HPV+ tumors vs. HPV– tumors (14% vs. 35%, $p < .001$). Smoking and nodal stage were prognostic. RPA for OS divided patients into three classes based on HPV status, smoking, and T and N stages: low risk (HPV-positive and ≤10 pack-years or HPV-positive, >10 pack-years, and N0–2a), intermediate risk (HPV-positive, >10 pack-years, and N2b–3 or HPV-negative, ≤10 pack-years, and T2–3), or high risk (HPV-negative, ≤10 pack-years, and T4 or >10 pack-years). **Conclusion: OS is dramatically higher in HPV+ disease.**

Can treatment intensity be safely reduced for HPV+ patients?

No standard regimen has been identified to date, but multiple trials are investigating deintensification for low-risk HPV+ patients. Given the inferior results of the three cetuximab trials above, treatment de-escalation should be reserved for patients treated on protocol until phase III data are available. MSKCC is investigating the role of hypoxia on locoregional control and is utilizing F-MISO PETs to better select those who may benefit from dose de-escalation. This has been investigated in T0–2/N1–2c HPV+ OPC patients s/p resection of the primary site (see below)[59] as well as in patients treated without surgery who received definitive CRT (results at ASCO 2024).[60]

Marur, ECOG 1308 (*JCO* 2017, PMID 28029303): Phase II trial of 80 patients evaluating whether clinical complete response (cCR) to induction CHT could select patients with HPV+ OPC who could receive deintensified therapy with the goal of reducing late toxicity. Eligibility criteria: stage III to IV, T1–3N0–N2b OPC, p16+ or HPV+, ≤10 pack-years smoking history. Treated with three cycles of induction CHT with cisplatin, paclitaxel, and cetuximab. If cCR of primary site, patients were treated with IMRT to 54 Gy with weekly cetuximab. If PR at primary site or nodes, patients were treated to 69.3 Gy to involved site and cetuximab. Primary endpoint was 2-year PFS. Seventy percent had primary site cCR and received low-dose RT; these patients had 2-year PFS of 80%. At 12 months, patients treated with RT ≤54 Gy had less difficulty swallowing solids (40% vs. 89%, $p = .011$) or impaired nutrition (10% vs. 44%, $p = .025$). Eight of nine failures in reduced-dose arm were locoregional. **Conclusion: For patients who respond to induction CHT, reduced-dose IMRT with concurrent cetuximab for favorable HPV+ patients may improve swallowing and nutritional status.**

Yom, NRG HN002 (*JCO* 2021, PMID 33507809): Phase II PRT of 306 eligible patients with T1–2N1–2b or T3N0–2b (AJCC 7th) OPC with ≤10 pack-years smoking history randomized to 60 Gy/30 fx + weekly cisplatin (IMRT + C) vs. accelerated IMRT alone to 60 Gy/30 fx delivered 6 fx/wk. Powered to detect acceptable prespecified 2-year PFS of ≥85% without worse swallowing QOL at 1 year per MD Anderson Dysphagia Index (MDADI) as co-primary endpoint. At MFU of 2.6 years, there were no differences in 2-year OS. The 2-year PFS for IMRT + C was 91% (lower confidence bound 86.6%), which met the prespecified PFS endpoint, while it was 88% for IMRT alone arm (lower confidence bound 83.3%), which failed to meet the prespecified PFS. The CRT arm had significantly less LRF (3% vs. 10%, $p = .02$) at the expense of higher acute grades 3 to 4 toxicities (80% vs. 52%, $p < .001$). Both arms passed the MDADI dysphagia threshold. No differences in late toxicity were observed. **Conclusion: Deintensification of CRT for HPV+ OPC with 60 Gy/30 fx and weekly cisplatin warrants phase III comparison with 70 Gy, leading to NRG HN005. However, this arm was closed early due to interim futility analysis showing that concurrent CRT to 60 Gy did not meet prespecified noninferiority threshold.**

Tsai, MSKCC (*JAMA Oncol* 2022, PMID 35050342): Retrospective cohort study of 276 patients with HPV+ OPC treated with de-escalated RT of 30 Gy/15 fx to the elective neck with a cone-down boost of 40 Gy/20 fx to gross disease with concurrent CHT. Bilateral levels IB/V and contralateral retropharyngeal nodes were spared if uninvolved. Seventy-seven percent of patients received bolus cisplatin. Most patients were AJCC 8th edition T1 (25%) or T2 (40%) and N0–1 (76%). At MFU of 26 months, eight patients developed LRR, of which seven were in the 70 Gy volume. The 2-year LRC was 97%, PFS was 88%, DMFS was 95%, and OS was 95%. **Conclusion: Dose de-escalation to the elective neck is feasible for HPV+ OPC.**

Lee, MSKCC (*JCO* 2024, PMID 38241600): Phase II trial of 152 eligible patients investigating the importance of tumor hypoxia in patients with T0–2/N1–2c HPV+ OPC undergoing resection at the primary site (but not gross disease in neck) followed by CRT to the postoperative primary site, gross neck nodes, and elective neck. CHT was cisplatin 100 mg/m^2 or carboplatin/5-FU weeks 1 and 4. Tumor hypoxia was measured via 18F-fluoromisonidazole (F-MISO) PET at baseline and at 1 to 2 weeks during RT. Patients with nonhypoxic tumors received CRT with 30 Gy/15 fx and those with hypoxic tumors received a cone-down boost of 40 Gy/20 fx to gross disease (total dose of 70 Gy/35 fx). Of the patients, 128 received 30 Gy and 24 received 70 Gy. At MFU of 38 months, 2-year PFS (94% vs. 96%) and 2-year OS (100% vs. 96%) were similar between the 30 Gy and 70 Gy cohort, respectively. There were fewer acute grades 3 to 4 toxicities in the dose-reduced cohort (32% vs. 58%, p = .02). There were no grades 3 to 4 late toxicities in the 30 Gy arm, while 4.5% of the 70 Gy arm had grades 3 to 4 dysphagia. **Conclusion: Hypoxia-directed dose de-escalated CRT to the postoperative primary site and neck reduces toxicity without impacting tumor control.**

What are the expected outcomes with TORS? Who are the ideal candidates?

TORS and TLM have transformed the morbidity associated with surgical resection of OPC. FDA approval was obtained for the DaVinci robot in resection of T1–2 OPC in 2009, and the NCCN guidelines allow for TORS as option for select patients.[10] Series from multiple institutions have established the safety and efficacy of TORS.[61–68] For now, TORS remains institution- and surgeon-dependent and comparative data are limited to QOL as shown in the ORATOR trial below.

Nichols, ORATOR (*Lancet Oncol* 2019, PMID 31416685; Update *JCO* 2022, PMID 34995124; Update *JCO* 2024, PMID 39303189): Multicenter phase II PRT of 68 patients with T1–2N0–2 (≤4 cm) oropharynx SCC comparing TORS + neck dissection vs. RT (70 Gy/35 fx). CHT added to RT if N1–2; PORT with 60 Gy/30 fx (<2 mm margin, pT3/4, N+, LVSI) or CRT with 64 Gy/30 fx and concurrent CHT (positive margins or ECE) added to TORS based on pathology. Primary endpoint was swallowing-related QOL at 1 year using MDADI score, powered to detect clinically meaningful improvement in TORS group compared with RT group. MDADI scores at 1 year for TORS vs. RT did not meet clinically meaningful threshold, although patients treated with RT demonstrated statistically significant improvement in swallowing-related QOL scores. Of the TORS patients, 47% received PORT and 24% received adjuvant CRT. At the 5-year update, MDADI scores converged and were not significantly different across the follow-up period. Worse dry mouth, neutropenia, and hearing loss in the RT arm, and more dysphagia and other pain in the TORS arm. No differences in OS or PFS. One death was recorded due to bleeding after TORS. **Conclusion: Patients treated with RT did not have a clinically meaningful change in swallowing compared with those who underwent TORS. Discussion of toxicity profiles of TORS and RT/CRT should occur with patients.**

Palma, ORATOR II (*JAMA Oncol* 2022, PMID 35482348): Phase II PRT of 61 patients with T1–2N0–2 HPV+ oropharyngeal SCC randomized to de-escalated CRT with 60 Gy and concurrent weekly cisplatin vs. TORS and neck dissection followed by risk-adapted, reduced-dose RT depending on pathologic findings. Primary endpoint was OS; secondary endpoints included PFS, QOL using MDADI, and toxicity. Trial closed early due to excessive toxicity in the TORS arm, including two treatment-related deaths (one hemorrhage, one cervical osteomyelitis). While survival outcomes remain immature at MFU of 17 months and were not reported in official publication, the results at ASTRO 2021 for RT and TORS demonstrated 2-year OS of 100% vs. 89%, respectively, and 2-year PFS of 100% vs. 84%, respectively. Grades 2 to 5 toxicities occurred in 67% of RT arm and 71% of TORS arm. Mean MDADI total scores at 1 year were similar between the arms. **Conclusion: Primary TORS +/– RT was associated with upfront risk of treatment-related mortality and suboptimal PFS, while de-escalated CRT demonstrated excellent oncologic outcomes with moderate toxicity.**

Can RT to the primary site be avoided after TORS?

Select patients have favorable LC when avoiding deliberate RT to primary site per AVOID trial.

Swisher-McClure, AVOID (*IJROBP* 2019, PMID 31785337): Single-arm, phase II, prospective trial of 60 patients pT1–2N1–3, HPV+ OPC treated with TORS and selective neck dissection. Trial investigated avoiding RT to primary site in patients who had favorable pathologic features at primary site (negative margins ≥2mm, no PNI, no LVSI), but who required adjuvant RT to the neck (60–66 Gy for involved neck, 54 Gy for uninvolved neck). The 2-year LC was 98%, with one patient experiencing recurrence at primary site with successful surgical salvage. The 2-year LRFS was 98% and OS was 100%. Mean RT dose to primary site was 36.9 Gy (standard deviation 10.3 Gy). **Conclusion: De-intensification of postop RT in a select group of patients is safe and worthy of further study.**

REFERENCES

1. Semprini J, Pagedar NA, Boakye EA, Osazuwa-Peters N. Head and neck cancer incidence in the United States before and during the COVID-19 pandemic. *JAMA Otolaryngol Head Neck Surg*. 2024;150(3):193–200. doi:10.1001/jamaoto.2023.4322

2. Van Dyne EA, Henley SJ, Saraiya M, Thomas CC, Markowitz LE, Benard VB. Trends in human papillomavirus-associated cancers—United States, 1999–2015. *MMWR Morb Mortal Wkly Rep*. 2018;67(33):918–924. doi:10.15585/mmwr.mm6733a2

3. Louredo BVR, Prado-Ribeiro AC, Brandao TB, et al. State-of-the-science concepts of HPV-related oropharyngeal squamous cell carcinoma: a comprehensive review. *Oral Surg Oral Med Oral Pathol Oral Radiol*. 2022;134(2):190–205. doi:10.1016/j.oooo.2022.03.016

4. Lechner M, Liu J, Masterson L, Fenton TR. HPV-associated oropharyngeal cancer: epidemiology, molecular biology and clinical management. *Nat Rev Clin Oncol*. 2022;19(5):306–327. doi:10.1038/s41571-022-00603-7

5. Damgacioglu H, Sonawane K, Zhu Y, et al. Oropharyngeal cancer incidence and mortality trends in all 50 States in the US, 2001-2017. *JAMA Otolaryngol Head Neck Surg*. 2022;148(2):155–165. doi:10.1001/jamaoto.2021.3567

6. Salama JK, Gillison ML, Brizel DM. Oropharynx. In: Halperin EC, Wazer DE, Perez CA, Brady LW, eds. *Principles and Practice of Radiation Oncology*. 6th ed. Lippincott Williams & Wilkins; 2013:817–832.

7. Chaturvedi AK, Engels EA, Pfeiffer RM, et al. Human papillomavirus and rising oropharyngeal cancer incidence in the United States. *J Clin Oncol*. 2011;29(32):4294–4301. doi:10.1200/jco.2011.36.4596

8. Gillison ML, Broutian T, Pickard RK, et al. Prevalence of oral HPV infection in the United States, 2009–2010. *JAMA*. 2012;307(7):693–703. doi:10.1001/jama.2012.101

9. Gillison ML, Zhang Q, Jordan R, et al. Tobacco smoking and increased risk of death and progression for patients with p16-positive and p16-negative oropharyngeal cancer. *J Clin Oncol*. 2012;30(17):2102–2111. doi:10.1200/jco.2011.38.4099

10. Ang KK, Trotti A, Brown BW, et al. Randomized trial addressing risk features and time factors of surgery plus radiotherapy in advanced head-and-neck cancer. *Int J Radiat Oncol Biol Phys*. Nov 01 2001;51(3):571–578. doi:10.1016/s0360-3016(01)01690-x

11. Bagnardi V, Rota M, Botteri E, et al. Light alcohol drinking and cancer: a meta-analysis. *Ann Oncol*. 2013;24(2):301–308. doi:10.1093/annonc/mds337

12. Drake VE, Fakhry C, Windon MJ, et al. Timing, number, and type of sexual partners associated with risk of oropharyngeal cancer. *Cancer*. 2021;127(7):1029–1038. doi:10.1002/cncr.33346

13. Cannon GM, Harari PM, Gentry LR, Avey GD, Siu LL. Oropharyngeal cancer. In: Gunderson L, Tepper J, eds. *Clinical Radiation Oncology*. 3rd ed. Elsevier; 2012:585–617.

14. Lewis JS, Jr., Beadle B, Bishop JA, et al. Human papillomavirus testing in head and neck carcinomas: guideline from the College of American Pathologists. *Arch Pathol Lab Med*. 2018;142(5):559–597. doi:10.5858/arpa.2017-0286-CP

15. Mehanna H, Taberna M, von Buchwald C, et al. Prognostic implications of p16 and HPV discordance in oropharyngeal cancer (HNCIG-EPIC-OPC): a multicentre, multinational, individual patient data analysis. *Lancet Oncol*. 2023;24(3):239–251. doi:10.1016/S1470-2045(23)00013-X

16. Kreimer AR, Clifford GM, Boyle P, Franceschi S. Human papillomavirus types in head and neck squamous cell carcinomas worldwide: a systematic review. *Cancer Epidemiol Biomarkers Prev*. 2005;14(2):467–475. doi:10.1158/1055-9965.EPI-04-0551

17. Chung CH, Gillison ML. Human papillomavirus in head and neck cancer: its role in pathogenesis and clinical implications. *Clin Cancer Res*. 2009;15(22):6758–6762. doi:10.1158/1078-0432.ccr-09-0784

18. Chera BS, Kumar S, Shen C, et al. Plasma circulating tumor HPV DNA for the surveillance of cancer recurrence in HPV-associated oropharyngeal cancer. *J Clin Oncol*. 2020;38(10):1050–1058. doi:10.1200/jco.19.02444

19. **National Comprehensive Cancer Network (NCCN).** *NCCN Clinical Practice Guidelines in Oncology: Head and Neck Cancers*. Version [insert version number]; 2024. Accessed April 16, 2024. https://www.nccn.org/professionals/physician_gls/pdf/head-and-neck.pdf

20. Mehanna H, Wong WL, McConkey CC, et al. PET-CT surveillance versus neck dissection in advanced head and neck cancer. *N Engl J Med*. 2016;374(15):1444–1454. doi:10.1056/NEJMoa1514493

21. Broughman JR, Xiong DD, Moeller BJ, et al. Rethinking the 10-pack-year rule for favorable human papillomavirus-associated oropharynx carcinoma: a multi-institution analysis. *Cancer*. 2020;126(12):2784–2790. doi:10.1002/cncr.32849

22. Ang KK, Harris J, Wheeler R, et al. Human papillomavirus and survival of patients with oropharyngeal cancer. *N Engl J Med*. 2010;363(1):24–35. doi:10.1056/NEJMoa0912217

23. Schwartz DL, Harris J, Yao M, et al. Metabolic tumor volume as a prognostic imaging-based biomarker for head-and-neck cancer: pilot results from Radiation Therapy Oncology Group protocol 0522. *Int J Radiat Oncol Biol Phys*. 2015;91(4):721–729. doi:10.1016/j.ijrobp.2014.12.023

24. Huang SH, Xu W, Waldron J, et al. Refining American joint committee on cancer/union for international cancer control TNM stage and prognostic groups for human papillomavirus-related oropharyngeal carcinomas. *J Clin Oncol.* 2015;33(8):836–845. doi:10.1200/jco.2014.58.6412

25. Beitler JJ, Muller S, Grist WJ, et al. Prognostic accuracy of computed tomography findings for patients with laryngeal cancer undergoing laryngectomy. *J Clin Oncol.* 2010;28(14):2318–2322. doi:10.1200/jco.2009.24.7544

26. O'Sullivan B, Huang SH, Siu LL, et al. Deintensification candidate subgroups in human papillomavirus-related oropharyngeal cancer according to minimal risk of distant metastasis. *J Clin Oncol.* 2013;31(5):543–550. doi:10.1200/jco.2012.44.0164

27. Kramer S, Gelber RD, Snow JB, et al. Combined radiation therapy and surgery in the management of advanced head and neck cancer: final report of study 73-03 of the radiation therapy oncology group. *Head Neck Surg.* 1987;10(1):19–30. doi:10.1002/hed.2890100105

28. Nichols AC, Theurer J, Prisman E, et al. Randomized trial of radiotherapy versus transoral robotic surgery for oropharyngeal squamous cell carcinoma: long-term results of the ORATOR trial. *J Clin Oncol.* 2022;40(8):866–875. doi:10.1200/JCO.21.01961

29. Garrel R, Poissonnet G, Moyà Plana A, et al. Equivalence randomized trial to compare treatment on the basis of sentinel node biopsy versus neck node dissection in operable T1-T2N0 oral and oropharyngeal cancer. *J Clin Oncol.* 2020;38(34):4010–4018. doi:10.1200/jco.20.01661

30. Gillison ML, Trotti AM, Harris J, et al. Radiotherapy plus cetuximab or cisplatin in human papillomavirus-positive oropharyngeal cancer (NRG Oncology RTOG 1016): a randomised, multicentre, non-inferiority trial. *Lancet.* 2019;393(10166):40–50. doi:10.1016/s0140-6736(18)32779-x

31. Mehanna H, Robinson M, Hartley A, et al. Radiotherapy plus cisplatin or cetuximab in low-risk human papillomavirus-positive oropharyngeal cancer (De-ESCALaTE HPV): an open-label randomised controlled phase 3 trial. *Lancet.* 2019;393(10166):51–60. doi:10.1016/S0140-6736(18)32752-1

32. Bonner JA, Harari PM, Giralt J, et al. Radiotherapy plus cetuximab for squamous-cell carcinoma of the head and neck. *N Engl J Med.* 2006;354(6):567–578. doi:10.1056/NEJMoa053422

33. Haddad R, O'Neill A, Rabinowits G, et al. Induction chemotherapy followed by concurrent chemoradiotherapy (sequential chemoradiotherapy) versus concurrent chemoradiotherapy alone in locally advanced head and neck cancer (PARADIGM): a randomised phase 3 trial. *Lancet Oncol.* 2013;14(3):257–264. doi:10.1016/S1470-2045(13)70011-1

34. Vermorken JB, Remenar E, van Herpen C, et al. Cisplatin, fluorouracil, and docetaxel in unresectable head and neck cancer. *N Engl J Med.* 2007;357(17):1695–1704. doi:10.1056/NEJMoa071028

35. Lee NY, Ferris RL, Psyrri A, et al. Avelumab plus standard-of-care chemoradiotherapy versus chemoradiotherapy alone in patients with locally advanced squamous cell carcinoma of the head and neck: a randomised, double-blind, placebo-controlled, multicentre, phase 3 trial. *Lancet Oncol.* 2021;22(4):450–462. doi:10.1016/S1470-2045(20)30737-3

36. Machiels JP, Tao Y, Licitra L, et al. Pembrolizumab plus concurrent chemoradiotherapy versus placebo plus concurrent chemoradiotherapy in patients with locally advanced squamous cell carcinoma of the head and neck (KEYNOTE-412): a randomised, double-blind, phase 3 trial. *Lancet Oncol.* 2024;doi:10.1016/S1470-2045(24)00100-1

37. Tao Y, Biau J, Sun XS, et al. Pembrolizumab versus cetuximab concurrent with radiotherapy in patients with locally advanced squamous cell carcinoma of head and neck unfit for cisplatin (GORTEC 2015-01 PembroRad): a multicenter, randomized, phase II trial. *Ann Oncol.* 2023;34(1):101–110. doi:10.1016/j.annonc.2022.10.006

38. Mell LK, Torres-Saavedra P, Wong S, et al. Radiotherapy with Durvalumab vs. Cetuximab in patients with locoregionally advanced head and neck cancer and a contraindication to cisplatin: phase II results of NRG-HN004. *Int J Radiat Oncol Biol Phys.* 2022;114(5):945–954. doi:10.1016/j.ijrobp.2022.08.020

39. Garden AS, Harris J, Eisbruch A, et al. Final report of NRG Oncology RTOG 0022: a phase 1/2 study of conformal and intensity modulated radiation for oropharyngeal cancer. *Int J Radiat Oncol Biol Phys.* 2023;117(2):333–340. doi:10.1016/j.ijrobp.2023.02.057

40. Eisbruch A, Harris J, Garden AS, et al. Multi-institutional trial of accelerated hypofractionated intensity-modulated radiation therapy for early-stage oropharyngeal cancer (RTOG 00-22). *Int J Radiat Oncol Biol Phys.* 2010;76(5):1333–1338. doi:10.1016/j.ijrobp.2009.04.011

41. Ferris RL, Flamand Y, Weinstein GS, et al. Phase II randomized trial of transoral surgery and low-dose intensity modulated radiation therapy in resectable p16+ locally advanced oropharynx cancer: an ECOG-ACRIN cancer research group trial (E3311). *J Clin Oncol.* 2022;40(2):138–149. doi:10.1200/JCO.21.01752

42. Videtic GMM, Woody N, Vassil AD. *Handbook of Treatment Planning in Radiation Oncology.* 2nd. ed. Demos Medical; 2015:249.

43. Lassen P, Eriksen JG, Krogdahl A, et al. The influence of HPV-associated p16-expression on accelerated fractionated radiotherapy in head and neck cancer: evaluation of the randomised DAHANCA 6&7 trial. *Radiother Oncol.* 2011;100(1):49–55. doi:10.1016/j.radonc.2011.02.010

44. Rosenthal DI, Harari PM, Giralt J, et al. Association of human papillomavirus and p16 status with outcomes in the IMCL-9815 phase III registration trial for patients with locoregionally advanced oropharyngeal squamous cell carcinoma of the head and neck treated with radiotherapy with or without cetuximab. *J Clin Oncol.* 2015;33(17):1980–1987. doi:10.1200/jco.2015.62.5970

45. Gebre-Medhin M, Brun E, Engstrom P, et al. ARTSCAN III: A randomized phase III study comparing chemoradiotherapy with cisplatin versus cetuximab in patients with locoregionally advanced head and neck squamous cell cancer. *J Clin Oncol.* 2021;39(1):38–47. doi:10.1200/JCO.20.02072

46. Rischin D, King M, Kenny L, et al. Randomized trial of radiation therapy with weekly cisplatin or cetuximab in low-risk HPV-associated oropharyngeal cancer (TROG 12.01) - a trans-tasman radiation oncology group study. *Int J Radiat Oncol Biol Phys.* 2021;111(4):876–886. doi:10.1016/j.ijrobp.2021.04.015

47. Gupta T, Ghosh-Laskar S, Agarwal JP. Resource-sparing curative-intent hypofractionated-accelerated radiotherapy in head and neck cancer: more relevant than ever before in the COVID era. *Oral Oncol.* 2020;111:105045. doi:10.1016/j.oraloncology.2020.105045

48. Lorch JH, Goloubeva O, Haddad RI, et al. Induction chemotherapy with cisplatin and fluorouracil alone or in combination with docetaxel in locally advanced squamous-cell cancer of the head and neck: long-term results of the TAX 324 randomised phase 3 trial. *Lancet Oncol.* 2011;12(2):153–159. doi:10.1016/S1470-2045(10)70279-5

49. Posner MR, Hershock DM, Blajman CR, et al. Cisplatin and fluorouracil alone or with docetaxel in head and neck cancer. *N Engl J Med.* 2007;357(17):1705–1715. doi:10.1056/NEJMoa070956

50. Cohen EE, Karrison TG, Kocherginsky M, et al. Phase III randomized trial of induction chemotherapy in patients with N2 or N3 locally advanced head and neck cancer. *J Clin Oncol.* 2014;32(25):2735–2743. doi:10.1200/JCO.2013.54.6309

51. Yom S. Interim futility results of NRG-HN005, a randomized, phase II/III non-inferiority trial for non-smoking p16+ oropharyngeal cancer patients. *Int J Radiat Oncol Biol Phys.* 2024;120(2):S2–S3. doi:10.1016/j.ijrobp.2024.08.014

52. Chronowski GM, Garden AS, Morrison WH, et al. Unilateral radiotherapy for the treatment of tonsil cancer. *Int J Radiat Oncol Biol Phys.* 2012;83(1):204–209. doi:10.1016/j.ijrobp.2011.06.1975

53. Al-Mamgani A, van Rooij P, Fransen D, Levendag P. Unilateral neck irradiation for well-lateralized oropharyngeal cancer. *Radiother Oncol.* 2013;106(1):69–73. doi:10.1016/j.radonc.2012.12.006

54. Liu C, Dutu G, Peters LJ, Rischin D, Corry J. Tonsillar cancer: the Peter MacCallum experience with unilateral and bilateral irradiation. *Head Neck.* 2014;36(3):317–322. doi:10.1002/hed.23297

55. Taku N, Chronowski G, Brandon Gunn G, et al. Unilateral radiation therapy for tonsillar cancer: treatment outcomes in the era of human papillomavirus, positron-emission tomography, and intensity modulated radiation therapy. *Int J Radiat Oncol Biol Phys.* 2022;113(5):1054–1062. doi:10.1016/j.ijrobp.2022.04.035

56. Razavian NB, D'Agostino RB Jr, Steber CR, Helis CA, Hughes RT. Association of unilateral radiotherapy with contralateral lymph node failure among patients with squamous cell carcinoma of the tonsil: a systematic review and meta-analysis. *JAMA Netw Open.* 2023;6(2):e2255209. doi:10.1001/jamanetworkopen.2022.55209

57. Tsai CJ, Galloway TJ, Margalit DN, et al. Ipsilateral radiation for squamous cell carcinoma of the tonsil: American Radium Society appropriate use criteria executive summary. *Head Neck.* 2021;43(1):392–406. doi:10.1002/hed.26492

58. Ludwig R, Hoffmann JM, Pouymayou B, et al. Detailed patient-individual reporting of lymph node involvement in oropharyngeal squamous cell carcinoma with an online interface. *Radiother Oncol.* 2022;169:1–7. doi:10.1016/j.radonc.2022.01.035

59. Lee NY, Sherman EJ, Schoder H, et al. Hypoxia-directed treatment of human papillomavirus-related oropharyngeal carcinoma. *J Clin Oncol.* 2024;42(8):940–950. doi:10.1200/JCO.23.01308

60. Lee NY, et al. Intra-treatment hypoxia directed major radiation de-escalation as definitive treatment for human papillomavirus-related oropharyngeal cancer. *J Clin Oncol.* 2024;42(8):940–950. doi: 10.1200/JCO.23.01308

61. de Almeida JR, Li R, Magnuson JS, et al. Oncologic outcomes after transoral robotic surgery: a multi-institutional study. *JAMA Otolaryngol Head Neck Surg.* 2015;141(12):1043–1051. doi:10.1001/jamaoto.2015.1508

62. Hutcheson KA, Holsinger FC, Kupferman ME, Lewin JS. Functional outcomes after TORS for oropharyngeal cancer: a systematic review. *Eur Arch Otorhinolaryngol.* 2015;272(2):463–471. doi:10.1007/s00405-014-2985-7

63. Leonhardt FD, Quon H, Abrahão M, O'Malley BW Jr, Weinstein GS. Transoral robotic surgery for oropharyngeal carcinoma and its impact on patient-reported quality of life and function. *Head Neck.* 2012;34(2):146–154. doi:10.1002/hed.21688

64. Park YM, Kim WS, Byeon HK, Lee SY, Kim SH. Oncological and functional outcomes of transoral robotic surgery for oropharyngeal cancer. *Br J Oral Maxillofac Surg.* 2013;51(5):408–412. doi:10.1016/j.bjoms.2012.08.015

65. Weinstein GS, O'Malley BW Jr, Snyder W, Sherman E, Quon H. Transoral robotic surgery: radical tonsillectomy. *Arch Otolaryngol Head Neck Surg.* 2007;133(12):1220–1226. doi:10.1001/archotol.133.12.1220

66. Weinstein GS, Quon H, O'Malley BW Jr, Kim GG, Cohen MA. Selective neck dissection and deintensified postoperative radiation and chemotherapy for oropharyngeal cancer: a subset analysis of the University of Pennsylvania transoral robotic surgery trial. *Laryngoscope*. 2010;120(9):1749–1755. doi:10.1002/lary.21021

67. Weinstein GS, O'Malley BW Jr, Magnuson JS, et al. Transoral robotic surgery: a multicenter study to assess feasibility, safety, and surgical margins. *Laryngoscope*. 2012;122(8):1701–1707. doi:10.1002/lary.23294

68. Desai SC, Sung CK, Jang DW, Genden EM. Transoral robotic surgery using a carbon dioxide flexible laser for tumors of the upper aerodigestive tract. *Laryngoscope*. 2008;118(12):2187–2189. doi:10.1097/MLG.0b013e31818379e4

69. Mell LK, Torres-Saavedra PA, Wong SJ, et al. Radiotherapy with cetuximab or durvalumab for locoregionally advanced head and neck cancer in patients with a contraindication to cisplatin (NRG-HN004): an open-label, multicentre, parallel-group, randomised, phase 2/3 trial. *Lancet Oncol*. 2024;25(12):1576–1588. doi:10.1016/S1470-2045(24)00507-2

12 ORAL CAVITY CANCER

Adannia N. Ufondu, Kailin Yang, Bindu V. Rusia, and Neil M. Woody

QUICK HIT Oral cavity SCC is commonly associated with smoking and alcohol use. Primary management of oral cavity cancers is generally surgical resection with selective neck dissection (levels IB–III, others as indicated by primary site location and stage), followed by risk-adapted postoperative RT (PORT) with or without concurrent CHT (Table 12.1). Depth of invasion (DOI) is incorporated into staging and decision-making for nodal assessment and adjuvant therapy in oral cavity cancers.

Table 12.1 General Treatment Paradigm for Oral Cavity Squamous Cell Carcinoma	
cT1–2N0	Surgical resection with elective neck dissection (ipsilateral vs. bilateral depending on tumor thickness [4–5 mm] and location of primary) PORT (60–66 Gy) for T2 disease with ≥5 mm DOI, close margins (<5 mm), PNI, LVSI, or LN >3 cm
cT3–4 and/or N1–3	Surgical resection with neck dissection PORT (60–66 Gy) or concurrent CRT (60–66 Gy with cisplatin) if positive margins or ECE OR Definitive CRT (if unresectable)

EPIDEMIOLOGY: In 2020, estimated incidence of 35,000 and 7,000 deaths in the United States, comprising 30% of all H&N malignancies. Male to female ratio is approximately 2:1.[1] The most common sites for oral cavity cancer in the United States are the lip and tongue. Incidence is markedly higher internationally (20-fold increase in South Asia likely related to betel nut exposure).[2]

RISK FACTORS: Smoking and alcohol are primary risk factors for oral cavity squamous cell carcinoma (OC-SCC). Other risk factors include chewing tobacco, poor oral hygiene, periodontal disease, chronic irritation from ill-fitting dentures, betel nut, chronic sun exposure (for lip cancer), and immune suppression (HIV or solid organ transplant). Unlike oropharyngeal cancer, majority of OC-SCC are negative for HPV, unless near circumvallate papillae.[3] Genetic syndromes associated with OC-SCC include Fanconi anemia and dyskeratosis congenita.[4,5]

ANATOMY: See Table 12.2. Oral cavity boundaries: anterior border: junction of skin and vermilion border of lip; posterior border: junction of hard and soft palate; posterior/inferior border: circumvallate papillae of tongue; lateral border: anterior tonsillar pillars/buccal mucosa. Atlases are available for neck nodal level definition.[6] CN XII controls motor function of the tongue. Pharyngeal branch of CN X controls motor function of the palatoglossus muscle. Lingual branch of CN V3 carries sensory (touch) to the anterior tongue. Chorda tympani branch of CN VII (travels along the lingual nerve) controls taste to the anterior two-thirds of the tongue. Taste and sensory of the posterior one-third of the tongue is controlled by CN IX.

Table 12.2 Oral Cavity Anatomic Definition		
Site	**Key Features**	**Pattern of Drainage**
Mucosal lip	Bordered by the upper and lower lip vermillion. Upper lip innervated by infraorbital nerve (V2) and lower lip innervated by mental nerve (V3).	IA (lower lip), IB, II, III, facial lymphatics (upper lip)
Buccal mucosa	Mucosa of the inner cheek and lips to the attachment of mucosa of alveolar ridge and pterygomandibular raphe.	IB, parotid LN, II–IV
Alveolar ridges	Mucosa overlying the alveolar process of maxilla (upper) and mandible (lower). Posterior margin of the upper alveolar ridge is the pterygopalatine arch and posterior margin of the lower alveolar ridge is the ascending ramus of mandible.	IB, II–IV

(continued)

Table 12.2 Oral Cavity Anatomic Definition (*continued*)		
Site	Key Features	Pattern of Drainage
Retromolar trigone	Mucosa overlying the ascending ramus of mandible, from the posterior surface of the last molar tooth to tuberosity of maxilla.	IB, II–IV
Floor of mouth	Mucosa overlying the mylohyoid and hyoglossus muscles, extending from the inner surface of the lower alveolar ridge to the dorsal surface of tongue.	IA, IB, II–IV
Hard palate	Mucosa extending from the inner surface of the superior alveolar ridge to the posterior edge of palatine bone of maxillae.	II–IV
Oral tongue (anterior two-thirds of the tongue)	Mobile portion of tongue from circumvallate papillae to dorsal surface of tongue at the junction of floor of mouth. Sensation is from lingual nerve (V3), taste is from chorda tympani (CN VII), and motor function is from hypoglossal nerve (CN XII).	Three routes of drainage: Tip of tongue: submental nodes Lateral tongue: IB Medial tongue: deep cervical LN II–IV 15% drain to levels III and IV skipping II

PATHOLOGY: SCC comprises 95% of oral cavity cancers.[7] Less common histologies include minor salivary gland carcinomas, mucosal melanoma, lymphoma, and sarcoma. Basal cell carcinomas can arise from the vermillion border of the lip. Routine HPV testing is not recommended, and p16 is not specific to HPV infection in oral cavity. Note that DOI is not synonymous with tumor thickness (definition published in AJCC 8th ed.). DOI is measured by creating a horizon from the adjacent mucosal basement membrane and dropping a "plumb line" to measure deep tumor extent (does not take into consideration the exophytic component). Tumor thickness measurements are made independent of the basement membrane and can underestimate tumor size for ulcerated lesions.

GENETICS: Mutations in *TP53*, *CDKN2A*, *Rb* loss of function, and increased expression of *EGFR* are associated with worse prognosis.[4,5] *TP53* mutation was found in ~50% of SCCs of the H&N, and disruptive *TP53* mutations are associated with worse survival after surgical management.[8] Next-generation sequencing has identified subgroups of oral cavity tumors genetically distinct from other HPV-negative H&N cancers.[9]

SCREENING: Currently, there is no effective screening program established for OC-SCC in the United States. One study of 4,611 tobacco users >40 years old who were screened with systematic inspection of oral mucosa showed abnormal findings in >70% of patients, but cancer was only diagnosed in 3%.[10] One study in India suggested a 33% reduction in risk of oral cancer death with screening by physical examination.[11] Careful examination of the oral mucosal surfaces alongside dental care is recommended.

CLINICAL PRESENTATION: Symptoms include pain, nonhealing ulcer, bleeding, dysphagia, ill-fitting dentures, halitosis, and new-onset speech difficulty. Advanced lesions can present with symptoms of facial numbness, difficulty with protrusion of tongue, and trismus. Sharp shooting pains, taste changes, or numbness may be associated with perineural involvement. On examination, it may present as a visible, palpable mass or ulceration in the oral cavity or as palpable cervical lymphadenopathy.

WORKUP: H&P including visual inspection of the tumor noting the size and location, palpation of tumor borders, cranial nerve examination, and cervical LN examination. Exam should include flexible nasopharyngolaryngoscopy to determine the extent of disease and to rule out second primary neoplasm.

Imaging: CT neck with contrast. MRI if concern for perineural spread. PET is challenging to interpret in oral cavity, but it remains useful for nodal and distant staging.

Pathology: If safe, an in-office punch biopsy can be performed, but EUA with biopsy may be required.

Other: Dental, nutrition, speech, and audiometric evaluation as indicated.

PROGNOSTIC FACTORS: Age, smoking, tumor location, stage, and pathologic features (histologic grade, DOI [not to be confused with tumor thickness], worst pattern of invasion 5 [WPOI5], perineural invasion [PNI], margin status, number and size of LNs, extracapsular extension [ECE]) have been associated with worse prognosis. LN involvement was shown to be the most important prognostic factor for OC-SCC.[12] One study determined oral tongue to be associated with higher rate of LF, DM, and lower OS compared with other oral cavity subsites, while other studies have suggested no significant difference in prognosis.[13,14] Treatment package time (from day of surgery to last fraction of RT) >90 days predicts for worse OS in patients with extranodal extension (ENE) or positive margins.[15] Recommend all patients with ENE have medical oncology discussion.

STAGING: See Table 12.3.

Table 12.3 AJCC 8th Edition (2017): Staging for Oral Cavity									
N T/M		cN0	cN1	cN2a	cN2b	cN2c	cN3a	cN3b
T1	• ≤2 cm and DOI ≤5 mm	I						
T2	• ≤2 cm and DOI 5.1–10 mm • 2.1–4 cm and DOI ≤10 mm	II	III		IVA			
T3	• >4 cm with DOI ≤10 mm • 2.1–4 cm and DOI >10 mm							
T4a lip	• Invasion[1]							
T4a oral cavity	• >4 cm and DOI >10 mm • Invasion[2]							
T4b oral cavity	• Invasion[3]				IVB			
M1	• Distant metastasis				IVC			

Note: Invasion[1] = invasion into cortical bone or involves inferior alveolar nerve, floor of mouth, or skin of face. Invasion[2] = invasion through cortical bone of mandible/maxilla, into maxillary sinus, or skin of face. Invasion[3] = invasion into masticator space, pterygoid plates, or skull base, and/or encases internal carotid artery.
cN1: single ipsilateral LN (≤3 cm) and –ENE; cN2a: single ipsilateral LN (3.1–6 cm) and –ENE; cN2b: multiple ipsilateral LNs (≤6 cm) and –ENE; cN2c: bilateral or contralateral LNs (≤6 cm) and –ENE; cN3a: LN (>6 cm) and –ENE; cN3b: clinically overt ENE.
pN1: single LN (≤3 cm) and –ENE; pN2a: single ipsilateral or contralateral LN (≤3 cm) and +ENE or single ipsilateral LN (3.1–6 cm) and –ENE; pN2b: multiple ipsilateral LNs (≤6 cm) and –ENE; pN2c: bilateral or contralateral LNs (≤6 cm) and –ENE; pN3a: LN (>6 cm) and –ENE; pN3b: LN (>3 cm) and +ENE or multiple LNs any with +ENE or a single contralateral node with +ENE.

NATURAL HISTORY: Premalignant changes (white plaques known as leukoplakia—clinical diagnosis) are often present before the development of invasive carcinoma. The risk of leukoplakia developing into invasive carcinoma is ~1% to 20% in 10 years.[16] Risk of erythroplakia (red velvety patch) converting to SCC is higher and ~30%. Oral lichen planus and oral submucous fibrosis are also premalignant lesions whose rate of progression to malignancy is less clear. The 5-year OS for stage I to II OC-SCC is ~83% and stage III to IVa is 55%.[17,18] Compared with other H&N sites, OC-SCC has higher rates of LR after definitive therapy. The most frequent sites of DM are lung and bone.

TREATMENT PARADIGM

Surgery: Initial surgical resection is standard of care. Randomized trials comparing upfront surgery vs. RT demonstrated significantly worse OS with RT alone.[19,20] Achieving negative surgical margins is critical, and if feasible repeat resection of positive margin (CIS or invasive carcinoma at margin) is preferred. Standard transoral or open approaches are used for OC-SCC.[21] Hemiglossectomy, maxillectomy, and mandibulotomy are often required for locally advanced disease and will require reconstruction. A mandibulotomy uses incision in the mandible to expose tumors in the deep oral cavity and oropharynx. A marginal mandibulectomy allows the jawbone to remain continuous and does not require extensive reconstruction. A segmental mandibulectomy requires a full thickness cut leaving the mandible discontinuous and in need of reconstruction.

Surgical Management of the Neck

Elective dissection of the at-risk cN0 neck is indicated for tumors with a DOI >2 mm. Primary site and cN status define the extent and location of the neck to be dissected per ASCO guidelines.[22] Patients with primary tumors near or involving midline should be managed with bilateral neck dissection. Well-lateralized cancers (buccal, alveolar ridge, select oral tongue) could be considered for unilateral neck dissection. Early-stage lip, hard palate, and maxillary alveolar cancers are lower risk and may consider omission. An adequate elective lymph node dissection (LND) includes ³18 LN based on surgical quality data. Sentinel biopsy is an evolving strategy.[23]

Chemotherapy: Combined analysis of two PRTs demonstrated significant LRC, DFS, and OS benefits with the addition of concurrent CHT to PORT in patients with ECE and positive margin (see Chapter 17 for details).[24] A phase III noninferiority trial was conducted comparing once weekly (30 mg/m²) vs. bolus cisplatin (100 mg/m²) every 3 weeks. Weekly cisplatin led to worse 2-year LRC (59% vs. 73%, $p = .014$); OS endpoint not yet reached for bolus cisplatin. Acute grade 3 toxicity higher in the bolus arm (72% vs. 85%, $p = .006$).[25] Two PRTs examining the role of preoperative CHT demonstrated no OS improvement with induction cisplatin and 5-FU or docetaxel, cisplatin, and 5-FU (TPF).[26,27]

Radiation

Indications: Typical indications include pT3–T4a, pN2–3, or pT1–2N0–1 AND one or more of the following: PNI, LVSI, close/positive margins, or T2 with ≥5 mm DOI (can consider 4 mm based on Ganly et al. data).[28] Per NCCN, a close surgical margin is <5 mm from the resected margin. However, an RR demonstrated local recurrence-free survival was significantly higher with margins ≥2.2 mm, suggesting a possible new definition for close margin.[29]

MSKCC and Princess Margaret Hospital nomograms can be used to assess potential benefits of PORT.[30,31] PORT should start 4 to 6 weeks after surgery. See Chapter 17 for details.

For select nonoperative cases, definitive CRT is a feasible and viable approach based on a retrospective series from the University of Chicago (140 patients, 1994–2014, stage III–IV, maximum dose of 70–75 Gy, 5-year OS and LRC 63% and 79%).[32]

EBRT Dose: 60 Gy for negative margins, 64 to 66 Gy for microscopically positive, and 70 Gy for gross residual disease. Elective neck 54 Gy. See Table 12.2 for elective LN coverage. Sites that can be treated ipsilaterally include buccal mucosa, retromolar trigone, and alveolar ridge. See Chapter 17 for more details. The HYPO-ART study evaluated the feasibility of hypofractionated PORT, 50 Gy over 4 weeks, and found acceptable toxicity with similar oncologic outcomes.[33]

Toxicity: Acute: mucositis, loss of taste, xerostomia, thrush, dermatitis, dysphagia, odynophagia. Late: xerostomia, lifelong need for fluoride prophylaxis, risk for dental caries, osteoradionecrosis.

Intraoral Cone RT: Classic technique for small tumors (<3 cm) of floor of mouth. Preserves salivary gland function and decreases risk of osteoradionecrosis. Intraoral cone RT uses 100 to 250 kVp x-rays or 6 MeV electrons. LC rate ~85%.[34]

Brachytherapy: HDR or LDR interstitial implant can be used alone or in combination with EBRT for treatment of oral tongue, floor of mouth, or buccal mucosa. For tumor thickness <1 cm, single-plane implant is adequate, otherwise double-plane or volumetric implant is used. Surface mold brachytherapy can be used for select superficial (<1 cm depth) initial or recurrent superficial lesions of the hard palate, lower gingiva, and floor of mouth.

Procedure: See *Handbook of Treatment Planning in Radiation Oncology*, Chapter 4.[35]

EVIDENCE-BASED Q&A

Why is initial surgical resection preferred over definitive RT for management of OC-SCC?

Two PRTs, as well as several retrospective studies, suggest an LRC and OS benefit for surgical resection compared with definitive RT.[19,20]

Iyer, Singapore (*Cancer* 2015, PMID 25639864): PRT of 119 patients with stage III to IV H&N SCC randomized to surgery followed by PORT vs. concurrent CRT. MFU 13 years. There was no SS difference in 5-year OS (45% vs. 35%, p = .262) or 5-year DFS (56% vs. 46%, p = .637) for the entire cohort for surgery vs. RT alone, respectively. For patients with OC-SCC, upfront surgery significantly improved 5-year DSS (68% vs. 12%, p = .038). **Conclusion: DSS is significantly improved with surgery and PORT compared with RT alone for OC-SCC but not for other sites of H&N.**

Is there benefit for elective neck dissection, or can the neck be observed with imaging?

Randomized data suggest a survival benefit to upfront neck dissection, which increases the use of adjuvant RT by detecting microscopic disease. The ASCO 2019 guidelines consider an adequate dissection to include ≥18 LNs, as survival advantage has been reported in multiple studies.[22]

D'Cruz, India (*NEJM* **2015, PMID 26027881):** PRT of 596 patients with lateralized T1–2 OC-SCC randomized to elective ipsilateral neck dissection vs. salvage neck dissection at the time of nodal recurrence. Evaluation of LN involvement was performed with ultrasonography. MFU 39 months. At 3 years, elective neck dissection demonstrated significantly improved OS (80% vs. 68%, p = .01) and DFS (70% vs. 46%, p < .001) compared with therapeutic neck dissection. Overall rate of pathologic nodal positivity in cN0 neck was 30%. Rates of adverse events were 6.6% and 3.6% in elective neck dissection and therapeutic neck dissection arms, respectively. **Conclusion: Ipsilateral elective neck dissection provides OS and DFS benefit in patients with early stage, well-lateralized OC-SCC compared with therapeutic neck dissection. Comment: The use of adjuvant RT after surgery increased from 34% to 49% with elective neck dissection, which may account for the survival benefit of END.**

What is the role of SLNB vs. LND?

SLNB is an area of active investigation. Results from Senti-MERORL trial demonstrated oncologic equivalence of SLNB compared with LND for operable T1–T2 N0 patients.[23] *Phase II/III NRG-HN006 is currently investigating this question with primary endpoints of neck and shoulder function and related QOL (phase II) and DFS (phase III).*

Garrel, Senti-MERORL (*JCO* **2020, PMID 33052754):** Phase III PRT of 307 patients with oral cavity and oropharyngeal cancer randomized to SLNB vs. neck LND. The 2-year neck PFS (primary endpoint) was 91% (SLNB) vs. 90% (LND), confirming equivalence. No statistically significant difference for 5-year neck PFS or 2-/5-year OS or DSS. **Conclusion: This study demonstrated oncologic equivalence between SLNB and neck LND approaches.**

At what DOI should neck dissection be performed in early-stage (cT1–2N0) oral tongue cancer?

Several retrospective studies have demonstrated DOI as a significant predictor for locoregional recurrence. DOI ≥4 to 5 mm has been suggested as cutoff for neck dissection. The D'Cruz study cited above supports a 4-mm cutoff; others cited below.

Huang, Princess Margaret Meta-Analysis (*Cancer* **2009, PMID 19197973):** Meta-analysis of 16 studies investigating the NPV of DOI from 3 to 6 mm for cT1–2N0 oral cavity cancer to determine an optimal cutoff that is predictive of cervical LN involvement. There was a significant increase in nodal positivity between 4 and 5 mm DOI (p = .007). **Conclusion: DOI strongly predicts for cervical LN involvement. Elective neck dissection should be considered in patients with cN0 disease and DOI >4 mm.**

Ganly, MSKCC and PMH Combined Analysis (*Cancer* **2013, PMID 23184439):** Combined analysis of 164 patients from MSKCC and PMH with pT1–2N0 oral tongue cancer treated with partial glossectomy and ipsilateral elective LND (no PORT). MFU 66 months. Locoregional recurrence-free survival at 5 years was 80%. Regional recurrence was ipsilateral in 61% of cases and contralateral in 39% of cases. Regional recurrence was 6% for tumors with <4 mm DOI and 24% ≥4 mm DOI. MVA demonstrated that tumor thickness ≥4 mm was significantly associated with regional recurrence-free survival (p = .02). Patients with regional recurrence had significantly worse DSS (33% vs. 97%, p < .0001). **Conclusion: Neck recurrence was significantly higher with DOI ≥4 mm. The 5-year locoregional recurrence-free survival was 80%, and ~40% of the failures were from contralateral neck.**

What are the indications and benefits of PORT for OC-SCC?

Many historical H&N studies included patients with OC-SCC (although lip subsite was often excluded).[24,36,37] *Typical indications for PORT include pT3–T4a, pN2–3, pT1–2N0–1, AND one or more of the following:*

PNI, LVSI, close margin <5 mm, or T2 with ≥5 mm DOI (can consider 4 mm based on Ganly et al. data).[28] These are inclusion criteria for RTOG 0920, investigating the role of PORT ± cetuximab. These features have also been identified in various retrospective studies as significantly associated with inferior LRC, increased DMs, and inferior OS.[38,39] Observation to the cN0 contralateral neck can be considered in small lateralized OC-SCC (T1–T2), given the low contralateral neck failure rate (4% at 5 years) from a recent multi-institutional retrospective study.[40]

What are the indications and benefits for the addition of CHT to PORT?

The combined analysis of Bernier and Cooper (EORTC 22931 and RTOG 9501) suggests that ECE and positive margins are indications for postoperative concurrent CRT (see Chapter 17). One recent trial at Tata Memorial in India (see below) also addressed this question suggesting only a high-risk population T3–T4N2–3 with ECE benefits from the addition of CHT.

Laskar, OCAT (*Eur J Cancer* 2023, PMID 36669426): Phase III PRT of 900 patients with resected stage III/IV OC-SCC with ≥1 adverse pathologic features randomized to PORT only (56–60 Gy in 5 fx/wk; Arm A), PORT with concurrent weekly cisplatin (30 mg/m²; Arm B), or accelerated PORT (6 fx/wk; Arm C). MFU 95.9 months. There was no difference between the three arms, although an unplanned subset analysis demonstrated significantly improved LRC, DFS, and OS for patients with high-risk features (T3–T4, N2–3, and ECE) treated with intensified therapy (Table 12.4). **Conclusion: Only a high-risk subset of patients (T3–T4N2–3 with ECE) with OC-SCC benefit from intensification of therapy with concurrent CHT or accelerated RT.** *Note that 65% to 72% of patients had gingivobuccal primaries in contrast to lip/tongue primaries that are more common in the United States, and ~90% of patients had T1–2 disease.*

Table 12.4 OCAT Data						
Arm	10-Yr LRC	10-Yr DFS	10-Yr OS	High-Risk 10-Yr LRC	High-Risk 10-Yr DFS	High-Risk 10-Yr OS
A (RT alone)	60%	37%	40%	36%	16%	15%
B (concurrent CRT)	61%	44%	47%	51%	35%	36%
C (accelerated RT, 6 fx/wk)	66%	40%	40%	58%	34%	35%
p value	NS	NS	NS	NS	.001	.001

Is there benefit to preoperative CHT, RT, or CRT prior to surgical resection in OC-SCC?

Several PRTs have investigated the role of induction CHT with cisplatin/5-FU or TPF with no improvement in OS.[27,41] Retrospective evidence suggests benefit to downstaging for patients who are unresectable. Clinical response rate to two cycles of induction TPF is ~80%, and in a small prospective series, neoadjuvant cisplatin/5-FU with concurrent 60 Gy demonstrated a 40% CR rate.[27,42] Preoperative CRT with cisplatin and 36 Gy/18 fx may have LRC and OS benefits to surgery alone.[43] While there is no proven survival benefit, induction therapy may enable mandibular preservation in those otherwise needing a segmental resection.[44]

Chaukar, Tata Memorial (*JCO* 2022, PMID 34871101): Phase II open-label PRT where 68 patients with cT2–4 N0/N+ M0 OC-SCC requiring mandibular resection were randomized 1:1 to upfront segmental resection then adjuvant therapy vs. neoadjuvant CHT (two cycles of TPF) followed by surgery dictated by post-CHT disease extent then adjuvant CRT. At MFU of 3.6 years, 16 out of 34 patients (47%) in the experimental arm had mandibular preservation. DFS and OS were similar between the arms. Toxicity was similar between the arms, although most patients in the experimental arm had CHT-induced AE (G3 41% and G4 32%). **Conclusion: While neoadjuvant CHT does not confer a survival benefit, it allows for mandibular preservation at the cost of increased CHT-related toxicity.**

What are the patterns of failure after PORT?

Retrospective series have demonstrated that contralateral neck failure is common after ipsilateral neck RT and majority of failures are local, within the high-dose RT field. In a retrospective study from the University of Iowa comprising 55 patients, 9 patients experienced locoregional failures, with only one occurring in the contralateral neck; otherwise, the rest failed within the high-dose RT field.[45] A Princess Margaret retrospective review of 180 patients with OC-SCC found that 68% of locoregional failures occurred in-field. Failure in the contralateral neck was more common in N2b disease, raising the possibility that this subgroup may benefit from elective RT of the bilateral neck.[46]

REFERENCES

1. Siegel RL, Miller KD, Jemal A. Cancer statistics, 2016. *CA Cancer J Clin.* 2016;66(1):7–30. doi:10.3322/caac.21332
2. Warnakulasuriya S. Global epidemiology of oral and oropharyngeal cancer. *Oral Oncol.* 2009;45(4–5):309–316. doi:10.1016/j.oraloncology.2008.06.002
3. Castellsague X, Alemany L, Quer M, et al. HPV involvement in head and neck cancers: comprehensive assessment of biomarkers in 3680 patients. *J Natl Cancer Inst.* 2016;108(6):djv403. doi:10.1093/jnci/djv403
4. Kiaris H, Spandidos DA, Jones AS, Vaughan ED, Field JK. Mutations, expression and genomic instability of the H-ras proto-oncogene in squamous cell carcinomas of the head and neck. *Br J Cancer.* 1995;72(1):123–128. doi:10.1038/bjc.1995.287
5. Zhu X, Zhang F, Zhang W, He J, Zhao Y, Chen X. Prognostic role of epidermal growth factor receptor in head and neck cancer: a meta-analysis. *J Surg Oncol.* 2013;108(6):387–397. doi:10.1002/jso.23406
6. Grégoire V, Ang K, Budach W, et al. Delineation of the neck node levels for head and neck tumors: a 2013 update. DAHANCA, EORTC, HKNPCSG, NCIC CTG, NCRI, RTOG, TROG consensus guidelines. *Radiother Oncol.* 2014;110(1):172–181. doi:10.1016/j.radonc.2013.10.010
7. Wolff KD, Follmann M, Nast A. The diagnosis and treatment of oral cavity cancer. *Dtsch Arztebl Int.* 2012;109(48):829–835. doi:10.3238/arztebl.2012.0829
8. Poeta ML, Manola J, Goldwasser MA, et al. TP53 mutations and survival in squamous-cell carcinoma of the head and neck. *N Engl J Med.* 2007;357(25):2552–2561. doi:10.1056/NEJMoa073770
9. Network CGA. Comprehensive genomic characterization of head and neck squamous cell carcinomas. *Nature.* 2015;517(7536):576–582. doi:10.1038/nature14129
10. Prout MN, Sidari JN, Witzburg RA, Grillone GA, Vaughan CW. Head and neck cancer screening among 4611 tobacco users older than forty years. *Otolaryngol Head Neck Surg.* 1997;116(2):201–208. doi:10.1016/s0194-59989770326-7
11. Sankaranarayanan R, Ramadas K, Thomas G, et al. Effect of screening on oral cancer mortality in Kerala, India: a cluster-randomised controlled trial. *Lancet.* 2005;365(9475):1927–1933. doi:10.1016/s0140-6736(05)66658-5
12. Shah JP, Cendon RA, Farr HW, Strong EW. Carcinoma of the oral cavity. factors affecting treatment failure at the primary site and neck. *Am J Surg.* 1976;132(4):504–507. doi: 10.1016/0002-9610(76)90328-7
13. Zelefsky MJ, Harrison LB, Fass DE, et al. Postoperative radiotherapy for oral cavity cancers: impact of anatomic subsite on treatment outcome. *Head Neck.* 1990;12(6):470–475. doi:10.1002/hed.2880120604
14. Bell RB, Kademani D, Homer L, Dierks EJ, Potter BE. Tongue cancer: is there a difference in survival compared with other subsites in the oral cavity? *J Oral Maxillofac Surg.* 2007;65(2):229–236. doi:10.1016/j.joms.2005.11.094
15. I Ghanem A, Woody NM, Schymick MA, et al. Influence of treatment package time on outcomes in high-risk oral cavity carcinoma in patients receiving adjuvant radiation and concurrent systemic therapy: a multi-institutional oral cavity collaborative study. *Oral Oncol.* 2022;126:105781. doi:10.1016/j.oraloncology.2022.105781
16. Lee JJ, Hong WK, Hittelman WN, et al. Predicting cancer development in oral leukoplakia: ten years of translational research. *Clin Cancer Res.* 2000;6(5):1702–1710. PMID: 10815888
17. Luryi AL, Chen MM, Mehra S, Roman SA, Sosa JA, Judson BL. Treatment factors associated with survival in early-stage oral cavity cancer: analysis of 6830 cases from the national cancer data base. *JAMA Otolaryngol Head Neck Surg.* 2015;141(7):593–598. doi:10.1001/jamaoto.2015.0719
18. Liao CT, Chang JT, Wang HM, et al. Survival in squamous cell carcinoma of the oral cavity: differences between pT4 N0 and other stage IVA categories. *Cancer.* 2007;110(3):564–571. doi:10.1002/cncr.22814
19. Robertson AG, Soutar DS, Paul J, et al. Early closure of a randomized trial: surgery and postoperative radiotherapy versus radiotherapy in the management of intra-oral tumours. *Clin Oncol.* 1998;10(3):155–160. doi:10.1016/s0936-6555(98)80055-1
20. Iyer NG, Tan DS, Tan VK, et al. Randomized trial comparing surgery and adjuvant radiotherapy versus concurrent chemoradiotherapy in patients with advanced, nonmetastatic squamous cell carcinoma of the head and neck: 10-year update and subset analysis. *Cancer.* 2015;121(10):1599–1607. doi:10.1002/cncr.29251
21. Boudreaux BA, Rosenthal EL, Magnuson JS, et al. Robot-assisted surgery for upper aerodigestive tract neoplasms. *Arch Otolaryngol Head Neck Surg.* 2009;135(4):397–401. doi:10.1001/archoto.2009.24

22.   Koyfman SA, Ismaila N, Crook D, et al. Management of the neck in squamous cell carcinoma of the oral cavity and oropharynx: ASCO Clinical Practice Guideline. *J Clin Oncol*. 2019;37(20):1753–1774. doi:10.1200/JCO.18.01921

23.   Garrel R, Poissonnet G, Moyà Plana A, et al. Equivalence randomized trial to compare treatment on the basis of sentinel node biopsy versus neck node dissection in operable T1-T2N0 oral and oropharyngeal cancer. *J Clin Oncol*. 2020;38(34):4010–4018. doi:10.1200/jco.20.01661

24.   Bernier J, Cooper JS, Pajak TF, et al. Defining risk levels in locally advanced head and neck cancers: a comparative analysis of concurrent postoperative radiation plus chemotherapy trials of the EORTC (#22931) and RTOG (# 9501). *Head Neck*. 2005;27(10):843–850. doi:10.1002/hed.20279

25.   Noronha V, Joshi A, Patil VM, et al. Once-a-week versus once-every-3-weeks cisplatin chemoradiation for locally advanced head and neck cancer: a phase III randomized noninferiority trial. *J Clin Oncol*. 2018;36(11):1064–1072. doi:10.1200/JCO.2017.74.9457

26.   Bossi P, Lo Vullo S, Guzzo M, et al. Preoperative chemotherapy in advanced resectable OCSCC: long-term results of a randomized phase III trial. *Ann Oncol*. 2014;25(2):462–466. doi:10.1093/annonc/mdt555

27.   Zhong LP, Zhang CP, Ren GX, et al. Randomized phase III trial of induction chemotherapy with docetaxel, cisplatin, and fluorouracil followed by surgery versus up-front surgery in locally advanced resectable oral squamous cell carcinoma. *J Clin Oncol*. 2013;31(6):744–751. doi:10.1200/JCO.2012.43.8820

28.   Ganly I, Goldstein D, Carlson DL, et al. Long-term regional control and survival in patients with "low-risk," early stage oral tongue cancer managed by partial glossectomy and neck dissection without postoperative radiation: the importance of tumor thickness. *Cancer*. 2013;119(6):1168–1176. doi:10.1002/cncr.27872

29.   Zanoni DK, Migliacci JC, Xu B, et al. A proposal to redefine close surgical margins in squamous cell carcinoma of the oral tongue. *JAMA Otolaryngol Head Neck Surg*. 2017; 43(6):555–560. doi:10.1001/jamaoto.2016.4238

30.   Gross ND, Patel SG, Carvalho AL, et al. Nomogram for deciding adjuvant treatment after surgery for oral cavity squamous cell carcinoma. *Head Neck*. 2008;30(10):1352–1360. doi:10.1002/hed.20879

31.   Wang SJ, Patel SG, Shah JP, et al. An oral cavity carcinoma nomogram to predict benefit of adjuvant radiotherapy. *JAMA Otolaryngol Head Neck Surg*. 2013;139(6):554–559. doi:10.1001/jamaoto.2013.3001

32.   Foster CC, Melotek JM, Brisson RJ, et al. Definitive chemoradiation for locally-advanced oral cavity cancer: a 20-year experience. *Oral Oncol*. 2018;80:16–22. doi:10.1016/j.oraloncology.2018.03.008

33.   Verma M KD, Chakrabarti D, et al. A phase I/II study evaluating the feasibility and safety of delivering adjuvant hypofractionated radiotherapy in resected oral cavity cancers (HYPO-ART study). *Oral Oncology Reports*. 2024;10(100540). doi:10.1016/j.oor.2024.100540

34.   Wang CC, Doppke KP, Biggs PJ. Intra-oral cone radiation therapy for selected carcinomas of the oral cavity. *Int J Radiat Oncol Biol Phys*. 1983;9(8):1185–1189. doi:10.1016/0360-3016(83)90178-5

35.   Videtic GMM VA, Woody NM. *Handbook of Treatment Planning in Radiation Oncology*. 3rd ed. Springer; 2021.

36.   Bernier J, Domenge C, Ozsahin M, et al. Postoperative irradiation with or without concomitant chemotherapy for locally advanced head and neck cancer. *N Engl J Med*. 2004;350(19):1945–1852. doi:10.1056/NEJMoa032641

37.   Cooper JS, Pajak TF, Forastiere AA, et al. Postoperative concurrent radiotherapy and chemotherapy for high-risk squamous-cell carcinoma of the head and neck. *N Engl J Med*. 2004;350(19):1937–1944. doi:10.1056/NEJMoa032646

38.   Ang KK, Trotti A, Brown BW, et al. Randomized trial addressing risk features and time factors of surgery plus radiotherapy in advanced head-and-neck cancer. *Int J Radiat Oncol Biol Phys*. 2001;51(3):571–578. doi:10.1016/s0360-3016(01)01690-x

39.   Peters LJ, Goepfert H, Ang KK, et al. Evaluation of the dose for postoperative radiation therapy of head and neck cancer: first report of a prospective randomized trial. *Int J Radiat Oncol Biol Phys*. 1993;26(1):3–11. doi:10.1016/0360-3016(93)90167-t

40.   Liu HY, Tam L, Woody NM, et al. Failure rate in the untreated contralateral node negative neck of small lateralized oral cavity cancers: a multi-institutional collaborative study. *Oral Oncol*. 2021;115:105190. doi:10.1016/j.oraloncology.2021.105190

41.   Licitra L, Grandi C, Guzzo M, et al. Primary chemotherapy in resectable oral cavity squamous cell cancer: a randomized controlled trial. *J Clin Oncol*. 2003;21(2):327–333. doi:10.1200/JCO.2003.06.146

42.   von der Grün J, Winkelmann R, Burck I, et al. Neoadjuvant chemoradiotherapy for oral cavity cancer: predictive factors for response and interim analysis of the prospective INVERT-Trial. *Front Oncol*. 2022;12:817692. doi:10.3389/fonc.2022.817692

43.   Mohr C, Bohndorf W, Carstens J, et al. Preoperative radiochemotherapy and radical surgery in comparison with radical surgery alone. A prospective, multicentric, randomized DOSAK study of advanced squamous cell carcinoma of the oral cavity and the oropharynx (a 3-year follow-up). *Int J Oral Maxillofac Surg*. 1994;23(3):140–148. doi:10.1016/s0901-5027(05)80288-7

44.   Chaukar D, Prabash K, Rane P, et al. Prospective phase II open-label randomized controlled trial to compare mandibular preservation in upfront surgery with neoadjuvant chemotherapy followed by surgery in operable oral cavity cancer. *J Clin Oncol*. 2022;40(3):272–281. doi:10.1200/jco.21.00179

45. Yao M, Chang K, Funk GF, et al. The failure patterns of oral cavity squamous cell carcinoma after intensity-modulated radiotherapy-the university of iowa experience. *Int J Radiat Oncol Biol Phys*. 2007;67(5):1332–1341. doi:10.1016/j.ijrobp.2006.11.030

46. Chan AK, Huang SH, Le LW, et al. Postoperative intensity-modulated radiotherapy following surgery for oral cavity squamous cell carcinoma: patterns of failure. *Oral Oncol*. 2013;49(3):255–260. doi:10.1016/j.oraloncology.2012.09.006

35. Ang KK, Chang C, et al. Randomized trial addressing risk features and time factors of surgery plus radiotherapy in advanced head-and-neck cancer. Int J Radiat Oncol Biol Phys. 2001;51(3):571–578.

36. Chao KS, Ozyigit G, Low DA, et al. Intensity-modulated radiation therapy in the treatment of oropharyngeal carcinoma: impact of tumor volume. Int J Radiat Oncol Biol Phys. 2004;59(1):43–50.

13 NASOPHARYNGEAL CANCER

Erik M. Davies, Christopher W. Fleming, Nikhil P. Joshi, and Jacob A. Miller

QUICK HIT   Nasopharyngeal cancer (NPC) is rare in the United States, with high prevalence in endemic regions (South China, Southeast Asia, North Africa). Most U.S. cases (and nearly all cases in endemic areas) are related to EBV, and use of EBV DNA as a biomarker to guide therapy is under active investigation. Treatment is typically nonoperative (Table 13.1). RT targets and CHT sequence can be risk-adapted according to clinical features of the disease.

Table 13.1 General Treatment Paradigm for Nasopharyngeal Cancer[1,2]	
	Treatment Options
T1N0M0	Definitive IMRT (70 Gy/35 fx) + elective neck irradiation (ENI)
T2–3N0M0, T0–2N1	CRT vs. RT alone if no adverse features* are present Consider induction CHT for T3N0 with adverse features
T4N0, T3N+, or any N2–3	Induction CHT + definitive CRT OR definitive CRT + adjuvant CHT
M1	CHT ± locoregional RT (70 Gy) based on response

*No adverse features = nodes <3 cm, no low-neck involvement (IV, Vb), no ENE, EBV DNA <4,000 copies/mL.[3]
Source: Adapted from National Comprehensive Cancer Network. *NCCN Clinical Practice Guidelines in Oncology: Head and Neck Cancers.* Version 2.2025. https://www.nccn.org/professionals/physician_gls/pdf/head-and-neck.pdf; Chen YP, Ismaila N, Chua MLK, et al. Chemotherapy in combination with radiotherapy for definitive-intent treatment of stage II-IVA nasopharyngeal carcinoma: CSCO and ASCO guideline. *J Clin Oncol.* 2021;39(7):840–859. doi:10.1200/JCO.20.03237.

EPIDEMIOLOGY: A total of 3,200 cases per year in the United States (0.5–2 per 100,000). Endemic in South China, Hong Kong, Southeast Asia, and North Africa (rates as high as 25 per 100,000). Estimated 51,000 deaths worldwide. More common in males (2.3:1 ratio).[4] In endemic areas, incidence peaks at 50 to 59 years of age; otherwise, in low-risk populations, incidence appears to increase with age.[5]

RISK FACTORS: EBV, salt-preserved fish, preserved foods, low fruit/vegetable diet, tobacco smoke, family history, HPV.[5]

ANATOMY: The nasopharynx is a cuboidal space bordered anteriorly by the choanae, posteriorly by the clivus and cervical vertebrae (C1–2), superiorly by the skull base (sphenoid sinus), and inferiorly by the soft palate. The lateral walls consist of the Eustachian tube orifice bounded by the torus tubarius. The fossa of Rosenmüller, where most NPCs arise, is the fold between the torus tubarius and posterior wall.[6] First-echelon nodal drainage is to the retropharyngeal LNs (RPNs), then levels II, III, and VA in the upper neck. Lower neck (levels IV and Vb) is at lower risk, and skip metastases are rare.[7]

PATHOLOGY: WHO classification is divided into three groups: *keratinizing* squamous cell carcinoma (SCC), *nonkeratinizing* carcinoma (further subdivided into differentiated and undifferentiated subgroups), and *basaloid* SCC (see Table 13.2).

Table 13.2 WHO Classification for Nasopharyngeal Cancer[8–10]			
WHO Classification	**U.S. Incidence**	**Endemic Incidence**	**Notes**
Keratinizing	25%	1%	WHO type I (SCC), associated with smoking and occasionally HPV
Nonkeratinizing • Differentiated • Undifferentiated	12%	3%	WHO type II (transitional cell carcinoma)
	63%	95%	WHO type III (lymphoepithelial carcinoma), endemic, associated with EBV, most favorable prognosis

(continued)

Table 13.2 WHO Classification for Nasopharyngeal Cancer[8–10] (*continued*)			
WHO Classification	**U.S. Incidence**	**Endemic Incidence**	**Notes**
Basaloid	–	<0.2%	Aggressive clinical course, poor survival

Source: Data from Stelow EB, Wenig BM. Update From The 4th edition of the world health organization classification of head and neck tumours: nasopharynx. *Head Neck Pathol.* 2017;11(1):16–22. doi:10.1007/s12105-017-0787-0; Wei WI, Sham JS. Nasopharyngeal carcinoma. *Lancet.* 2005;365(9476):2041–2054. doi:10.1016/S0140-6736(05)66698-6; Amin MB, Edge SB, Greene FL, et al, eds. *AJCC Cancer Staging Manual.* 8th ed. Springer International Publishing; 2017.

SCREENING: Screening methods have been studied in endemic areas (e.g., IgA to EBV viral capsid antigen, circulating plasma EBV DNA), although population-based screening remains limited to clinical trials.[11]

CLINICAL PRESENTATION: The most common presentations are painless neck mass, nasal or ear symptoms, headache, diplopia, or facial numbness.[1] Other common symptoms include nasal obstruction with epistaxis and otitis media. Diplopia occurs due to local invasion, with CN VI often compressed first. Jacod's triad of vision loss, ophthalmoplegia, and trigeminal neuralgia results from cavernous sinus invasion. Dysphagia, hoarseness, Horner syndrome, and CN XI deficits can occur from lateral RPN compression on CNs IX to XII (Villaret syndrome) or from invasion into the jugular foramen (Vernet syndrome). LN involvement is extremely common at diagnosis (75%–90%, bilateral in 50%). Metastatic disease at diagnosis is present in 5% to 11%. The most common sites for DM are bone, lung, and liver.[12–14]

WORKUP: H&P with attention to cranial nerves and neck adenopathy; nasopharyngoscopy. Dental, nutritional, speech and swallowing, and audiology exam as clinically indicated. Ophthalmologic and endocrine evaluation as clinically indicated. Smoking cessation should be advised.

Labs: Routine CBC, CMP, as well as plasma quantitative EBV DNA testing. Pretreatment plasma EBV DNA levels (quantitative EBV PCR) are prognostic.[1] Other terminology: EBV antibody testing is available for diagnosis of EBV infection but not useful in oncologic management. EBER in situ hybridization (ISH) is available for testing tissue specimens (biopsy slides) for EBV; an alternative test in tissue is IHC for latent membrane protein (LMP).

Imaging: MRI (face/orbits with and without contrast) and CT with contrast evaluating the base of skull and regional node involvement. PET/CT for distant disease, especially for T3–4 or N+ patients, as well as those with high plasma EBV viral load ≥4,000 copies/mL.

PROGNOSTIC FACTORS: Performance status, stage, WHO classification (keratinizing worse, EBV-associated better), pre/post-RT EBV DNA.[9]

STAGING: See Table 13.3.

Table 13.3 AJCC 8th Edition (2017): Staging for Nasopharynx Cancer		cN0	cN1	cN2	cN3
T0	No primary tumor, but EBV-positive cervical node (unknown primary)				
T1	Confined to nasopharynx or extension to oropharynx/nasal cavity	I	II	III	IVA
T2	Extension to parapharyngeal space and/or medial pterygoid, lateral pterygoid, prevertebral muscles				
T3	Infiltration of bony structures[1]				
T4	Extension[2]				
M1	Distant metastasis	IVB			

Note: Infiltration of bony structures[1] = skull base, cervical vertebrae, pterygoid plates, paranasal sinuses.
Extension[2] = intracranial extension and/or involvement of cranial nerves, hypopharynx, orbit, parotid gland, soft tissue beyond lateral surface of lateral pterygoid muscle.
cN1: unilateral cervical LNs and/or unilateral or bilateral metastasis in RPNs (≤6 cm), above caudal border of cricoid; cN2: bilateral cervical LNs (≤6 cm), above caudal border of cricoid; cN3: unilateral or bilateral LNs (>6 cm) and/or LNs below caudal border of cricoid cartilage.

TREATMENT PARADIGM

Surgery: Surgery is not routine in upfront setting but rather reserved as salvage option in select patients with resectable LR. Persistent nodal disease after primary therapy or nodal recurrence may be treated with neck dissection.

Chemotherapy

Concurrent CRT with adjuvant CHT has historically been the standard treatment regimen in the United States for patients with stage II to IVA disease. More recently, induction CHT is preferred to adjuvant with the advantage of potentially reducing RT volumes (see Evidence-Based Q&A section).

Concurrent: Cisplatin is given concurrently with RT as 100 mg/m^2 bolus at weeks 1, 4, and 7 or 40 mg/m^2 weekly. Addition of sintilimab (PD-1 inhibitor) to concurrent regimen showed improved EFS on the CONTINUUM trial, although at the expense of more adverse events.[15]

Adjuvant: Cisplatin (80 mg/m^2) and 5-FU (1,000 mg/m^2 continuous infusion for 4 days) q4 weeks × 3 cycles beginning 4 weeks after completion of RT (considered if no induction was delivered).

Induction: Cisplatin (80 mg/m^2 day 1) and gemcitabine (1 gm/m^2 days 1 and 8) q3 weeks × 3 cycles. The gemcitabine/cisplatin regimen was studied primarily among endemic cases; therefore, some consider TPF (docetaxel, cisplatin, and 5-FU) for nonendemic cases or cisplatin with 5-FU. Results from NPC-0501 suggest safety of replacing 5-FU with capecitabine.[16]

Immunotherapy: Addition of toripalimab to CHT improves PFS and OS in recurrent and metastatic disease on the basis of the JUPITER-02 trial and is a Category 1 recommendation in the 2025 NCCN guidelines.[1,17] A separate phase III trial demonstrated a PFS benefit in recurrent/metastatic disease with camrelizumab.[18]

Radiation

Indications: Stage I disease (T1N0M0) is generally treated with RT alone. Stage II to IVA NPC is treated with concurrent CRT ± induction/adjuvant CHT; however, may omit concurrent CHT in stage II and T3N0 patients with low-risk features (see Evidence-Based Q&A). Induction CHT is indicated for T3N+, N2–3, or T4 disease.

Dose: Treat primary site to 70 Gy/35 fx or 69.96 Gy/33 fx. Treat clinically involved nodes to 66 to 70 Gy. Elective nodal RT (high risk 60–62 Gy, low risk 54–56 Gy) to bilateral RPNs (including retrostyloid) and levels II, III, and VA in cN0 patients. If cN+, add IV and VB on involved side or bilaterally if both sides of the neck are involved. Treat level IB in cN+ patients or those with primary tumor extension to nasal cavity, hard palate, or maxillary sinus. The following at-risk sites are also included in the elective volume: entirety of the nasopharynx, anterior one-third of the clivus (the entire clivus if involved), foramen ovale, foramen rotundum, pterygopalatine fossae, parapharyngeal space, inferior sphenoid sinus (entire sphenoid sinus if T3–4), posterior fourth of the nasal cavity, and maxillary sinuses. Consider coverage of the cavernous sinus for T3–4 tumors.

Toxicity: Acute: xerostomia, dysphagia, odynophagia, nausea, weight loss. Late: hearing loss, dental caries, trismus, brainstem necrosis, temporal lobe necrosis, optic neuritis, endocrinopathy (hypopituitarism), cranial nerve palsies, stroke.

Procedure: See *Handbook of Treatment Planning in Radiation Oncology*, Chapter 4.[19]

EVIDENCE-BASED Q&A

What is the role of CHT in the treatment of nasopharyngeal cancer?

Concurrent CRT followed by adjuvant CHT has been the standard of care in the United States. Historically, most patients were treated with RT alone, until the Intergroup Al-Sarraf trial demonstrated OS benefit to concurrent and adjuvant CHT compared with definitive RT alone in patients with stage III to IV NPC (AJCC, 4th ed.). These results were initially controversial, particularly in Asia. Critics argued outcomes in the definitive RT alone arm were worse than historical standards. In addition, a high proportion of WHO type I patients (22%) may account for poor outcomes and need for CHT. WHO type I histology is more common in the United States compared with endemic regions. Since then, multiple randomized trials have defined the benefit of concurrent CHT, and the MAC-NPC meta-analysis demonstrated absolute survival benefit of 6% at 5 years with concomitant CHT. Induction CHT followed by concurrent CRT has since emerged as the standard of care for select high-risk patients, with the MAC-NPC meta-analysis finding a superior OS benefit to induction CHT over adjuvant CHT.[20] Note that all trials of induction CHT are among EBV-related disease cohorts, so adjuvant CHT may be appropriate in some populations.

Al-Sarraf, Intergroup 0099 (*JCO* 1998, PMID 9552031): PRT of 193 patients with biopsy-proven stage III to IV (M0) NPC. Note that AJCC 4th edition included T1–2N1 patients in stage III (now stage II). Randomized to RT alone vs. RT with concurrent cisplatin and adjuvant CHT (cisplatin and 5-FU). Study was closed early after interim analysis of 147 patients demonstrated OS benefit in experimental arm (see Table 13.4). Sixty-three percent completed all concurrent CHT; 55% completed all cycles of adjuvant. **Conclusion: Concurrent and adjuvant CHT with RT improves OS for stage III to IV (and N1, 7th/8th edition stage II) NPC.**

Table 13.4 Results of Al-Sarraf INT 0099 Nasopharynx Trial		
	5-Yr PFS*	5-Yr OS*
RT	29%	37%
CRT + adjuvant CHT	58%	67%

*p < .001.

Blanchard, MAC-NPC Meta-Analysis (*IJROBP* 2006, PMID 16377415; Update *Lancet Oncol* 2015, PMID 25957714; Update *JAMA Oncol* 2023, PMID 37269842): Update with 8,214 patients. MFU 7.6 years; addition of CHT to RT improved OS with absolute benefit of 6% at 5 years (*SS*). CHT also improved PFS, LRC, distant control, and cancer mortality. Increase in OS was statistically significant for concomitant CHT (with and without adjuvant CHT), but not adjuvant CHT alone or induction CHT alone. The 2023 update found that induction CHT had a larger OS benefit (HR 0.75) than adjuvant CHT (HR 0.88). **Conclusion: Concurrent CHT improves OS in locally advanced NPC. Induction CHT has a larger OS benefit than adjuvant CHT.**

Is adjuvant CHT necessary?

This is an area of controversy. One trial from Chen et al. directly addresses this question and found no benefit to adjuvant CHT, but it is heavily criticized (see below). The 2025 NCCN guidelines favor induction over adjuvant CHT for locally advanced disease in light of current evidence suggesting a benefit for distant progression over adjuvant CHT. A major caveat to these data is that trials supporting induction have been within EBV-related disease. In some cases, adjuvant CHT may be appropriate. In the study by Miao et al. of adjuvant, "metronomic" low-dose capecitabine below demonstrating an FFS benefit among a high-risk population, the majority of patients had received induction CHT.[21]

Chen, Sun Yat-sen China (*Lancet Oncol* 2012, PMID 22154591): Chinese multi-institutional PRT of 508 patients with stage III/IV (T3–4N0 excluded) randomized to concurrent CRT ± adjuvant CHT (cisplatin 80 mg/m^2 and 5-FU 800 mg/m^2 for 120 hours q4 weeks × 3 cycles). Primary endpoint was FFS. The 2-year FFS rate was 84% in concurrent-only arm and 86% in concurrent + adjuvant arm (*p* = .13). **Conclusion: Adjuvant CHT did not improve FFS.** *Comment: Did not use noninferiority design; 18% randomized to adjuvant CHT did not receive it, nearly 60% did not complete concurrent CHT, 50% required RT dose reduction, and 70% had treatment delays.*

Miao (*JAMA Oncol* 2022, PMID 36227615): RCT of patients with locally advanced, high-risk stage III to IVB NPC with at least one of T3–4N2 or T1–4N3; plasma EBV DNA titer >20,000 copies/mL, gross tumor >30 cm^3; PET SUV >10; or multiple involved nodes and any >4 cm. Eighty-nine percent of these patients had at least two of these high-risk features. All patients received CRT with concurrent cisplatin (100 mg/m^2 q3 weeks for 2–3 cycles), then randomized to "metronomic" adjuvant capecitabine (1,000 mg/m^2 BID for 14 days q3 weeks for 8 cycles) or observation. Most patients received induction CHT. Primary endpoint was FFS. The 3-year FFS was 83% in the capecitabine group vs. 72% in the observation group (SS). G3 acute AEs were higher in the capecitabine arm (60%) than the control (51%). **Conclusion: Adjuvant capecitabine improves FFS among patients with locally advanced NPC with high-risk features. More investigation needed regarding indications with patients receiving induction.**

Which patients benefit from concurrent CHT?

Patients with stage I NPC can be treated with definitive RT alone. Majority of clinical trials demonstrating benefit with the addition of CHT to RT (including INT 0099) included patients with stage III to IV disease. Patients with stage II disease treated with RT alone have been found to have worse outcomes compared with stage I, with distant failure rates as high as 10% to 15% with N1 disease. RR from Taiwan suggested that addition of CHT in stage II patients resulted in similar outcomes to those found in stage I patients treated with RT alone.[22] This finding led to the phase III Sun Yat-sen trial below. Further evidence from Tang et al. (below) indicates that omission of concurrent CHT among patients with stage II and T3N0 disease without adverse features (nodes <3 cm, no low-neck involvement, no ENE, EBV DNA <4,000 copies/mL) is safe. Dai et al. published similarly compelling phase III data indicating that concurrent CHT may be omitted in patients with locally advanced stage III to IVB disease who received induction CHT.

Chen, Sun Yat-sen China (*JNCI*** 2011, PMID 22056739; 10-Yr Update *** Eur J Cancer*** 2019, PMID 30739837):** PRT of 230 patients with stage II NPC randomized to concurrent CRT with weekly cisplatin (30 mg/m^2) vs. RT alone (see Table 13.5). Concurrent CHT significantly improved OS, PFS, and DMFS at the expense of worse acute toxicity. OS advantage driven by improvement in DMFS; LRC unchanged. MVA showed that the number of CHT cycles delivered was the only factor associated with improved OS, PFS, and distant control. OS, PFS, and DMFS benefits sustained at 10 years. **Conclusion: Concurrent CHT improved survival for patients with stage II NPC.**

Table 13.5 Sun Yat-sen Trial (China) Investigating Concurrent CRT for NPC						
	5-Yr LRC	5-Yr PFS	5-Yr DMFS	5-Yr OS	Acute G3–4	Late G3–4
RT	91%	79%	84%	86%	40%	10%
CRT	93%	88%	95%	95%	64%	14%
p value	.29	.017	.007	.007	.001	NS

Tang (*JAMA*** 2022, PMID 35997729):** Phase III PRT of 341 patients at five Chinese hospitals with low-risk NPC (8th edition stage II or T3N0M0 without adverse features [all nodes <3 cm, no level IV/Vb nodes, no ENE, EBV DNA <4,000 copies/mL]). Randomized to IMRT alone vs. concurrent CRT (IMRT with cisplatin 100 mg/m^2 q3 weeks for 3 cycles). MFU 46 months. Primary endpoint 3-year FFS, 91% in IMRT-alone group vs. 92% for concurrent CRT (difference −1.4% and satisfied noninferiority threshold). No significant differences observed in OS, LRR, or DM. The IMRT-alone group experienced a significantly lower incidence of grades 3 to 4 adverse events (17% vs. 46%, SS), with significantly better QOL scores. **Conclusion: Among patients with low-risk NPC, treatment with IMRT alone resulted in 3-year FFS that was not inferior to concurrent CRT.**

Dai (*JAMA Oncol*** 2024, PMID 38329737):** Multicenter, noninferiority phase III RCT of patients with new diagnosis of stage III to IVB NPC who received three cycles of induction cisplatin/docetaxel/5-FU. Randomization was RT alone vs. cisplatin-based concurrent CRT. Primary endpoint was 3-year PFS with noninferiority margin of 10%. The 3-year PFS was 76% in the RT-alone arm and 77% in the CRT arm, satisfying the noninferiority criteria. Grade 3/4 AEs were fewer in the RT-alone arm. There was no difference in late effects. **Conclusion: Omission of concurrent CHT in patients with locally advanced NPC is noninferior to concurrent CRT in terms of PFS following induction CRT and mitigates acute AEs.**

What is the role of induction CHT?

Induction CHT added to CRT was explored as an alternative to adjuvant CHT due to the potential benefits of improved compliance and downstaging to allow for reduced RT volumes. Note that RT volume reduction is particularly helpful for NPC due to proximity to serial structures such as optic structures and brainstem. Phase IIR trial from Hong Kong demonstrated 27% absolute improvement in 3-year OS by adding induction cisplatin and docetaxel to CRT with no compromise in ability to deliver full course of CRT afterward.[23] However, phase IIR trial from Europe was negative.[24] The NPC-0501 (six-arm trial investigating induction–concurrent sequence, use of capecitabine, and accelerated fractionation) found no difference in outcomes based on RT acceleration; however, there may be superior clinical outcomes with induction CHT over adjuvant CHT.[16]

Zhang (*NEJM*** 2019, PMID 31150573; Update ***JCO*** 2022, PMID 35709465):** Multicenter PRT of 480 patients with stage III to IVB NPC with involved LNs randomized to induction cisplatin/gemcitabine followed by CRT vs. CRT alone. Induction CHT was cisplatin (80 mg/m^2 day 1) and gemcitabine (1 gm/m^2 days 1 and 8) q3 weeks × 3 cycles. Concurrent CHT was bolus cisplatin. Induction CHT improved 3-year RFS (85% vs. 77%; HR 0.51, 95% CI 0.34–0.77) and 3-year OS (95% vs. 90%; HR 0.43, CI 0.24–0.77). Vast majority of induction patients completed CHT (97%). G3+ acute toxicity increased with induction, 76% vs. 56%. Late G3+ toxicity was similar, 9% induction vs. 11% CRT. On the 5-year update, the OS benefit to induction held. The magnitude of tumor response to induction was significantly correlated with survival outcomes. Those with low pretreatment cell-free EBV DNA load (<4,000 copies/mL) might not benefit from induction CHT (5-year OS 91% in both groups). **Conclusion: Induction CHT with cisplatin and gemcitabine significantly improved RFS and OS over CRT alone. Patients with low cell-free EBV DNA may not benefit from an induction strategy. Comment: No adjuvant CHT used in comparison arm.**

Lee, NPC-0501 (*Cancer*** 2020, PMID 32497261):** Six-arm randomized trial (*n* = 803) of locally advanced stage III to IVB NPC exploring the utility of induction vs. adjuvant CHT, replacing 5-FU with capecitabine, and altered fractionation. Patients randomized to induction CHT vs. adjuvant CHT demonstrated superior 5-year PFS (78% vs. 62%, SS) and 5-year OS (84% vs. 72%, SS) when accounting for comparisons of various treatment arms. **Conclusion: Induction CHT may improve PFS and OS relative to adjuvant CHT. A dedicated head-to-head trial is needed.**

Can RT volumes be de-intensified based on clinical characteristics of the tumor?

The RPNs and high neck are at risk in all NPCs; however, the noninferiority trial below from Huang et al. provides robust evidence that the uninvolved low neck may be omitted from elective volumes without compromising clinical outcomes.[7] Additionally, the phase III trial from Xiang et al. indicates that tumor targets may be safely delineated from the postinduction volume rather than the (typically larger) preinduction volume.[25]

Huang, Sun Yat-sen (*Lancet Oncol*** 2022, PMID 35240053; Update ***JCO*** 2024, PMID 38507662):** Phase III multicenter RCT of patients with new diagnosis of NPC with N0–N1 disease randomized to deintensified upper neck irradiation (UNI) vs. standard whole neck irradiation (WNI). Patients with stage II to IVA disease were given concurrent cisplatin-based CHT. The primary tumor received 70 Gy, involved cervical nodes received 66 to 70 Gy, high-risk targets received 60 to 62 Gy, and low-risk targets received 54 to 56 Gy in 30 to 33 fractions. WNI consisted of the bilateral RPNs as well as levels II to VA/B. UNI omitted levels IV and VB either contralateral to the involved neck or bilaterally in patients with cN0 disease. MFU 74 months; primary endpoint was 5-year OS. The UNI and WNI showed similar 5-year OS (96% and 93%, respectively, NSS) and RRFS (95% in both arms, NSS). The UNI cohort had less hypothyroidism, neck tissue damage, dysphagia, and carotid artery stenosis on follow-up. **Conclusion: Omission of the low neck (levels IV and VB) from elective target volumes on uninvolved sides does not compromise OS or RRFS and leads to fewer late effects.**

Xiang (*JCO*** 2022, PMID 37356553):** Phase III noninferiority study of stage III to IVB patients with new diagnosis of NPC treated with two cycles of induction CHT (either paclitaxel/cisplatin or 5-FU and cisplatin). Patients were randomized to delineation of the GTV to either the pre- or postinduction volumes. MFU 82 months; primary endpoint was locoregional failure-free survival (LRFFS). At 5 years, LRFFS was 71% in the preinduction volumes vs. 78% in the postinduction volumes, meeting noninferiority criteria. The 5-year outcomes in terms of OS, PFS, and DMFS were similarly noninferior. G3 mucositis was significantly lower in the postinduction arm (21% vs. 9%, SS). **Conclusion: Reducing the IMRT target volume based on the postinduction GTV results in excellent long-term LRC with fewer late toxicities and better QOL.**

Is there a benefit to altered fractionation?

Altered fractionation is not indicated in the upfront setting (although it has a role in re-RT per below). Although NPC-9902 did show improvement in failure-free rates with accelerated RT and CHT, this was an underpowered trial with older RT techniques, and the majority of benefit was driven by improvement in DM. More recently, NPC-0501 discussed above found no benefit to acceleration and worse compliance with CHT.

What is the role of targeted therapies/immunotherapy?

In modern series of concurrent CRT using IMRT, LC is excellent (>90%), and therefore the primary pattern of failure is DM. Compliance with standard CHT regimens is challenging, making adding further systemic therapy with the goal of addressing distant disease difficult. As such, there has been significant interest in targeted therapies. The most prominent example is RTOG 0615, phase II trial of CRT (Al-Sarraf regimen) + concurrent and adjuvant bevacizumab.[26] The regimen was shown to be feasible, and 2-year DM-free interval was noted to be 91%. The VANCE trial was a phase III study of metastatic/locally recurrent EBV-positive NPC (with no other curative options) randomized to carboplatin + gemcitabine ± EBV-specific cytotoxic T-lymphocytes showing safety but no OS benefit.[27] KEYNOTE-028 demonstrated a 26% overall response rate in patients with PD-L1-positive recurrent or metastatic NPC. On this trial, patients had to have PD-L1 expression ≥1%.[28]

What is the best strategy to salvage recurrent disease?

Phase III data from China examined patients with locally recurrent, resectable NPC randomized to naso-pharyngectomy or IMRT (60–70 Gy/27–35 fx). The endoscopic arm showed significantly better survival at 3 years, 86% vs. 68%. While longer term follow-up is needed, the results indicate that surgery should be considered for resectable LR.[29] For unresectable disease, the randomized trial below provided evidence of a dramatic 3-year OS benefit to hyperfractionation with improved late toxicity over standard fractionation.

You, China (*Lancet* 2023, PMID 36842439): Phase III PRT conducted at three Chinese hospitals with 144 patients with recurrent, locally advanced NPC previously treated with RT. Patients were randomized to standard fractionation 54 Gy/27 fx vs. hyperfractionation 65 Gy/54 fx BID. Induction CHT at the treating physician's discretion. Co-primary endpoints were 3-year OS and incidence of late grades 3 to 5 complications. MFU 45.0 months. The hyperfractionated arm showed superior 3-year OS (75% vs. 55%, SS) and fewer grades 3 to 5 RT-induced toxicities (34% vs. 57%; SS). Fewer grade 5 late complications (mostly nasal hemorrhage) in the hyperfractionated cohort (7% vs. 24%). No significant difference in LRR and DMFS. **Conclusion: Hyperfractionated RT for locally advanced recurrent NPC results in superior OS with fewer late grades 3 to 5 toxicities.**

What is the role of serum EBV DNA levels?

EBV is the primary etiologic agent in the pathogenesis of NPC, and EBV levels both pre- and posttreatment are prognostic for survival. Patients with pretreatment values ranging from <1,500 EBV BamHI-W copies/mL to <4,000 copies/mL tend to have improved survival. Multiple studies have shown that detectable EBV after definitive RT is a poor prognostic marker.[30,31] NRG HN001 is a closed phase II/III study of individualized treatment for NPC based on posttreatment EBV DNA awaiting publication. Undetectable patients after CRT were randomized to adjuvant CHT vs. observation, while detectable patients were randomized between cisplatin/5-FU and gemcitabine/paclitaxel. Use caution when interpreting quantitative values of EBV DNA, as assays vary significantly among laboratories.

Do metastatic patients benefit from locoregional RT?

You, China (*JAMA Oncol* 2020, PMID 32701129): Phase III trial of 126 patients with metastatic NPC (not limited to oligometastatic disease) with PR/CR following three cycles of cisplatin + 5-FU randomized to CHT ± locoregional IMRT (70 Gy/35 fx + risk-adapted nodal volumes) to primary site. The addition of locoregional RT was associated with improved 2-year OS, 76% vs. 55% (*p* = .004). RT was associated with greater risk of grade 3+ dermatitis, mucositis, xerostomia, and late effects including hearing loss and trismus. **Conclusion: The addition of locoregional RT to palliative CHT in patients with CHT-sensitive synchronous metastatic NPC is associated with improved OS.**

How is pediatric NPC treated?

In the United States, induction CHT is the standard treatment paradigm. ARAR0331 was a single-arm prospective study by the COG. Pediatric patients with a median age of 15 received three cycles (later amended to two cycles) of induction cisplatin and 5-FU q3 weeks followed by CRT with concurrent cisplatin. The dose was adapted from 61.2 to 71.2 Gy based on response. The 5-year EFS and OS were 84% and 89%, establishing induction CHT followed by risk-adapted CRT as a reasonable treatment paradigm.[32]

REFERENCES

1. National Comprehensive Cancer Network. *NCCN Clinical Practice Guidelines in Oncology: Head and Neck Cancers*. Version 2.2025. https://www.nccn.org/professionals/physician_gls/pdf/head-and-neck.pdf

2. Chen YP, Ismaila N, Chua MLK, et al. Chemotherapy in combination with radiotherapy for definitive-intent treatment of stage II-IVA nasopharyngeal carcinoma: CSCO and ASCO guideline. *J Clin Oncol.* 2021;39(7):840–859. doi:10.1200/JCO.20.03237

3. Tang LL, Guo R, Zhang N, et al. Effect of radiotherapy alone vs radiotherapy with concurrent chemoradiotherapy on survival without disease relapse in patients with low-risk nasopharyngeal carcinoma: a randomized clinical trial. *JAMA.* 2022;328(8):728–736. doi:10.1001/jama.2022.13997

4. Ferlay J, Soerjomataram I, Dikshit R, et al. Cancer incidence and mortality worldwide: sources, methods and major patterns in GLOBOCAN 2012. *Int J Cancer.* 2015;136(5):E359-E386. doi:10.1002/ijc.29210

5. Chang ET, Adami HO. The enigmatic epidemiology of nasopharyngeal carcinoma. *Cancer Epidemiol Biomarkers Prev.* 2006;15(10):1765–1777. doi:10.1158/1055-9965.EPI-06-0353

6. Halperin EC, Perez CA, Brady LW, eds. *Principles and Practice of Radiation Oncology.* 6th ed. Lippincott Williams & Wilkins; 2013.

7. Huang CL, Zhang N, Jiang W, et al. Reduced-volume irradiation of uninvolved neck in patients with nasopharyngeal cancer: updated results from an open-label, noninferiority, multicenter, randomized phase III trial. *J Clin Oncol.* 2024;42(17):2021–2025. doi:10.1200/JCO.23.02086

8. Stelow EB, Wenig BM. Update From The 4th edition of the world health organization classification of head and neck tumours: nasopharynx. *Head Neck Pathol.* 2017;11(1):16–22. doi:10.1007/s12105-017-0787-0

9. Wei WI, Sham JS. Nasopharyngeal carcinoma. *Lancet.* 2005;365(9476):2041–2054. doi:10.1016/S0140-6736(05)66698-6

10. Amin MB, Edge SB, Greene FL, et al, eds. *AJCC Cancer Staging Manual.* 8th ed. Springer International Publishing; 2017.

11. Tabuchi K, Nakayama M, Nishimura B, Hayashi K, Hara A. Early detection of nasopharyngeal carcinoma. *Int J Otolaryngol.* 2011;2011:638058. doi:10.1155/2011/638058

12. Vokes EE, Liebowitz DN, Weichselbaum RR. Nasopharyngeal carcinoma. *Lancet.* 1997;350(9084):1087–1091. doi:10.1016/S0140-6736(97)07269-3

13. Hsu MM, Tu SM. Nasopharyngeal carcinoma in Taiwan. Clinical manifestations and results of therapy. *Cancer.* 1983;52(2):362–368. doi:10.1002/1097-0142(19830715)52:2<362::aid-cncr2820520230>3.0.co;2-v

14. Altun M, Fandi A, Dupuis O, Cvitkovic E, Krajina Z, Eschwege F. Undifferentiated Nasopharyngeal Cancer (UCNT): current diagnostic and therapeutic aspects. *Int J Radiat Oncol Biol Phys.* 1995;32(3):859–877. doi:10.1016/0360-3016(95)00516-2

15. Liu X, Zhang Y, Yang KY, et al. Induction-concurrent chemoradiotherapy with or without sintilimab in patients with locoregionally advanced nasopharyngeal carcinoma in China (CONTINUUM): a multicentre, open-label, parallel-group, randomised, controlled, phase 3 trial. *Lancet.* 2024;403(10445):2720–2731. doi:10.1016/S0140-6736(24)00594-4

16. Lee AWM, Ngan RKC, Ng WT, et al. NPC-0501 trial on the value of changing chemoradiotherapy sequence, replacing 5-fluorouracil with capecitabine, and altering fractionation for patients with advanced nasopharyngeal carcinoma. *Cancer.* 2020;126(16):3674–3688. doi:10.1002/cncr.32972

17. Mai HQ, Chen QY, Chen D, et al. Toripalimab or placebo plus chemotherapy as first-line treatment in advanced nasopharyngeal carcinoma: a multicenter randomized phase 3 trial. *Nat Med.* 2021;27(9):1536–1543. doi:10.1038/s41591-021-01444-0

18. Yang Y, Qu S, Li J, et al. Camrelizumab versus placebo in combination with gemcitabine and cisplatin as first-line treatment for recurrent or metastatic nasopharyngeal carcinoma (CAPTAIN-1st): a multicentre, randomised, double-blind, phase 3 trial. *Lancet Oncol.* 2021;22(8):1162–1174. doi:10.1016/S1470-2045(21)00302-8

19. Videtic GMM, Woody NM, Vassil AD. *Handbook of Treatment Planning in Radiation Oncology.* 3rd ed. Demos Medical; 2020.

20. Blanchard P, Lee A, Marguet S, et al. Chemotherapy and radiotherapy in nasopharyngeal carcinoma: an update of the MAC-NPC meta-analysis. *Lancet Oncol.* 2015;16(6):645–655. doi:10.1016/S1470-2045(15)70126-9

21. Miao J, Wang L, Tan SH, et al. Adjuvant Capecitabine Following Concurrent Chemoradiotherapy in Locoregionally Advanced Nasopharyngeal Carcinoma: A Randomized Clinical Trial. *JAMA Oncol.* 2022;8(12):1776–1785. doi:10.1001/jamaoncol.2022.4656

22. Cheng SH, Tsai SY, Yen KL, et al. Concomitant radiotherapy and chemotherapy for early-stage nasopharyngeal carcinoma. *J Clin Oncol.* 2000;18(10):2040–2045. doi:10.1200/JCO.2000.18.10.2040

23. Hui EP, Ma BB, Leung SF, et al. Randomized phase II trial of concurrent cisplatin-radiotherapy with or without neoadjuvant docetaxel and cisplatin in advanced nasopharyngeal carcinoma. *J Clin Oncol.* 2009;27(2):242–249. doi:10.1200/JCO.2008.18.1545

24. Fountzilas G, Ciuleanu E, Bobos M, et al. Induction chemotherapy followed by concomitant radiotherapy and weekly cisplatin versus the same concomitant chemoradiotherapy in patients with nasopharyngeal carcinoma: a randomized phase II study conducted by the Hellenic Cooperative Oncology Group (HeCOG) with biomarker evaluation. *Ann Oncol.* 2012;23(2):427–435. doi:10.1093/annonc/mdr116

25. Xiang L, Rong JF, Xin C, et al. Reducing target volumes of intensity modulated radiation therapy after induction chemotherapy in locoregionally advanced nasopharyngeal carcinoma: long-term results of a prospective, multicenter, randomized trial. *Int J Radiat Oncol Biol Phys.* 2023;117(4):914–924. doi:10.1016/j.ijrobp.2023.06.001

26. Lee NY, Zhang Q, Pfister DG, et al. Addition of bevacizumab to standard chemoradiation for locoregionally advanced nasopharyngeal carcinoma (RTOG 0615): a phase 2 multi-institutional trial. *Lancet Oncol.* 2012;13(2):172–180. doi:10.1016/S1470-2045(11)70303-5

27. Toh HC, Yang MH, Wang HM, et al. Gemcitabine, carboplatin, and Epstein-Barr virus-specific autologous cytotoxic T lymphocytes for recurrent or metastatic nasopharyngeal carcinoma: VANCE, an international randomized phase III trial. *Ann Oncol.* 2024;35(12):1181–1190. doi:10.1016/j.annonc.2024.08.2344

28. Hsu C, Lee SH, Ejadi S, et al. Safety and antitumor activity of pembrolizumab in patients with programmed death-ligand 1-positive nasopharyngeal carcinoma: results of the KEYNOTE-028 Study. *J Clin Oncol.* 2017;35(36):4050–4056. doi:10.1200/JCO.2017.73.3675

29. Liu YP, Wen YH, Tang J, et al. Endoscopic surgery compared with intensity-modulated radiotherapy in resectable locally recurrent nasopharyngeal carcinoma: a multicentre, open-label, randomised, controlled, phase 3 trial. *Lancet Oncol.* 2021;22(3):381–390. doi:10.1016/S1470-2045(20)30673-2

30. Lin JC, Wang WY, Chen KY, et al. Quantification of plasma Epstein-Barr virus DNA in patients with advanced nasopharyngeal carcinoma. *N Engl J Med.* 2004;350(24):2461–2470. doi:10.1056/NEJMoa032260

31. Leung SF, Zee B, Ma BB, et al. Plasma Epstein-Barr viral deoxyribonucleic acid quantitation complements tumor-node-metastasis staging prognostication in nasopharyngeal carcinoma. *J Clin Oncol.* 2006;24(34):5414–5418. doi:10.1200/JCO.2006.07.7982

32. Rodriguez-Galindo C, Krailo MD, Krasin MJ, et al. Treatment of childhood nasopharyngeal carcinoma with induction chemotherapy and concurrent chemoradiotherapy: results of the children's oncology group ARAR0331 study. *J Clin Oncol.* 2019;37(35):3369–3376. doi:10.1200/JCO.19.01276

14 LARYNGEAL CANCER

David S. Buchberger, Aditya Juloori, and Shauna R. Campbell

QUICK HIT Laryngeal cancer includes squamous cell carcinoma (SCC) originating from the supraglottis, glottis, or rarely the subglottis. The goal of treatment is to achieve disease control while maintaining organ function, defined as functional voice with intact swallowing. Early-stage glottic cancers can be managed with RT alone or microsurgery. Locoregionally advanced disease, defined as T3–4 or N+, frequently requires either total laryngectomy (with adjuvant RT as indicated) or definitive CRT to attempt organ preservation. For patients with T4a disease with extralaryngeal spread, total laryngectomy with PORT is preferred over definitive CRT (Table 14.1).

Table 14.1 General Treatment Paradigm for Larynx Cancer		
	Supraglottic	**Glottic**
Tis	Endoscopic surgery	
T1N0	Larynx-sparing surgery OR	Definitive RT (63 Gy/28 fx at 2.25 Gy/fx) OR larynx-sparing surgery
T2N0	Definitive RT (66–70 Gy) to primary tumor + elective LN levels II–IV	Definitive RT (65.25 Gy/29 fx at 2.25 Gy/fx) OR larynx-sparing surgery
T3 or N+	Larynx-sparing surgery with PORT OR definitive CRT (70 Gy/35 fx) to tumor + elective LN II–IV (V if LN+) with cisplatin	
T4a	Total laryngectomy (preferred for thyroid cartilage penetration or significant soft tissue extension) with adjuvant RT ± concurrent cisplatin as indicated OR Larynx preservation with concurrent CRT to 70 Gy/35 fx with cisplatin	

EPIDEMIOLOGY: A total of 12,650 new diagnoses of laryngeal cancer are expected in the United States, with an estimated 3,880 deaths in 2024. More common in men than women; incidence increases with age.[1]

RISK FACTORS: Smoking, alcohol, environmental exposures (asbestos, cement, wood dust, perchlorethylene).

ANATOMY: The major functions of the larynx are voice production, airway patency during breathing, and airway occlusion during swallowing. It spans from C3 to C6 vertebral bodies and is bordered superiorly by the hyoepiglottic ligament, inferiorly by the cricoid, anteriorly by the thyrohyoid membrane/thyroid cartilage, and posteriorly by the arytenoid cartilage. Preepiglottic and paraglottic spaces are one continuous space anterosuperiorly. Laryngeal muscles (with the exception of the cricothyroid) are innervated by the recurrent laryngeal nerve (branch of the vagus nerve). Damage to this nerve results in a fixed, midline cord. The cricothyroid muscle is innervated by the superior laryngeal nerve. Damage to this nerve results in mobile, "bowed" cords.

The larynx is divided into three segments:

1. *Supraglottis* (one-third of all laryngeal cancers[1]; mnemonic FAVEA: false vocal cords, arytenoids, ventricles, epiglottis, aryepiglottic folds): Bordered superiorly by the epiglottis, posteriorly by the arytenoids, anteriorly by the posterior edge of vallecula and anterior false cord, and inferiorly by the epithelium of the true vocal cord as it turns upward to form the apex of ventricle. More than 50% of patients with supraglottic primaries present with N+ disease due to presence of extensive lymphatics in this part of the larynx. Levels II to IV are primary drainage sites.
2. *Glottis* (two-thirds of all laryngeal cancers[2]): Consists of the true vocal cords and anterior and posterior commissures. Due to sparse lymphatics, early-stage disease rarely involves regional nodes. The true vocal cord is made up of the following layers: epithelial mucosa, basement membrane, superficial layer of lamina propria, and thyroarytenoid muscle.

3. *Subglottis* (1%–2% of all laryngeal cancers[3]): Starts 5 mm inferior to the margin of the vocal cords and extends to the inferior aspect of the cricoid cartilage. Subglottic tumors can drain to pretracheal (Delphian) nodes.

The hypopharynx is below the oropharynx and posterior to the larynx, representing a distinct H&N subsite. Anatomic subsites of the hypopharynx include the pyriform sinuses, postcricoid space, and posterior pharyngeal wall (PPW).

PATHOLOGY: Ninety-five percent of tumors are SCC. Carcinoma in situ occurs in vocal cords but is rare in the supraglottis. Rare malignancies: malignant minor salivary gland, small cell, lymphoma, plasmacytoma, carcinoid, soft tissue sarcoma, chondrosarcoma, osteosarcoma, malignant melanoma. HPV positivity has not been shown to be prognostic or predictive in laryngeal cancer.

CLINICAL PRESENTATION: Presenting clinical symptoms are classically related to the site of origin. Glottic cancers often present at an early stage with hoarseness, but as the disease progresses patients develop otalgia, dysphagia, cough, hemoptysis, and stridor. In the supraglottis, cancers are often detected later and commonly present with dysphagia, globus sensation, airway obstruction, and lymphadenopathy. Otalgia is due to referred pain to the auricular branch of Arnold (from vagus nerve).

WORKUP: H&P including flexible nasopharyngolaryngoscopy. Videostroboscopy can be used to evaluate mucosal wave of true cords. Pain with palpation of thyroid cartilage can be reflective of cartilage invasion.

Labs: Routine CBC and CMP.

Imaging: CT neck with contrast and PET/CT for stage III/IV disease. CT scan has high PPV for thyroid cartilage penetration (74%) and extralaryngeal spread (81%).[4]

Procedure: EUA with triple endoscopy (~4% incidence of second primary) and biopsy. Dental, nutrition, speech and swallow evaluation as indicated. Pre-CHT audiology exam.

STAGING: See Table 14.2.

Table 14.2 AJCC 8th Edition (2017): Staging for Larynx Cancer									
SUPRAGLOTTIS									
T/M ╲ **N**		**cN0**	**cN1**	**cN2a**	**cN2b**	**cN2c**	**cN3a**	**cN3b**	
T1	Limited to 1 subsite of supraglottis with normal vocal cord mobility	I							
T2	Invades mucosa of >1 adjacent subsite of supraglottis or glottis, or region outside supraglottis* without fixation of larynx	II	III	IVA			IVB		
T3	• Limited to larynx with vocal cord fixation • Invasion**								
T4	**a.** Moderately advanced local disease[†]								
	b. Very advanced local disease[††]								
M1	Distant metastasis	IVC							

Notes: *Regions include mucosa of BOT, vallecula, and medial wall of pyriform sinus.
**Postcricoid area, preepiglottic space, paraglottic space, and/or inner cortex of thyroid cartilage.
[†]Invades through thyroid cartilage outer cortex, trachea, soft tissues of neck, deep extrinsic muscles of tongue, strap muscles, thyroid, or esophagus.
[††]Invades prevertebral space, encases carotid artery, or invades mediastinal structures.
cN1: single ipsilateral LN (3 cm) and –ENE; cN2a: single ipsilateral LN (3.1–6 cm) and –ENE; cN2b: multiple ipsilateral LN (≤6 cm) and –ENE; cN2c: bilateral or contralateral LN (≤6 cm) and –ENE; cN3a: LN (>6 cm) and –ENE; cN3b: clinically overt ENE.
pN1: single LN (≤3 cm) and –ENE; pN2a: single ipsilateral or contralateral LN (≤3 cm) and +ENE or single ipsilateral LN (3.1–6 cm) and –ENE; pN2b: multiple ipsilateral LN (≤6 cm) and –ENE; pN2c: bilateral or contralateral LN (≤6 cm) and –ENE; pN3a: LN (>6 cm) and ENE; pN3b: LN (>3 cm) and +ENE.

GLOTTIS								
T/M \ **N**		cN0	cN1	cN2a	cN2b	cN2c	cN3a	cN3b
T1	**a.** Limited to 1 vocal cord with normal mobility	I	III	IVA			IVB	
	b. Involves 2 vocal cords with normal mobility	I	III	IVA			IVB	
T2	Extends to supraglottis and/or subglottis and/or with impaired vocal cord mobility*	II	III	IVA			IVB	
T3	• Limited to larynx with vocal cord fixation • Invades**	IVA					IVB	
T4	**a.** Moderately advanced local disease†	IVA					IVB	
	b. Very advanced local disease††	IVA					IVB	
M1	Distant metastasis	IVC						

Notes: *Unofficially, T2 can be divided into T2a (mobile cord) and T2b (impaired cord mobility).
**Paraglottic space and/or inner cortex of thyroid cartilage.
†Invades through thyroid cartilage outer cortex, trachea, soft tissues of neck, deep extrinsic muscles of tongue, strap muscles, thyroid, or esophagus.
††Invades prevertebral space, encases carotid artery, or invades mediastinal structures.
Refer to supraglottic larynx for nodal staging.

SUBGLOTTIS								
T/M \ **N**		cN0	cN1	cN2a	cN2b	cN2c	cN3a	cN3b
T1	Limited to subglottis	I	III	IVA			IVB	
T2	Extends to vocal cords with normal or impaired mobility	II	III	IVA			IVB	
T3	• Limited to larynx with vocal cord fixation • Invades*	IVA					IVB	
T4	**a.** Moderately advanced local disease**	IVA					IVB	
	b. Very advanced local disease†	IVA					IVB	
M1	Distant metastasis	IVC						

Notes: *Invasion of paraglottic space and/or inner cortex of thyroid cartilage.
**Invades through thyroid cartilage outer cortex, trachea, soft tissues of neck, deep extrinsic muscles of tongue, strap muscles, thyroid, or esophagus.
†Invades prevertebral space, encases carotid artery, or invades mediastinal structures.
Refer to supraglottic larynx for nodal staging.

TREATMENT PARADIGM

Surgery

Glottis: Modern surgical options for early glottic tumors focus on endoscopic resection with the aim of preserving laryngeal function and have largely replaced external approaches. Note that at least one mobile arytenoid complex must be preserved to maintain adequate function of the larynx. Endoscopic techniques can include mucosal stripping (for in situ disease), microdissection (including TORS), electrocautery, and CO_2 laser (TLM or TOLM), among others. Other voice-conserving options are as follows:

Vertical hemilaryngectomy: Removes up to one true vocal cord as well as one-third of the contralateral true cord. Appropriate for lesions with up to 1-cm anterior subglottic extension and 5-mm posterior subglottic extension.[5]

Supracricoid partial laryngectomy with cricohyoidopexy (SCPL–CHEP): Resection of true and false cords, paraglottic spaces, and the entire thyroid cartilage. Arytenoids and cricoid cartilage are preserved. CHEP is performed, which involves reconstruction by suturing the cricoid to the hyoid and epiglottis.

Supraglottis: Voice-preserving options include the following:

SGL: Swallow- and voice-preserving surgery that may be used for tumors of the epiglottis, single arytenoid, aryepiglottic fold, or false cord. Included in the resection: hyoid bone, epiglottis, superior half of thyroid cartilage, AE folds, and false cords.

SCPL–CHEP: Resection of both true and false cords, paraglottic space, preepiglottic space, epiglottis, and thyroid cartilage. Reconstruction includes suturing of the cricoid to the hyoid-cricohyoidopexy.

Total laryngectomy (TL): Removal of the larynx, reconstruction of the pharynx (often with free flap), and permanent stoma.

For patients treated with a primary surgical approach, elective neck dissection of bilateral levels II to IV is warranted for most patients with supraglottic cancer and for locally advanced glottic disease.

Systemic Therapy

Concurrent CHT is not routinely given for early-stage disease, but it is considered by some for unfavorable T2 disease (impaired mobility). In definitive CRT for T2b or stage III to IVB disease, concurrent cisplatin is the standard of care, given as 100 mg/m² bolus weeks 1, 4, and 7 (NCCN Category 1) OR 40 mg/m² weekly (NCCN category 2B). Cetuximab can be used for nonplatinum candidates, with loading dose of 400 mg/m² 1 week prior to RT followed by 250 mg/m² weekly during RT. Use of induction CHT is controversial but has been used to select patients for laryngectomy vs. preservation and consists of docetaxel, cisplatin, and 5-fluorouracil (TPF) q3 weeks × 4 cycles completed 4 to 7 weeks prior to RT. The use of immunotherapy for locally advanced laryngeal and hypopharyngeal cancer has been investigated in multiple randomized settings with negative results (see Chapter 11).

Radiation

Indications: Early-stage disease (cT1–T2N0) is typically treated with RT alone. Locally advanced disease is treated definitively (larynx preservation) or postoperatively (see Chapter 17). Nodal basins are not typically included in the elective RT volume in early-stage glottic patients unless supraglottic involvement is suspected, making the risk of occult nodal metastasis higher. Cervical LN levels II to IV are targeted bilaterally and level V is included for N+ hemineck or with primary tumor extension to BOT. Consider inclusion of level VIa for anterior thyroid cartilage/soft tissue extension or emergency tracheostomy with tumor cut-through. Consider level VIb with subglottic extension of primary tumor.

Dose: For T1N0 glottic cancers, accelerated hypofractionation has been shown to improve LC compared with standard fractionation. Recommended dose is 63 Gy/28 fx (2.25 Gy/fx). For T2aN0 disease, common dose is 65.25 Gy/29 fx. For patients with T2bN0 disease, LC is inferior with RT alone and thus alternative approaches including the addition of concurrent CHT or hyperfractionation are considered. For locally advanced disease, 70 Gy/35 fx with CHT is common.

Toxicity: Acute: fatigue, dysphagia, mucositis, hoarseness, xerostomia, odynophagia, RT dermatitis, dysgeusia, aspiration. Late: dysphagia, esophageal stricture, aspiration, hoarseness, neck fibrosis, stroke, hypothyroidism.

Procedure: See *Handbook of Treatment Planning in Radiation Oncology*, Chapter 4.[6]

EVIDENCE-BASED Q&A

EARLY-STAGE DISEASE

What is the general treatment paradigm for early-stage disease?

Both RT and laryngeal preservation surgery provide excellent outcomes for early-stage glottic cancer. Retrospective evidence demonstrates 5-year DFS above 90% for stage I disease and around 80% for stage II disease with either definitive RT or surgery[7]; however, randomized data are sparse. A small randomized trial published in 2014[8] did show less patient-reported hoarseness in those treated with RT compared with those treated with transoral laser surgery, but overall voice quality was similar. In general, voice quality is related to the amount of vocal cord resected.

What is the impact of larger fraction size for early-stage glottic cancer?

Mild hypofractionation and acceleration has shown consistent improvement in LC for early-stage glottic cancer.

Le, UCSF (*IJROBP* 1997, PMID 9300746): RR of 398 patients with T1–T2 glottic cancer (315 T1, 83 T2) treated with definitive RT to a median dose of 63 Gy. Overall, the 5-year LC was 85% for T1 patients and 70% for T2 patients. Anterior commissure involvement and earlier treatment era predicted for worse LC in T1 patients. See Table 14.3 for poor prognostic factors for LC in T2. **Conclusion: RT alone provides excellent LC for T1 lesions. Poor prognostic factors for LC in T2 disease include overall treatment time, smaller fraction size, lower total dose, impaired vocal cord (VC) mobility, and subglottic extension.**

Table 14.3 UCSF Experience in Early Larynx Cancer (cT2 patients)					
	5-Yr LC		**5-Yr LC**		**5-Yr LC**
Treatment time ≤43 days	100%	Fx size ≥ 2.25 Gy/day	100%	>65 Gy	78%
Treatment time >43 days	84%	Fx size < 1.8 Gy/day	44%	≤65 Gy	60%
p value	.003	*p* value	.003	*p* value	.01
No VC mobility impairment	79%	No subglottic extension	77%		
VC mobility impairment	45%	Subglottic extension	58%		
p value	.02	*p* value	.04		

Yamazaki, Japan (*IJROBP* 2006, PMID 16169681): PRT of 180 patients with T1N0 SCC of the glottis (80% T1a) treated with definitive RT and randomized to 2 Gy/fx or 2.25 Gy/fx. For the standard fractionation arm, patients were treated to 60 Gy for tumor length <⅔ of glottis and to 66 Gy for ≥⅔ of glottis. In the 2.25 Gy/fx arm, total dose was 56.25 for tumor length <⅔ and 63 Gy for tumor length ≥⅔ of glottis. The 5-year LC was 92% in hypofractionation arm compared with 77% in standard fractionation arm. Fraction size was an independent predictor for LC. Acute and late toxicities were equivalent. **Conclusion: Decreasing overall treatment time with larger fraction sizes improved LC without causing increased acute or late toxicity in patients with T1N0 glottic cancer.**

What is the impact of hyperfractionation (HFX) for early-stage glottic cancer?

RTOG 9512 demonstrated a modest but not statistically significant benefit in LC with use of HFX RT in patients with T2N0 glottic cancer. T2b was a negative prognostic factor.

Trotti, RTOG 9512 (*IJROBP* 2014, PMID 25035199): PRT of 250 patients with T2N0 SCC of the glottis treated with definitive RT randomized to HFX (79.2 Gy/66 fx at 1.2 Gy BID) or standard fractionation (70 Gy/35 fx). Primary endpoint was LC. Study powered to detect 15% absolute difference in 5-year LC. While there were trends toward improved outcomes with HFX, there were no significant differences in 5-year LC (78% vs. 70%, *p* = .14), 5-year DFS (49% vs. 40%, *p* = .13), or 5-year OS

(72% vs. 63%, *p* = .29). LC in T2b patients was relatively lower (70% T2b vs. 76% T2a, *p* = .1). No difference in rates of grades 3 to 4 late toxicities between treatment arms. **Conclusion: HFX modestly improves LC, although not statistically significant in this study.**

How should T2b glottic patients be treated?

T2b glottic cancer has not been adopted by the AJCC but has been described as the presence of a hypomobile cord. Patients with T2b disease had worse LC (70 vs. 76%, p = .10) and LRC (63% vs. 74%, p = .03) in RTOG 9512 as well as in other large retrospective series[9,10] and thus may benefit from alteration in standard treatment. Options to improve LC in this unfavorable subset include hyperfractionation, hypofractionation (e.g., 65.25 Gy/29 fx), or addition of concurrent CHT.[11]

Is there any role for IMRT in the early-stage population?

Early-stage glottic cancer is the last H&N subsite to adopt IMRT, with early series suggesting that carotid sparing is feasible without a detriment in LC.[12,13] The proposed rationale for the use of IMRT includes reducing late toxicity, particularly vascular toxicity with carotid sparing. Recently, a meta-analysis of 15 studies showed no difference in LC between IMRT and conventional RT, providing the strongest evidence for efficacy of IMRT in this population to date. Of note, SBRT for early-stage glottic cancer is being actively investigated. While data are mixed,[14-20] a recent phase II study showed acceptable rates of control and toxicity.[16]

Razavian, IMRT for Early-Stage Glottic Larynx Meta-Analysis (*IJROBP* 2023, PMID 37150263): Included 15 studies (14 retrospective, 1 prospective). 873 patients who received IMRT were compared with 738 patients who received conventional RT. There was no significant difference in local or regional failure between the two modalities. The pooled crude rate of regional failure post-IMRT was 1.5%. Increased rate of LF was associated with T2 disease and grades 2 to 3 histology. **Conclusion: IMRT is effective in early-stage glottic cancer and compares favorably to conventional techniques.**

LOCALLY ADVANCED DISEASE

What is the basis for larynx preservation for locally advanced disease?

While definitive surgery followed by PORT had been the traditional paradigm, the VA Larynx Study prospectively demonstrated equivalent survival rates with a nonoperative approach, and RTOG 91-11 demonstrated superior rates of larynx preservation with concurrent CRT compared with patients treated with either induction CHT followed by RT or RT alone. T4 patients had higher rates of salvage laryngectomy in the VA Larynx Study, and thus a large volume of T4 patients were excluded in RTOG 91-11. However, an NCDB analysis demonstrated that the majority of patients with T4a disease still undergo organ preservation in clinical practice, despite general guidelines, with inferior OS compared with those who had TL (median survival 61 vs. 39 months).[21] Multiple individual retrospective series have also identified tumor volume as prognostic of outcomes in addition to T stage.

Wolf, VA Larynx Study (*NEJM* 1991, PMID 2034244): PRT of 332 patients with stage III to IV locally advanced SCC of the larynx (63% supraglottis, 57% with vocal cord fixation) randomized to induction CHT followed by RT or TL followed by postop RT. Patients in the larynx preservation arm received cisplatin 100 mg/m^2 and 5-FU 1,000 mg/m^2/day × 5 days on days 1 and 22. Tumor response was assessed by exam and indirect laryngoscopy 18 to 21 days after the second cycle. Patients without at least PR in the larynx and those with any evidence of disease progression (including neck disease) underwent salvage laryngectomy. Patients with at least PR at the primary tumor site and no progression of any neck lymphadenopathy received the third cycle of CHT on day 43. Twelve weeks after completion of RT, tumor response was reassessed; patients with persistent disease in the larynx underwent salvage laryngectomy. Patients with persistent neck disease alone underwent neck dissection only. All patients randomized to initial TL underwent postop RT. MFU 33 months. See Table 14.4 for results. After 2C of induction CHT, 31% had CR and 54% had PR. Lack of response to induction CHT, however, was not associated with reduced OS. Rate of laryngeal preservation was 64%. Fifty-six percent of patients with T4 primary tumors required salvage laryngectomy (vs. 29% in the remainder of the study population). Rate of DM was lower in CHT arm, but LC was inferior. **Conclusion: Induction CHT followed by definitive RT can be effective in preserving the larynx in a high percentage of patients without compromising OS.**

Table 14.4 Results of VA Larynx Study

	2-Yr OS	2-Yr LC	Recurrence at Site of Primary	DM
Induction CHT + definitive RT	68%	80%	12%	11%
TL + PORT	68%	93%	2%	17%
p value	.9846	.001	.001	.001

Forastiere, RTOG 91-11 (*NEJM* 2003, PMID 14645636; Update *JCO* 2013, PMID 23182993): PRT of 518 patients with SCC of the supraglottic/glottic larynx, stage III to IV (T1 or T4 with tumor extending through the thyroid cartilage into the neck of soft tissue or >1 cm of BOT involvement was excluded) randomized to one of three arms: Arm 1 (induction, standard per VA Larynx): cisplatin 100 mg/m² day 1 + 5-FU 1,000 mg/m²/day for 5 days on day 1 and day 22 followed by response evaluation. Those with less than PR or progression proceeded to TL with PORT. Those with CR or PR continued to additional cycle of cisplatin/5-FU followed by RT alone, 70 Gy/35 fx. Arm 2 (CRT): cisplatin 100 mg/m² days 1, 22, and 43 concurrent with RT, 70 Gy/35 fx. Arm 3 (RT alone): 70 Gy/35 fx. Patients with single LN >3 cm or multiple LNs underwent neck dissection 8 weeks after completion of therapy. Seven endpoints were reported, but the primary endpoint was laryngectomy-free survival (LFS). In 2023 update (MFU 10.8 years), compared with induction, CRT improved larynx preservation (LP), LC, and LRC, but not LFS (primary endpoint), and trended to worse OS (*p* = .08), potentially suggestive of late effects from RT (see Table 14.5). **Conclusion: Concurrent CRT declared "winner" due to LRC and LP benefit, although LFS was similar.**

Table 14.5 Ten-Year Results of the RTOG 91-11 Larynx Preservation Trial

Arm	LFS (1°)	LP	LC	LRC	DC	DFS	OS
1. Induction	29%*	68%	54%	49%	83%	20%	39%
2. CRT	24%*	82%*†	69%*†	65%*†	84%	22%*	28%
3. RT alone	17%†	64%	50%	47%	76%	15%	32%

*Significant relative to RT alone.
†Significant relative to induction (standard arm).

What is the role of cetuximab in locally advanced laryngeal cancer?

The Bonner trial established a survival benefit with the addition of cetuximab to RT in patients with locally advanced HNSCC. While no statistically significant difference was noted in an unplanned secondary analysis of patients with laryngeal cancer,[22] cetuximab is still a Category 2B recommendation per NCCN and can be considered in those who are cisplatin-ineligible.

Bonner, Cetuximab Secondary Analysis (*JAMA Otolaryngol Head Neck Surg* 2016, PMID 27389475): Secondary analysis of the original Bonner trial investigating the role of concurrent cetuximab in LP. Arms included RT alone vs. RT + concurrent cetuximab; 168 patients with larynx or hypopharynx cancers were included in this subset (90 in cetuximab, 78 in RT alone). The 2-year rates of LP were 88% for cetuximab and 86% for RT alone (HR 0.57, 95% CI 0.23–1.42). HR for LFS was 0.78 (95% CI 0.54–1.11). No difference in OS. **Conclusion: There was not a statistically significant benefit to cetuximab with regard to larynx preservation and laryngectomy-free survival.** *Comment: Conclusions are limited by lack of power and nature of subset analysis.*

HYPOPHARYNX

What is the general treatment paradigm for hypopharynx cancer?

The hypopharynx represents a distinct H&N subsite. Below the oropharynx and posterior to the larynx, the hypopharynx is associated with a high risk of LN metastasis given the rich lymphatic drainage. Like larynx cancer, the goal of treatment is organ preservation due to the implications on speech and swallowing with radical resection. The standard nonoperative definitive treatment paradigm includes CRT, similar to other H&N subsites. Hypopharyngeal cancer has its own staging system outlined in the AJCC 8th edition,[23] with T staging including size and number of involved subsites. Similar to a larynx primary, early-stage disease (cT1–T2N0) is typically treated with RT alone or surgery. Locally advanced disease is treated definitively (larynx preservation) with either definitive CRT (typically to 70 Gy/35 fx with concurrent cisplatin) or induction CHT followed by CRT.[24] Due to rich lymphatic drainage, elective nodal irradiation includes bilateral retropharyngeal nodes and levels II to VI. Additional CTV margin is typically required along the PPW due to the contiguous nature without any natural barriers to spread.

REFERENCES

1. Siegel RL, Giaquinto AN, Jemal A. Cancer statistics, 2024. *CA Cancer J Clin.* 2024;74(1):12–49. doi:10.3322/caac.21820

2. Hoffman HT, Porter K, Karnell LH, et al. Laryngeal cancer in the United States: changes in demographics, patterns of care, and survival. *Laryngoscope.* 2006;116(9 Pt 2 Suppl 111):1–13. doi:10.1097/01.mlg.0000236095.97947.26

3. Dahm JD, Sessions DG, Paniello RC, Harvey J. Primary subglottic cancer. *Laryngoscope.* 1998;108(5):741–746. doi:10.1097/00005537-199805000-00022

4. Beitler JJ, Muller S, Grist WJ, et al. Prognostic accuracy of computed tomography findings for patients with laryngeal cancer undergoing laryngectomy. *J Clin Oncol.* May 10 2010;28(14):2318–2322. doi:10.1200/jco.2009.24.7544

5. Fein DA, Mendenhall WM, Parsons JT, Million RR. T1-T2 squamous cell carcinoma of the glottic larynx treated with radiotherapy: a multivariate analysis of variables potentially influencing local control. *Int J Radiat Oncol Biol Phys.* Mar 15 1993;25(4):605–611. doi:10.1016/0360-3016(93)90005-g

6. Videtic GMM, Woody NM, Vassil AD, eds. *Handbook of Treatment Planning in RT Oncology.* 3rd ed. Demos Medical; 2020.

7. Tamura Y, Tanaka S, Asato R, et al. Therapeutic outcomes of laryngeal cancer at Kyoto University Hospital for 10 years. *Acta Otolaryngol Suppl.* 2007;(557):62–65. doi:10.1080/00016480601067990

8. Aaltonen LM, Rautiainen N, Sellman J, et al. Voice quality after treatment of early vocal cord cancer: a randomized trial comparing laser surgery with radiation therapy. *Int J Radiat Oncol Biol Phys.* 2014;90(2):255–260. doi:10.1016/j.ijrobp.2014.06.032

9. Mendenhall WM, Amdur RJ, Morris CG, Hinerman RW. T1-T2N0 squamous cell carcinoma of the glottic larynx treated with radiation therapy. *J Clin Oncol.* 2001;19(20):4029–4036. doi:10.1200/JCO.2001.19.20.4029

10. Le QT, Fu KK, Kroll S, et al. Influence of fraction size, total dose, and overall time on local control of T1-T2 glottic carcinoma. *Int J Radiat Oncol Biol Phys.* 1997;39(1):115–126. doi:10.1016/s0360-3016(97)00284-8

11. Bhateja P, Ward MC, Hunter GH, et al. Impaired vocal cord mobility in T2N0 glottic carcinoma: suboptimal local control with radiation alone. *Head Neck.* 2016;38(12):1832–1836. doi:10.1002/hed.24520

12. Zumsteg ZS, Riaz N, Jaffery S, et al. Carotid sparing intensity-modulated radiation therapy achieves comparable locoregional control to conventional radiotherapy in T1-2N0 laryngeal carcinoma. *Oral Oncol.* 2015;51(7):716–723. doi:10.1016/j.oraloncology.2015.02.003

13. Ward MC, Pham YD, Kotecha R, Zakem SJ, Murray E, Greskovich JF. Clinical and dosimetric implications of intensity-modulated radiotherapy for early-stage glottic carcinoma. *Med Dosim.* 2016;41(1):64–69. doi:10.1016/j.meddos.2015.08.004

14. Al-Mamgani A, Kwa SL, Tans L, et al. Single vocal cord irradiation: image guided intensity modulated hypofractionated radiation therapy for T1a glottic cancer: early clinical results. *Int J Radiat Oncol Biol Phys.* 2015;93(2):337–343. doi:10.1016/j.ijrobp.2015.06.016

15. Sher DJ, Timmerman RD, Nedzi L, et al. Phase 1 fractional dose-escalation study of equipotent stereotactic radiation therapy regimens for early-stage glottic larynx cancer. *Int J Radiat Oncol Biol Phys.* 2019;105(1):110–118. doi:10.1016/j.ijrobp.2019.03.010

16. Sher DJ, Avkshtol V, Moon D, et al. Stereotactic ablative radiotherapy for T1 to T2 glottic larynx cancer: mature results from the phase 2 GLoTtic larynx-SABR trial. *Int J Radiat Oncol Biol Phys.* 2025;121(1):137–144. doi:10.1016/j.ijrobp.2024.07.2147

17. Kang BH, Yu T, Kim JH, et al. Early closure of a phase 1 clinical trial for SABR in early-stage glottic cancer. *Int J Radiat Oncol Biol Phys.* 2019;105(1):104–109. doi:10.1016/j.ijrobp.2019.03.011

18. Sanguineti G, Pellini R, Vidiri A, et al. Stereotactic body radiotherapy for T1 glottic cancer: dosimetric data in 27 consecutive patients. *Tumori.* 2021;107(6):514–524. doi:10.1177/03008916211000440

19. Sanguineti G, D'Urso P, Bottero M, et al. Stereotactic radiation therapy in 3 fractions for T1 glottic cancer. *Int J Radiat Oncol Biol Phys.* 2025;121(1):145–152. doi:10.1016/j.ijrobp.2024.09.051

20. Young MR, Decker RH. SBRT for early stage laryngeal cancer: progress, but not quite ready for prime time. *Int J Radiat Oncol Biol Phys.* 2019;105(1):121–123. doi:10.1016/j.ijrobp.2019.05.021

21. Grover S, Swisher-McClure S, Mitra N, et al. Total laryngectomy versus larynx preservation for T4a larynx cancer: patterns of care and survival outcomes. *Int J Radiat Oncol Biol Phys.* 2015;92(3):594–601. doi:10.1016/j.ijrobp.2015.03.004

22. Bonner J, Giralt J, Harari P, et al. Cetuximab and radiotherapy in laryngeal preservation for cancers of the larynx and hypopharynx: a secondary analysis of a randomized clinical trial. *JAMA Otolaryngol Head Neck Surg.* 2016;142(9):842–849. doi:10.1001/jamaoto.2016.1228

23. *AJCC Cancer Staging Manual.* 8th ed. Springer International Publishing; 2017.

24. Lefebvre JL, Andry G, Chevalier D, et al. Laryngeal preservation with induction chemotherapy for hypopharyngeal squamous cell carcinoma: 10-year results of EORTC trial 24891. *Ann Oncol.* 2012;23(10): 2708–2714. doi:10.1093/annonc/mds065

Jenna E. Kocsis, Sarah S. Kilic, and Shlomo A. Koyfman

QUICK HIT Salivary gland tumors are an uncommon group of benign and malignant neoplasms with natural histories that vary by histology. The most common benign histology is pleomorphic adenoma. The most common malignant histology depends on location: parotid gland, mucoepidermoid carcinoma; submandibular and minor salivary glands, adenoid cystic carcinoma. Surgery is the standard of care for all histologies, and the facial nerve should be preserved if possible. Postoperative RT should be considered for those at high risk of recurrence (Table 15.1). No benefit to CHT has been demonstrated prospectively.

Table 15.1 General Treatment Paradigm for Malignant Salivary Cancer				
Surgical Resection With Consideration of Adjuvant RT as Follows				
Primary Site			**Ipsilateral Neck**	
Stage I–II and no risk factors	Observation		**cN0 or pN0 and low risk**	Observation
T3–4, tumor spillage, PNI, deep lobe involvement, bone involvement, high grade, adenoid cystic histology, or recurrent disease	60 Gy		**pN0 with risk factors (see Terhaard and RTOG 1008): T3–4, high grade, facial nerve deficit, recurrent disease**	50–54 Gy levels II–IV
			Node-positive, resected	60 Gy levels Ib–V
Positive or close margins (<1 mm)	66 Gy		**ECE**	66 Gy
Gross disease	70 Gy		**Gross nodal disease**	70 Gy

EPIDEMIOLOGY: Salivary gland tumors are rare neoplasms that represent approximately 6% to 8% of H&N cancers,[1,2] with ~2,500 cases in the United States annually.[2] Benign and malignant histologies are slightly more common in females (mean age 52 for benign and 56 for malignant).[3] Histology is classified according to the WHO 5th edition published in 2022, with over 35 different histologies defined and more focus placed on molecular alterations.[4] The parotid gland is the most common site (60%–70% of all tumors, 70% of which are benign), with 32% in minor glands and 8% in submandibular glands.[1–3]

RISK FACTORS: Risk factors are not clearly defined. The strongest evidence is for RT exposure, as shown among Hiroshima/Nagasaki survivors.[5] Smoking is not a risk factor (except in Warthin's tumor). EBV has been implicated in lymphoepithelial carcinomas,[6] and other viruses such as HIV and HPV are under investigation.

Table 15.2 Characteristics of Salivary Tumors				
	Parotid	**Submandibular**	**Sublingual**	**Minor Glands**
Pathology[7,8]	75% benign, 25% malignant	50% benign, 50% malignant	75% malignant	
Frequency[7]	70%	8%	22%	
Salivary fluid[8,9]	Serous	Mixed	Mucous	
Associated nerves	CN VII (facial) with spread to V3 via chorda tympani	V3 (lingual) and XII (hypoglossal)	V3 (lingual)	Location-dependent

ANATOMY: Major salivary glands consist of parotid, submandibular, and sublingual gland (between mylohyoid and floor of mouth mucosa). The borders of parotid are the second maxillary molar (anterior), zygomatic arch (superior), internal jugular vein (deep), mastoid tip (posterior), and posterior digastric muscle (inferior). Parotid contributes primarily to stimulated serous saliva production, and submandibular to unstimulated mucous/serous saliva (and therefore RT-induced xerostomia).[10] Parotid lies behind the ramus of the mandible and is separated into superficial and deep lobes by facial nerve. Retromandibular vein is a common radiographic landmark for facial nerve. Stensen's duct drains to buccal mucosa. Facial nerve (CN VII) courses through parotid after exiting stylomastoid foramen. There are five branches of CN VII: temporal, zygomatic, buccal, marginal mandibular, and cervical. CN VII controls facial muscles and taste to oral tongue. Auriculotemporal nerve originates from V3, innervates parotid (salivation/parasympathetic), and can be route of perineural spread; if damaged during surgery, this can aberrantly regenerate to innervate skin, causing auriculotemporal syndrome (preauricular sweating and flushing), also called Frey syndrome.[10] Submandibular gland is innervated by the chorda tympani, and perineural spread can be to CN XII, to CN V via lingual nerve, or to CN VII via chorda tympani. Minor salivary glands are distributed throughout aerodigestive epithelium. Multiple contouring guides are available to aid in the anatomy of cranial nerves when PNI is present.[11,12]

PATHOLOGY: Characteristics of salivary tumors are outlined in Table 15.2. The most common histologies are listed in Tables 15.3 and 15.4, in order of decreasing incidence. Grade is prognostic of mucoepidermoid carcinoma, adenocarcinoma (ACA), salivary duct carcinoma, and acinic cell carcinoma.[2] Adenoid cystic carcinoma (ACC) is graded by percentage of solid component (high grade if >30% solid).

Table 15.3 Benign Salivary Tumor Histologies	
Pleomorphic adenoma	Most common salivary gland tumor, two-thirds of parotid tumors, two-thirds are females in their 40s. Treatment is surgery, with <5% risk of recurrence, but beware of tumor spillage, in which case recurrence can be up to 45%. Risk of second recurrence is 46%. Can transform into carcinoma *ex* pleomorphic adenoma (CExP). Rate of transformation is <1% in patients without recurrence; 4% with recurrence.[9] Consider RT to 50–60 Gy for multiple recurrences, deep involvement, or large tumors.[13]
Warthin's tumor	Often of parotid and often bilateral (6%).[14] Associated with smoking, more common in men.[15] Can be highly PET-avid and is often an incidental finding. Malignant degeneration is rare (<1%)[8]; observation is reasonable.
Basal cell adenoma	~2% of salivary tumors.[8] May be confused with basal cell of skin metastatic to parotid LN.
Oncocytoma	1% of salivary tumors. Slowly progressive parotid tumor in older patients.

Table 15.4 Malignant Salivary Tumor Histologies	
Mucoepidermoid	Most common parotid malignancy. Grade is prognostic.
Adenoid cystic carcinoma (ACC)	Almost always demonstrates PNI and can track along cranial nerves. Tubular pattern is most favorable, cribriform is intermediate, and solid is least favorable. >30% solid pattern is considered high-grade. Long natural history. Risk of nodal involvement classically thought to be <5%, but recent data as high as 37% in oral cavity and 19% in major glands.[16,17] Indolent DM to lungs in up to 50%.[8] Late recurrences (>20 years) can be seen. Most benefit from adjuvant RT.[18]
Adenocarcinoma, NOS	Grade is prognostic, nodal metastases seen in 50%–60% of high-grade lesions.[17]
Acinic cell carcinoma	Low-grade, slowly progressive tumors, 80% within parotid. Submandibular tumors are uncommon and most aggressive.[8] Can undergo high-grade transformation, which should be treated aggressively with multimodality therapy.[19,20]
Carcinoma *ex* pleomorphic adenoma (CExP)	4% of salivary tumors, 12% of malignancies. Degenerated pleomorphic adenoma. More than 80% of patients do not have history of known pleomorphic adenoma.[8]
Salivary duct carcinoma	9% of salivary malignancies. More common in males (4:1). Aggressive, high-grade, similar to high-grade breast ductal carcinoma.[8] Androgen receptor and HER2 amplification common.

(continued)

Table 15.4 Malignant Salivary Tumor Histologies (*continued*)	
Metastasis to salivary gland	5% of salivary malignancies[8]; incidence varies by region based on frequency of skin cancer. Squamous histology is assumed to be a metastasis from a cutaneous primary until proven otherwise, as primary squamous of the parotid is very rare.
Epithelial– myoepithelial	Only 1% of salivary tumors, twice as common in women, 60% parotid, typically slow-growing. Can have high rates of LR, 30%–50% of patients.[21,22]

GENETICS: EGFR, c-kit, HER2, NTRK fusion, and androgen receptor positivity have all been described, most commonly in salivary duct carcinomas,[23] but no standard role for targeted or hormonal agents in the nonmetastatic setting.

CLINICAL PRESENTATION: Most present initially as a slowly progressive painless mass. ACC may present initially as neuropathic pain (misdiagnosis as trigeminal neuralgia) and progress to facial nerve motor deficit.

WORKUP: H&P, including H&N exam with cranial nerve exam. Ultrasound can be helpful to differentiate between benign and malignant prior to biopsy. FNA sensitivity and specificity are 80% and >95%, respectively.[13] Contrast-enhanced MRI is critical for evaluation of perineural spread in malignant histologies. CT chest for malignant histologies. PET is not standard, but it may be performed for advanced stage high-grade tumors.[24] Dental, nutrition, speech, and swallow evaluation as indicated.

PROGNOSTIC FACTORS: Stage, grade, histology, recurrence, positive margins, bone invasion, positive LNs, facial nerve palsy.[13,25,26] Staging outlined in Table 15.5.

TREATMENT PARADIGM

Observation: Observation can be appropriate for benign histologies other than pleomorphic adenoma. Pleomorphic adenoma should be treated upfront in healthy patients due to risk of malignant transformation. Malignant histologies should always be treated.

Surgery: Surgical resection of the primary tumor is the standard of care for all technically resectable salivary gland tumors warranting treatment. Care should be taken to minimize risk of tumor spillage; enucleation should not be performed. Partial superficial parotidectomy is appropriate for superficial T1 or T2 low-grade tumors, and at least a superficial parotidectomy with consideration of a total or subtotal parotidectomy should be performed for any high-grade or T3–4 parotid cancer.[24] Preservation of functional cranial nerves should be attempted. Microscopic margins are preferred over facial nerve sacrifice, although not at the expense of residual gross disease.[27] Consider nerve grafting for reconstruction of sacrificed cranial nerve. For all locations and histologies, cN+ neck should be dissected. For parotid tumors, elective nodal dissection of ipsilateral levels II to III, and possibly IV, may be recommended, and is surgeon-dependent based on risk factors (size, stage, grade, histology, location). For submandibular tumors, elective ipsilateral dissection of levels I to III is surgeon-dependent. For parotid tumors, levels I and V may be at risk only if levels II to IV are involved.[13]

Table 15.5 AJCC 8th Edition (2017): Staging for Salivary Gland Cancer			cN0	cN1	cN2a	cN2b	cN2c	cN3a	cN3b
T/M	N								
T1	• ≤2 cm		I						
T2	• 2.1–4 cm		II	III		IVA			
T3	• >4 cm and/or extraparenchymal extension								
T4a	• Invasion[1]								
T4b	• Invasion[2]					IVB			
M1	• Distant metastasis					IVC			

Notes: Invasion[1] = invasion of skin, mandible, ear canal, or facial nerve. Invasion[2] = invasion of skull base, pterygoid plates, and/or encasing carotid artery. Nodal classification is similar to other non-HPV-associated H&N cancers; see Table 11.4 for clinical and pathologic nodal categories. Minor salivary cancers are staged according to their site of origin.

Chemotherapy: The addition of CHT for high-risk lesions is investigational and retrospective data are inconsistent.[28–30] The results of RTOG 1008 are pending as of publication (phase II/III study of adjuvant RT 60–66 Gy vs. adjuvant RT 60–66 Gy with concurrent cisplatin 40 mg/m2 weekly). RTOG 1008 included nonmetastatic patients with resected intermediate- or high-grade ACA, intermediate- or high-grade mucoepidermoid carcinoma, high-grade salivary duct carcinoma, high-grade acinic cell carcinoma, and high-grade (>30% solid component) ACC with any of the following risk factors: T3–T4, N+, or T1–T2 AND positive/close (≤1 mm) margins.

For inoperable primary tumors, recurrent tumors, and metastatic disease, systemic therapy has shown varying success rates.[31] Early studies using targeted agents (imatinib,[32] lapatinib,[33] and dasatinib[34]) have had disappointing results. However, the tyrosine kinase inhibitors (TKIs) larotrectinib and entrectinib have shown encouraging response rates (>75%) for NTRK fusion-positive tumors across various primary sites,[35] and axitinib was shown to improve 6-month PFS when compared with observation (73% vs. 23%) in patients with recurrent or metastatic ACC.[36] Phase I/II studies of androgen blockade (for androgen receptor-positive salivary duct carcinomas),[37] lenvatinib (for ACC),[38] and pembrolizumab (for any PD-L1-positive histology)[39] have shown some promise. Trastuzumab + docetaxel in locally advanced, recurrent, or metastatic salivary duct carcinoma was shown to have an overall response rate of 70% with mPFS of 8.9 months.[40] Ongoing trials investigating the role of T-DM1 in HER2-amplified salivary gland tumors.

Radiation

Indications and Dose: Consider PORT for pT3–4 disease, close or positive margins, high-grade, recurrent disease, positive LN, PNI, LVSI, or bone invasion. ACCs typically display significant PNI, and RT should be offered.[24] NCCN recommends 60 Gy to primary site and 54 Gy to elective neck (if included via SIB). Dose should be escalated to 66 Gy for positive margins or ECE, and to 70 Gy for gross disease.[13,41] Treatment of ipsilateral neck for pathologically node-positive disease is required, and elective nodal coverage should be considered for pT3–4, high-grade, facial nerve deficits, or recurrent disease. Hypofractionated RT using 50 Gy/20 fx has been studied retrospectively with excellent 2-year locoregional control, low mucosal doses, and no acute or late grade 4 or 5 toxicities.[42] Definitive RT up to 70 Gy can be considered for those who are medically inoperable or those with unresectable disease. Proton therapy has been shown to have low rates of acute mucosal toxicity (grade ≥2 mucositis 14%) and high rates of LC (2-year 96%).[43] For all cases with extensive facial nerve invasion or ACC histology, cover facial nerve pathway (or other involved cranial nerves) up to the base of skull.[44] If the stylomastoid foramen is involved, target the facial nerve to the geniculate ganglion. Similarly, if CN V is involved at the foramen rotundum or ovale, treat proximally to include the Gasserian ganglion in Meckel's cave. If Meckel's cave is involved, cover the entirety of the nerve root as it exits the brainstem.

Procedure: See *Handbook of Treatment Planning in Radiation Oncology*, Chapter 4.[45]

Complications: Oral mucositis, odynophagia, skin erythema, altered taste, partial xerostomia, trismus, hypothyroidism, and ear complications (secretory otitis media or partial hearing loss). Limit contralateral parotid and submandibular dose to <5 Gy and aggressively spare midline structures (oral cavity, larynx, constrictors, spinal cord) to a mean of <20 Gy if possible.

Neutrons: Higher LC, but more late effects than photons.[27] RBE is >2.6. Neutrons lack skin sparing, are less affected by hypoxia, and are less cell cycle-dependent than photons. Consider for unresectable or recurrent tumors, particularly ACC. In one small series of tumors involving the base of the skull, 3-year LC doubled (from 39% to 82%) with SRS boost following neutron treatment, without increased toxicity.[46] Complications include osteoradionecrosis, fibrosis, cervical myelopathy, CNS necrosis, optic neuritis, palatal fistula, retinopathy, and glaucoma.

EVIDENCE-BASED Q&A

What are the indications for postoperative RT?

Because salivary cancer is relatively rare, no prospective trials have been performed. Therefore, indications for PORT are based on retrospective evidence.[47–50] In general, adjuvant RT indications include pT3–4 disease, close or positive margins, high-grade, recurrent disease, positive LN, PNI, LVSI, or bone invasion.

Terhaard, Netherlands (*Head & Neck* 2005, PMID 15629600): RR of 498 patients treated for salivary cancers between 1984 and 1995; 386 patients received RT to a median dose of 62 Gy (60.7 Gy for negative margins, 62.4 Gy for close, and 64 Gy for positive). Forty percent received elective nodal RT. Results summarized in Table 15.6. The 10-year LC improved for those with T3–4 tumors, close (<5 mm) and positive margins, PNI, and bone invasion. Unresectable patients showed dose response, with 5-year LC of 0% for <66 Gy and 50% for ≥66 Gy. **Conclusion: Postoperative RT is indicated for T3–4 disease, close or positive margins, bone invasion, and PNI. Risk of nodal disease was defined using T stage and histology.**

Table 15.6 Results of Terhaard et al.[47]

10-Yr Local Control	No RT	RT	Risk of Positive Neck Nodes (%) by Score and Primary Location				
			T Score + Histology Score*	Parotid	Submandibular	Oral Cavity	Other
T3–4 tumor	18%	84%	2	4%	0%	4%	0%
Close margins	55%	95%	3	12%	33%	13%	29%
Positive margins	44%	82%	4	25%	57%	19%	56%
Bone invasion	54%	86%	5	33%	60%	–	–
PNI	60%	88%	6	38%	50%	–	–
All results statistically significant.			*Scoring: T1 = 1, T2 = 2, T3–4 = 3. Acinic/adenoid cystic/CExP = 1, MucoEp = 2, Squamous/Undifferentiated = 3.				

Source: Data from Terhaard CH, Lubsen H, Rasch CR, et al. The role of radiotherapy in the treatment of malignant salivary gland tumors. *Int J Radiat Oncol Biol Phys.* 2005;61(1):103–111. doi:10.1016/j.ijrobp.2004.03.018.

Cho, Korea (*Ann Surg Oncol* **2016, PMID 27342828):** RR of 179 patients with low-grade salivary gland cancers. The 10-year OS was 97% and RFS was 90%. Adjuvant RT improved RFS for patients with N+, PNI, LVSI, extraparenchymal extension, positive margin, or T3–4. Close margins (<5 mm) did not increase risk of recurrence. T1–2 patients without risk factors had low risk of recurrence after surgery alone. **Conclusion: Adjuvant RT improves RFS for low-grade salivary tumors, with risk factors including T3–4, positive margin, N+, PNI, LVSI, or extraparenchymal extension. Those without risk factors have good outcomes after surgery alone.**

Sajisevi, AHNS (*JAMA H&N Surgery* **2023, PMID 38095911):** RR of 865 patients with low- and intermediate-grade salivary carcinomas with close or positive margins treated from 2010 to 2019 at 41 centers. Ninety-three percent had parotid carcinoma and 86% had low-grade tumors. Seventy-eight percent had an R0 resection, 19% with R1, and 3% with R2. Close margins (defined as ≤1 mm) seen in 79% of those with R0. A total of 305 patients (35%) underwent PORT. Of all patients, 4% had an LR with MFU of 35.3 months. In patients with close margins as the sole risk factor for recurrence, LR rates were similar in those who underwent PORT (0%) vs. observation (2%). Patients with clear margins had no recurrences. LRR with R1 and R2 margins was improved with PORT (2% vs. 20%; HR 0.05, 95% CI 0.01–0.24). **Conclusion: In those with low- and intermediate-grade salivary gland carcinoma with close surgical margins (≤1 mm) as the only risk factor for LR, observation may be considered.**

Which patients are at higher risk of nodal metastasis?

High-grade, vascular invasion, facial nerve palsy, histology, and higher T stage appear to predict risk for nodal metastases. The three most common histologies with occult nodal metastases are ACA, CExP, and salivary duct carcinoma.

Xiao, NCDB Analysis (*Otolaryngol Head Neck Surg* **2016, PMID 26419838):** NCDB analysis of 22,653 cases of primary parotid cancer with pathologic LN evaluation. N0 patients had improved 5-year OS compared with N+ (79% vs. 40%, $p < .001$). Patients with low-grade tumors had improved 5-year OS vs. high-grade (88% vs. 69%, $p < .001$). Overall incidence of nodal and occult disease by histology outlined in Table 15.7. Incidence of N+ independently predicted by high grade (51% vs. 9% in low grade) and high T stage. **Conclusion: Incidence of occult nodal disease varies by histology. High T stage and grade predict nodal disease in most histologies.**

Table 15.7 Incidence of Nodal Metastases in Parotid Malignancies			
Primary Parotid Cancer Histology	cN+ (%)	Occult N+ (%)	Occult N+ (% if High-Grade/T4)
Salivary ductal carcinoma	54	24	36/40
Adenocarcinoma NOS	45	20	32/32
Carcinoma *ex* pleomorphic adenoma	24	12	19/36
Mucoepidermoid carcinoma	20	9	22/22
Adenoid cystic carcinoma	14	7	10/13
Acinar cell carcinoma	10	4	25/12
Basal cell ACA	9	6	7/22
Epithelial–myoepithelial carcinoma	5	2	0/0
Average	24.4	10.2	

Warshavsky, Meta-Analysis (*Ann Surg Oncol* 2021, PMID 33175260): Meta-analysis of nine retrospective studies from 1980 to 2019 of patients with parotid malignancies who underwent elective neck dissection. Using a random-effect model for each LN level, the risk of occult N+ in level 1 ranged from 0% to 9%, level 2 from 3% to 28%, level 3 from 0% to 22%, level 4 from 0% to 17%, and level 5 from 0% to 12%. The three most common tumors with occult nodal metastases were ACA, CExP, and salivary duct carcinoma. **Conclusion: The rate of occult nodal metastases is low in parotid tumors, with neck level 2 being the most commonly involved.**

Can salivary cancer be treated with RT alone?

Based on retrospective evidence, surgery is essential for LC and is the accepted standard of care for medically operable and technically resectable patients.

Mendenhall, University of Florida (*Cancer* 2005, PMID 15880750): RR of 224 patients treated from 1964 to 2003 with RT alone ($n = 64$) or surgery with RT ($n = 160$). Median dose was 74 Gy for RT alone and 66 Gy for postoperative. LRC was significantly worse with RT alone (stages I–III 89% vs. 70%, $p = .01$; stage IV 66% vs. 24%, $p = .002$; overall 81% vs. 40%, $p < .0001$). In patients with technically unresectable disease treated with RT alone, the 10-year LRC was 20%. **Conclusion: RT alone is inferior to surgery combined with RT in terms of LRC.**

Does the addition of adjuvant CRT improve outcomes compared with adjuvant RT alone?

Several small retrospective analyses have demonstrated promising control rates.[28–30] Conversely, an NCDB analysis actually revealed inferior survival with adjuvant CRT compared with RT alone.[51] RTOG 1008 is a phase II/III RCT that aims to answer this question in high-risk salivary gland cancer.

Amini, NCDB (*JAMA Otolaryngol Head Neck Surg* 2016, PMID 27541166): NCDB analysis of 2,210 patients with salivary gland cancer s/p resection comparing adjuvant CRT with adjuvant RT alone. Included those with grade 2 or 3 disease and ≥1 adverse feature (T3–4, N+, or positive margins). Eighty-three percent received RT and 17% received CRT. At MFU of 39 months, the 5-year OS was inferior with CRT compared with RT alone (39% vs. 54%, $p < .001$). OS with CRT was inferior on MVA (HR 1.22, $p = .02$) and trended to inferiority on propensity score matched analysis (HR 1.20, $p = .08$). **Conclusion: In high-risk salivary gland cancer, adjuvant CRT was not associated with improved OS compared with adjuvant RT alone and may actually worsen outcomes.**

Does neutron therapy offer improved control or survival outcomes?

LC is improved, but without a survival benefit. Cost and toxicity are significant with neutron therapy.

Laramore, RTOG 8001-MRC Trial (*IJROBP* 1993, PMID 8407397): PRT in England and the United States of 25 patients with inoperable or unresectable salivary cancer randomized to photon/electron therapy or neutron therapy. CR was more frequent in neutron arm. LC was significantly improved in neutron arm (56% vs. 17%, $p = .009$), leading to early closure of trial. No difference in OS (15% vs. 25%, $p = NS$). However, severe late complications were seen in 69% of neutron patients vs. 15% of photon patients ($p = .07$). **Conclusion: Neutron RT improves LC but not survival, with significant long-term toxicity.**

Douglas, University of Washington (*Arch Otolaryngol Head Neck Surg* 2003, PMID 12975266): RR of 279 patients treated with fast neutrons for salivary gland cancers, 263 of whom had evidence of gross disease at the time of treatment. MFU 36 months. Total dose delivered between 17.4 and 20.7 nGy, with fractions given three to four times per week. CSS and LRC were 67% and 59% at 6 years, respectively. Grades 3 to 4 RTOG toxicity at 6 years was 10%. **Conclusion: For gross residual disease, neutrons offer modest LC and good survival outcomes.**

Is modern RT as effective as neutron therapy with less toxicity?

This was suggested by a small RR from MSKCC, although data are limited.

Spratt, MSKCC (*Radiol Oncol* 2014, PMID 24587780): RR of 27 patients with unresectable salivary cancer treated with photons to a median dose of 70 Gy with IMRT or 3D-CRT. Eighteen patients also received CHT. At MFU of 52 months, the 5-year LRC was 47%, which compared favorably to the neutron arm of RTOG 8001. **Conclusion: Modern photon therapy with or without CHT may be a reasonable alternative to neutrons with less toxicity.**

Is there a role for carbon ion therapy in the treatment of salivary gland tumors?

Jensen, COSMIC Trial (*IJROBP* 2015, PMID 26279022): *German prospective phase II trial of 53 patients with malignant salivary gland tumors. All patients treated with 24 Gy (RBE) C12 followed by IMRT 50 Gy. MFU 42 months. At 3 years, LC was 82%, PFS 58%, and OS 78%. High rates of long-term hearing impairment (25%) and "adverse events of the eye" (20%).* **Conclusion: Carbon ion + IMRT treatment offered good control outcomes but with significant late toxicities.**

REFERENCES

1. El-Naggar AK, Chan JKC, Grandis JR, Takata T, Slootweg PJ, eds. *World Health Organization Classification of Tumours of Head and Neck.* 4th ed. Vol 9. IARC; 2017.
2. Guzzo M, Locati LD, Prott FJ, Gatta G, McGurk M, Licitra L. Major and minor salivary gland tumors. *Crit Rev Oncol Hematol.* 2010;74(2):134–148. doi:10.1016/j.critrevonc.2009.10.004
3. Alsanie I, Rajab S, Cottom H, et al. Distribution and frequency of salivary gland tumours: an international multicenter study. *Head Neck Pathol.* 2022;16(4):1043–1054. doi:10.1007/s12105-022-01459-0
4. Skalova A, Hyrcza MD, Leivo I. Update from the 5th edition of the World Health Organization classification of head and neck tumors: salivary glands. *Head Neck Pathol.* 2022;16(1):40–53. doi:10.1007/s12105-022-01420-1
5. Saku T, Hayashi Y, Takahara O, et al. Salivary gland tumors among atomic bomb survivors, 1950–1987. *Cancer.* 1997;79(8):1465–1475.
6. Leung SY, Chung LP, Yuen ST, Ho CM, Wong MP, Chan SY. Lymphoepithelial carcinoma of the salivary gland: in situ detection of Epstein-Barr virus. *J Clin Pathol.* 1995;48(11):1022–1027. doi:10.1136/jcp.48.11.1022
7. Spiro RH. Salivary neoplasms: overview of a 35-year experience with 2,807 patients. *Head Neck Surg.* 1986;8(3):177–184. doi:10.1002/hed.2890080309
8. Fang P. Internal mammary misfortune. *Int J Radiat Oncol Biol Phys.* 2017;97(3):447. doi:10.1016/j.ijrobp.2016.10.032
9. Andreasen S, Therkildsen MH, Bjorndal K, Homoe P. Pleomorphic adenoma of the parotid gland 1985-2010: a Danish nationwide study of incidence, recurrence rate, and malignant transformation. *Head Neck.* 2016;38(suppl 1):E1364–E1369. doi:10.1002/hed.24228
10. Motz KM, Kim YJ. Auriculotemporal syndrome (Frey syndrome). *Otolaryngol Clin North Am.* 2016;49(2):501–509. doi:10.1016/j.otc.2015.10.010
11. Gluck I, Ibrahim M, Popovtzer A, et al. Skin cancer of the head and neck with perineural invasion: defining the clinical target volumes based on the pattern of failure. *Int J Radiat Oncol Biol Phys.* 2009;74(1):38–46. doi:10.1016/j.ijrobp.2008.06.1943
12. Ko HC, Gupta V, Mourad WF, et al. A contouring guide for head and neck cancers with perineural invasion. *Pract Radiat Oncol.* 2014;4(6):e247–e258. doi:10.1016/j.prro.2014.02.001
13. Halperin EC, Brady LW, Perez CA, Wazer DE. *Perez & Brady's Principles and Practice of Radiation Oncology.* Lippincott Williams & Wilkins; 2013.
14. Maiorano E, Lo Muzio L, Favia G, Piattelli A. Warthin's tumour: a study of 78 cases with emphasis on bilaterality, multifocality and association with other malignancies. *Oral Oncol.* 2002;38(1):35–40. doi:10.1016/s1368-8375(01)00019-7

15. Pinkston JA, Cole P. Cigarette smoking and Warthin's tumor. *Am J Epidemiol.* 1996;144(2):183–187. doi:10.1093/oxfordjournals.aje.a008906

16. Amit M, Binenbaum Y, Sharma K, et al. Incidence of cervical lymph node metastasis and its association with outcomes in patients with adenoid cystic carcinoma. An international collaborative study. *Head Neck.* 2015;37(7):1032–1037. doi:10.1002/hed.23711

17. Xiao CC, Zhan KY, White-Gilbertson SJ, Day TA. Predictors of nodal metastasis in parotid malignancies: a National Cancer Data Base study of 22,653 patients. *Otolaryngol Head Neck Surg.* 2016;154(1):121–130. doi:10.1177/0194599815607449

18. Lee A, Givi B, Osborn VW, Schwartz D, Schreiber D. Patterns of care and survival of adjuvant radiation for major salivary adenoid cystic carcinoma. *Laryngoscope.* 2017;127(9):2057–2062. doi:10.1002/lary.26516

19. Stanley RJ, Weiland LH, Olsen KD, Pearson BW. Dedifferentiated acinic cell (acinous) carcinoma of the parotid gland. *Otolaryngol Head Neck Surg.* 1988;98(2):155–161. doi:10.1177/019459988809800210

20. Chintakuntlawar AV, Shon W, Erickson-Johnson M, et al. High-grade transformation of acinic cell carcinoma: an inadequately treated entity? *Oral Surg Oral Med Oral Pathol Oral Radiol.* 2016;121(5):542–549.e1. doi:10.1016/j.oooo.2016.01.011

21. Seethala RR, Barnes EL, Hunt JL. Epithelial-myoepithelial carcinoma: a review of the clinicopathologic spectrum and immunophenotypic characteristics in 61 tumors of the salivary glands and upper aerodigestive tract. *Am J Surg Pathol.* 2007;31(1):44–57. doi:10.1097/01.pas.0000213314.74423.d8

22. Nakaguro M, Nagao T. Epithelial-myoepithelial carcinoma. *Surg Pathol Clin.* 2021;14(1):97–109. doi:10.1016/j.path.2020.10.002

23. Can NT, Lingen MW, Mashek H, et al. Expression of hormone receptors and HER-2 in benign and malignant salivary gland tumors. *Head Neck Pathol.* 2018;12(1):95–104. doi:10.1007/s12105-017-0833-y

24. Geiger JL, Ismaila N, Beadle B, et al. Management of salivary gland malignancy: ASCO guideline. *J Clin Oncol.* 2021;39(17):1909–1941. doi:10.1200/JCO.21.00449

25. Carrillo JF, Vazquez R, Ramirez-Ortega MC, Cano A, Ochoa-Carrillo FJ, Onate-Ocana LF. Multivariate prediction of the probability of recurrence in patients with carcinoma of the parotid gland. *Cancer.* 2007;109(10):2043–2051. doi:10.1002/cncr.22647

26. Storey MR, Garden AS, Morrison WH, Eicher SA, Schechter NR, Ang KK. Postoperative radiotherapy for malignant tumors of the submandibular gland. *Int J Radiat Oncol Biol Phys.* 2001;51(4):952–958. doi:10.1016/s0360-3016(01)01724-2

27. Douglas JG, Koh WJ, Austin-Seymour M, Laramore GE. Treatment of salivary gland neoplasms with fast neutron radiotherapy. *Arch Otolaryngol Head Neck Surg.* 2003;129(9):944–948. doi:10.1001/archotol.129.9.944

28. Pederson AW, Salama JK, Haraf DJ, et al. Adjuvant chemoradiotherapy for locoregionally advanced and high-risk salivary gland malignancies. *Head Neck Oncol.* 2011;3:31. doi:10.1186/1758-3284-3-31

29. Schoenfeld JD, Sher DJ, Norris CM Jr, et al. Salivary gland tumors treated with adjuvant intensity-modulated radiotherapy with or without concurrent chemotherapy. *Int J Radiat Oncol Biol Phys.* 2012;82(1):308–314. doi:10.1016/j.ijrobp.2010.09.042

30. Tanvetyanon T, Qin D, Padhya T, et al. Outcomes of postoperative concurrent chemoradiotherapy for locally advanced major salivary gland carcinoma. *Arch Otolaryngol Head Neck Surg.* 2009;135(7):687–692. doi:10.1001/archoto.2009.70

31. Cohen EE, Karrison TG, Kocherginsky M, et al. Phase III randomized trial of induction chemotherapy in patients with N2 or N3 locally advanced head and neck cancer. *J Clin Oncol.* 2014;32(25):2735–2743. doi:10.1200/JCO.2013.54.6309

32. Hotte SJ, Winquist EW, Lamont E, et al. Imatinib mesylate in patients with adenoid cystic cancers of the salivary glands expressing c-kit: a Princess Margaret Hospital phase II consortium study. *J Clin Oncol.* 2005;23(3):585–590. doi:10.1200/JCO.2005.06.125

33. Agulnik M, Cohen EW, Cohen RB, et al. Phase II study of lapatinib in recurrent or metastatic epidermal growth factor receptor and/or erbB2 expressing adenoid cystic carcinoma and non adenoid cystic carcinoma malignant tumors of the salivary glands. *J Clin Oncol.* 2007;25(25):3978–3984. doi:10.1200/JCO.2007.11.8612

34. Wong SJ, Karrison T, Hayes DN, et al. Phase II trial of dasatinib for recurrent or metastatic c-KIT expressing adenoid cystic carcinoma and for nonadenoid cystic malignant salivary tumors. *Ann Oncol.* 2016;27(2):318–323. doi:10.1093/annonc/mdv537

35. Cocco E, Scaltriti M, Drilon A. NTRK fusion-positive cancers and TRK inhibitor therapy. *Nat Rev Clin Oncol.* 2018;15(12):731–747. doi:10.1038/s41571-018-0113-0

36. Kang EJ, Ahn MJ, Ock CY, et al. Randomized phase II study of axitinib versus observation in patients with recurred or metastatic adenoid cystic carcinoma. *Clin Cancer Res.* 2021;27(19):5272–5279. doi:10.1158/1078-0432.CCR-21-1061

37. Fushimi C, Tada Y, Takahashi H, et al. A prospective phase II study of combined androgen blockade in patients with androgen receptor-positive metastatic or locally advanced unresectable salivary gland carcinoma. *Ann Oncol.* 2018;29(4):979–984. doi:10.1093/annonc/mdx771

38. Tchekmedyian V, Sherman EJ, Dunn L, et al. Phase II study of lenvatinib in patients with progressive, recurrent or metastatic adenoid cystic carcinoma. *J Clin Oncol.* 2019;37(18):1529–1537. doi:10.1200/JCO.18.01859

39. Cohen RB, Delord JP, Doi T, et al. Pembrolizumab for the treatment of advanced salivary gland carcinoma: findings of the phase 1b KEYNOTE-028 study. *Am J Clin Oncol.* 2018;41(11):1083–1088. doi:10.1097/COC.0000000000000429

40. Takahashi H, Tada Y, Saotome T, et al. Phase II trial of trastuzumab and docetaxel in patients with human epidermal growth factor receptor 2-positive salivary duct carcinoma. *J Clin Oncol.* 2019;37(2):125–134. doi:10.1200/JCO.18.00545

41. National Comprehensive Cancer Network. *NCCN Clinical Practice Guidelines in Oncology: Head and Neck Cancers.* Accessed April 16, 2024. https://www.nccn.org/professionals/physician_gls/pdf/head-and-neck.pdf

42. Mayo ZS, Ilori EO, Matia B, et al. Limited toxicity of hypofractionated intensity modulated radiation therapy for head and neck cancer. *Anticancer Res.* 2022;42(4):1845–1849. doi:10.21873/anticanres.15660

43. Hanania AN, Zhang X, Gunn GB, et al. Proton therapy for major salivary gland cancer: clinical outcomes. *Int J Part Ther.* 2021;8(1):261–272. doi:10.14338/IJPT-20-00044.1

44. Bakst RL, Glastonbury CM, Parvathaneni U, Katabi N, Hu KS, Yom SS. Perineural invasion and perineural tumor spread in head and neck cancer. *Int J Radiat Oncol Biol Phys.* 2019;103(5):1109–1124. doi:10.1016/j.ijrobp.2018.12.009

45. Videtic GMM, Woody NM, Vassil AD. *Handbook of Treatment Planning in Radiation Oncology.* 3rd ed. Demos Medical; 2020.

46. Douglas JG, Goodkin R, Laramore GE. Gamma knife stereotactic radiosurgery for salivary gland neoplasms with base of skull invasion following neutron radiotherapy. *Head Neck.* 2008;30(4):492–496. doi:10.1002/hed.20729

47. Terhaard CH, Lubsen H, Rasch CR, et al. The role of radiotherapy in the treatment of malignant salivary gland tumors. *Int J Radiat Oncol Biol Phys.* 2005;61(1):103–111. doi:10.1016/j.ijrobp.2004.03.018

48. Armstrong JG, Harrison LB, Spiro RH, Fass DE, Strong EW, Fuks ZY. Malignant tumors of major salivary gland origin. A matched-pair analysis of the role of combined surgery and postoperative radiotherapy. *Arch Otolaryngol Head Neck Surg.* 1990;116(3):290–293. doi:10.1001/archotol.1990.01870030054008

49. North CA, Lee DJ, Piantadosi S, Zahurak M, Johns ME. Carcinoma of the major salivary glands treated by surgery or surgery plus postoperative radiotherapy. *Int J Radiat Oncol Biol Phys.* 1990;18(6):1319–1326. doi:10.1016/0360-3016(90)90304-3

50. Cho JK, Lim BW, Kim EH, et al. Low-grade salivary gland cancers: treatment outcomes, extent of surgery and indications for postoperative adjuvant radiation therapy. *Ann Surg Oncol.* 2016;23(13):4368–4375. doi:10.1245/s10434-016-5353-6

51. Amini A, Waxweiler TV, Brower JV, et al. Association of adjuvant chemoradiotherapy vs radiotherapy alone with survival in patients with resected major salivary gland carcinoma: data from the National Cancer Data Base. *JAMA Otolaryngol Head Neck Surg.* 2016;142(11):1100–1110. doi:10.1001/jamaoto.2016.2168

16 CARCINOMA OF UNKNOWN PRIMARY OF THE HEAD AND NECK

Jana M. Kobeissi, Monica E. Shukla, Jeffrey A. Kittel, and Shauna R. Campbell

QUICK HIT H&N carcinoma of unknown primary represents ~3% of H&N cancers. Diagnostic workup to identify a primary source for malignancy must include comprehensive H&P, fiberoptic laryngoscopy, analysis of histology and anatomic disease distribution (nodal levels), presence/absence of biomarkers (p16, HPV DNA, EBV DNA, TMB), advanced imaging (e.g., contrast-enhanced CT and PET/CT), and diagnostic surgical procedures (e.g., palatine tonsillectomy). Biopsy showing adenocarcinoma in the low neck should prompt evaluation for a salivary, thyroid, thoracic, or abdominopelvic primary. Squamous cell carcinomas of unknown primary (SCCUP) despite thorough workup are assumed to arise from H&N sites (mucosal or skin) and are treated based on the probability of the primary site given anatomic location of nodal involvement and presence/absence of biomarkers. Two broad treatment approaches exist: primary surgery (with risk-adapted adjuvant RT ± CHT) and definitive RT (± CHT; Table 16.1).

Table 16.1 General Treatment Paradigm for Unknown Primary Presenting as SCC of H&N Lymph Nodes	
	Treatment Options
cT0N1	Option 1: Neck dissection (at least levels II–IV), ipsilateral palatine tonsillectomy, and if negative ipsilateral lingual tonsillectomy (optional). Bilateral palatine tonsillectomy can be considered. • Adjuvant treatment based on pathologic risk factors (see Chapter 17). Option 2: RT alone with consideration of concurrent CHT for one LN >3 cm.
cT0N2–3	Option 1: Definitive CRT (favored for bilateral/bulky presentation or radiographic concern for ENE to avoid trimodality therapy). Option 2: For unilateral nodal involvement, ipsilateral neck dissection (at least levels II–IV), ipsilateral palatine tonsillectomy, and if negative ipsilateral lingual tonsillectomy. Bilateral palatine tonsillectomy can be considered. For bilateral nodal involvement, bilateral neck dissection and lingual tonsillectomy on the side with the greatest nodal burden can be done. If negative, contralateral lingual tonsillectomy can be performed. Neck dissection (± TORS lingual tonsillectomy). • Adjuvant treatment based on pathologic risk factors (see Chapter 17).

EPIDEMIOLOGY: Carcinoma of unknown primary represents 2% to 3% of all newly diagnosed H&N carcinomas, with incidence rising over time as incidence of HPV-associated disease has increased.[1] Median age at diagnosis is 50 to 70 years, with male predominance (M:F of 4:1). The majority of head and neck SCCUP (HNSCCUP) in the United States are now HPV-associated.[2,3]

RISK FACTORS: Standard risk factors for H&N cancer apply, as do those of other primaries that spread to cervical LNs. *General:* alcohol, tobacco, betel and areca nuts, Plummer–Vinson syndrome. *Oropharyngeal:* HPV infection. *Nasopharyngeal:* EBV infection, salt-cured foods, occupational smoke/dust exposure. *Sinonasal:* nickel, wood dust, leather tanning agents. *Cutaneous:* UV exposure.

ANATOMY: Pattern of nodal involvement on physical exam helps direct further workup toward potential sites of the occult primary.

PATHOLOGY: The most common pathology of H&N cancer of unknown primary (HNCUP) is squamous cell carcinoma (SCC). Adenocarcinoma (ACA) and neuroendocrine carcinomas are less common. Lymphoma, sarcoma, thyroid, melanoma, and germ cell tumors may also be encountered.

CLINICAL PRESENTATION: Classic presentation is unilateral painless neck mass in level II (~50%) ± level III. N1 presentation occurs in ~25%. With the rise of HPV-related cancers, some centers have noted a higher incidence of HNSCCUP,[3] with the hypothesis that HPV-related disease often presents with a small primary tumor,[4] which can be difficult to identify against a background of often irregular-appearing lymphoid tissue.

WORKUP: Comprehensive H&P: Attention to history of malignancy (including skin cancers) and risk factors. Exam should include direct inspection of the mucosal surfaces of the upper aerodigestive tract (including flexible nasopharyngolaryngoscopy to visualize surfaces not able to be evaluated on standard exam, e.g., nasal cavity, nasopharynx, posterior/inferior oropharynx, larynx, and hypopharynx), digital exam of high-risk sites to evaluate for palpable abnormalities (without a visual correlate), and thorough exam of the skin of the H&N. Anatomic location of the pathologic LN and histology will provide clues as to the primary site (Table 16.2).

Table 16.2 Lymph Node Levels* and Correlation With Possible Primary Site		
Level	**Anatomic Correlation**	**Possible Primary Site**
Ia	Submental	Anterior oral cavity/lower lip
Ib	Submandibular	Oral cavity (upper and lower lip, cheek, nose) and skin (lip, nose, medial canthus)
II	Upper jugular	Oropharynx, hypopharynx, oral cavity, larynx
III	Middle jugular	Oropharynx, larynx, hypopharynx, thyroid
IV	Lower jugular	Larynx, hypopharynx, thyroid, cervical esophagus, trachea
V	Posterior cervical triangle	Nasopharynx, skin of posterior neck, scalp, hypopharynx
VI	Anterior cervical (prelaryngeal [Delphian], pre/paratracheal, tracheoesophageal)	Larynx, thyroid
VII	Lateral retropharyngeal and retrostyloid	Nasopharynx, oropharyngeal wall or soft palate, hypopharynx, paranasal sinuses
Supraclavicular	Medial SCV (IVa) and lateral SCV (Vc)	Thyroid, cervical esophagus, infraclavicular primary (e.g., lung, gastrointestinal or gynecologic)
VIII	Intra/periparotid	Skin

*Cervical LN levels as per Robbins et al.[5]
Source: Adapted from Robbins KT, Clayman G, Levine PA, et al. Neck dissection classification update: revisions proposed by the American Head and Neck Society and the American Academy of Otolaryngology-Head and Neck Surgery. *Arch Otolaryngol Head Neck Surg.* Jul 2002;128(7):751–758. doi:10.1001/archotol.128.7.751.

Labs: CBC, CMP (thyroglobulin and calcitonin if ACA).

Biopsy: FNA of pathologic LN for initial sampling (unless suspicious for lymphoma). If FNA is nondiagnostic, proceed to core needle biopsy. Excisional biopsy is a less favored alternative; if done, ideally with planned neck dissection to follow. Excisional biopsy alone is not recommended due to disruption of tissue planes, which can alter lymphatic drainage (nononcologic resection). In the current era, testing of viral and other biomarkers from the biopsy specimen is essential in directing the search for a primary tumor (Table 16.3). IHC for p16 protein or another HPV-specific test should be performed on every SCCUP with levels II to III LN involvement ± other levels as clinically indicated. If p16 and HPV are negative, other markers (e.g., EBV) should be performed. Consider PAX8 and thyroid transcription factor testing for ACA and anaplastic/undifferentiated tumors. Primary H&N cutaneous SCC has demonstrated higher TMB compared with primary oral SCC.[6]

Table 16.3 Pathologic Markers and Correlation With Possible Primary Site	
Marker	**Possible Primary Site**
EBV DNA ISH+ or EBER ISH+	Nasopharynx
p16+, HPV DNA/RNA ISH+	Oropharynx
p16+/−, HPV DNA/RNA ISH−, high TMB[6]	Skin[38]
Adenocarcinoma, thyroid transcription factor	Thyroid, lung

Imaging: Contrast-enhanced CT is the primary imaging modality for evaluation of cervical lymphadenopathy. PET/CT is the next test of choice if CT and clinical exam (including scope) are unrevealing for a primary site. MRI is not clearly superior to CT, although it could help guide biopsies in the setting of substantial metal artifact, iodine contrast allergy, or if a nasopharynx primary is suspected.[7] Imaging should be performed prior to panendoscopy to guide selection of biopsy sites and to avoid uncertainties of interpretation due to false-positive FDG avidity at sites manipulated during endoscopy. PET detection rate of primary tumor is ~30% in patients with HNCUP after standard workup.[8]

Procedures: Following PET/CT, the next step is EUA with panendoscopy with directed biopsies of suspicious areas. With panendoscopy, the primary site is identified in 50% to 65% of patients with suspicious radiographic or physical findings, but only in 15% to 29% of those without.[9,10] Utility of random biopsies in the absence of PET/CT or clinical suspicion is very low and no longer recommended.[11] If LN levels I to III are involved, ipsilateral palatine tonsillectomy is recommended and increases detection of the primary tumor by about 10-fold as compared with tonsillar biopsy alone (30% vs. 3%).[12,13] Particularly in the p16+ setting, consider lingual tonsillectomy if palatine tonsillectomy is negative. Meta-analyses of lingual tonsillectomy a.k.a. "tongue base mucosectomy" with transoral approach (via TORS or TLM) demonstrated 78% of patients had a primary site in the base of tongue (BOT) after negative comprehensive workup.[14] Palatine and/or lingual tonsillectomies can be unilateral if there is only unilateral LN involvement.[11] If bilateral LNs are involved, the primary site is more likely to be in the BOT than the palatine tonsil. Consider unilateral lingual tonsillectomy on the side with greatest nodal burden and contralateral lingual tonsillectomy if frozen sections are negative. Consider unilateral palatine tonsillectomy if lingual tonsillectomy is negative, but avoid bilateral palatine tonsillectomy combined with bilateral lingual tonsillectomy due to morbidity.[11] Tissue specimens taken during diagnostic evaluation are ideally anatomically oriented with margin evaluation performed.

PROGNOSTIC FACTORS: Histology, number of LNs, LN level (upper vs. lower/SCV), KPS, extracapsular extension, and grade, among others.

NATURAL HISTORY: Mucosal emergence rates, historically, are low after comprehensive RT. Retrospective series suggest rates of 25% after neck dissection alone and rates from 8% to 14% with RT.[15] These rates may be lower in the modern era with improved imaging. Regional failure in the neck and DM is more common at 20% to 35%.[15]

STAGING: T classification for cancer of unknown primary is T0 (not TX, which implies incomplete workup). Staging for SCC is per standard H&N staging (see Chapter 11 for details). EBV-associated unknown primary follows nasopharyngeal staging (see Chapter 13 for details).

TREATMENT PARADIGM: Initial treatment can follow a paradigm of primary surgery (with risk-adapted adjuvant RT ± CHT as indicated) or primary RT (± CHT as indicated). Results have generally been comparable with either approach, and institutional preference often determines treatment algorithm.[16–18] Treatment strategy should take into account toxicities of each therapy.[19] In general, HPV-positive tumors are managed as oropharyngeal, and EBV-positive are managed as nasopharyngeal.

Surgery: Surgery/neck dissection is primarily recommended for HNSCCUP with N1 disease and may be considered for N2–N3.[12] It is also recommended for all ACAs that are both thyroglobulin- and calcitonin-negative.[20] Typically, selective dissection is performed with levels IIA to IV routinely dissected ± other levels based on anatomic location of involved nodes, nodal burden, and suspected primary site.[11] Potential complications of neck dissection include hematoma, seroma, chyle leak, lymphedema, wound infection/dehiscence, fistula, cranial nerve damage (e.g., CN XI), and carotid rupture. The major potential complication of lingual tonsillectomy is hemorrhage, occurring in 5% of patients.[14] After surgery, adjuvant RT ± CHT should be offered based on standard recommendations for H&N cancer (see Chapter 17 for details).

Chemotherapy: Concurrent CHT with RT is recommended for patients with either (a) extranodal extension (ENE) or positive margin after a neck dissection or (b) >1 positive LN treated nonoperatively. These concepts are largely extrapolated from major definitive and postop studies in the setting of known H&N primaries (see Chapters 11–15 and 17). Small observational studies have shown good outcomes with CRT for patients with unknown primary and N2–N3 nodal disease.[19,21–23] If delivered,

CHT dosing strategy is similar to that of other H&N sites, commonly high-dose cisplatin 100 mg/m^2 on days 1, 22, and 43 or cisplatin 40 mg/m^2 weekly. If there is a high suspicion for a skin primary, adjuvant RT without concurrent CHT is preferred after resection of LN metastases due to lack of benefit seen on TROG 05.01[24] (although some consider concurrent CHT in the definitive setting).

Radiation

Indications: RT can be employed in either (a) high-risk postoperative setting or (b) definitive setting. Following neck dissection, RT indications mimic standard indications for PORT in the H&N: >1 positive LN, one LN >3 cm, or ENE. Adjuvant RT may be omitted in the case of a single LN <3 cm without ENE, given dissection is of high quality and no primary lesion is found.[11] In the definitive setting, RT can be delivered alone or with concurrent CHT (e.g., cN2–3; see the preceding text). Most commonly, RT is delivered to putative mucosal sites along with the bilateral neck, unless skin primary is suspected.

- Primary: Guidelines for coverage of putative primary sites are similar whether in the adjuvant or in the definitive setting.[11] Classically, comprehensive RT for likely mucosal primaries included the nasopharynx, oropharynx, and hypopharynx, with exclusion of the oral cavity and larynx (sites that can be easily visualized). Potential gain with comprehensive RT in controlling primary should be weighed against its effects on QOL/toxicity. Target volumes have evolved and are often modified by HPV/EBV status and diagnostic interventions (e.g., palatine or lingual tonsillectomy). Guidelines now recommend targeting only the oropharynx for HPV+ disease; for unilateral adenopathy, target ipsilateral tonsil, ipsilateral soft palate, and bilateral BOT, modified by prior surgical diagnostic interventions; for bilateral adenopathy, target bilateral oropharynx.[11] For HPV– disease in unilateral levels II to III, consider the ipsilateral tonsil, bilateral BOT, ipsilateral fossa of Rosenmüller, and ipsilateral pyriform sinus to be at risk. Consider treating only the nasopharynx for EBV+ disease. Omitting putative mucosal sites after comprehensive surgical diagnostics (at least ipsilateral palatine tonsillectomy and high-quality bilateral lingual tonsillectomy) is investigational.
- Neck/lymphatics: Most treat bilateral neck levels II to IV and retropharyngeal nodes, although other levels (IB, V) should be included as indicated by presumed primary location (e.g., include V with EBV+ presumed nasopharyngeal primary) or bulky nodal burden. Unilateral nodal treatment for suspected mucosal primaries is controversial and should only be considered with involvement of a single node (unless concerned for a nasopharyngeal primary, in which bilateral coverage is recommended).[11]

Dose: As in target delineation, dosing is heterogeneous. An acceptable dose scheme in the definitive setting is 70 Gy/35 fx to gross disease, 56–63 Gy/35 fx to mucosal sites at risk, and 56 Gy/35 fx to the uninvolved neck. Postoperatively, an acceptable dose regimen is 66 Gy/30–33 fx to areas harboring ENE (or gross residual disease), 60 Gy/30 fx to the postoperative bed and pathologically involved nodal levels, and 54 Gy/30 fx to the uninvolved neck. For fractionations other than 30 or 35 fx, a radiobiological equivalent dose should be used.

Toxicity: Acute: mucositis, skin erythema/desquamation, odynophagia, dysphagia, fatigue, aspiration, xerostomia/thickened secretions, taste alterations. Late: xerostomia, taste alteration, fibrosis, trismus, decreased hearing, hypothyroidism, submental lymphedema, dysphagia, esophageal strictures, bone/soft tissue necrosis, secondary malignancy.

EVIDENCE-BASED Q&A

Does association with HPV carry the same implications in HNCUP as it does in oropharyngeal cancer?

Yes. HPV-associated HNCUPs have a better prognosis relative to their p16-negative counterparts, independent of nodal status.[25] In one study, 5-year OS was 85% in HPV+ disease vs. 44% in HPV– disease (p < .0001).[26] HPV positivity also leads practitioners to target only likely primary sites (i.e., oropharynx), which may decrease toxicity of treatment.

What is the role of transoral lingual tonsillectomy in the workup of HNCUP?

TORS is used to perform lingual tonsillectomy in search of occult primary and appears to increase the likelihood of detecting a primary site when added to the standard diagnostic algorithm.[27,28]

Farooq, Meta-Analysis (*Oral Oncol* 2019, PMID 30926070): Meta-analysis including 21 studies evaluating TORS or TLM in identifying the primary site in HNSCCUP. In patients with negative exam, conventional imaging, and PET/CT, tongue base mucosectomy identified the primary in 64% of cases, which rose to 78% in patients who also had a negative EUA and tonsillectomy. **Conclusion: BOT mucosectomy performed by TORS or TLN is effective at identifying the unknown primary site.**

Does bilateral neck RT improve outcomes as compared with unilateral treatment?

Unilateral treatment is controversial considering that occult primary tumors presumed to be arising from the oropharynx often reside in the BOT, which is a midline structure. Several older studies have investigated unilateral treatment, but they are limited by either a very small sample size, application of 2D techniques only, and/or comparison of ipsilateral RT without mucosal coverage with comprehensive RT.[29–34] A more recent multi-institutional cohort study with a larger sample size has suggested similar oncologic outcomes between unilateral and bilateral nodal coverage, as detailed below.[35] Less controversy exists in the setting of a single LN without clinical or radiologic evidence of ENE, in which case it is reasonable to consider unilateral neck RT with coverage of putative mucosal sites.[11]

Pflumio, Multicenter in France and Italy (*Eur J Cancer* 2019, PMID 30826659): Retrospective cohort study of 297 patients with HNSCCUP, of whom 21% had unilateral disease and received unilateral nodal RT, while 52% had unilateral disease and received bilateral nodal RT. The rest had bilateral adenopathy and bilateral RT. Among patients with unilateral disease only, there were no significant difference in the 3-year regional relapse (8% vs. 17%, $p = .17$), 3-year local relapse (4% vs. 11%, $p = .32$), or cancer-specific mortality (9% vs. 16%, $p = .92$) in those who received bilateral vs. unilateral RT, respectively. Bilateral RT was associated with significantly higher acute toxicities, including dysphagia ($p < .01$) and pain ($p = .03$), as well as higher late toxicities, such as xerostomia ($p < .01$). Of note, the majority of patients also received RT to mucosal sites, and mucosal RT was itself a prognostic factor for LR on MVA. **Conclusion: Bilateral RT has nonsignificant better LC but higher acute and late toxicities.**

Can TORS allow omission of mucosal sites (pharyngeal-sparing) in the radiation field?

While omitting the oropharynx and/or contralateral neck is controversial, early evidence suggests TORS may help identify patients in whom volume deintensification is possible. The studies below are in addition to other similar studies for early-stage oropharynx cancer with a known primary post-TORS.[36,37]

De Almeida, FIND Trial (*JAMA Otolaryngol Head Neck Surg* 2024, PMID 38602692): Phase II non-RCT of 22 patients with p16+ HNSCCUP who underwent either diagnostic or therapeutic TORS followed by definitive or adjuvant RT, respectively. Pharyngeal-sparing RT was offered to patients with negative margins or those with no primary tumor on pathology (pT0), while unilateral neck RT was offered to patients with unilateral neck involvement and in whom TORS either showed a lateralized primary or pT0. The 2-year OS, LRC, and DM control rates were 100%, 100%, and 95% respectively. Pharyngeal-sparing RT spared the superior constrictors as well as the swallowing function to a greater extent. **Conclusion: In p16+ HNSCCUP patients, TORS allows for pharyngeal-sparing in the RT volumes without a significant change in oncologic outcomes.** *Note: Among the 22 patients, 17 were found to have an oropharyngeal primary tumor on TORS, and only 5 had an unknown primary at the time of RT. Hence, the above results may not apply to those with true HNCUP, given the low representation in the trial.*

Grewal, UPenn (*Laryngoscope* 2020, PMID 31411747): Retrospective study including 45 patients with HNCUP who had pT0 on TORS. Of those, 49% received pharyngeal-sparing RT, while the rest received pharyngeal targeted RT. While not randomized, both groups were similar in terms of N stage, HPV positivity (55% vs. 43%), rates of neck dissection, and receipt of CHT. However, MFU was slightly longer in the pharyngeal targeted RT group (28 vs. 24 months, $p = .04$). There were no significant differences in the 2-year RFS (86% vs. 74%, $p = .3$) and 2-year OS (91% vs. 74%, $p = .31$) among the pharyngeal-sparing and pharyngeal targeted RT groups, respectively. Patients who received pharyngeal-sparing RT had significantly less toxicity, including grade 2+ mucositis (18% vs. 91%, $p < .01$), opioid needs (27% vs. 91%, $p < .01$), and feeding tube requirements (5% vs. 43%, $p < .01$). **Conclusion: Pharyngeal-sparing RT after TORS results in less toxicity without a significant change in oncologic outcomes.** *Note: The study included both HPV-positive and negative patients with no subgroup analysis, so the potential role of HPV status cannot be extrapolated. Being a retrospective study with a small sample size, confounding factors should be considered.*

REFERENCES

1. Cummings MA, Ma SJ, Van Der Sloot P, Milano MT, Singh DP, Singh AK. Squamous cell carcinoma of the head and neck with unknown primary: trends and outcomes from a hospital-based registry. *Ann Transl Med.* 2021;9(4):284. doi:10.21037/atm-20-4631

2. Keller LM, Galloway TJ, Holdbrook T, et al. p16 status, pathologic and clinical characteristics, biomolecular signature, and long-term outcomes in head and neck squamous cell carcinomas of unknown primary. *Head Neck.* 2014;36(12):1677–1684. doi:10.1002/hed.23514

3. Motz K, Qualliotine JR, Rettig E, Richmon JD, Eisele DW, Fakhry C. Changes in unknown primary squamous cell carcinoma of the head and neck at initial presentation in the era of human papillomavirus. *JAMA Otolaryngol Head Neck Surg.* 2016;142(3):223–228. doi:10.1001/jamaoto.2015.3228

4. Huang SH, Perez-Ordonez B, Liu FF, et al. Atypical clinical behavior of p16-confirmed HPV-related oropharyngeal squamous cell carcinoma treated with radical radiotherapy. *Int J Radiat Oncol Biol Phys.* 2012;82(1):276–283. doi:10.1016/j.ijrobp.2010.08.031

5. Robbins KT, Clayman G, Levine PA, et al. Neck dissection classification update: revisions proposed by the American Head and Neck Society and the American Academy of Otolaryngology-Head and Neck Surgery. *Arch Otolaryngol Head Neck Surg.* 2002;128(7):751–758. doi:10.1001/archotol.128.7.751

6. Gupta R, Strbenac D, Satgunaseelan L, et al. Comparing genomic landscapes of oral and cutaneous squamous cell carcinoma of the head and neck: quest for novel diagnostic markers. *Mod Pathol.* 2023;36(8):100190. doi:10.1016/j.modpat.2023.100190

7. Ruhlmann V, Ruhlmann M, Bellendorf A, et al. Hybrid imaging for detection of carcinoma of unknown primary: a preliminary comparison trial of whole-body PET/MRI versus PET/CT. *Eur J Radiol.* 2016;85(11):1941–1947. doi:10.1016/j.ejrad.2016.08.020

8. Johansen J, Buus S, Loft A, et al. Prospective study of 18FDG-PET in the detection and management of patients with lymph node metastases to the neck from an unknown primary tumor. Results from the DAHANCA-13 study. *Head Neck.* 2008;30(4):471–478. doi:10.1002/hed.20734

9. Cianchetti M, Mancuso AA, Amdur RJ, et al. Diagnostic evaluation of squamous cell carcinoma metastatic to cervical lymph nodes from an unknown head and neck primary site. *Laryngoscope.* 2009;119(12):2348–2354. doi:10.1002/lary.20638

10. Mendenhall WM, Mancuso AA, Parsons JT, Stringer SP, Cassisi NJ. Diagnostic evaluation of squamous cell carcinoma metastatic to cervical lymph nodes from an unknown head and neck primary site. *Head Neck.* 1998;20(8):739–744. doi:10.1002/(sici)1097-0347(199812)20:8<739::aid-hed13>3.0.co;2-0

11. Maghami E, Ismaila N, Alvarez A, et al. Diagnosis and management of squamous cell carcinoma of unknown primary in the head and neck: ASCO guideline. *J Clin Oncol.* 2020;38(22):2570–2596. doi:10.1200/JCO.20.00275

12. National Comprehensive Cancer Network. Head and neck cancers (version 1.2025). Accessed December 27, 2024. https://www.nccn.org/professionals/physician_gls/pdf/head-and-neck.pdf

13. Waltonen JD, Ozer E, Schuller DE, Agrawal A. Tonsillectomy vs. deep tonsil biopsies in detecting occult tonsil tumors. *Laryngoscope.* 2009;119(1):102–106. doi:10.1002/lary.20017

14. Farooq S, Khandavilli S, Dretzke J, et al. Transoral tongue base mucosectomy for the identification of the primary site in the work-up of cancers of unknown origin: systematic review and meta-analysis. *Oral Oncol.* 2019;91:97–106. doi:10.1016/j.oraloncology.2019.02.018

15. Nieder C, Ang KK. Cervical lymph node metastases from occult squamous cell carcinoma. *Curr Treat Options Oncol.* 2002;3(1):33–40. doi:10.1007/s11864-002-0039-7

16. Demiroz C, Vainshtein JM, Koukourakis GV, et al. Head and neck squamous cell carcinoma of unknown primary: neck dissection and radiotherapy or definitive radiotherapy. *Head Neck.* 2014;36(11):1589–1595. doi:10.1002/hed.23479

17. Christiansen H, Hermann RM, Martin A, Nitsche M, Schmidberger H, Pradier O. Neck lymph node metastases from an unknown primary tumor retrospective study and review of literature. *Strahlenther Onkol.* 2005;181(6):355–362. doi:10.1007/s00066-005-1338-2

18. Balaker AE, Abemayor E, Elashoff D, St John MA. Cancer of unknown primary: does treatment modality make a difference? *Laryngoscope.* 2012;122(6):1279–1282. doi:10.1002/lary.22424

19. Chen AM, Farwell DG, Lau DH, Li BQ, Luu Q, Donald PJ. Radiation therapy in the management of head-and-neck cancer of unknown primary origin: how does the addition of concurrent chemotherapy affect the therapeutic ratio? *Int J Radiat Oncol Biol Phys.* 2011;81(2):346–352. doi:10.1016/j.ijrobp.2010.06.031

20. Galloway TJ, Ridge JA. Management of squamous cancer metastatic to cervical nodes with an unknown primary site. *J Clin Oncol.* 2015;33(29):3328–3337. doi:10.1200/JCO.2015.61.0063

21. Sher DJ, Balboni TA, Haddad RI, et al. Efficacy and toxicity of chemoradiotherapy using intensity-modulated radiotherapy for unknown primary of head and neck. *Int J Radiat Oncol Biol Phys.* 2011;80(5):1405–1411. doi:10.1016/j.ijrobp.2010.04.029

22. Argiris A, Smith SM, Stenson K, et al. Concurrent chemoradiotherapy for N2 or N3 squamous cell carcinoma of the head and neck from an occult primary. *Ann Oncol.* 2003;14(8):1306–1311. doi:10.1093/annonc/mdg330

23. Shehadeh NJ, Ensley JF, Kucuk O, et al. Benefit of postoperative chemoradiotherapy for patients with unknown primary squamous cell carcinoma of the head and neck. *Head Neck.* 2006;28(12):1090–1098. doi:10.1002/hed.20470

24. Porceddu SV, Bressel M, Poulsen MG, et al. Postoperative concurrent chemoradiotherapy versus postoperative radiotherapy in high-risk cutaneous squamous cell carcinoma of the head and neck: the randomized phase III TROG 05.01 trial. *J Clin Oncol.* 2018;36(13):1275–1283. doi:10.1200/JCO.2017.77.0941

25. Lee MY, Fowler N, Adelstein D, Koyfman S, Prendes B, Burkey BB. Detection and oncologic outcomes of head and neck squamous cell carcinoma of unknown primary origin. *Anticancer Res.* 2020;40(8):4207–4214. doi:10.21873/anticanres.14421

26. Hardman JC, Constable J, Dobbs S, et al. Survival outcomes in head and neck squamous cell carcinoma of unknown primary: a national cohort study. *Clin Otolaryngol.* 2024;49(5):604–620. doi:10.1111/coa.14167

27. Mehta V, Johnson P, Tassler A, et al. A new paradigm for the diagnosis and management of unknown primary tumors of the head and neck: a role for transoral robotic surgery. *Laryngoscope.* 2013;123(1):146–151. doi:10.1002/lary.23562

28. Patel SA, Magnuson JS, Holsinger FC, et al. Robotic surgery for primary head and neck squamous cell carcinoma of unknown site. *JAMA Otolaryngol Head Neck Surg.* 2013;139(11):1203–1211. doi:10.1001/jamaoto.2013.5189

29. Reddy SP, Marks JE. Metastatic carcinoma in the cervical lymph nodes from an unknown primary site: results of bilateral neck plus mucosal irradiation vs. ipsilateral neck irradiation. *Int J Radiat Oncol Biol Phys.* 1997;37(4):797–802. doi:10.1016/S0360-3016(97)00025-4

30. Grau C, Johansen LV, Jakobsen J, Geertsen P, Andersen E, Jensen BB. Cervical lymph node metastases from unknown primary tumours. Results from a national survey by the Danish Society for Head and Neck Oncology. *Radiother Oncol.* 2000;55(2):121–129. doi:10.1016/S0167-8140(00)00172-9

31. Ligey A, Gentil J, Créhange G, et al. Impact of target volumes and radiation technique on loco-regional control and survival for patients with unilateral cervical lymph node metastases from an unknown primary. *Radiother Oncol.* 2009;93(3):483–487. doi:10.1016/j.radonc.2009.08.027

32. Fakhrian K, Thamm R, Knapp S, et al. Radio(chemo)therapy in the management of squamous cell carcinoma of cervical lymph nodes from an unknown primary site. A retrospective analysis. *Strahlenther Onkol.* 2012;188(1):56–61. doi:10.1007/s00066-011-0017-8

33. Cuaron J, Rao S, Wolden S, et al. Patterns of failure in patients with head and neck carcinoma of unknown primary treated with radiation therapy. *Head Neck.* 2016;38(suppl 1):E426–E431. doi:10.1002/hed.24013

34. Perkins SM, Spencer CR, Chernock RD, et al. Radiotherapeutic management of cervical lymph node metastases from an unknown primary site. *Arch Otolaryngol Head Neck Surg.* 2012;138(7):656–661. doi:10.1001/archoto.2012.1110

35. Pflumio C, Troussier I, Sun XS, et al. Unilateral or bilateral irradiation in cervical lymph node metastases of unknown primary? A retrospective cohort study. *Eur J Cancer.* 2019;111:69–81. doi:10.1016/j.ejca.2019.01.004

36. Anderson JD, DeWees TA, Ma DJ, et al. A prospective study of mucosal sparing radiation therapy in resected oropharyngeal cancer patients. *Int J Radiat Oncol Biol Phys.* 2023;115(1):192–201. doi:10.1016/j.ijrobp.2022.06.057

37. Swisher-McClure S, Lukens JN, Aggarwal C, et al. A phase 2 trial of Alternative Volumes of Oropharyngeal Irradiation for De-intensification (AVOID): omission of the resected primary tumor bed after transoral robotic surgery for human papilloma virus-related squamous cell carcinoma of the oropharynx. *Int J Radiat Oncol Biol Phys.* 2020;106(4):725–732. doi:10.1016/j.ijrobp.2019.11.021

38. McDowell LJ, Young RJ, Johnston ML, et al. p16-positive lymph node metastases from cutaneous head and neck squamous cell carcinoma: no association with high-risk human papillomavirus or prognosis and implications for the workup of the unknown primary. *Cancer.* 2016;122(8):1201–1208. doi:10.1002/cncr.29901

17 POSTOPERATIVE RADIATION FOR HEAD AND NECK CANCER

Bryn M. Myers, Timothy D. Smile, Carryn M. Anderson, and Jacob A. Miller

QUICK HIT Surgery is the preferred initial management of resectable head and neck (H&N) cancers of the oral cavity, salivary gland, nasal cavity/paranasal sinuses, and thyroid, and some oropharynx and larynx cancers. Organ preservation is utilized in nasopharynx cancer and in many oropharynx, larynx, and hypopharynx cancers. Oncologic surgery alone is often sufficient treatment for T1–T2N0–1 tumors when resected with negative margins. Adjuvant RT (PORT) is recommended for specific pathologic risk factors, with concurrent CHT indicated for positive margins and/or extracapsular extension (ECE) in mucosal head and neck squamous cell carcinoma (HNSCC). See Table 17.1 for a summary of PORT indications and dosing.

Table 17.1 PORT Indications and Dosing Summary		
Risk Group	**Treatment**	**Patient Characteristics**
Low risk	Observation	pT1–T2, 0–1 pathologically involved nodes, –PNI, –LVSI, –margins, –ECE
Intermediate risk	60 Gy	pT3–T4, pN2–3 disease, PNI, LVSI, close margins (<5 mm), or DOI >4 mm in oral tongue[1]
	66 Gy	Consider multiple of above risk factors
High risk	66 Gy + CHT	+ECE, microscopic positive margins[2]
	70 Gy + CHT	Residual gross disease

EPIDEMIOLOGY: HNSCC is the seventh most common cancer in the world, with a worldwide estimated yearly incidence of 890,000.[3] Estimated U.S. 2024 incidence of 71,100 cases and 16,110 deaths, not including skin cancer.[4] Male-to-female ratio 3:1. Cancers of the tongue, tonsil, and oropharynx have been increasing in incidence, with a rate of 2.3% per year in the last decade.[4]

RISK FACTORS: Tobacco (cigarettes and chew, 5–25× increased risk), alcohol (dose-dependent and synergistic with tobacco), HPV infection (oropharyngeal), HIV, immunosuppressed from transplant drugs or autoimmune diseases, betel nut chewing (oral cavity), previous RT, occupational/environmental exposures.

ANATOMY: See Chapters 11–15 and 19 for site-specific anatomy.

PATHOLOGY: The most common histology is SCC (~95%). "Keratin pearls" are seen in well-differentiated SCC, often associated with classic HNSCC related to smoking/alcohol misuse. Nonkeratinizing, poorly differentiated, "basaloid" squamous cancers are often associated with HPV-related p16+ oropharyngeal SCC. Other histologies (<5%) include those arising from minor salivary glands (mucoepidermoid carcinoma, adenoid cystic carcinoma), adenosquamous, adenocarcinoma, acinic cell, lymphoma, lymphoepithelial carcinoma, and mucosal melanoma.

GENETICS: Mutation of p53, CDKN2A, Rb loss of function, and increased expression of EGFR are associated with worse prognosis in oral cavity cancers.[5,6]

SCREENING: No established role for screening. See Chapters 13 and 14 for further discussion of screening investigations.

CLINICAL PRESENTATION: Dependent on primary site. Many patients are asymptomatic from their primary disease and present with adenopathy, most commonly level II jugulodigastric node. Paranasal sinus/nasal cavity/nasopharynx: nasal obstruction, epistaxis, lateral gaze palsy, unilateral hearing loss, epiphora. Oropharynx: dysphagia, trismus, otalgia, odynophagia. Oral cavity:

nonhealing ulceration, dysarthria, loose teeth. Larynx: hoarseness, stridor, dysphagia, odynophagia, otalgia. Hypopharynx: dysphagia, hoarseness, weight loss.

WORKUP: H&P including flexible nasopharyngolaryngoscopy or mirror examination.

Labs: Routine labs including CBC and CMP.

Imaging: CT neck with contrast, PET/CT for stage III/IV patients, CT chest to screen for metastasis or second primary if PET/CT not obtained, MRI for select primary sites (paranasal sinuses, salivary gland, suspicion for PNI). If unknown primary by office exam and imaging, obtain PET/CT prior to panendoscopy/exam under anesthesia.[7]

Pathology: FNA of neck node and/or biopsy of primary site. See Chapters 11 to 15 and 19 for site-specific workup. Optimally, multidisciplinary consult should be performed prior to resection.

Other: Dental, nutrition, speech, and audiometric evaluation as indicated.

PROGNOSTIC FACTORS: Positive margins and ECE are the most important pathologic prognostic factors. Other pathologic risk factors for locoregional recurrence include close margins, perineural invasion (PNI), lymphovascular space invasion (LVSI), tumor size, depth of invasion (DOI; oral tongue in particular), nodal involvement, poor differentiation, and worst pattern of invasion (WPOI). HPV-associated oropharynx cancers (OPC) have a better prognosis overall. In HPV-associated OPC, ECE and advanced nodal stage do not have the same degree of negative impact on survival when compared with their HPV-negative counterparts, as reflected in AJCC's 8th edition of the Staging Manual. ECE ranges from microscopic (small break in capsule, desmoplastic stromal reaction) to macroscopic (visible to eye at surgery), to gross soft tissue deposits (no evidence of LN architecture, which likely represents complete LN replacement).[8] Recurrence rates double when ECE is present. CT can predict ECE with frequent false-negatives (sensitivity/specificity/PPV/NPV: 43%, 97%, 82%, and 87%).[7] Nodes <2.5 cm on CT imaging have ~6% rate of pathologic ECE as compared with larger nodes with ~32% rate.[9]

NATURAL HISTORY: Majority of disease-related recurrences will be locoregional and occur within the first 2 years of treatment completion. The most common site of distant metastasis (DM) is the lung, with bone the second most common. HPV-associated cancers have been known to spread to less common sites such as the liver, skin, soft tissues, brain, and leptomeninges.[10]

STAGING: See Chapters 11 to 16 and 18 to 19 for staging details.

TREATMENT PARADIGM

Observation: Observation is appropriate following surgery for low-risk patients, generally defined as pT1–2, zero to one pathologically involved LN (<3 cm), without LVSI, PNI, ECE, DOI <4 mm (especially oral tongue), and negative margins (>5 mm ideally).

Surgery: Resection of primary should be performed with least morbidity possible. Free flap reconstruction may be necessary for larger tumors (hemiglossectomy, total glossectomy, mandibular reconstruction, laryngopharyngectomy, etc.). Free flaps typically include the radial forearm, anterolateral thigh, or fibula (when bone is required). Minimally invasive techniques such as transoral robotic surgery (TORS) and transoral laser microsurgery (TLM) are evolving. TORS is performed using a robotic platform, suggested for oropharynx and possibly larynx/hypopharynx primaries, and is FDA-approved for cT1–2 tumors. TLM is piecemeal removal of tumor through laryngoscope using CO_2 laser aimed via a micromanipulator attached to a microscope (only available at a few specialized centers). Both are suggested as a possible method to improve toxicity through lower RT doses and to intensify treatment for advanced disease (see terminated RTOG 1221). Given lack of long-term outcomes, specific issues related to TORS/TLM have been discussed and include optimal patient selection and its impact on adjuvant therapy indications.[11,12] For sinonasal tumors, endoscopic surgery is preferred and is performed in a piecemeal manner. Neck dissection is typically performed at the time of surgery (see Table 17.2).

Chemotherapy: CHT can be added concurrently to RT in the postoperative setting to escalate treatment for high-risk tumors. Bolus cisplatin is the most evidence-based regimen from prospective clinical trials, given at 100 mg/m[2] on days 1, 22, and 43. Weekly cisplatin 40 mg/m[2] is considered an acceptable alternative.[13] Further, RTOG 1216 is an ongoing trial investigating the role of alternative

Table 17.2 Neck Dissection Types for H&N Cancer	
Radical neck dissection	All LN groups I–V, CN XI, IJ vein, SCM
Modified radical neck dissection	All LN groups I–V, preserves ≥1 of CN XI, IJ, SCM
Selective neck dissection (SND)	Preservation of ≥1 LN group
Supraomohyoid	SND of only I–III, considered for oral cavity cases
Lateral neck dissection	SND II–IV (oropharynx, hypopharynx, larynx, thyroid)
Central neck dissection (thyroid cancer)	SND VI

multiagent regimens for high-risk patients. RTOG 0920 defined the relative benefit of concurrent cetuximab for intermediate-risk tumors.[14]

Radiation

Indications: Risk-adapted approach to RT is used to escalate therapy in the postoperative setting. Indications for PORT are described (Table 17.1) by loosely defined risk groups of low (observation), intermediate (RT alone, defined by RTOG 0920), and high (CRT, defined by RTOG 1216). For sinonasal tumors, PORT is almost always recommended (except for T1 ethmoid). RT should be initiated within 6 weeks of surgery for optimal LRC and OS.[15]

Dose: In the era of IMRT with SIB, doses of 66, 59.4, and 56.1 Gy in 33 fx to areas of high risk (microscopic margin positive, ECE, or multiple primary site risk factors), intermediate risk (postop bed or undissected neck at risk), and low risk (elective lower risk nodal areas), respectively, are commonly used. In cases with only "intermediate" features, 60 Gy/30 fx is delivered to involved postop bed simultaneously with 54 to 56 Gy to the high-risk undissected/low-risk neck. RTOG 0920 protocol can be used for further guidance on target volumes and dose constraints.[14]

Toxicity: Acute: mucositis, hoarseness, dysgeusia, xerostomia, dysphagia, weight loss, erythema/hyperpigmentation of skin, hair loss. Late: laryngeal edema, soft tissue or bone necrosis, dysphagia requiring PEG tube ± dilatation, silent aspiration, xerostomia, change/loss of taste, dental caries, hypothyroidism, soft tissue fibrosis, secondary malignancy.

EVIDENCE-BASED Q&A

What evidence suggests that PORT is effective?

Most evidence is retrospective, although there are two older RCTs demonstrating improved LRC with PORT compared with observation.[16,17]

Historically, what evidence suggests postoperative RT is superior to preoperative RT?

Tupchong, RTOG 7303 (*IJROBP* 1991, PMID 1993628): Phase III PRT of preoperative RT vs. PORT for supraglottic larynx and hypopharynx cancer. Preoperative RT was 50 Gy, PORT was 60 Gy; 277 patients, follow-up from 9 to 15 years. LRC improved in PORT group compared with preoperative RT (70% vs. 58%, $p = .04$). No difference in OS ($p = .15$). **Conclusion: PORT improves LRC compared with preoperative RT. Because of this trial, PORT has become standard in H&N cancer patients managed with primary surgery.**

What data support current standard dosing for PORT?

All patients require a minimum dose of 57.6 Gy at 1.8 Gy/fx to the entire operative bed. High-risk areas of two or more adverse factors or ECE require 63 Gy at 1.8 Gy/fx.

Peters, MD Anderson (*IJROBP* 1993, PMID 8482629): PRT of stage III/IV SCC of the oral cavity, oropharynx, hypopharynx, and larynx stratified by risk factors. Lower risk patients randomized to 52.2 to 57.6 Gy vs. 63 Gy and higher risk patients randomized to 63 Gy vs. 68.4 Gy, all in 1.8 Gy fx. On interim analysis, patients who received dose of ≤54 Gy had significantly higher primary failure rate and the dose group was increased to 57.6 Gy, improving LRF ($p = .02$). Overall, no dose response was demonstrated. However, if ECE was present, recurrence was significantly higher at 57.6 Gy than at ≥63 Gy. ECE was the only independent variable prognostic of LRR. Having two or more of the following was progressively prognostic: oral cavity primary, mucosal margins close or positive, nerve invasion, ≥2 positive LNs, largest node ≥3 cm, treatment delay >6 weeks, and Zubrod performance status ≥2. **Conclusion: Minimum dose of 57.6 Gy to the whole operative bed should be delivered with boost of 63 Gy to sites of increased risk (e.g., ECE). Treatment should be started as soon as possible after surgery. Dose escalation above 63 Gy does not appear to improve therapeutic ratio. This trial defined the most common dosing regimens used today (60–66 Gy).**

What data support risk-adapted approach to PORT?

Ang, MD Anderson (*IJROBP* 2001, PMID 11597795): Multi-institutional PRT of 213 patients with advanced HNSCC of the oral cavity, oropharynx, larynx, and hypopharynx assessing the role of risk stratification and PORT scheduling (concomitant boost vs. standard). Patients received therapy predicated on a set of pathologic risk features: oral cavity site, mucosal margin status, nerve invasion, one positive node, more than one positive nodal group, largest node >3 cm, ECE, and treatment delay of >6 weeks (see Table 17.3). **Conclusion: Dosing based on risk stratification is a legitimate approach to PORT for H&N cancer.** (*See altered fractionation in the following for the second conclusion.*)

Table 17.3 Results of MD Anderson Risk-Adapted PORT for H&N Cancer			
Risk Group	**PORT**	**5-Yr LRC**	**5-Yr OS**
Low risk: no adverse factors	None	90%	83%
Intermediate risk: one adverse factor other than ECE	57.6 Gy/6.5 weeks	94%	66%
High risk: ≥2 adverse factors or ECE	63 Gy/5 or 7 weeks (± concomitant boost)	68%	42%

With definitive RT, altered fractionation improves control (RTOG 9003). Should we accelerate patients receiving PORT?

No benefit for most patients; however, acceleration may compensate for delay in PORT after surgery beyond 6 weeks.

Sanguineti, Italy (*IJROBP* 2005, PMID 15708255): Phase III trial of PORT 60 Gy/6 weeks (CF) or altered fractionation (AF) with "biphasic concomitant boost" schedule, with boost delivered during the first and last weeks of treatment (64 Gy/5 weeks); 2-year LRC CF 80% vs. AF 78% (*p* = .52), trend to benefit for patients with RT delay >7 weeks; 2-year OS 67% vs. 64% (*p* = .84). Toxicity: Confluent mucositis CF 27% vs. AF 50% (*p* = .006), duration same. Late toxicity 18% vs. 27% (NS). **Conclusion: Accelerated fractionation is not beneficial overall, but it might be an option for patients who delay starting RT.**

Ang, MD Anderson (*IJROBP* 2001, PMID 11597795): Same trial as detailed earlier. Regarding hyperfractionation, only "trend" to benefit when comparing 5 weeks vs. 7 weeks in high-risk patients (LRC *p* = .11, OS *p* = .08). However, when looking at interval from surgery to PORT initiation for high-risk patients, acceleration seemed to make up for delay. **Conclusion: Hyperfractionation may be beneficial, particularly in patients with treatment delay >6 weeks from surgery.**

CHEMOTHERAPY

Which patients benefit from treatment escalation with concurrent CRT?

In high-risk patients, those with ECE or positive margins seem to benefit from the addition of CHT based on combined RTOG 9501/EORTC 22931 analyses. A phase III study from Tata Memorial found that patients with high-risk oral cavity SCC may benefit from intensified adjuvant CRT[18] (see Chapter 12).

Bernier, EORTC 22931 (*NEJM* 2004, PMID 15128894): PRT of 334 patients with HNSCC (oral cavity, oropharynx, hypopharynx, or larynx) s/p primary surgical resection with high-risk features comparing PORT alone (66 Gy/33 fx) vs. CRT (cisplatin 100 mg/m^2 on days 1, 22, and 43 with same RT). Eligible patients included pT3–4 and any N (except pT3N0 of the larynx with negative margins), or T1–2 and N2–3, or T1–2N0–1 with unfavorable pathologic findings (ENE, +margins, PNI, or vascular tumor embolism), or oral cavity/oropharynx tumors with levels IV to V LNs. Overall, 67% had pT3–4, 57% had pN2–3, 28% had +margins, and 54% had ≥2 positive LNs. MFU 60 months (see Table 17.4). Acute grades 3 to 4 mucosal adverse effects were worse with CRT (41% vs. 21%, p = .001), while cumulative incidence of late effects was not. **Conclusion: Postop CRT improves survival over RT alone for patients with locally advanced HNSCC (with unfavorable clinical and pathologic factors) without high incidence of late effects.**

Table 17.4 Results of Bernier EORTC CHT Trial

	mPFS	5-Yr PFS	MS	5-Yr OS	5-Yr LRR	5-Yr DM
Postop RT	23 months	36%	32 months	40%	31%	25%
Postop CRT	55 months	47%	72 months	53%	18%	21%
p value	.04		.02		.007	.61

Cooper, RTOG 9501 (*NEJM* 2004, PMID 15128893; Update *IJROBP* 2012, PMID 22749632): PRT of 416 patients (update 410 patients) with HNSCC (oral cavity, oropharynx, hypopharynx, or larynx) s/p macroscopic complete resection with high-risk features (any or all of ≥2 LNs, ECE, or +margins) comparing RT alone (60–66 Gy/30–33 fx) vs. CRT (cisplatin 100 mg/m^2 on days 1, 22, and 43). Overall, 18% had positive margins and 82% had two or more LNs or ECE. MFU 6.1 years; update 9.4 years for survivors (see Table 17.5). Incidence of acute adverse effects grade ≥3 was 34% and 77% in the RT and CRT arms, respectively ($p < .001$). In the first report, CHT improved LRF and DFS but not OS. With long-term follow-up, CHT improved LRF in patients with ECE or +margins. **Conclusion: ECE and positive margins are indications for concurrent CHT and PORT.**

Table 17.5 Results of RTOG 9501 Postoperative CHT Trial

	Original Report (2004)			Long-Term Update (2012)		
	2-Yr LRC	2-Yr DFS	2-Yr OS	10-Yr LRF, All	10-Yr LRF, ECE, or +Margins	10-Yr OS, ECE, or +Margins
PORT	72%			29%	33%	20%
Postop CRT	82%	HR 0.78	HR 0.84	22%	21%	27%
p value	.01	.04	.19	.10	.02	.07

Bernier, Pooled Analysis of EORTC and RTOG (*Head Neck* 2005, PMID 16161069): Data from EORTC 22931 and RTOG 9501 were pooled for comparative analysis. ECE and/or microscopically positive margins were the only risk factors with significant impact from CRT in both trials. **Conclusion: Positive margins and ECE are the most significant prognostic factors for poor outcomes, and postoperative CRT compared with RT alone improves outcomes in patients with one or both of these risk factors.**

Does the schedule of cisplatin (bolus vs. weekly) influence outcomes?

Weekly cisplatin may be an acceptable alternative to bolus cisplatin. In the definitive CRT setting, NRG-HN009, a phase II/III RCT, is comparing concurrent weekly vs. bolus cisplatin.

Noronha, India (*JCO* 2018, PMID 22920295): PRT of 300 patients with stage III to IV SCC of the oral cavity, oropharynx, hypopharynx, larynx, or unknown primary, randomized to weekly cisplatin (30 mg/m^2) vs. bolus high-dose cisplatin (100 mg/m^2 q3 weeks). High-dose cisplatin resulted in higher 2-year LRC (59% vs. 73%, p = .014) and higher G3+ toxicity (72% vs. 85%, p = .006). OS 39.5 months in weekly arm vs. not reached in high-dose arm (HR 1.14, 95% CI 0.79–1.65). **Conclusion: High-dose cisplatin q3 weeks should remain the preferred CHT regimen.**

Kiyota, JCOG1008 (*JCO* 2022, PMID 35230884): PRT noninferiority trial of 261 patients with stage III to IV SCC of the oral cavity, oropharynx, hypopharynx, or larynx with pathologic microscopic positive margins (≤5 mm of margin) or ENE randomized to concurrent CRT with either weekly cisplatin (40 mg/m^2) or bolus cisplatin (100 mg/m^2 q3 weeks). At MFU of 2.2 years, weekly cisplatin was noninferior to bolus cisplatin (HR 0.69, 99.1% CI 0.374–1.273) and had fewer G3+ hematologic AE and less renal/hearing impairment. **Conclusion: Weekly cisplatin is an acceptable alternative to bolus cisplatin, although longer follow-up is needed.**

How much ECE should trigger the addition of CHT?

Randomized data included any ECE. Recent data show survival detriment proportional to the amount of ECE.[19,20] There does not appear to be a level of ECE low enough to omit CHT, and levels with gross ECE have inferior survival even with CHT. For HPV-associated patients, this is evolving, with multiple trials investigating the omission of CHT for those with minor ECE (≤1 mm).

Is there a role for cetuximab with RT for intermediate-risk patients?

Machtay, RTOG 0920 (*JCO*, PMID 39841939): Phase III RCT evaluating the benefit of the addition of cetuximab (loading dose: 400 mg/m^2; weekly dose ×6: 250 mg/m^2; post-RT weekly dose ×4: 250 mg/m^2) to standard postoperative IMRT (60 Gy/30 fx) for patients with one or more risk factors warranting PORT. At MFU of 7.2 years, DFS was significantly improved in the RT + cetuximab arm (71.7 vs. 63.6 months, *p* = .02), but OS was not significantly improved. Grades 3 to 4 acute toxicity rate was 70% (cetuximab + RT) vs. 40% (RT alone; *p* < .0001), mostly related to skin and/or mucosal effects. **Conclusion: In resected, intermediate-risk HNSCC, RT + cetuximab did not improve OS, but the addition of cetuximab did significantly improve DFS compared with RT alone. Grades 3 to 4 acute toxicities were significantly higher in the RT + cetuximab arm.**

MANAGEMENT OF LOW-RISK PATIENTS

Is PORT necessary in N1 patients?

A microscopic single node without other risk factors was not sufficient to receive PORT in the preceding Ang MD Anderson trial. However, any node positivity was an indication for PORT in the Tata Memorial study of oral cavity patients, which may have contributed to the difference in OS (see Chapter 12).[18,21] It is likely that carefully selected pN1 (single node) nonoral cavity patients, in the absence of other risk factors and after adequate neck dissection, can be observed.[22,23]

Can treatment volumes be decreased in PORT?

A small phase II study (mixture of primary sites, selected group) omitting the pN0 neck demonstrated favorable LC.[24] Other phase II data support the omission of a resected primary in HPV-associated N+ oropharynx cancer (OPC). These are early data and should be approached with caution off study.

Contreras (*JCO* 2019, PMID 31246526): Phase II study of 72 patients who underwent resection of the primary and bilateral neck dissection (six patients were unable to undergo contralateral neck dissection), with high-risk features warranting PORT. The pN0 neck was not irradiated (if patient had bilateral pN0, only the primary was irradiated). Primary endpoint was rate of recurrence in unirradiated pN0 neck (aimed to demonstrate <10% failure). Sites included oral cavity (20%), oropharynx (51%), hypopharynx (6%), larynx (22%), and unknown primary (1%). No patients had contralateral neck RT; 24% of patients received RT to the primary only. Two patients had a failure in the pN0 unirradiated neck; unirradiated neck control was 97%. The 5-year LC, LRC, PFS, and OS rates were 84%, 93%, 60%, and 64%, respectively. **Conclusion: In this small study, eliminating PORT to the pN0 neck had favorable LC rates.**

Swisher-McClure, AVOID (*IJROBP* 2020, PMID 31785337): Single-arm, phase II prospective trial of 60 stage pT1–2 N1–3 HPV-associated OPC patients treated with TORS and selective neck dissection at a single institution. Patients had favorable features at the primary site (negative surgical margins ≥2 mm, no PNI, and no LVSI) but required adjuvant therapy based on LN involvement. PORT to at-risk areas in the involved neck (60–66 Gy) and uninvolved neck (54 Gy). The resected primary site was treated as an active avoidance structure. Concurrent CHT given for ECE. MFU 2.4 years. A single patient recurred at the primary site; 2-year LC was 98%. One patient (1.7%) developed a regional neck recurrence, and two patients (3.3%) developed DMs; 2-year LRFS was 98%. OS was 100% at the time of analysis. The mean RT dose to the primary site was 36.9 Gy. **Conclusion:**

Deintensified PORT that avoids the resected primary tumor site for selected patients with HPV-associated OPC appears safe and is worthy of further study.

Can PORT dose be deintensified after surgery for HPV+ OPC patients?

There are select patients for whom reduced dose PORT without CHT seems sufficient based on ECOG/ACRIN 3311.[25] For post-TORS patients with negative margins, <5 involved nodes, and minimal ENE (<1 mm), reduced-dose PORT with 50 Gy had similar 2-year PFS to 60 Gy (95% vs. 98.6%, respectively). Phase II data from Mayo Clinic suggest comparable LRC rates to historical controls using 30 to 36 Gy PORT after transoral surgery (provided no ECE, which portends worse outcomes with reduced dose).[26] TORS with de-escalated PORT should be evaluated in a phase III trial.

Ma, Mayo MC1273 (*JCO* 2019, PMID 31163012; Update *IJROBP* 2022, PMID 35675850): Single-arm, phase II trial of RT de-escalation after transoral surgery. Included patients with p16-positive oropharyngeal SCC, smoking history of <10 pack-years, and negative margins. Cohort A (intermediate risk) received 30 Gy (1.5 Gy/fx given BID) with 15 mg/m² docetaxel weekly. Cohort B included patients with ECE who received the same treatment plus an SIB to nodal levels with ECE to 36 Gy in 1.8 Gy fx, given BID. MFU 36 months. The 2-year LRC rate was 96%, with PFS of 91% and OS of 99%. Grade 3+ toxicity at pre-RT, 1 year, and 2 years post-RT was 2.5%, 0%, and 0%. Swallowing function improved slightly between pre-RT and 12 months post-RT, with one patient requiring temporary feeding tube. **Conclusion: Aggressive RT de-escalation resulted in locoregional tumor control rates comparable to those of historical controls, low toxicity, and little decrement in swallowing function or QOL.** Note: *Caution advised when adopting single-institution results off the trial, particularly when ECE is present.[26]*

Ferris, ECOG 3311 (*JCO* 2021, PMID 34699271): Randomized phase II trial of TORS followed by low-dose vs. standard-dose IMRT in stage III to IVA (AJCC 7th) p16+ OPC. Primary goals were feasibility of prospective multi-institutional study of TORS for HPV+ OPC and oncologic efficacy (2-year PFS) of TORS and adjuvant therapy in intermediate-risk patients after resection. Arms and 2-year PFS per Table 17.6. **Conclusion: Primary TORS with de-escalated PORT is a reasonable strategy for intermediate-risk patients as defined by pathologic tumor characteristics.**

Table 17.6 Results of ECOG 3311 De-Escalated PORT trial			
Risk Category	**Pathologic Criteria**	**Intervention**	**2-Yr PFS**
Low risk (A)	T1–2N0–1, margins ≥3 mm, no ECE	Observation	97%
Intermediate risk (B and C)	Close (<3 mm) margins, ≤1 mm ECE, 2–4 LN+, PNI/LVI	Arm B: 50 Gy/25 fx	B: 95%*
		Arm C: 60 Gy/30 fx	C: 96%*
High risk (D)	>1 mm ECE, ≥5 LNs, +margins	66 Gy/33 fx + concurrent cisplatin (40 mg/m² weekly)	D: 91%

*No statistically significant difference.

REFERENCES

1. Ganly I, Goldstein D, Carlson DL, et al. Long-term regional control and survival in patients with "low-risk," early stage oral tongue cancer managed by partial glossectomy and neck dissection without postoperative radiation: the importance of tumor thickness. *Cancer.* 2013;119(6):1168–1176. doi:10.1002/cncr.27872

2. Bernier J, Cooper JS, Pajak TF, et al. Defining risk levels in locally advanced head and neck cancers: a comparative analysis of concurrent postoperative radiation plus chemotherapy trials of the EORTC (#22931) and RTOG (#9501). *Head Neck.* 2005;27(10):843–850. doi:10.1002/hed.20279

3. Barsouk A, Aluru JS, Rawla P, Saginala K, Barsouk A. Epidemiology, risk factors, and prevention of head and neck squamous cell carcinoma. *Med Sci (Basel).* 2023;11(2):42. doi:10.3390/medsci11020042

4. Siegel RL, Giaquinto AN, Jemal A. Cancer statistics, 2024. *CA Cancer J Clin.* 2024;74(1):12–49. doi:10.3322/caac.21820

5. Kiaris H, Spandidos DA, Jones AS, Vaughan ED, Field JK. Mutations, expression and genomic instability of the H-ras proto-oncogene in squamous cell carcinomas of the head and neck. *Br J Cancer.* 1995;72(1):123–128. doi:10.1038/bjc.1995.287

6. Zhu X, Zhang F, Zhang W, He J, Zhao Y, Chen X. Prognostic role of epidermal growth factor receptor in head and neck cancer: a meta-analysis. *J Surg Oncol.* 2013;108(6):387–397. doi:10.1002/jso.23406

7. Mani N, George MM, Nash L, Anwar B, Homer JJ. Role of 18-Fludeoxyglucose positron emission tomography-computed tomography and subsequent panendoscopy in head and neck squamous cell carcinoma of unknown primary. *Laryngoscope.* 2016;126(6):1354–1358. doi:10.1002/lary.25783

8. Lewis JS Jr, Carpenter DH, Thorstad WL, Zhang Q, Haughey BH. Extracapsular extension is a poor predictor of disease recurrence in surgically treated oropharyngeal squamous cell carcinoma. *Mod Pathol.* 2011;24(11):1413–1420. doi:10.1038/modpathol.2011.105

9. Prabhu RS, Magliocca KR, Hanasoge S, et al. Accuracy of computed tomography for predicting pathologic nodal extracapsular extension in patients with head-and-neck cancer undergoing initial surgical resection. *Int J Radiat Oncol Biol Phys.* 2014;88(1):122–129. doi:10.1016/j.ijrobp.2013.10.002

10. Trosman SJ, Koyfman SA, Ward MC, et al. Effect of human papillomavirus on patterns of distant metastatic failure in oropharyngeal squamous cell carcinoma treated with chemoradiotherapy. *JAMA Otolaryngol Head Neck Surg.* 2015;141(5):457–462. doi:10.1001/jamaoto.2015.136

11. Ward MC, Koyfman SA. Transoral robotic surgery: the radiation oncologist's perspective. *Oral Oncol.* 2016;60:96–102. doi:10.1016/j.oraloncology.2016.07.008

12. Huang SH, Hansen A, Rathod S, O'Sullivan B. Primary surgery versus (chemo)radiotherapy in oropharyngeal cancer: the radiation oncologist's and medical oncologist's perspectives. *Curr Opin Otolaryngol Head Neck Surg.* 2015;23(2):139–147. doi:10.1097/MOO.0000000000000141

13. Kiyota N, Tahara M, Mizusawa J, et al. Weekly cisplatin plus radiation for postoperative head and neck cancer (JCOG1008): a multicenter, noninferiority, phase II/III randomized controlled trial. *J Clin Oncol.* 2022;40(18):1980–1990. doi:10.1200/JCO.21.01293

14. Machtay M, Torres-Saavedra P, Thorstad WL, et al. Randomized phase III trial of postoperative radiotherapy with or without cetuximab for intermediate-risk Squamous Cell Carcinoma of the Head and Neck (SCCHN): NRG/RTOG 0920. *J Clin Oncol.* 2025;43(12):1474–1487. doi:10.1200/JCO-24-01829

15. Tribius S, Donner J, Pazdyka H, et al. Survival and overall treatment time after postoperative radio(chemo)therapy in patients with head and neck cancer. *Head Neck.* 2016;38(7):1058–1065. doi:10.1002/hed.24407

16. Mishra RC, Singh DN, Mishra TK. Post-operative radiotherapy in carcinoma of buccal mucosa, a prospective randomized trial. *Eur J Surg Oncol.* 1996;22(5):502–504. doi:10.1016/S0748-7983(96)92969-8

17. Kokal WA, Neifeld JP, Eisert D, et al. Postoperative radiation as adjuvant treatment for carcinoma of the oral cavity, larynx, and pharynx: preliminary report of a prospective randomized trial. *J Surg Oncol.* 1988;38(2):71–76. doi:10.1002/jso.2930380202

18. Laskar SG, Chaukar D, Deshpande M, et al. Oral Cavity Adjuvant Therapy (OCAT)—a phase III, randomized controlled trial of surgery followed by conventional RT (5 fr/wk) versus concurrent CT-RT versus accelerated RT (6 fr/wk) in locally advanced, resectable, squamous cell carcinoma of oral cavity. *Eur J Cancer.* 2023;181:179–187. doi:10.1016/j.ejca.2022.12.016

19. Prabhu RS, Hanasoge S, Magliocca KR, et al. Extent of pathologic extracapsular extension and outcomes in patients with nonoropharyngeal head and neck cancer treated with initial surgical resection. *Cancer.* 2014;120(10):1499–1506. doi:10.1002/cncr.28596

20. Greenberg JS, Fowler R, Gomez J, et al. Extent of extracapsular spread: a critical prognosticator in oral tongue cancer. *Cancer.* 2003;97(6):1464–1470. doi:10.1002/cncr.11202

21. D'Cruz AK, Vaish R, Kapre N, et al. Elective versus therapeutic neck dissection in node-negative oral cancer. *N Engl J Med.* 2015;373(6):521–529. doi:10.1056/NEJMoa1506007

22. Schmitz S, Machiels JP, Weynand B, Gregoire V, Hamoir M. Results of selective neck dissection in the primary management of head and neck squamous cell carcinoma. *Eur Arch Otorhinolaryngol.* 2009;266(3):437–443. doi:10.1007/s00405-008-0767-9

23. Jäckel MC, Ambrosch P, Christiansen H, Martin A, Steiner W. Value of postoperative radiotherapy in patients with pathologic N1 neck disease. *Head Neck.* 2008;30(7):875–882. doi:10.1002/hed.20794

24. Contreras JA, Spencer C, DeWees T, et al. Eliminating postoperative radiation to the pathologically node-negative neck: long-term results of a prospective phase II study. *J Clin Oncol.* 2019;37(28):2548–2555. doi:10.1200/JCO.19.00186

25. Ferris RL, Flamand Y, Weinstein GS, et al. Phase II randomized trial of transoral surgery and low-dose intensity modulated radiation therapy in resectable p16+ locally advanced oropharynx cancer: an ECOG-ACRIN Cancer Research Group Trial (E3311). *J Clin Oncol.* 2022;40(2):138–149. doi:10.1200/JCO.21.01752

26. Ma DM, PK, Moore EJ, et al. MC1675, a phase III evaluation of De-escalated Adjuvant Radiation Therapy (DART) vs standard adjuvant treatment for human papillomavirus associated oropharyngeal squamous cell carcinoma. *Int J Radiat Oncol Biol Phys.* 2021;111(5):1324. doi:10.1016/j.ijrobp.2021.09.012

18 THYROID CANCER

David S. Buchberger, Nikhil P. Joshi, and Neil M. Woody

QUICK HIT Papillary thyroid cancer (PTC), medullary thyroid cancer (MTC), and follicular thyroid cancer (FTC) are forms of differentiated thyroid cancer that are treated with surgical resection (thyroid lobectomy and isthmusectomy vs. total thyroidectomy) followed by adjuvant therapy dependent upon ATA risk group. Radioactive iodine (RAI) is delivered to ablate residual thyroid tissue and microscopic disease in iodine-avid disease (common in FTC and PTC). MTC is a neuroendocrine thyroid tumor that produces calcitonin and CEA and is associated with MEN2 syndrome. Adjuvant EBRT is used infrequently for differentiated/medullary thyroid cancers, but it may be indicated after resection of recurrent disease at high risk for additional unresectable recurrence (positive margins, gross extrathyroidal extension [ETE], gross and extensive extracapsular nodal extension [ENE], insular or poorly differentiated, tall cell, hobnail, or other high-risk histology).

Anaplastic thyroid cancer (ATC) is an aggressive disease with treatment that is rapidly evolving, with an emerging potential role for neoadjuvant immunotherapy and targeted therapy dependent on BRAF status. When mutations are absent, resection for nonmetastatic disease followed by CRT vs. definitive CRT vs. palliative RT and targeted therapy as applicable. RAI is not effective in MTC or ATC.

EPIDEMIOLOGY: There were an estimated 44,020 new cases (PTC 60%, FTC 25%, MTC 5%, ATC <5%) and 2,170 deaths in the United States in 2024.[1]

RISK FACTORS: Previous radiation exposure particularly during childhood.[2] Approximately 85% of RT-induced thyroid cancers are well-differentiated PTC. Other factors include iodine deficiency, family history of thyroid cancer, and female gender.

GENETICS: MEN2 is a rare, autosomal-dominant syndrome in which nearly all patients develop MTC due to mutations in the RET proto-oncogene. BRAF and TERT mutations are commonly present in high-risk PTC, and BRAF status is important in ATC.

ANATOMY: Bilobed gland joined near the lower pole by the isthmus, crossing the trachea anteriorly just below the cricoid cartilage. Thyroid gland is composed of follicles or acini, each with a basement membrane lined with a single layer of follicular cells responsible for thyroid hormone synthesis. Each contains a central space with thyroglobulin (Tg), the molecule upon which the thyroid hormones are synthesized and stored prior to release by TSH stimulation. *Lymphatics*: LN spread has more prognostic significance in MTC than for the well-differentiated subtypes. The first echelon is paratracheal, paralaryngeal, and prelaryngeal (Delphian) nodes of level VI. Secondary spread is to the mid/lower jugular (levels III–IV) and supraclavicular LNs. *Physiology*: Hypothalamus secretes thyrotropin-releasing hormone, which stimulates the anterior pituitary to secrete TSH, which stimulates the thyroid to make T3 (triiodothyronine) and T4 (thyroxine), which control cellular metabolic activity in all cellular tissues and exert negative feedback on the hypothalamus and pituitary. Tg is a storage form of T3 and T4. Nearly 90% of well-differentiated thyroid cancers secrete Tg, and 60% take up radioiodine detectable on imaging. Thus, radioiodine is used in diagnosis/treatment of differentiated thyroid cancers, under maximal TSH stimulation. T3 half-life ~2.5 days. T4 half-life ~6.5 days.

PATHOLOGY: Four major subtypes (see Table 18.1); rare histologies include lymphoma or metastasis (usually breast, colon, renal, or melanoma).

Table 18.1 Thyroid Cancer Subtypes	
Subtype	**Description**
Papillary	• Accounts for 60% of thyroid cancer cases. • Well-differentiated. Arise from follicular cells. Produce and secrete T3, T4 (RAI effective). • Associated with psammoma bodies; slow-growing, indolent; multifocal in 75%; metastasizes locally to LNs, less commonly DM. Better long-term prognosis than follicular. • Good prognostic variants: papillary microcarcinoma (<1 cm), encapsulated, solid, and follicular. • Poor prognostic variants: high-grade transformation, poorly differentiated, de-differentiated, tall cell, hobnail, columnar cell, and diffuse sclerosing. These variants often do not concentrate ^{131}I to a degree that is curative.
Follicular	• Accounts for 25% of thyroid cancer cases. • Well-differentiated. Arise from follicular cells. Produce and secrete T3, T4 (RAI effective). • Metastasizes hematogenously to lung and bone. Compared with PTC, has lower predilection for LN spread and occurs in older population. • Hurthle cell variant has a worse prognosis and is less likely to uptake [131]I. Need ≥75% Hurthle cells present (characterized by abundant eosinophilic granular content).
Medullary	• Accounts for 5% of thyroid cancer cases. • Arise from parafollicular or C cells (neural crest, i.e., neuroendocrine). • Produce and secrete calcitonin and CEA. • RAI ineffective.
Poorly differentiated thyroid cancers	• Accounts for <5% of thyroid cancers. • Represents an aggressive, often RAI insensitive tumor. • May be a de-differentiated variant from less aggressive variants.
Anaplastic	• Accounts for <5% of thyroid cancer cases, but 40% of all thyroid cancer deaths.[3] • Extremely aggressive. Always classified as stage IV regardless of size, invasion, nodal status, or DM. • RAI ineffective. • 20% have history of differentiated thyroid cancer. • Variants include spindle cell, squamoid, and pleomorphic giant cell. • 45% have DM at diagnosis, most often to lung and bone.

CLINICAL PRESENTATION: Commonly presents as palpable nodule or hoarseness if recurrent laryngeal nerve is involved or as an incidental finding. ATC presents as rapidly enlarging neck mass. Differential diagnosis includes thyroid lymphoma, metastasis, benign thyroid nodule, and thyroiditis.

WORKUP: H&P. US and/or MRI (preferred over CT to avoid iodine contamination from contrast for PTC/FTC, but neither is reliable at distinguishing malignant nodules). Laryngoscopy for vocal cord movement. If nodule is present, US criteria are used to define risks and necessity of proceeding to FNA. Genetic sequencing classifier may be employed on thyroid biopsy to further classify risks of malignancy. [131]I scan can be performed to see if the thyroid nodule is functioning/hot (97% benign) or nonfunctioning/cold (10% malignant). If cold, proceed to FNA.[4] Hurthle cell cancers have poor ^{131}I uptake and are better seen by Tc-99m sestamibi scan. PET may be used for poorly differentiated tumors with elevated Tg level and a negative ^{131}I scan. For the possibility of MTC, calcitonin and CEA levels should be checked preop and if MTC is identified repeated postop. Consider serum calcium and urinary excretion of metanephrines and catecholamines to evaluate for possible MEN syndrome in cases of MTC. For ATC, recommend US neck, CT neck, PET/CT, and CT or MRI brain.

PROGNOSTIC FACTORS: Tumor size (>1.5 cm), age (<20 or >55 years is worse), male sex (worse), extent of local and distant spread including ETE, stage, extent of surgery, response to RAI, and histology.[5] Unilateral LN spread does not impact OS, but bilateral or mediastinal LN involvement has poor prognosis. Elevated serum Tg correlates with recurrence postop (most sensitive when hypothyroid with high TSH).

STAGING: See Table 18.2.

Table 18.2 AJCC 8th Edition (2017): Staging for Papillary, Follicular, Poorly Differentiated, Hurthle Cell, and Anaplastic Thyroid Carcinoma						
T/M	N	N0a	N0b	N1a	N1b
T1	a. ≤1 cm, limited to the thyroid	I (see note*)		II (see note*)	
	b. 1.1–2 cm, limited to the thyroid				
T2	2.1–4 cm, limited to the thyroid				
T3	a. >4 cm, limited to the thyroid				
	b. Gross extension[1]				
T4	a. Gross extension[2]	III (see note*)			
	b. Gross extension[3]	IVA (see note*)			
M1	Distant metastasis	IVB (see note*)			

Notes: Extension[1] = extension invading only strap muscles (sternohyoid, sternothyroid, thyrohyoid, or omohyoid muscles). Extension[2] = extension invading subcutaneous soft tissue, larynx, trachea, esophagus, or recurrent laryngeal nerve. Extension[3] = extension invading prevertebral fascia or encasing the carotid artery or mediastinal vessels. Solitary tumor (s) or multifocal tumor (m) identifiers may be used.
N0a: ≥1 pathologically confirmed benign LNs; N0b: no radiologic or clinical evidence of LNs; N1a: unilateral or bilateral metastasis to level VI or VII LNs; N1b: unilateral, bilateral, or contralateral metastasis to levels I–V or retropharyngeal LNs.
*Only for patients ≥55 years. In patients <55 years, M0 disease is stage I and M1 disease is stage II, regardless of T and N staging. Anaplastic thyroid carcinoma uses same TNM stage, but separate group staging with T1–3aN0 stage IVA and all T3b–T4 or N+ as IVB and metastatic as IVC.

TREATMENT PARADIGM

Well-Differentiated Thyroid Cancer (PTC or FTC)

Surgery: Surgery is the primary treatment for well-differentiated thyroid cancer. Options include thyroid lobectomy plus isthmusectomy vs. total thyroidectomy. Very favorable tumors may be observed and not require resection in select cases (see Table 18.3 for the ATA's risk classification). Thyroid hormone (T4, levothyroxine) replacement therapy is required following total thyroidectomy to prevent hypothyroidism and to minimize potential TSH stimulation of tumor growth. Lobectomy plus isthmusectomy is an option for select patients unable or unwilling to undergo lifelong thyroid hormone replacement. Total thyroidectomy is recommended for patients with tumors ≥4 cm, ETE, cervical node involvement, DM, or poorly differentiated or anaplastic histology. Consider regional nodal dissection for clinically involved nodes, tumor >4 cm, or extrathyroidal invasion.[6]

Table 18.3 American Thyroid Association (ATA) 2016 Risk of Recurrence for Differentiated Thyroid Cancer	
Low risk	• PTC histology and all of the following: organ-confined disease, completely resected, no aggressive histologic variants, no vascular invasion, no ^{131}I uptake outside the thyroid bed posttreatment, clinical N0 or ≤5 pathologic N1 micrometastases • Follicular variant of PTC: intrathyroidal, encapsulated • Well-differentiated follicular thyroid cancer with capsular invasion and <4 foci of vascular invasion • Papillary microcarcinoma, unifocal or multifocal (including BRAF V600E mutated if known)
Intermediate risk	*Any are present:* • Local soft tissue microscopic invasion • Cervical lymph node metastases or ^{131}I-avid metastatic foci in the neck posttreatment • Aggressive histology or vascular invasion • Clinical N1 or >5 pathologic N1 with all involved lymph nodes <3 cm in largest dimension • Multifocal papillary thyroid microcarcinoma with extrathyroidal extension (including BRAF V600E mutated if known)

(continued)

Table 18.3 American Thyroid Association (ATA) 2016 Risk of Recurrence for Differentiated Thyroid Cancer (*continued*)	
High risk	*Any are present:* • Gross (macroscopic) invasion of local structures • Incomplete tumor resection with gross residual disease • Distant metastases • Elevated postoperative serum thyroglobulin (suggestive of distant metastases) • Lymph node ≥3 cm in largest dimension • Follicular thyroid cancer with extensive vascular invasion (>4 foci of vascular invasion)

Source: Adapted from Haugen BR, et al. 2015 American Thyroid Association management guidelines for adult patients with thyroid nodules and differentiated thyroid cancer: the American Thyroid Association Guidelines Task Force on thyroid nodules and differentiated thyroid cancer. *Thyroid.* Jan 2016;26(1):1–133. doi:10.1089/thy.2015.0020.

Radioiodine: TSH stimulates radioiodine uptake into follicular cells through sodium-iodide transporters. This leads to acute thyroid cell death by emission of short path-length (1–2 mm) β particles. ^{131}I must be taken up by thyroid tissue to be effective and is of no value to thyroid cancers that do not concentrate iodide (i.e., MTC, ATC). A radioactive uptake study using ^{123}I is typically performed prior to ^{131}I administration to ensure adequate iodine uptake. ^{123}I is a γ emitter used for imaging only. Patients are instructed to follow a low-iodine diet, avoid IV iodinated contrast, and temporarily stop thyroid hormone replacement prior to administration to ensure adequate uptake. The entire body is imaged ~1 week after ^{131}I administration to document the quality of treatment.

Indications: Postoperatively for ATA intermediate- and high-risk patients as well as select low-risk patients (Table 18.4).

Table 18.4 Indications for ^{131}I Ablation Based on ATA Risk Group[6]			
Surgical resection	ATA Risk Group	^{131}I Ablation (RAI)	Goal TSH (mU/L) via T4 Replacement
	Low	Do not routinely give ^{131}I.	0.5–2.0 (if Tg undetectable); 0.1–0.5 (if Tg detectable)
	Intermediate	Consider ^{131}I.	0.1–0.5
	High	Give ^{131}I.	<0.1

Source: Data from Haugen BR, Alexander EK, Bible KC, et al. 2015 American thyroid association management guidelines for adult patients with thyroid nodules and differentiated thyroid cancer: the American thyroid association guidelines task force on thyroid nodules and differentiated thyroid cancer. *Thyroid.* 2016;26(1):1–133. doi:10.1089/thy.2015.0020.

Radiation: There is no consensus on the role of adjuvant EBRT, although it may be considered for patients with residual disease unlikely to respond to RAI (absent or inadequate radioiodine avidity), unresectable residual disease, at high risk for residual disease (age ≥55, positive margins, gross ETE, insular or poorly differentiated histology), or recurrent disease. Consider omitting EBRT in patients under age 45 who may not benefit from treatment and may be at risk for late effects (second malignancies). Dose is 60 to 66 Gy in 30 to 33 fx. Consideration should be made for histologic subtypes less likely to respond to RAI (especially with high-risk features), and nomograms exist to help guide these decisions.

MTC

Surgery: All should undergo total thyroidectomy if possible. Completeness of surgical removal is the most important prognostic factor for long-term survival.[7] Central compartment neck dissection (level VI) is indicated, with sampling of cervical and mediastinal nodes. Consider lateral neck (levels III–V) and/or mediastinal dissection if positive. Radical neck dissection does not improve prognosis and is not indicated. Serum calcitonin and CEA should be measured 2 to 3 months after surgery to detect the presence of residual disease. Patients with normal calcitonin and CEA are considered biochemically cured and should continue surveillance. Patients with postop calcitonin levels detectable but <150 pg/mL (2–6 months after surgery) should have neck imaging (US ± CT or MRI) to identify persistent locoregional disease. Patients with postop calcitonin levels ≥150 pg/mL (2–6 months after surgery) should undergo additional imaging (CT or MRI neck, CT C/A/P, bone scan, or bone MRI in patients suspected of having skeletal metastases) to identify possible DM.[8]

Radioiodine: Not indicated because the tumor cells do not concentrate iodine.

Thyroid Hormone Replacement: Thyroxine (T4, levothyroxine) replacement therapy should be started immediately after surgery. The goal of T4 therapy is to restore and maintain euthyroidism. Suppression of serum TSH is not indicated with MTC because C cells are not TSH-responsive.

Radiation: Indications are similar to those of well-differentiated thyroid tumors. Some consider EBRT for persistently elevated calcitonin/CEA levels following surgery without evidence of gross disease or DM, although not routine. Dose is 63 Gy and 56 Gy in 35 fx or 66 Gy and 59.4 Gy in 33 fx and can be delivered similar to RTOG 0912.

Systemic Therapy: Reserved for patients with DM. Patients with asymptomatic small and slow-growing DM can be observed. RET mutation testing is important to guide systemic treatment (selpercatinib). Multikinase inhibitors like cabozantinib and vandetanib are used for non-RET mutated MTC.

ATC

Typically presents with a rapidly enlarging neck mass, and the cause of death is often asphyxiation. DM at presentation is common.

Systemic Therapy: BRAF status assessed immediately on diagnosis. Emerging paradigm for neo-adjuvant therapy (typically dabrafenib/trametinib +/– IO) when positive. For BRAF-negative disease, surgery is recommended for resectable disease, which is followed by adjuvant therapy. For unresectable disease, definitive CRT for locoregional control. Optimal concurrent agent with RT is controversial, with low-dose doxorubicin an option. For patients without mutations, RTOG 0912 offers a paradigm that delivers 66 Gy and 59.4 Gy in 33 fx with concurrent paclitaxel.[9] Note aggressive locoregional therapy (surgery + RT) is indicated even when DM is present given risk of asphyxiation.

Radioiodine: RAI is not indicated.

EVIDENCE-BASED Q&A

What are the indications for EBRT in differentiated thyroid cancer?

The role of adjuvant EBRT in patients with well-differentiated thyroid cancer has been studied only retrospectively, and many of the studies included patients at low risk of recurrence who were unlikely to benefit from the therapy. Recently, institutional nomograms have been generated suggesting a particular benefit in aggressive histologies less responsive to RAI (tall cell, hobnail). The addition of EBRT to patients with recurrent or high-risk differentiated thyroid cancer can lead to LC and OS outcomes comparable to historical controls. EBRT can improve outcomes in patients with gross residual disease,[10] but it may need to be given in partnership with RAI[11] and the outcomes overall may be worse.[12] EBRT seems to be well-tolerated.[13]

Wu, Adjuvant RT Nomogram (*JAMA Otolaryn* 2023, PMID 36454559): All cases of PTC with tall cell morphology (TCM) from 1997 to 2018 treated at a single institution underwent an outcomes analysis. 365 patients were evaluated. The vast majority (92%) underwent total thyroidectomy. Nineteen (5%) received adjuvant RT with two LRFs. The 5-year LRFS, DRFS, and OS rates were 82%, 92%, and 93% respectively. pT3/T4, pN+, positive surgical margins, LVSI, and tumor size ≥1.5 cm were each associated with worse 5-year LRFS and DRFS. On MVA, positive surgical margins (HR 3.5, 95% CI 2.0–6.3), pN+ (HR 2.8, 1.4–5.8), and primary tumor ≥3 cm vs. <1.5 cm (HR 3.3, 1.4–7.8) were identified as independent predictors of significantly inferior LRFS. **Conclusion: Intensified locoregional therapy should be considered in patients with PTC with tall cell morphology who have positive margins, pN+, and tumor size ≥3 cm.**

Tam, MDACC Matched Pair Analysis (*JAMA Otolaryn* 2017, PMID 29098272): Matched-pair analysis of 88 patients with surgically resected T4a differentiated thyroid cancer comparing RAI vs. RAI + EBRT; 5-year DFS was 43% in the RAI-alone group compared with 57% in RAI + EBRT (effect size = 14%; 95% CI –7% to 33%). RAI alone had increased LRF. Age and esophageal invasion predicted worse DFS. **Conclusion: Addition of EBRT to RAI results in good disease control for locally advanced differentiated thyroid cancer.**

ATA 2015 Guidelines (*Thyroid* 2016, PMID 26462967): Recommend EBRT (in combination with surgery and RAI) in patients with aerodigestive invasive disease. Recommend against routine adjuvant EBRT in patients who have had initial complete surgical resection. However, the use of EBRT in this latter setting is controversial. Selective use of EBRT may be considered in patients with initial complete surgical resection who have locally advanced disease and in patients >60 years with ETE. It is unknown whether EBRT reduces the risk of recurrence in patients with aggressive histologic subtypes who have adequate initial surgery and/or RAI.

What is the recommended follow-up for thyroid cancer patients?

Most recurrences occur within the first 5 years, but recurrences can happen even decades after PTC diagnosis. US has been particularly useful at identifying malignant cervical LNs, the most common site of recurrent PTC. Serum Tg is a useful marker of persistent or recurrent tumor in patients after thyroidectomy and ablation of residual normal thyroid tissue. If initial surgery and thyroid-remnant ablation are successful, the serum Tg concentration should be very low, both during thyroxine therapy and after it is discontinued or stimulated by recombinant human TSH. A stimulated Tg value of ≥2 ng/mL suggests disease is present and more extensive evaluation is indicated. Antithyroglobulin antibodies, present initially in ~25% of patients with thyroid cancer, may interfere with assays for Tg, and antithyroglobulin antibodies should be tested for prior to measuring serum Tg.

What is the standard treatment regimen for patients with anaplastic thyroid cancer?

Given the rare nature of the disease, data to guide treatment are limited. Historically, series utilized surgery (if possible) and concurrent CRT. RTOG 0912 (below) investigated the use of the targeted agent pazopanib with concurrent CRT finding no survival benefit.[9] Over the past decade, the use of targeted therapy (dabrafenib/trametinib) ± IO for BRAF-mutated ATC has improved outcomes and created a paradigm shift in the treatment of this disease (below).[14-18] A recent consensus statement from MD Anderson Cancer Center recommends neoadjuvant dabrafenib, trametinib, and pembrolizumab for stage IVB/IVC patients followed by surgery in patients with an appropriate response and postoperative CRT for resected stage IVB patients.[14] Palliative treatment is appropriate for urgent airway compromise, and tracheostomy should be considered as needed. However, recent guidelines also advocate for the consideration of expedited BRAF testing in the setting of a tenuous airway, with rapid initiation of targeted therapy as a potential means of avoiding tracheostomy.[14]

Hamidi, MD Anderson BRAF Cohort (*Thyroid* 2024, PMID 38226606): RR of BRAF-mutated ATC patients treated with dabrafenib/trametinib ± pembrolizumab. Three groups were evaluated: (a) patients treated with dabrafenib/trametinib alone ("DT"; 23 patients), (b) patients treated with upfront dabrafenib/trametinib/pembrolizumab or upfront dabrafenib/trametinib plus IO at progression ("DTP"; 48 patients), and (c) neoadjuvant dabrafenib/trametinib followed by definitive surgery with pembrolizumab added before or after surgery ("exploratory neoadjuvant group"; 23 patients). Median OS for the DTP group was 17 months vs. 9 months in the DT group (*p* = .037). Median PFS was 11 months for the DTP group vs. 4 months for DT alone (*p* = .049). For the 23 patients who fell into the exploratory neoadjuvant group, median OS was 63 months. No G5 events in any group; 32% rate of immune AEs. **Conclusion: In BRAF-mutated ATC, neoadjuvant dabrafenib/trametinib with IO has promising outcomes and may improve survival. Surgery appears to confer an additional survival benefit.**

Sherman, RTOG 0912 (*Lancet Oncol* 2022, PMID 36681089): Multicenter, prospective, randomized phase II clinical trial investigating the addition of pazopanib vs. placebo to concurrent CRT in ATC (all TNM stages included). CRT consisted of paclitaxel given concurrently with 66 Gy/33 fx. Patients were randomized to receive concurrent pazopanib or placebo. Primary endpoint OS. Seventy-one patients were evaluated with an MFU of 2.9 years. There was no difference in OS between the two groups, with an mOS of 5.7 months in the pazopanib group and 7.3 months in the placebo group (*p* = .28). The 1-year OS was 37% in the pazopanib group vs. 29% in the placebo group. Post-hoc analysis adjusted by M stage yielded similar results. No difference in LRF or grades 3 to 5 adverse events between the two groups. **Conclusion: The addition of pazopanib to concurrent CRT in the treatment of ATC did not improve survival.**

Sherman, MSKCC (*R&O* 2011, PMID 21981877): RR of 37 patients treated with weekly doxorubicin (10 mg/m^2) and RT to a median of 57.6 Gy; 1-year OS was 28%. **Conclusion: Weekly doxorubicin is feasible, although outcomes remain poor.**

What are the indications for EBRT in medullary thyroid cancer?

Data are limited and retrospective. See below for the results from one large multi-institutional series.

Groen, MSKCC Multi-Institutional Review of PORT for MTC (*J Surg Oncol* 2020, PMID 31733124): RR of 297 patients with MTC treated with surgery from 2000 to 2016 at MSKCC and University Medical Center Groningen; 46 received PORT. In the surgery-only cohort, the rates of 5- and 10-year LRF were 20% and 30%, respectively. The 5- and 10-year OS rates were 89% and 76%. In the PORT cohort, the rates of 5- and 10-year LRF were 14% and 17%, respectively. The 5- and 10-year OS rates were 44% and 38%. On univariable analysis, T4 disease, ETE, N stage, ENE, and residual disease were associated with a decreased LRFS. **Conclusion: LRF is ~30% at 10 years with surgery alone; for high-risk patients, PORT results in effective locoregional control.** *Comment: PORT was performed in patients with higher risk at baseline—a propensity matched analysis was attempted to better compare high-risk patients receiving PORT vs. surgery alone, but it was unable to be completed as the two groups were so fundamentally different.*

REFERENCES

1. Siegel RL, Giaquinto AN, Jemal A. Cancer statistics, 2024. *CA Cancer J Clin.* 2024;74(1):12–49. doi:10.3322/caac.21820
2. Schneider AB, Sarne DH. Long-term risks for thyroid cancer and other neoplasms after exposure to radiation. *Nat Clin Pract Endocrinol Metab.* 2005;1(2):82–91. doi:10.1038/ncpendmet0022
3. Are C, Shaha AR. Anaplastic thyroid carcinoma: biology, pathogenesis, prognostic factors, and treatment approaches. *Ann Surg Oncol.* 2006;13(4):453–464. doi:10.1245/ASO.2006.05.042
4. Cabanillas ME, McFadden DG, Durante C. Thyroid cancer. *Lancet.* 2016;388(10061):2783–2795. doi:10.1016/S0140-6736(16)30172-6
5. Duntas L, Grab-Duntas BM. Risk and prognostic factors for differentiated thyroid cancer. *Hell J Nucl Med.* 2006;9(3):156–162. PMID: 17160155
6. Haugen BR, Alexander EK, Bible KC, et al. 2015 American thyroid association management guidelines for adult patients with thyroid nodules and differentiated thyroid cancer: the American thyroid association guidelines task force on thyroid nodules and differentiated thyroid cancer. *Thyroid.* 2016;26(1):1–133. doi:10.1089/thy.2015.0020
7. Momin S, Chute D, Burkey B, Scharpf J. Prognostic variables affecting primary treatment outcome for medullary thyroid cancer. *Endocr Pract.* 2017;23(9):1053–1058. doi:10.4158/EP161684.OR
8. Wells SA Jr, Asa SL, Dralle H, et al. Revised American Thyroid Association guidelines for the management of medullary thyroid carcinoma. *Thyroid.* 2015;25(6):567–610. doi:10.1089/thy.2014.0335
9. Sherman EJ, Harris J, Bible KC, et al. Radiotherapy and paclitaxel plus pazopanib or placebo in anaplastic thyroid cancer (NRG/RTOG 0912): a randomised, double-blind, placebo-controlled, multicentre, phase 2 trial. *Lancet Oncol.* 2023;24(2):175–186. doi:10.1016/S1470-2045(22)00763-X
10. Chow SM, Law SC, Mendenhall WM, et al. Papillary thyroid carcinoma: prognostic factors and the role of radioiodine and external radiotherapy. *Int J Radiat Oncol Biol Phys.* 2002;52(3):784–795. doi:10.1016/S0360-3016(01)02686-4
11. Lutz ST, Jones J, Chow E. Role of radiation therapy in palliative care of the patient with cancer. *J Clin Oncol.* 2014;32(26):2913–2919. doi:10.1200/JCO.2014.55.1143
12. Schwartz DL, Lobo MJ, Ang KK, et al. Postoperative external beam radiotherapy for differentiated thyroid cancer: outcomes and morbidity with conformal treatment. *Int J Radiat Oncol Biol Phys.* 2009;74(4):1083–1091. doi:10.1016/j.ijrobp.2008.09.023
13. Kwon J, Wu HG, Youn YK, Lee KE, Kim KH, Park DJ. Role of adjuvant postoperative external beam radiotherapy for well differentiated thyroid cancer. *Radiat Oncol J.* 2013;31(3):162–170. doi:10.3857/roj.2013.31.3.162
14. Hamidi S, Dadu R, Zafereo ME, et al. Initial management of BRAF V600E-variant anaplastic thyroid cancer: the FAST multidisciplinary group consensus statement. *JAMA Oncol.* 2024;10(9):1264–1271. doi:10.1001/jamaoncol.2024.2133
15. Hamidi S, Iyer PC, Dadu R, et al. Checkpoint inhibition in addition to dabrafenib/trametinib for BRAF(V600E)-mutated anaplastic thyroid carcinoma. *Thyroid.* 2024;34(3):336–346. doi:10.1089/thy.2023.0573
16. Cabanillas ME, Ferrarotto R, Garden AS, et al. Neoadjuvant BRAF- and immune-directed therapy for anaplastic thyroid carcinoma. *Thyroid.* 2018;28(7):945–951. doi:10.1089/thy.2018.0060
17. Wang JR, Zafereo ME, Dadu R, et al. Complete surgical resection following neoadjuvant dabrafenib plus trametinib in BRAF(V600E)-mutated anaplastic thyroid carcinoma. *Thyroid.* 2019;29(8):1036–1043. doi:10.1089/thy.2019.0133
18. Subbiah V, Kreitman RJ, Wainberg ZA, et al. Dabrafenib plus trametinib in patients with BRAF V600E-mutant anaplastic thyroid cancer: updated analysis from the phase II ROAR basket study. *Ann Oncol.* 2022;33(4):406–415. doi:10.1016/j.annonc.2021.12.014

19 SINONASAL TUMORS

Katherine R. Amarell, Timothy D. Smile, and Jacob A. Miller

QUICK HIT Sinonasal tumors include a range of malignancies arising in complex locations. Squamous cell carcinoma (SCC) and adenocarcinoma (ACA) of the maxillary sinus, nasal cavity, and the ethmoid sinus are the most common. Typical management includes surgery and postoperative RT, although induction CHT and definitive CRT both have a role depending on histology, stage, and proximity to critical OARs (Table 19.1).

Table 19.1 General Treatment Paradigm for Sinonasal Tumors	
Stage	**Treatment Options**
Stage I/II	Surgical resection (preferred) followed by observation (only select T1 tumors), RT, or CRT based on postoperative risk factors OR definitive RT
Stage III/IVA*	Surgical resection (preferred) followed by RT or CRT based on postoperative risk factors OR definitive CRT OR induction CHT (if requiring orbital/skull base resection)
Stage IVB*	CRT OR induction CHT followed by CRT OR RT alone

*Incorporate histology in decision; consider upfront surgery for more resistant histologies (i.e., adenocarcinoma) and induction CHT or CRT for more CHT or RT sensitive histologies (i.e., SCC, SNUC, esthesioneuroblastoma, poorly differentiated carcinoma).

EPIDEMIOLOGY: Sinonasal cancers comprise a range of rare malignancies and account for ~3% of all H&N cancers, with an annual incidence of 1 case per 100,000 people worldwide (~2,000 cases).[1] M:F ratio of 1.8:1. Tumors generally develop after age 40 and between the ages of 60 and 70. The maxillary sinus is the most common site of paranasal sinus cancer (60%–70%), followed by nasal cavity (20%–30%), ethmoid sinus (10%–15%), and frontal and sphenoid sinuses (1%–2%). Prevalence is higher in Asia and Africa.

RISK FACTORS: Occupational exposure (including leather tanners, textile, wood dust, and formaldehyde), air pollution, and tobacco smoke. There are data suggesting viral infections may be associated with sinonasal tumors, specifically HPV with degeneration of inverted papilloma and EBV with lymphoma of the sinonasal tract.[2,3] Chronic sinusitis is not causative.

ANATOMY: The paranasal sinuses are air-filled spaces that are located within the bones of the skull and face. They are centered on the nasal cavity and consist of four sets of paired sinuses: maxillary, frontal, sphenoid, and ethmoid. For maxillary sinus tumors, one important landmark is Ohngren's line: extends from the medial canthus of the eye to the angle of mandible. Anteroinferior/infrastructures have good prognosis, whereas superoposterior/suprastructures have poor prognosis and have early extension into the eye, skull base, pterygoids, and infratemporal fossa.

Maxillary Sinus: Largest paranasal sinus in the shape of a pyramid with the base along the nasal wall and the apex pointing laterally toward the zygoma. The anterior maxillary sinus wall houses the infraorbital nerve, which runs through the infraorbital canal along the roof of the sinus and sends branches to the soft tissues of the cheek. The roof of the maxillary sinus is the floor of the orbit. The posteromedial wall of the maxillary sinus is adjacent to the pterygopalatine fossa, and the posterolateral wall is adjacent to the infratemporal fossa. The maxillary sinus is innervated by the branches of V2 (infraorbital nerve and the greater palatine nerves).

Frontal Sinus: Located in the frontal bone superior to the orbits in the forehead. The posterior wall of the frontal sinus separates the sinus from the anterior cranial fossa (much thinner than the anterior wall). It is innervated by the supraorbital and supratrochlear nerves of V1.

Sphenoid Sinus: Located in the center of the head in the sphenoid bone and may extend posteriorly as far as the foramen magnum. Innervation of the sphenoid sinus is from V1 and V2 branches.

Ethmoid Sinus: Air cells between the orbits in the ethmoid bone. The ethmoid cells are shaped like pyramids and are divided by thin septa. The lamina papyracea (paper-thin bony plate) separates ethmoid cells from the orbit.

PATHOLOGY: The most common histology of sinonasal tract tumors is SCC (~80% of cases). Other common histologies include ACA, adenoid cystic carcinoma, and mucoepidermoid carcinoma. Other more rare histologies include SNUC, olfactory neuroblastoma (esthesioneuroblastoma), HPV-related multiphenotypic carcinomas, angiosarcoma, rhabdomyosarcoma, lymphoma, mucosal melanoma, NUT-midline carcinoma, teratocarcinosarcoma, meningioma, plasmacytoma, and metastasis. Benign etiologies include sinonasal polyposis, choanal polyps, and juvenile angiofibromas. Inverted papilloma is benign but associated with SCC in ~5% of cases and can be locally invasive.

CLINICAL PRESENTATION: Most patients are asymptomatic or have nonspecific sinonasal symptoms until the tumor invades an adjacent structure and prompts a more detailed evaluation. Therefore, most patients have locally advanced disease at presentation. A triad of facial asymmetry, palpable or visible tumor in the oral cavity, and visible intranasal disease occurs in ~50% of patients. Patients can initially present with facial or dental pain, nasal obstruction, and epistaxis. Other symptoms include cranial nerve deficits, chronic sinusitis, facial swelling, headaches, rhinorrhea, and hyposmia.

WORKUP: H&P with particular attention to cranial nerves and assessing for local invasion. Nasal endoscopy as clinically indicated. Dental consult.

Labs: CBC and CMP.

Imaging: CT sinuses and MRI are both performed to evaluate disease extent and distinguish from benign etiologies (infection, retained secretions, granulation of scar tissue). CT chest for stage I/II disease and PET/CT for stage III/IV disease. CT of the sinuses provides information about bone invasion, and MRI provides information about the involvement of soft tissues, nerves, skull base, and brain, and better differentiation of fluid from solid tumor.

Biopsy: Endoscopic biopsy is typically performed unless tumor is protruding through the nasal cavity, oral cavity, or skin. Maxillary sinus lesions may also be biopsied through gingivobuccal sulcus if tumor extends through the anterior maxilla.

PROGNOSTIC FACTORS: The 5-year OS is 50% for those with local disease, 30% with regional disease, and 15% with distant metastatic disease. Favorable prognostic factors: earlier T stage, cN0, ACA histology, and maxillary sinus location. Poor prognostic factors: intracranial extension, infiltration into the pterygopalatine fossa, skull base, dura, cribriform plate, or orbits. There is no AJCC 8th edition staging system for frontal or sphenoid sinus tumors.

STAGING: See Tables 19.2 and 19.3.

Table 19.2 AJCC 8th Edition (2017): Staging for Maxillary Sinus Tumors								
T/M	N	cN0	cN1	cN2a	cN2b	cN2c	cN3a	cN3b
T1	Tumor limited to maxillary sinus mucosa with no erosion or destruction of bone	I		IVA				
T2	Extension	II	III					
T3	Invasion[1]							
T4a	Invasion[2]							
T4b	Invasion[3]		IVB					
M1	Distant metastasis		IVC					

Notes: Extension = bone erosion or extension into the hard palate and/or middle nasal meatus, except extension to posterior wall of maxillary sinus and pterygoid plates. Invasion[1] = invasion of posterior wall of maxillary sinus, subcutaneous tissues, floor or medial wall of orbit, pterygoid fossa, or ethmoid sinuses. Invasion[2] = invasion of anterior orbital contents, skin of cheek, pterygoid plates, infratemporal fossa, cribriform plate, sphenoid or frontal sinuses. Invasion[3] = invasion of orbital apex, dura, brain, middle cranial fossa, cranial nerves other than V2, nasopharynx, or clivus.
N1: single ipsilateral LN ≤3 cm without extranodal extension (ENE); N2a: single ipsilateral LN 3–6 cm without ENE; N2b: multiple ipsilateral LNs ≤6 cm without ENE; N2c: bilateral or contralateral LN ≤6 cm without ENE; N3a: LN >6 cm without ENE; N3b: any node with clinically overt ENE. Similar to oral cavity cancers, pathologic nodal staging is identical to clinical nodal staging, with the exception of pN2a for single ipsilateral LN ≤3 cm with extranodal extension (ENE) present.

T/M	N	cN0	cN1	cN2a	cN2b	cN2c	cN3a	cN3b
Table 19.3 AJCC 8th Edition (2017): Staging for Nasal Cavity and Ethmoid Sinus Tumors								
T1	Tumor limited to any one subsite, with or without bony invasion	I						
T2	Invasion[1]	II	III		IVA			
T3	Extension							
T4a	Invasion[2]							
T4b	Invasion[3]			IVB				
M1	Distant metastasis			IVC				

Notes: Invasion[1] = invasion of two subsites in a single region or extending to involve an adjacent region within the nasoethmoidal complex, with or without bony invasion. Extension = invading the medial wall or floor of the orbit, maxillary sinus, palate, or cribriform plate. Invasion[2] = invasion of anterior orbital contents, skin of nose or cheek, minimal extension to anterior cranial fossa, pterygoid plates, sphenoid or frontal sinuses. Invasion[3] = invasion of orbital apex, dura, brain, middle cranial fossa, cranial nerves other than V2, nasopharynx, or clivus. Clinical and pathologic nodal staging identical to maxillary sinus tumors.

TREATMENT PARADIGM

In general, no randomized trials exist to optimize and define standard treatment paradigms for this disease as it remains rare and encompasses a wide range of histology, locations, and prognoses.

Surgery: Open or endoscopic surgery with attempted GTR of involved bone and soft tissue. Image-guided endoscopic techniques are becoming increasingly popular and are performed by both ENT and neurosurgery with lower frequencies of surgical complications and decreased morbidity. The endoscopic method was historically criticized because it involves piecemeal resection (vs. en bloc resection). However, negative margin status is now known to be the most important factor for LC and is equivalent between open and endoscopic approaches. Advantages of endoscopic approach include no facial incision, no craniotomy, no facial bone osteotomy, shorter hospital stay, and faster recovery time. Endoscopic sinus surgery alone can be used for early-stage lesions or in combination with open craniofacial surgery for locally advanced cases. Contraindications to endoscopic surgery include extensive dural involvement or extension into facial or orbital soft tissues. Prior to surgery, it is important to evaluate the extent of disease including orbital involvement. There are three grades of orbital invasion:

- Grade I—destruction of the medial orbital wall.
- Grade II—invasion of the periorbital fat, extraconal.
- Grade III—invasion of the medial rectus, optic nerve bulb, or eyelid skin, which implies breaching of the periorbita/periosteum.

Orbital exenteration is generally performed for those with grade III invasion. In cases of incomplete periosteal invasion, most surgeons prefer orbital preservation with periosteal resection given comparable survival and functional eye preservation.[4] After resection, most patients undergo surgical and/or prosthetic reconstruction to improve cosmesis, function, and quality of life. Complications of surgery include meningitis, hemorrhage, wound infection, abscess, CSF leak, pneumocephalus, trismus, and blindness. Cervical LN metastases are less common for patients with sinonasal cancers. Neck management (RT or neck dissection) should be performed in patients who have documented cervical LN involvement or locally advanced disease (T3/T4).

Chemotherapy: Indications for CHT extrapolated from other H&N SCC. Cisplatin-based CHT given concurrently with RT is recommended in cases of unresectable disease or postoperatively in patients with positive margins and extracapsular spread and can be considered for multiple intermediate risk factors (appropriate for SCC or ACA, but benefit is unclear for other histologies). For patients with borderline resectable disease and CHT-sensitive histology (SCC, SNUC, poorly differentiated carcinoma), induction CHT (TPF is category 1) can decrease tumor size to facilitate surgery or definitive RT.

Radiation: Typically, postoperative RT (started within 6 weeks of surgery) is used after maximum surgical resection and reconstruction. Definitive (C)RT is recommended for medically inoperable patients or those with unresectable disease. It can also be considered after clinical CR to induction CHT. Extrapolating from other H&N sites: 60 Gy for GTR, 66 Gy for positive margins, and 70 Gy for unresectable or gross residual disease. In the paranasal sinus area, 1.8 Gy/fraction can be considered if multiple neural structures are treated or if escalating dose to >70 Gy. Elective neck coverage is personalized and not always mandatory. Risk of nodal recurrence is driven by histology (higher risk: neuroendocrine carcinoma, SNUC, poorly differentiated SCC, SCC, and advanced esthesioneuroblastoma), T classification (higher risk: T3–T4b), tumor site (higher risk: maxillary sinus), and extension to adjacent tissues (orbit, dural, infratemporal fossa, palate, nasopharynx). Tumors arising from the paranasal sinuses often drain to levels IB, II, III, and retropharyngeal LN. Anterior extension through the maxilla or anterior nasal cavity can drain to facial lymphatics (level IX).[5] Refer to Chapter 17 for more detailed information.

Toxicity: Acute: See Chapter 11. Chronic: Visual complications (chronic pain/keratopathy and vision loss), pituitary dysfunction, osteoradionecrosis, frontal/temporal lobe necrosis. IMRT has resulted in a decline in these complications without sacrificing LC or OS. Proton beam therapy is gaining increasing interest.[6]

EVIDENCE-BASED Q&A

SINONASAL TUMORS

What is the risk of lymph node involvement?

In general, LN involvement is uncommon (<15%–20%) at the time of diagnosis for patients with sinonasal tumors. However, in patients with SCC or poorly differentiated histology, this could be as high as 30%. The risk of LN involvement correlates with advanced T stage and inferior involvement of the alveolar ridge, gingivobuccal sulcus, and palate. In retrospective series, adjuvant elective nodal RT is associated with improved LC and RFS in these subgroups.[7–9] Nasal, ethmoidal, sphenoid, and frontal sinus cancers rarely metastasize regionally. The most commonly involved LN levels are ipsilateral Ib and II, but consider retropharyngeal and parotid for cancers of the mid-face or those with lateral extension; contralateral involvement is rare.

Wang, China (*IJROBP* 2023, PMID 38862085): RR of 368 patients who were cN0 at diagnosis, 75% of which had maxillary or nasal cavity tumors and 68% had T4 disease. 217 (59%) patients received elective nodal radiation (ENI), 16 of which had neck recurrence. ENI reduced the regional failure rate (8% in patients without ENI vs. 2% with ENI). Maxillary tumor origin, T4 disease, and poorly differentiated histology exhibited higher cumulative incidences of regional failures without ENI (2% vs. 14%, *p* = .025 for maxillary; 2% vs. 9%, *p* = .028 for T4; 2% vs. 14%, *p* = .029 for poorly differentiated). There was no survival benefit with ENI. **Conclusion: ENI is safe and may decrease rates of regional failure, especially in those with maxillary disease, T4 disease, and poorly differentiated histology.**

What are the treatment options for locally advanced T3–T4 patients?

Management decisions must consider both tumor histology and anatomic location with consideration to resectability, reconstruction, and functional deficits. Although surgery is typically the treatment of choice for sinonasal cancers, definitive RT/CRT appears to have similar oncologic outcomes to surgical intervention for T3–4 disease. Induction CHT and response-based local therapy with surgery and/or RT are also increasingly used.

Kim, South Korea (*IJROBP* 2023, PMID 37245536): RR of 155 patients who underwent definitive RT (63) or surgical resection (92). Of these, 91% vs. 39% of patients had T3–4 disease in the RT group and surgery group, respectively. Among the T3–4 patients, the 3-year OS, local PFS, and PFS rates for RT alone vs. surgery were 65.1% vs. 64.8%, 57.4% vs. 56.8%, and 43.2% vs. 46.5%, respectively (all not SS). **Conclusion: Definitive RT can be an option for patients with locally advanced disease and has similar oncologic outcomes to surgery.**

Is there a role for induction CHT in patients with sinonasal cancer?

Induction is feasible. Response to induction CHT may be predictive of treatment outcome and prognosis for those with locally advanced disease, and favorable response is associated with improved OS and possibility of organ preservation.[10]

Resteghini, SINTART 1 (*Eur J Cancer* 2023, PMID 37164774): Phase II nonrandomized trial of 35 patients with inoperable sinonasal tumors who received five cycles of induction CHT (ICT) followed by either CRT (if >80% reduction in the tumor was seen) or surgery with adjuvant (chemo)RT. The 5-year PFS of the entire cohort was 38% and the 5-year OS was 46%. The 3-year PFS for large volume responders to ICT vs. lack of response was 82% vs. 28%, with OS of 92% vs. 36%. **Conclusion: Treatment decisions driven by induction response are feasible and may suggest a role for induction.**

Contrera, MDACC (ASCO Abstract 2023): Phase II, single-institution trial of 31 patients with locally advanced, poorly differentiated carcinoma of the nasal cavity or paranasal sinuses treated with two cycles of induction CHT followed by clinical and radiographic assessment. Those who responded underwent a third cycle of CHT followed by CRT (79%), while those who did not respond underwent surgery with PORT (21%). Overall response rate was 82% and the 2-year LC was 54%. **Conclusion: Induction CHT is a valid treatment approach and can guide further treatment for those with locally advanced disease.**

Is there a role for proton beam therapy (PBT) and other charged particle therapy (CPT) in the treatment of sinonasal cancer?

PBT has been observed to be safe and efficacious in multiple retrospective series, but prospective validation has yet to be published. It is important to consider PBT when the high-dose RT volume approaches critical OARs. Yu et al. reviewed 69 patients who underwent definitive PBT (27 were re-RT) for sinonasal tumors from 2010 to 2016 and found excellent 3-year OS rates and FFLR rates in de novo patients with reduced efficacy in the re-RT setting. Late toxicity was observed in 15%, with no grade >3 toxicities.[11] Mayo Arizona published a meta-analysis reviewing 41 studies of patients with nasal cavity and paranasal sinus tumors treated with CPT (proton and carbon) and photon therapy. At 5 years, DFS was significantly higher for CPT, but this did not differ at the longest follow-up. Locoregional control did not differ at 5 years, but it was higher for CPT at the longest follow-up.[12]

SNUC

SNUC is a rare, poorly differentiated, rapidly growing malignancy that arises from the mucosa of the nasal cavity or paranasal sinuses. SNUC historically accounted for 3% to 5% of sinonasal carcinomas, but retrospective pathology review has changed SNUC to a diagnosis of exclusion.[13,14] SNUC is associated with a poor prognosis, generally presenting with locally advanced disease (80% are T4 at presentation) and a high frequency of DM, even when local disease control can be achieved. There are no prospective randomized clinical trials, and historically treatment has involved surgery with adjuvant CRT or definitive CRT. There is a prospective series from MD Anderson evaluating induction CHT followed by response-adapted local therapy, which found that patients with favorable response to induction CHT should be treated with CRT and those with a poor response to induction CHT should be treated with surgery to improve disease control and OS.

What are the outcomes with multimodality therapy in SNUC?

A recent meta-analysis shows bimodality and trimodality therapy are both used, although trimodality therapy does not show a survival benefit when compared with bimodality therapy. An NCDB analysis also suggests combined modality therapy, either CRT alone or surgery combined with CRT, yields the best survival rates.

See, Singapore (*Clin Otolaryngol* 2024, PMID 37859617): Meta-analysis of 17 studies, 208 total patients with SNUC treated from 1993 to 2020. The overall cumulative survival was 30% at 95 months. Cumulative OS in low vs. high stage was not significantly different (*p* = .69). Those who were treated with CRT had the highest rate of cumulative survival (42% at 40 months), and definitive CRT was associated with improved disease survival rate. There was no significant difference in mortality outcomes for patients treated with bimodality vs. trimodality therapy. **Conclusion: Patients should be treated aggressively independent of stage. Trimodality therapy does not offer survival advantage when compared with bimodality therapy.**

Kuo, NCDB (*Otol Head Neck Surg* 2017, PMID 27703092): Retrospective NCDB analysis of 435 patients treated from 2004 to 2012. Multivariate Cox regression evaluated OS based on treatment when adjusting for other prognostic factors (age, primary site, sex, race, comorbidity, insurance, and TNM stage). OS was 42%. On MVA, surgery + CRT was associated with significantly higher OS compared with surgery + RT and RT alone. Surgery + CRT was not significantly different from CRT alone. **Conclusion: Combined modality therapy (CRT or surgery + CRT) is associated with improved OS vs. other treatment modalities in patients with SNUC.**

Is there a benefit to induction CHT in SNUC?

The following study from MD Anderson is the only prospective study to guide therapy for patients with SNUC.

Amit, MDACC (*JCO* 2019, PMID 30615549): Prospective cohort study of 95 patients with treatment-naive SNUC undergoing induction CHT prior to definitive locoregional therapy with either definitive CRT or surgery followed by RT or CRT. The 5-year DSS was 59% for the entire cohort. For patients with PR or CR after induction CHT, the 5-year DSS estimates for patients treated with CRT vs. surgery with postop RT or CRT (not randomized) were 81% and 54%, respectively (*p* = .001). For patients without at least PR after induction CHT, the 5-year DSS estimates for CRT vs. surgery with postop RT or CRT were 0% and 39%, respectively (HR 5.68, 95% CI 2.89–9.36). **Conclusion: For patients with favorable response after induction CHT, CRT was associated with improved OS compared with surgery. However, for patients without favorable response to induction CHT, surgery was associated with improved disease control and OS.**

How should the neck be managed in SNUC?

While prospective data are lacking, a meta-analysis of 12 studies demonstrated fewer regional recurrences with elective neck treatment in patients with cN0, specifically showing regional failures in 4% of patients undergoing elective neck therapy vs. 26% in those without (OR 0.2, 95% CI 0.08–0.49).[15]

RARE SINONASAL CANCER SUBTYPES

What are the histologic subtypes of sinonasal malignancies?

There are several emerging rare histologies of sinonasal malignancies characterized in the pathology literature,[16] and some of them have not been distinctly classified by the World Health Organization.

HPV-related multiphenotypic sinonasal carcinoma (HMSC): Rare entity characterized by indolent clinical course despite aggressive-appearing histologic morphology with high rates of LR. Mediated by HPV subtype 33 rather than 16, which is common in oropharyngeal HPV-related SCC. A retrospective case series of 57 patients demonstrated LR rate of 36% among all patients, with LR rates of 40% if PNI+ and 60% if bone invasion.[17] Despite these high rates of LR, there were no nodal recurrences and no cases of disease-specific mortality. In a more recent retrospective review from the Middle East, the rate of nodal metastasis was 35% and was associated with expression of VEGF, TERT, EGFR, and other mutations.[18]

NUT-midline carcinoma: Arises from translocation of the nuclear protein on the testis called *NUTM1* on chromosome 15q14.6. These tumors represent ~2% of sinonasal carcinomas and are observed more in teens and young adults. These are aggressive tumors, with half of patients presenting with locoregional or DM. Treatment involves surgery with adjuvant cisplatin-based CRT. Prognosis is poor and is almost uniformly fatal with MS of 9 months.

SMARCB1 (INI-1)-deficient sinonasal carcinoma: Locally aggressive tumor usually presenting as T4 disease. Name is derived from the deletion of the tumor-suppressor gene *SMARCB1* found on chromosome 22. Often arise in the ethmoid sinus and can demonstrate local invasion into the orbit or anterior cranial fossa. Imaging can demonstrate calcifications and "hair on end" phenomenon suggestive of aggressive periosteal reaction.

Olfactory neuroblastoma (esthesioneuroblastoma): Small, round, blue cell tumor arising from the olfactory epithelium. See Table 19.4 for histologic grading system. General treatment paradigm includes aggressive locoregional therapy with endoscopic resection followed by adjuvant RT for Kadish stage B through D patients (Table 19.5). Kadish stage A patients may be observed postoperatively. Standard postop RT dosing recommended with minimum dose of 54 Gy. The risk of cervical nodal metastasis at diagnosis is 5%, but delayed cervical LN metastasis is common. Prophylactic vs. salvage management of the neck is controversial, but patients with Kadish stage C or Hyams grade III or IV disease are thought to be at higher risk of LN relapse.[19] NCDB analysis demonstrated that prognosis is good for Kadish A to C patients (5-year OS 80%, 88%, and 77% for stage A, B, and C, respectively) but worse for stage D (5-year OS 50%).[20] However, a meta-analysis and SEER study demonstrate higher risk of DM and worse OS correlating with higher Hyams grade, suggesting grade is more prognostic than stage.[21,22] Adjuvant CRT with cisplatin/etoposide is indicated for positive margins or extranodal extension.

Table 19.4 Hyams Histologic Grading System: Esthesioneuroblastoma

Grade I	Prominent fibrillary matrix, tumor cells with uniform nuclei, absent mitotic activity, and no necrosis
Grade II	Some fibrillary matrix, moderate nuclear pleomorphism with some mitotic activity, and no necrosis
Grade III	Minimal fibrillary matrix, Flexner-type rosettes present, more prominent mitotic activity and nuclear pleomorphism, and some necrosis possible
Grade IV	No fibrillary matrix or rosettes, marked nuclear pleomorphism, increased mitotic activity, and frequent necrosis

Table 19.5 Kadish Staging System: Esthesioneuroblastoma

Stage	Definition
A	Confined to the nasal cavity
B	Involves the nasal cavity and one or more paranasal sinuses
C	Extending beyond the nasal cavity or paranasal sinuses
D	Regional lymph node or distant metastasis

REFERENCES

1. Siegel RL, Miller KD, Jemal A. Cancer statistics, 2020. *CA Cancer J Clin.* 2020;70(1):7–30. doi:10.3322/caac.21590

2. Re M, Gioacchini FM, Bajraktari A, et al. Malignant transformation of sinonasal inverted papilloma and related genetic alterations: a systematic review. *Eur Arch Otorhinolaryngol.* 2017;274(8):2991–3000. doi:10.1007/s00405-017-4571-2

3. Mitarnun W, Suwiwat S, Pradutkanchana J. Epstein-Barr virus-associated extranodal non-Hodgkin's lymphoma of the sinonasal tract and nasopharynx in Thailand. *Asian Pac J Cancer Prev.* 2006;7(1):91–94. PMID: 16629523

4. Carrau RL, Segas J, Nuss DW, et al. Squamous cell carcinoma of the sinonasal tract invading the orbit. *Laryngoscope.* 1999;109(2 Pt 1):230–235. doi:10.1097/00005537-199902000-00012

5. Siddiqui F, Smith RV, Yom SS, et al. ACR appropriateness criteria® nasal cavity and paranasal sinus cancers. *Head Neck.* 2017;39(3):407–418. doi:10.1002/hed.24639

6. Madani I, Bonte K, Vakaet L, Boterberg T, De Neve W. Intensity-modulated radiotherapy for sinonasal tumors: Ghent University Hospital update. *Int J Radiat Oncol Biol Phys.* 2009;73(2):424–432. doi:10.1016/j.ijrobp.2008.04.037

7. Jiang GL, Ang KK, Peters LJ, Wendt CD, Oswald MJ, Goepfert H. Maxillary sinus carcinomas: natural history and results of postoperative radiotherapy. *Radiother Oncol.* 1991;21(3):193–200. doi:10.1016/0167-8140(91)90037-h

8. Bristol IJ, Ahamad A, Garden AS, et al. Postoperative radiotherapy for maxillary sinus cancer: long-term outcomes and toxicities of treatment. *Int J Radiat Oncol Biol Phys.* 2007;68(3):719–730. doi:10.1016/j.ijrobp.2007.01.032

9. Le QT, Fu KK, Kaplan MJ, Terris DJ, Fee WE, Goffinet DR. Lymph node metastasis in maxillary sinus carcinoma. *Int J Radiat Oncol Biol Phys.* 2000;46(3):541–549. doi:10.1016/s0360-3016(99)00453-8

10. Hanna EY, Cardenas AD, DeMonte F, et al. Induction chemotherapy for advanced squamous cell carcinoma of the paranasal sinuses. *Arch Otolaryngol Head Neck Surg.* 2011;137(1):78–81. doi:10.1001/archoto.2010.231

11. Yu NY, Gamez ME, Hartsell WF, et al. A multi-institutional experience of proton beam therapy for sinonasal tumors. *Adv Radiat Oncol.* 2019;4(4):689–698. doi:10.1016/j.adro.2019.07.008

12. Patel SH, Wang Z, Wong WW, et al. Charged particle therapy versus photon therapy for paranasal sinus and nasal cavity malignant diseases: a systematic review and meta-analysis. *Lancet Oncol.* 2014;15(9):1027–1038. doi:10.1016/S1470-2045(14)70268-2

13. Llorente JL, Lopez F, Suarez C, Hermsen MA. Sinonasal carcinoma: clinical, pathological, genetic and therapeutic advances. *Nat Rev Clin Oncol.* 2014;11(8):460–472. doi:10.1038/nrclinonc.2014.97

14. Frierson HF Jr, Mills SE, Fechner RE, Taxy JB, Levine PA. Sinonasal undifferentiated carcinoma. An aggressive neoplasm derived from schneiderian epithelium and distinct from olfactory neuroblastoma. *Am J Surg Pathol.* 1986;10(11):771–779. PMID: 2430477

15. Faisal M, Seemann R, Lill C, et al. Elective neck treatment in sinonasal undifferentiated carcinoma: systematic review and meta-analysis. *Head Neck*. 2020;42(5):1057–1066. doi:10.1002/hed.26077

16. Contrera KJ WN, Rahman M, Sindwani R, Burkey BB. Clinical management of emerging sinonasal malignancies. *Head Neck*. 2020;42(8):2202–2212. doi:10.1002/hed.26150

17. Ward ML KM, Willson TJ. HPV-related multiphenotypic sinonasal carcinoma: a case report and literature review. *Laryngoscope*. 2020;131(1):106–110. doi:10.1002/lary.28598

18. Alabiad MA, Said WMM, Adim AMA, et al. Evaluation of some prognostic biomarkers in human papillomavirus-related multiphenotypic sinonasal carcinoma. *Iran J Med Sci*. 2024;49(3):156–166. doi:10.30476/IJMS.2023.97341.2906

19. Jiang W, Mohamed ASR, Fuller CD, et al. The role of elective nodal irradiation for esthesioneuroblastoma patients with clinically negative neck. *Pract Radiat Oncol*. 2016;6(4):241–247. doi:10.1016/j.prro.2015.10.023

20. Konuthula N IA, Miles B, et al. Prognostic significance of Kadish staging in esthesioneuroblastoma: an analysis of the National Cancer Database. *Head Neck*. 2017;39(10):1962–1968. doi:10.1002/hed.24770

21. Dulguerov P AA, Calcaterra TC. Esthesioneuroblastoma: a meta-analysis and review. *Lancet Oncol*. 2001;2(11):683–690. doi:10.1016/S1470-2045(01)00558-7

22. Tajudeen BA AA, Suh JD, St et al. Importance of tumor grade in esthesioneuroblastoma survival: a population-based analysis. *JAMA Otolaryngol Head Neck Surg*. 2014;140(12):1124–1129. doi:10.1001/jamaoto.2014.2541

PART III: Skin

PART III: Skin

20 CUTANEOUS SQUAMOUS CELL CARCINOMA AND BASAL CELL CARCINOMA

Bryn M. Myers, Timothy D. Smile, Nikhil P. Joshi, Neil M. Woody, and Shlomo A. Koyfman

QUICK HIT Nonmelanomatous skin cancer, of which basal cell carcinoma (BCC) and squamous cell carcinoma (SCC) represent the majority of cases, is the most commonly diagnosed cancer. Most patients present with low-risk disease and are effectively treated with surgical excision or other focal therapy alone. Infrequently, lesions may be classified as high or very high risk, and benefit from surgery followed by adjuvant RT. Definitive RT is an option for unresectable lesions/nonsurgical candidates. Systemic therapies such as checkpoint inhibitors for SCC and BCC and hedgehog inhibitors for BCC have an increasing role in locally advanced and metastatic disease. Treatment options are provided in Table 20.1.

Table 20.1 General Treatment Paradigm for SCC and BCC	
Low risk	Surgical resection (Mohs, WLE for noncosmetic areas) OR definitive RT (nonsurgical) For superficial BCC or SCC in situ, may additionally consider topical imiquimod, 5-FU, electrodessication and curettage, cryotherapy
High risk/very high risk	Surgery (WLE or Mohs) with consideration of SLNB + adjuvant RT (indications: >4 cm, deep tissue invasion, extensive PNI or large nerve [>0.1 mm] involvement, vascular invasion, +margins, recurrent disease, N+) OR Definitive RT (nonsurgical candidates) For SCC, consider addition of neoadjuvant cemiplimab (indications: borderline resectable, high anticipated surgical morbidity, in-transit disease, bulky nodal disease)
Node-positive	Nodal dissection followed by adjuvant RT (pN2 or greater, pN1 controversial); consider neoadjuvant cemiplimab for bulky nodal disease (N3, gross ECE)
Locally advanced or unresectable	Neoadjuvant systemic therapy followed by surgery or RT OR Systemic therapy alone

EPIDEMIOLOGY: Prevalence in North America was estimated to be 5.4 million cases in 2022. BCC accounts for 80% of cases, while SCC accounts for 20%.[1] SCC occurs mostly in older adults (highest incidence in the eighth decade) and the male-to-female ratio is ~2:1.

RISK FACTORS: Older age, higher UV exposure (UVB 290–320 nm is higher risk than UVA), fair complexion, prior RT exposure, chemical exposure (arsenic, coal tar), prior phototherapy, steroid use, and chronic ulcers/scars/inflammation. Of note, chronic inflammation increases the risk of SCC significantly more than the risk of BCC. SCC is a major contributor to morbidity and mortality in immune-suppressed patients (65× risk[2]; organ transplant patients on calcineurin inhibitors [tacrolimus, cyclosporine] have higher risk than on mTOR inhibitor sirolimus; see the following for details).

ANATOMY: The skin is the largest organ in the body and is composed of two primary layers: epidermis superficially (devoid of lymphatics) and dermis, which contains superficial lymphatic plexus. Dermis is composed of papillary region superficially connecting with epidermis and reticular region below. Beneath the dermis is the subdermis (or hypodermis), composed primarily of fat and connective tissue. Basement membrane separates the epidermis from the dermis. Tumors of skin may be characterized by Clark's levels—level 1: tumor confined to epidermis (in situ); level 2: invasion into papillary dermis; level 3: invasion into junction of papillary and reticular dermis; level 4: invasion into reticular dermis; and level 5: invasion into subcutaneous fat.

PATHOLOGY

BCC: Arises from the basal layer of the epidermis. Histology shows nests of basaloid cells with peripheral palisading.

SCC: Histology demonstrates pleomorphism, numerous and atypical mitoses, dyskeratosis, and "horn pearl" formation.

GENETICS: Basal cell nevus syndrome (Gorlin syndrome) is a disorder of the PTCH gene, which results in macrocephaly, frontal bossing, bifid ribs, palmar and plantar pitting, medulloblastoma, and bone cysts. PTCH is in the sonic hedgehog (SHH) signaling pathway. BCC is also associated with Bazex–Dupré–Christol syndrome, which is an X-linked dominant syndrome characterized by multiple BCCs and pitting or "ice pick" scars of skin (follicular atrophoderma). Others: xeroderma pigmentosum (XP) with 57% lifetime incidence of skin cancer (autosomal recessive disorder associated with mutations in seven identified genes [XPA to XPG] resulting in impaired ability to correct UV-related DNA damage with nucleotide excision repair), albinism with 35% lifetime incidence of skin cancer, Bloom syndrome, epidermolysis bullosa, and Fanconi anemia. Muir–Torre syndrome (autosomal dominant disorder characterized by sebaceous skin tumors [eyelid] ± keratoacanthoma and internal malignancies [GI/GU]) is associated with germline mutation of DNA mismatch repair genes: MSH-1 and MLH-1 exhibiting microsatellite instability.

PREVENTION: Two PRTs confirm that application of sunscreen reduces the incidence of actinic keratosis (AK), BCC, and SCC.[3,4] In a phase III, placebo-controlled trial, oral nicotinamide led to lower rates of BCC, AK, and SCC at 12 months.[5] However, oral nicotinamide does not reduce the incidence of AK or SCC in immunosuppressed transplant recipients.[6] Retrospective studies have shown that low-dose acitretin significantly reduces the incidence of new SCC and BCC in immunosuppressed solid organ transplant recipients; however, there can be a rebound effect upon discontinuation.[7]

SCREENING: Patients with prior diagnosis of BCC or SCC should be screened by dermatologists at regular intervals to detect new skin cancers. The American Academy of Dermatology provides guidelines for patient self-surveillance, while the USPSTF suggests there is insufficient evidence to recommend routine screening of asymptomatic patients.

CLINICAL PRESENTATION

BCC: Has three presentations. Nodular subtype accounts for 60% of cases and presents with pink- or flesh-colored papule. These may become ulcerated and hence the term "noduloulcerative" ("rodent ulcer"). Superficial subtype accounts for 30% of cases and demonstrates red, scaly macule. Morpheaform subtype accounts for 5% to 10% of cases and presents as light-colored macules, or shiny, atrophic lesions with indistinct margins; it is more likely to have infiltrating growth. Rare subtypes include infiltrative and basosquamous subtypes, which are more aggressive, with basosquamous behaving similarly to SCC.

SCC: Lesions often begin as round to irregular, plaque-like or nodular, and overlaid with warty keratotic scale or conical keratinized protrusion ("cutaneous horn"). May also see as ulcer or induration and propensity to bleed. Bowen disease: SCC in situ; red-brown epidermal plaque in sun-exposed sites. Known as "erythroplasia of Queyrat" if on glans penis.

WORKUP: H&P including history of prior operations, procedures, or prior RT to involved area or other history of skin cancers or premalignant lesions. Complete skin examination with investigation for skip lesions and regional nodal examination. Review for any neurologic symptoms suggestive of perineural invasion (PNI). Punch, shave, or excisional biopsy confirmation is recommended.

Imaging: MRI with and without contrast should be considered for lesions involving the periorbital structures, skull base, symptoms suspicious for PNI, or lesions fixed to underlying muscle, bone, or fascia. CT with contrast of the nodal basin should be done in the setting of suspicious LNs or locally advanced primary tumors. FDG-PET/CT for high-risk or N+ patients to rule out metastatic disease.

PROGNOSTIC FACTORS: Tumor size, depth of invasion, immunosuppression, location (high-risk sites include scalp, temple, ear, and lip), development within an ulcer or wound (i.e., Marjolin's ulcer), prior RT, presence of PNI or lymphovascular invasion (LVI), neurologic symptoms, recurrent tumor, and histologic poor differentiation. NCCN stratifies BCC into low and high risk, and stratifies SCC into low, high, and very high risk (see Tables 20.2 and 20.3).[8,9] Only one high- or very high-risk factor is necessary to place them within that category.

Table 20.2 NCCN Risk Stratification for BCC (NCCN 3.2024)[10]		
	Low Risk	**High Risk**
Tumor location and size	Trunk, extremities <2 cm	• Trunk/extremities ≥2 cm; or any size on head, neck, hands, feet, pretibial skin, or anogenital region
Clinical margins	Clearly defined	Poorly defined
Recurrence status	Primary lesion	Recurrent lesion
Immune status	Immunocompetent	Immunosuppressed
Histologic subtype	Nodular or superficial	Infiltrative, basosquamous, sclerosing/morpheaform, micronodular subtypes; or carcinosarcomatous differentiation.
Perineural invasion	Absent	Present
Site of prior RT	No previous radiation at site	Previously-irradiated site

Source: Adapted from NCCN Clinical Practice Guidelines in Oncology: Basal Cell Skin Cancer. 2024.

Table 20.3 NCCN Risk Stratification for SCC (NCCN 1.2024)[11]			
Risk Group	**Low Risk**	**High Risk**	**Very High Risk**
	Clinical Criteria		
Tumor Location/size	Trunk, extremities ≤2 cm	Trunk/extremities >2, or ≤4 cm on high-risk sites (e.g., head/neck, feet, hands, pretibial, anogenital)	>4 cm in any location
Clinical extent	Well-defined	Poorly defined	
Primary vs. recurrent	Primary	Recurrent	
Immune status	Immunocompetent	Immunocompromised	
Prior radiation or chronic inflammation	Absent	Present	
Tumor growth rate	Slow	Rapid	
Neurologic symptoms	Absent	Present	
	Pathologic Criteria		
Differentiation	Well to moderately differentiated		Poorly differentiated
Histology	Conventional	Acantholytic (adenoid), adenosquamous (showing mucin production), or metaplastic (carcinosarcomatous) subtypes	Desmoplastic subtype
Depth of invasion	<2 mm thick and confined above subcutaneous fat	2–6 mm depth	>6 mm or invasion beyond subcutaneous fat
Perineural involvement	Absent	Present in small (<0.1 mm) and/or superficial nerves	Involvement of nerves deeper than the dermis or larger than 0.1 mm
Lymphatic or vascular invasion	Absent	Absent	Present

Source: Adapted from NCCN Clinical Practice Guidelines in Oncology: Squamous Cell Skin Cancer. 2024.

STAGING: BCC and SCC of the H&N are staged according to AJCC 8th edition staging system (Table 20.4), with the exception of SCC of the eyelid, which is staged separately.[2] A second staging system known as the Brigham and Women's Hospital staging system has been proposed for SCC (Table 20.5). This T-staging system was found to better discriminate prognosis of patients in an internal cohort than the AJCC staging system.[12]

Table 20.4 AJCC 8th Edition (2017): Staging System for Cutaneous Carcinoma of H&N (BCC and SCC)[2]									
T/M	N	cN0	cN1	cN2a	cN2b	cN2c	cN3a	cN3b
T1	• ≤2 cm	I						
T2	• 2.1–4 cm	II	III					
T3	• >4 cm • 1 high-risk feature[1]				IV			
T4a	• Gross cortical bone invasion							
T4b	• Invasion into skull base							
M1	• Distant metastasis							

Notes: 1 high risk feature[1] = minor bone erosion, PNI (nerve measuring ≥0.1 mm), or deep invasion (beyond subcutaneous fat or >6 mm depth). Nodal category definition is similar to other non–HPV-associated H&N cancers; see Chapter 11 for clinical and pathologic nodal categories.

Table 20.5 Brigham and Women's Hospital Staging System for Cutaneous SCC[13,14]				
		LR	High-Risk Factors	
T1	0 high-risk factor	2.7%	Tumor ≥2 cm	
T2a	1 high-risk factor	7.5%	Poor differentiation	
T2b	2–3 high-risk factors	15.7%	PNI ≥0.1 mm	
T3	≥4 high-risk factors	33.5%	Tumor beyond fat (bone invasion automatically T3)	

TREATMENT PARADIGM: General treatment paradigm for low-risk SCC and BCC lesions is surgical excision or alternative focal therapy. For high-risk lesions or LN involvement, resection followed by adjuvant therapy may be indicated.

Surgery: Surgical resection has two forms: wide local excision (WLE) and complete circumferential peripheral and deep margin assessment (CCPDMA), the most common form of which is Mohs surgery. WLE is appropriate for small BCC and SCC in noncritical areas. Surgical margin should be 3 to 5 mm with BCC and 4 to 6 mm with SCC. Alternatively, Mohs surgery provides on-site *comprehensive* margin assessment and is preferred for lesions located in cosmetically critical areas for which larger surgery would be disfiguring. During Mohs, horizontal layers of tissue are serially excised at an oblique angle and systematically mapped with particular attention to peripheral and deep margins. The location of positive margins during the excision process is generated and can help inform planning of adjuvant RT. The goal of Mohs resection is to obtain negative margins with maximal sparing of normal tissue. It involves comprehensive margin assessment, where 100% of the margin is pathologically assessed. This contrasts with standard pathologic assessment using "bread loafing" technique, which typically examines 3% to 5% of tissue. Mohs surgery is associated with cure rates for BCC around 99% for primary and 95% for recurrent tumors; cure rates for SCC are 92% to 99% and 90% for recurrent tumors.[9,15] There is an evolving role for SLNB in SCC, although identifying the subpopulation most likely to benefit has been a challenge.

Other Local Therapies: Local therapies are appropriate for small low-risk BCC and SCC lesions. Cryotherapy with liquid nitrogen for two to three applications can be employed for low-risk lesions with cell kill resulting from hypertonic damage. Cryotherapy is both convenient and inexpensive but provides no histologic diagnosis, no margin assessment, and can be associated with subsequent hypopigmentation. Curettage and electrodessication, where the tumor is scraped with curette and the base electrodessicated, is a procedure guided by "feel" of the tumor vs. the dermis with the goal of achieving 3- to 4-mm margin on curetting. It may have superior cosmetic outcomes to cryotherapy but is contraindicated in patients with pacemakers or other electronic implants and is not recommended in hair-bearing areas where feel of the tumor vs. normal tissue is more difficult due to hair follicles. Topical CHT with 5-FU is applied twice daily for 5–6, or sometimes up to 10, weeks depending on clinical response. Topical 5-FU is often employed for preinvasive lesions including Bowen disease, AKs, and cases of Gorlin syndrome. Imiquimod is an immune response modifier thought to promote apoptosis and/or stimulate release of tumoricidal mediated immunity factors from monocytes/macrophages. Cure rates are as high as 90% for low-risk BCC, but only 75% for nodular BCC. It is also effective for SCC in situ.

Systemic Therapy: For SCC, immunotherapy (IO) with cemiplimab or pembrolizumab is recommended for DM or locally advanced or recurrent disease not amenable to curative surgery or RT.[16–18] For patients not eligible for checkpoint inhibitors or clinical trials, consider cisplatin ± 5-FU, EGFR inhibitors (e.g., cetuximab), or carboplatin ± paclitaxel.[11]

For BCC, a SHH pathway inhibitor such as vismodegib or sonidegib is the systemic therapy of choice, with response rates of 49% to 67% after induction vismodegib and up to 83% after concurrent vismodegib and RT.[19–22] Many patients have AEs associated with vismodegib leading to discontinuation (alopecia, loss of taste, weight loss, muscle cramps, fatigue); patients progressing on or intolerant to SHH pathway inhibitors are treated with cemiplimab (response rates 20%–30%).[23]

Radiation

Indications: RT is indicated as definitive therapy for unresectable, inoperable, or cosmetically unacceptable cases[24] For lesions of the eyelid, external ear, nose, or lip, RT is often preferred. Indications for PORT are outlined in Table 20.6.

Table 20.6 NCCN Indications for PORT[10,11]	
SCC	BCC
Gross perineural spread that is clinically or radiologically apparent, positive margins not amenable to further surgery, recurrence after prior margin-negative resection, tumor diameter ≥6 cm.[25]	
BWH T2b or higher, especially in the setting of chronic immunosuppression. AJCC T3 or T4. Multiple nodes positive. Multiply recurrent.	Locally advanced or neglected tumors involving bone or infiltrating muscle.

In cases of PNI (particularly clinically symptomatic PNI), multiply recurrent tumor, or bone/cartilage invasion, consider treating the entire nerves up to the base of skull and certainly if major named nerves are clinically/radiographically involved. Ipsilateral LNs should be treated in cases of parotid LN involvement or N2/3 disease.[26] RT has the advantages of being noninvasive and cosmetically favorable, although RT cosmesis outcomes worsen with time and are increased with use of larger fraction sizes.

DecisionDx-SCC is a 40-gene expression profile test that was developed and further validated to stratify patients with SCC into three classes, namely class 1 (low risk), class 2A (high risk), and class 2B (highest risk), with corresponding 3-year metastasis-free survival rates of 91%, 81%, and 44% respectively.[27] Such genetic tests may be useful to use in combination with current staging systems to better select high-risk patients for adjuvant treatment.

Dose: ACR Appropriateness Criteria[28] recommend the following as curative regimens for cutaneous SCC and BCC: 60–70 Gy/30–35 fx, 50–55 Gy/17–20 fx, 40–44 Gy/10 fx, 40 Gy/5 fx (twice weekly), 30 Gy/3 fx (once weekly), or 20–25 Gy/1 fx (small volumes only). In areas where target volumes exist in close proximity to critical structures or cosmetically sensitive areas (overlying cartilage), more protracted RT courses are recommended. For adjuvant therapy to the primary site, NCCN guidelines[11] recommend BED10 of 60 to 79 Gy for conventional fractionation and 56 to 70 Gy for hypofractionation. NCCN guidelines also note that isotope-based brachytherapy is an effective option for certain disease sites. For adjuvant therapy to LNs, consider standard H&N dosing schemes at 2 Gy/fx.

Toxicity: Acute: fatigue, erythema, RT dermatitis, hypo/hyperpigmentation, alopecia/epilation, others location-dependent. Late: hypo/hyperpigmentation, fibrosis, ulceration, alopecia/epilation, lymphedema, others location-dependent.

EVIDENCE-BASED Q&A

What are the outcomes of definitive RT for BCC and SCC?

Retrospective studies show good response with definitive RT. LRC is between 80% and 90%.[29,30] Increasing T stage is associated with higher LR risk, 26% for T3/4 tumors.[30]

How does definitive RT compare with surgical resection?

A PRT using older RT techniques of contact therapy, orthovoltage RT, and Ir-192 brachytherapy showed inferior LC compared with Mohs (4-year failure rate 0.7% vs. 7.5%, p = .003).[31] More recent data using electronic brachytherapy found excellent control rates with RT compared with Mohs.[32]

Patel, CA (*J Contemp Brachy* 2017, PMID 28951753): Matched-pair cohort study of 369 patients with BCC or SCC treated with electronic brachytherapy (EBT) or Mohs. Most lesions were located on the head and were >1 cm and ≤2 cm. At a mean of 3.4 years posttreatment, freedom from recurrence was 99.5% in the EBT group and 100% in the Mohs group (NS). **Conclusion: EBT is an effective nonsurgical option for the treatment of BCC or SCC.**

What are the advantages of Mohs surgery over conventional excision?

Smeets, Netherlands (*Lancet* 2004, PMID 15541449): PRT of 612 BCCs (408 primary, 204 recurrent) of Mohs vs. WLE. Mohs trended to better 2-year LC at 98% vs. 97% for primary and 98% vs. 92% for recurrent. WLE with worse cosmesis and more likely to have +margins (in 18% of primary and 32% of recurrent), especially with aggressive histology, high-risk location (except lips and preauricular), and recurrent tumor. **Conclusion: Mohs surgery may permit better cosmesis and reduce +margin rate for tumors in difficult locations or recurrent tumors.**

What studies have defined worse prognosis of immunosuppressed SCC patients?

Manyam, Multi-Institution (*Cancer* 2017, PMID 28171708): Multi-institutional RR of 205 patients investigating the effect of immune status on disease outcomes in patients with primary or recurrent stage I to IV cutaneous HNSCC who underwent surgery and received PORT between 1995 and 2015; 138 patients (67%) were immunocompetent and 67 (33%) were immunosuppressed (chronic hematologic malignancy, HIV/AIDS, or had received immunosuppressive therapy for organ transplantation ≥6 months before diagnosis). Locoregional RFS (47% vs. 86%, p < .0001) and PFS (39% vs. 72%, p = .002) were significantly lower in immunosuppressed patients at 2 years; 2-year OS rate in immunosuppressed patients demonstrated similar trend (61% vs. 78%, p = .135) but did not meet significance. On MVA, immunosuppressed status, recurrent disease, poor differentiation, and PNI were significantly associated with LRR. **Conclusion: Immunosuppression led to dramatically inferior outcomes compared with immunocompetent status, despite receiving bimodality therapy.**

Can alteration of specific immunosuppressive agents prevent recurrent SCC?

mTOR inhibitors (sirolimus) improve outcomes in immunosuppressed patients compared with calcineurin inhibitors (tacrolimus, cyclosporine).

Euvrard, TUMORAPA (*NEJM* 2012, PMID 22830463): Multicenter PRT in kidney transplant patients with history of at least one cSCC while on calcineurin inhibitors randomized to either the same therapy (56 patients) vs. switching to sirolimus (64 patients). Primary endpoint was survival free of SCC at 2 years. Secondary endpoints included time until onset of new SCC, occurrence of other skin tumors, graft function, and problems with sirolimus. Survival free of SCC was significantly longer in the sirolimus group than in the calcineurin inhibitor group. Overall, new SCC developed in 14 patients (22%) in the sirolimus group (6 after withdrawal of sirolimus) and in 22 (39%) in the calcineurin inhibitor group (median time until onset, 15 vs. 7 months, p = .02), with relative risk reduction in the sirolimus group of 0.56 (95% CI 0.32–0.98); 60 serious AEs in the sirolimus group, as compared with 14 events in the calcineurin inhibitor group (average, 0.938 vs. 0.250). **Conclusion: Switching from calcineurin inhibitors to sirolimus had antitumoral effect among kidney transplant patients with previous SCC. These observations may have implications concerning immunosuppressive treatment of patients with SCC.**

What data guide the treatment of patients with node-positive SCC or those at risk of node-positive disease?

Patients with parotid or cervical LN metastases have higher rates of locoregional recurrence even with adjuvant RT. Spread to multiple nodes and single modality treatment predict worse OS.[26]

Moore, MDACC (*Laryngoscope* 2005, PMID 16148695): Prospective cohort evaluation of 193 patients with cSCC in H&N. Forty patients (21%) found to have LN or parotid metastases at presentation. Thirty-seven of these patients received adjuvant RT to a median dose of 60 Gy. Recurrent tumor, poorly differentiated histology, LVSI, inflammation, and invasion beyond subcutaneous fat were all associated with nodal metastases. Thirty-seven percent of lesions >4 cm and 31% of lesions invading >8 mm were LN-positive. **Conclusion: Patients with ipsilateral neck or parotid LN metastasis from SCC should receive adjuvant RT regardless of clinical nodal status.** *Exception may be single node <3 cm without ECE/PNI. Patients with direct invasion of parotid, tumor >2 cm, PNI, or recurrence in tissue adjacent to parotid or immune-compromised state should be considered for LN dissection and may also benefit from adjuvant RT.*

Which patients with cutaneous SCC/BCC of the H&N are most likely to benefit from adjuvant RT?

Harris (*JAMA Otol HNS* 2019, PMID 30570645): RR of 349 H&N cSCC patients at two tertiary care centers treated with primary resection with or without RT. A subset analysis was conducted for tumors with PNI and for patients with regional disease (N2 or greater nodal disease). In tumors with PNI, adjuvant RT was associated with improved OS (HR 0.44, 95% CI 0.24–0.86). In patients with regional disease, adjuvant RT was associated with improved OS (HR 0.30, 0.15–0.61). **Conclusion: Adjuvant RT was associated with improved OS in those with PNI and regional disease.**

Ruiz (*JAAD* 2022, PMID 35364211): Matched-pair analysis comparing observation with adjuvant RT in 508 BWH T2b/T3 lesions after negative margin resection. Adjuvant RT improved the 5-year LRR among BWH T2b/T3 lesions (4% vs. 9%) and a high-risk subgroup (17% vs. 31%) defined as BWH T3, recurrent, or diameter ≥6 cm. **Conclusion: Adjuvant RT halves the risk of LRR in high T-stage tumors following R0 resection.**

What is the importance of clinical and microscopic PNI in SCC?

Two RRs of patients with cutaneous H&N cancer showed increased LR with clinical PNI compared with microscopic PNI.[33,34]

Gluck, Michigan (*IJROBP* 2009, PMID 18938044): Patterns of failure study of 11 patients with clinical PNI treated with 3D-CRT or IMRT who recurred. Most patients had single nerve involved initially, while all patients recurred with involvement of multiple nerves, indicating substantial cross communication between the nerve branches of cranial nerves V and VII. **Conclusion: In cases of PNI, it is crucial to cover the involved nerve proximally to cavernous sinus.** *For CN VII, cover nerve to brainstem and distally, skin innervated by nerve, major communicating branches, and compartment in which it is embedded/innervates (e.g., orbit for V1 or V2 involvement; masticator space for V3 involvement; parotid gland for VII involvement).*

Massey (*JAMA Dermatol* 2023, PMID 37851425): Retrospective cohort study comparing four PNI measures (nerve caliber, number of involved nerves per section, PNI maximal depth, and PNI location) in the pathology specimens of 140 patients with cSCC to assess prognostic utility. The study found that the only PNI measure associated with poor outcomes was involvement of multiple nerves. PNI of ≥5 distinct nerves, denoted as extensive PNI (ePNI), was independently associated with increased LR (HR 13.83, 95% CI 3.50–54.6). **Conclusion: ePNI should be considered as a high-risk factor in SCC.**

What is the significance of satellitosis or in-transit metastasis in cutaneous SCC?

Although satellitosis or in-transit metastasis (S-ITM) is not incorporated into the AJCC staging system for SCC, retrospective data suggest these patients have clinical outcomes comparable to those with N+ or meta-static disease with an increased risk of recurrence and worse survival compared with patients who have T3 and T4 disease.

Smile (*JAMA Derm* 2022, PMID 35195668): RR of 518 patients with S-ITM, AJCC 8th T3, T4, N+, or M1 cutaneous SCC. The 5-year DSS was 76% for T3, 64% for T4, 41% for S-ITM, and 39% for N+. Compared with the S-ITM cohort, DSS was significantly higher in the T3N0 (HR 0.23, 95% CI 0.15–0.35) and T4N0 (HR 0.37, 0.19–0.76) cohorts, but not significantly different in the N+ (HR 0.77, 0.84–3.93) and M1 cohorts (HR 1.81, 0.84–3.93). **Conclusion: S-ITM is an important prognostic factor and portends outcomes similar to N+ or M1 disease.**

Is there a role for concurrent CRT in the treatment of high-risk cutaneous SCC?

Porceddu, TROG 05.01 (*JCO* 2018, PMID 29537906): PRT of 321 patients with high-risk (T3–T4, ITM, intraparotid metastases, or cervical nodal metastases either ≥3 cm or ≥2 involved nodes or with ECE) cSCC of the H&N randomized to adjuvant RT (60 or 66 Gy) ± CHT (carboplatin AUC 2 × 6 cycles). Primary endpoint was LC and secondary endpoints were DFS and OS. Results: 238 patients (77%) had high-risk nodal disease, 59 patients (19%) had high-risk primary or in-transit disease, and 13 patients (4%) had both; 84% completed all six cycles of CHT. The 2- and 5-year LRC rates were 88% and 83%, respectively, for RT and 89% and 87% (p = .58), respectively, for CRT. No differences in DFS or OS. Locoregional failure was the most common site of failure, and dis-tant-only failure occurred in 7% of patients in both arms. **Conclusion: No benefit to the addition of carboplatin to RT for the adjuvant management of high-risk cSCC.**

Is there a role for concurrent CRT in the treatment of locally advanced, unresectable BCC?

Barker (*JCO* 2024, PMID 38630954): Multicenter, phase II, single-arm study of 24 unresectable locally advanced BCC patients who received 12 weeks of induction vismodegib followed by RT with 7 weeks of concurrent vismodegib. MFU 5.7 years; 1-year LRC 91%, 5-year PFS 78%, and 5-year OS 83%. There were no grades 4 to 5 treatment-related AEs. **Conclusion: Induction and concurrent vismodegib with RT yields high rates of LRC and PFS.**

Is immunotherapy effective in the management of cutaneous SCC/BCC?

Recent phase I and II studies have shown the safety and efficacy of cemiplimab and pembrolizumab for patients with locally advanced or metastatic cutaneous SCC.[16,17,35] Overall response rate with cemiplimab was 50% for metastatic disease and 44% in locally advanced disease. Cemiplimab has also been tested in the neoadjuvant setting for advanced cSCC patients, with over half of patients demonstrating complete patho-logic response.[36] For locally advanced/metastatic BCC, cemiplimab has emerged as a second-line treatment option. KEYNOTE-630 was a phase III PRT evaluating the role of adjuvant pembrolizumab after surgery and RT in high-risk cSCC; however, it was recently closed for futility.[37] An RR from MDACC[38] showed that checkpoint inhibitors in patients with prior solid organ transplant lead to high allograft rejection rates with high mortality rates.

Stratigos (*Lancet Oncol* 2021, PMID 34000246): Multicenter, phase II PRT of 84 patients with locally advanced/metastatic BCC after first-line SHH inhibitor therapy who received cemiplimab. At MFU of 15 months, 5 (6%) patients had a CR and 21 (25%) patients a PR. Grade 3+ toxicity in 40 (48%) patients with no treatment-related deaths. **Conclusion: Cemiplimab demonstrated antitu-mor activity in a quarter of patients with acceptable safety profile for locally advanced/meta-static BCC.**

Gross (*NEJM* 2022, PMID 36094839): Phase II nonrandomized study of 79 patients with resectable stage II to IV cSCC receiving preoperative neoadjuvant cemiplimab administered q3 weeks for up to four doses before undergoing surgery. Forty patients (51%) demonstrated complete pathologic response, with grade 3 toxicity rate of 18%. **Conclusion: Neoadjuvant therapy with cemiplimab was associated with complete pathologic response in half of patients with advanced cSCC patients.**

Hanna, Brigham and Women's (*JCO* 2024, PMID 38252908): Phase I study of 12 kidney transplant recipients with locally advanced or metastatic cSCC who received cemiplimab after being cross-tapered to an mTOR inhibitor and pulsed-dose corticosteroids. At MFU of 6.8 months (range 0.7–29.8), no kidney rejection or loss was observed. Five patients (42%) had grade 3+ treatment-related adverse events. One patient died of angioedema and anaphylaxis attributed to mTOR inhibitor cross-taper. **Conclusion: In kidney transplant recipients with advanced cutaneous SCC receiving cemiplimab, mTOR inhibitors with corticosteroids are a favorable concurrent immunosuppressive regimen.**

Is there any role for superficial RT in the management of early-stage nonmelanoma skin cancer?

Image-guided superficial radiation therapy (IGSRT): Common technique in outpatient dermatology practices with favorable outcomes.[39] The use of IGSRT in early nonmelanoma skin cancer provides excellent control but may be excessively involved and costly for these early lesions.

Electronic brachytherapy: There have been several single-center, short-term studies demonstrating the effectiveness of electronic brachytherapy in the treatment of early-stage disease. Typical fractionation schemes range from 36 Gy/3 fx to 40–42 Gy/7–8 fx delivered by specialized HDR electronic brachytherapy surface applicators. While there is a lack of long-term outcomes, LC is good with rates of 98% at 1 year, with 85% to 94% of patients achieving excellent cosmesis.[40,41]

REFERENCES

1. Roky AH, Islam MM, Ahasan AMF, et al. Overview of skin cancer types and prevalence rates across continents. *Cancer Pathog Ther.* 2024;3(2):89–100. doi:10.1016/j.cpt.2024.08.002
2. *AJCC Cancer Staging Manual,* 8th ed. Springer Publishing Company; 2017.
3. Green A, Williams G, Neale R, et al. Daily sunscreen application and betacarotene supplementation in prevention of basal-cell and squamous-cell carcinomas of the skin: a randomised controlled trial. *Lancet.* 1999;354(9180):723–729. doi:10.1016/S0140-6736(98)12168-2
4. Thompson SC, Jolley D, Marks R. Reduction of solar keratoses by regular sunscreen use. *N Engl J Med.* 1993;329(16):1147–1151. doi:10.1056/NEJM199310143291602
5. Chen AC, Martin AJ, Choy B, et al. A Phase 3 randomized trial of nicotinamide for skin-cancer chemoprevention. *N Engl J Med.* 2015;373(17):1618–1626. doi:10.1056/NEJMoa1506197
6. Allen NC, Martin AJ, Snaidr VA, et al. Nicotinamide for skin-cancer chemoprevention in transplant recipients. *N Engl J Med.* 2023;388(9):804–812. doi:10.1056/NEJMoa2203086
7. Solomon-Cohen E, Reiss-Huss S, Hodak E, Davidovici B. Low-dose acitretin for secondary prevention of keratinocyte carcinomas in solid-organ transplant recipients. *Dermatology.* 2022;238(1):161–166. doi:10.1159/000515496
8. Wang DM, Kraft S, Rohani P, et al. Association of nodal metastasis and mortality with vermilion vs cutaneous lip location in cutaneous squamous cell carcinoma of the lip. *JAMA Dermatol.* 2018;154(6):701–707. doi:10.1001/jamadermatol.2018.0792
9. Rowe DE, Carroll RJ, Day CL, Jr. Prognostic factors for local recurrence, metastasis, and survival rates in squamous cell carcinoma of the skin, ear, and lip. Implications for treatment modality selection. *J Am Acad Dermatol.* 1992;26(6):976–990. doi:10.1016/0190-9622(92)70144-5
10. *NCCN Clinical Practice Guidelines in Oncology: Basal Cell Skin Cancer.* 2024.
11. *NCCN Clinical Practice Guidelines in Oncology: Squamous Cell Skin Cancer.* 2024.
12. Karia PS, Jambusaria-Pahlajani A, Harrington DP, Murphy GF, Qureshi AA, Schmults CD. Evaluation of American joint committee on cancer, international union against cancer, and brigham and women's hospital tumor staging for cutaneous squamous cell carcinoma. *J Clin Oncol.* 2014;32(4):327–334. doi:10.1200/JCO.2012.48.5326
13. Karia PS, Jambusaria-Pahlajani A, Harrington DP, Murphy GF, Qureshi AA, Schmults CD. Evaluation of American joint committee on cancer, international union against cancer, and brigham and women's hospital tumor staging for cutaneous squamous cell carcinoma. *J Clin Oncol.* 2014;32(4):327–334. doi:10.1200/jco.2012.48.5326
14. Zakhem GA, Qiblawi S, Shelton E, Xu YG. Prevalence of poor outcomes in cutaneous squamous cell carcinoma by AJCC and BWH tumor stages: a systematic review and meta-analysis. *J Am Acad Dermatol.* 2025;S0190–9622(25)00151-3. doi:10.1016/j.jaad.2024.11.082
15. Rowe DE, Carroll RJ, Day CL, Jr. Long-term recurrence rates in previously untreated (primary) basal cell carcinoma: implications for patient follow-up. *J Dermatol Surg Oncol.* 1989;15(3):315–328. doi:10.1111/j.1524-4725.1989.tb03166.x

16. Migden MR, Rischin D, Schmults CD, et al. PD-1 Blockade with cemiplimab in advanced cutaneous squa-mous-cell carcinoma. *N Engl J Med*. 2018;379(4):341–351. doi:10.1056/NEJMoa1805131

17. Grob JJ, Gonzalez R, Basset-Seguin N, et al. Pembrolizumab monotherapy for recurrent or metastatic cuta-neous squamous cell carcinoma: a single-arm phase II trial (KEYNOTE-629). *J Clin Oncol*. 2020;38(25):2916–2925. doi:10.1200/JCO.19.03054

18. Rischin D, Hughes BGM, Basset-Seguin N, et al. High response rate with extended dosing of cemiplimab in advanced cutaneous squamous cell carcinoma. *J Immunother Cancer*. 2024;12(3):e008325. doi:10.1136/jitc-2023-008325

19. Barker CA, Dufault S, Arron ST, et al. Phase II, single-arm trial of induction and concurrent vismodegib with curative-intent radiation therapy for locally advanced, unresectable basal cell carcinoma. *J Clin Oncol*. 2024;42(19):2327–2335. doi:10.1200/jco.23.01708

20. Basset-Seguin N, Hauschild A, Kunstfeld R, et al. Vismodegib in patients with advanced basal cell carci-noma: primary analysis of STEVIE, an international, open-label trial. *Eur J Cancer*. Nov 2017;86:334-348. doi:10.1016/j.ejca.2017.08.022

21. Sekulic A, Migden MR, Basset-Seguin N, et al . Long-term safety and efficacy of vismodegib in patients with advanced basal cell carcinoma: final update of the pivotal ERIVANCE BCC study. *BMC cancer*. 2017;17(1):332. doi:10.1186/s12885-017-3286-5

22. Dummer R, Guminski A, Gutzmer R, et al. The 12-month analysis from Basal Cell Carcinoma Outcomes with LDE225 Treatment (BOLT): a phase II, randomized, double-blind study of sonidegib in patients with advanced basal cell carcinoma. *J Am Acad Dermatol*. 2016;75(1):113–125 e5. doi:10.1016/j.jaad.2016.02.1226

23. Stratigos AJ, Sekulic A, Peris K, et al. Cemiplimab in locally advanced basal cell carcinoma after hedgehog inhibitor therapy: an open-label, multi-centre, single-arm, phase 2 trial. *Lancet Oncol*. 2021;22(6):848–857. doi:10.1016/S1470-2045(21)00126-1

24. Mendenhall WM, Amdur RJ, Hinerman RW, Cognetta AB, Mendenhall NP. Radiotherapy for cutane-ous squamous and basal cell carcinomas of the head and neck. *Laryngoscope*. 2009;119(10):1994–1999. doi:10.1002/lary.20608

25. Ruiz ES, Kus KJB, Smile TD, et al. Adjuvant radiation following clear margin resection of high T-stage cutaneous squamous cell carcinoma halves the risk of local and locoregional recurrence: A dual-center retrospective study. *J Am Acad Dermatol*. 2022;87(1):87–94. doi:10.1016/j.jaad.2022.03.044

26. Veness MJ, Morgan GJ, Palme CE, Gebski V. Surgery and adjuvant radiotherapy in patients with cutaneous head and neck squamous cell carcinoma metastatic to lymph nodes: combined treatment should be consid-ered best practice. *Laryngoscope*. 2005;115(5):870–875. doi:10.1097/01.MLG.0000158349.64337.ED

27. Wysong A, Newman JG, Covington KR, et al. Validation of a 40-gene expression profile test to predict met-astatic risk in localized high-risk cutaneous squamous cell carcinoma. *J Am Acad Dermatol*. 2021;84(2):361–369. doi:10.1016/j.jaad.2020.04.088

28. Koyfman SA, Cooper JS, Beitler JJ, et al. ACR appropriateness criteria((R)) aggressive nonmelanomatous skin cancer of the head and neck. *Head Neck*. 2016;38(2):175–182. doi:10.1002/hed.24171

29. Su W, Anstadt EJ, Gupta N, et al. Definitive radiation therapy is a viable treatment for locally advanced basal cell carcinoma otherwise requiring radical or disfiguring resection. *Int J Radiat Oncol Biol Phys*.2024;doi:10.1016/j.ijrobp.2024.09.034

30. Krausz AE, Ji-Xu A, Smile T, Koyfman S, Schmults CD, Ruiz ES. A systematic review of primary, adjuvant, and salvage radiation therapy for cutaneous squamous cell carcinoma. *Dermatol Surg*. 2021;47(5):587–592. doi:10.1097/DSS.0000000000002965

31. Avril MF, Auperin A, Margulis A, et al. Basal cell carcinoma of the face: surgery or radiotherapy? Results of a randomized study. *Br J Cancer*. 1997;76(1):100–106. doi:10.1038/bjc.1997.343

32. Patel R, Strimling R, Doggett S, et al. Comparison of electronic brachytherapy and Mohs micrographic surgery for the treatment of early-stage non-melanoma skin cancer: a matched pair cohort study. *J Contemp Brachytherapy*. 2017;9(4):338–344. doi:10.5114/jcb.2017.68480

33. Garcia-Serra A, Hinerman RW, Mendenhall WM, et al. Carcinoma of the skin with perineural invasion. *Head Neck*. 2003;25(12):1027–1033. doi:10.1002/hed.10334

34. Jackson JE, Dickie GJ, Wiltshire KL, et al. Radiotherapy for perineural invasion in cutaneous head and neck carcinomas: toward a risk-adapted treatment approach. *Head Neck*. 2009;31(5):604–610. doi:10.1002/hed.20991

35. Migden MR, Khushalani NI, Chang ALS, et al. Cemiplimab in locally advanced cutaneous squamous cell carcinoma: results from an open-label, phase 2, single-arm trial. *Lancet Oncol*. 2020;21(2):294–305. doi:10.1016/S1470-2045(19)30728-4

36. Gross ND, Miller DM, Khushalani NI, et al. Neoadjuvant Cemiplimab for Stage II to IV Cutaneous Squamous-Cell Carcinoma. *N Engl J Med*. 2022;387(17):1557–1568. doi:10.1056/NEJMoa2209813

37. Schenker M, Klochikhin M, Kirtbaya D, et al. The KEYNOTE-630 trial: a phase 3 study of adjuvant pem-brolizumab in high-risk locally advanced (LA) cutaneous squamous cell carcinoma (cSCC). *Int J Radiat Oncol Biol Phys*. 2024;118(5):e81–e82. doi:10.1016/j.ijrobp.2024.01.180

38. Abdel-Wahab N, Safa H, Abudayyeh A, et al. Corrections to: Checkpoint inhibitor therapy for cancer in solid organ transplantation recipients: an institutional experience and a systematic review of the literature. *J Immunother Cancer.* 2019;7(1):158. doi:10.1186/s40425-019-0639-4

39. Tran A, Moloney M, Kaczmarski P, et al. Analysis of image-guided superficial radiation therapy (IGSRT) on the treatment of early-stage non-melanoma skin cancer (NMSC) in the outpatient dermatology setting. *J Cancer Res Clin Oncol.* 2023;149(9):6283–6291. doi:10.1007/s00432-023-04597-2

40. Paravati AJ, Hawkins PG, Martin AN, et al. Clinical and cosmetic outcomes in patients treated with high-dose-rate electronic brachytherapy for nonmelanoma skin cancer. *Pract Radiat Oncol.* 2015;5(6):e659–664. doi:10.1016/j.prro.2015.07.002

41. Gauden R, Pracy M, Avery AM, Hodgetts I, Gauden S. HDR brachytherapy for superficial non-melanoma skin cancers. *J Med Imaging Radiat Oncol.* 2013;57(2):212–217. doi:10.1111/j.1754-9485.2012.02466.x

21 MERKEL CELL CARCINOMA

Katherine R. Amarell, Ian W. Winter, Nikhil P. Joshi, and Shlomo A. Koyfman

QUICK HIT   Merkel cell carcinoma (MCC) is a rare primary neuroendocrine malignancy of skin that can be aggressive with rapid regional, in-transit, marginal, and distant recurrence. Management is primarily surgical with WLE + SLNB (depending on site and nodal drainage) followed by wide-field (3- to 4-cm margin) adjuvant RT. Small node-negative lesions <1 cm excised with widely negative margins can be observed. Definitive RT is an alternative option for patients for whom surgery would be disfiguring or excessively morbid (Table 21.1). Immunotherapy has high activity in this disease and is standard of care in advanced/metastatic disease and has an increasing role in the neoadjuvant setting for locally advanced disease.

Table 21.1 General Treatment Paradigm for Nonmelanoma Skin Cancer	
Localized disease	WLE + SLNB followed by wide-field adjuvant RT to primary site, with inclusion of regional nodes in cases of nodal involvement (can consider omitting nodal RT if SLNB negative or single positive node without ENE after full dissection)
Locoregionally advanced disease	WLE with LN dissection followed by adjuvant RT vs. definitive RT in nonsurgical candidates
Recurrent/metastatic	Immunotherapy (pembrolizumab, avelumab, nivolumab), can consider CHT if checkpoint inhibitors contraindicated

EPIDEMIOLOGY: MCC is considered a nonmelanomatous skin cancer. MCC represents a small percentage of nonmelanomatous skin cancer cases with an incidence of ~0.7 per 100,000 and occurs mostly in older adults (average age 74–76) with fair skin; M:F ratio approximately 2:1.[1,2]

RISK FACTORS: Risk factors for MCC include light skin, older age, UV exposure, immunosuppression, organ transplant (×24 risk),[3] CLL, melanoma, and myeloma.[4] Merkel cell polyomavirus is ubiquitous and can be detected in normal skin flora as well as tumors, but clonal integration of viral DNA provides evidence of causal relationship.[5]

ANATOMY: The skin is the largest organ in the body and is composed of two primary layers: epidermis superficially, which is devoid of lymphatics; and the dermis, which contains the superficial lymphatic plexus. The dermis is composed of the papillary region superficially connecting with the epidermis and reticular region below. Beneath the dermis is the subdermis (or hypodermis), composed primarily of fat and connective tissue. Basement membrane separates epidermis from dermis. Tumors of the skin may be characterized by Clark's levels—level 1: tumor confined to epidermis (in situ); level 2: invasion into papillary dermis; level 3: invasion into junction of papillary and reticular dermis; level 4: invasion into reticular dermis; and level 5: invasion into subcutaneous fat. Normal Merkel cells exist in the basal epidermis and around hair follicles, and they act as mechanoreceptors. MCC is most common in sun-exposed areas (43% H&N, 24% upper limb, 15% lower limb as per NCDB).[6]

PATHOLOGY: MCC is a small round blue cell tumor of uncertain origin. Merkel cell polyomavirus is detected in >80% of MCC.[7,8] Theories of origin include sensory cells in skin mechanoreceptors or skin stem cells that undergo malignant differentiation.[9,10] Three subtypes exist (small cell type, trabecular type, and intermediate type), but these are not thought to be prognostic. Immunostaining includes perinuclear dot-like CK20 positivity, as well as TTF1 and CK7 (negative in MCC, positive in SCLC).

GENETICS: Genetic counseling is generally recommended in patients <50 years old. Common germline mutations that may be associated with MCC include MAGT1, ATM, BRCA1/BRCA2, and TP53 mutations.[11]

SCREENING: Routine screening skin checks by a dermatologist at regular intervals can detect new skin abnormalities. The American Academy of Dermatology provides guidelines for patient self-surveillance, while the USPSTF suggests there is insufficient evidence to recommend routine screening of asymptomatic patients.

CLINICAL PRESENTATION: MCCs typically present as firm, painless, rapidly growing, single red or purple cutaneous dome-shaped nodules. Sixty-five percent present with localized disease.[6]

WORKUP: H&P including history of prior skin cancers/premalignant lesions, prior operations/procedures, or prior RT to the involved area. Complete skin examination with investigation for skip lesions; regional nodal examination. Biopsy confirmation is recommended, and approaches include punch, shave, or excisional biopsy. SLNB is generally recommended.

Imaging: PET/CT is recommended for regional and distant staging. Other studies can include MRI with contrast of primary tumor as clinically indicated to assess for deep/adjacent structure invasion, as well as MRI brain for clinical suspicion.

PROGNOSTIC FACTORS: Presence of nodal disease is the most important prognostic factor. The 5-year OS for local disease without nodal involvement, regional disease, and distant disease is 56%, 35%, and 14%, respectively.[6] Merkel cell polyoma virus antigen expression and presence of tumor-infiltrating lymphocytes are associated with favorable prognosis.[12] LVI, large tumor size, infiltrating pattern, deep invasion, ECE, and older age are associated with unfavorable prognosis.[13] Anti-VP1 (Merkel polyomavirus) antibody titer >10,000 copies is associated with favorable prognosis.[14] Local and nodal failure is common. Recurrences can occur early (start RT early after surgery), with median time to recurrence of 9 months. Nodal failure is the most common site of first failure (55% of failures), followed by distant (29% of failures), local (15% of failures), and in transit (9% of failures).[15]

STAGING: MCC staging is outlined in Table 21.2.

Table 21.2 AJCC 8th Edition (2017): Staging for MCC[16]									
T/M \ N		cN0	cN1	pN1a(sn)	pN1a	pN1b	c/pN2	c/pN3
T1	• ≤2 cm	I	IIIA				IIIB		
T2	• 2.1–5 cm	IIA							
T3	• >5 cm								
T4	• Invasion[1]	IIB							
M1a	• Distant skin • Subcutaneous tissue • Distant LN	IV							
M1b	• Lung								
M1c	• Any other visceral sites								

Notes: Invasion[1] = invasion into fascia, cartilage, bone, or muscle.
cN1: metastasis in regional LN(s); pN1a(sn): clinically occult regional LN identified by SLNB only; pN1a: clinically occult regional LN following LN dissection; pN1b: clinically and/or radiologically detected regional LN with microscopic confirmation; c/pN2: in-transit metastasis (ITM; discontinuous from primary tumor, located between primary tumor and draining LN basin), without LN metastasis; c/pN3: ITM with LN metastasis.
Source: Adapted from NCCN. NCCN Clinical Practice Guidelines: Merkel Cell Carcinoma. 2023;1.2024.

TREATMENT PARADIGM: The general treatment paradigm for nonmetastatic MCC is surgical resection followed by adjuvant RT.

Surgery: Surgical resection has two forms: WLE and Mohs surgery. WLE is the mainstay of treatment in MCC, and surgical margin should be 1 to 2 cm. Alternatively, Mohs surgery provides on-site comprehensive margin assessment and is preferred for lesions located in critical areas for which larger surgery would be disfiguring (see Chapter 20 for further discussion on Mohs surgery). For cN0 patients, SLNB should be performed (SLNB controversial in H&N locations). For cN+ patients, either regional LN dissection should be performed or biopsy should be obtained (FNA appropriate) with subsequent regional nodal RT. If surgery to primary would be disfiguring or otherwise morbid, definitive RT may be appropriate.

Systemic Therapy: There is no clear role for concurrent or adjuvant CHT for locoregionally confined disease, although phase II data do exist with concurrent cisplatin/etoposide.[17] Emerging data have shown a DFS benefit of adjuvant immunotherapy in completely resected disease (see Evidence-Based Q&A section). In the metastatic setting, phase II data suggest response rates of >50% to PD-1 or PD-L1 inhibition.[18–21]

Radiation

Indications: RT is indicated postoperatively to the primary site (can consider observation for small <1 cm tumors widely excised without any of the following risk factors: chronic immunosuppression, HIV, CLL, prior history of transplant, or LVI). Nodal RT can also be omitted if a full nodal dissection is performed and is negative or only one positive LN without ENE or if SLNB is negative (without high-risk features for a false-negative). Other indications for RT may include definitive therapy for unresectable cases, inoperable cases, or those for whom surgery would be disfiguring or excessively morbid.[16] There is limited evidence suggesting that RT reduces LRR. Risk factors for recurrence include LVI, immune suppression, and positive margins (further resection not possible).[16,22] PORT for MCC should be initiated without delay (~4 weeks) as rapid recurrences can occur.

Dose: Adjuvant dosing varies by margin status and nodal involvement (Table 21.3).

Table 21.3 Adjuvant RT Dosing for Postoperative Treatment of MCC[16]			
Primary Lesion		**Regional Lymph Nodes**	
Negative margins	50–56 Gy/25–28 fx	**Negative SLNB**	Observe (*unless accuracy of SLNB is in question, such as in H&N*)
Microscopic positive margins	56–60 Gy/28–30 fx	**Microscopic node-positive**	50–56 Gy (*or observation after full dissection with only one positive node*)
Gross residual or definitive RT	60–66 Gy/30–33 fx	**Extracapsular extension**	56–60 Gy

Source: Adapted from NCCN. NCCN Clinical Practice Guidelines: Merkel Cell Carcinoma. 2023;1.2024.

Toxicity: Acute: fatigue, erythema, RT dermatitis, hypo/hyperpigmentation, alopecia/epilation, others location-dependent. Late: hypo/hyperpigmentation, fibrosis, ulceration, alopecia/epilation, lymphedema, others location-dependent.

Procedure: See *Handbook of Treatment Planning in Radiation Oncology*, Chapter 4.[23]

EVIDENCE-BASED Q&A

Does RT improve survival for early-stage MCC?

Although adjuvant RT is standard of care, the exact benefit is controversial given contradicting results on retrospective SEER and NCDB analyses. SEER analysis by Mojica et al. in 2007 found adjuvant RT was associated with an improved OS and was particularly important for tumors >2 cm.[24] Follow-up SEER analysis by Kim and Choi found that when eliminating patients with <4 months survival, adjuvant RT improved OS but not MCC-specific survival.[25] NCDB analysis by Bhatia et al. in 2016 found that adjuvant RT was associated with an improved OS in stage I to II MCC but not in stage III patients.[26] Further NCDB analysis showed that best OS was associated with WLE + adjuvant RT.[27]

Is RT to lymph nodes indicated in stage I patients?

In the pre-SLNB and pre-PET/CT era, RT improved nodal recurrence rates. In the modern era, omission of nodal RT is recommended for patients with negative SLNB. For patients with positive SLNB but no nodal dissection, RT is recommended. For patients with complete nodal dissection, RT is recommended for multiple positive nodes or ECE.[16]

Jouary, France (*Ann Oncol* 2012, PMID 21750118): PRT from 1993 to 2005 including patients with stage I MCC treated with WLE + RT to primary tumor bed, then randomized to observation of regional nodes vs. prophylactic RT. Notably excluded patients with unclear nodal drainage (median head and trunk), immune suppression, and for delay in RT initiation over 6 weeks. RT consisted of 50 Gy to primary bed and nodal region with 3-cm margin. Powered to detect 20% gain in OS ($n = 105$). Study stopped early as SLNB became common in France, and this was not permitted per protocol. No difference in OS. Regional recurrence 17% vs. 0% favoring nodal RT ($p = .007$). PFS 90% vs. 81% favoring nodal RT ($p = .4$). **Conclusion: In the pre-SLNB and pre-PET/CT era, nodal RT improved the rate of nodal recurrence.**

What is the optimal dose for definitive treatment of MCC?

Retrospective evidence suggests that doses >50 Gy are necessary to achieve locoregional control.[28] NCDB supports doses ranging from 50 to 55 Gy, although selection bias may factor into doses above 55 Gy.[29] Furthermore, impressive results have been observed in the metastatic setting from 8 Gy/1 fx, with complete response rates of up to 45%.[30] This suggests that there may be an immune–system interaction. Further work is ongoing.

What treatment margins should be used around the tumor bed?

Given proclivity for in-transit recurrences and lymphovascular spread, wide margins of 3 to 4 cm are generally recommended.[28] Treat regional lymphatics in continuity (same field) with primary lesion if tolerable (the TROG 9607 trial defined "tolerable" as less than 20 cm with cone down).[17]

Are there any anatomic locations that may benefit from primary site RT in the absence of other risk factors?

Postoperative RT reduces local recurrence of MCC of the H&N regardless of risk factors. For sites outside of the H&N, omitting RT can be considered in the setting of low-risk disease.

Bierma, University of Washington (*Adv Radiat Oncol* 2023, PMID 38189056): RR of 147 patients with low-risk MCC defined as T1 tumor with negative margins and negative LN with no history of immunosuppression or prior systemic therapy. Patients received PORT ($n = 79$) or surgery alone ($n = 68$). Local recurrence at 5 years was 0% vs. 9.5% for PORT and surgery-alone arm, respectively ($p = .004$). Specifically, PORT reduced recurrence in H&N locations. Conversely, in sites outside of the H&N, there were no recurrences observed. **Conclusion: For low-risk stage I MCC, LC with surgery alone was excellent for locations outside of the H&N (extremities and trunk).**

What is the role of adjuvant RT in resected stage III disease?

Pairawan, NCDB (*JAMA Surg* 2024, PMID 38231528): NCDB analysis of 3,683 patients with pathologic stage III MCC who underwent resection. Sixty-seven percent received adjuvant RT and 18% received adjuvant RT to nodal basins. Seventy-seven percent did not receive CHT. Median OS of patients who received adjuvant RT was 60.6 vs. 38.7 months for those who did not receive RT. Use of adjuvant RT was associated with age <70 years, 2+ positive LNs, and ≤T2 disease. **Conclusion: Adjuvant RT is associated with a large survival benefit in stage III resected disease and should be considered.**

Is there benefit to the addition of concurrent CHT with RT?

Concurrent CRT has been studied but is not standard given good responses seen with RT alone and unclear benefit of CHT.

Poulsen, TROG 9607 (*JCO* 2003, PMID 14645427): Single-arm phase II of 53 nonmetastatic MCC patients with either high-risk postoperative (gross residual, tumor >1 cm, involved nodes) occult primary with positive nodes or recurrent disease. Twenty-eight percent treated definitively, 72% adjuvant. Patients treated to 50 Gy/25 fx; 45 Gy with boost to 50 Gy (shrinking field) was possible for large fields and 45 Gy alone recommended if 50 Gy was felt to be intolerable. Four cycles of concurrent and adjuvant carboplatin AUC 4.5 and etoposide 80 mg/m²/day for 3 days were delivered on weeks 1, 4, 7, and 10. The 3-year OS, LRC, and DC rates were 76%, 75%, and 76%, respectively. Tumor location and presence of nodes were associated with LC and OS. **Conclusion: High levels of LC and OS were achieved compared with historical controls; further study is warranted.**

Is there a role for immunotherapy in the treatment of MCC?

NCCN guidelines suggest immunotherapy as a treatment option in the metastatic or recurrent setting. Immunotherapy can also be used neoadjuvantly for those with locally advanced disease if curative surgery/RT is not feasible. Adjuvant systemic therapy is currently not recommended outside of a clinical trial.[16] A phase II study of patients with metastatic or recurrent MCC treated with pembrolizumab showed a 56% response rate, with 24% having a CR. Durable antitumor activity was sustained with MS and median duration of response not reached after MFU of 15 months.[19,21] Avelumab and pembrolizumab are approved for metastatic MCC and are considered standard monotherapies for metastatic/recurrent disease.[18–21] Recent update to the JAVELIN Merkel 200 study showed continued survival benefit with the use of avelumab.[31] Combination of ipilimumab and nivolumab has been investigated with the addition of SBRT for recurrent, advanced, and metastatic disease. CheckMate 358 and the recent phase II ADMEC-O study show potential for the use of immunotherapy in resectable disease. The STAMP trial is an ongoing phase III trial investigating adjuvant pembrolizumab for resected stage I to III MCC.

Kim, Moffitt (*Lancet* 2023, PMID 36108657): Phase II trial of 50 patients with unresectable, recurrent, or stage IV MCC with at least two lesions on imaging randomized to receive ipilimumab and nivolumab with or without SBRT to at least one tumor site (24 Gy/3 fx). Primary outcome was objective response rate (ORR), which was defined as the proportion of patients with CR or PR. There was no difference in ORR between the SBRT and the no-SBRT arm (72% vs. 52%, respectively, *p* = .26). Patients were also stratified by prior use of immune checkpoint inhibitors (ICI). Of those who were ICI-naive, 100% of patients had an ORR, compared with 31% in patients with prior ICI exposure. **Conclusion: Combined ipilimumab and nivolumab showed clinical benefit even in those with prior ICI exposure. The addition of SBRT did not improve objective response rate.**

Becker, ADMEC-O (*Lancet* 2023, PMID 37451295): Multicenter phase II trial of 179 patients with completely resected MCC randomized to adjuvant nivolumab for 1 year vs. observation. Adjuvant RT was more common in the observation group (74% vs. 50%). At 2 years, DFS for nivolumab vs. the observation group was 84% and 73%, respectively. **Conclusion: Adjuvant nivolumab confers an absolute risk reduction of 10% in DFS at 2 years.**

Topalian, CheckMate 358 Trial (*JCO*, PMID 32324435): Phase I/II study of 39 patients with stage IIA to IV resectable MCC who received nivolumab on days 1 and 15 followed by planned surgery on day 29. Among those who underwent surgery, 18 (55%) had tumor reductions greater than 30%. For those with a pCR at the time of surgery, none had tumor relapse during follow-up (MFU of 20.3 months). **Conclusion: Nivolumab was well-tolerated and showed good response in over half of treated patients. Patients with pCR or significant tumor regression had improved RFS.**

REFERENCES

1. Rogers HW, Weinstock MA, Feldman SR, Coldiron BM. Incidence estimate of nonmelanoma skin cancer (Keratinocyte Carcinomas) in the U.S. population, 2012. *JAMA Dermatol.* 2015;151(10):1081–1086. doi:10.1001/jamadermatol.2015.1187
2. Paulson KG, Park SY, Vandeven NA, et al. Merkel cell carcinoma: current US incidence and projected increases based on changing demographics. *J Am Acad Dermatol.* 2018;78(3):457–463 e2. doi:10.1016/j.jaad.2017.10.028
3. Clarke CA, Robbins HA, Tatalovich Z, et al. Risk of merkel cell carcinoma after solid organ transplantation. *J Natl Cancer Inst.* 2015; 107(2):dju382. doi:10.1093/jnci/dju382
4. Howard RA, Dores GM, Curtis RE, Anderson WF, Travis LB. Merkel cell carcinoma and multiple primary cancers. *Cancer Epidemiol Biomarkers Prev.* 2006;15(8):1545–1549. doi:10.1158/1055-9965.EPI-05-0895
5. Feng H, Shuda M, Chang Y, Moore PS. Clonal integration of a polyomavirus in human Merkel cell carcinoma. *Science.* 22 2008;319(5866):1096–1100. doi:10.1126/science.1152586
6. Harms KL, Healy MA, Nghiem P, et al. Analysis of prognostic factors from 9387 merkel cell carcinoma cases forms the basis for the new 8th edition AJCC staging system. *Ann Surg Oncol.* 2016;23(11):3564–3571. doi:10.1245/s10434-016-5266-4
7. Santos-Juanes J, Fernandez-Vega I, Fuentes N, et al. Merkel cell carcinoma and Merkel cell polyomavirus: a systematic review and meta-analysis. *Br J Dermatol.* 2015;173(1):42–49. doi:10.1111/bjd.13870
8. Rodig SJ, Cheng J, Wardzala J, et al. Improved detection suggests all Merkel cell carcinomas harbor Merkel polyomavirus. *J Clin Invest.* 2012;122(12):4645–4653. doi:10.1172/JCI64116
9. Tilling T, Moll I. Which are the cells of origin in merkel cell carcinoma? *J Skin Cancer.* 2012;2012:680410. doi:10.1155/2012/680410

10. Ratner D, Nelson BR, Brown MD, Johnson TM. Merkel cell carcinoma. *J Am Acad Dermatol*. 1993;29(2 Pt 1): 143–56. doi:10.1016/0190-9622(93)70159-q

11. Mohsin N, Hunt D, Yan J, et al. Genetic risk factors for early-onset merkel cell carcinoma. *JAMA Dermatol*. 2024;160(2):172–178. doi:10.1001/jamadermatol.2023.5362

12. Paulson KG, Iyer JG, Tegeder AR, et al. Transcriptome-wide studies of merkel cell carcinoma and validation of intratumoral CD8+ lymphocyte invasion as an independent predictor of survival. *J Clin Oncol*. 2011;29(12):1539–1546. doi:10.1200/JCO.2010.30.6308

13. Sihto H, Kukko H, Koljonen V, Sankila R, Bohling T, Joensuu H. Merkel cell polyomavirus infection, large T antigen, retinoblastoma protein and outcome in Merkel cell carcinoma. *Clin Cancer Res*. 2011;17(14): 4806–13. doi:10.1158/1078-0432.CCR-10-3363

14. Touze A, Le Bidre E, Laude H, et al. High levels of antibodies against merkel cell polyomavirus identify a subset of patients with merkel cell carcinoma with better clinical outcome. *J Clin Oncol*. 2011;29(12): 1612–1619. doi:10.1200/JCO.2010.31.1704

15. Allen PJ, Bowne WB, Jaques DP, Brennan MF, Busam K, Coit DG. Merkel cell carcinoma: prognosis and treatment of patients from a single institution. *J Clin Oncol*. 2005;23(10):2300–2309. doi:10.1200/JCO.2005.02.329

16. NCCN. NCCN Clinical Practice Guidelines: Merkel Cell Carcinoma. 2023;1.2024. Accessed December 2024. https://www.nccn.org/professionals/physician_gls/pdf/mcc.pdf

17. Poulsen M, Rischin D, Walpole E, et al. High-risk Merkel cell carcinoma of the skin treated with synchronous carboplatin/etoposide and radiation: a Trans-Tasman Radiation Oncology Group Study--TROG 96:07. *J Clin Oncol*. 2003;21(23):4371–4376. doi:10.1200/JCO.2003.03.154

18. Winkler JK, Bender C, Kratochwil C, Enk A, Hassel JC. PD-1 blockade: a therapeutic option for treatment of metastatic Merkel cell carcinoma. *Br J Dermatol*. 2017;176(1):216–219. doi:10.1111/bjd.14632

19. Nghiem PT, Bhatia S, Lipson EJ, et al. PD-1 blockade with pembrolizumab in advanced merkel-cell carcinoma. *N Engl J Med*. 2016;374(26):2542–2552. doi:10.1056/NEJMoa1603702

20. Kaufman HL, Russell J, Hamid O, et al. Avelumab in patients with chemotherapy-refractory metastatic Merkel cell carcinoma: a multicentre, single-group, open-label, phase 2 trial. *Lancet Oncol*. 2016;17(10):1374–1385. doi:10.1016/S1470-2045(16)30364-3

21. Nghiem P, Bhatia S, Lipson EJ, et al. Durable tumor regression and overall survival in patients with advanced merkel cell carcinoma receiving pembrolizumab as first-line therapy. *J Clin Oncol*. 2019;37(9):693–702. doi:10.1200/JCO.18.01896

22. Decker RH, Wilson LD. Role of radiotherapy in the management of merkel cell carcinoma of the skin. *J Natl Compr Canc Netw*. 2006;4(7):713–718. doi:10.6004/jnccn.2006.0061

23. Videtic GNM WN, Vassil AD. *Handbook of Treatment Planning in Radiation Oncology*. 3rd ed. Demos Medical; 2020.

24. Mojica P, Smith D, Ellenhorn JD. Adjuvant radiation therapy is associated with improved survival in Merkel cell carcinoma of the skin. *J Clin Oncol*. 2007;25(9):1043–1047. doi:10.1200/JCO.2006.07.9319

25. Kim JA, Choi AH. Effect of radiation therapy on survival in patients with resected Merkel cell carcinoma: a propensity score surveillance, epidemiology, and end results database analysis. *JAMA Dermatol*. 2013;149(7):831–838. doi:10.1001/jamadermatol.2013.409

26. Bhatia S, Storer BE, Iyer JG, et al. Adjuvant radiation therapy and chemotherapy in merkel cell carcinoma: survival analyses of 6908 cases from the national cancer data base. *J Natl Cancer Inst*. 2016;108(9):djw042. doi:10.1093/jnci/djw042

27. Vargo JA, Ghareeb ER, Balasubramani GK, Beriwal S. RE: Adjuvant radiation therapy and chemotherapy in merkel cell carcinoma: survival analyses of 6908 cases from the National Cancer Data Base. *J Natl Cancer Inst*. 2017;109(10). doi:10.1093/jnci/djx052

28. Veness M, Foote M, Gebski V, Poulsen M. The role of radiotherapy alone in patients with merkel cell carcinoma: reporting the Australian experience of 43 patients. *Int J Radiat Oncol Biol Phys*. 2010;78(3):703–709. doi:10.1016/j.ijrobp.2009.08.011

29. Patel SA, Qureshi MM, Mak KS, et al. Impact of total radiotherapy dose on survival for head and neck Merkel cell carcinoma after resection. *Head Neck*. 2017;39(7):1371–1377. doi:10.1002/hed.24776

30. Iyer JG, Parvathaneni U, Gooley T, et al. Single-fraction radiation therapy in patients with metastatic Merkel cell carcinoma. *Cancer Med*. 2015;4(8):1161–1170. doi:10.1002/cam4.458

31. D'Angelo SP, Lebbe C, Mortier L, et al. First-line avelumab treatment in patients with metastatic Merkel cell carcinoma: 4-year follow-up from part B of the JAVELIN Merkel 200 study. *ESMO Open*. 2024;9(5):103461. doi:10.1016/j.esmoop.2024.103461

22 MALIGNANT CUTANEOUS MELANOMA

Cole Billena, Sarah S. Kilic, Nikhil P. Joshi, and Neil M. Woody

QUICK HIT Melanoma is increasing in incidence. Primary treatment is either surgical excision with lymph node evaluation (SLNB vs. complete dissection) or neoadjuvant immunotherapy (IO) followed by surgery. IO and targeted therapies are the mainstay of systemic treatment in the neoadjuvant, adjuvant, unresectable, and metastatic settings. The role of adjuvant RT is controversial, although it may be considered in patients with multiple risk factors to improve local and/or regional control. Definitive RT can be used for lentigo maligna melanoma when surgery would be disfiguring (Table 22.1).

Table 22.1 Indications for Adjuvant RT of Malignant Melanoma After Resection	
Primary site	Desmoplastic neurotropic histology Ulceration Satellitosis Breslow depth >4 mm Positive margins Locally recurrent disease
Regional lymph nodes	Gross ECE Multiple positive LNs (see Burmeister et al.; criteria vary by site) Size ≥3–4 cm

EPIDEMIOLOGY: Rising incidence over the past 30 years; 100,640 new diagnoses and 8,290 deaths estimated in the United States in 2024.[1] Incidence increases with age (median age at diagnosis 63). In patients younger than 45, melanoma is more commonly diagnosed in females, but by age 65 the incidence is twice as high in men; 20 times more common in Caucasians than Black individuals.[2] Roughly 84% present with localized disease, 9% with regional disease, and 4% with distant metastatic disease.[3]

RISK FACTORS: Fair skin (particularly Fitzpatrick skin types I and II), red/blonde hair, high-density freckling, light eyes (green/hazel/blue), increased lifetime exposure to sunlight (natural or artificial), family history of melanoma or dysplastic nevi, immunosuppression (congenital or acquired).[4] UVB (intermittent exposure, sunburn during early ages) is higher risk than UVA (tanning beds, PUVA therapy); 10% of cases are familial with mutations in *CDKN2A*, *CDK4*, *XP*, or *BRCA2* genes.[5]

ANATOMY: Human skin is composed of, from superficial to deep, epidermis, dermis, and hypodermis (subcutis). The hypodermis contains collagen and fat cells. The dermis consists of a superficial papillary layer and a deep reticular layer and contains sweat glands, vessels, lymphatics, pain and touch receptors, and follicles, and is highly collagenized. The epidermis is subdivided into five layers, which are, from superficial to deep, stratum corneum (dead, fully keratinized anucleate keratinocytes), stratum lucidum (highly keratinized), stratum granulosum (cells contain keratin precursors), stratum spinosum (contains dendritic cells), and stratum basale (contains melanocytes and mitotically active keratinocyte progenitors that contribute to constant regeneration of the overlying layers). Malignant melanoma originates from the neoplastic proliferation of melanocytes, the melanin pigment-producing cells of the skin that arise from the neural crest during embryonic development and migrate to the stratum basale. Melanocytes are present in the skin, eye, sinonasal tract, and upper respiratory, GI, and GU tracts, and thus malignant melanoma can arise in cutaneous, conjunctival/uveal, and mucosal sites.

PATHOLOGY: The most common subtype is superficial spreading, comprising 70% of melanoma.[6] These usually occur in the trunk and extremities and are commonly related to sun exposure. The nodular melanoma subtype makes up 15% to 30% of cases.[6] The lentigo maligna subtype commonly occurs in older patients in sun-damaged areas of skin and often presents as a mildly pigmented macule.[7] The least common subtype is acral lentiginous melanoma, which comprises <5% of cases.[6]

Acral lentiginous melanoma is the most common subtype in patients of Asian origin and in those with dark skin; most commonly arises in the palms of hand and soles of feet. Mucosal melanoma is rare and makes up ~1% of all melanoma cases. These most commonly occur in H&N, anorectum, vagina, and vulva.[8] *BRAF* mutation status can help guide systemic therapy; targetable mutations include V600E and V600K.

SCREENING: Clinician skin exams may reduce the risk of advanced melanoma, but no prospective randomized evidence exists to suggest decreased mortality/morbidity with clinical exams. Per 2023 USPSTF recommendations, there is insufficient evidence to recommend either for or against routine screening for the general population. The AAD recommends that everyone perform regular skin self-examinations, especially those at high risk (strong family history of melanoma or personal history of multiple clinically atypical moles), and receive routine physician exams at the discretion of their dermatologist depending on individual risk factors. The ABCDE system is useful for screening: **a**symmetry, **b**order irregularities, **c**olor variegation (different colors in same region), **d**iameter >6 mm, **e**nlargement or evolution of color change, shape, or symptoms. Genetic counseling should be considered for those with a strong family history.[5]

WORKUP: H&P with full-body skin exam and thorough LN evaluation; 20% of clinically node-negative patients have metastatic involvement, while 20% of clinically node-positive patients are pathologically negative.

Pathology: Excisional biopsy of lesion with at least 1- to 3-mm margins. Alternatively, clinician can consider full-thickness punch or incisional biopsy depending on location (palm/sole, digit, face, ear) or size. If clinical suspicion is low, shave biopsy may be used, but this may complicate depth assessment if malignancy is identified. Per 2024 NCCN guidelines, SLNB is routinely recommended for patients with clinical stage IB (T1b–T2a) or II (T2b or higher) disease, namely patients with Breslow depth <0.8 mm with ulceration or lesion depth >0.8 mm regardless of ulceration. Patients with Breslow depth >0.5 mm and additional risk factors, such as age ≤42 years, H&N location, lymphovascular invasion, and/or mitotic index ≥2/mm^2, can be considered for SLNB. SLNB may be less accurate after a prior wide excision, rotation flap, or skin graft closure, but these are not contraindications to attempting the procedure. Historically important features on pathology include Breslow depth (thickness of the lesion, measured to the tenth of a millimeter) and Clark level (scored 1 through 5 based on the deepest involved layer of the skin, with 1 being confined to the epidermis and 5 invading into the hypodermis).

Imaging: Cross-sectional imaging (CT, PET, and MRI brain) is considered for patients with a single clinically occult positive node identified on SLNB alone (pathologic stage IIIA). It should be performed for all patients with clinically positive nodes or more extensive nodal disease (pIIIB–D) and for any patient with symptoms suspicious for locoregional or distant metastatic disease.[9]

PROGNOSTIC FACTORS: SLNB status is the most important predictor for LR and DSS. Extracapsular extension (ECE), number of LN, LN size, anatomic region, pathologic factors, and margins are used to determine benefit of adjuvant RT to nodes or primary site. Historically, important pathologic features were Breslow thickness and Clark level; Breslow is more prognostic than Clark, but both have been supplanted by AJCC 8th staging.

STAGING: See Table 22.2.

Table 22.2 AJCC 8th Edition: Clinical Staging for Cutaneous Malignant Melanoma											
T/N	N	cN0	cN1a	cN1b	cN1c	cN2a	cN2b	cN2c	cN3a	cN3b	cN3c
T1a	<0.8 mm thick with no ulceration	IA									
T1b	<0.8 mm thick with ulceration; 0.8–1.0 mm thick	IB				III					
T2a	1–2 mm with no ulceration										

(continued)

T/N		N	cN0	cN1a	cN1b	cN1c	cN2a	cN2b	cN2c	cN3a	cN3b	cN3c
T2b	1–2 mm with ulceration		IIA									
T3a	2–4 mm with no ulceration											
T3b	2–4 mm with ulceration		IIB									
T4a	>4 mm with no ulceration											
T4b	>4 mm with ulceration		IIC									
M1a	Skin, muscle, nonregional LNs							IV				
M1b	Lung											
M1c	Non-CNS visceral											
M1d	CNS											

Table 22.2 AJCC 8th Edition: Clinical Staging for Cutaneous Malignant Melanoma (*continued*)

cN1a: 1 clinically occult LN (detected by SLN biopsy); cN1b: 1 clinically detected LN; cN1c: negative regional LN, with in-transit, satellite, or microsatellite metastasis; cN2a: 2–3 clinically occult LNs; cN2b: 2–3 LNs, at least one of which clinically detected; cN2c: 1 clinically occult or clinically detected LN with in-transit, satellite, or microsatellite metastasis; cN3a: ≥4 clinically occult LNs; cN3b: ≥4 LNs, at least one of which was clinically detected or presence of any number of matted nodes without in-transit, satellite, or microsatellite metastasis; cN3c: ≥2 clinically occult or clinically detected LNs and/or presence of any number of matted nodes with presence of in-transit, satellite, or microsatellite metastasis.

TREATMENT PARADIGM

Surgery: Surgical excision is the primary treatment for melanoma. Wide local excision (WLE) is recommended, with margin requirement based on thickness of tumor. NCCN 2024 guidelines outline the margin requirements (Table 22.3) based on findings from multiple randomized surgical trials, although these can be modified for individual anatomic or functional needs.[9]

Table 22.3 NCCN-Recommended Clinical Margins for Malignant Melanoma	
Tumor Thickness	**NCCN-Recommended Clinical Margins**
In situ	0.5–1.0 cm
≤1.0 mm	1.0 cm
1–2 mm	1–2 cm
2.01–4 mm	2.0 cm
>4 mm	2.0 cm

SLNB is recommended for patients based on lesion thickness and other pathologic features, as discussed earlier. Historically, completion lymphadenectomy was recommended if positive SLNB[9,10]; however, the MSLT-II trial randomized patients with positive SLNB to immediate completion dissection or nodal observation with ultrasound and found that patients who underwent completion dissection had favorable regional disease control, although there was no improvement in melanoma-specific survival despite a 5% improvement in regional control.[11] Complete dissection is required for any clinically N+ patient. Adequate dissections require >10 LNs in the groin and >15 LNs in the axilla and neck.

Systemic Therapy: Previously, adjuvant high-dose interferon for at least 1 year was standard of care after multiple randomized trials demonstrated improved DFS. However, targeted therapies and modern IO have replaced interferon as the systemic treatment of choice in the neoadjuvant, adjuvant, unresectable, and metastatic setting. The 2024 NCCN guidelines provide recommendations for targeted therapies and immune checkpoint inhibitors in these settings. IO is increasingly employed neoadjuvantly, particularly in the clinically N+ setting. Assessment of response at the time of surgery may also help guide adjuvant therapy.

Radiation

Definitive: For lentigo maligna melanoma, definitive RT is used when surgery would be disfiguring. There is no standard dose, but 50 Gy/20 fx with electrons is commonly used.[12]

Adjuvant: Per NCCN guidelines, indications for treating primary tumor include pure desmoplastic histologic subtype, extensive neurotropic features, close margins without the ability to re-resect, H&N location, and locally recurrent disease. For positive margins, re-resection is preferred, but adjuvant RT can be employed if resection to a negative margin is not feasible. Potential indications for treating regional LNs include multiple positive LNs (≥1 parotid node, ≥2 cervical or axillary nodes, ≥3 inguinofemoral nodes, ≥3 cm cervical or axillary nodes, and/or ≥4 cm inguinofemoral nodes), ECE, SLN involvement without complete or inadequate LND, and recurrent disease.[9] Indications for RT are stronger if multiple risk factors are present. However, with the increasing application of adjuvant IO, RT may be often reserved for salvage therapy following re-resection. Adjuvant RT should be carefully considered in patients with marginal pathologic response to neoadjuvant IO and in patients who are unable to receive IO due to intolerance or risks such as prior organ transplant.

Dose: 48 Gy/20 fx over 4 weeks (see Burmeister; consider 50 Gy/21 fx for positive margins) or 30 Gy/5 fx over 2.5 weeks (see Ang).

Toxicity: Acute: fatigue, RT dermatitis, others location-dependent. Late: fibrosis, hypo/hyperpigmentation, lymphedema, others location-dependent.

EVIDENCE-BASED Q&A

Which patients benefit from adjuvant RT to regional nodal basin?

Even with adequate lymphadenectomy, recurrence in nodal basin is relatively common and quite morbid, negatively impacting quality of life. This led to multiple prospective studies evaluating nodal RT (as summarized in the following), which were generally completed before the era of modern IO/targeted therapy. Given that regional failure is low (10%–20%) with modern adjuvant systemic therapy, the role of adjuvant RT has become more controversial in the modern era.[13,14] The decision regarding adjuvant RT should be undertaken in a comprehensive multidisciplinary manner to ensure selection of patients who are most likely to benefit from treatment. Patients who present with LRR after adjuvant systemic treatment are likely to benefit from adjuvant RT after salvage surgery.

Ang, MDACC (*IJROBP* 1994, PMID 7960981; Update *Cancer* 2003, PMID 12655537): Phase II study of 160 patients managed with one of the following: (a) elective RT after WLE of lesions >1.5 mm thick/Clark level IV/V, (b) adjuvant RT after WLE/LND with pN+ (stage II/III), or (c) RT for nodal only relapse s/p nodal dissection. RT was 30 Gy/5 fx over 2.5 weeks. MFU 78 months; 10-year LC and LRC of 94% and 91%. Authors recommended adjuvant RT for ECE, LN ≥3 cm (in axilla or inguinal region), LN ≥2 cm (cervical), involvement of multiple LNs (≥4 nodes in axilla or inguinal region, ≥2 if cervical), recurrent disease, or selective LND (rather than modified radical or radical LND). **Conclusion: Hypofractionated RT (30 Gy/5 fx) is safe and effective for adjuvant treatment of melanoma, with excellent 10-year LRC and rare toxicity.**

Burmeister, ANZMTG 01.02/TROG 02.01 (*Lancet* 2012, PMID 22575589; Update *Lancet* 2015, PMID 26206146): PRT of 250 patients with clinically N+ melanoma after LND with specific high-risk features (≥1 parotid, ≥2 cervical or axillary, or ≥3 groin nodes, ENE, maximum metastatic node diameter ≥3 cm in neck or ≥4 cm in groin/axilla) randomized to adjuvant RT (48 Gy/20 fx over 4 weeks) or observation. For margin-positive patients, dose was escalated to 50 Gy/21 fx. Previous phase II study described the regional fields used in detail.[15] Patients in the observation group who recurred received resection and RT at that time. At 6 years, LN field relapse significantly improved with RT (21% vs. 36%, *p* = .021). OS and RFS similar between the groups; 22% of patients experienced grades 3 to 4 toxicities, mostly skin/subcutaneous. **Conclusion: Adjuvant nodal RT reduces nodal recurrence in select patients with high-risk features after nodal dissection.** *Comment: Trial was performed prior to systemic therapy/IO era (<5% received interferon); 23 of 26 patients in the observation group with regional failure underwent salvage surgery with similar 5-year OS to overall cohort.*

What should the field extent be for patients treated with axillary nodal RT?

In patients with axillary metastasis, limiting RT field to the axilla rather than extending it to the supraclavicular region provided equivalent LC rates, and extended-field RT was associated with significantly higher rate of treatment-related complications.

Beadle, MDACC (*Cancer* 2009, PMID 18774657): RR of 200 patients with melanoma metastatic to axillary LN region who had high-risk features and received PORT. High risk was defined as LN ≥3 cm in size, ≥4 positive LNs, presence of ECE, or recurrent disease after initial resection; 48% of patients were treated to axilla only and 52% were treated to axilla and supraclavicular fossa. Dose was 30 Gy/5 fx. MFU 59 months; 5-year axillary control was 89% for axilla only vs. 84% for axilla and supraclavicular fossa (NS). OS, DSS, and DMFS were not significantly different. On MVA, extended-field RT was associated with increased risk of complications. **Conclusion: Limiting RT field to the axilla rather than extending to the adjacent SCV nodal area provides equivalent control with decreased toxicity.**

Which patients benefit from adjuvant RT to the primary site?

The data for primary site RT are sparse. Risk factors associated with a higher risk of LR in surgical series include increased tumor thickness, ulceration, H&N location, and desmoplastic/neurotropic features, and therefore adjuvant RT to the primary site is sometimes considered for patients with one or more of these features. Desmoplastic melanoma is a rare subtype that tends to be locally aggressive, with increased incidence of LR rather than nodal or DM. It has a neurotropic predilection and tends to spread along large named nerves, especially in the H&N, where wide surgical margins are difficult to achieve. Phase II data from Mayo Clinic and retrospective evidence from MDACC suggest that the use of PORT significantly reduces LR in patients with desmoplastic melanoma.[16,17] RTN2 Trial 01.09, evaluating adjuvant RT vs. observation in patients with cutaneous neurotropic melanoma of the H&N following resection with ≥5 mm margins, closed prematurely due to slow accrual during the COVID-19 pandemic, but in the 50 patients available to be randomized (23 observation, 27 RT), there were three local relapses in the observation arm and one in the RT arm (HR 0.29, p = .2).[18] G3+ toxicity occurred in 12.5% of the RT arm and 10% observation. TROG (TROG 08.09)/ANZ Melanoma Trials Group (ANZMTG 01.09) is an ongoing randomized trial that prospectively evaluates the impact of adjuvant RT in this population.

What is the role of SLNB in the surgical management of melanoma?

The MSLT trials investigated this question and found that SLNB is useful for prognostication but does not improve DSS in most patients; additionally, in patients with a positive SLNB, completion dissection does not improve DSS.

Morton, MSLT-I (*NEJM* 2014, PMID 24521106): PRT of 1,661 patients with cN0 cutaneous melanoma s/p WLE randomized to upfront SLNB (followed by immediate lymphadenectomy if positive SLNB) or observation (with lymphadenectomy at nodal recurrence); 16% of patients in the SLNB arm had positive LN; 17% of patients in the observation arm had eventual nodal recurrence. For the entire cohort, no difference in 10-year DSS between SLNB and observation. However, in intermediate-thickness tumors, those with positive SLNB had improved melanoma-specific survival (MSS) compared with those initially observed who later developed nodal metastases. In patients with intermediate (1.2–3.5 mm) or thick (>3.5 mm) tumors, 10-year MSS was significantly lower in patients with a positive SLNB (intermediate: 62% vs. 85%; thick: 48% vs. 66%) compared with those who had negative biopsy. **Conclusion: SLNB is useful for staging and prognostication. However, SLNB does not improve melanoma-specific survival.**

Faries, MSLT-II (*NEJM* 2017, PMID 28591523): PRT of 1,934 patients with cutaneous melanoma s/p WLE and positive SLNB randomized to completion dissection or nodal observation. No difference in 3-year MSS between groups. At 3 years, regional nodal control (92% vs. 77%, p < .001) and nodal recurrence (HR 0.31, 95% CI 0.24–0.41) were improved in the completion dissection group. Significantly more lymphedema in the completion dissection group (24% vs. 6%, p < .001). **Conclusion: Completion dissection improves nodal disease control but does not improve melanoma-specific survival and is associated with a higher rate of lymphedema.** *Comment: Most patients had a low disease burden (70% had only one positive sentinel node; 12% had only RT-PCR evidence of nodal disease); some feel results may not apply to higher disease burden.*

Can RT replace neck dissection?

Single-institution retrospective data from MDACC suggest that patients with stage I/II cutaneous melanoma who did not have SLNB or LND and had subsequent adjuvant treatment with hypofractionated regional nodal RT had good outcomes (89% 5- and 10-year actuarial regional controls and 10-year symptomatic complication rate of 6%).[19] This is not standard of care and is limited by retrospective analysis and selection bias. If the sentinel node does not map, a multidisciplinary decision between observation, adjuvant IO, and nodal dissection will be required—elective RT is not common.

When is definitive RT considered?

Definitive RT is not appropriate for most cases. RT alone is considered in patients with superficial lentigo maligna (confined to epidermis) and lentigo maligna melanoma (invasive into dermis). These patients are often older adults and can present with large superficial lesions on the face; therefore, nonsurgical options can offer better function and cosmesis. In this setting, dose fractionation schedules vary widely, but generally, good LC outcomes have been observed (70%–90%).[20] The RADICAL trial randomizing 126 patients with lentigo maligna who are not surgical candidates or who refuse surgery to definitive RT or imiquimod was recently presented in abstract form at ASCO 2024 and found the recurrence rate within 24 months was 24% in the RT arm and 10.5% in the imiquimod arm (OR 2.68, p = .06) and the conclusion was that both options are valid.[21]

REFERENCES

1. Siegel RL, Giaquinto AN, Jemal A. Cancer statistics, 2024. *CA Cancer J Clin*. 2024;74(1):12–49. doi:10.3322/caac.21820
2. Bradford PT. Skin cancer in skin of color. *Dermatol Nurs*. 2009;21(4):170–177. PMID:19691228
3. Harlan LC, Lynch CF, Ballard-Barbash R, Zeruto C. Trends in the treatment and survival for local and regional cutaneous melanoma in a US population-based study. *Melanoma Res*. 2011;21(6):547–554. doi:10.1097/CMR.0b013e32834b58e4
4. Rastrelli M, Tropea S, Rossi CR, Alaibac M. Melanoma: epidemiology, risk factors, pathogenesis, diagnosis and classification. *In Vivo*. 2014;28(6):1005–1011. PMID:25398793
5. Leachman SA, Lucero OM, Sampson JE, et al. Identification, genetic testing, and management of hereditary melanoma. *Cancer Metastasis Rev*. 2017;36(1):77–90. doi:10.1007/s10555-017-9661-5
6. Goldsmith LA, Katz SI, Gilchrest BA, Paller AS, Leffell DJ, Wolff K. *Fitzpatrick's Dermatology in General Medicine*. 8th ed. The McGraw-Hill Companies; 2012.
7. Star P, Guitera P. Lentigo maligna, macules of the face, and lesions on sun-damaged skin: confocal makes the difference. *Dermatol Clin*. 2016;34(4):421–429. doi:10.1016/j.det.2016.05.005
8. Chang AE, Karnell LH, Menck HR. The national cancer data base report on cutaneous and noncutaneous melanoma: a summary of 84,836 cases from the past decade. The American college of surgeons commission on cancer and the American Cancer Society. *Cancer*. 1998;83(8):1664–1678. doi:10.1002/(sici)1097-0142(19981015)83:8<1664::aid-cncr23>3.0.co;2-g
9. Cascinelli N, Bombardieri E, Bufalino R, et al. Sentinel and nonsentinel node status in stage IB and II melanoma patients: two-step prognostic indicators of survival. *J Clin Oncol*. 2006;24(27):4464–4471. doi:10.1200/jco.2006.06.3198
10. Lee JH, Essner R, Torisu-Itakura H, Wanek L, Wang H, Morton DL. Factors predictive of tumor-positive nonsentinel lymph nodes after tumor-positive sentinel lymph node dissection for melanoma. *J Clin Oncol*. 2004;22(18):3677–3684. doi:10.1200/jco.2004.01.012
11. Faries MB, Thompson JF, Cochran AJ, et al. Completion dissection or observation for sentinel-node metastasis in melanoma. *N Engl J Med*. 2017;376(23):2211–2222. doi:10.1056/NEJMoa1613210
12. Fogarty GB, Hong A, Economides A, Guitera P. Experience with treating lentigo maligna with definitive radiotherapy. *Dermatol Res Pract*. 2018;2018:7439807. doi:10.1155/2018/7439807
13. Eggermont AMM, Kicinski M, Blank CU, et al. Five-year analysis of adjuvant pembrolizumab or placebo in stage III melanoma. *NEJM Evid*. 2022;1(11):EVIDoa2200214. doi:10.1056/EVIDoa2200214
14. Long GV, Hauschild A, Santinami M, et al. Final results for adjuvant dabrafenib plus trametinib in stage III melanoma. *N Engl J Med*. 2024;391(18):1709–1720. doi:10.1056/NEJMoa2404139
15. Burmeister BH, Mark Smithers B, Burmeister E, et al. A prospective phase II study of adjuvant postoperative radiation therapy following nodal surgery in malignant melanoma-Trans Tasman Radiation Oncology Group (TROG) Study 96.06. *Radiother Oncol*. 2006;81(2):136–142. doi:10.1016/j.radonc.2006.10.001
16. Rule WG, Allred JB, Pockaj BA, et al. Results of NCCTG N0275 (Alliance)–a phase II trial evaluating resection followed by adjuvant radiation therapy for patients with desmoplastic melanoma. *Cancer Med*. 2016;5(8):1890–1896. doi:10.1002/cam4.783

17. Guadagnolo BA, Prieto V, Weber R, Ross MI, Zagars GK. The role of adjuvant radiotherapy in the local management of desmoplastic melanoma. *Cancer*. 2014;120(9):1361–1368. doi:10.1002/cncr.28415

18. Pinkham MB, Herschtal A, Hong AM, et al. Randomized trial of postoperative radiation therapy after wide excision of neurotropic melanoma of the head and neck (RTN2 Trial 01.09). *Ann Surg Oncol*. 2024;31(9):6088–6096. doi:10.1245/s10434-024-15569-2

19. Bonnen MD, Ballo MT, Myers JN, et al. Elective radiotherapy provides regional control for patients with cutaneous melanoma of the head and neck. *Cancer*. 2004;100(2):383–389. doi:10.1002/cncr.11921

20. Hendrickx A, Cozzio A, Plasswilm L, Panje CM. Radiotherapy for lentigo maligna and lentigo maligna melanoma–a systematic review. *Radiat Oncol*. 2020;15(1):174. doi:10.1186/s13014-020-01615-2

21. Hong AM, Lo SN, Fogarty GB, et al. A randomised, controlled, multicentre trial of imiquimod versus radiotherapy for lentigo maligna. *J Clin Oncol*. 2024;42(16_suppl):9502. doi:10.1200/JCO.2024.42.16_suppl.9502

23 MYCOSIS FUNGOIDES

Anirudh Bommireddy, Matthew C. Ward, and Gregory M. M. Videtic

QUICK HIT Mycosis fungoides (MF) is the most common cutaneous lymphoma in the United States and originates from the T-cell. The final diagnosis is often revealed by skin biopsies since it is often confused with other entities. Appropriate imaging and LN biopsies are utilized to evaluate for extracutaneous disease. Treatments tend to be localized (skin-directed therapy, phototherapy, and localized superficial RT) for early stages of disease and systemic for more advanced or refractory disease (Table 23.1).

Table 23.1 General Treatment Paradigm for Mycosis Fungoides[1]	
Stage I	Observation, skin-directed therapy, phototherapy, TSEBT
Stage II	Observation, skin-directed therapy, phototherapy, TSEBT, interferon alpha
Stage III	TSEBT, photopheresis, interferon alpha, phototherapy, methotrexate
Stage IV	CHT, TSEBT, oral bexarotene, interferon alpha, vorinostat, romidepsin, low-dose methotrexate, clinical trials

Source: Data from Trautinger F, Eder J, Assaf C, et al. European organisation for research and treatment of cancer consensus recommendations for the treatment of mycosis fungoides/Sezary syndrome–Update 2017. *Eur J Cancer.* 2017;77:57–74. doi:10.1016/j.ejca.2017.02.027.

EPIDEMIOLOGY: In the United States and Europe, six cases of MF are diagnosed annually per million people. The disease accounts for ~4% of all NHL diagnoses. It affects men almost twice as often as women and has a higher prevalence in the Black population.[2] Median age at diagnosis is 55 to 60.[3]

RISK FACTORS: Risk factors for MF are unclear. Although HTLV1 has been found in skin lesions of patients with MF, there are also studies providing evidence against the role of HTLV1 as a risk factor.[4]

ANATOMY: Lesions can present anywhere on the body, but are most commonly seen in a truncal distribution.[5] In rare cases, malignant T-cells can be found in peripheral blood, and in advanced stages the disease may present in regional or distant LN, or other organ systems, most commonly in the lungs, oral cavity, pharynx, or CNS.[3,6]

PATHOLOGY: Pathogenesis of MF is currently unclear. On histology, skin biopsies show Pautrier's abscesses (pathognomonic, present in 38% of cases), haloed lymphocytes, exocytosis, disproportionate epidermotropism, epidermal lymphocytes larger than dermal lymphocytes, hyperconvoluted intraepidermal lymphocytes, and lymphocytes aligned within the basal layer.[7] Disease can also present with circulating malignant T-cells (Sézary cells) that usually possess CD4+/CD7– or CD4+/CD26– immunophenotype.[8] The two main histopathologic grading systems for LNs in MF are the NCI/VA classification system and the Dutch system, with the main difference residing in the criteria defining "abnormal" lymphocytes.[8]

CLINICAL PRESENTATION: Typical clinical presentation is preceded by a premycotic period, defined by nonspecific, slightly scaling lesions, accompanied by nondiagnostic skin biopsies. As deposition of malignant T-cells becomes more persistent, the disease presents with heterogeneous patches that may evolve into plaques, and then finally cutaneous tumors. MF commonly presents with debilitating pruritus.[9]

WORKUP: H&P including percentage of body surface area affected by patches, plaques, or tumor lesions. Laboratory studies should include CBC, CMP, LFTs, and serum LDH, as well as evaluation for Sézary cells (PCR/flow cytometry). Skin biopsies should be taken from at least two sites and should be assessed with H&E staining, immunostaining for surface marker expression profiles, and

PCR for clonal TCR rearrangement. If only one biopsy can be obtained, the lesion with the greatest induration should be chosen.[8] Chest x-ray or nodal ultrasound is sufficient for patients with early-stage disease. However, CT scan of the chest, abdomen, and pelvis or whole-body integrated PET/CT should be performed for patients with T2b disease or greater in order to rule out any lymphadenopathy or visceral involvement.[10]

PROGNOSTIC FACTORS: Advanced clinical stage, large cell histology, folliculotropic disease, age >60, increased LDH, and extracutaneous involvement have worse prognosis.[11]

STAGING: Current standard for staging MF utilizes the TNMB system proposed by ISCL/EORTC as summarized in Table 23.2 and Table 23.3.[8]

Table 23.2 ISCL/EORTC Revision to Staging of Mycosis Fungoides and Sézary Syndrome[8]	
Skin	**Characteristics**
T1	Limited patches, papules, and/or plaques covering <10% of skin surface; may further stratify into T1a (patch only) vs. T1b (plaque ± patch)
T2	Patches, papules, or plaques covering ≥10% of skin surface; may further stratify into T2a (patch only) vs. T2b (plaque ± patch)
T3	≥1 tumor (≥1 cm diameter)
T4	Confluence of erythema covering ≥80% of body surface area
Node	**Characteristics**
N0	No clinically abnormal peripheral LNs; biopsy not required
N1	Clinically abnormal peripheral LNs; histopathology Dutch grade 1 or NCI LN0–2
N1a	Clone negative
N1b	Clone positive
N2	Clinically abnormal peripheral LNs; histopathology Dutch grade 2 or NCI LN3
N2a	Clone negative
N2b	Clone positive
N3	Clinically abnormal peripheral LNs; histopathology Dutch grades 3–4 or NCI LN4; clone positive or negative
Nx	Clinically abnormal peripheral LNs; no histologic confirmation
Visceral	**Characteristics**
M0	No visceral organ involvement
M1	Visceral involvement (must have pathology confirmation, and organ involved should be specified)
Peripheral Blood Involvement	**Characteristics**
B0	Absence of significant blood involvement: ≤5% of peripheral blood lymphocytes are atypical (Sézary) cells
B0a	Clone negative
B0b	Clone positive
B1	Low blood-tumor burden: >5% of peripheral blood lymphocytes are atypical (Sézary) cells but does not meet criteria of B2
B1a	Clone negative
B1b	Clone positive
B2	High blood-tumor burden: ≥1,000/µL Sézary cells with positive clone

Source: From Olsen E, Vonderheid E, Pimpinelli N, et al. Revisions to the staging and classification of mycosis fungoides and Sézary syndrome: a proposal of the International Society for Cutaneous Lymphomas (ISCL) and the Cutaneous Lymphoma Task Force of the European Organization of Research and Treatment of Cancer (EORTC). *Blood.* 2007;110(6):1713–1722. doi:10.1182/blood-2007-03-055749.

T/B/M \ N	N0	N1	N2	N3
T1	IA	IIA		IVA2
T2	IB			
T3	IIB			
T4	IIIA (if B0) or IIIB (if B1)			
B2	IVA1			
M1	IVB			

Table 23.3 TNMB Clinical Staging System

TREATMENT PARADIGM

Observation: Expectant observation is recommended for informed patients with stage IA disease but requires attentive monitoring and proper patient education.[1]

Medical: Various skin-directed therapies should be considered as first-line treatment in early disease and supplemental treatment in more advanced disease. Preferred initial skin-directed therapies are topical corticosteroids, topical nitrogen mustard (e.g., carmustine), and topical retinoids.[1] Pruritus is common and should be treated according to general guidelines for managing pruritus.

Surgery: There is no clear role for surgical resection in MF.

Chemotherapy: Although skin-directed therapies should be attempted initially in patients with early disease, CHT should be considered early in patients with extensive, advanced, or refractory disease. Common CHT regimens include low-dose methotrexate, pegylated liposomal doxorubicin, gemcitabine, pralatrexate, fludarabine with cyclophosphamides, fludarabine with interferon alpha, CHOP (cyclophosphamide, doxorubicin, vincristine, and prednisone), and EPOCH (etoposide, prednisone, vincristine, cyclophosphaimde, doxorubicin).[12] Other systemic therapies include retinoids, histone deacetylase inhibitors, brentuximab vedotin, mogamulizumab (anti-CCR4), pembrolizumab, and bortezimib.[1,13,14]

Radiation: Localized RT is indicated for patients with stage IA disease presenting with one to three lesions that are in close enough proximity to be targeted by single or abutting RT fields.[15] It is also indicated as palliative treatment for patients with advanced disease. Photons as well as electron beam may be used. Local superficial RT for curative treatment of unilesional stage IA disease should be dosed at least 20 to 30 Gy at 2 Gy per fx with 5 fx per week, and palliative treatment for advanced disease can be dosed at 8 to 20 Gy given in 1 to 5 fxs.[16,17] Adverse effects include mild dermatitis, local alopecia, and pigmentation changes.[15]

TSEBT: In TSEBT, electrons are calibrated to penetrate the skin to limited depth, targeting the epidermis, adnexal structures, and dermis. It can be considered in all stages of disease. Historically, treatment dosed to 26 to 36 Gy to 4- to 6-mm depth (surface dose 31–36 Gy), given in 30 to 36 treatments (2 days per fx) over 9 weeks, 4 days per week. Recent evidence suggests shorter course of 12 Gy may be effective, with shorter duration of control. During treatment, some symptoms such as pruritus and cutaneous erythema may be exacerbated. In addition, alopecia, temporary nail stasis, peripheral edema, epistaxis, blisters of fingers and feet, anhidrosis, parotitis, gynecomastia, corneal tears, chronic nail dystrophy, chronic xerosis, and fingertip dysesthesias may occur.[18] For technical details regarding both local superficial RT and TSEBT, see the *Handbook of Treatment Planning in Radiation Oncology*, Chapter 10.[19]

Other Modalities: Phototherapy may be used in the treatment of MF, including UVB and PUVA. More recently, treatments also include UVA1 and excimer laser.[20] In cases refractory to other modalities, allogenic hematopoietic stem cell transplant may be considered.[21]

EVIDENCE-BASED Q&A

Do patients benefit from early aggressive therapy?

While CR is higher in those undergoing aggressive therapy with TSEBT and CHT, there is no benefit in DFS or OS, with a significantly increased toxicity rate.

Kaye (*NEJM* 1989, PMID 2594037): RCT of 103 patients w/ MF randomized to 30 Gy TSEBT w/ CHT (cyclophosphamide, doxorubicin, etoposide, and vincristine) vs. sequential topical treatment. Higher rate of CR in patients treated with combination therapy (38% vs. 18%, $p = .03$) but no difference in DFS or OS after 75 months of MFU. Increased toxicity in combination therapy group including hospitalization for fever/neutropenia and CHF. **Conclusion: Early aggressive therapy with RT and CHT does not improve prognosis for patients with MF as compared with conservative treatment beginning with sequential topical therapies.**

What dose should be used for localized disease?

When using standard fractionation, doses of 20 to 30 Gy are necessary for durable response. However, doses as low as 7 Gy single fraction have been shown to be effective for local palliation.

Cotter (*IJROBP* 1983, PMID 6195138): RR of 110 lesions from 14 patients with MF who underwent RT with Co-60 or electrons. Doses ranged from 6 to 40 Gy; 53% of lesions were plaques, 20% were tumors ≤3 cm in diameter, and 27% were tumors >3 cm in diameter. CR in 95% of plaques, 95% of tumors ≤3 cm, and 93% in tumors >3 cm in diameter. CR in all tumors receiving >20 Gy. In lesions having CR, 42% had in-field recurrence if they received <10 Gy, 32% for 10 to 20 Gy, 21% for 20 to 30 Gy, and 0% for >30 Gy, with mean time to first recurrence of 5 months, 10 months, and 16 months, respectively, for each dose range. Of 30 recurrences, 83% were within 1 year, while 100% were within 2 years of treatment. **Conclusion: Tumor doses equivalent to at least 30 Gy at 2 Gy per fraction, 5 fractions per week, are suggested for adequate LC of cutaneous MF lesions.**

Wilson, Yale (*IJROBP* 1998, PMID 9422565): RR of 21 patients with 32 lesions receiving curative local superficial RT (LSRT) for stage IA MF; nine patients received prior focal therapy (steroids, PUVA, BCNU, UVB) and six received adjuvant therapy after local RT (PUVA, steroids). MFU was 36 months. Median surface dose was 20 Gy (6–40 Gy) with a median of 5 fx. For fields receiving >20 Gy, median fraction number was 10. CR was 97% overall, with one patient having PR, treated with 6 Gy. Three patients had LR. The 10-year DFS was 91% for those receiving ≥20 Gy, with 91% LC. **Conclusion: Patients should be offered choice of LSRT alone, without adjuvant therapies, to a dose of 20 Gy or greater with a minimum margin of 1 to 2 cm around target.**

Thomas, Northwestern University (*IJROBP* 2013, PMID 22818412): RR of 270 patients treated with single-fraction RT dose of ≥7 Gy or more. MFU 41.3 months. CR in 94% of patients, PR in 4%, conversion to CR after second treatment in 2%, and no response in 0.4%. **Conclusion: Single fraction of 7 to 8 Gy is sufficient to provide palliation for cutaneous T-cell lymphoma lesions.**

Can de-escalated RT provide adequate palliation?

When giving local palliative RT for MF lesions, dose de-escalation to 4 Gy/2 fx results in inferior response rates.

Neelis, Dutch (*IJROBP* 2009, PMID 18834672): RR of 31 patients with 82 symptomatic sites of MF treated with palliative local RT, initially with 4 Gy/2 fx ($n = 17$) and later with 8 Gy/2 fx ($n = 65$). CR rates were lower with 4 Gy/2 fx compared with the 8 Gy/2 fx cohort (30% vs. 92%). Those in the lower dose group who failed treatment were salvaged with 20 Gy/8 fx re-RT. **Conclusion: Palliative RT with 4 Gy/2 fx is inadequate for treating MF, but low-dose local RT with 8 Gy/2 fx can induce a high response rate.**

What dose should be used for TSEBT?

TSEBT is conventionally dosed to at least 30 Gy, yielding greater CR rates and lower rates of disease recurrence. However, phase II studies suggest 12 Gy can provide rapid reduction of disease burden for a sustained period of time and reduce toxicity.

Hoppe, Stanford (*IJROBP* 1977, PMID 591404): A total of 176 patients with MF treated with TSEBT from 1958 to 1975 with varying doses. CR rates increased with decreased skin involvement, ranging from 86% in limited plaques to 44% in tumors. Survival was also related to the extent of disease with 10-year OS of 76%, 44%, and 6% in those with limited plaques, generalized plaques, and tumors, respectively. Stage was also correlated with survival, exemplified by 5-year OS of 80% and 51% for stage I and stage II patients, respectively, along with lack of stage III/IV long-term survivors. CR was directly related to initial dose of TSEBT, with 18% CR for 8 to 9.9 Gy, 55% for 10 to 19.9 Gy, 66% for 20 to 24.9 Gy, 75% for 25 to 29.9 Gy, and 94% for 30 to 36 Gy. Thirty-nine percent (20 patients) of those who had CR after TSEBT >30 Gy remained without disease 3 to 14 years after completion. **Conclusion: Patients receiving TSEBT dose of at least 30 Gy experienced the greatest rates of CR and had lower rates of disease recurrence.**

Hoppe, Stanford (*J Am Acad Dermatol* 2015, PMID 25476993): Pooled data from three clinical trials using low-dose (12 Gy) TSEBT. All trials involved TSEBT-naive patients with stage IB to IIIA MF. Treatment was 12 Gy, 1 Gy per fraction over 3 weeks. Primary endpoint was clinical response rate; 33 patients enrolled; 18 males. Stages were 22 IB, 2 IIA, 7 IIB, and 2 IIIA. Overall response rate was 88% (29/33), including nine patients with CR. Median time to response was 7.6 weeks (3–12.4 weeks). Median duration of clinical benefit was 70.7 weeks (95% CI 41.8–133.8). **Conclusion: Low-dose TSEBT provides reliable and rapid reduction of MF, can be administered safely multiple times during the course of a patient's disease, and has acceptable toxicity profile.**

Morris (*IJROBP* 2017, PMID 28843374): Prospective cohort study of 103 patients with MF treated with low-dose TSEBT (12 Gy/8 fx). Stages were 54 IB, 33 IIB, 12 III, and 4 IV. CR in 18% and PR in 69%. Eighty percent of patients had stable disease and 5% progressed on treatment. In patients with CR, median time to relapse was 7.3 months and median response duration was 11.8 months. Median PFS for the whole cohort was 13.2 months. **Conclusion: Low-dose TSEBT of 12 Gy in 8 fractions is effective and well-tolerated.**

REFERENCES

1. Trautinger F, Eder J, Assaf C, et al. European organisation for research and treatment of cancer consensus recommendations for the treatment of mycosis fungoides/Sézary syndrome–Update 2017. *Eur J Cancer.* 2017;77:57–74. doi:10.1016/j.ejca.2017.02.027
2. Criscione VD, Weinstock MA. Incidence of cutaneous T-cell lymphoma in the United States, 1973–2002. *Arch Dermatol.* 2007;143(7):854–859. doi:10.1001/archderm.143.7.854
3. Willemze R, Cerroni L, Kempf W, et al. The 2018 update of the WHO-EORTC classification for primary cutaneous lymphomas. *Blood.* 2019;133(16):1703–1714. doi:10.1182/blood-2018-11-881268
4. Wood GS, Salvekar A, Schaffer J, et al. Evidence against a role for human T-cell Lymphotrophic Virus type I (HTLV-I) in the pathogenesis of American cutaneous T-cell lymphoma. *J Invest Dermatol.* 1996;107(3): 301–307. doi:10.1111/1523-1747.ep12363010
5. Pimpinelli N, Olsen EA, Santucci M, et al. Defining early mycosis fungoides. *J Am Acad Dermatol.* 2005;53(6):1053–1063. doi:10.1016/j.jaad.2005.08.057
6. Kim YH, Liu HL, Mraz-Gernhard S, Varghese A, Hoppe RT. Long-term outcome of 525 patients with mycosis fungoides and Sézary syndrome: clinical prognostic factors and risk for disease progression. *Arch Dermatol.* 2003;139(7):857–866. doi:10.1001/archderm.139.7.857
7. Smoller BR, Bishop K, Glusac E, Kim YH, Hendrickson M. Reassessment of histologic parameters in the diagnosis of mycosis fungoides. *Am J Surg Pathol.* 1995;19(12):1423–1430. doi:10.1097/00000478-199512000-00009
8. Olsen E, Vonderheid E, Pimpinelli N, et al. Revisions to the staging and classification of mycosis fungoides and Sézary syndrome: a proposal of the International Society for Cutaneous Lymphomas (ISCL) and the cutaneous lymphoma task force of the European Organization of Research and Treatment of Cancer (EORTC). *Blood.* 2007;110(6):1713–1722. doi:10.1182/blood-2007-03-055749
9. Olsen EA, Whittaker S, Kim YH, et al. Clinical end points and response criteria in mycosis fungoides and Sézary syndrome: a consensus statement of the international society for cutaneous lymphomas, the United States cutaneous lymphoma consortium, and the cutaneous lymphoma task force of the European organisation for research and treatment of cancer. *J Clin Oncol.* 2011;29(18):2598–2607. doi:10.1200/JCO .2010.32.0630
10. Tsai EY, Taur A, Espinosa L, et al. Staging accuracy in mycosis fungoides and Sézary syndrome using integrated positron emission tomography and computed tomography. *Arch Dermatol.* 2006;142(5):577–584. doi:10.1001/archderm.142.5.577

11. Scarisbrick JJ, Prince HM, Vermeer MH, et al. Cutaneous lymphoma international consortium study of outcome in advanced stages of mycosis fungoides and Sézary syndrome: effect of specific prognostic markers on survival and development of a prognostic model. *J Clin Oncol.* 2015;33(32):3766–3773. doi:10.1200/JCO.2015.61.7142

12. Hughes CF, Khot A, McCormack C, et al. Lack of durable disease control with chemotherapy for mycosis fungoides and Sézary syndrome: a comparative study of systemic therapy. *Blood.* 2015;125(1):71–81. doi:10.1182/blood-2014-07-588236

13. Larocca C, Kupper T. Mycosis fungoides and Sézary syndrome: an update. *Hematol Oncol Clin North Am.* 2019;33(1):103–120. doi:10.1016/j.hoc.2018.09.001

14. Kim YH, Bagot M, Pinter-Brown L, et al. Mogamulizumab versus vorinostat in previously treated cutaneous T-cell lymphoma (MAVORIC): an international, open-label, randomised, controlled phase 3 trial. *Lancet Oncol.* 2018;19(9):1192–1204. doi:10.1016/S1470-2045(18)30379-6

15. Wilson LD, Kacinski BM, Jones GW. Local superficial radiotherapy in the management of minimal stage IA cutaneous T-cell lymphoma (Mycosis Fungoides). *Int J Radiat Oncol Biol Phys.* 1998;40(1):109–115. doi:10.1016/s0360-3016(97)00553-1

16. Cotter GW, Baglan RJ, Wasserman TH, Mill W. Palliative radiation treatment of cutaneous mycosis fungoides–a dose response. *Int J Radiat Oncol Biol Phys.* 1983;9(10):1477–1480. doi:10.1016/0360-3016(83)90321-8

17. Neelis KJ, Schimmel EC, Vermeer MH, Senff NJ, Willemze R, Noordijk EM. Low-dose palliative radiotherapy for cutaneous B- and T-cell lymphomas. *Int J Radiat Oncol Biol Phys.* 2009;74(1):154–158. doi:10.1016/j.ijrobp.2008.06.1918

18. Jones GW, Kacinski BM, Wilson LD, et al. Total skin electron radiation in the management of mycosis fungoides: consensus of the European Organization for Research and Treatment of Cancer (EORTC) cutaneous lymphoma project group. *J Am Acad Dermatol.* 2002;47(3):364–370. doi:10.1067/mjd.2002.123482

19. Videtic GMM, Woody N, Vassil AD. *Handbook of Treatment Planning in Radiation Oncology.* 3rd ed. Demos Medical; 2020.

20. Olsen EA, Hodak E, Anderson T, et al. Guidelines for phototherapy of mycosis fungoides and Sézary syndrome: a consensus statement of the United States cutaneous lymphoma consortium. *J Am Acad Dermatol.* 2016;74(1):27–58. doi:10.1016/j.jaad.2015.09.033

21. Duarte RF, Boumendil A, Onida F, et al. Long-term outcome of allogeneic hematopoietic cell transplantation for patients with mycosis fungoides and Sézary syndrome: a European society for blood and marrow transplantation lymphoma working party extended analysis. *J Clin Oncol.* 2014;32(29):3347–3348. doi:10.1200/JCO.2014.57.5597

PART IV: Breast

Katherine R. Amarell, Kailin Yang, Rahul D. Tendulkar, and Chirag Shah

QUICK HIT For early-stage breast cancer, treatment typically involves surgical resection followed by adjuvant therapy (CHT, RT, and/or endocrine therapy) depending on pathologic features and tumor biology/assays. Breast conserving surgery (BCS) + adjuvant RT is an equivalent alternative (LC and OS) to mastectomy for most patients with unifocal cancers who desire organ preservation. Whole breast irradiation (WBI) after BCS improves LR rates (from 26% to 7% at 5 years) and OS by 5% at 15 years.[1] Conventional WBI dose is 45 to 50 Gy, followed by a tumor bed boost of 10 to 16 Gy in some patients. Hypofractionated WBI regimens (40–42.5 Gy/15–16 fx or 26–28.5 Gy/5 fx) have replaced conventional WBI for most patients. In patients with limited axillary nodal involvement on SLNB, a completion ALND is not necessary, provided the patient undergoes WBI ± RNI. Lower risk patients (e.g., older age, T1N0, ER+, negative margins) may be eligible for partial breast irradiation (PBI) or endocrine therapy alone after lumpectomy.

EPIDEMIOLOGY: Worldwide, breast cancer is the most frequently diagnosed and leading cause of cancer death in women. In the United States, >300,000 new diagnoses in 2024 and >40,000 deaths were reported.[2] Lifetime risk is one in eight women (~1 in 50 by age 50). Median age at diagnosis is 61. About two-thirds of new diagnoses have no significant risk factors. Males account for 1% (associated with Klinefelter syndrome and BRCA2; 90% are ER+).

RISK FACTORS

Estrogen Exposure: Female gender, older age, early menarche, nulliparity, older age at first birth (>30 years), lack of breastfeeding, late menopause (>55 years), hormone replacement therapy.

Family History: Risk increases with the number of first-degree relatives.

Genetics (5%–10% Hereditary): BRCA1: AD (17q21), 60% to 80% lifetime risk of breast cancer, 30% to 50% lifetime risk of ovarian cancer, higher risk of triple-negative (ER–/PR–/HER2–); BRCA2: AD (13q12), 50% to 60% lifetime risk of breast cancer, 10% to 20% lifetime risk of ovarian cancer, male breast cancer, prostate, bladder, endometrial, and pancreatic cancers; Li–Fraumeni: AD (17p), p53, associated with sarcoma, leukemia, brain tumors, adrenocortical carcinoma; Cowden syndrome: AD (10q23), PTEN, associated with hamartomas of the skin and oral cavity; ataxia–telangiectasia: AR (11q22), ATM; Peutz–Jeghers.

Personal History of Breast Disease: Prior breast cancer, DCIS, LCIS, atypical ductal hyperplasia, dense breast tissue, history of RT during youth (age <30 years).

Lifestyle/Exposure: High-fat diet, postmenopausal obesity, sedentary lifestyle.

ANATOMY: The breast overlies the pectoralis major muscle, extends from approximately the second to the sixth rib and from the lateral sternum to the anterior axillary fold. The axillary tail of Spence extends laterally into the low axilla. Glandular tissue is arranged in 15 to 20 lobes with a system of lactiferous ducts that open at the nipple. UOQ contains the greatest volume of glandular tissue (most common location of breast cancers). The least common location is the LIQ. Breast is supported by Cooper's ligaments, which are fibrous septae joining the superficial fascia (skin) and deep fascia covering the pectoralis major muscle. Lymphatic drainage is primarily to the axilla. ALN levels I, II, and III are, respectively, located inferolateral, deep, and superomedial to the pectoralis minor, which inserts on the coracoid process of the scapula. Rotter's nodes are located between the pectoralis major and minor (anterior to level II). Internal mammary nodes (IMNs) are situated along the internal mammary (IM) vessels adjacent to the sternum in the first three intercostal spaces, about 2 to 3 cm lateral to midline and 2 to 3 cm deep. Approximately 30% of medial tumors and 15% of lateral tumors drain to the IMNs.

PATHOLOGY: Breast carcinomas arise from epithelial elements and comprise a diverse group of lesions with differing biological behavior, although they are often discussed as a single disease with similar management guidelines. ER and/or PR are expressed in 70% of tumors (more common in postmenopausal patients). HER2/neu (c-ERbB-2 or human epidermal growth factor receptor 2) is a receptor tyrosine kinase, with HER2 amplification seen in 25% to 30% of invasive cancers. Triple-negative breast cancer (TNBC) is an aggressive entity in which tumors do not express ER, PR, or HER2, accounting for ~15% of cases, and is more commonly found in BRCA mutation carriers.

Invasive Ductal Carcinoma (IDC): 80% of cases, firm mass with desmoplastic reaction, solid cords of cells.

Invasive Lobular Carcinoma (ILC): 5% to 10% of cases, rubbery texture, less visible on mammogram (better imaged with MRI), "Indian filing" histology, often bilateral/multicentric, >80% ER+, spreads to unusual locations such as meninges, serosal surfaces, BM, ovary, and retroperitoneum.

Rarer Subtypes (Need >90% Predominant Pattern): *Tubular*: small, well-differentiated variant of IDC, >75% tubules, usually ER+/PR+. *Medullary*: associated with BRCA1, presents at younger age (<50 years), LNs are large/hyperplastic, most are triple-negative. *Mucinous/colloid*: older patients, favorable. *Papillary*: older patients, often multifocal/diffuse, often LN+ even when small size. *Cribriform*: ER+/PR+. Other uncommon variants include metaplastic (poor prognosis), squamous cell, invasive micropapillary, adenoid cystic, mucoepidermoid, secretory, apocrine, spindle cell, lymphoma, neuroendocrine small cell, and clear cell. Mammary carcinoma is a mixture of invasive ductal and lobular carcinoma.

Extensive Intraductal Component (EIC): Defined as ≥25% DCIS within the invasive carcinoma specimen and extending beyond edges of tumor. Originally identified as a risk factor for LR after breast-conserving therapy (BCT), but no longer considered the case provided margins are negative.[3]

Paget Disease: Chronic eczematous changes of the nipple–areolar complex, with an underlying intraepidermal adenocarcinoma (ACA) of the nipple (in 95%). About 50% have a palpable mass (>90% are invasive cancer) and 50% have no mass (typically DCIS). Low risk of axillary nodal mets.

Cystosarcoma Phyllodes: Fibroepithelial, "leaf-like," large, encapsulated tumors, most frequently benign but can also be qualified as borderline or malignant. Can grow slowly and then have sudden rapid increase in size. Uncommonly malignant and nodal mets and distant metastases are rare.

GENETICS: A number of gene expression profiling models exist, including the Amsterdam 70-gene good-versus-poor outcome model (low signature vs. high signature),[4] the 21-gene recurrence score model,[5] and the intrinsic subtype model.[6] The 21-gene recurrence score (Oncotype DX) was developed for patients with LN-negative, ER+ breast cancers receiving tamoxifen ± CHT on NSABP B-14, and is stratified into low risk (<18 score), intermediate risk (18–30), and high risk (>30) of recurrence in order to estimate the relative benefit of CHT in addition to hormonal therapy.[5] Rates of distant recurrence in the low-risk, intermediate-risk, and high-risk groups were 7%, 14%, and 31% at 10 years. The TAILORx study showed noninferiority of endocrine therapy alone over endocrine + CHT in women with intermediate risk (revised score of 11–25).[7] There are four main intrinsic subtypes: luminal A (best prognosis), luminal B, HER2-enriched (HER2+), and basal-like (worst prognosis).[6] *Luminal A-like*: ER+/HER2– with either low Ki-67 (<14%) or combination of PR+ (≥20%) and intermediate Ki-67 (14%–19%); *luminal B-like*: ER+/HER2– with either high Ki-67 (≥20%) or combination of intermediate Ki-67 (14%–19%) with PR– or low (<20%), or ER+/PR+ with HER2+; *basal-like*: usually triple-negative (~70%–80% correlation), high prevalence in young Black women and BRCA mutation carriers; *HER2-enriched*: usually ER–/PR–, HER2+, high Ki-67.[8] The luminal subtypes, while usually HER2–, can be HER2+. Higher response rates to neoadjuvant CHT (pCR rates of ~60%) are seen with basal-like and HER2-enriched cancers.[9]

SCREENING: Yearly mammography is associated with ~40% relative reduction of dying from breast cancer within 10 years and 25% reduction in the rate of advanced breast cancer.[10] Forty percent of breast lesions are detected by mammogram only, but 10% have palpable tumors that are not visualized.

■ *ACR Appropriateness Guidelines*[11]: Begin annual screening at 40 years; screen at 25 to 30 years for BRCA mutation carriers and untested first-degree relatives of carriers; screen at 25 to 30 years or 10 years earlier than first-degree relatives (whichever is later) with lifetime risk for breast cancer

≥20%. Screen 8 years after or at 25 years (whichever is later) for women who received mantle RT/thoracic RT between 10 and 30 years old. Screen annually for women with biopsy-proven lobular neoplasia, atypical ductal hyperplasia, or personal history of breast cancer beginning at age of diagnosis, but not when <30 years. Supplemental screening may be necessary in women with genetic predisposition to disease and/or dense breasts. Clinical breast examination is not recommended in average-risk women.

- *USPSTF*[12]: Recommends biennial screening for ages 40 to 74. High-risk women should begin screening 10 years before the age of the youngest first-degree relative diagnosed. Insufficient evidence for benefit/harm of clinical exam; however, recommend against teaching breast self-examination.
- *ACS Guidelines:* Recommend screening MRI for women with 20% to 25% or greater lifetime risk of breast cancer, including women with hereditary mutations (BRCA, Li–Fraumeni, Cowden), strong family history of breast/ovarian cancer, and women who received prior thoracic RT for Hodgkin disease before 30 years of age.[13,14]

CLINICAL PRESENTATION: Typically detected by screening mammogram (~90%), self-breast exam, and/or clinical exam (~10%).[15] The most common presentation is a painless mass, but can occasionally present with pain (~5%), nipple discharge (although usually benign), nipple retraction, or axillary lymphadenopathy with occult primary. A mass is less concerning for malignancy if associated with changes in menstrual cycle. The most common location is UOQ (40%), followed by the central area (30%), UIQ (15%), LOQ (10%), and LIQ (5%). Bilateral disease in 1% to 3% of cases. Risk of developing contralateral cancer after primary diagnosis is 0.75% per year. *Multifocal* defined as ≥2 cancer foci in the same quadrant (typically eligible for breast conservation). *Multicentric:* ≥2 foci in different quadrants or >5 cm apart (historically not considered for breast conservation). *Differential Diagnosis*: Fibroadenoma (solitary mass, well-defined, mobile), cysts (more diffuse and less firm, suspicious if blood in aspirate or contents reaccumulate quickly), infection (mastitis or abscess), Mondor's cord (thrombophlebitis of superficial breast veins), fat necrosis, intraductal papilloma (common cause of bloody discharge), sclerosing adenosis (nodular benign condition consisting of hyperplastic lobules of acinar tissue), lactocele.

WORKUP

H&P: Full H&P with attention to breast and LN exam (axilla and SCV).

Imaging: Mammogram (Table 24.1) and ultrasound are typical first steps.[16] Systemic staging workup is not routinely indicated per NCCN for anatomic stages I to II in the absence of suspicious symptoms, physical exam findings, or lab abnormalities (e.g., elevated ALP or LFTs). If suspicious, studies may include PET/CT or CT chest/abdomen/pelvis and bone scan, ± MRI brain.

Table 24.1 Breast Imaging and Reporting Data System Classification[16]			
BI-RADS	**Description**	**Malignancy**	**Follow-Up**
0	Incomplete	1%	Completion of imaging or review of previous imaging not previously available
1	Negative	<1%	Routine annual screening
2	Benign lesion	<1%	Routine annual screening
3	Probably benign	<2%	Short interval follow-up (6 months)
4a	Low suspicion for malignancy	2%–10%	Biopsy
4b	Moderate suspicion for malignancy	10%–50%	Biopsy
4c	High suspicion for malignancy	50%–95%	Biopsy
5	Highly suggestive of malignancy	>95%	Biopsy
6	Biopsy-proven malignancy	100%	Appropriate treatment per stage

Source: Vanel D. The American College of Radiology (ACR) Breast Imaging and Reporting Data System (BI-RADS): a step towards a universal radiological language? *Eur J Radiol.* 2007;61(2):183. doi:10.1016/j.ejrad.2006.08.030.

- *Mammography*: On craniocaudal (CC) view, the lateral edge of the film is typically marked "CC." On mediolateral oblique (MLO) view, assess for image quality by ensuring inclusion of the pectoralis muscle. Concerning mammographic findings: calcifications 100 to 300 microns, >10 clustered linear calcifications, and spiculated lesions. Spot compression views are useful for suspicious masses (vs. disappearance of dense breast tissue on compression), and magnification views are used for evaluation of calcifications.

- *Ultrasound (US):* Helps distinguish solid from cystic masses (but not useful for calcifications) and evaluates nonpalpable masses identified on mammogram. Can also be used to evaluate the axilla.
- *MRI:* Higher sensitivity (>90%) than mammography, but lower specificity (39%–95%) due to false-positives. Suspicious features for malignancy: strong, rapid contrast enhancement, spiculated margins, rim enhancement, heterogeneous appearance. Potential indications for MRI include an obscured breast (silicone implants), suspicious masses with negative mammogram and ultrasound, evaluation of poorly imaged tumors such as ILC or DCIS without microcalcifications, or patients presenting with positive axillary nodes of unknown primary (MRI detects primary tumor 80%–90% of the time). MRI can change surgical management in 25% of cases but does not reduce positive margins, re-excision rates, or LR rates.[17–19]

Procedures: Core biopsy, needle aspirate (if cystic on ultrasound). FNA may detect abnormal cells, but it cannot distinguish DCIS from IDC and cannot identify ER/PR/HER2 status; thus, core biopsy is preferred. US core biopsy for palpable masses. Stereotactic core biopsy or needle localization if nonpalpable/visualizable of suspicious calcifications. MRI-guided biopsy if only visible on MRI. Punch biopsy for Paget or if suspicious of dermal involvement (e.g., suspected inflammatory breast cancer).

PROGNOSTIC FACTORS: Poor prognostic factors include LN+ (strongest factor), young age, ER/PR negativity, HER2/neu amplification (in the absence of HER2-directed therapy), high grade, LVSI+, and basal-like subtype.[20]

STAGING: See Table 24.2.

Table 24.2 AJCC 8th Edition (2017): Staging for Breast Cancer				
cT/pT		**cN**		**pN**
Tis	• Carcinoma in situ	**N0**	• No LNs by imaging or clinical exam	**N0** (i–) negative ITC
				(i+) positive ITC (≤0.2 mm)
				(mol–) negative RT-PCR
				(mol+) positive RT-PCR
T1mic	• ≤0.1 cm	**N1**	• Mobile ipsilateral level I/II axillary LNs	**N1** (mi) >0.2 mm and/or >200 cells, but ≤2 mm
				a. 1–3 axillary LNs
				b. IM LN+ pathologically, but not clinically
				c. pN1a + pN1b
T1	a. >0.1 cm and ≤0.5 cm	**N2a**	• Fixed/matted ipsilateral level I/II axillary LNs	**N2** a. 4–9 axillary LNs
	b. >0.5 cm and ≤1 cm			
	c. >1 cm and ≤2 cm			b. IM LNs+ clinically with negative axillary LNs
T2	• >2 cm and ≤5 cm	**N2b**	• Clinically detected ipsilateral IM LNs, without axillary LNs	**N3** a. ≥10 axillary LNs or positive infraclavicular LNs
				b. Clinically positive IM LNs with positive axillary LNs; or pathologically, but not clinically positive IM LNs with >3 axillary LNs
				c. Ipsilateral SCV LNs
T3	• >5 cm	**N3a**	• Ipsilateral infraclavicular LNs	**Group Staging**

(continued)

Table 24.2 AJCC 8th Edition (2017): Staging for Breast Cancer (*continued*)				
cT/pT		**cN**		**Stage**	

cT/pT		**cN**		**Stage**	
T4	a. Extension to chest wall (except pectoralis major)	**N3b**	• Ipsilateral IM and axillary LNs	**0**	Tis
				IA	T1N0M0
	b. Peau d'orange, ulcer, or satellite skin nodules			**IB**	T0–1N1miM0
				IIA	T0–1N1M0, T2N0M0
	c. Both T4a and T4b			**IIB**	T2N1M0, T3N0M0
	d. Inflammatory carcinoma			**IIIA**	T0–3N2M0, T3N1M0
M0(i+)	• Circulating tumor cells in bone marrow	**N3c**	• Ipsilateral supraclavicular LNs	**IIIB**	T4N0–2M0
				IIIC	Any T, N3M0
M1	• Distant metastasis			**IV**	M0(i+), M1

Note: In addition to the preceding anatomic staging, prognostic group staging was developed in the AJCC 8th edition, which includes grade and ER/PR/HER2 status and is preferred over the historical anatomic group staging.

TREATMENT PARADIGM: Local therapy options include modified radical mastectomy (MRM) or BCT composed of lumpectomy ± RT (see Table 24.3 for surgical options). There are no significant differences in LR (with negative margins), distant DFS, or OS between MRM and BCT at extended follow-up in at least six prospective randomized trials. CHT, if needed, is delivered either neoadjuvantly or postoperatively, but generally before RT.[21,22] Hormonal therapy is indicated for hormone receptor-positive cancers and usually follows all other therapies. Breast cancer is both a local and a distant disease and optimizing both LC and systemic therapy can provide the best outcomes.

Prevention: Tamoxifen as chemoprevention reduces the risk of noninvasive and invasive cancers in high-risk women by up to 50% (NSABP P-1).[23] Raloxifene is as effective as tamoxifen, but with lower rates of thromboembolic events (NSABP P-2 "STAR").[24] Prophylactic mastectomy reduces breast cancer risk by >90% in those with a strong family history and may improve survival in BRCA carriers.[25] Prophylactic oophorectomy decreases risk in BRCA carriers by 50% if before 40 years of age.[26] No conclusive evidence of a benefit from special dietary changes; however, alcohol/obesity is associated with increased risk of developing breast cancer.

Surgery: See Table 24.3.

Table 24.3 Surgical Options for Breast Cancer	
Radical mastectomy (RM)	Popularized by Halsted starting in 1894. Involves en bloc removal of the breast, overlying skin, pectoralis major, pectoralis minor, and level I, II, and III LNs; there are currently no absolute indications for this procedure.
Modified radical mastectomy (MRM)	Complete removal of breast tissue, pectoralis fascia, and level I and II LNs (preserves pectoralis major, lateral pectoral nerve, and level III nodes).
Total mastectomy (TM)	Removal of breast tissue only (preservation of both pectoralis muscles and axillary LNs).
Skin-sparing mastectomy	Resection of biopsy scar, breast parenchyma, and/or skin immediately overlying the tumor. Preservation of majority of breast skin for reconstruction.
Nipple-sparing mastectomy	Skin-sparing mastectomy with preservation of the nipple–areolar complex.
Lumpectomy or partial mastectomy	Removal of only part of the breast containing the cancer (i.e., BCS). Margins are considered negative if there is "no tumor on ink."[27]
Axillary lymph node dissection	Typical level I and II ALND yields ~15 LNs. A complete ALND with removal of level III nodes is generally unnecessary unless grossly positive. Incidence of skip metastases to level III LNs without involved level I LNs is <3%.
Sentinel lymph node biopsy	Tc-99m sulfur colloid and/or isosulfan blue dye are injected into the breast (peritumoral, subareolar, or subdermal) for 3–7 minutes, and gamma camera identifies SLNs. False-negative rate is 8%–10% after negative SLNB (less when dual tracers are used).[28,29] Less lymphedema, less pain, and better arm mobility compared with ALND.

Chemotherapy: Considered pre- or postop for LN+ patients (based on tumor biology, or gene assays for N1 disease in the adjuvant setting), ER−, HER2+, and for women with multiple adverse features (e.g., young age or high Oncotype DX scores). Neoadjuvant CHT has equivalent survival as adjuvant (NSABP B-18) but may allow for less extensive surgery while also allowing for adjustment of adjuvant therapies based on response (e.g., capecitabine, TDM-1). For patients with ER+ and N0–N1, gene expression assays such as Oncotype DX and MammaPrint can be considered to assist with decision-making regarding the addition of adjuvant CHT to endocrine therapy.[7,30] Note: The role of CHT is unclear in women >70 years because this age group was excluded from early clinical trials. Trastuzumab has OS advantage for HER2+ patients in addition to cytotoxic CHT.[31] Trastuzumab is not given concurrently with Adriamycin because of cardiotoxicity concerns but is safe to give with RT. Trastuzumab-related cardiac effects are reversible, so obtain cardiac echo q3 months to monitor. Pertuzumab has been added to trastuzumab to provide dual anti-HER2 therapy, which results in pCR rates of 50% to 60% in the neoadjuvant setting. Common CHT regimens include the following:

- AC: Adriamycin 60 mg/m^2 + cyclophosphamide (CYC) 600 mg/m^2 q3 weeks × 4 cycles.
- AC → T: Adriamycin 60 mg/m^2 + CYC 600 mg/m^2 q3 weeks × 4 cycles followed by paclitaxel 175 mg/m^2 q3 weeks × 4 cycles or 80 mg/m^2 q1 week × 12 weeks (dose-dense regimen is q2 weeks with filgrastim or pegfilgrastim for support).
- AC → TH: Same as AC → T, with the addition of trastuzumab 4 mg/kg loading dose followed by 2 mg/kg per week concurrently with paclitaxel, then trastuzumab monotherapy (6 mg/kg q3 weeks) for 1 year.
- TC: Docetaxel 75 mg/m^2 and CYC 600 mg/m^2.
- TCHP: Nonanthracycline regimen consisting of docetaxel 75 mg/m^2 + carboplatin (AUC 6 mg/mL/min) q3 weeks × 6 cycles + trastuzumab (8 mg/kg loading dose followed by 6 mg/kg q3 weeks for 1 year) + pertuzumab (840 mg loading dose followed by 420 mg q3 weeks).
- Pembrolizumab per KEYNOTE 522: First neoadjuvant treatment: pembro (200 mg) q3 weeks × 4C + paclitaxel (80 mg/m^2) weekly + carboplatin (AUC 5 mg/mL/min) q3 weeks or carboplatin (AUC 1.5 mg/mL/min) weekly for 12 weeks, followed by second neoadjuvant treatment 4C pembrolizumab + doxorubicin (60 mg/m^2) or epirubicin (90 mg/m^2) + cyclophosphamide (600 mg/m^2) q3 weeks for 12 weeks, followed by adjuvant pembro q3 weeks up to 9C.[32]

The addition of a taxane has OS benefit for LN+ patients compared with AC alone.[33,34] Dose-dense regimens (q2 weeks instead of q3 weeks) offer OS advantage for high-risk patients as well.[35] TC provides OS benefit compared with AC.[36] Other CHT regimens include the following: TAC (docetaxel, adriamycin, and CYC), CMF (CYC, methotrexate, 5-FU), FAC (5-FU, doxorubicin, CYC), and FEC (5-FU, epirubicin, CYC). Please see Chapter 25 for more on systemic therapy.

Hormone Therapy: Indicated for essentially all ER+ or PR+ patients, unless a specific contraindication exists. Tamoxifen is a partial estrogen agonist that functions as a competitive inhibitor. Premenopausal women are typically treated with tamoxifen 20 mg daily for 5 years, although 10 years of therapy was found to further reduce recurrence and breast cancer mortality by approximately one-third in the first 10 years following diagnosis and by approximately half subsequently.[37] Side effects include hot flashes, vaginal discharge/bleeding, cataracts, retinopathy, thromboembolic events (1%), endometrial cancer (relative risk 2–7×), and uterine sarcomas. Aromatase inhibitors (AI) such as anastrozole or letrozole block conversion of androgens to estrogen in fat, liver, and muscle and are ineffective in premenopausal women (due to ovarian production of estrogen). However, AI + ovarian suppression or ablation in premenopausal patients can be considered and is a Category 1 recommendation per NCCN.[38] Postmenopausal women are typically treated with anastrozole 1 mg daily for 5 years. Compared with tamoxifen in postmenopausal women, AIs improve DFS and have higher rates of myalgias, arthralgias, and osteoporosis, but less risk of endometrial cancer and DVTs.[39,40]

Radiation: WBI after lumpectomy significantly lowers the risk of LRR when compared with lumpectomy alone and improves 15-year OS by reducing breast cancer mortality (BCM).[1]

Indications: WBI is indicated in most patients following BCS. Favorable subgroups (e.g., older patients with T1N0 ER+ breast cancers) may be treated with PBI or adjuvant endocrine therapy alone.

Absolute Contraindications to BCS: Persistently positive resection margins after re-excision attempts, historically multicentric tumors (although the ASCOSOG trial showed multiple lumpectomies are feasible[41]), diffuse malignant-appearing mammographic microcalcifications, and inflammatory breast cancer.

Relative Contraindications to BCS: Pregnancy (can perform BCS in third trimester and defer RT until after delivery), active scleroderma, large tumor in a small breast (cosmetic outcome may not be satisfactory), prior RT to the breast or chest wall. BRCA mutation carriers are not contraindicated to receive RT; however, their risk of developing new primary cancers remains high after BCT, so bilateral mastectomies are commonly performed.

Dose: Conventional WBI (45–50.4 Gy in 1.8–2 Gy/fx, typically with boost of 10–16 Gy) is no longer appropriate in most cases of early breast cancer. Moderately hypofractionated regimens (typically 40–42.5 Gy at 2.66 Gy/fx with consideration of boost) are the current standard.[42] Other WBI regimens include ultra-hypofractionated approaches including 28.5 Gy/5 fx once weekly or 26 Gy/5 fx once daily. Regimens for PBI include 30 Gy/5 fx and 38.5 Gy/10 fx BID with external beam and 34 Gy/10 fx BID with brachytherapy.[43]

Timing: RT usually starts within 4 to 6 weeks of completion of surgery or CHT; delaying RT for longer than 16 weeks after surgery is associated with higher breast relapse rates.[44]

Procedure: See *Handbook of Treatment Planning in Radiation Oncology*, Chapter 5.[45]

Toxicity: Acute effects: erythema, pruritus, tenderness, desquamation. Late effects: hyperpigmentation, volume loss, fibrosis, rib fracture, lymphedema, pulmonary fibrosis, secondary malignancies (<1% at 10 years, with angiosarcoma being the most common), cardiac effects.[46]

EVIDENCE-BASED Q&A

Is there a role for radical mastectomy in the modern era?

NSABP B-04 established there is no advantage to radical mastectomy vs. total mastectomy ± RT.

Fisher, NSABP B-04 (*NEJM* **2002, PMID 12192016):** PRT of nonfixed, operable tumors confined to the breast/axilla (*n* = 1079 LN− and *n* = 586 LN+). Randomization of cN0 patients to RM vs. TM + RT (50 Gy/25 fx tangents + PAB; 45 Gy/25 fx IM + SCV; boost if LN+) vs. TM alone; cN+ patients were randomized to RM vs. TM + RT. No significant differences between the three arms of LN− patients or between the two arms of LN+ patients for DFS, RFS, or OS. ALN status is a strong prognostic indicator, but no survival advantage to removing occult positive nodes at surgery. Forty percent of cN0 women had pathologically positive nodes in the RM arm; 18% of TM-alone patients needed delayed ALND for axillary failure, usually within the first 2 years. **Conclusion: RM not necessary for operable breast cancer.**

How does mastectomy compare with breast conservation?

At least six randomized trials have demonstrated no significant differences in OS between BCT and mastectomy (Table 24.4). Two trials, which did not require negative margin lumpectomies (e.g., 48% in the EORTC trial had positive margins), found higher LR rates with BCT, likely due to inadequate surgery.[47,48] At 20-year follow-up in the Milan trial, there were higher rates of LR in the BCT arm (9% after quadrantectomy [Q] vs. 2% after RM), likely due to new primary tumors (two-thirds of recurrences were in other quadrants and only one-third occurred in the index quadrant scar).[49] A 1992 NCI consensus statement declared both mastectomy and BCT to be acceptable standards of care for operable breast cancer.

Table 24.4 Prospective Randomized Trials of Breast Conservation Therapy vs. Mastectomy									
Trial	Years	N	Stage	Surgery	Adjuvant	F/U	OS % (*p*)	DFS % (*p*)	LR % (*p*)
Milan[49]	1973–1980	701	I	Q/RM	CMF	20 yrs	58/59 (NS)		9/2 (<.001)
Gustave-Roussy[50]	1972–1980	179	I	WE/MRM	None	15 yrs	73/65 (.19)		9/14 (NS)
NSABP B-06[51]	1976–1984	1,851	I–II	WE/MRM	MF	20 yrs	46/47 (.74)	35/36 (.95)	2.7/10.2
NCI[52]	1979–1987	237	I–II	WE/MRM	AC	25 yrs	38/44 (.38)	56/29 (.0017)	22/1.0 (<.001)
EORTC 10801[53]	1980–1986	868	I–II	LE/MRM	CMF	22 yrs	39/45 (NS)		20/12 (.01)
Danish[54]	1983–1989	904	I–III	Q, WE/MRM	CMF, Tam	6 yrs	79/82 (NS)	70/66 (NS)	3/4 (NS)

What is the role of adjuvant WBI after breast-conserving surgery?

Up to 40% of women after surgical resection of gross tumor will have residual microscopic disease that can develop into a recurrence. The Holland study demonstrated that 43% of unifocal cancers in mastectomy specimens had tumor foci >2 cm from the index lesion.[55] NSABP B-06 showed that 20-year LR rates were reduced from 39% to 14% with the addition of RT.[51] The EBCTCG meta-analysis was the first study large enough to demonstrate that adjuvant WBI improves OS—the individual trials were not sufficiently powered. RT decreased 15-year risk of death from breast cancer from 31% to 26% for LN– patients and 55% to 48% for LN+.[1] The EBCTCG meta-analysis suggested a "4:1 ratio"—one breast cancer death was avoided by year 15 for every four LRs prevented by year 5 and for every 4 overall recurrences prevented by year 10.[56] There has been no subgroup (age, grade, size, hormone status) that has not been shown to benefit from RT.

Fisher, NSABP B-06 (*NEJM*** 2002, PMID 12393820):** PRT of 1,851 patients from 1976 to 1984 with stage I to II, mobile tumor ≤4 cm, mobile axillary LNs, and negative margins randomized to MRM vs. lumpectomy vs. lumpectomy + WBI 50 Gy/25 fx. ALND was levels I to II. Patients with +LNs received CHT (5-FU and melphalan). Similar DFS and OS observed between MRM and BCT (Table 24.5). The 20-year IBTR rate was 39% after lumpectomy alone and 14% after lumpectomy + RT, with significant benefit to RT in both LN+ and LN–. **Conclusion: Mastectomy and BCT have similar long-term outcomes. Adjuvant WBI after lumpectomy reduces IBTR by approximately two-thirds.**

Table 24.5 Results of NSABP B-06

NSABP B-06	5-Yr IBTR	5-Yr DFS	5-Yr OS	20-Yr IBTR	20-Yr DFS	20-Yr OS
MRM (TM + ALND)		67%	82%		36%	47%
Lumpectomy	28%	64%	83%	39%	35%	46%
Lumpectomy + RT	8%	71%	84%	14%	35%	46%

EBCTCG 2005 Meta-Analysis (*Lancet*** 2005, PMID 16360786):** Meta-analysis of 42,080 women with breast cancer treated on 78 randomized trials that began by 1995. Studies included RT vs. no RT (*n* ~23,500), more vs. less surgery (*n* ~9,300), and more surgery vs. RT (*n* ~9,300). In 10 trials, 7,311 patients were treated with BCS + RT vs. BCS alone. Overall, RT reduces the risk of 5-year LR by 70% (Table 24.6). The absolute 19% reduction in LR at 5 years translated to a 5% reduction in BCM at 15 years. **Conclusion: For every four LRs prevented, one death was avoided with the addition of RT to BCS.**

Table 24.6 2005 EBCTCG Meta-Analysis

	All Patients (N = 7,311)			LN– (N = 6,097)		LN+ (N = 1,214)	
	5-Yr LR	15-Yr BCM	15-Yr OS	5-Yr LR	15-Yr BCM	5-Yr LR	15-Yr BCM
BCS + RT	7%	31%	65%	7%	26%	11%	48%
BCS alone	26%	36%	60%	23%	31%	41%	55%
p value	<.00001	.0002	.005	SS	.006	SS	.01

EBCTCG 2011 Meta-Analysis (*Lancet*** 2011, PMID 22019144):** Meta-analysis of 10,801 early-stage breast cancer patients s/p BCS from 17 PRTs, 67% pN0. RT reduced the 10-year risk of any recurrence by approximately half (Table 24.7). With addition of RT to BCS, about one breast cancer death was avoided by year 15 for every four overall recurrences avoided at 10 years, another 4:1 ratio. **Conclusion: Adjuvant RT after BCS halves the rate of disease recurrence and reduces breast cancer death rate.**

Table 24.7 2011 EBCTCG Meta-Analysis

	10-Yr Recurrence (Any)			15-Yr BCM		
	All	pN0	pN+	All	pN0	pN+
BCS + RT	19%	16%	43%	21%	17%	43%
BCS alone	35%	31%	64%	25%	21%	51%
p value	<.0001	<.0001	<.0001	<.0001	.005	.01

Williams, Scottish Breast Conservation Trial, 30-Year Update (*Lancet* 2024, PMID 39127062): 589 patients with T1–2N0 breast cancer who underwent BCS were randomized to ± RT (50 Gy/25 fx). ER+ patients received adjuvant tamoxifen and ER-negative patients received adjuvant CHT. There was no difference in median survival (19.2 with RT vs. 18.7 years without RT, *p* = .43) or 30-year OS (24% vs. 28%, *p* = .43). Death from breast cancer was lower with adjuvant RT (37% vs. 46%, *p* = .054), but there was a higher rate of death from other cancers in the RT arm (20% vs. 11%, *p* = .012). IBTR was lower with RT (16% vs. 36%, *p* < .0001). In the RT arm, there was a 0.5% increase in recurrence per year vs. a 2% to 3% recurrence risk per year without RT in the first 10 years. After 10 years, the recurrence risks were similar in both arms. **Conclusion: The IBTR benefit of RT is predominantly in the first 10 years.**

Does completion ALND after a positive SLNB benefit cN0 patients? Can RT replace ALND in select cN0 patients?

NSABP B-04 demonstrated that not all undissected nodal disease results in clinical recurrence. Several randomized trials have since shown similar rates of axillary recurrence and DFS between SLNB and ALND among cN0 patients, most of whom received adjuvant RT. ACOSOG Z0011, IBCSG 23-01, and SENOMAC showed that completion ALND after SLNB offered no improvement over SLNB alone in SLN+ patients receiving BCS and WBI, for both macrometastases and micrometastases in patients with cT1–3N0 disease. The AMAROS trial evaluated ALND vs. axillary RT after a positive SLNB and found no difference in recurrence rates, but ALND had twice the rate of lymphedema (28% vs. 14%). Patients undergoing mastectomy were not well-represented in AMAROS, but common practice is to extrapolate to these patients and offer PMRT.

Guiliano, ACOSOG Z0011 (*JAMA* 2011, PMID 21304082; Lucci, *JCO* 2007, PMID 17485711; Jagsi, *JCO* 2014 PMID 25135994; Giuliano, *Ann Surg* 2016, PMID 27513155; Giuliano, *JAMA* 2017, PMID 28898379): PRT of 891 patients with cT1–T2N0 BC who underwent lumpectomy and SLNB with 1 to 2 LN+ randomized to ± completion ALND. All patients received WBI, without node-directed RT (per protocol). Patients were excluded for >2 LN+, matted LNs, gross ENE, received neoadjuvant CHT, or underwent mastectomy. Target enrollment was 1,900 but closed early due to very low event rate. Approximately 96% of patients received systemic therapy in both arms. Primary endpoint of OS was similar in both arms. Median 17 ALNs removed in the ALND arm vs. 2 in the SLNB arm (*p* < .001). In the ALND arm, 27% had additional metastases in dissected LNs, and 14% had ≥4 LN+. The ALND arm had higher rates of subjective lymphedema, wound infections, axillary seromas, and paresthesias than SLNB alone. While standard tangent fields were specified by protocol, ~50% utilized high tangents (defined as ≤2 cm from humeral head) and 19% received RNI to include at least SCV nodes. At 10-year update, nodal recurrences were 0.5% in the ALND arm vs. 1.5% in the SLNB arm, and 10-year IBTR was 6% vs. 4% (*p* = NS; Table 24.8). **Conclusion: Completion ALND is not necessary in patients with 1 to 2 SLN metastases who receive WBI and systemic therapy.**

Table 24.8 ACOSOG Z0011 Results					
	10-Yr IBTR	**Nodal Recurrence**	**Lymphedema**	**10-Yr DFS**	**10-Yr OS**
BCS + ALND + RT	6%	0.5%	13%	78%	84%
BCS + SLNB + RT	4%	1.5%	2%	80%	86%
p value	.13	NS	<.001	.32	.02 (noninferiority)

Galimberti, *IBCSG* 23-01 (*Lancet Oncol* 2013, PMID 23491275; Update *Lancet Oncol* 2018, PMID 30196031): PRT of 931 patients with cT1–2N0 who underwent SLNB and had ≤1 micrometastatic (≤2 mm) SLN without ECE randomized to ± completion ALND (noninferiority design). Ninety-one percent underwent BCT, 9% had mastectomy. Median 21 LNs removed at ALND, and 13% had additional nodal metastases. The 10-year DFS was 77% in the SLNB arm vs. 75% in the ALND arm (*p* = .24); 10-year OS was also similar (91% in the SLNB arm and 88% in the ALND arm). **Conclusion: Supports omission of completion ALND for micrometastases.**

Boniface, SENOMAC Trial (*NEJM* 2024, PMID 38598571): Phase III PRT of 2,540 patients with one to two positive SLNs with >0.2 cm tumor randomized to ± completion ALND. Adjuvant RT was up to physician discretion (90% of patients in both arms received adjuvant RT to some level of nodal targets). Similar to ACOSOG Z0011 by randomization but included patients undergoing mastectomy, SLNs with ECE, T3 tumors, and men. The 5-year RFS was 89% in the axillary dissection group and 90% in the omission group. **Conclusion: Omission of axillary dissection was noninferior to completion dissection in patients with cN0 breast cancer with SLN+ macrometastatic disease who received adjuvant RT.**

Donker, AMAROS/EORTC 10981/22023 (*Lancet* **2014, PMID 25439688;** *JCO* **2023, PMID 36383926**): Phase III trial of 4,806 patients with cT1–2N0 BC randomized preoperatively prior to SLNB; 1,425 patients (30% of initial cohort) with SLN+ received axillary RT (*n* = 681) vs. completion ALND (*n* = 744) in a noninferiority design. Axillary RT to levels I to III and SCV fossa to 50 Gy/25 fx. Eighty-two percent underwent BCT and 18% mastectomy. Thirty-three percent of those undergoing ALND had additional LN+. Primary endpoint was 5-year axillary recurrence rate, which was 0.43% after ALND vs. 1% with axillary RT (NS). In comparison, nonrandomized patients with negative SLNB had similar axillary recurrence rate of 0.8%. OS and DFS rates similar between ALND and RT; however, lymphedema more frequent after ALND (Table 24.9). **Conclusion: For SLN+ patients, axillary RT provides similar control with less risk of lymphedema compared with ALND.**

Table 24.9 AMAROS Trial Results			
	5-Yr Lymphedema	10-Yr DFS	10-Yr OS
ALND	28%	82%	85%
RT	14%	78%	81%
p value	<.001	.18	.34

Is axillary sampling necessary for everyone at the time of surgery?

SLNB is the standard of care for early-stage breast cancer. However, questions have arisen regarding the need for any surgical staging of the axilla. The SOUND trial investigated the safety of omitting SLNB in patients with early-stage breast cancer with negative ultrasound. Given low risk, the Choosing Wisely Campaign recommends against routine SLNB in women >70 years of age with ER+ breast cancer.[57]

Gentilini, SOUND (*JAMA* **2023, PMID 37733364**): Phase III PRT of 1,405 patients randomized to ± SLNB at the time of surgery. Patients had to have a small breast cancer focus (median tumor size of 1.1 cm) with negative preop axillary ultrasound with a plan to undergo BCS and RT. Most were ER-positive (87%) and 84% of patients in the SLNB group and 81% of patients in the no axillary surgery group received WBI. The 5-year distant DFS was 97.7% in the SLNB arm and 98% in the no SLNB arm (noninferiority *p* = .02). Rates of LRR, DM, and deaths were similar in both groups. **Conclusion: Omission of SLNB can be considered for patients with small early-stage breast cancers with negative axillary ultrasound who receive adjuvant RT. These findings were corroborated by the INSEMA trial** (*NEJM* **2024, PMID 39665649**).

What is the role of regional nodal irradiation (RNI) in breast conservation patients undergoing axillary dissection?

After lumpectomy, RNI should be considered for N+ patients, with less data available to include for high-risk node-negative patients. The NCIC MA.20 and EORTC 22922/10925 trials showed an improvement in LRR, DM, and DFS and a trend toward OS with the use of comprehensive nodal radiation, while the EBCTG meta-analysis showed a survival advantage with the addition of RNI.[58,59] *It remains an area of controversy which patients may be adequately treated without RNI. See Chapter 25 for additional details.*

Whelan, MA.20/NCIC-CTG (*NEJM* **2015, PMID 26200977**): PRT of 1,832 patients who underwent BCT and SLNB or ALND found to be pN+ or pN0 with high-risk features (tumor ≥5 cm, or tumor ≥2 cm with <10 ALNs removed and at least one of the following: grade 3, ER–, LVSI). All patients received adjuvant systemic therapy with CHT, endocrine therapy, or both. Exclusion: T4, cN2–3, M1. Patients randomized to WBI only (50 Gy/25 fx ± boost) ± RNI. RNI included IM nodes in the first three intercostal spaces + SCV + axilla (covered levels I + II if <10 axillary nodes removed or >3 LN+) with optional PAB. Primary endpoint was OS. MFU 9.5 years; 85% had 1–3 +LNs, 5% had ≥4 +LNs, and 10% were LN–. Absolute magnitude of benefit is variable across the population and suggests need for risk-stratified approach to these patients (Table 24.10). In a subgroup of ER-negative patients, DFS was significantly improved with RNI (82% vs. 71%, *p* = .04) and OS approached significance (81% vs. 74%; HR 0.69, 95% CI 0.47–1.00, *p* = .05). **Conclusion: RNI improved DFS, locoregional DFS, and distant DFS in high-risk patients after BCT, but no OS benefit was observed.**

Table 24.10 NCIC MA.20 Results							
10-Yr Results	DFS	Locoregional DFS	Distant DFS	BCM	OS	Pneumonitis	Lymphedema
BCS + CHT + WBI + RNI	82%	95%	86%	10%	83%	1%	8%
BCS + CHT + WBI	77%	9%	82%	12%	82%	0.2%	5%
p value	.01	.009	.03	.11	.38	<.001	<.001

EBCTCG, 2023 Meta-Analysis (*Lancet* 2023, PMID 37931633): Individual patient-level meta-analysis of 14,324 women with early-stage breast cancer on 16 eligible trials evaluating the role of RNI. Trials were classified as newer (after 1989) or older. Among patients treated on eight RCTs after 1989, RNI significantly reduced recurrence risk, DM, BCM, and ACM. There was also no difference in nonbreast cancer mortality. The benefit of RNI for any recurrence was 2% for node-negative patients (19% vs. 21%), 3% for 1 to 3 LNs (26% vs. 29%), and 4% for ≥4 LNs (51% vs. 47%). BCM at 15 years increased with increasing burden of nodal disease, with a 2% BCM reduction with RNI for N0 patients (11% vs. 13%), 3% BCM reduction for 1 to 3 nodes (20% vs. 23%), and 4.5% BCM reduction for ≥4 LNs (40.5% vs. 45%). In trials before 1989, RNI did not improve BCM and increased the risk of non-BCM. **Conclusion: The addition of RNI in the modern treatment era reduces the rate of recurrence and improves mortality. The benefit of RNI increases as nodal burden increases.**

For patients with early breast cancer, can treatment duration be reduced via hypofractionation?

At least four randomized trials from the United Kingdom and Canada (Table 24.11) have demonstrated similar outcomes between conventionally fractionated and moderately hypofractionated WBI with respect to IBTR, cosmesis, toxicity, and OS (some trials demonstrated less toxicity with moderate hypofractionation). Moderate hypofractionation is the standard of care for early-stage (pT1–2N0) breast cancer and should be strongly considered for most patients receiving RNI (see Chapter 25).[60] Recently, randomized trials have presented 10-year outcomes with ultra-hypofractionated WBI regimens of five fractions delivered once weekly over 5 weeks (UK FAST) or over 5 consecutive days (UK FAST-Forward).

Table 24.11 Summary of Hypofractionated Whole Breast Irradiation Trials			
	Dose	% Boost	10-Yr LRR
RMH/GOC[61]*	50 Gy/25 fx 42.9 Gy/13 fx QOD 39 Gy/13 fx QOD	74% 75% 74%	12% 10% 15%
START A[62]*	50 Gy/25 fx 41.6 Gy/13 fx QOD 39 Gy/13 fx QOD	60% 61% 61%	7% 6% 9%
START B[62]	50 Gy/25 fx 40 Gy/15 fx	41% 44%	6% 4%
Whelan, Canadian OCOG 93-010[63]	50 Gy/25 fx 42.56 Gy/16 fx	0% 0%	7% 6%
FAST[64]	50 Gy/25 fx 30 Gy/5 fx (once weekly) 28.5 Gy/ 5 fx (once weekly)	0% 0% 0%	1.0% 1.3% 1.3%
FAST-Forward[65]	40 Gy/15 fx 27 Gy/5 fx QD 26 Gy/5 fx QD	25% 25% 24%	4% 3% 2%

*All schedules in RMH/GOC and START A trials delivered over 5 weeks.

Haviland, START A and B (*Lancet Oncol* 2013, PMID 24055415; Update *Radiother Oncol* 2018, PMID 29153463): Two UK PRTs that enrolled women with pT1–T3 N0–1 s/p complete excision (without immediate breast reconstruction) from 1999 to 2002. **START A:** 2,236 patients randomized to 50 Gy/25 fx over 5 weeks vs. 41.6 Gy (3.2 Gy/fx) or 39 Gy (3.0 Gy/fx) in 13 fx QOD. Eighty-five percent underwent BCT (of whom 61% received RT boost); 29% LN+; 14% underwent RNI. MFU 9.3 years. No difference in 10-year LRR between 41.6 Gy and 50 Gy (6% vs. 7%; HR 0.91, 95% *0.59–1.38*) or 39 Gy and 50 Gy (9% vs. 7%; HR 1.18, 0.79–1.76). **START B:** 2,215 patients randomized to 50 Gy/25 fx over 5 weeks vs. 40 Gy/15 fx over 3 weeks. Ninety-two percent underwent BCT; 23% LN+; 7% underwent RNI. MFU 9.9 years. No difference in 10-year LRR between 40 Gy and 50 Gy (4% vs. 6%; HR 0.77, 0.51–1.16). Breast shrinkage, telangiectasia, and breast edema significantly less common with 40 Gy than 50 Gy; 15% of patients received hypofractionated RNI with no long-term risk of arm and shoulder dysfunction. **Conclusion: Moderately hypofractionated WBI is safe and effective for patients with early breast cancer.**

Whelan, Canadian OCOG 93-010 (*NEJM* 2010, PMID 20147717; Bane, *Annals Oncol* 2014, PMID 24562444): PRT of 1,234 patients with pT1–2 pN0 BC, negative margins, separation <25 cm, s/p lumpectomy/ALND randomized to 42.5 Gy/16 fx (2.66 Gy/fx) vs. 50 Gy/25 fx. RT was two opposed tangents with 2D planning and wedges; no boost, no RNI. MFU 12 years. Twenty-five percent were <50 years. CHT used in only 11%, tamoxifen in 41%. Grade 3 skin toxicity or fibrosis at 10 years was 3% to 4% in both arms. No grade 4 ulceration or necrosis. No difference in outcomes between arms, including LR, OS, and cosmesis (Table 24.12). On initial subgroup analysis, LR of high-grade tumors in the hypofractionation arm was 16% vs. 5% in the conventional arm (*p* = .01). An updated subgroup analysis found HER2+ was the most significant predictor of IBTR, regardless of fractionation. **Conclusion: Moderately hypofractionated WBI is similar to conventionally fractionated RT for women with negative-margin BCS, pN0, and breast separation <25 cm.**

Table 24.12 Ontario Cooperative Oncology Group 93-010 Hypofractionation Trial Results					
	10-Yr LR	Excellent/Good Cosmesis	Grade 3 Skin Toxicity	10-Yr DSS	10-Yr OS
42.5 Gy/16 fx	6.2%	70%	2.5%	87%	84%
50 Gy/25 fx	6.7%	71%	2.7%	87%	84%

Murray Brunt, FAST (*JCO* 2020, PMID 32663119): PRT of 915 patients with pT1–2 pN0 IDC, age ≥50, randomized to WBI 50 Gy/25 fx (5 weeks), 30 Gy/5 fx (once weekly), or 28.5 Gy/5 fx (once weekly). MFU 9.9 years. Normal tissue effect (NTE) rates were comparable between 28.5 Gy/5 fx (19%) and 50 Gy/25 fx (18%), but higher with 30 Gy/5 fx (25%). Similar rates of IBTR: 1.0% (50 Gy), 1.3% (30 Gy), and 1.3% (28.5 Gy). **Conclusion: Once-weekly schedule of WBI 28.5 Gy/5 fractions appears to be radiobiologically comparable for NTE to conventional fractionation.**

Murray Brunt, FAST-Forward (*Lancet* 2020, PMID 32580883; 10-yr data ESTRO 2025): PRT of 4,096 patients with pT1–3 pN0–1 IDC, after BCS or mastectomy, randomized to WBI 40 Gy/15 fx (over 3 weeks), 27 Gy/5 fx (over 1 week), or 26 Gy/5 fx (over 1 week). MFU 71.5 months. The 5-year IBTR was not statistically different among the three arms: 2.1% (40 Gy), 1.7% (27 Gy), and 1.4% (26 Gy); 10 year rates of IBTR were 3.6% (40 Gy), 3.0% (27 Gy), and 2.0% (26 Gy). Number of moderate or marked events was not statistically different between 40 Gy/15 fx (11%) vs. 26 Gy/5 fx (12%), but higher in 27 Gy/5 fx (16%), with similar findings at 10 years. **Conclusion: 26 Gy/5 fx over 1 week is noninferior to standard 40 Gy/15 fx (over 3 weeks) for LC and NTE at 10 years.**

Which patients benefit from a tumor bed boost?

The EORTC 22881 and Lyon trials demonstrated that a tumor bed boost reduces IBTR compared with WBI alone. The relative risk reduction was observed in all age subsets proportionally, although the absolute risk reduction was greatest in younger women.[66,67] A boost does not improve DFS or OS and is associated with an increase in fibrosis and telangiectasia rates.[68] Predictive factors of IBTR include younger age, high grade, and associated DCIS.[69] The 2018 ASTRO guideline recommended tumor bed boost for patients ≤50 years old with any grade, age 51 to 70 years with high grade, or positive margin.[42]

Bartelink, EORTC 22881 (*NEJM* 2001, PMID 11794170; Update *JCO* 2007, PMID 17577015; Update *Lancet Oncol* 2015, PMID 25500422; Update *JAMA Oncol* 2017, PMID 27607734): PRT of 5,569 patients with stage I to II (T1–2, N0–1), age ≤70, and treated with lumpectomy + RT (50 Gy). For negative margins (95%), patients randomized to either no boost or 16 Gy boost to tumor bed + 1.5 cm margin (by electrons, tangential photons, or Ir-192 implant). For positive margins (5%), patients randomized to low-dose boost (10 Gy) or high-dose boost (26 Gy); however, these patients were excluded from this analysis. 90% cN0, 78% pN0. Patients with negative margins treated with a boost had a significantly lower rate of LR (4% vs. 7% at 5 years, $p < .0001$; 6% vs. 10% at 10 years, $p < .0001$). Boost reduced the number of salvage mastectomies by 41%. DMFS and OS similar in both groups. All age subsets benefitted proportionally from a boost, although the ARR was greatest in younger women (Table 24.13). At 20-year follow-up, IBTR rates were 17% without a boost vs. 12% with boost ($p < .001$). Young age and presence of DCIS adjacent to the invasive tumor were associated with increased risk for IBTR. **Conclusion: Tumor bed boost can reduce the risk of LR, especially in those <50 years of age.**

Table 24.13 EORTC Boost Trial Results						
10-Yr LR rates	**Overall**	**Age ≤40**	**41–50**	**51–60**	**61–70**	**Fibrosis**
No boost	10%	24%	13%	8%	7%	2%
16 Gy boost	6%	14%	9%	5%	4%	4%
p value	<.0001	.0014	.0099	.0157	.0008	<.0001

Romestaing, Lyon Trial (*JCO* 1997, PMID 9060534): PRT of 1,024 patients <70 years with breast cancers ≤3 cm, treated with lumpectomy (1-cm surgical margin) + WBI (50 Gy/20 fx) and randomized to ± electron boost (10 Gy/4 fx); 98% had negative margins. Patients treated with boost had significantly lower LR at 3.3 years (3.6% vs. 4.5%, $p = .044$). No difference in self-reported cosmetic outcomes (>90% good/excellent), but higher rates of telangiectasias. **Conclusion: Tumor bed boost significantly reduces the risk of early LR without significant deterioration in cosmesis.**

Is there a difference between sequential and concurrent boost with WBI following lumpectomy?

RTOG 1005 was presented at ASTRO 2022 and demonstrated that concomitant boost resulted in similar oncologic outcomes to sequential boost, with no differences in cosmesis. The recently published IMPORT HIGH trial also compared WBI with sequential boost vs. SIB and found no differences in oncologic and cosmetic outcomes when an SIB to the tumor bed of 48 Gy was used (similar dose as RTOG 1005). They did find increased breast induration with a dose-escalated boost of 53 Gy.

Vicini, RTOG 1005 (ASTRO 2022): Phase III PRT of 2,262 women with early stage, high-risk breast cancer randomized to either (a) 50 Gy/25 fx or 42.7 Gy/16 fx with sequential 12–14 Gy/6–7 fx boost or (b) 40 Gy/15 fx with concomitant boost of 8 Gy/15 fx (0.53 Gy/day). Thirty-four percent of patients were stage II, 52% grade 3, 30% ER-negative, and 17% had close or positive margins. At 7 years, concomitant boost was noninferior in terms of IBTR (2.6% vs. 2.2%). There were no differences in grade 3+ toxicity (3.5% vs. 3.3%) or good to excellent cosmesis (86% vs. 84%). **Conclusion: Hypofractionated RT with concomitant boost should be a standard treatment option for early-stage breast cancer patients requiring boost.**

Krug, HYPOSIB-Trial (ASTRO 2024): Phase III RCT of 2,179 patients who received WBI with a sequential vs. SIB technique (40 Gy to whole breast and 48 Gy to lumpectomy cavity over 16 fx). The 5-year LC was 98.2% with SIB and 98.0% with sequential boost ($p = .48$). Cumulative incidence of grade 2+ fibrosis at 5 years was similar, 7% in the SIB arm vs. 8% in the sequential boost arm ($p = .32$). The rate of grade 2+ telangiectasia was 1.5% in both arms. **Conclusion: Moderately hypofractionated WBI with SIB is safe and effective.**

Coles, IMPORT HIGH (*Lancet* 2023, PMID 37302395): Phase III noninferiority trial of patients who underwent BCS were randomized to one of three groups: (a) 36 Gy/15 fx to the whole breast with 16 Gy/8 fx sequential boost; (b) 36 Gy/15 fx to the whole breast, 40 Gy/15 fx to partial breast, and 48 Gy/15 fx concomitant boost; (c) 36 Gy/15 fx to the whole breast, 40 Gy/15 fx to partial breast, and 53 Gy/15 fx concomitant boost. The 5-year IBTR was lower than the expected 5% among all groups (1.9%, 2.0%, 3.2%), with low toxicity rates. With a dose of 53 Gy SIB, there was an increased rate of breast induration. **Conclusion: SIB is safe, effective, and reduces patient visits.**

What is the role of IMRT in early-stage breast cancer?

Compared with older 2D techniques, IMRT improves dosimetry and is associated with lower acute toxicity. A randomized trial showed a negative change in breast appearance by photographs in 58% of patients randomized to 2D vs. 40% with IMRT.[70] Another randomized trial of IMRT vs. 2D showed improved dose homogeneity and reduced moist desquamation with IMRT.[71] However, no trial has compared inverse-planned IMRT with 3D-CRT field in field techniques, and 3D-CRT with field in field is likely sufficient to provide adequate dose homogeneity in most patients.

What is the role of cardiac-sparing RT techniques?

Darby et al. found that rates of major coronary events (MI, coronary revascularization, or death from ischemic heart disease) after breast RT increased linearly with mean heart dose (relative risk increased by 7% per Gy MHD) with no apparent threshold.[72] Cardiac-sparing techniques for left-sided breast RT include selective use of a heart block (as long as target coverage is not compromised), deep inspiration breath hold (DIBH), and prone positioning. In current trials, MHD <4 Gy is ideal (<5 Gy acceptable) for left-sided cancer (<2 Gy on the right), although the "ALARA" principles apply. In a series using older RT techniques, left-sided breast cancer patients had higher risk of cardiac mortality.[73] Using modern RT techniques, laterality does not appear to influence survival.[74] With the adoption of DIBH and prone positioning, MHD <1 Gy and <2 Gy can be achieved for WBI in right and left breast cancers, respectively.[75]

What is the role of endocrine therapy in BCT? Are there some patients in whom RT may be omitted after lumpectomy?

NSABP B-21 showed that adjuvant tamoxifen alone is inferior to RT alone, but together they act synergistically to reduce IBTR in low-risk patients undergoing BCT; of note, no difference in DMs was noted with the addition of tamoxifen in this low-risk cohort. Omission of RT may be considered in carefully selected patients with T1N0, ER+/PR+, HER2–, negative margins, who are older (>65–70 years) or with reduced life expectancy, and who are committed to taking 5 years of endocrine therapy (~30%–40% discontinue endocrine therapy before completion of 5 years). Multiple trials (Table 24.14) have studied the omission of RT in patients at low risk for recurrence—none were powered to observe a difference in DFS or OS, and there remains an increased risk of IBTR in the absence of RT.[76–81] Overall, careful consideration of risks/benefits and life expectancy is required, and patients who decline adjuvant RT must be willing to accept a higher risk of IBTR and commit to taking endocrine therapy for at least 5 years. Given the concern for low compliance rate of endocrine therapy, the EUROPA trial (NCT04134598) is examining PBI vs. endocrine therapy with interim analysis demonstrating improved QOL with PBI as compared to endocrine therapy.

Table 24.14 Trials Summarizing RT Omission in Early-Stage Breast Cancer						
Trial	N	Reported Follow-Up	Eligibility	Treatment	IBTR/LR	OS
NSABP B-21[76]	1,009	8 years	≤1 cm, N0	BCS + tamoxifen BCS + WBI BCS + WBI + tamoxifen	17% 9% 3%	93% 94% 93%
PMH[79]	769	8 years	≥50, T1–2N0	BCS + tamoxifen BCS + tamoxifen + WBI	12% 4%	89% 89%
CALBG 9343[77]	636	10 years	≥70 yrs, T1N0, ER+	BCS + tamoxifen BCS + tamoxifen + WBI	10% 2%	66% 67%
PRIME II[78]	1,326	10 years	≥65 yrs, T1–2 (≤3 cm), negative margins (≥1 mm)	BCS + tamoxifen BCS + tamoxifen + WBI	10% 1%	81% 81%
LUMINA[82]	500	5 years	≥55 yrs, T1N0 grade 1 or 2 luminal A	BCS + endocrine therapy	2%	97%
IDEA[83]	200	5 years	50-69 yrs, T1N0, margins ≥2 mm, ER+/PR+/HER–, Oncotype DX ≤18	BCS + endocrine therapy	1%	100%

What is the role of IORT in early breast cancer?

Two large prospective RCTs have demonstrated higher rates of LR following IORT compared with WBI. Advantages to IORT include improved patient convenience and less acute skin erythema due to rapid dose falloff. Disadvantages to IORT include lack of long-term efficacy data, no pathology information available at the time of treatment, inability to visualize dose to normal structures, longer anesthesia time, and limited availability. Some are concerned that the dose falloff with 50 kV x-rays may be too steep, as evidenced by the increased risk of LR, and no trials have proven a benefit to IORT over endocrine therapy alone. Current ASTRO guidelines do not recommend low-energy IORT (i.e., TARGIT) outside of prospective studies. ABS guidelines do not recommend IORT outside of prospective studies.[84,85]

Vaidya, TARGIT-A (*Lancet* 2010, PMID 20570343; Update *Lancet* 2014, PMID 24224997; Update *JAMA Oncol* 2020, PMID 32239210; Update *BMJ* 2020, PMID 32816842): Phase III noninferiority trial of WBI vs. IORT in 3,451 patients ≤45 years with clinically unifocal IDC. Patients stratified by timing: patients randomized before surgery (prepathology, immediate IORT) and those after final pathology, in which case IORT was given in a second procedure (postpathology, delayed IORT). For prepathology patients, if final pathology revealed high-risk disease (ILC, EIC, or a site-specific criterion such as grade III, LN+, or LVI+), WBI was given, omitting the tumor bed boost (after re-excision to achieve negative margins if applicable). For postpathology patients, high-risk pathologic features were excluded, and thus only lower risk women were randomized. WBI varied by center (typically 40–56 Gy ± boost of 10–16 Gy). IORT was 20 Gy to cavity surface (~5–7 Gy at 1 cm) with 50 kV photons. Fifteen percent of patients randomized to IORT received WBI (22% prepathology, 4% postpathology). Long-term outcomes for the entire IORT cohort are not available. No statistically significant difference was seen between WBI and prepathology IORT for LR, DM, and OS. The 5-year IBTR was higher with delayed IORT in postpathology patients (4% vs. 1%; *non*inferiority not met). **Conclusion: For selected low-risk patients with early-stage breast cancer, delayed IORT is not recommended. Given increased rates of LR and lack of data for the entire cohort being presented, IORT remains investigational.**

Veronesi, ELIOT Trial (*Lancet Oncol* 2013, PMID 24225155; *Lancet Oncol* 2021, PMID 33845035): A total of 1,305 patients aged 48 to 75 years with unicentric tumors <2.5 cm s/p quadrantectomy were randomized to WBI (50 Gy/25 fx + 10 Gy boost) vs. ELIOT (21 Gy/1 fx IORT prescribed to 90% IDL using 3–12 MeV electrons). Equivalence trial design with primary endpoint of IBTR. Eighty-nine percent received endocrine therapy. The 5- and 10-year event rates for IBTR were 4% and 13% for the ELIOT group vs. 0.5% and 2% in the WBI arm ($p < .0001$). The 15-year OS was 83% vs. 84%. Overall toxicity favored the ELIOT group ($p = .0002$) due to lower incidence of skin erythema ($p < .0001$), dry skin ($p = .04$), hyperpigmentation ($p = .0004$), breast edema ($p = .004$), and breast itching ($p = .002$). However, ELIOT had higher fat tissue necrosis. **Conclusion: ELIOT has higher rate of IBTR than WBI.**

In whom is partial breast irradiation (PBI) acceptable?

The rationale for PBI is that the majority of recurrences after BCT are seen at or near the tumor bed (~80%), and irradiation of this region alone instead of the entire breast may eradicate residual disease while maintaining acceptable cosmesis and improving toxicity outcomes.[86–88] In addition, the prolonged course of conventional WBI has been an obstacle for compliance.[89] Advantages of PBI include shorter treatment time of ~5 to 15 days and potentially better cosmesis (depending on technique).[88] Disadvantages of PBI include potentially worse cosmetic outcomes with 3D-CRT techniques and invasive procedures with brachytherapy. Accepted PBI selection criteria are listed in Tables 24.15 and 24.16.[84,85]

Table 24.15 Eligibility Criteria for PBI Based on Professional Society Recommendations			
	ABS	**ASBS**	**NSABP B-39/RTOG 0413**
Age	45 yrs	Invasive 45 yrs; DCIS 50 yrs	18 yrs
Histology	IDC, DCIS	IDC, DCIS	Unifocal IDC, DCIS
Size	≤3 cm	≤3 cm	≤3 cm
Margins	Negative	Negative	Negative
Nodes	N0	N0	0–3 +LN
LVSI	No	–	–
Estrogen receptor	Positive or negative	–	–

Table 24.16 2024 ASTRO Consensus Guidelines for APBI Suitability[90]			
Recommended	**Conditionally Recommended***	**Conditionally Not Recommended**	**Not Recommended**
Age ≥40 yrs T1 (≤2 cm) Grades 1–2 ER positive DCIS: low-intermediate grade, age ≥40 yrs and size ≤2 cm	Grade 3 disease ER negative >2 and ≤3 cm DCIS: high grade or >2 and ≤3 cm	HER2+ and not receiving anti-HER2 therapy LVSI Lobular histology	Age <40 yrs Positive LNs Positive surgical margins Known BRCA1 or 2 mutation DCIS: same as invasive guidelines

*PBI may not be appropriate when multiple of these factors are present given higher risk of recurrence.
Source: Adapted from Shaitelman SF, Anderson BM, Arthur DW, et al. Partial breast irradiation for patients with early-stage invasive breast cancer or ductal carcinoma in situ: an ASTRO clinical practice guideline. *Pract Radiat Oncol.* 2024;14(2): 112–132. doi:10.1016/j.prro.2023.11.001.

Is PBI safe and effective compared with standard WBI?

To date, more than seven modern randomized trials evaluating various techniques of PBI compared with WBI have been reported (Table 24.17), and all have demonstrated similar rates of IBTR between PBI and WBI. The GEC-ESTRO trial found no difference in IBTR rates or cosmetic outcomes, with reduced late grades 2 to 3 skin toxicities with PBI.[91–93] The RAPID trial utilized PBI by 3D-CRT (38.5 Gy/10 fx BID) and found an increase in moderate late toxicity and adverse cosmesis with PBI compared with WBI.[94] Concerns regarding toxicity outcomes from 3D-CRT APBI using similar BID dose fractionation were noted in other institutional series as well.[95–97] PBI by IMRT with or without altered fractionation (daily RT as in IMPORT LOW or every other day in the University of Florence trial) may improve outcomes further.[98]

NSABP B-39/RTOG 0413 is the largest PRT completed to date, with over 4,300 patients with stage 0 to II (≤3 cm) breast cancer or DCIS s/p lumpectomy with negative margins and 0 to 3 LN+ randomized to WBI (50 Gy with optional 10 Gy boost) vs. PBI via either multicatheter brachytherapy (34 Gy/10 fx BID), intracavity brachytherapy (MammoSite 34 Gy/10 fx BID), or 3D-CRT (38.5 Gy/10 fx BID), but the trial did not meet equivalence.

Table 24.17 Randomized Trials of APBI vs. Whole Breast Irradiation							
	N; FU	**Eligibility**	**PBI Technique**	**Dose**	**IBTR**	**Toxicity**
Hungary Polgar, 2013 (20-yr update)[99]	258; 17 yrs	pT1, pN0–1mi, G1–2, nonlobular, negative margins, age >40	Interstitial brachytherapy or electrons	36.4 Gy/7 fx (brachytherapy) 50 Gy/25 fx (electrons)	10% vs. 8%	PBI improved cosmesis (81% vs. 63%)
GEC-ESTRO Strnad 2016 (10-yr update)[100]	1,184; 10 yrs	pT1–2 (<3 cm), pN0–1mi, IDC/ILC/DCIS, margins >2 mm, no LVSI, age >40	Interstitial	32 Gy/8 fx or 30.2 Gy/7 fx (HDR), 50 Gy (PDR)	3.5% vs. 1.6%	PBI reduced breast pain, less late grades 2–3 skin toxicities
Florence Meattini (2020)[98]	520; 10.7 yrs	pT1–2 (<2.5 cm), negative margins, clips in cavity, age >40	IMRT	30 Gy/5 fx QOD	2.5% vs. 3.7%	PBI less toxicity
Barcelona Rodriguez (2013)[101]	102; 5.0 yrs	pT1–2 (<3 cm), N0, grades 1–2, IDC, negative margins, age >60	3D-CRT	37.5 Gy/10 fx	0%	Lower rates of late toxicity with PBI, no difference in cosmesis

(continued)

Table 24.17 Randomized Trials of APBI vs. Whole Breast Irradiation (*continued*)

	N; FU	Eligibility	PBI Technique	Dose	IBTR	Toxicity
IMPORT LOW Coles (2017)[102]	2,018; 6.0 yrs	pT1–2 (<3 cm), N0–1, IDC, margins ≤2 mm, age ≤50	IMRT	40 Gy/15 fx WBI vs. 36 Gy WBI + 40 Gy PBI vs. 40 Gy/15 PBI	1.1% vs. 0.2% vs. 0.5%	Reduced toxicity in both experimental arms
RAPID Whelan (2019)[94]	2,135; 10.2 yrs	pT1–2 (<2 cm), pN0, IDC/DCIS, negative margins, age >40	3D-CRT	38.5 Gy/10 fx BID	4% vs. 3%	PBI group: grade 3 10%, no grades 4–5
NSABP B-39 Vicini (2019)[43]	4,216; 10.2 yrs	pT1–2 (<3 cm), pN0–1 (no ECE, cN0), IDC or DCIS, negative margins, age >18	3D-CRT or brachytherapy (interstitial/applicator)	38.5 Gy/10 fx BID (3D), 34 Gy/10 fx BID (brachy)	3.9% vs. 4.6% (non-equivalent)	PBI: grade 3 10%, no grades 4–5
DBCG Offersen (2022)[103]	886; 7.6 yrs (LRR); 5.0 yrs morbidity	pT1N0 (<2.1 cm), IDC, margins >2 mm, age >60	3D-CRT	40 Gy/15 fx WBI vs. 40 Gy/15 fx APBI	3% vs. 2% (9 yrs)	Gr 2–3 Induration: 10% vs. 5%
IMRA Meduri (2023)[104]	3,309; 5 yrs morbidity	pT1N0 (<3 cm), margins >2 mm, pN0–N1	3D-CRT or IMRT	50 Gy/25 fx or 42.56/16 fx or 45/18 fx or 40/15 fx vs. 38.5/10 Gy BID		5-yr fair/poor cosmesis: 14% PBI vs. 10% WBI

What PBI techniques are available and how do they differ?

PBI can be delivered via interstitial brachytherapy, intracavitary brachytherapy, or EBRT. See Table 24.18 for details.

Table 24.18 Techniques of PBI

Interstitial brachytherapy	PBI technique with the longest follow-up.[105,106] Catheters are placed through the breast tissue in 1- to 1.5-cm intervals. Primary limitation is technical complexity, with few practitioners having expertise. *Dose:* 34 Gy/10 fx, 32 Gy/8 fx, or 36.4 Gy/7 fx, usually delivered BID with 6-hour interfraction interval. *Target:* PTV = tumor cavity + 15 mm and limited by 5 mm from skin and posterior breast tissue.
Intracavity brachytherapy	MammoSite was the first intracavitary device approved by the FDA in May 2002.[107] A silicone balloon is connected to a double-lumen catheter with an inflation channel and port for passage of the HDR source. A cavity evaluation device can be placed in the cavity at the time of surgery, which is replaced by the treatment device postoperatively (after pathology confirmation) under ultrasound guidance. The balloon is filled with saline (30–70 mL) and mixed with a small amount of contrast (1–2 mL) to achieve a diameter of 4–6 cm to allow for visualization for treatment planning. The most robust data with applicator PBI come from the MammoSite registry, which demonstrated a 5-yr LR rate of 4% with low toxicity.[108,109] Multi-lumen and strut applicators have been developed, which can improve target coverage and allow for smaller skin spacing. Studies evaluating these options have demonstrated good clinical outcomes and low toxicity rates.[110,111] *Dose:* 34 Gy/10 fx BID with 6-hour interfraction interval.

(continued)

Table 24.18 Techniques of PBI (*continued*)	
EBRT	Noninvasive technique, with advantages including widespread availability, fewer technical/QA demands, and potentially better dose homogeneity. *Dose*: 38.5 Gy/10 fx BID, 40 Gy/15 fx QD, or 30 Gy/5 fx QOD or QD (IMRT). *Target*: per NSABP B39, CTV = tumor cavity + 15 mm (limited by 5 mm from skin and posterior breast tissue), PTV = CTV + 10 mm, excluding volume outside breast and 5 mm from skin, and beyond posterior breast[43]; per Florence trial, CTV = tumor cavity + 10 mm (limited to 3 mm from skin), PTV = CTV + 10 mm, allowing 4 mm inside ipsilateral lung and limited to 3 mm from skin.[98]

REFERENCES

1. Clarke M, Collins R, Darby S, et al. Effects of radiotherapy and of differences in the extent of surgery for early breast cancer on local recurrence and 15-year survival: an overview of the randomised trials. *Lancet*. 2005;366(9503):2087–2106. doi:10.1016/S0140-6736(05)67887-7

2. Siegel RL, Giaquinto AN, Jemal A. Cancer statistics, 2024. *CA Cancer J Clin*. 2024;74(1):12–49. doi:10.3322/caac.21820

3. Jacquemier J, Kurtz JM, Amalric R, Brandone H, Ayme Y, Spitalier JM. An assessment of extensive intraductal component as a risk factor for local recurrence after breast-conserving therapy. *Br J Cancer*. 1990;61(6):873–876. doi:10.1038/bjc.1990.195

4. van de Vijver MJ, He YD, van't Veer LJ, et al. A gene-expression signature as a predictor of survival in breast cancer. *N Engl J Med*. 2002;347(25):1999–2009. doi:10.1056/NEJMoa021967

5. Paik S, Shak S, Tang G, et al. A multigene assay to predict recurrence of tamoxifen-treated, node-negative breast cancer. *N Engl J Med*. 2004;351(27):2817–2826. doi:10.1056/NEJMoa041588

6. Perou CM, Sorlie T, Eisen MB, et al. Molecular portraits of human breast tumours. *Nature*. 2000;406(6797): 747–752. doi:10.1038/35021093

7. Sparano JA, Gray RJ, Makower DF, et al. Adjuvant chemotherapy guided by a 21-gene expression assay in breast cancer. *N Engl J Med*. 2018;379(2):111–121. doi:10.1056/NEJMoa1804710

8. Maisonneuve P, Disalvatore D, Rotmensz N, et al. Proposed new clinicopathological surrogate definitions of luminal A and luminal B (HER2-negative) intrinsic breast cancer subtypes. *Breast Cancer Res*. 2014; 16(3):R65. doi:10.1186/bcr3679

9. Sjostrom M, Chang SL, Fishbane N, et al. Clinicogenomic radiotherapy classifier predicting the need for intensified locoregional treatment after breast-conserving surgery for early-stage breast cancer. *J Clin Oncol*. 2019;37(35):3340–3349. doi:10.1200/JCO.19.00761

10. Duffy SW, Tabar L, Yen AM, et al. Mammography screening reduces rates of advanced and fatal breast cancers: results in 549,091 women. *Cancer*. 2020;126(13):2971–2979. doi:10.1002/cncr.32859

11. Expert Panel on Breast Imaging, Niell BL, Jochelson MS, et al. ACR Appropriateness Criteria® female breast cancer screening: 2023 update. *J Am Coll Radiol*. 2024;21(6S):S126–S143. doi:10.1016/j.jacr.2024.02.019

12. Force USPST, Nicholson WK, Silverstein M, et al. Screening for breast cancer: US preventive services task force recommendation statement. *JAMA*. 2024;331(22):1918–1930. doi:10.1001/jama.2024.5534

13. Saslow D, Boetes C, Burke W, et al. American cancer society guidelines for breast screening with MRI as an adjunct to mammography. *CA Cancer J Clin*. 2007;57(2):75–89. doi:10.3322/canjclin.57.2.75

14. Oeffinger KC, Fontham ET, Etzioni R, et al. Breast cancer screening for women at average risk: 2015 guideline update from the American cancer society. *JAMA*. 2015;314(15):1599–1614. doi:10.1001/jama.2015.12783

15. Smart CR, Hartmann WH, Beahrs OH, Garfinkel L. Insights into breast cancer screening of younger women. Evidence from the 14-year follow-up of the breast cancer detection demonstration project. *Cancer*. 1993;72(4 Suppl):1449–1456. doi:10.1002/1097-0142(19930815)72:4+<1449::aid-cncr2820721406>3.0.co;2-c

16. Vanel D. The American College of Radiology (ACR) Breast Imaging and Reporting Data System (BI-RADS): a step towards a universal radiological language? *Eur J Radiol*. 2007;61(2):183. doi:10.1016/j.ejrad.2006.08.030

17. Tillman GF, Orel SG, Schnall MD, Schultz DJ, Tan JE, Solin LJ. Effect of breast magnetic resonance imaging on the clinical management of women with early-stage breast carcinoma. *J Clin Oncol*. 2002;20(16):3413–3423. doi:10.1200/JCO.2002.08.600

18. Houssami N, Turner R, Morrow M. Preoperative magnetic resonance imaging in breast cancer: meta-analysis of surgical outcomes. *Ann Surg*. 2013;257(2):249–255. doi:10.1097/SLA.0b013e31827a8d17

19. Houssami N, Turner R, Macaskill P, et al. An individual person data meta-analysis of preoperative magnetic resonance imaging and breast cancer recurrence. *J Clin Oncol*. 2014;32(5):392–401. doi:10.1200/JCO.2013.52.7515

20. Hattangadi-Gluth JA, Wo JY, Nguyen PL, et al. Basal subtype of invasive breast cancer is associated with a higher risk of true recurrence after conventional breast-conserving therapy. *Int J Radiat Oncol Biol Phys*. 2012;82(3):1185–1191. doi:10.1016/j.ijrobp.2011.02.061

21. Recht A, Come SE, Henderson IC, et al. The sequencing of chemotherapy and radiation therapy after conservative surgery for early-stage breast cancer. *N Engl J Med*. 1996;334(21):1356–1361. doi:10.1056/NEJM199605233342102

22. Bellon JR, Come SE, Gelman RS, et al. Sequencing of chemotherapy and radiation therapy in early-stage breast cancer: updated results of a prospective randomized trial. *J Clin Oncol*. 2005;23(9):1934–1940. doi:10.1200/JCO.2005.04.032

23. Fisher B, Costantino JP, Wickerham DL, et al. Tamoxifen for the prevention of breast cancer: current status of the national surgical adjuvant breast and bowel project P-1 study. *J Natl Cancer Inst*. 2005;97(22):1652–1662. doi:10.1093/jnci/dji372

24. Vogel VG, Costantino JP, Wickerham DL, et al. Update of the national surgical adjuvant breast and bowel project Study of Tamoxifen and Raloxifene (STAR) P-2 trial: preventing breast cancer. *Cancer Prev Res (Phila)*. 2010;3(6):696–706. doi:10.1158/1940-6207.CAPR-10-0076

25. Hartmann LC, Schaid DJ, Woods JE, et al. Efficacy of bilateral prophylactic mastectomy in women with a family history of breast cancer. *N Engl J Med*. 1999;340(2):77–84. doi:10.1056/NEJM199901143400201

26. Eisen A, Lubinski J, Klijn J, et al. Breast cancer risk following bilateral oophorectomy in BRCA1 and BRCA2 mutation carriers: an international case-control study. *J Clin Oncol*. 2005;23(30):7491–7496. doi:10.1200/JCO.2004.00.7138

27. Moran MS, Schnitt SJ, Giuliano AE, et al. Society of surgical oncology-American society for radiation oncology consensus guideline on margins for breast-conserving surgery with whole-breast irradiation in stages I and II invasive breast cancer. *Int J Radiat Oncol Biol Phys*. 2014;88(3):553–564. doi:10.1016/j.ijrobp.2013.11.012

28. Veronesi U, Paganelli G, Viale G, et al. Sentinel-lymph-node biopsy as a staging procedure in breast cancer: update of a randomised controlled study. *Lancet Oncol*. 2006;7(12):983–990. doi:10.1016/S1470-2045(06)70947-0

29. Caudle AS, Yang WT, Krishnamurthy S, et al. Improved axillary evaluation following neoadjuvant therapy for patients with node-positive breast cancer using selective evaluation of clipped nodes: implementation of targeted axillary dissection. *J Clin Oncol*. 2016;34(10):1072–1078. doi:10.1200/JCO.2015.64.0094

30. Cardoso F, van't Veer LJ, Bogaerts J, et al. 70-gene signature as an aid to treatment decisions in early-stage breast cancer. *N Engl J Med*. 2016;375(8):717–729. doi:10.1056/NEJMoa1602253

31. Smith I, Procter M, Gelber RD, et al. 2-year follow-up of trastuzumab after adjuvant chemotherapy in HER2-positive breast cancer: a randomised controlled trial. *Lancet*. 2007;369(9555):29–36. doi:10.1016/S0140-6736(07)60028-2

32. Schmid P, Cortes J, Pusztai L, et al. Pembrolizumab for early triple-negative breast cancer. *N Engl J Med*. 2020;382(9):810–821. doi:10.1056/NEJMoa1910549

33. Henderson IC, Berry DA, Demetri GD, et al. Improved outcomes from adding sequential Paclitaxel but not from escalating Doxorubicin dose in an adjuvant chemotherapy regimen for patients with node-positive primary breast cancer. *J Clin Oncol*. 2003;21(6):976–983. doi:10.1200/JCO.2003.02.063

34. Martin M, Pienkowski T, Mackey J, et al. Adjuvant docetaxel for node-positive breast cancer. *N Engl J Med*. 2005;352(22):2302–2313. doi:10.1056/NEJMoa043681

35. Citron ML, Berry DA, Cirrincione C, et al. Randomized trial of dose-dense versus conventionally scheduled and sequential versus concurrent combination chemotherapy as postoperative adjuvant treatment of node-positive primary breast cancer: first report of intergroup trial C9741/cancer and leukemia group B trial 9741. *J Clin Oncol*. 2003;21(8):1431–1439. doi:10.1200/JCO.2003.09.081

36. Jones S, Holmes FA, O'Shaughnessy J, et al. Docetaxel with cyclophosphamide is associated with an overall survival benefit compared with doxorubicin and cyclophosphamide: 7-year follow-up of US oncology research trial 9735. *J Clin Oncol*. 2009;27(8):1177–1183. doi:10.1200/JCO.2008.18.4028

37. Davies C, Pan H, Godwin J, et al. Long-term effects of continuing adjuvant tamoxifen to 10 years versus stopping at 5 years after diagnosis of oestrogen receptor-positive breast cancer: ATLAS, a randomised trial. *Lancet*. 2013;381(9869):805–816. doi:10.1016/S0140-6736(12)61963-1

38. NCCN Clinical Practice Guidelines in Oncology: Breast Cancer. Accessed April 24, 2024. https://www.nccn.org/professionals/physician_gls/pdf/breast.pdf

39. Baum M, Budzar AU, Cuzick J, et al. Anastrozole alone or in combination with tamoxifen versus tamoxifen alone for adjuvant treatment of postmenopausal women with early breast cancer: first results of the ATAC randomised trial. *Lancet*. 2002;359(9324):2131–2139. doi:10.1016/s0140-6736(02)09088-8

40. Early Breast Cancer Trialists' Collaborative Group (EBCTCG). Aromatase inhibitors versus tamoxifen in early breast cancer: patient-level meta-analysis of the randomised trials. *Lancet*. 2015;386(10001):1341–1352. doi:10.1016/S0140-6736(15)61074-1

41. Boughey JC, Rosenkranz KM, Ballman KV, et al. Local recurrence after breast-conserving therapy in patients with multiple ipsilateral breast cancer: results from ACOSOG Z11102 (Alliance). *J Clin Oncol*. 2023;41(17):3184–3193. doi:10.1200/JCO.22.02553

42. Smith BD, Bellon JR, Blitzblau R, et al. Radiation therapy for the whole breast: executive summary of an American Society for Radiation Oncology (ASTRO) evidence-based guideline. *Pract Radiat Oncol*. 2018;8(3):145–152. doi:10.1016/j.prro.2018.01.012

43. Vicini FA, Cecchini RS, White JR, et al. Long-term primary results of accelerated partial breast irradiation after breast-conserving surgery for early-stage breast cancer: a randomised, phase 3, equivalence trial. *Lancet*. 2019;394(10215):2155–2164. doi:10.1016/S0140-6736(19)32514-0

44. Recht A, Come SE, Gelman RS, et al. Integration of conservative surgery, radiotherapy, and chemotherapy for the treatment of early-stage, node-positive breast cancer: sequencing, timing, and outcome. *J Clin Oncol*. 1991;9(9):1662–1667. doi:10.1200/JCO.1991.9.9.1662

45. Videtic GMM, Woody NM, Vassil AD. *Handbook of Treatment Planning in Radiation Oncology*. 3rd ed. Demos Medical; 2020.

46. Buchholz TA. Radiation therapy for early-stage breast cancer after breast-conserving surgery. *N Engl J Med*. 2009;360(1):63–70. doi:10.1056/NEJMct0803525

47. Jacobson JA, Danforth DN, Cowan KH, et al. Ten-year results of a comparison of conservation with mastectomy in the treatment of stage I and II breast cancer. *N Engl J Med*. 1995;332(14):907–911. doi:10.1056/NEJM199504063321402

48. van Dongen JA, Voogd AC, Fentiman IS, et al. Long-term results of a randomized trial comparing breast-conserving therapy with mastectomy: European organization for research and treatment of cancer 10801 trial. *J Natl Cancer Inst*. 2000;92(14):1143–1150. doi:10.1093/jnci/92.14.1143

49. Veronesi U, Cascinelli N, Mariani L, et al. Twenty-year follow-up of a randomized study comparing breast-conserving surgery with radical mastectomy for early breast cancer. *N Engl J Med*. 2002;347(16):1227–1232. doi:10.1056/NEJMoa020989

50. Arriagada R, Le MG, Rochard F, Contesso G. Conservative treatment versus mastectomy in early breast cancer: patterns of failure with 15 years of follow-up data. Institut Gustave-Roussy Breast Cancer Group. *J Clin Oncol*. 1996;14(5):1558–1564. doi:10.1200/JCO.1996.14.5.1558

51. Fisher B, Anderson S, Bryant J, et al. Twenty-year follow-up of a randomized trial comparing total mastectomy, lumpectomy, and lumpectomy plus irradiation for the treatment of invasive breast cancer. *N Engl J Med*. 2002;347(16):1233–1241. doi:10.1056/NEJMoa022152

52. Simone NL, Dan T, Shih J, et al. Twenty-five year results of the national cancer institute randomized breast conservation trial. *Breast Cancer Res Treat*. 2012;132(1):197–203. doi:10.1007/s10549-011-1867-6

53. Litiere S, Werutsky G, Fentiman IS, et al. Breast conserving therapy versus mastectomy for stage I-II breast cancer: 20 year follow-up of the EORTC 10801 phase 3 randomised trial. *Lancet Oncol*. 2012;13(4):412–419. doi:10.1016/S1470-2045(12)70042-6

54. Blichert-Toft M, Rose C, Andersen JA, et al. Danish randomized trial comparing breast conservation therapy with mastectomy: six years of life-table analysis. Danish breast cancer cooperative group. *J Natl Cancer Inst Monogr*. 1992;(11):19–25. PMID:1627427

55. Holland R, Veling SH, Mravunac M, Hendriks JH. Histologic multifocality of Tis, T1-2 breast carcinomas. Implications for clinical trials of breast-conserving surgery. *Cancer*. 1985;56(5):979–990. doi:10.1002/1097-0142(19850901)56:5<979::aid-cncr2820560502>3.0.co;2-n

56. Early Breast Cancer Trialists' Collaborative Group (EBCTCG), Darby S, McGale P, et al. Effect of radiotherapy after breast-conserving surgery on 10-year recurrence and 15-year breast cancer death: meta-analysis of individual patient data for 10,801 women in 17 randomised trials. *Lancet*. 2011;378(9804):1707–1716. doi:10.1016/S0140-6736(11)61629-2

57. Grossi S, Le J, Armani A. Omitting axillary staging in selected patients: rationale of choosing wisely in breast cancer treatment. *Surgery*. 2023;174(2):413–415. doi:10.1016/j.surg.2023.03.023

58. Whelan TJ, Olivotto IA, Parulekar WR, et al. Regional nodal irradiation in early-stage breast cancer. *N Engl J Med*. 2015;373(4):307–316. doi:10.1056/NEJMoa1415340

59. Poortmans PM, Collette S, Kirkove C, et al. Internal mammary and medial supraclavicular irradiation in breast cancer. *N Engl J Med*. 2015;373(4):317–327. doi:10.1056/NEJMoa1415369

60. Smith BD, Bentzen SM, Correa CR, et al. Fractionation for whole breast irradiation: an American Society for Radiation Oncology (ASTRO) evidence-based guideline. *Int J Radiat Oncol Biol Phys*. 2011;81(1):59–68. doi:10.1016/j.ijrobp.2010.04.042

61. Yarnold J, Ashton A, Bliss J, et al. Fractionation sensitivity and dose response of late adverse effects in the breast after radiotherapy for early breast cancer: long-term results of a randomised trial. *Radiother Oncol*. 2005;75(1):9–17. doi:10.1016/j.radonc.2005.01.005

62. Haviland JS, Owen JR, Dewar JA, et al. The UK standardisation of breast radiotherapy (START) trials of radiotherapy hypofractionation for treatment of early breast cancer: 10-year follow-up results of two randomised controlled trials. *Lancet Oncol*. 2013;14(11):1086–1094. doi:10.1016/S1470-2045(13)70386-3

63. Whelan TJ, Pignol JP, Levine MN, et al. Long-term results of hypofractionated radiation therapy for breast cancer. *N Engl J Med*. 2010;362(6):513–520. doi:10.1056/NEJMoa0906260

64. Brunt AM, Haviland JS, Sydenham M, et al. Ten-year results of FAST: a randomized controlled trial of 5-fraction whole-breast radiotherapy for early breast cancer. *J Clin Oncol*. 2020;38(28):3261–3272. doi:10.1200/JCO.19.02750

65. Murray Brunt A, Haviland JS, Wheatley DA, et al. Hypofractionated breast radiotherapy for 1 week versus 3 weeks (FAST-Forward): 5-year efficacy and late normal tissue effects results from a

multicentre, non-inferiority, randomised, phase 3 trial. *Lancet.* 2020;395(10237):1613–1626. doi:10.1016/S0140-6736(20)30932-6

66. Bartelink H, Horiot JC, Poortmans PM, et al. Impact of a higher radiation dose on local control and survival in breast-conserving therapy of early breast cancer: 10-year results of the randomized boost versus no boost EORTC 22881-10882 trial. *J Clin Oncol.* 2007;25(22):3259–3265. doi:10.1200/JCO.2007.11.4991

67. Romestaing P, Lehingue Y, Carrie C, et al. Role of a 10-Gy boost in the conservative treatment of early breast cancer: results of a randomized clinical trial in Lyon, France. *J Clin Oncol.* 1997;15(3):963–968. doi:10.1200/JCO.1997.15.3.963

68. Bartelink H, Maingon P, Poortmans P, et al. Whole-breast irradiation with or without a boost for patients treated with breast-conserving surgery for early breast cancer: 20-year follow-up of a randomised phase 3 trial. *Lancet Oncol.* 2015;16(1):47–56. doi:10.1016/S1470-2045(14)71156-8

69. Vrieling C, van Werkhoven E, Maingon P, et al. Prognostic factors for local control in breast cancer after long-term follow-up in the EORTC boost vs no boost trial: a randomized clinical trial. *JAMA Oncol.* 2017;3(1):42–48. doi:10.1001/jamaoncol.2016.3031

70. Donovan E, Bleakley N, Denholm E, et al. Randomised trial of standard 2D radiotherapy (RT) versus intensity modulated radiotherapy (IMRT) in patients prescribed breast radiotherapy. *Radiother Oncol.* 2007;82(3):254–264. doi:10.1016/j.radonc.2006.12.008

71. Pignol JP, Olivotto I, Rakovitch E, et al. A multicenter randomized trial of breast intensity-modulated radiation therapy to reduce acute radiation dermatitis. *J Clin Oncol.* 2008;26(13):2085–2092. doi:10.1200/JCO.2007.15.2488

72. Darby SC, Ewertz M, McGale P, et al. Risk of ischemic heart disease in women after radiotherapy for breast cancer. *N Engl J Med.* 2013;368(11):987–998. doi:10.1056/NEJMoa1209825

73. Darby SC, McGale P, Taylor CW, Peto R. Long-term mortality from heart disease and lung cancer after radiotherapy for early breast cancer: prospective cohort study of about 300,000 women in US SEER cancer registries. *Lancet Oncol.* 2005;6(8):557–565. doi:10.1016/S1470-2045(05)70251-5

74. Rutter CE, Chagpar AB, Evans SB. Breast cancer laterality does not influence survival in a large modern cohort: implications for radiation-related cardiac mortality. *Int J Radiat Oncol Biol Phys.* 2014;90(2):329–334. doi:10.1016/j.ijrobp.2014.06.030

75. Karimi AM, Tom MC, Manyam BV, et al. Evaluating improvements in cardiac dosimetry in breast radiotherapy and comparison of cardiac sparing techniques. *J Radiat Oncol.* 2019;8:305–310. doi:10.1007/s13566-019-00400-3

76. Fisher B, Bryant J, Dignam JJ, et al. Tamoxifen, radiation therapy, or both for prevention of ipsilateral breast tumor recurrence after lumpectomy in women with invasive breast cancers of one centimeter or less. *J Clin Oncol.* 2002;20(20):4141–4149. doi:10.1200/JCO.2002.11.101

77. Hughes KS, Schnaper LA, Bellon JR, et al. Lumpectomy plus tamoxifen with or without irradiation in women age 70 years or older with early breast cancer: long-term follow-up of CALGB 9343. *J Clin Oncol.* 2013;31(19):2382–2387. doi:10.1200/JCO.2012.45.2615

78. Kunkler IH, Williams LJ, Jack WJ, Cameron DA, Dixon JM, investigators PI. Breast-conserving surgery with or without irradiation in women aged 65 years or older with early breast cancer (PRIME II): a randomised controlled trial. *Lancet Oncol.* 2015;16(3):266–273. doi:10.1016/S1470-2045(14)71221-5

79. Fyles AW, McCready DR, Manchul LA, et al. Tamoxifen with or without breast irradiation in women 50 years of age or older with early breast cancer. *N Engl J Med.* 2004;351(10):963–970. doi:10.1056/NEJMoa040595

80. Winzer KJ, Sauerbrei W, Braun M, et al. Radiation therapy and tamoxifen after breast-conserving surgery: updated results of a 2 × 2 randomised clinical trial in patients with low risk of recurrence. *Eur J Cancer.* 2010;46(1):95–101. doi:10.1016/j.ejca.2009.10.007

81. Potter R, Gnant M, Kwasny W, et al. Lumpectomy plus tamoxifen or anastrozole with or without whole breast irradiation in women with favorable early breast cancer. *Int J Radiat Oncol Biol Phys.* 2007;68(2):334–340. doi:10.1016/j.ijrobp.2006.12.045

82. Whelan TJ, Smith S, Parpia S, et al. Omitting radiotherapy after breast-conserving surgery in luminal a breast cancer. *N Engl J Med.* 2023;389(7):612–619. doi:10.1056/NEJMoa2302344

83. Jagsi R, Griffith KA, Harris EE, et al. Omission of radiotherapy after breast-conserving surgery for women with breast cancer with low clinical and genomic risk: 5-year outcomes of IDEA. *J Clin Oncol.* 2024; 42(4):390–398. doi:10.1200/JCO.23.02270

84. Shah C, Vicini F, Shaitelman SF, et al. The American brachytherapy society consensus statement for accelerated partial-breast irradiation. *Brachytherapy.* 2018;17(1):154–170. doi:10.1016/j.brachy.2017.09.004

85. Correa C, Harris EE, Leonardi MC, et al. Accelerated partial breast irradiation: executive summary for the update of an ASTRO evidence-based consensus statement. *Pract Radiat Oncol.* 2017;7(2):73–79. doi:10.1016/j.prro.2016.09.007

86. Gage I, Recht A, Gelman R, et al. Long-term outcome following breast-conserving surgery and radiation therapy. *Int J Radiat Oncol Biol Phys.* 1995;33(2):245–251. doi:10.1016/0360-3016(95)02001-R

87. Vicini FA, Kestin LL, Goldstein NS. Defining the clinical target volume for patients with early-stage breast cancer treated with lumpectomy and accelerated partial breast irradiation: a pathologic analysis. *Int J Radiat Oncol Biol Phys*. 2004;60(3):722–730. doi:10.1016/j.ijrobp.2004.04.012

88. Vicini F, Shah C, Tendulkar R, et al. Accelerated partial breast irradiation: an update on published level I evidence. *Brachytherapy*. 2016;15(5):607–615. doi:10.1016/j.brachy.2016.06.007

89. Morrow M, White J, Moughan J, et al. Factors predicting the use of breast-conserving therapy in stage I and II breast carcinoma. *J Clin Oncol*. 2001;19(8):2254–2262. doi:10.1200/JCO.2001.19.8.2254

90. Shaitelman SF, Anderson BM, Arthur DW, et al. Partial breast irradiation for patients with early-stage invasive breast cancer or ductal carcinoma in situ: an ASTRO clinical practice guideline. *Pract Radiat Oncol*. 2024;14(2):112–132. doi:10.1016/j.prro.2023.11.001

91. Polgar C, Fodor J, Major T, Sulyok Z, Kasler M. Breast-conserving therapy with partial or whole breast irradiation: ten-year results of the Budapest randomized trial. *Radiother Oncol*. 2013;108(2):197–202. doi:10.1016/j.radonc.2013.05.008

92. Polgar C, Ott OJ, Hildebrandt G, et al. Late side-effects and cosmetic results of accelerated partial breast irradiation with interstitial brachytherapy versus whole-breast irradiation after breast-conserving surgery for low-risk invasive and in-situ carcinoma of the female breast: 5-year results of a randomised, controlled, phase 3 trial. *Lancet Oncol*. 2017;18(2):259–268. doi:10.1016/S1470-2045(17)30011-6

93. Strnad V, Ott OJ, Hildebrandt G, et al. 5-year results of accelerated partial breast irradiation using sole interstitial multicatheter brachytherapy versus whole-breast irradiation with boost after breast-conserving surgery for low-risk invasive and in-situ carcinoma of the female breast: a randomised, phase 3, non-inferiority trial. *Lancet*. 2016;387(10015):229–238. doi:10.1016/S0140-6736(15)00471-7

94. Whelan TJ, Julian JA, Berrang TS, et al. External beam accelerated partial breast irradiation versus whole breast irradiation after breast conserving surgery in women with ductal carcinoma in situ and node-negative breast cancer (RAPID): a randomised controlled trial. *Lancet*. 2019;394(10215):2165–2172. doi:10.1016/S0140-6736(19)32515-2

95. Liss AL, Ben-David MA, Jagsi R, et al. Decline of cosmetic outcomes following accelerated partial breast irradiation using intensity modulated radiation therapy: results of a single-institution prospective clinical trial. *Int J Radiat Oncol Biol Phys*. 2014;89(1):96–102. doi:10.1016/j.ijrobp.2014.01.005

96. Hepel JT, Tokita M, MacAusland SG, et al. Toxicity of three-dimensional conformal radiotherapy for accelerated partial breast irradiation. *Int J Radiat Oncol Biol Phys*. 2009;75(5):1290–1296. doi:10.1016/j.ijrobp.2009.01.009

97. Chafe S, Moughan J, McCormick B, et al. Late toxicity and patient self-assessment of breast appearance/satisfaction on RTOG 0319: a phase 2 trial of 3-dimensional conformal radiation therapy-accelerated partial breast irradiation following lumpectomy for stages I and II breast cancer. *Int J Radiat Oncol Biol Phys*. 2013;86(5):854–859. doi:10.1016/j.ijrobp.2013.04.005

98. Meattini I, Marrazzo L, Saieva C, et al. Accelerated partial-breast irradiation compared with whole-breast irradiation for early breast cancer: long-term results of the randomized phase III APBI-IMRT-florence trial. *J Clin Oncol*. 2020;38(35):4175–4183. doi:10.1200/JCO.20.00650

99. Polgar C, Major T, Takacsi-Nagy Z, Fodor J. Breast-conserving surgery followed by partial or whole breast irradiation: twenty-year results of a phase 3 clinical study. *Int J Radiat Oncol Biol Phys*. 2021;109(4):998–1006. doi:10.1016/j.ijrobp.2020.11.006

100. Strnad V, Polgar C, Ott OJ, et al. Accelerated partial breast irradiation using sole interstitial multicatheter brachytherapy compared with whole-breast irradiation with boost for early breast cancer: 10-year results of a GEC-ESTRO randomised, phase 3, non-inferiority trial. *Lancet Oncol*. 2023;24(3):262–272. doi:10.1016/S1470-2045(23)00018-9

101. Rodriguez N, Sanz X, Dengra J, et al. Five-year outcomes, cosmesis, and toxicity with 3-dimensional conformal external beam radiation therapy to deliver accelerated partial breast irradiation. *Int J Radiat Oncol Biol Phys*. 2013;87(5):1051–1057. doi:10.1016/j.ijrobp.2013.08.046

102. Coles CE, Griffin CL, Kirby AM, et al. Partial-breast radiotherapy after breast conservation surgery for patients with early breast cancer (UK IMPORT LOW trial): 5-year results from a multicentre, randomised, controlled, phase 3, non-inferiority trial. *Lancet*. 2017;390(10099):1048–1060. doi:10.1016/S0140-6736(17)31145-5

103. Offersen BV, Alsner J, Nielsen HM, et al. Partial breast irradiation versus whole breast irradiation for early breast cancer patients in a randomized phase III trial: the danish breast cancer group partial breast irradiation trial. *J Clin Oncol*. 2022;40(36):4189–4197. doi:10.1200/JCO.22.00451

104. Meduri B, Baldissera A, Iotti C, et al. Cosmetic results and side effects of accelerated partial-breast irradiation versus whole-breast irradiation for low-risk invasive carcinoma of the breast: the randomized phase III IRMA trial. *J Clin Oncol*. 2023;41(12):2201–2210. doi:10.1200/JCO.22.01485

105. Polgar C, Major T, Fodor J, et al. Accelerated partial-breast irradiation using high-dose-rate interstitial brachytherapy: 12-year update of a prospective clinical study. *Radiother Oncol*. 2010;94(3):274–279. doi:10.1016/j.radonc.2010.01.019

106. Shah C, Antonucci JV, Wilkinson JB, et al. Twelve-year clinical outcomes and patterns of failure with accelerated partial breast irradiation versus whole-breast irradiation: results of a matched-pair analysis. *Radiother Oncol.* 2011;100(2):210–214. doi:10.1016/j.radonc.2011.03.011

107. Benitez PR, Keisch ME, Vicini F, et al. Five-year results: the initial clinical trial of MammoSite balloon brachytherapy for partial breast irradiation in early-stage breast cancer. *Am J Surg.* 2007;194(4):456–462. doi:10.1016/j.amjsurg.2007.06.010

108. Shah C, Badiyan S, Ben Wilkinson J, et al. Treatment efficacy with Accelerated Partial Breast Irradiation (APBI): final analysis of the American society of breast surgeons MammoSite(®) breast brachytherapy registry trial. *Ann Surg Oncol.* 2013;20(10):3279–3285. doi:10.1245/s10434-013-3158-4

109. Shah C, Khwaja S, Badiyan S, et al. Brachytherapy-based partial breast irradiation is associated with low rates of complications and excellent cosmesis. *Brachytherapy.* 2013;12(4):278–284. doi:10.1016/j.brachy.2013.04.005

110. Cuttino LW, Arthur DW, Vicini F, Todor D, Julian T, Mukhopadhyay N. Long-term results from the Contura multilumen balloon breast brachytherapy catheter phase 4 registry trial. *Int J Radiat Oncol Biol Phys.* 2014;90(5):1025–1029. doi:10.1016/j.ijrobp.2014.08.341

111. Yashar C, Attai D, Butler E, et al. Strut-based accelerated partial breast irradiation: report of treatment results for 250 consecutive patients at 5 years from a multicenter retrospective study. *Brachytherapy.* 2016;15(6):780–787. doi:10.1016/j.brachy.2016.07.002

Adannia N. Ufondu, Yvonne D. Pham, Rahul D. Tendulkar, and Chirag Shah

QUICK HIT Locally advanced breast cancer (LABC) is characterized by advanced tumor (T3 or T4) or nodal stage (N2 or N3), generally including clinical stage IIB (T3N0) to stage III. Patients are commonly treated with neoadjuvant CHT, followed by surgery and adjuvant RT (Table 25.1). Inflammatory breast cancer (IBC) represents an aggressive subset of LABC.

Table 25.1 General Treatment Paradigm of LABC	
Neoadjuvant chemotherapy (NACT)	Associated with high rates (up to 60%) of pCR for certain biological subsets and can allow for cosmetically acceptable surgery, but it has similar DFS and OS compared with adjuvant CHT; pCR associated with improved outcomes. For HER2+ disease, add trastuzumab and pertuzumab to CHT. In TNBC, neoadjuvant and adjuvant pembrolizumab has been shown to improve OS, pCR rates, and EFS. Response to neoadjuvant therapy directs need and agents for adjuvant treatment.
Surgery	Performed 3–6 weeks after completing NACT. Usually, TM with ALND, although LABC is not a contraindication to breast-conserving therapy (BCT) or SLNB, when appropriate.
RT	Initiated ~4–6 weeks following surgery (or CHT if given adjuvantly). Indications for postmastectomy radiation therapy (PMRT) are generally based on initial clinical stage rather than response to neoadjuvant CHT. However, with results of B-51, omission of RNI can be considered in those with cN1 disease who convert to ypN0. PMRT is indicated for clinical or pathologic stage III and is controversial for stage II (N1 or T3 alone).

EPIDEMIOLOGY: Approximately 25% of new breast cancer diagnoses are locally advanced at presentation.[1] From 2012 to 2019, the incidence of LABC declined by 0.8% per year, which may reflect a shift toward earlier stage at diagnosis.[2] LABC includes heterogeneous presentations. Some LABC cases present between routine screening mammograms and represent disease with a rapid growth rate. This is particularly true for IBC, which accounts for ~2% of all new breast malignancies and is slightly more common in African Americans than in Caucasians.[3] LABC also includes patients with slow-growing, neglected tumors that have become extensive over time. With this heterogeneous group, there are no clear unique risk factors. However, young/premenopausal women and African Americans are more likely to present with LABC.[4]

RISK FACTORS, ANATOMY, PATHOLOGY, GENETICS, SCREENING: See Chapter 24 for details.

CLINICAL PRESENTATION: Breast masses are typically found by self-breast exam, mammogram, or clinical exam, and are rarely painful (~5%). Lesions present late (T3/T4) usually due to lack of screening, delay due to patient neglect or misdiagnosis, or aggressive tumor biology. Other signs may include axillary adenopathy, skin erythema, dimpling, nipple retraction, bloody discharge, or change in size or shape of the breast. IBC is a clinical diagnosis that requires erythema and dermal edema (peau d'orange) of ≥⅓ of the breast, which develops in ≤6 months and includes rapid enlargement of the breast, generalized induration in the presence or absence of a distinct breast mass, and a biopsy-proven carcinoma. The pathologic hallmark for IBC is tumor emboli within the dermal lymphatics (present in 50%–75% of cases), but it is neither sufficient nor required for diagnosis of IBC. Occult dermal lymphatic invasion without clinical signs of IBC is unusual (<2% of cases).[5] Patients with IBC are more frequently hormone receptor-negative and HER2+ than other breast cancers; most are LN-positive and ~30% present with DM.

WORKUP: H&P with attention to extent of disease, especially the extent of skin involvement if IBC (photo documentation), assess mobility/fixation of the tumor and LNs. As many patients will receive NACT, it is important to assess and document extent of disease prior to therapy.

Labs: CBC, CMP, alkaline phosphatase.

Imaging: Bilateral mammograms and ultrasound as necessary. MRI of the breast is commonly performed to assess the locoregional extent of disease. For clinical stage IIIA and higher (T3N1, T4, or N2) or triple-negative stage II (i.e., T2N1) patients, order CT chest/abdomen/pelvis and bone scan or PET/CT for identifying unsuspected regional nodal disease and/or DM.[6] Additional imaging may include an MRI brain if neurologic symptoms are present, and plain films of areas of increased uptake on bone scan.

Procedures: Core needle biopsy (full thickness of skin for IBC) rather than FNA for determination of ER/PR and HER2 status.

Other: Echocardiography to evaluate left ventricular ejection fraction (LVEF) prior to anthracycline CHT (Adriamycin contraindicated with LVEF <30%–35%; cardiotoxicity seen after cumulative dose of 450–500 mg/m²) and trastuzumab-containing regimens.[7]

PROGNOSTIC FACTORS: Negative prognostic factors include LN involvement (most important), young age, smoking, African American race, presentation in pregnancy, palpable mass, extensive erythema, IBC, high grade, LVSI, positive margins, high Oncotype DX 21-gene Recurrence Score®, ER-negative, incomplete response to NACT.

STAGING: See Chapter 24 for AJCC staging system.

TREATMENT PARADIGM

In general, CHT and RT are indicated for almost all LABC cases. CHT is commonly delivered neoadjuvantly, while RT is reserved for the adjuvant setting, outside of unresectable situations. For IBC, treat with trimodality therapy including NACT, mastectomy, and PMRT (regardless of response to NACT).

Chemotherapy: Nodal positivity was generally an indication for cytotoxic CHT. However, Oncotype DX 21-gene Recurrence Score® has shown to be predictive of benefit of CHT for hormone-positive, HER2– patients, and has been incorporated into current guidelines.[8,9] The RxPONDER (SWOG S1007) trial included over 5,000 pre- and postmenopausal women with hormone receptor-positive, HER2– breast cancer with one to three positive axillary nodes and a recurrence score of ≤25, randomizing them to endocrine therapy only or to adjuvant CHT + endocrine therapy. In postmenopausal women, there was no benefit derived from CHT, but in premenopausal women, 5-year invasive DFS was improved in CHT-endocrine group (94% vs. 89%) conferring a distant RFS benefit of 2.5% for CHT.[10]

Neoadjuvant CHT/IO: There is no difference in DFS or OS between NACT or adjuvant CHT,[11,12] but NACT may help make upfront inoperable disease more amenable to surgery, improve cosmetic outcomes following surgery, and direct adjuvant therapy based on response to neoadjuvant therapy. Patients who are diagnosed during pregnancy and unable to have surgery may also benefit from NACT. The choice of a specific NACT regimen is based on tumor biology. A common regimen for hormone receptor-positive/HER2– patients is dose-dense AC-T, which consists of doxorubicin and cyclophosphamide (CYC) q2 weeks for four cycles followed by weekly paclitaxel for 12 weeks. Docetaxel and CYC (TC) is an option for patients with contraindications to anthracyclines. Docetaxel and carboplatin are used in combination with trastuzumab and pertuzumab (TCHP) for HER2+ patients. For stage II/III TNBC patients, the addition of neoadjuvant and adjuvant pembrolizumab to NACT improves OS, pCR rates, and EFS per the KEYNOTE-522 trial. The response is independent of PD-L1 status.[13–15] TNBC and HER2+ subtypes have the highest likelihood of pCR, generally 50% to 60%,[16,17] while ER-positive tumors have pCR rates closer to 15% to 25%.[18] Patients with pCR have significant improvements in DFS (HR 0.48) and OS (HR 0.48) compared with those with residual disease.[19,20] Patients without pCR to NACT may undergo additional adjuvant systemic therapy.

Adjuvant CHT: Following NACT and surgery, adjuvant CHT is based on biology and response to NACT. In patients with hormone receptor+/HER2– disease and pCR, no adjuvant systemic therapy is indicated. In patients with the hormone receptor+/HER2– disease without pCR, consider CDK4/6 inhibitors where eligible. Options include ribociclib, abemaciclib, and palbociclib.

In patients with HER2+ disease (regardless of hormone receptor status) with pCR, trastuzumab ± pertuzumab is indicated (if N+ at initial staging, then include pertuzumab). In HER2+ patients with residual disease, the KATHERINE trial found adjuvant trastuzumab emtansine (T-DM1) improved invasive DFS.[21] In patients with TNBC, adjuvant pembrolizumab is indicated, as discussed above per KEYNOTE-522 trial. In HER2– patients without pCR who did not receive neoadjuvant CHT/IO, consider the use of capecitabine per the CREATE-X trial, which found an OS benefit to six to eight cycles of adjuvant capecitabine (benefit was greatest in TNBC).[22] Olaparib is used in patients with germline BRCA1/2 mutation in the adjuvant or recurrent setting.

Surgery: Radio-opaque clips should be placed in the tumor to aid in planning of locoregional treatment and subsequent pathologic assessment (facilitates locoregional treatment should a CR to CHT occur). For suspicion of an involved axillary LN, perform FNA and/or core needle biopsy with placement of a radio-opaque clip.

Surgery is typically performed 3 to 6 weeks after completing NACT and usually consists of mastectomy with axillary surgery (either SLNB or ALND based on clinical extent of axillary disease and pathologic nodal status). ALND involves levels I and II; level III may be dissected if disease is apparent in level I or II. For the initially cN0 axilla, a negative SLNB is generally sufficient.[23] Clinically N1 women with CR to NACT may be considered for SLNB alone to avoid ALND, assuming SLNB shows no residual nodal disease and multiple SLNs map.[24] If SLNB is positive after NACT, ALND should be performed. LABC is not a contraindication to BCT, but it must be undertaken with caution. At least one PRT has shown BCT after NACT does not decrease OS, but IBTR is higher in patients who were downstaged to be eligible for BCT.[25]

Radiation

Indications: Indications for PMRT generally include clinical stage III prior to NACT (can consider omission of RNI in cN1 patients who convert to ypN0 after NACT per B-51), residual LN+ after NACT, or pathologic stage III. PMRT is controversial for pT3N0 or pT1–2N1 patients who do not undergo NACT.[26] PMRT generally includes RT to the chest wall as well as comprehensive regional nodal irradiation (RNI) to the axilla, supraclavicular LNs, and internal mammary nodes (IMNs). Historical indications for treating the full axilla with a posterior axillary boost (PAB) are based on risk factors for subsequent axillary recurrence: gross extranodal extension, ≥10 +LNs, >50% +LN nodal ratio, or undissected axilla. IM nodal RT has historically been controversial over the rarity of documented IM nodal failures and concerns about cardiotoxicity, but it was performed in all the classic PMRT trials. Updated data from the Danish trial and from a meta-analysis show improved OS with IMN RT for patients with pN+ disease, without significant increases in cardiac or pneumonitis events.[27–29] Indications for IMN RT may include clinically positive IM nodes, central/medial tumor location, and/or axillary LN+ disease. Risk of IM nodal positivity rules of thumb: medial tumor with (+) axilla: 50%; lateral with (+) axilla: 25%; medial with (–) axilla: 15%; lateral with (–) axilla: 5%. RT usually initiated 4 to 6 weeks following surgery or CHT (whichever is last) provided adequate healing has taken place. In the KATHERINE trial, patients receiving adjuvant T-DM1 received concurrent RT, while CREATE-X allowed for RT to be delivered either before or after capecitabine. Both allowed concurrent use of endocrine therapy with RT.

Dose: Conventional dose to chest wall and regional LNs is 50 Gy/25 fx; however, a Chinese randomized trial demonstrated noninferiority with moderately hypofractionated PMRT (43.5 Gy/15 fx) in patients without breast reconstruction,[30] and the Alliance A221505/RT CHARM trial (results presented at ASTRO 2024) demonstrated a moderately hypofractionated course (42.56 Gy/16 fx) was noninferior with regard to reconstruction complications, consistent with the FABREC trial data.[31,32] Given these studies, there is no clear role for conventional fractionation in the postmastectomy setting outside of IBC or gross residual disease requiring boosts. Recent retrospective data and ESTRO consensus recommendations demonstrate that the use of bolus is not associated with increased LC.[33,34] Clinical indications for bolus include mastectomy for DCIS or invasive cancer with positive anterior margin without overlying skin removed, skin involvement or IBC, chest wall recurrence, inoperable breast cancer, or fungating mass. If margins are close or positive, consider boost to 60 Gy (conventional fractionation) and boost gross residual (unresectable) disease to ≥66 Gy.

Procedure: See *Handbook of Treatment Planning in Radiation Oncology,* Chapter 5.

EVIDENCE-BASED Q&A

What are the current indications for PMRT?

Based on ASCO guidelines[35] from 2001, in the setting of adjuvant CHT, PMRT is recommended for patho-logic stage III patients: T3N1, N2–N3, T4. The most recent guidelines from ASCO/ASTRO/SSO published in 2016 are outlined below and recommend PMRT in patients with axillary nodal involvement after neoad-juvant systemic therapy and consideration of PMRT in patients with T1–2 breast cancer with 1 to 3 +LNs. NCCN recommends PMRT for patients with ≥4 axillary LNs (stage pN2–N3), positive margins if re-resec-tion is not feasible, multiple high-risk recurrence factors including central/medial tumors or tumors ≥2 cm, and at least one of the following: grade 3, ER-negative, or LVI. NSABP B-51 showed similar 5-year invasive breast cancer RFS in patients with node-positive breast cancer who converted to node-negative after NACT regardless of RNI (see below).

Recht, ASCO/ASTRO/SSO Guidelines (*JCO* 2016, PMID 27646947): PMRT for patients with pT1–2N1 reduces LRF, any recurrence, and BCM, but PMRT should be used only if expected ben-efits outweigh potential toxicity risks. PMRT indicated for patients who are ypN+ (any T) after NACT. For patients who are cN0 before NACT or have a pCR in the axilla, there is insufficient evidence to recommend for or against PMRT, and it is recommended to enroll these patients into clinical trials (see updated info on B-51). When PMRT is used, it should routinely include the chest wall/reconstructed breast, supraclavicular-axillary apical nodes, and IMNs, although there are subgroups that may not derive benefit from treating all nodal regions.

What are the classic data on recurrence patterns after mastectomy and adjuvant CHT?

There were two landmark pooled analyses (EORTC and NSABP) that defined high-risk factors for recur-rence and patterns of failure after mastectomy and adjuvant CHT for LN+ patients. The common risk fac-tors between these two trials were large tumors and ≥4 LN+. The ECOG pooled analysis (trials from 1978 to 1982)[36] demonstrated the following risk factors as portending at least 10% risk of LRR within 3 years: tumor >5 cm, ≥4 LN+, ER-negative, tumor necrosis, and pectoral fascia involvement. The NSABP pooled analysis (notably 90% received doxorubicin-based CHT ± tamoxifen) also demonstrated large tumors and ≥4 LN+ as high-risk factors as well as age, premenopausal status, and number of dissected LN. Of the recurrences, ≥50% were in the chest wall, 23% in the SCV LN, 12% in the axilla, and <1% in the parasternal/subclav-icular areas.[37] In 2023, an analysis of EORTC 22922 was published in which the locations of the local and regional recurrences were mapped and analyzed by treatment type. At 15 years, the LR rate was 7% for BCS and 3% for mastectomy. Overall, the absolute benefit of RT in preventing LRR increased with stage and less extensive surgery. After RNI, recurrence location was found to be distributed as follows: axilla: 1.7%; supraclavicular: 1.6%; IMN: 0.2%. Without RNI, recurrence distribution: axilla: 2.4%; supraclavicular: 2.5%; IMN: 0.8%.[38]

What is the benefit of PMRT after adjuvant CHT?

In historical trials using older CHT regimens (British Columbia Cancer Agency, Danish Breast Cancer Cooperative Group 82b/82c), PMRT was demonstrated to have a survival benefit in high-risk patients and particularly those with N+ disease.[39–43] An older EBCTCG meta-analysis reviewing 22 RCTs from 1964 to 1986 found that PMRT improved 10-year LRR and 20-year BCM in pN+ patients, but there was no benefit to PMRT in node-negative patients.[44,45] In the modern era, the risk of LRR in pT1–2N1 patients without PMRT is less (<10%) compared with historical series (20%–30%), and so this remains a contro-versial subgroup. One large multi-institutional review/nomogram found a benefit to PMRT with respect to LRR and overall recurrence. In addition, new data show a survival advantage to RNI for pN1 and pN2 patients.[46]

Sittenfeld, Multi-Institutional Nomogram (*Cancer* 2022, PMID 35713598): RR of 3,532 patients with pT1–2N1M0 breast cancer after mastectomy without neoadjuvant CHT. At MFU of 6.8 years, 61% of patients had received PMRT and these patients had significantly more adverse risk factors than those who did not receive PMRT. PMRT was found to have a benefit in LRR and overall recurrence on competing risk regression analysis (HR 0.21 and 0.76, respectively, SS). **Conclusion: PMRT is associated with decreased LRR and overall recurrence in patients with pT1–2N1 breast cancer after accounting for competing risks.** *Comment: Adverse risk factors were defined as younger age, larger tumors, more positive LNs, LVI, ECE, and positive margins.*

EBCTCG Meta-Analysis (*Lancet* 2023, PMID 37931633): Meta-analysis of 16 trials, consisting of 14,324 participants, showed that RNI significantly reduced recurrence in those receiving PORT to the breast or chest wall, especially distant recurrence, as well as reduced BCM and ACM. The 15-year BCM reduction with RNI was 1.6% in patients with 0 positive nodes, 2.7% in patients with 1 to 3 nodes, and 4.5% for those with ≥4 nodes. Of note, the benefits seen in the meta-analysis were observed in the newer trials included in the study. The older trials (1961–1978) showed no benefit to RNI. **Conclusion: RNI significantly improves mortality in patients receiving PORT to the breast or chest wall.**

Do some N0 patients benefit from PMRT?

The utility of PMRT for pT3N0 patients is controversial. Conflicting evidence shows some cohorts with LRF rates <10% after mastectomy and systemic therapy, while others show elevated risk. The MGH cohort defined several risk factors for LRR (T >2 cm, margin <2 mm, premenopausal status, LVI); however, other studies did not include these variables in their analyses. See Table 25.2 for further details.

Table 25.2 Studies Evaluating Benefit of PMRT in Node-Negative LABC				
Study	Population (*N*, Stage)	MFU	Outcome	Recommendation
MGH, Jagsi (2005)[47]	877, N0	8 yrs	10-yr LRR 6% without PMRT (range 1%–41% depending on number of risk factors)	N0 patients with multiple risk factors may benefit from PMRT. Risk factors: close margins, T2+, premenopausal status, LVI.
NSABP Pooled Analysis, Taghian (2006)[48]	313, T3N0	15 yrs	10-yr cumulative incidence isolated LRF 7% without PMRT; 6% in those who received CHT	LRF remains low; PMRT should not be routinely used.
MGH, Floyd (2006)[49]	70, T3N0	7 yrs	5-yr LRF 8% without PMRT; LVI associated with LRF, OS, and DFS	PMRT not indicated, can consider in patients with LVI.
Canadian, Goulart (2011)[50]	100, T3N0	10 yrs	10-yr LRR 2% in PMRT group and 9% in no-PMRT group (NS); all patients with LRR in no-PMRT group had G3 disease and no hormonal therapy	PMRT not indicated; consider for G3 and those not getting hormones.
MDACC, Nagar (2011)[51]	162, cT3N0	6 yrs	5-yr LRR 4% in PMRT group vs. 24% in no-PMRT group (SS); ypN+ associated with LRR	PMRT reduces LRR and should be considered **45% of patients were found to have residual ypN+ disease even after NACT.*
SEER, Johnson (2014)[52]	2,525, T3N0	8 yrs	PMRT improved OS (77% vs. 62%, SS) and CSS (85% vs. 84%, S)	PMRT should be considered.

What is the role of PMRT for patients with a TNBC molecular subtype?

Women with TNBC have an aggressive clinical course (early relapse, higher incidence of visceral and brain metastases, and relatively poor prognosis compared with other subtypes), so some consider PMRT in these patients even with earlier stage disease.

Wang, China (*Radiother Oncol* 2011, PMID 21852010): Multicenter PRT of 681 women with TNBC stage I to II (82% N0) s/p mastectomy randomized to systemic CHT ± PMRT (50 Gy/25 fx ± RNI as clinically indicated). At MFU of 7.2 years, PMRT improved the 5-year RFS (75%–88%, *p* = .02) and 5-year OS (79% vs. 90%, *p* = .03). **Conclusion: Adjuvant CHT plus RT was more effective than CHT alone in women with early-stage TNBC after mastectomy.** *Comment: Independent confirmation would be valuable to confirm the role of PMRT in LN-negative TNBC.*

What is the preferred sequencing of CHT, neoadjuvant or adjuvant?

There is no difference in DFS or OS between neoadjuvant or adjuvant CHT. NACT is associated with high rates of pathologic response and a higher likelihood for allowing a cosmetically acceptable surgery. With NACT, there is downstaging of the tumor and involved axillary LNs with an increased opportunity for BCT, as well as allows for response-based adjuvant systemic therapy.

Fisher, NSABP B-18 (*JCO* 1997, PMID 9215816; Update *JCO* 1998, PMID 9704717; Wolmark, *J Natl Cancer Inst Monogr* 2001, PMID 11773300; Rastogi, *JCO* 2008, PMID 18258986): PRT of 1,523 patients with operable breast cancer (T1–3N0–1M0) randomized to preop AC × 4C vs. postop AC × 4C (q3 weeks). Tamoxifen (10 mg BID × 5 years) was given to all patients ≥50 years regardless of ER status (status unknown for many patients). All patients who had a lumpectomy received RT to 50 Gy. The results are in Table 25.3. Breast tumor size decreased in 80% of patients after preoperative therapy; 36% clinical CR, 43% clinical PR, and 13% pathologic CR (pCR). Patients with pCR had significantly improved DFS (HR 0.47, $p < .0001$) and OS (HR 0.32, $p < .0001$) vs. patients who did not have a pCR. MVA showed that posttreatment pathologic nodal status was also a strong predictor of OS and DFS ($p < .0001$). IBTR was greater in the preop group who had BCT due to downstaging vs. patients who were planned to have BCT (15% vs. 7%, $p = .04$).[18] **Conclusion: Preoperative CHT is equivalent to adjuvant CHT in regard to OS and DFS.**

Table 25.3 NSABP B-18 Results (16-Yr Data)					
	pN+	BCS Rate	IBTR	DFS	OS
Preop CHT	42%	68%	13%	42%	55%
Postop CHT	58%	60%	10%	39%	55%
p value	.001	.001	.21	.27	.90

Van Der Hage, EORTC 10902 (*JCO* 2001, PMID 11709566; Update Van Nes, *Breast Cancer Res Treat* 2009, PMID 18484198): PRT of 698 patients with operable breast cancer (T1c–T3, T4b, N0–1M0) comparing preop FEC (5-FU, epirubicin, cyclophosphamide) × 4C vs. postop FEC × 4C. All patients who had BCT received RT to 50 Gy to breast and 45 Gy to IM nodes and SCV. Tamoxifen 20 mg QD given to all patients ≥50 years regardless of ER status. Tumors were assessed by clinical and mammographic evaluation. MFU at 10 years. No difference in OS, DFS, or LRR between groups. NACT improves the rate of BCT compared with adjuvant CHT (35% vs. 22%, respectively). **Conclusion: NACT does not lead to a detriment in OS or DFS compared with adjuvant CHT.**

Which patients are at increased risk for LRR after NACT?

Mamounas, Combined NSABP B-18 and B-27 (*JCO* 2012, PMID 23032615): Combined analysis of NSABP B-18 and B-27; included 3,088 patients with cT1–3, N0–N1 patients. NACT was either AC alone or AC followed by neoadjuvant/adjuvant docetaxel. Lumpectomy patients received breast RT alone, while mastectomy patients did not undergo PMRT. The 10-year cumulative LRR rate in mastectomy patients was 12% (9% local; 3% regional); predictors of LRR on MVA included clinical tumor size >5 cm (before NACT), clinical N+ (before NACT), and incomplete pathologic response in the breast or axillary LNs. For lumpectomy patients, the LRR was 10% (8% local; 2% regional); predictors of LRR included age <50, clinical N+ (before NACT), and incomplete pathologic response in the breast or axillary LNs. **Conclusion: The 10-year risk of LRR is significant after NACT (≥10%). Tumor size >5 cm, positive axillary LNs, younger age, and incomplete response to NACT portend a higher risk of LRR and can be used to optimize use of adjuvant RT.**

In those groups with an increased risk for LRR after NACT, which studies show a benefit to adding RT?

Huang, MDACC (*JCO* 2004, PMID 15570071): RR of 542 patients treated on six consecutive prospective trials with NACT followed by mastectomy and PMRT compared with 134 patients on same trials who did not receive PMRT. PMRT reduced 10-year LRR from 22% to 11% ($p = .0001$). On MVA, PMRT improved 10-year LRR in the following groups: cT3–4, clinical stage IIB or higher, pT2–4, and pN2–3. For patients with pCR to NACT, PMRT improved LRR for clinical stage III or higher (33% vs. 3%, p = .006). PMRT improved CSS in the following groups: cT4, pN2–3, clinical stage IIIB or higher. **Conclusion: PMRT improves LRC and CSS in high-risk groups after NACT.**

Krug, Meta-Analysis of Gepar Trials (*Ann Surg Oncol* 2019, PMID 31350646): Pooled analysis of the randomized NACT trials GeparTrio, GeparQuattro, and GeparQuinto; included 817 patients who underwent mastectomy after NACT; 83% received RT. The 5-year cumulative incidence of LRR was 15% in patients treated without RT and 11% in patients treated with RT (p = .23). On MVA, RT was associated with a lower risk of LRR (HR 0.51, p = .05). This effect was shown especially in patients with cT3–4 tumors, as well as in patients who were cN+ before NACT, including those with pCR. **Conclusion: RT reduces LRR rates in breast cancer patients who undergo mastectomy after NACT, including those with pCR to NACT.**

For patients with a complete response to NACT, is there benefit to further RT?

Per NSABP B-51/RTOG 1304, the omission of RT in patients with clinical T1–T3N1 breast cancer who converted to node-negative after neoadjuvant CHT led to no difference in invasive breast cancer recurrence-free interval (RFI) or OS at 5-year follow-up. Limitations to the study include short follow-up (5 years, trend toward increased LRF [p = .08], and far fewer events occurred than projected [109 vs. 172]).

NSABP B-51/RTOG 1304 (*NEJM* 2025, PMID 40466065): Phase III RCT evaluating whether PMRT + RNI after mastectomy or WBI + RNI after lumpectomy significantly improves invasive breast cancer RFI (primary endpoint) in cT1–T3N1 patients who are ypN0 after NACT. Patients could get ALND or SLNB ± ALND based on physician discretion. MFU 59.5 months. Approximately 20% of patients had TNBC and 20% had pCR in nodes but not in the breast. There was no improvement in 5-year invasive breast cancer RFI with RNI (93% vs. 92%, p = .51), distant recurrences, or OS. There was a trend toward increased LRR in the no-RNI group, but fewer events occurred than were expected. Exploratory subset analysis suggests that RNI is favored in ER+/HER2– patients, while no RNI is favored in TNBC. **Conclusion: In biopsy-proven N1 axillary node patients who convert to ypN0 after NACT, omission of adjuvant RNI can be considered given no improvement in 5-year invasive breast cancer RFI; however, there is only 5-year follow-up at this time.**

For patients with an incomplete response to NACT, is there benefit to further systemic therapy?

Masuda, CREATE-X (*NEJM* 2017, PMID 28564564): PRT of 910 patients with HER2– breast cancer with residual disease after NACT randomized to standard adjuvant therapy ± capecitabine, 1,250 mg/m^2 BID on days 1 to 14 q3 weeks for 6 to 8 cycles. RT was delivered as needed, either before or after capecitabine; 68% hormone-positive, 32% TNBC. Capecitabine improved 5-year DFS (74% vs. 68%, p = .01) and 5-year OS (89% vs. 84%, p = .01). For TNBC patients, DFS 70% vs. 56% (HR 0.58, 95% CI 0.39–0.87) and OS 79% vs. 70% (HR 0.52, 0.30–0.90). For hormone-positive patients, DFS 76% vs. 73% (HR 0.81, 0.55–1.17) and OS 93% vs. 90% (HR 0.73, 0.38–1.40). **Conclusion: In HER2– patients with residual disease after NACT, adjuvant capecitabine prolongs DFS and OS, particularly in those with TNBC.**

Von Minckwitz, KATHERINE (*NEJM* 2019, PMID 30516102): PRT of 1,486 HER2+ patients with residual disease after NACT containing a taxane and trastuzumab randomized to adjuvant T-DM1 or trastuzumab for 14 cycles. If indicated, PMRT was delivered concurrently. T-DM1 improved 3-year DFS (88% vs. 77%, p < .001). **Conclusion: In HER2+ patients with residual disease after NACT, adjuvant T-DM1 prolongs DFS. RT is safe to give concurrently with T-DM1.**

Can hypofractionated RT be delivered to the chest wall and regional nodes?

Although Ragaz's British Columbia randomized study evaluating the role of PMRT utilized a moderately hypofractionated regimen (37.5 Gy/16 fx), the majority of PMRT studies have used regimens of either 1.8 or 2 Gy per day.[41,42,44] A study from the Chinese Academy of Medical Sciences evaluated the efficacy and tolerance of hypofractionated RT in the modern era in patients without reconstruction. Long-term toxicity results from the minority of patients (~15%) on the START A/B trials who received hypofractionated RNI were reported in 2017 showing safety according to patient and physician-assessed arm and shoulder symptoms.[53] Receipt of any PMRT increases complication rates after breast reconstruction, although recent trials support the use of moderately hypofractionated PMRT after reconstruction without higher rates of reconstruction complications.[32]

Wang, China (*Lancet Oncol* 2019, PMID 30711522): Noninferiority trial comparing 50 Gy/25 fx vs. 43.5 Gy/15 fx (all 2D planning) in 820 patients with pT3–4 or pN2+ s/p mastectomy enrolled between 2008 and 2016. RT delivered to chest wall and regional nodes. For both arms, 5-year LRR was 8%. No significant difference in acute and late toxicities other than fewer patients in the hypofractionated group experienced grade 3 acute skin toxicity (3% vs. 8%, $p < .0001$). **Conclusion: Hypofractionated PMRT was noninferior to conventional PMRT in both efficacy and toxicity.**

Wong, FABREC (*JAMA Oncol* 2024, PMID 39115975): Multicenter prospective RCT of women with immediate tissue expander or implant placement after mastectomy randomized to hypof-ractionation (HF) 42.56 Gy/16 fx vs. conventional fractionation (CF) 50 Gy/25 fx to the chest wall ± axillary/supraclavicular LNs (boost not permitted, bolus per physician discretion). The primary endpoint was improvement in the Physical Well-Being (PWB) domain of FACT-B at 6 months in all age groups as well as preplanned subgroups stratified by age (<45 and ≥45 years). 330 patients had PWB scores at baseline and 6 months. MFU 40.4 months. No difference in the change in PWB between the study arms ($p = .80$), but there was a significant interaction between age group and study arm ($p = .03$). Patients <45 years had higher 6-month absolute PWB with HF rather than CR ($p = .047$). There was also no difference in chest wall toxicity between the two groups (19 CF vs. 20 HF, $p = .58$). There were no differences in oncologic outcomes including LR, distant recurrence, and death. **Conclusion: Hypofractionated PMRT resulted in comparable QOL and toxicity as CF in patients with implants or tissue-expander reconstruction.**

RT Charm, Alliance A221505 (ASTRO 2024): Prospective multi-institutional noninferiority RCT of patients with unilateral breast cancer who were planning delayed or immediate breast recon-struction and PMRT randomized to 50 Gy/25 fx (CF) vs. 42.56 Gy/16 fx (HF). Noninferiority design with a margin of 10% assuming a complication rate of 25% in the CF arm. 572 patients completed reconstruction: 45% immediate, 55% delayed; 57% implant alone, 43% autologous ± implant. The 24-month incidence of reconstruction complications was 14% with HF vs. 12% with CF (SS, confirm-ing noninferiority). Complication rate was decreased in both arms with autologous vs. implant only reconstruction (OR 0.50, $p = .006$). No significant differences in acute and late toxicity between the arms. Similar 36-month local and regional recurrences, ~2% in both arms. **Conclusion: HF-PMRT is noninferior to CF-PMRT; however, rates of complications remain higher for implant only reconstruction compared with autologous.**

Naoum, Harvard (*IJROBP* 2019, PMID 31756414): RR of 1,286 patients who underwent 1,814 breast reconstructions ± PMRT. Evaluated rates of reconstruction complications in those who underwent two-stage tissue expander/implant (TE/I), single-stage direct to implant (DTI), and autologous tissue reconstructions; 5-year cumulative incidence of any reconstruction complication with and without PMRT: autologous 15% vs. 11%, DTI 18% vs. 13%, TE/I 37% vs. 20%. **Conclusion: Complication rates after TE/I are high with PMRT. DTI and autologous reconstructions have significantly lower complications rates than TE/I.**

Should the SCV and/or IM nodes be included in the RT field?

IMNs were included in three randomized PMRT trials (British Columbia,[39] DBCCG 82b/82c[41,42]), although isolated recurrence in the IMN is low (≤1%). The incidence of IMN involvement in extended radical mas-tectomy series was based on the location and size of the primary tumor along with the extent of axillary involvement. Hennequin et al. showed no OS benefit (although underpowered) with the inclusion of IMNs, while a Danish prospective nonrandomized cohort study suggested an OS benefit. The EORTC 22922 trial demonstrated a DFS benefit to including IMN-SCV fields over omitting them, although it remains unclear whether the benefit was achieved by inclusion of the IMN or SCV fields (or both). The NCIC MA.20 trial[54] included IMNs, SCV, and axilla in the RNI field and showed an improvement in DFS, but no OS benefit with RNI (see Chapter 24 for more details).

Hennequin, French Trial (*IJROBP* 2013, PMID 23664327): PRT of 1,334 patients with axillary LN+ or central/medial tumors (irrespective of axillary involvement). All patients underwent MRM with ALND of levels I and II. No IMN dissection allowed. PMRT delivered to chest wall + SCV. For pN+ cases, levels I + II covered, mainly 50 Gy/25 fx. Randomized between ± IMN RT (included the first five intercostal spaces) to a dose of 45 Gy/18 fx (2.5 Gy/fx) using mixed photon and electron fields. MFU 11.3 years; 10-year OS 59% without IMNs vs. 63% with IMNs ($p = .8$). IMN RT did not signifi-cantly improve OS for any subgroup. **Conclusion: No benefit to including IMNs in PMRT.** *Comment:*

Included node-negative patients (25%) who have lower risk for IMN involvement; used 2D planning, which may have underestimated the coverage of IMNs; study was powered for a 10% survival benefit, which is likely optimistic given that the British Columbia/Danish trials of PMRT vs. no RT showed a ~10% OS benefit.

Poortmans, EORTC 22922–10925 (*NEJM* 2015, PMID 26200978; Update *Lancet Oncol* 2020, PMID 33152277): PRT of 4,004 patients with axillary LN+ and/or a medially located primary tumor (irrespective of axillary involvement) randomized between ± IMN and medial SCV irradiation (IM-MSV); 7% of control vs. 8% in IM-MSV group received axillary RT. BCT in 76%; mastectomy in 24%. After mastectomy, chest wall RT was given to 73% in both arms; 44% were node-negative. Updated MFU 15.7 years; any breast cancer recurrence and BCM were reduced with IM-MSV RT, although OS, DFS, and DMFS were not (Table 25.4). **Conclusion: The inclusion of IMNs and medial SCV LNs in the PMRT field significantly reduced BCM and any breast cancer recurrence. However, no OS difference was noted.**

Table 25.4 EORTC 22922 Results						
15-Yr Results	**DFS**	**Any Breast Recurrence**	**BCM**	**OS**	**Pulmonary Fibrosis**	**Cardiac Disease**
Surgery + IM-MS RT	61%	25%	16%	73%	4%	7%
Surgery	60%	27%	20%	71%	2%	6%
p value	.18	.024	.0055	.36	*NR*	*NR*

Thorsen, DBCG-IMN/DBCG-IMN2 (*JCO* 2015, PMID 26598752; *JCO* 2022, PMID 35394824): Prospective population-based cohort study of 3,089 patients with unilateral LN+ breast cancer who underwent mastectomy or BCS with ALND (levels I–II) from 2003 to 2007. Included pT1–T3 and pN1–3. Patients with right-sided disease received IMN RT, while left-sided disease did not (due to concerns of RT-induced heart disease). RT to breast/chest wall, scar, SCV, infraclavicular (level III), and axillary levels I to II to 48 Gy/24 fx. IMN RT included intercostal spaces 1 to 4 treated with anterior electron field or included in tangential photon fields. Primary endpoint OS. MFU 8.9 years. Three percent of right-sided did not receive IMN RT, while 10% of left-sided received IMN RT. OS (76% vs. 72%, *p* = .005) and BCM (21% vs. 23%, *p* = .03) benefits were noted with IMN RT, with equal number of cardiac deaths in two groups. Subgroup analysis showed lateral tumors with ≥4 LNs had OS benefit with IMN RT (HR 0.71, 95% CI 0.57–0.89). The 15-year update of patients treated from 2007 to 2014 revealed improvements in OS, BCM, and decreased risk of developing distant recurrence with the addition of IMN RT (Table 25.5). **Conclusion: IMN RT improves OS in LN+ breast cancer.** *Comment: Not a randomized trial and excluded patients unfit for standard RT, which may potentially lead to overestimation of IMN RT effect.*

Table 25.5 DBCG-IMN Results			
DBCG-IMN 15-Yr Results	**OS**	**BCM**	**DM**
With IMN RT	60%	32%	36%
Without IMN RT	55%	34%	39%
p value	.007	.05	.04

Kim, KROG 08-06 (*JAMA Oncol* 2022, PMID 34695841): Phase III prospective RCT of 735 women in South Korea with pN+ breast cancer after BCS or mastectomy with ALND randomized to breast or chest wall RT with RNI ± IMN RT. Neoadjuvant treatment was not allowed. The primary endpoint was DFS at 7 years. At MFU of 100.4 months, there was no difference in 7-year DFS for IMN RT vs. no IMN RT (85% vs. 82%, respectively). An ad hoc subgroup analysis demonstrated higher 7-year DFS with IMN RT among patients with mediocentrally located tumors, 92% vs. 82% (*p* = .008), with 7-year BCM rates of 10% vs. 5% favoring IMN RT (*p* = .04). There were no differences between the groups in AEs, including cardiac toxicity and radiation pneumonitis. **Conclusion: Inclusion of IMNs with RNI did not significantly improve DFS in patients with node-positive breast cancer; however, patients with medial or central tumors may benefit from IMNI.**

REFERENCES

1. Breast Cancer Facts & Figures 2024–2025. *American Cancer Society*. 2024 American Cancer Society. Accessed July 11, 2024. https://www.cancer.org/content/dam/cancer-org/research/cancer-facts-and-statistics/breast-cancer-facts-and-figures/2024/breast-cancer-facts-and-figures-2024.pdf

2. Breast Cancer Facts & Figures 2019–2020. *American Cancer Society*. 2019 Atlanta: American Cancer Society. Accessed December 30, 2024. https://www.cancer.org/content/dam/cancer-org/research/cancer-facts-and-statistics/breast-cancer-facts-and-figures/breast-cancer-facts-and-figures-2019-2020.pdf

3. Levine PH, Steinhorn SC, Ries LG, Aron JL. Inflammatory breast cancer: the experience of the surveillance, epidemiology, and end results (SEER) program. *J Natl Cancer Inst*. 1985;74(2):291–297. PMID:3856043

4. Li CI, Malone KE, Daling JR. Differences in breast cancer hormone receptor status and histology by race and ethnicity among women 50 years of age and older. *Cancer Epidemiol Biomarkers Prev*. 2002;11(7):601–607. PMID:12101106

5. Gruber G, Ciriolo M, Altermatt HJ, Aebi S, Berclaz G, Greiner RH. Prognosis of dermal lymphatic invasion with or without clinical signs of inflammatory breast cancer. *Int J Cancer*. 2004;109(1):144–148. doi:10.1002/ijc.11684

6. NCCN. Breast Cancer (Version 6.2024). Accessed January 6, 2025, https://www.nccn.org/professionals/physician_gls/pdf/breast.pdf

7. NCCN Survivorship Guidelines. Vol. Version 2.2024. 2024.

8. Mamounas EP, Russell CA, Lau A, Turner MP, Albain KS. Clinical relevance of the 21-gene Recurrence Score® assay in treatment decisions for patients with node-positive breast cancer in the genomic era. *NPJ Breast Cancer*. 2018;4:27. doi:10.1038/s41523-018-0082-6

9. NCCN. Breast Cancer (Version 6.2024). Accessed January 6, 2025, https://www.nccn.org/professionals/physician_gls/pdf/breast.pdf

10. Kalinsky K, Barlow WE, Gralow JR, et al. 21-gene assay to inform chemotherapy benefit in node-positive breast cancer. *N Engl J Med*. 2021;385(25):2336–2347. doi:10.1056/NEJMoa2108873

11. Fisher B, Brown A, Mamounas E, et al. Effect of preoperative chemotherapy on local-regional disease in women with operable breast cancer: findings from national surgical adjuvant breast and bowel project B-18. *J Clin Oncol*. 1997;15(7):2483–2493. doi:10.1200/JCO.1997.15.7.2483

12. van der Hage JA, van de Velde CJ, Julien JP, Tubiana-Hulin M, Vandervelden C, Duchateau L. Preoperative chemotherapy in primary operable breast cancer: results from the European organization for research and treatment of cancer trial 10902. *J Clin Oncol*. 2001;19(22):4224–4237. doi:10.1200/JCO.2001.19.22.4224

13. Schmid P, Cortes J, Dent R, et al. Overall survival with pembrolizumab in early-stage triple-negative breast cancer. *N Engl J Med*. 2024;391(21):1981–1991. doi:10.1056/NEJMoa2409932

14. Schmid P, Cortes J, Dent R, et al. Event-free survival with pembrolizumab in early triple-negative breast cancer. *N Engl J Med*. 2022;386(6):556–567. doi:10.1056/NEJMoa2112651

15. Schmid P, Cortes J, Pusztai L, et al. Pembrolizumab for early triple-negative breast cancer. *N Engl J Med*. 2020;382(9):810–821. doi:10.1056/NEJMoa1910549

16. Gianni L, Pienkowski T, Im YH, et al. Efficacy and safety of neoadjuvant pertuzumab and trastuzumab in women with locally advanced, inflammatory, or early HER2-positive breast cancer (NeoSphere): a randomised multicentre, open-label, phase 2 trial. *Lancet Oncol*. 2012;13(1):25–32. doi:10.1016/S1470-2045(11)70336-9

17. Schneeweiss A, Chia S, Hickish T, et al. Pertuzumab plus trastuzumab in combination with standard neoadjuvant anthracycline-containing and anthracycline-free chemotherapy regimens in patients with HER2-positive early breast cancer: a randomized phase II cardiac safety study (TRYPHAENA). *Ann Oncol*. 2013;24(9):2278–2284. doi:10.1093/annonc/mdt182

18. Bear HD, Anderson S, Brown A, et al. The effect on tumor response of adding sequential preoperative docetaxel to preoperative doxorubicin and cyclophosphamide: preliminary results from national surgical adjuvant breast and bowel project protocol B-27. *J Clin Oncol*. 2003;21(22):4165–4174. doi:10.1200/JCO.2003.12.005

19. Mieog JS, van der Hage JA, van de Velde CJ. Preoperative chemotherapy for women with operable breast cancer. *Cochrane Database Syst Rev*. 2007;2007(2):CD005002. doi:10.1002/14651858.CD005002.pub2

20. Untch M, Fasching PA, Konecny GE, et al. Pathologic complete response after neoadjuvant chemotherapy plus trastuzumab predicts favorable survival in human epidermal growth factor receptor 2-overexpressing breast cancer: results from the TECHNO trial of the AGO and GBG study groups. *J Clin Oncol*. 2011;29(25):3351–3357. doi:10.1200/JCO.2010.31.4930

21. von Minckwitz G, Huang CS, Mano MS, et al. Trastuzumab emtansine for residual invasive HER2-positive breast cancer. *N Engl J Med*. 2019;380(7):617–628. doi:10.1056/NEJMoa1814017

22. Masuda N, Lee SJ, Ohtani S, et al. Adjuvant capecitabine for breast cancer after preoperative chemotherapy. *N Engl J Med*. 2017;376(22):2147–2159. doi:10.1056/NEJMoa1612645

23. Geng C, Chen X, Pan X, Li J. The feasibility and accuracy of sentinel lymph node biopsy in initially clinically node-negative breast cancer after neoadjuvant chemotherapy: a systematic review and meta-analysis. *PLoS One*. 2016;11(9):e0162605. doi:10.1371/journal.pone.0162605

24. El Hage Chehade H, Headon H, El Tokhy O, Heeney J, Kasem A, Mokbel K. Is sentinel lymph node biopsy a viable alternative to complete axillary dissection following neoadjuvant chemotherapy in women with node-positive breast cancer at diagnosis? An updated meta-analysis involving 3,398 patients. *Am J Surg*. 2016;212(5):969–981. doi:10.1016/j.amjsurg.2016.07.018

25. Fisher B, Bryant J, Wolmark N, et al. Effect of preoperative chemotherapy on the outcome of women with operable breast cancer. *J Clin Oncol*. 1998;16(8):2672–2685. doi:10.1200/JCO.1998.16.8.2672

26. Recht A, Comen EA, Fine RE, et al. Postmastectomy radiotherapy: an American society of clinical oncology, American society for radiation oncology, and society of surgical oncology focused guideline update. *Ann Surg Oncol*. 2017;24(1):38–51. doi:10.1245/s10434-016-5558-8

27. Shaikh PM, Mulherkar R, Khasawneh MT, et al. Treatment of internal mammary nodes is associated with improved overall survival in breast cancer: a meta-analysis. *Am J Clin Oncol*. 2024;47(2):81–87. doi:10.1097/COC.0000000000001060

28. Thorsen LB, Offersen BV, Dano H, et al. DBCG-IMN: a population-based cohort study on the effect of internal mammary node irradiation in early node-positive breast cancer. *J Clin Oncol*. 2016;34(4):314–320. doi:10.1200/JCO.2015.63.6456

29. Thorsen LBJ, Overgaard J, Matthiessen LW, et al. Internal mammary node irradiation in patients with node-positive early breast cancer: fifteen-year results from the danish breast cancer group internal mammary node study. *J Clin Oncol*. 2022;40(36):4198–4206. doi:10.1200/JCO.22.00044

30. Wang SL, Fang H, Song YW, et al. Hypofractionated versus conventional fractionated postmastectomy radiotherapy for patients with high-risk breast cancer: a randomised, non-inferiority, open-label, phase 3 trial. *Lancet Oncol*. 2019;20(3):352–360. doi:10.1016/S1470-2045(18)30813-1

31. Wong JS, Uno H, Tramontano AC, et al. Hypofractionated vs conventionally fractionated postmastectomy radiation after implant-based reconstruction: a randomized clinical trial. *JAMA Oncol*. 2024;10(10):1370–1378. doi:10.1001/jamaoncol.2024.2652

32. Poppe MM, Le-Rademacher J, Haffty Jr BG, Hansen EK. A randomized trial of hypofractionated Post-Mastectomy Radiation Therapy (PMRT) in women with breast reconstruction (RT CHARM, Alliance A221505). *Int J Radiat Oncol Biol Phys*. 2024;120(2):S11. doi:10.1016/j.ijrobp.2024.07.002

33. Kaidar-Person O, Dahn HM, Nichol AM, et al. A delphi study and international consensus recommendations: the use of bolus in the setting of postmastectomy radiation therapy for early breast cancer. *Radiother Oncol*. 2021;164:115–121. doi:10.1016/j.radonc.2021.09.012

34. Nichol A, Narinesingh D, Raman S, et al. The effect of bolus on local control for patients treated with mastectomy and radiation therapy. *Int J Radiat Oncol Biol Phys*. 2021;110(5):1360–1369. doi:10.1016/j.ijrobp.2021.01.019

35. Recht A, Edge SB, Solin LJ, et al. Postmastectomy radiotherapy: clinical practice guidelines of the American society of clinical oncology. *J Clin Oncol*. 2001;19(5):1539–1569. doi:10.1200/JCO.2001.19.5.1539

36. Fowble B, Gray R, Gilchrist K, Goodman RL, Taylor S, Tormey DC. Identification of a subgroup of patients with breast cancer and histologically positive axillary nodes receiving adjuvant chemotherapy who may benefit from postoperative radiotherapy. *J Clin Oncol*. 1988;6(7):1107–1117. doi:10.1200/JCO.1988.6.7.1107

37. Taghian A, Jeong JH, Mamounas E, et al. Patterns of locoregional failure in patients with operable breast cancer treated by mastectomy and adjuvant chemotherapy with or without tamoxifen and without radiotherapy: results from five national surgical adjuvant breast and bowel project randomized clinical trials. *J Clin Oncol*. 2004;22(21):4247–4254. doi:10.1200/jco.2004.01.042

38. Kaidar-Person O, Giasafaki P, Boersma L, et al. Mapping the location of local and regional recurrences according to breast cancer surgery and radiation therapy: results from EORTC 22922/10925. *Radiother Oncol*. 2023;185:109698. doi:10.1016/j.radonc.2023.109698

39. Ragaz J, Jackson SM, Le N, et al. Adjuvant radiotherapy and chemotherapy in node-positive premenopausal women with breast cancer. *N Engl J Med*. 1997;337(14):956–962. doi:10.1056/nejm199710023371402

40. Ragaz J, Olivotto IA, Spinelli JJ, et al. Locoregional radiation therapy in patients with high-risk breast cancer receiving adjuvant chemotherapy: 20-year results of the British Columbia randomized trial. *J Natl Cancer Inst*. 2005;97(2):116–126. doi:10.1093/jnci/djh297

41. Overgaard M, Hansen PS, Overgaard J, et al. Postoperative radiotherapy in high-risk premenopausal women with breast cancer who receive adjuvant chemotherapy. danish breast cancer cooperative group 82b trial. *N Engl J Med*. 1997;337(14):949–955. doi:10.1056/NEJM199710023371401

42. Overgaard M, Jensen MB, Overgaard J, et al. Postoperative radiotherapy in high-risk postmenopausal breast-cancer patients given adjuvant tamoxifen: danish breast cancer cooperative group DBCG 82c randomised trial. *Lancet*. 1999;353(9165):1641–1648. doi:10.1016/s0140-6736(98)09201-0

43. Overgaard M, Nielsen HM, Overgaard J. Is the benefit of postmastectomy irradiation limited to patients with four or more positive nodes, as recommended in international consensus reports? A subgroup analysis of the DBCG 82 b&c randomized trials. *Radiother Oncol*. 2007;82(3):247–253. doi:10.1016/j.radonc.2007.02.001

44. Clarke M, Collins R, Darby S, et al. Effects of radiotherapy and of differences in the extent of surgery for early breast cancer on local recurrence and 15-year survival: an overview of the randomised trials. *Lancet.* 2005;366(9503):2087–2106. doi:10.1016/S0140-6736(05)67887-7

45. Early Breast Cancer Trialists' Collaborative Group, McGale P, Taylor C, et al. Effect of radiotherapy after mastectomy and axillary surgery on 10-year recurrence and 20-year breast cancer mortality: meta-analysis of individual patient data for 8135 women in 22 randomised trials. *Lancet.* 2014;383(9935):2127–2135. doi:10.1016/S0140-6736(14)60488-8

46. Early Breast Cancer Trialists' Collaborative Group. Radiotherapy to regional nodes in early breast cancer: an individual patient data meta-analysis of 14 324 women in 16 trials. *Lancet.* 2023;402(10416):1991–2003. doi:10.1016/S0140-6736(23)01082-6

47. Jagsi R, Raad RA, Goldberg S, et al. Locoregional recurrence rates and prognostic factors for failure in node-negative patients treated with mastectomy: implications for postmastectomy radiation. *Int J Radiat Oncol Biol Phys.* 2005;62(4):1035–1039. doi:10.1016/j.ijrobp.2004.12.014

48. Taghian AG, Jeong JH, Mamounas EP, et al. Low locoregional recurrence rate among node-negative breast cancer patients with tumors 5 cm or larger treated by mastectomy, with or without adjuvant systemic therapy and without radiotherapy: results from five national surgical adjuvant breast and bowel project randomized clinical trials. *J Clin Oncol.* 2006;24(24):3927–3932. doi:10.1200/JCO.2006.06.9054

49. Floyd SR, Buchholz TA, Haffty BG, et al. Low local recurrence rate without postmastectomy radiation in node-negative breast cancer patients with tumors 5 cm and larger. *Int J Radiat Oncol Biol Phys.* 2006;66(2):358–364. doi:10.1016/j.ijrobp.2006.05.001

50. Goulart J, Truong P, Woods R, Speers CH, Kennecke H, Nichol A. Outcomes of node-negative breast cancer 5 centimeters and larger treated with and without postmastectomy radiotherapy. *Int J Radiat Oncol Biol Phys.* 2011;80(3):758–764. doi:10.1016/j.ijrobp.2010.02.014

51. Nagar H, Mittendorf EA, Strom EA, et al. Local-regional recurrence with and without radiation therapy after neoadjuvant chemotherapy and mastectomy for clinically staged T3N0 breast cancer. *Int J Radiat Oncol Biol Phys.* 2011;81(3):782–787. doi:10.1016/j.ijrobp.2010.06.027

52. Johnson ME, Handorf EA, Martin JM, Hayes SB. Postmastectomy radiation therapy for T3N0: a SEER analysis. *Cancer.* 2014;120(22):3569–3574. doi:10.1002/cncr.28865

53. Haviland JS, Mannino M, Griffin C, et al. Late normal tissue effects in the arm and shoulder following lymphatic radiotherapy: results from the UK START (Standardisation of Breast Radiotherapy) trials. *Radiother Oncol.* 2018;126(1):155–162. doi:10.1016/j.radonc.2017.10.033

54. Whelan TJ, Olivotto IA, Parulekar WR, et al. Regional nodal irradiation in early-stage breast cancer. *N Engl J Med.* 2015;373(4):307–316. doi:10.1056/NEJMoa1415340

26 DUCTAL CARCINOMA IN SITU

Sean M. Parker, Timothy D. Smile, Rahul D. Tendulkar, and Chirag Shah

QUICK HIT Ductal carcinoma in situ (DCIS) represents ~15% of all BCs. Without treatment, up to 25% to 30% of DCIS cases can progress to invasive breast cancer (BC) over 30 years. Standard treatment involves either breast conservation therapy (BCT: lumpectomy plus adjuvant RT) or mastectomy. After lumpectomy, adjuvant RT results in a 50% relative risk reduction in LR (with approximately half of recurrences being invasive cancers) but no improvement in OS. The absolute risk of ipsilateral breast tumor recurrence (IBTR) depends on grade, histologic subtype, size, ER status, and margin status. Lobular carcinoma in situ (LCIS) is a distinct entity from DCIS with negative margin excision reserved only for nonclassic variants (e.g., pleomorphic, florid), and there is no clear role for adjuvant RT.

EPIDEMIOLOGY: Over 50,000 cases of DCIS are diagnosed in the United States annually compared with ~310,000 cases of invasive BC.[1,2] Incidence increased fivefold with the introduction of mammography. Left untreated, ~25% to 30% of patients with DCIS develop invasive cancer over 30 years.[3–5]

RISK FACTORS: Similar to invasive BC: female gender, older age, BRCA status, family history (first-degree relative), unopposed estrogen (includes early menarche, late menopause, nulliparity, late age at first birth, hormone replacement), obesity, alcohol (dose-dependent), prior RT, atypical ductal hyperplasia.

PATHOLOGY: DCIS implies that the basement membrane is preserved despite CIS cells arising from the ductal epithelium. Typically grows toward the nipple. Five histologic subtypes (mnemonic: C^{2}PMS): cribriform, comedo (worst prognosis), papillary, micropapillary, solid (second worst prognosis). Among DCIS cases, 75% to 80% are ER-positive and up to 35% are HER2-amplified.

Overall, there are three main categories of grading:

- *Grade 1 (low grade):* Monomorphic nuclei with inconspicuous nucleoli and diffuse chromatin. Typically, ER- and PR-positive, have a low proliferative rate, and rarely (if ever) show abnormalities of the HER2 or p53 oncogenes.
- *Grade 2 (intermediate grade):* Neither grade 1 nor grade 3.
- *Grade 3 (high grade):* Large and pleomorphic nuclei, >1 nucleolus per cell, irregular chromatin. Typically exhibit aneuploidy, more frequently ER- and PR-negative, high proliferative rate, angiogenesis in surrounding stroma, overexpression of HER2, and can have p53 mutations.

LCIS: A noninfiltrating lobular proliferation characterized by loose, noncohesive epithelial cells filling the acinar space.[6] The presence of LCIS increases the risk of developing invasive disease (~7% at 10 years in either breast) but is not considered a premalignant condition.[7] The most common morphologic variants of LCIS are classic, pleomorphic, and florid. Pleomorphic and florid LCIS possess more aggressive architectural features and genetic aberrations compared with classic LCIS.[8,9]

GENETICS: The genetics underlying DCIS are heterogenous, and identification of a specific genetic profile that confers higher risk of progression to invasive disease has proved difficult. The DCISionRT assay includes seven markers and four clinicopathologic factors and is prognostic for recurrence (overall and invasive) and is predictive of RT benefit. The Oncotype Dx DCIS Score is a multigene expression assay that attempts to stratify risk through analysis of 12 genes and has demonstrated utility as a prognostic biomarker for recurrence but is not predictive of RT benefit.[10,11]

SCREENING: Mammographic screening reduces BC mortality.[12–15] ACS, ACR, AMA, and NCCN recommend initiation of annual screening at age 40, whereas the USPSTF recommends screening every other year starting at age 40. See Chapter 24 for additional details on screening modalities.

CLINICAL PRESENTATION: In situ breast disease is generally asymptomatic and is usually detected on mammography. On occasion, DCIS may be palpable. It may also be discovered incidentally during investigation of a nearby breast mass or asymmetry (benign or malignant).

WORKUP: H&P with breast and LN exam.

Imaging: Bilateral diagnostic mammograms with spot compression views (to evaluate masses) and magnification (to evaluate calcifications) as necessary. Concerning findings on mammography include 100 to 300 μm clustered or linear calcifications, spiculated lesions, or new lesions. Linear/branching calcifications are associated with high-grade DCIS and necrosis, whereas fine/granular calcifications are associated with low-grade DCIS.[16] Ninety percent of DCIS present with calcifications, and 80% of lesions with calcifications contain DCIS.[16,17] BI-RADS is the standard mammographic terminology (further detailed in Chapter 24). MRI may be superior to mammography in detecting DCIS (especially high-grade or multicentric disease) and identifying candidates for breast-conserving surgery (BCS). However, it is not clear if this increased sensitivity significantly impacts disease outcomes.[18,19]

Biopsy Technique: FNA is inadequate to distinguish DCIS from invasive cancer, and therefore stereotactic core or excisional biopsy is recommended. Consider stereotactic guided "bracketing" of the suspicious areas to help facilitate excision. Use ultrasound guidance for masses. Atypical ductal hyperplasia on core biopsy requires complete excision as ~20% of patients are upstaged.[20]

PROGNOSTIC FACTORS: Higher risk of recurrence for young age, high grade, comedonecrosis, multifocality, large tumor size, positive surgical margins, ER negativity, and HER2 amplification.[21] The Van Nuys Prognostic Index (VNPI) quantifies prognostic factors for LR in patients with DCIS (low score 4–6, intermediate 7–9, and high 10–12; see Table 26.1).[22,23] Note that VNPI has not been prospectively validated.[24,25] Over the last decade, genomic (Oncotype DX DCIS) and tumor (DCISionRT) assays have demonstrated increased utility as independent prognostic tools for estimating the risk of recurrence.

Table 26.1 Updated VNPI			
	1	**2**	**3**
Size	≤15 mm	16–40 mm	>40 mm
Margin	≥10 mm	1–9 mm	<1 mm
Grade	Grade 1/2 without necrosis	Grade 1/2 with necrosis	Grade 3
Age	>60	40–60	<40

STAGING: T classification is Tis, and stage is 0 for all DCIS. LCIS is no longer included in AJCC staging.

TREATMENT PARADIGM: Options include observation if short life expectancy, lumpectomy alone, lumpectomy ± adjuvant RT ± tamoxifen/anastrozole (based on menopausal and ER– status), or mastectomy. A risk-based patient-specific assessment is necessary.

Prevention: Tamoxifen and raloxifene both reduce the risk of BC (invasive and noninvasive) by ~50% in high-risk populations.[26,27] However, this benefit is only seen in ER-positive tumors.

Surgery: Either lumpectomy (LR reduced by adjuvant RT) or simple mastectomy (LR 1%–2% without RT).[28] Skin-sparing mastectomy can be considered.[29] No randomized trials have compared BCT with mastectomy. Data from the Netherlands show only 8% of DCIS is present beyond 1 cm from the initial focus.[30] SLNB should not be performed in the absence of invasive cancer but may be considered if there is clinicopathologic suggestion of invasion.[31] SLNB should be considered in those undergoing mastectomy given the limitation of future sampling if invasion is demonstrated on final pathology. Among patients diagnosed with DCIS on biopsy, 10% to 20% will have invasive cancer identified at surgery.[32,33] Follow-up radiograph prior to RT is useful to confirm complete excision of the suspicious calcifications. Among patients with LCIS, surgical excision alone is recommended for nonclassic pleomorphic/florid variants and for extensive LCIS involving >4 terminal ductal lobular units on core biopsy.[34]

Chemotherapy: No indication in DCIS/LCIS. The NSABP B-43/RTOG 0974 trial demonstrated that for patients with HER2+ DCIS after lumpectomy, concurrent trastuzumab and RT compared with RT alone did not improve ipsilateral breast tumor recurrence (IBTR) rates.

Hormonal Therapy: Consider adjuvant tamoxifen given 20 mg/day or anastrozole 1 mg/day for 5 years after excision of ER-positive DCIS. NCCN recommends tamoxifen for patients with ER-positive DCIS treated with excision alone or in those treated with lumpectomy + RT.[31] Low-dose tamoxifen (5 mg/day) for 3 years is also an option based on the TAM01 trial.[35] For postmenopausal patients, consider anastrozole given improved breast cancer-free interval on B-35.[36]

Radiation

Indications: RT after surgery is indicated for most patients choosing BCS. Five randomized controlled trials have demonstrated a LC benefit to RT, although CSS and OS are similar to lumpectomy alone. NCCN guidelines suggest either mastectomy or BCT as level 1 treatment options and lumpectomy alone as 2B.[31]

Whole Breast Irradiation (WBI): Treat whole breast using opposed tangents to 40.05–42.5 Gy/15–16 fx. Prospective and retrospective series have demonstrated similar outcomes between hypofractionation and standard fractionation.[37] Per most recent ASTRO guidelines, boost (10–16 Gy in 5–8 fx) can be considered for high-risk DCIS patients (age ≤50 years, high grade, <2 mm margin or positive margins).[38] Prospective data from the BIG 3–07/TROG 07.01 trial have demonstrated that the addition of boost for non–low-risk DCIS patients decreases LR but also worsens cosmesis and increases breast pain.[37] Other WBI regimens include ultra-hypofractionated approaches including 28.5 Gy/5 fx once weekly or 26 Gy/5 fx once daily.[39,40] RT following BCS for nonclassic variants of LCIS remains controversial and is not currently recommended by the NCCN.

Partial Breast Irradiation (PBI): Current ASTRO, ABS, and ASBS guidelines support the use of PBI for select patients with DCIS (not recommended for positive margins, BRCA 1/2 mutation, size ≥3 cm, and age <40 per ASTRO).[41–43] Rationale: approximately 80% to 90% of LR occur at/near lumpectomy site, underutilization of BCT due to treatment duration. Modalities: applicator brachytherapy, multicatheter interstitial, or EBRT.

Intraoperative RT (IORT): Higher rates of LR in two randomized trials for invasive BC; however, limited data in DCIS.[44] IORT is not recommended for DCIS off protocol.

BCT Contraindications: Absolute: persistently positive surgical margins despite maximal re-excision, diffuse malignant-appearing calcifications, inability to receive postop RT (prior chest/breast RT, pregnancy). Relative: active connective tissue disease (scleroderma, lupus), ataxia telangiectasia, risk of poor cosmesis (large tumor [>4–5 cm] in small breast).

Toxicity: Acute effects: erythema, pruritus, tenderness, desquamation. Late effects: altered pigmentation, volume loss, fibrosis, rib fracture, lymphedema, pulmonary fibrosis, secondary malignancies, cardiac toxicity.

EVIDENCE-BASED Q&A

Can RT reduce the risk of recurrence after lumpectomy?

Four large PRTs (NSAPBP B-17, SweDCIS, EORTC 10853, and UK ANZ) have consistently demonstrated a ~50% relative reduction in the risk of DCIS recurrence and invasive recurrence with the addition of WBI to lumpectomy (Table 26.2).[45–48] EBCTCG and Cochrane Database meta-analyses of these trials confirmed a statistically significant reduction in ipsilateral breast events, DCIS recurrences, and invasive recurrences with the addition of RT among all subgroups including those with favorable risk factors (complete excision, age >50 years, absence of comedonecrosis, and small tumor size).[21,49] None of the individual trials or meta-analyses demonstrate a difference in DM, BCSM, or OS with the addition of RT. Long-term outcomes of a combined analysis of B-17/B-24 (detailed below) suggest invasive IBTRs following treatment for DCIS are associated with increased breast cancer mortality.[47]

Wapnir, NSABP-B17/24 Long-Term Outcomes (*JNCI* 2011, PMID 21398619): Combined analysis of two NSABP trials enrolling patients with DCIS; B-17 comparing lumpectomy only vs. lumpectomy

+ RT and B-24 comparing lumpectomy + RT with or without tamoxifen. Of 490 IBTR events, 54% were invasive. RT reduced invasive IBTR by 52%. Invasive IBTR was associated with increased mortality risk (HR 1.75, 95% CI 1.45–2.96). After invasive IBTR, 22 of 39 deaths were attributed to BC. **Conclusion: Half of DCIS recurrences are invasive and increase the risk of mortality. RT reduces the risk of invasive IBTR by approximately half.**

Table 26.2 Summary of DCIS Trials Evaluating RT vs. No RT

	EBCTG 10-Yr		NSABP-B17 15-Yr		SweDCIS 20-Yr		EORTC 10853 15-Yr		UK/ANZ RT Arm 12.7-Yr	
	RT	No RT	RT	No RT	RT	No RT	RT	No RT	RT	No RT
IBE (%)	13*	28%	20*	35	20*	32	17*	30	7*	19
Invasive recurrence (%)	NR	NR	11*	20	15	20	10*	16	3*	9
CSS (%)	96	96	95	97	96	96	96	95	NR	NR
OS (%)	92	92	83	84	77	73	88	90	NR	NR

*Statistically significant difference.
IBE, ipsilateral breast events; NR, not reported.

What factors predict for recurrence?

A combined analysis of B-17 and B-24 demonstrated that younger age, clinically detected DCIS, comedone-crosis, and positive margins are associated with a higher risk of recurrence.[47] On SweDCIS, grade 3 histology and necrosis were predictors of recurrence.[50] Additional RRs have shown that younger age and multifocality may also be associated with higher rates of recurrence.[51,52]

Is there a subset of patients at a low enough absolute risk of recurrence that RT can be omitted?

Given no clear survival benefit with the addition of RT, there has been much interest in identifying patients who may be able to safely omit RT. Single-arm trials from Harvard and ECOG of lower risk cohorts (based on grade, size, and margins) demonstrate that LR rates after lumpectomy in the absence of RT are ~1% per year for low-intermediate grade and ~2% per year for high-grade DCIS.[53,54] However, a low-risk subset that does not benefit from RT with respect to LC has not been clearly defined with clinicopathologic features alone (although can consider genomic assays) and remains a patient-specific decision based on life expectancy and patient wishes.

Solin, ECOG 5194 (*JCO* 2009, PMID 19826126; *JCO* 2015, PMID 26371148): Single-arm trial of 711 DCIS patients (grades 1–2 and ≤2.5 cm or grade 3 and ≤1 cm) treated with local excision only (margins ≥3 mm; 30% received tamoxifen). The 12-year IBE was 14% for grades 1 to 2 and 25% for grade 3. The 12-year IBR was 8% for grades 1 to 2 and 13% for grade 3. **Conclusion: Rate of recurrence increases without plateau (~1% per year for grades 1–2 and 2% per year for grade 3).**

McCormick, RTOG 9804 (*JCO* 2015, PMID 25605856; *JCO* 2021 PMID 34406870): PRT of "low-risk" DCIS (grades 1–2, size <2.5 cm, mammographically detected with margins ≥3 mm) randomized to WBI 50 Gy/25 fx vs. observation; 636 patients enrolled of a planned 1,790. MFU 13.9 years; 62% received tamoxifen (optional). Primary endpoint was IBTR. At 15 years, IBTR was 7% with RT vs. 15% with observation (*p* = .007). **Conclusion: RT reduces IBTR even in a very low-risk cohort.**

What other assays can be used to guide prognosis and treatment for DCIS patients?

Over the last decade, genomic and tumor assays have demonstrated increased utility as independent prognostic tools for estimating the risk of recurrence. The Oncotype DX DCIS multigene assay is associated with IBTR and has received prognostic validation.[10,11] However, the test's cost-effectiveness is uncertain.[55] The DCISionRT tumor assay has been validated as both prognostic and predictive of RT benefit.[56,57]

Solin, Albert Einstein (*JNCI* 2013, PMID 23641039): Molecular profiling of patients with negative margins treated without RT on the ECOG 5194 study (grades 1–2 and ≤2.5 cm or grade 3 and ≤1 cm; margins ≥3 mm; 30% received tamoxifen). Oncotype DX DCIS multigene assay was performed on a subset of 327 patients. Identified three groups (70% low risk, 16% intermediate, and 14% high) with

IBTR risks of 11%, 27%, and 26% at 10 years, respectively. Invasive recurrence risks were 4%, 12%, and 19% for low, intermediate, and high risk, respectively. Prognostic value persisted on MVA. **Conclusion: Oncotype for DCIS adds independent value; however, even in the low-risk group, the LR risk may be high enough to offer RT.**

Wärnberg, DCISionRT SweDCIS Cohort (*Cancers* 2021, PMID 34885211): DCISionRT testing was performed on a validation cohort of 504 women with negative margins from the SweDCIS trial; the assay includes seven biomarkers (COX-2, FOXA1, HER2, Ki-67, p16/INK4A, PR, and SIAH2) and four clinicopathologic factors (age at diagnosis, tumor size, palpability, and surgical margin status). In the elevated risk group (DS >3.0), RT significantly decreased 10-year IBTR and invasive recurrence, whereas no benefit with the addition of RT was observed in the low-risk cohort (DS <3.0). When using a cutoff of DS >2.8, RT was predictive of benefit with regard to recurrences ($p = .038$). **Conclusion: Incorporation of this DS biosignature into this randomized validation cohort was both prognostic and predictive of RT benefit.**

Vicini, DS Biosignature (*IJROBP* 2022, PMID 36115740): Analysis of 926 patients with DCIS undergoing BCS ± RT using the DS Biosignature (DCISionRT) identified three risk groups: a "low-risk" group with low 10-year IBTR rates with or without RT (5% RT vs. 6% no RT, $p = .78$); an "elevated-risk" group that benefitted from the addition of RT (5% RT vs. 21% no RT, $p < .001$); and a "residual-risk" group that benefitted from RT (15% RT vs. 42% no RT, $p < .001$) but still had significantly high risk to consider treatment escalation. **Conclusion: This biosignature identifies low-risk patients who may be able to forego RT and residual risk patients who still may need treatment escalation after RT.**

What surgical margins are necessary?

Margins ≥2 mm are ideal when RT is delivered based on data from two large meta-analyses and supported by consensus guidelines. However, margins from 0 to 2 mm require clinical discussion.

Dunne, Ireland (*JCO* 2009, PMID 19255332). Study-level meta-analysis of 4,660 patients on 22 trials of BCT in DCIS looking at IBTR and margin status. Median time to IBTR 5 years. Negative margins had lower IBTR than positive (64% less), close (41% less), or unknown margins (44% less) after RT. No significant difference in IBTR with 2-mm vs. >5-mm margins. **Conclusion: Margins of ≥2 mm are sufficient when RT is used.**

Morrow, SSO/ASTRO/ASCO Consensus Guideline (*JCO* 2016, PMID 27528719): Multidisciplinary consensus guidelines derived from published literature and a meta-analysis of margin width and IBTR rates from 20 studies including 7,883 patients. Negative margins (no DCIS on ink) halved the risk of IBTR compared with positive margins. When WBI is given, a 2-mm margin minimizes the risk of IBTR compared with smaller negative margins (OR 0.51). Margins ≥2 mm up to 10 mm do not have significantly decreased IBTR compared with 2-mm margins (with WBI). **Conclusion: Negative margins greatly reduce the risk of IBTR. The use of a ≥2-mm margin after surgery is sufficient when RT is delivered.**

Is adjuvant tamoxifen beneficial? Who should receive it? What is the optimal dose?

Tamoxifen lowers the incidence of ipsilateral and contralateral breast events (B24 and UK/ANZ) but does not affect ipsilateral invasive recurrences and therefore is not a substitute for RT (UK/ANZ; Table 26.3). Tamoxifen benefits only ER-positive patients (B-24).

Fisher, NSABP B-24 (*Lancet* 1999, PMID 10376613; *JNCI* 2011, PMID 21398619): PRT of 1,798 DCIS patients comparing BCS + RT with or without tamoxifen delivered 10 mg BID within 56 days of lumpectomy for 5 years. RT given within 8 weeks of lumpectomy using tangents to 50 Gy/25 fx. Thirty-one percent stopped tamoxifen due to side effects or other reasons. Any BC event was decreased with tamoxifen (13% vs. 8% at 5 years, $p = .0009$), as was the rate of invasive BC (7% vs. 4%, $p = .004$). ER status was initially not reported, but an unplanned subgroup analysis determined the benefits of tamoxifen were restricted to ER-positive tumors.[58] **Conclusion: Addition of tamoxifen reduces the incidence of any breast event and on subgroup analysis only demonstrated efficacy for ER-positive patients.**

Houghton, UK/ANZ Trial (*Lancet* 2003, PMID 12867108; *Lancet Oncol* 2011, PMID 21145284): PRT of 1,694 DCIS patients after lumpectomy randomized using a 2 × 2 design: ± RT and ±

tamoxifen; microinvasion was allowed. RT was 50 Gy/25 fx without a boost. Tamoxifen was 20 mg QD for 5 years. Patients could choose the four-way randomization or one of the two-way randomizations. Only patients randomized to a treatment were analyzed for that arm. At 10 years, the risk of any breast event with no adjuvant treatment was 32%, tamoxifen alone 24%, RT alone 13%, and RT and tamoxifen 10%. Tamoxifen had no effect on ipsilateral invasive disease (HR 0.95, 95% CI 0.66–1.38). **Conclusion: Both tamoxifen and RT significantly decreased the risk of IBTR. Tamoxifen did not affect invasive recurrences and therefore is not a substitute for RT.**

Table 26.3 Summary of DCIS Trials Evaluating Tamoxifen vs. No Tamoxifen

	NSABP B24 15 Yrs			UK/ANZ Tamoxifen Randomization 12.7 Yrs		
	Tam	No Tam	HR	Tam	No Tam	HR
IBE (%)	13	17	0.68*	16	20	0.78*
Invasive recurrence (%)	7	9	NR	7	7	0.95
CBE (%)	5	8	0.68*	2	4	0.44*
BCSM (%)	97.7	97.3	NR	NR	NR	NR

*Statistically significant difference.
IBE, ipsilateral breast event; CBE, contralateral breast event.

DeCensi, TAM01 (*JCO* 2019, PMID 30973790): PRT of 500 patients ≤75 years with ER+ DCIS randomized to low-dose tamoxifen (5 mg/day) or placebo for 3 years. MFU 5.1 years. The low-dose tamoxifen arm had fewer cumulative breast events (6% vs. 11%, p = .02) and CBEs (1% vs. 5%, p = .02). No difference in patient-reported outcomes except for slight increase in daily hot flashes with tamoxifen (p = .02). **Conclusion: Low-dose tamoxifen decreased CBEs by 75% with limited toxicity.**

Since tamoxifen prevents contralateral recurrences in the preceding trials, can we use it to prevent BC in high-risk patients?

The NSABP P-1 trial showed that tamoxifen reduces the risk of ER-positive invasive BC but increases the side effects along with the risk of endometrial cancer.[59] The NSABP P-2 trial found that raloxifene had similar efficacy as tamoxifen but with a lower rate of thromboembolic events among postmenopausal women.[60]

Is anastrozole superior to tamoxifen for DCIS?

The NSABP B-35 trial found that anastrozole 1 mg/day improves breast cancer-free interval compared with tamoxifen 20 mg/day for 5 years among postmenopausal women with ER- or PR-positive DCIS.[36]

Is hypofractionation appropriate for DCIS?

Many early prospective DCIS trials treated to 50 Gy/25 fx without a boost. Given the efficacy and safety in invasive BC, most consider hypofractionation to be appropriate for DCIS. Hypofractionation for DCIS has been prospectively studied in the TROG trial below. DCIS also accounted for 22% of the MDACC hypofractionation trial (42.56 Gy/16 fx) and 13% of the DBCG HYPO trial (40 Gy/15 fx), which demonstrated no difference in recurrence and similar-to-improved cosmesis with hypofractionation.[61,62]

BIG 3–07/TROG 07.01 (*Lancet* 2022, PMID 35934006): Phase III PRT of 1,608 women with unilateral non–low-risk DCIS (age <50, symptomatic, palpable, size ≥1.5 cm, grades 2–3, central necrosis, comedo-histology, or margin <1 mm) treated with BCS randomized to one of four groups: conventional (50 Gy/25 fx) or hypofractionated WBI (42.5 Gy/16 fx) with or without tumor bed boost (16 Gy/8 fx). MFU 6.6 years. LR at 5 years was not significantly different between conventional (94.4%) and hypofractionated (93.7%) groups. LR at 5 years was improved with boost (97% vs. 93%; HR 0.47, 95% CI 0.31–0.72). The boost group had higher rates of grade ≥2 breast pain (10% no boost vs. 14% boost, p = .003) and induration (6% no boost vs. 14% boost, p < .001). **Conclusion: Hypofractionation is appropriate for DCIS. Tumor bed boost improves LR rates in non–low-risk DCIS with an increase in acute and chronic toxicity.**

Is it necessary to boost the tumor bed for DCIS?

Boost was performed in a small minority of patients on historical prospective trials (5%–9% NSABP B-17/EORTC, not recommended on SweDCIS/UK/ANZ/RTOG 9804). A retrospective meta-analysis of *nonrandomized studies suggested reduced IBTR with boost.[63] ASTRO whole breast guidelines from 2018 conditionally recommend tumor bed boost in DCIS patients with age ≤50 years, high grade, or close (<2 mm) or positive margins.[38] More recently the BIG 3–07/TROG 07.01 trial (detailed above) prospectively demonstrated improved LC with the addition of boost for non–low-risk DCIS at the cost of worse cosmesis and breast pain.[37]*

Are there any patients who require RT after a mastectomy for DCIS?

PMRT for DCIS may reduce the risk of recurrence, particularly in those with positive margins, but it is not standard given conflicting poor-quality data. Two retrospective series demonstrate low recurrence rates (<2% all patients and <4% high-grade) after mastectomy with close/positive margins.[64,65] In another retrospective study of skin-sparing mastectomy, LR was 11% (2/19 patients) in those with close margins (<1 mm).[29]

Is PBI appropriate for patients with DCIS?

Multiple studies support the use of PBI in appropriately selected patients.[66–68] Current ASTRO, ABS, and ASBS guidelines support the use of PBI for select patients with DCIS.[41–43] ASTRO 2024 Consensus Guidelines[43] recommend PBI for DCIS patients if they meet the following criteria: low-intermediate grade, age ≥40, and size ≤2 cm. PBI is conditionally recommended for high-grade DCIS patients with tumor size >2 and ≤3 cm. PBI is not recommended for patients with positive surgical margins, BRCA1/2 mutation, or age <40. The RAPID trial of WBI (42.5 Gy/16 fx) vs. PBI (38.5 Gy/10 fx BID) included 18% DCIS patients and showed noninferior IBTR.[69] The NSABP B-39/RTOG 0413 trial included 24% DCIS patients and showed similar IBTR outcomes between standard fractionation and PBI without meeting prespecified CI threshold for equivalence.[70] Refer to Chapter 24 for further details on PBI.

Is there a role for IORT in the treatment of DCIS?

IORT has been shown to have higher rates of LR in two randomized trials (TARGIT-A and ELIOT).[71,72] Limited data are available for patients with DCIS[44] and thus IORT is not recommended off protocol at this time.

REFERENCES

1. Siegel RL, Giaquinto AN, Jemal A. Cancer statistics, 2024. *CA Cancer J Clin.* 2024;74(1):12–49. doi:10.3322/caac.21820

2. Giaquinto AN, Sung H, Miller KD, et al. Breast Cancer Statistics, 2022. *CA Cancer J Clin.* 2022;72(6):524–541. doi:10.3322/caac.21754

3. Collins LC, Tamimi RM, Baer HJ, Connolly JL, Colditz GA, Schnitt SJ. Outcome of patients with ductal carcinoma in situ untreated after diagnostic biopsy: results from the Nurses' Health Study. *Cancer.* 2005;103(9):1778–1784. doi:10.1002/cncr.20979

4. Sanders ME, Schuyler PA, Dupont WD, Page DL. The natural history of low-grade ductal carcinoma in situ of the breast in women treated by biopsy only revealed over 30 years of long-term follow-up. *Cancer.* 2005;103(12):2481–2484. doi:10.1002/cncr.21069

5. Eusebi V, Feudale E, Foschini MP, et al. Long-term follow-up of in situ carcinoma of the breast. *Semin Diagn Pathol.* 1994;11(3):223–235. PMID:7831534

6. Rosen PP, Lieberman PH, Braun DW Jr, Kosloff C, Adair F. Lobular carcinoma in situ of the breast Detailed analysis of 99 patients with average follow-up of 24 years. *Am J Surg Pathol.* 1978;2(3):225–252. doi:10.1097/00000478-197809000-00001

7. Chuba PJ, Hamre MR, Yap J, et al. Bilateral risk for subsequent breast cancer after lobular carcinoma-in-situ: analysis of surveillance, epidemiology, and end results data. *J Clin Oncol.* 2005;23(24):5534–5541. doi:10.1200/jco.2005.04.038

8. Harrison BT, Nakhlis F, Dillon DA, et al. Genomic profiling of pleomorphic and florid lobular carcinoma in situ reveals highly recurrent ERBB2 and ERRB3 alterations. *Mod Pathol.* 2020;33(7):1287–1297. doi:10.1038/s41379-020-0459-6

9. Shamir ER, Chen YY, Chu T, Pekmezci M, Rabban JT, Krings G. Pleomorphic and florid lobular carcinoma in situ variants of the breast. *Am J Surg Pathol.* 2019;43(3):399–408. doi:10.1097/pas.0000000000001191

10. Rakovitch E, Nofech-Mozes S, Hanna W, et al. A population-based validation study of the DCIS Score predicting recurrence risk in individuals treated by breast-conserving surgery alone. *Breast Cancer Res Treat.* 2015;152(2):389–398. doi:10.1007/s10549-015-3464-6

11. Solin LJ, Gray R, Baehner FL, et al. A multigene expression assay to predict local recurrence risk for ductal carcinoma in situ of the breast. *J Natl Cancer Inst.* 2013;105(10):701–710. doi:10.1093/jnci/djt067

12. Independent UK Panel on Breast Cancer Screening. The benefits and harms of breast cancer screening: an independent review. *Lancet*. 2012;380(9855):1778–1786. doi:10.1016/s0140-6736(12)61611-0

13. Duffy S, Vulkan D, Cuckle H, et al. Annual mammographic screening to reduce breast cancer mortality in women from age 40 years: long-term follow-up of the UK Age RCT. *Health Technol Assess*. 2020;24(55):1–24. doi:10.3310/hta24550

14. Duffy SW, Tabar L, Yen AM, et al. Mammography screening reduces rates of advanced and fatal breast cancers: results in 549,091 women. *Cancer*. 2020;126(13):2971–2979. doi:10.1002/cncr.32859

15. Duffy SW, Vulkan D, Cuckle H, et al. Effect of mammographic screening from age 40 years on breast cancer mortality (UK Age trial): final results of a randomised, controlled trial. *Lancet Oncol*. 2020;21(9):1165–1172. doi:10.1016/S1470-2045(20)30398-3

16. Holland R, Stekhoven JHS, Hendriks JHCL, Verbeek ALM, Mravunac M. Extent, distribution, and mammographic/histological correlations of breast ductal carcinoma in situ. *Lancet*. 1990;335(8688):519–522. doi:10.1016/0140-6736(90)90747-s

17. Dershaw DD, Abramson A, Kinne DW. Ductal carcinoma in situ: mammographic findings and clinical implications. *Radiology*. 1989;170(2):411–415. doi:10.1148/radiology.170.2.2536185

18. Kuhl CK, Schrading S, Bieling HB, et al. MRI for diagnosis of pure ductal carcinoma in situ: a prospective observational study. *Lancet*. 2007;370(9586):485–492. doi:10.1016/s0140-6736(07)61232-x

19. Fancellu A, Turner RM, Dixon JM, Pinna A, Cottu P, Houssami N. Meta-analysis of the effect of preoperative breast MRI on the surgical management of ductal carcinoma in situ. *Br J Surg*. 2015;102(8):883–893. doi:10.1002/bjs.9797

20. McGhan LJ, Pockaj BA, Wasif N, Giurescu ME, McCullough AE, Gray RJ. Atypical ductal hyperplasia on core biopsy: an automatic trigger for excisional biopsy? *Ann Surg Oncol*. 2012;19(10):3264–3269. doi:10.1245/s10434-012-2575-0

21. Group EBCTC, Correa C, McGale P, et al. Overview of the randomized trials of radiotherapy in ductal carcinoma in situ of the breast. *J Natl Cancer Inst Monogr*. 2010;2010(41):162–177. doi:10.1093/jncimonographs/lgq039

22. Silverstein MJ. An argument against routine use of radiotherapy for ductal carcinoma in situ. *Oncology (Williston Park)*. 2003;17(11):1511–1533. PMID:14682107

23. Silverstein MJ, Lagios MD. Choosing treatment for patients with ductal carcinoma in situ: fine tuning the University of Southern California/Van Nuys Prognostic Index. *J Natl Cancer Inst Monogr*. 2010;2010(41):193–196. doi:10.1093/jncimonographs/lgq040

24. MacAusland SG, Hepel JT, Chong FK, et al. An attempt to independently verify the utility of the Van Nuys Prognostic Index for ductal carcinoma in situ. *Cancer*. 2007;110(12):2648–2653. doi:10.1002/cncr.23089

25. Whitfield R, Kollias J, de Silva P, Turner J, Maddern G. Management of ductal carcinoma in situ according to Van Nuys Prognostic Index in Australia and New Zealand. *ANZ J Surg*. 2012;82(7–8):518–523. doi:10.1111/j.1445-2197.2012.06133.x

26. Fisher B, Costantino JP, Wickerham DL, et al. Tamoxifen for prevention of breast cancer: report of the national surgical adjuvant breast and bowel project P-1 study. *J Natl Cancer Inst*. 1998;90(18):1371–1388. doi:10.1093/jnci/90.18.1371

27. Vogel VG, Costantino JP, Wickerham DL, et al. Effects of tamoxifen vs raloxifene on the risk of developing invasive breast cancer and other disease outcomes: the NSABP Study of Tamoxifen and Raloxifene (STAR) P-2 trial. *JAMA*. 2006;295(23):2727–2741. doi:10.1001/jama.295.23.joc60074

28. Hwang ES. The impact of surgery on ductal carcinoma in situ outcomes: the use of mastectomy. *J Natl Cancer Inst Monogr*. 2010;2010(41):197–199. doi:10.1093/jncimonographs/lgq032

29. Carlson GW, Page A, Johnson E, Nicholson K, Styblo TM, Wood WC. Local recurrence of ductal carcinoma in situ after skin-sparing mastectomy. *J Am Coll Surg*. 2007;204(5):1074–1078. doi:10.1016/j.jamcollsurg.2007.01.063

30. Faverly DR, Burgers L, Bult P, Holland R. Three dimensional imaging of mammary ductal carcinoma in situ: clinical implications. *Semin Diagn Pathol*. 1994;11(3):193–198. PMID:7831530

31. Gradishar WJ, Moran MS, Abraham J, et al. Breast cancer, version 3.2024, NCCN clinical practice guidelines in oncology. *J Natl Compr Cancer Netw*. 2024;22(5):331–357. doi:10.6004/jnccn.2024.0035

32. Kurniawan ED, Rose A, Mou A, et al. Risk factors for invasive breast cancer when core needle biopsy shows ductal carcinoma in situ. *Arch Surg*. 2010;145(11):1098–1104. doi:10.1001/archsurg.2010.243

33. Yen TWF, Hunt KK, Ross MI, et al. Predictors of invasive breast cancer in patients with an initial diagnosis of ductal carcinoma in situ: a guide to selective use of sentinel lymph node biopsy in management of ductal carcinoma in situ. *J Am Coll Surg*. 2005;200(4):516–526. doi:10.1016/j.jamcollsurg.2004.11.012

34. Breast Cancer Screening and Diagnosis, Version 2.2024, NCCN Clinical Practice Guidelines in Oncology. National Comprehensive Cancer Network; 2024. Accessed December 1, 2024. https://www.nccn.org/professionals/physician_gls/pdf/breast-screening.pdf

35. Lazzeroni M, Puntoni M, Guerrieri-Gonzaga A, et al. Randomized placebo controlled trial of low-dose tamoxifen to prevent recurrence in breast noninvasive neoplasia: a 10-year follow-up of TAM-01 study. *J Clin Oncol*. 2023;41(17):3116–3121. doi:10.1200/jco.22.02900

36. Margolese RG, Cecchini RS, Julian TB, et al. Anastrozole versus tamoxifen in postmenopausal women with ductal carcinoma in situ undergoing lumpectomy plus radiotherapy (NSABP B-35): a randomised, double-blind, phase 3 clinical trial. *Lancet*. 2016;387(10021):849–856. doi:10.1016/S0140-6736(15)01168-X

37. Chua BH, Link EK, Kunkler IH, et al. Radiation doses and fractionation schedules in non-low-risk ductal carcinoma in situ in the breast (BIG 3–07/TROG 07.01): a randomised, factorial, multicentre, open-label, phase 3 study. *Lancet*. 2022;400(10350):431–440. doi:10.1016/s0140-6736(22)01246-6

38. Smith BD, Bellon JR, Blitzblau R, et al. Radiation therapy for the whole breast: executive summary of an American Society for Radiation Oncology (ASTRO) evidence-based guideline. *Pr Radiat Oncol*. 2018;8(3): 145–152. doi:10.1016/j.prro.2018.01.012

39. Brunt AM, Haviland JS, Sydenham M, et al. Ten-year results of FAST: a randomized controlled trial of 5-fraction whole-breast radiotherapy for early breast cancer. *J Clin Oncol*. 2020;38(28):3261–3272. doi:10.1200/JCO.19.02750

40. Murray Brunt A, Haviland JS, Wheatley DA, et al. Hypofractionated breast radiotherapy for 1 week versus 3 weeks (FAST-Forward): 5-year efficacy and late normal tissue effects results from a multicentre, non-inferiority, randomised, phase 3 trial. *Lancet*. 2020;395(10237):1613–1626. doi:10.1016/S0140-6736(20)30932-6

41. Anderson B, Arthur D, Hannoun-Levi JM, et al. Partial breast irradiation: an updated consensus statement from the American brachytherapy society. *Brachytherapy*. 2022;21(6):726–747. doi:10.1016/j.brachy.2022.07.004

42. Correa C, Harris EE, Leonardi MC, et al. Accelerated partial breast irradiation: executive summary for the update of an ASTRO evidence-based consensus statement. *Pract Radiat Oncol*. 2017;7(2):73–79. doi:10.1016/j.prro.2016.09.007

43. Shaitelman SF, Anderson BM, Arthur DW, et al. Partial breast irradiation for patients with early-stage invasive breast cancer or ductal carcinoma in situ: an ASTRO clinical practice guideline. *Pract Radiat Oncol*. 2024;14(2):112–132. doi:10.1016/j.prro.2023.11.001

44. Rivera R, Banks A, Casillas-Lopez A, et al. Targeted intraoperative radiotherapy for the management of ductal carcinoma in situ of the breast. *Breast J*. 2016;22(1):63–74. doi:10.1111/tbj.12516

45. Cuzick J, Sestak I, Pinder SE, et al. Effect of tamoxifen and radiotherapy in women with locally excised ductal carcinoma in situ: long-term results from the UK/ANZ DCIS trial. *Lancet Oncol*. 2011;12(1):21–29. doi:10.1016/s1470-2045(10)70266-7

46. Donker M, Litière S, Werutsky G, et al. Breast-conserving treatment with or without radiotherapy in ductal carcinoma in situ: 15-year recurrence rates and outcome after a recurrence, from the EORTC 10853 randomized phase III trial. *J Clin Oncol*. 2013;31(32):4054–4059. doi:10.1200/jco.2013.49.5077

47. Wapnir IL, Dignam JJ, Fisher B, et al. Long-term outcomes of invasive ipsilateral breast tumor recurrences after lumpectomy in NSABP B-17 and B-24 randomized clinical trials for DCIS. *J Natl Cancer Inst*. 2011;103(6):478–488. doi:10.1093/jnci/djr027

48. Wärnberg F, Garmo H, Emdin S, et al. Effect of radiotherapy after breast-conserving surgery for ductal carcinoma in situ: 20 years follow-up in the randomized SweDCIS trial. *J Clin Oncol*. 2014;32(32):3613–3618. doi:10.1200/jco.2014.56.2595

49. Goodwin A, Parker S, Ghersi D, Wilcken N. Post-operative radiotherapy for ductal carcinoma in situ of the breast. *Cochrane Database Syst Rev*. 2013;(11):CD000563. doi:10.1002/14651858.cd000563.pub7

50. Ringberg A, Nordgren H, Thorstensson S, et al. Histopathological risk factors for ipsilateral breast events after breast conserving treatment for ductal carcinoma in situ of the breast–results from the Swedish randomised trial. *Eur J Cancer*. 2007;43(2):291–298. doi:10.1016/j.ejca.2006.09.018

51. Meijnen P, Bartelink H. Multifocal ductal carcinoma in situ of the breast: a contraindication for breast-conserving treatment? *J Clin Oncol*. 2007;25(35):5548–5549. doi:10.1200/jco.2007.13.9121

52. Vicini FA, Recht A. Age at diagnosis and outcome for women with ductal carcinoma-in-situ of the breast: a critical review of the literature. *J Clin Oncol*. 2002;20(11):2736–2744. doi:10.1200/jco.2002.07.137

53. Solin LJ, Gray R, Hughes LL, et al. Surgical excision without radiation for ductal carcinoma in situ of the breast: 12-year results from the ECOG-ACRIN E5194 study. *J Clin Oncol*. 2015;33(33):3938–3944. doi:10.1200/jco.2015.60.8588

54. Wong JS, Chen YH, Gadd MA, et al. Eight-year update of a prospective study of wide excision alone for small low- or intermediate-grade Ductal Carcinoma In Situ (DCIS). *Breast Cancer Res Treat*. 2014;143(2): 343–350. doi:10.1007/s10549-013-2813-6

55. Raldow AC, Sher D, Chen AB, Recht A, Punglia RS. Cost effectiveness of the oncotype DX DCIS score for guiding treatment of patients with ductal carcinoma in situ. *J Clin Oncol*. 2016;34(33):3963–3968. doi:10.1200/jco.2016.67.8532

56. Bremer T, Whitworth P, Patel R, et al. A biologic signature for breast ductal carcinoma in situ to predict Radiation Therapy (RT) benefit and assess recurrence risk. *Clin Cancer Res*. 2018;24(23):5895–5901. doi:10.1158/1078-0432.ccr-18-0842

57. Wärnberg F, Karlsson P, Holmberg E, et al. Prognostic risk assessment and prediction of radiotherapy benefit for women with Ductal Carcinoma In Situ (DCIS) of the breast, in a randomized clinical trial (SweDCIS). *Cancers*. 2021;13(23):6103. doi:10.3390/cancers13236103

58. Allred DC, Anderson SJ, Paik S, et al. Adjuvant tamoxifen reduces subsequent breast cancer in women with estrogen receptor–positive ductal carcinoma in situ: a study based on NSABP protocol B-24. *J Clin Oncol.* 2012;30(12):1268–1273. doi:10.1200/jco.2010.34.0141

59. Fisher B, Costantino JP, Wickerham DL, et al. Tamoxifen for prevention of breast cancer: report of the national surgical adjuvant breast and bowel project P-1 study. *J Natl Cancer Inst.* 1998;90(18):1371–1388. doi:10.1093/jnci/90.18.1371

60. Vogel VG, Costantino JP, Wickerham DL, et al. Effects of tamoxifen vs raloxifene on the risk of developing invasive breast cancer and other disease outcomesthe NSABP Study of Tamoxifen and Raloxifene (STAR) P-2 trial. *JAMA.* 2006;295(23):2727–2741. doi:10.1001/jama.295.23.joc60074

61. Offersen BV, Alsner J, Nielsen HM, et al. Hypofractionated versus standard fractionated radiotherapy in patients with early breast cancer or ductal carcinoma in situ in a randomized phase III trial: the DBCG HYPO trial. *J Clin Oncol.* 2020;38(31):3615–3625. doi:10.1200/jco.20.01363

62. Shaitelman SF, Schlembach PJ, Arzu I, et al. Acute and short-term toxic effects of conventionally fractionated vs hypofractionated whole-breast irradiation: a randomized clinical trial. *JAMA Oncol.* 2015;1(7):931–941. doi:10.1001/jamaoncol.2015.2666

63. Moran MS, Zhao Y, Ma S, et al. Association of radiotherapy boost for ductal carcinoma in situ with local control after whole-breast radiotherapy. *JAMA Oncol.* 2017;3(8):1060–1068. doi:10.1001/jamaoncol.2016.6948

64. Chan LW, Rabban J, Hwang ES, et al. Is radiation indicated in patients with ductal carcinoma in situ and close or positive mastectomy margins? *Int J Radiat Oncol Biol Phys.* 2011;80(1):25–30. doi:10.1016/j.ijrobp.2010.01.044

65. Childs SK, Chen YH, Duggan MM, et al. Impact of margin status on local recurrence after mastectomy for ductal carcinoma in situ. *Int J Radiat Oncol Biol Phys.* 2013;85(4):948–952. doi:10.1016/j.ijrobp.2012.07.2377

66. Shah C, Badiyan S, Wilkinson JB, et al. Treatment efficacy with Accelerated Partial Breast Irradiation (APBI): final analysis of the American society of breast surgeons mammosite® breast brachytherapy registry trial. *Ann Surg Oncol.* 2013;20(10):3279–3285. doi:10.1245/s10434-013-3158-4

67. Strnad V, Ott OJ, Hildebrandt G, et al. 5-year results of accelerated partial breast irradiation using sole interstitial multicatheter brachytherapy versus whole-breast irradiation with boost after breast-conserving surgery for low-risk invasive and in-situ carcinoma of the female breast: a randomised, phase 3, non-inferiority trial. *Lancet.* 2016;387(10015):229–238. doi:10.1016/s0140-6736(15)00471-7

68. Vicini F, Shah C, Wilkinson JB, Keisch M, Beitsch P, Lyden M. Should Ductal Carcinoma-In-Situ (DCIS) be removed from the ASTRO consensus panel cautionary group for off-protocol use of Accelerated Partial Breast Irradiation (APBI)? A pooled analysis of outcomes for 300 patients with DCIS treated with APBI. *Ann Surg Oncol.* 2013;20(4):1275–1281. doi:10.1245/s10434-012-2694-7

69. Whelan TJ, Julian JA, Berrang TS, et al. External beam accelerated partial breast irradiation versus whole breast irradiation after breast conserving surgery in women with ductal carcinoma in situ and node-negative breast cancer (RAPID): a randomised controlled trial. *Lancet.* 2019;394(10215):2165–2172. doi:10.1016/s0140-6736(19)32515-2

70. Vicini FA, Cecchini RS, White JR, et al. Long-term primary results of accelerated partial breast irradiation after breast-conserving surgery for early-stage breast cancer: a randomised, phase 3, equivalence trial. *Lancet.* 2019;394(10215):2155–2164. doi:10.1016/s0140-6736(19)32514-0

71. Vaidya JS, Bulsara M, Baum M, et al. Long term survival and local control outcomes from single dose targeted intraoperative radiotherapy during lumpectomy (TARGIT-IORT) for early breast cancer: TARGIT-A randomised clinical trial. *BMJ.* 2020;370:m2836. doi:10.1136/bmj.m2836

72. Orecchia R, Veronesi U, Maisonneuve P, et al. Intraoperative irradiation for early breast cancer (ELIOT): long-term recurrence and survival outcomes from a single-centre, randomised, phase 3 equivalence trial. *Lancet Oncol.* 2021;22(5):597–608. doi:10.1016/S1470-2045(21)00080-2

Zachary S. Mayo and Chirag Shah

QUICK HIT Patients with isolated locoregional recurrence (LRR) of breast cancer harbor an increased risk of DM and mortality. The majority of LRRs occur in the ipsilateral breast or chest wall (CW) within 10 years of initial treatment. Patients with LRR represent a heterogenous group, and data are limited to guide management. Treatment is often dependent upon the initial management and the location of recurrence (Table 27.1). Therapy is directed toward maximizing LC with a curative intent utilizing surgery and/or RT with consideration for CHT and/or endocrine therapy. RT may be given with concurrent hyperthermia (HYP) or CHT.

Table 27.1 General Treatment Paradigm for Locoregionally Recurrent Breast Cancer		
LR only	Initial BCS + RT	Total mastectomy ± repeat SLN/ALND (if level I/II dissection not previously done); can consider repeat BCT; consider CHT either preop or postop
	Initial mastectomy only	Surgery if possible ± repeat SLN/ALND (if not previously done) + RT; consider CHT either preop or postop
	Initial mastectomy + ALN I/II dissection + RT	Surgery if possible; ± re-RT and/or CHT
Regional ± LR	ALN recurrence	Surgery, ± CHT, ± RT/re-RT (sequence pending clinical scenario)
	SCV or IMN recurrence	CHT, consideration for surgery and/or RT/re-RT if possible

EPIDEMIOLOGY: It is estimated that there are over four million breast cancer survivors in the United States.[1] LRR occurs in 5% to 15%, with decreasing rates in modern studies.[2–5] Most LRRs occur within 10 years of diagnosis, with recurrences after mastectomy occurring earlier than after BCT (~1.2 years earlier).[6] Following LRR, the 5-year OS varies widely, ranging from 25% to 75%.[6–9]

RISK FACTORS: Younger age, premenopausal status, larger tumor size, higher BMI, increasing number of LN+, decreased number of dissected LN, ER-negative, HER2+ not treated with trastuzumab, high grade, LVSI, positive margins, not receiving endocrine therapy, BCS without RT, and mastectomy without RT when indicated.[10–15] Genetic susceptibility (BRCA1 or BRCA2) increases the risk of a new primary cancer.

ANATOMY: Following BCT, LRR occurs most commonly in the ipsilateral breast. Following mastectomy, LRR occurs most commonly on the CW (~60%) > SCV (~20%) > ALN (~10%).[10]

CLINICAL PRESENTATION: LRR is usually detected via mammography (following BCT), physical exam, or other imaging. Symptoms can include palpable mass, skin changes, new-onset lymphedema, palpable LN, skin changes, or brachial plexopathy.[16–18]

WORKUP

Labs: CBC, LFTs, alkaline phosphatase, creatinine.

Imaging: Mammogram/ultrasound of breast (if following BCS), CT chest/abdomen/pelvis and bone scan, or PET/CT. MRI brain if symptomatic. X-rays of symptomatic bones or suspicious areas noted on bone scan. Consider breast MRI for those with intact breast and MRI of the brachial plexus for those with brachial plexopathy symptoms.

Other: Biopsy with comparison to original pathology, receptor status evaluation, genetic counseling (if high risk).[19]

PROGNOSTIC FACTORS: Prognosis is better if LRR is isolated in the CW/axilla/IM nodes only (5-year OS 44%–49%) vs. SCV/multiple sites (5-year OS 21%–24%).[20] Negative prognostic factors: LRR within 2 years of initial treatment, LRR after mastectomy (vs. BCT), skin involvement, larger primary tumor, initial multiple LN+, older age, or higher BMI.[8,13,20,21]

STAGING: Assign a recurrent TNM (rTNM) stage per AJCC (see Chapter 24 for staging).

TREATMENT PARADIGM

Surgery: Surgical options are dependent on the location of the recurrence, previous surgery performed, and feasibility of resection (ability to obtain negative margins). In general, in-breast recurrences after previous lumpectomy may be salvaged with mastectomy. Repeat breast conservation is becoming more commonly utilized with prospective data available and can be considered in patients who wish to avoid mastectomy. CW recurrences and nodal recurrences should be excised if feasible, often after cytoreductive systemic therapy.

Chemotherapy: Choices of systemic therapy are determined by the tumor receptor status (ER, PR, HER2) and previous therapy received. CHT concurrent with RT may be considered in select patients and is typically utilized in patients with gross residual disease. Consider CHT after maximum LC achieved for ER-negative cancers (per the CALOR trial).[22]

Radiation: In the RT-naïve patient, adjuvant RT to the CW with doses of 50 to 60 Gy is appropriate using standard fractionation, with increasing data supporting moderate hypofractionation. For positive margins, doses of 60 to 66 Gy or higher are recommended. For gross disease, doses of 66 to 70 Gy are recommended, with consideration of concurrent CHT (capecitabine). Many different regimens have been used for re-RT. One option for repeat breast conservation includes 45 Gy at 1.5 Gy/fx BID to the partial breast (RTOG 1014).[23] Conventionally fractionated RT with 45 Gy/25 fx given daily has also been reported.[24] For re-RT following mastectomy, consider concurrent HYP to improve LC. Sequelae can include fatigue, radiation dermatitis, fibrosis, lymphedema, brachial plexopathy, CW pain, rib fracture, pneumonitis, wound healing issues, and cardiotoxicity.

Hyperthermia (HYP): Typically given to superficial CW recurrences concurrent with re-RT to temperature of 43°C. When used in conjunction with RT, HYP impairs the cell's ability to repair RT-induced DNA damage resulting in more effective tumor cell kill. At 43°C, there is a dramatic decrease in the cell survival slope (Arrhenius plot). HYP dosing is frequently described in terms of CEM43°C T90, which represents the number of cumulative equivalent minutes at 43°C exceeded by 90% of the monitored points within the tumor. HYP-related damage is cell cycle nonspecific (as opposed to RT, which is most damaging during G2/M and least effective in S). However, cells may develop thermotolerance (resistance to subsequent HYP), which is a phenomenon thought to be due to the production of heat shock proteins, and therefore HYP is not delivered daily.[25] A commonly used RT dosing regimen is 32 to 40 Gy in 8 to 10 fx delivered twice weekly with concurrent HYP as per the ESHO 5–88 trial published in 1996 as well as other series,[26] with more recent data using this regimen published by Dutch investigators in 2015.[27] HYP techniques include microwave heating, regional perfusional HYP, ultrasound, and wrapping.

EVIDENCE-BASED Q&A

How are true recurrences and new primaries differentiated? How does this change prognosis?

Characteristics of a new primary include different histology, change in receptor status, different location, loss of heterozygosity (LOH), and change from aneuploid to diploid when compared with the original tumor. The risk of new primary is higher if BRCA 1 or 2 positive. Tumor recurrences and true primaries occur at a similar rate until 8 years; subsequently, new primaries occur more frequently. A new primary has a more favorable prognosis compared with a true recurrence (10-year OS 75% vs. 55%).[28–30]

Can an SLNB be repeated for LRR breast cancer?

Yes. A 2018 meta-analysis found repeat SLNB was feasible, accurate, spares patients from unnecessary ALND, and provides information that can alter management. It included 1,761 patients who had prior SLNB or ALND who underwent repeat SLNB. An SLN was identified in 64% (more successful if no prior ALND), with 18% node-positive. Aberrant drainage was seen more frequently in those with prior ALND.

The negative predictive value was 97%. There was no statistical difference between those with previous RT vs. those without.[31]

LOCAL RECURRENCE AFTER BCT

What is the preferred treatment for LRR after initial BCT? Is salvage BCS an option?

Many clinicians prefer salvage mastectomy given the higher observed LR rates following salvage BCS (4%–25% vs. 7%–49%, respectively).[32] However, no prospective trials have compared the two strategies. Approximately 80% to 95% of patients with LR after BCT are suitable mastectomy candidates.[33,34] After salvage mastectomy, LR ranges from 4% to 25%, with 5-year OS ranging from 57% to 100% and 10-year OS rates of 40% to 80%.[32,34–39] LR is much higher in patients undergoing excision alone and can be as high as 49%.[40] PMRT in patients with prior RT is reserved for those with high-risk features, including T3, multiple LN involved, or positive margins. Retrospective studies show that following primary BCT with a subsequent IBTR, salvage mastectomy vs. salvage BCS had no difference in OS,[34] with the caveat that the Milan study showed increased IBTR with repeat BCS.[35] RTOG 1014 is a phase II study that provides a framework for repeat BCS with re-RT.[23]

After initial BCT, is re-RT safe and feasible?

Although data are limited, repeat BCT is becoming more common. A German RR of 83 patients with recurrent breast cancer treated with mastectomy (followed by mastectomy scar RT) or lumpectomy (followed by partial breast RT) reported a recurrence rate of 14.5% at MFU of 34 months. RT dose was 45 Gy/25 fx and no grade 3+ toxicities were reported.[24] RTOG 1014 evaluated repeat BCS followed by 45 Gy/30 fx (3D partial breast re-RT) delivered BID, with data demonstrating excellent LC with a 5-year recurrence rate of 5%. However, one must consider its stringent entrance criteria.[23]

Arthur, RTOG 1014 (*JAMA Oncol* 2019, PMID 31750868): Phase II single-arm trial investigating 3D conformal partial breast re-RT (PBrI) following repeat lumpectomy for IBTR after previous BCS + WBI. Patients included those with a recurrent unifocal tumor <3 cm in the ipsilateral breast more than 1 year following initial treatment with WBI. PBrI was delivered 45 Gy/30 fx BID using 3D-CRT with a 1.5-cm CTV and 1-cm PTV. Of the initial recurrences, 40% were noninvasive and 60% were invasive. Among invasive recurrences, 7% were HER-2+ and 23% were triple-negative. Ninety-one percent of patients had tumors 2 cm or smaller, median size 1.0 cm. At MFU of 5.5 years for 58 evaluable patients, there were four IBTRs (5-year cumulative incidence 5%). The 5-year incidence of ipsilateral mastectomy was 10%. The 5-year DMFS and OS rates were both 95%. The rate of late grade 3 toxicity was 7%, and no late grade 4 toxicities were seen. **Conclusion: For patients with IBTR after BCT, repeat BCT is a reasonable alternative to mastectomy, with a low risk of second recurrence and a 5-year freedom from mastectomy rate of 90%.**

Is interstitial brachytherapy after LRR safe and feasible?

Yes. Multiple studies have found repeat lumpectomy plus multicatheter brachytherapy (MCB) is safe and effective in preventing second LR with at least equivalent OS to salvage mastectomy. The 10-year rates of second LR, DM, and OS with lumpectomy and MCB were 7%, 19%, and 76%, respectively.[41] A GEC-ESTRO matched cohort analysis of salvage mastectomy vs. lumpectomy plus brachytherapy found no differences in OS or a third breast event.[42]

Hannoun-Levi, GEC-ESTRO (*IJROBP* 2021, PMID 33383125): Propensity score-matched analysis of patients with a second breast event treated with mastectomy or lumpectomy plus brachytherapy. Among 1,327 analyzed patients, 754 (377 each arm) were matched. There were no differences in 5-year OS (88% vs. 87%) or incidence of third breast event (2% vs. 3%). In patients treated with re-RT, 4% required mastectomy. Grade 3 or worse toxicity was seen in 10%. **Conclusion: Lumpectomy with brachytherapy for IBTR provides similar oncologic outcomes compared with mastectomy.**

Hannoun-Levi, GEC-ESTRO (*IJROBP* 2023, PMID 37459998): RR of 508 patients with IBTR following primary BCT (lumpectomy + ALND/SLNB + RT) re-treated with lumpectomy followed by interstitial MCB. MFU 61 months. The 5-year cumulative incidence was 4% for local relapse and 5% for DM. The 5-year DFS and OS rates were 89% and 91%, respectively. The rate of grade 3 toxicity was 12%. **Conclusion: Lumpectomy plus partial breast brachytherapy is feasible and effective in preventing second LR with acceptable toxicity.**

LOCAL RECURRENCE AFTER MASTECTOMY

How should local/CW recurrences after mastectomy be treated?

In patients undergoing upfront mastectomy with negative margins, CW recurrences are rare but can be seen in up to 20% in high-risk patients.[43] NCCN guidelines recommend surgical resection followed by RT to the CW and regional LN (if feasible).[19] If possible, aggressive RT after resection is preferred (see Halverson) with consideration of CHT afterwards per the CALOR study (see below) for receptor-negative cancers. Consider neoadjuvant CHT based on biopsy and extent of tumor recurrence.

Halverson, Washington U. (IJROBP 1990, PMID 2211253): RR of 244 patients with LRR following mastectomy alone. Based on the findings, the authors had four recommendations: (a) Large-field RT (i.e., entire CW) improved control compared with localized RT (i.e., lesion + 1–2 cm margin). The 10-year freedom from CW re-recurrence was 63% vs. 18% (*p* < .01). (b) Elective RT to SCV nodes 46 to 50 Gy reduced SCV failure from 16% to 6% (*p* = .05). (c) Elective RT to uninvolved CW to >50 Gy. Patients with SCV or ALN disease failed in CW 29% and 21%, respectively. RT to uninvolved CW decreased recurrence from 27% to 17% (*p* = .32). (d) Treatment to >50 Gy for completely excised recurrences and >60 Gy for incompletely excised <3 cm recurrences (tumors <3 cm control with ≥60 Gy vs. <60 Gy was 100% vs. 76%). Tumor control for >3 cm lesions was only 50% despite doses of 70 Gy.

Is re-RT in the postmastectomy setting safe and feasible?

The Wahl study included 31 patients s/p mastectomy and demonstrated that re-RT to the CW appears safe. Acute/late toxicity occurred at acceptable rates, and included lymphedema or skin toxicity (e.g., dermatitis, fibrosis, skin infection). The risk of pneumonitis is low with modern techniques.[44] However, one must account for the risk of brachial plexopathy, which has been shown to increase significantly with cumulative doses above 95 Gy and with re-RT intervals less than 1 year.[45] Consider HYP in addition to RT.

REGIONAL RECURRENCE TO AXILLARY LN OR SUPRACLAVICULAR LN

Following mastectomy, LRR occurs in the CW (~60%) > SCV (~20%) > ALN (~10%).[11] For patients with an axillary recurrence and history of prior SLNB, completion ALND is recommended. For those with a prior ALND presenting with an axillary recurrence, resection should be attempted. Postsurgical comprehensive nodal RT should also be considered. If the patient is unable to undergo surgery, consider concurrent capecitabine with RT.[46] Prognosis is better if LRR is isolated to CW/ALNs/IMNs alone (5-year OS 44%–49%) vs. SCV/multiple sites (5-year OS 21%–24%).[20]

What are the outcomes after treatment for supraclavicular recurrence?

SCV recurrence (SCVr) is associated with a poor prognosis. However, long-term survival is possible and aggressive treatment may be beneficial. Consider RT doses ≥60 Gy as this improves RFS and OS in the upfront setting compared with doses <60 Gy.[47]

Reddy, MD Anderson (IJROBP 2011, PMID 21168284): RR of 140 patients with LRR following initial MRM and CHT, 47 patients with recurrence involving SCV (23 isolated SCVr). Patients with SCVr had worse 3-year DMFS and OS than those without SCV involvement. However, those with isolated SCVr had similar outcomes to those with isolated CW recurrences, with 5-year OS of ~25%. **Conclusion: SCVr carries a poor prognosis, but those with isolated SCVr can achieve long-term OS (25% >5 years).**

How should isolated internal mammary nodal recurrences be managed?

There are little data available to guide management of IMN recurrences. For patients who underwent initial mastectomy without RT, comprehensive RT to the CW, SCV, and IM nodes with consideration of IM boost is recommended. If prior history of RT, consider CHT followed by restaging. RT options in this scenario may include SBRT vs. hyperfractionation.[48–51] Can consider thoracoscopic resection at institutions with experience, although data are limited.

Are there any techniques to reduce the incidence of lymphedema in patients with recurrent breast cancer?

Lymphovenous bypass surgery can be considered in select patients to reduce the risk of lymphedema, particularly in those undergoing ALND and/or regional nodal RT. In an RR of 58 patients who underwent ALND (52 also had regional nodal RT) and lymphovenous bypass surgery, only 2 had symptomatic lymphedema.[52]

What is the role of chemotherapy for locoregional recurrence?

For ER-negative recurrences, consider CHT after maximum local control is achieved or preoperatively to facilitate a GTR.

Aebi, CALOR Trial (*Lancet Oncol* 2014, PMID 24439313; Wapnir, *JCO* 2018, PMID 29443653): PRT of 162 patients with isolated LRR s/p radical resection (R0 or R1) randomized to adjuvant multiagent CHT or observation. All could receive hormone/HER2 therapy or RT. Excluded SCVr. The CHT used was not standardized and left to clinician discretion. MFU 9 years. For ER-negative patients, 10-year DFS 70% vs. 34% for CHT vs. no CHT, with HR 0.29 (95% CI 0.13–0.67). In ER-positive patients, the 10-year DFS 50% vs. 59% for CHT vs. no CHT, with HR 1.07 (95% CI 0.32–1.55). OS was not significantly different between groups regardless of ER status. **Conclusion: Following complete resection for isolated LRR, adjuvant CHT should be recommended for those with ER-negative disease to improve DFS.**

Does RT with hyperthermia (HYP) improve complete response (CR) rates compared with RT alone?

Yes. Two prospective studies and a meta-analysis of patients with unresectable disease show significantly improved CR rates with RT + HYP compared with RT alone (~40% vs. ~60%) and favorable CR rates (~66%) for re-RT with HYP.

Datta, Meta-Analysis (*IJROBP* 2016, PMID 26899950): Meta-analysis of RT + HYP in locally recurrent breast cancers treated without surgery or CHT; 34 studies (8 two-arm, 26 single-arm). Treatment was a median of seven HYP sessions at an average of 42.5°C, with a mean RT dose of 38.2 Gy (26–60 Gy). In the two-arm studies (627 patients), RT + HYP had CR in 60% vs. RT alone 38% (SS). In the single-arm studies, RT + HYP had CR rate of 63%. Among the 779 patients with previous RT, RT + HYP had CR of 67%. Mean acute and late grade 3/4 toxicities with RT + HYP were 14% and 5%, respectively. **Conclusion: In locally recurrent breast cancer, RT + HYP improves CR rates compared with RT alone. For re-RT + HYP, CR was achieved in 67% of patients.**

REFERENCES

1. Miller KD, Nogueira L, Devasia T, et al. Cancer treatment and survivorship statistics, 2022. *CA Cancer J Clin.* 2022;72(5):409–436. doi:10.3322/caac.21731
2. Fisher B, Anderson S, Bryant J, et al. Twenty-year follow-up of a randomized trial comparing total mastectomy, lumpectomy, and lumpectomy plus irradiation for the treatment of invasive breast cancer. *N Engl J Med.* 2002;347(16):1233–1241. doi:10.1056/NEJMoa022152
3. Ragaz J, Jackson SM, Le N, et al. Adjuvant radiotherapy and chemotherapy in node-positive premenopausal women with breast cancer. *N Engl J Med.* 1997;337(14):956–962. doi:10.1056/nejm199710023371402
4. Overgaard M, Nielsen HM, Overgaard J. Is the benefit of postmastectomy irradiation limited to patients with four or more positive nodes, as recommended in international consensus reports? A subgroup analysis of the DBCG 82 b&c randomized trials. *Radiother Oncol.* 2007;82(3):247–253. doi:10.1016/j.radonc.2007.02.001
5. Overgaard M, Jensen MB, Overgaard J, et al. Postoperative radiotherapy in high-risk postmenopausal breast-cancer patients given adjuvant tamoxifen: danish breast cancer cooperative group DBCG 82c randomised trial. *Lancet.* 1999;353(9165):1641–1648. doi:10.1016/s0140-6736(98)09201-0
6. van Tienhoven G, Voogd AC, Peterse JL, et al. Prognosis after treatment for loco-regional recurrence after mastectomy or breast conserving therapy in two randomised trials (EORTC 10801 and DBCG-82TM). EORTC breast cancer cooperative group and the danish breast cancer cooperative group. *Eur J Cancer.* 1999;35(1):32–38. doi:10.1016/s0959-8049(98)00301-3
7. Wapnir IL, Anderson SJ, Mamounas EP, et al. Prognosis after ipsilateral breast tumor recurrence and locoregional recurrences in five national surgical adjuvant breast and bowel project node-positive adjuvant breast cancer trials. *J Clin Oncol.* 2006;24(13):2028–2037. doi:10.1200/jco.2005.04.3273
8. Anderson SJ, Wapnir I, Dignam JJ, et al. Prognosis after ipsilateral breast tumor recurrence and locoregional recurrences in patients treated by breast-conserving therapy in five national surgical adjuvant breast and bowel project protocols of node-negative breast cancer. *J Clin Oncol.* 2009;27(15):2466–2473. doi:10.1200/jco.2008.19.8424

9. Reddy JP, Levy L, Oh JL, et al. Long-term outcomes in patients with isolated supraclavicular nodal recurrence after mastectomy and doxorubicin-based chemotherapy for breast cancer. *Int J Radiat Oncol Biol Phys.* 2011;80(5):1453–1457. doi:10.1016/j.ijrobp.2010.04.015

10. Taghian A, Jeong JH, Mamounas E, et al. Patterns of locoregional failure in patients with operable breast cancer treated by mastectomy and adjuvant chemotherapy with or without tamoxifen and without radiotherapy: results from five national surgical adjuvant breast and bowel project randomized clinical trials. *J Clin Oncol.* 2004;22(21):4247–4254. doi:10.1200/jco.2004.01.042

11. Recht A, Gray R, Davidson NE, et al. Locoregional failure 10 years after mastectomy and adjuvant chemotherapy with or without tamoxifen without irradiation: experience of the Eastern Cooperative Oncology Group. *J Clin Oncol.* 1999;17(6):1689–700. doi:10.1200/JCO.1999.17.6.1689

12. Cheng SH, Horng CF, Clarke JL, et al. Prognostic index score and clinical prediction model of local regional recurrence after mastectomy in breast cancer patients. *Int J Radiat Oncol Biol Phys.* 2006;64(5):1401–1409. doi:10.1016/j.ijrobp.2005.11.015

13. Nielsen HM, Overgaard M, Grau C, Jensen AR, Overgaard J. Loco-regional recurrence after mastectomy in high-risk breast cancer–risk and prognosis. An analysis of patients from the DBCG 82 b&c randomization trials. *Radiother Oncol.* 2006;79(2):147–155. doi:10.1016/j.radonc.2006.04.006

14. Wo JY, Taghian AG, Nguyen PL, et al. The association between biological subtype and isolated regional nodal failure after breast-conserving therapy. *Int J Radiat Oncol Biol Phys.* 2010;77(1):188–196. doi:10.1016/j.ijrobp.2009.04.059

15. Warren LE, Ligibel JA, Chen YH, Truong L, Catalano PJ, Bellon JR. Body mass index and locoregional recurrence in women with early-stage breast cancer. *Ann Surg Oncol.* 2016;23(12):3870–3879. doi:10.1245/s10434-016-5437-3

16. Dershaw DD, McCormick B, Osborne MP. Detection of local recurrence after conservative therapy for breast carcinoma. *Cancer.* 1992;70(2):493–496. doi:10.1002/1097-0142(19920715)70:2<493::aid-cncr2820700219>3.0.co;2-3

17. Montgomery DA, Krupa K, Jack WJ, et al. Changing pattern of the detection of locoregional relapse in breast cancer: the Edinburgh experience. *Br J Cancer.* 2007;96(12):1802–1807. doi:10.1038/sj.bjc.6603815

18. Montgomery DA, Krupa K, Cooke TG. Follow-up in breast cancer: does routine clinical examination improve outcome? A systematic review of the literature. *Br J Cancer.* 2007;97(12):1632–1641. doi:10.1038/sj.bjc.6604065

19. NCCN Clinical Practice Guidelines in Oncology: Breast Cancer. Accessed April 24, 2024. https://www.nccn.org/professionals/physician_gls/pdf/breast.pdf

20. Halverson KJ, Perez CA, Kuske RR, Garcia DM, Simpson JR, Fineberg B. Survival following locoregional recurrence of breast cancer: univariate and multivariate analysis. *Int J Radiat Oncol Biol Phys.* 1992;23(2):285–291. doi:10.1016/0360-3016(92)90743-2

21. Gage I, Schnitt SJ, Recht A, et al. Skin recurrences after breast-conserving therapy for early-stage breast cancer. *J Clin Oncol.* 1998;16(2):480–486. doi:10.1200/JCO.1998.16.2.480

22. Wapnir IL, Price KN, Anderson SJ, et al. Efficacy of chemotherapy for ER-negative and ER-positive isolated locoregional recurrence of breast cancer: final analysis of the CALOR trial. *J Clin Oncol.* 2018;36(11):1073–1079. doi:10.1200/jco.2017.76.5719

23. Arthur DW, Winter KA, Kuerer HM, et al. Effectiveness of breast-conserving surgery and 3-dimensional conformal partial breast reirradiation for recurrence of breast cancer in the ipsilateral breast: the NRG Oncology/RTOG 1014 phase 2 clinical trial. *JAMA Oncol.* 2019;6(1):75–82. doi:10.1001/jamaoncol.2019.4320

24. Janssen S, Rades D, Meyer A, et al. Local recurrence of breast cancer: conventionally fractionated partial external beam re-irradiation with curative intention. *Strahlenther Onkol.* 2018;194(9):806–814. doi:10.1007/s00066-018-1315-1

25. Hall EJ, Giaccia AJ. *Radiobiology for the Radiologist.* 8th ed. Wolters Kluwer; 2019:597.

26. Vernon CC, Hand JW, Field SB, et al. Radiotherapy with or without hyperthermia in the treatment of superficial localized breast cancer: results from five randomized controlled trials. International Collaborative Hyperthermia Group. *Int J Radiat Oncol Biol Phys.* 1996;35(4):731–744. doi:10.1016/0360-3016(96)00154-x

27. Linthorst M, Baaijens M, Wiggenraad R, et al. Local control rate after the combination of re-irradiation and hyperthermia for irresectable recurrent breast cancer: results in 248 patients. *Radiother Oncol.* 2015;117(2):217–222. doi:10.1016/j.radonc.2015.04.019

28. Smith TE, Lee D, Turner BC, Carter D, Haffty BG. True recurrence vs. new primary ipsilateral breast tumor relapse: an analysis of clinical and pathologic differences and their implications in natural history, prognoses, and therapeutic management. *Int J Radiat Oncol Biol Phys.* 2000;48(5):1281–1289. doi:10.1016/s0360-3016(00)01378-x

29. Huang E, Buchholz TA, Meric F, et al. Classifying local disease recurrences after breast conservation therapy based on location and histology: new primary tumors have more favorable outcomes than true local disease recurrences. *Cancer.* 2002;95(10):2059–2067. doi:10.1002/cncr.10952

30. McGrath S, Antonucci J, Goldstein N, et al. Long-term patterns of in-breast failure in patients with early stage breast cancer treated with breast-conserving therapy: a molecular based clonality evaluation. *Am J Clin Oncol.* 2010;33(1):17–22. doi:10.1097/COC.0b013e31819cccc3

31. Poodt IGM, Vugts G, Schipper RJ, Nieuwenhuijzen GAP. Repeat sentinel lymph node biopsy for ipsilateral breast tumor recurrence: a systematic review of the results and impact on prognosis. *Ann Surg Oncol.* 2018;25(5):1329–1339. doi:10.1245/s10434-018-6358-0

32. Shah C, Wilkinson JB, Jawad M, et al. Outcome after ipsilateral breast tumor recurrence in patients with early-stage breast cancer treated with accelerated partial breast irradiation. *Clin Breast Cancer.* 2012;12(6): 392–397. doi:10.1016/j.clbc.2012.09.006

33. Kurtz JM, Jacquemier J, Amalric R, et al. Is breast conservation after local recurrence feasible? *Eur J Cancer.* 1991;27(3):240–244. doi:10.1016/0277-5379(91)90505-8

34. Alpert TE, Kuerer HM, Arthur DW, Lannin DR, Haffty BG. Ipsilateral breast tumor recurrence after breast conservation therapy: outcomes of salvage mastectomy vs. salvage breast-conserving surgery and prognostic factors for salvage breast preservation. *Int J Radiat Oncol Biol Phys.* 2005;63(3):845–851. doi:10.1016/j.ijrobp.2005.02.035

35. Salvadori B, Marubini E, Miceli R, et al. Reoperation for locally recurrent breast cancer in patients previously treated with conservative surgery. *Br J Surg.* 1999;86(1):84–87. doi:10.1046/j.1365-2168.1999.00961.x

36. Voogd AC, van Tienhoven G, Peterse HL, et al. Local recurrence after breast conservation therapy for early stage breast carcinoma: detection, treatment, and outcome in 266 patients. Dutch Study Group on Local Recurrence after Breast Conservation (BORST). *Cancer.* 1999;85(2):437–446. doi:10.1002/(sici)1097-0142(19990115)85:2<437::aid-cncr23>3.0.co;2-1

37. Chen SL, Martinez SR. The survival impact of the choice of surgical procedure after ipsilateral breast cancer recurrence. *Am J Surg.* 2008;196(4):495–499. doi:10.1016/j.amjsurg.2008.06.018

38. Doyle T, Schultz DJ, Peters C, Harris E, Solin LJ. Long-term results of local recurrence after breast conservation treatment for invasive breast cancer. *Int J Radiat Oncol Biol Phys.* 2001;51(1):74–80. doi:10.1016/s0360-3016(01)01625-x

39. Shen J, Hunt KK, Mirza NQ, et al. Predictors of systemic recurrence and disease-specific survival after ipsilateral breast tumor recurrence. *Cancer.* 2005;104(3):479–490. doi:10.1002/cncr.21224

40. Ofuchi T, Amemiya A, Hatayama J. Salvage surgery for patients with ipsilateral breast tumor recurrence after breast-conserving treatment. *Nihon Rinsho.* 2007;65(suppl 6):439–444. PMID:17682190

41. Hannoun-Levi JM, Resch A, Gal J, et al. Accelerated partial breast irradiation with interstitial brachytherapy as second conservative treatment for ipsilateral breast tumour recurrence: multicentric study of the GEC-ESTRO breast cancer working group. *Radiother Oncol.* 2013;108(2):226–231. doi:10.1016/j.radonc.2013.03.026

42. Hannoun-Levi JM, Gal J, Van Limbergen E, et al. Salvage mastectomy versus second conservative treatment for second ipsilateral breast tumor event: a propensity score-matched cohort analysis of the GEC-ESTRO breast cancer working group database. *Int J Radiat Oncol Biol Phys.* 2021;110(2):452–461. doi:10.1016/j.ijrobp.2020.12.029

43. Lim GH, Alcantara VS, Ng RP, et al. Patterns of breast cancer second recurrences in patients after mastectomy. *Breast Cancer Res Treat.* 2022;196(3):583–589. doi:10.1007/s10549-022-06772-4

44. Wahl AO, Rademaker A, Kiel KD, et al. Multi-institutional review of repeat irradiation of chest wall and breast for recurrent breast cancer. *Int J Radiat Oncol Biol Phys.* 2008;70(2):477–484. doi:10.1016/j.ijrobp.2007.06.035

45. Chen AM, Yoshizaki T, Velez MA, Mikaeilian AG, Hsu S, Cao M. Tolerance of the brachial plexus to high-dose reirradiation. *Int J Radiat Oncol Biol Phys.* 2017;98(1):83–90. doi:10.1016/j.ijrobp.2017.01.244

46. Woodward WA, Fang P, Arriaga L, et al. A phase 2 study of capecitabine and concomitant radiation in women with advanced breast cancer. *Int J Radiat Oncol Biol Phys.* 2017;99(4):777–783. doi:10.1016/j.ijrobp.2017.04.030

47. Diao K, Andring LM, Barcenas CH, et al. Contemporary outcomes after multimodality therapy in patients with breast cancer presenting with ipsilateral supraclavicular node involvement. *Int J Radiat Oncol Biol Phys.* 2022;112(1):66–74. doi:10.1016/j.ijrobp.2021.08.026

48. Fang P. Internal Mammary Misfortune. *Int J Radiat Oncol Biol Phys.* 2017;97(3):447. doi:10.1016/j.ijrobp.2016.10.032

49. Melotek JM, Chmura SJ. Oligometastasis-directed ablative therapy: a clinical trial question. *Int J Radiat Oncol Biol Phys.* 2017;97(3):448. doi:10.1016/j.ijrobp.2016.10.023

50. Rahimi A, Timmerman R. Ablative therapy: a reasonable approach. *Int J Radiat Oncol Biol Phys.* 2017;97(3): 448–449. doi:10.1016/j.ijrobp.2016.10.028

51. Angervall L, Enzinger FM. Extraskeletal neoplasm resembling Ewing's sarcoma. *Cancer.* 1975;36(1): 240–251. doi:10.1002/1097-0142(197507)36:1<240::aid-cncr2820360127>3.0.co;2-h

52. Schwarz GS, Grobmyer SR, Djohan RS, et al. Axillary reverse mapping and lymphaticovenous bypass: lymphedema prevention through enhanced lymphatic visualization and restoration of flow. *J Surg Oncol.* 2019;120(2):160–167. doi:10.1002/jso.25513

PART V: Thoracic

Salem Alfaifi, Gaurav Marwaha, Kevin L. Stephans, and Gregory M. M. Videtic

QUICK HIT   Surgical resection is the standard of care for operable early-stage NSCLC. For medically inoperable patients, SBRT is the standard of care. For high-risk operable patients, given the absence of completed randomized trials, there is controversy regarding whether surgery or SBRT is the preferred option with regard to the endpoint of overall survival. See Table 28.1 for general treatment paradigm.

Table 28.1 General Treatment Paradigm for Early-Stage NSCLC				
	Operable			**Medically Inoperable** (FEV1 <40%, DLCO <40%)
	Surgery	**CHT†**	**RT**	
Stage IA (*cT1a–bN0*)	Segmentectomy* + mediastinal LND	No (unless in Japan)	No PORT (except for positive margins or pN2‡)	SBRT *Peripheral:* 54 Gy/3 fx, 50 Gy/5 fx, 48 Gy/4 fx, 34 Gy/1 fx *Central:* 50 (–60) Gy/5 fx *Ultracentral:* 56 Gy/8 fx, 60 Gy/8 fx
Stage IB (*cT2aN0*)	Lobectomy + mediastinal LND	Debatable (per LACE meta-analysis[1])		
IIA and select IIB (*cT2bN0, cT3N0*)		Yes (per LACE meta-analysis[1])		

*Only for peripheral lung tumors.
†See Evidence-Based Q&A for the role of adjuvant targeted therapies.
‡Controversial given results of LungART[2]; see Chapter 29.

EPIDEMIOLOGY: Lung cancer is the most common noncutaneous cancer worldwide, the second most common in the United States, and the leading cause of cancer mortality in the United States with ~234,580 new cases and ~125,070 deaths annually.[3] NSCLC comprises ~80% of all lung cancers, and 20% to 30% of NSCLC patients present with early-stage disease.

RISK FACTORS: Smoking, radon, asbestos, family history, pulmonary fibrosis, occupational exposures (silica, cadmium, arsenic, beryllium, diesel exhaust, coal soot).

ANATOMY: Lobes in both lungs are separated by the oblique fissure, and the right lung is also separated by the horizontal fissure. Trachea starts at C3/4, carina at T5. Nodal stations range from 1 to 14; see atlas by Lynch et al.[4]

PATHOLOGY

- *Adenocarcinoma (ACA)*: Most common histology, ~40% of all lung cancers. The majority are peripheral. Bronchioloalveolar carcinoma (subtype of ACA) arises from type II pneumocytes, grows along the alveolar septa, and has a long natural history.
- *Squamous cell carcinoma (SCC)*: ~20% of all lung cancers. The majority are central.
- *Small-cell carcinoma*: ~15% of all lung cancers, almost always associated with smoking (see Chapter 30).
- *Other*: Consists of other rare histologies and other neuroendocrine carcinomas such as large cell or carcinoid.

GENETICS: Greater than 95% of clinically relevant mutations are found in ACAs. *EGFR* is a transmembrane tyrosine kinase mutated in ~17% of NSCLC. These mutants are targetable with tyrosine kinase inhibitors (TKIs) such as osimertinib, erlotinib, gefitinib, and afatinib. *ALK* rearrangements are found in ~5% of NSCLC. These mutants are associated with younger age and never smokers; they respond to TKIs like crizotinib, alectinib, and ceritinib. *ROS-1* mutations are seen in 1% to 2% of NSCLC and can respond to crizotinib.[3] *BRAF V600E, MET, RET, and KRAS* are emerging driver mutations that are thought to respond to vemurafenib, crizotinib, cabozantinib, and sotorasib, respectively.

SCREENING: USPSTF criteria: Screen with low-dose CT for patients ages 50 to 80 and ≥20 pack-year smoker and cessation <15 years ago. Recent data from the International Lung Screening Trial suggest that a model incorporating 11 predictors including features such as age, race, education, and BMI may be more sensitive than the current USPSTF criteria.[5]

CLINICAL PRESENTATION: Cough, dyspnea, wheeze, stridor, hemoptysis, anorexia, weight loss, decline in performance status, paraneoplastic syndromes such as hypercalcemia from PTHrP (SCC) or hypertrophic osteoarthropathy.

WORKUP: H&P. ACCP guidelines define the standard for PFT evaluation and recommend FEV1 and DLCO be measured in all patients who are being considered for surgery.[6] SBRT trials define medical inoperability using the Indiana University criteria: baseline FEV1 <40% predicted, predicted postop FEV1 <30% predicted, DLCO <40% predicted, pO_2 <70 mmHg, pCO_2 >50 mmHg, exercise oxygen consumption <50% predicted. Preoperative cardiac workup if necessary.

Labs: CBC, CMP.

Imaging: CT chest (with contrast if evaluating nodes); consider CT abdomen for metastatic workup but at least review liver and adrenal on CT chest. PET scan. "Pathologic" LNs defined as short-axis diameter >1.0 cm and "bulky" lymphadenopathy as short axis >3.0 cm, multiple matted nodes, radiographic ECE or ≥3 stations involved. MRI of thoracic inlet for superior sulcus tumors and octreotide scan for carcinoid. MRI brain for stage II or higher (NCCN 2024); consider MRI brain for central stage IB (NCCN 2024 optional recommendation); otherwise, brain imaging unnecessary unless neurologic symptoms are present. CT brain with contrast is sufficient if MRI is not feasible.[7]

Procedures: Biopsy indicated (EBUS, CT-guided, or thoracentesis depending on location/presence of effusion; sputum pathology is unreliable but at least three needed to be negative). EBUS/mediastinoscopy to confirm positive nodes on CT or PET and for all T3 or central T1–2 tumors. EBUS allows sampling of stations 2, 4, 7, and 10. Mediastinoscopy allows sampling of 2, 4, and 7. Chamberlain procedure or VATS is required to reach stations 5 and 6. EUS required for stations 8 and 9.

PROGNOSTIC FACTORS: Stage, weight loss >5% in 3 months, KPS <90, age >70, +LVSI, marital status.

STAGING: See Table 28.2.

Table 28.2 AJCC 8th Edition (2017): Staging for Lung Cancer						
T/M	N	cN0	cN1	cN2	cN3
T1	a: ≤1 cm[1]	IA1	IIB	IIIA	IIIB
	b: 1.1–2 cm	IA2			
	c: 2.1–3 cm	IA3			
T2[2]	a: 3.1–4 cm	IB			
	b: 4.1–5 cm	IIA			
T3	• 5.1–7 cm • Invasion[3] • Separate nodule(s) in the same lobe	IIB	IIIA	IIIB	IIIC
T4	• >7 cm • Invasion[4] • Separate nodule(s) in a different ipsilateral lobe				

(continued)

T/M		N	cN0	cN1	cN2	cN3
M1a	• Separate nodule(s) in contralateral lobe • Pleural or pericardial nodules • Malignant pleural/pericardial effusion		IVA			
M1b	• Single extrathoracic metastasis in a single organ (including single nonregional LN)					
M1c	• Multiple extrathoracic metastases		IVB			

Table 28.2 AJCC 8th Edition (2017): Staging for Lung Cancer (*continued*)

Notes: ≤1 cm[1]: or rare superficial, spreading tumor with invasive component limited to bronchial wall. T2[2]: or involves main bronchus (but not carina), invades visceral pleura, or associated with atelectasis or obstructive pneumonitis extending to hilar region. Invasion[3]: invasion of parietal pleura, chest wall, phrenic nerve, or parietal pericardium. Invasion[4]: invasion of diaphragm, mediastinum, heart, great vessels, trachea, carina, recurrent laryngeal nerve, esophagus, or vertebral body. cN1: ipsilateral peribronchial and/or ipsilateral hilar LNs and intrapulmonary nodes (stations 10–14). cN2: ipsilateral mediastinal and/or subcarinal LNs (stations 2–9). cN3: contralateral mediastinal, hilar, or any scalene or supraclavicular LNs (station 1).

TREATMENT PARADIGM

Observation: "Active surveillance" is not an established option for NSCLC because even in medically inoperable patients, lung cancer-specific mortality is 53%.[8] Therefore, postponement of treatment is generally inappropriate unless the lesion is too small to diagnose (see following). That said, there is a subset of early-stage low-grade ACAs whose indolent biological behavior can support discussions regarding observation only.

Solitary Pulmonary Nodule: Discrete opacity in lung parenchyma ≤3 cm (>3 cm is "mass," and malignancy until proven otherwise). Differential includes granuloma, abscess, fungal infection, hamartoma, tuberculosis, metastasis, lymphoma, and carcinoid. Factors associated with malignancy: faster growth rate, lack of calcifications, greater size, spiculated (vs. smooth or lobulated) margins, air bronchograms, solid appearance (vs. ground glass), contrast enhancement, high SUV. If ≥8 mm, consider PET/CT or biopsy; see NCCN guidelines for additional size-specific follow-up guidelines. Lung-RADS is an evolving standardization system for follow-up of indeterminate nodules on lung cancer screening CT reporting.[9]

Surgery: Standard treatment for medically operable patients. Lobectomy remains superior in terms of oncologic outcomes for most early-stage NSCLC cases but at the cost of higher functional morbidity. Wedge and segmentectomy are alternatives for high-risk patients or those with compromised lung function, particularly when the tumor is small and peripheral.[10,11] VATS lobectomy is comparable to open lobectomy.[12] For accurate staging, mediastinal LN dissection should be performed. Preoperative medical workup including PFTs (see Workup) and cardiac clearance is necessary.

Systemic Therapy: See Evidence-Based Q&A. Generally, no role for adjuvant CHT in stage I NSCLC, but it should be considered for stage II. Adjuvant osimertinib and alectinib were shown to improve oncologic outcomes in resected EGFR-mutant and ALK-positive stage IB to IIIA NSCLC, respectively.[13,14]

Radiofrequency Ablation (RFA): Placement of electrode in tumor with ablative heating. Retrospective series have reported complete radiographic responses from 38% to 93% with relapse rates from 8% to 43%. Factors associated with CR include smaller tumors, metastases, and ablation zone 4× tumor diameter. Pneumothorax is a risk associated with the procedure.

Radiation

Indications: Historically, fractionated RT was the standard treatment for medically inoperable patients, with results inferior to surgery. SBRT, however, may be comparable to surgery and is now the treatment of choice (rather than wedge or RFA) for medically inoperable patients. Adjuvant RT is not indicated in completely resected stage I/II patients (although Italian trial by Trodella et al.[15] does show benefit; other trials have not).

Dose: Common fractionation schemes for SBRT vary, and tumor location, histology, and size may influence choice.

- Peripheral: 54 Gy/3 fx (60 Gy without heterogeneity correction) given with an interfraction interval of 40 hours to 7 days, with an overall treatment time of 8 to 14 days; 50 Gy/5 fx, 48 Gy/4 fx, 34 Gy/1 fx.
- Central: 50 (–60) Gy/5 fx (RTOG 0813[16]).
- Ultracentral: 56 Gy/8 fx (HILUS[17]), 60 Gy/8 fx (SUNSET[18]).

Postop dose is 54 to 60 Gy for microscopically (R1) positive margins and ≥60 Gy for macroscopically (R2) positive margins.[19]

Toxicity: Acute: mainly fatigue. Rarely, cough, pneumonitis, esophagitis, subacute chest wall pain. Late: radiation pneumonitis, chest wall pain. On average, PFTs remain stable (some improve, some decrease, often related to baseline comorbidity).

Procedure: See *Handbook of Treatment Planning in Radiation Oncology*, Chapter 6.[20]

EVIDENCE-BASED Q&A

SCREENING AND STAGING

Is there benefit to routine radiographic screening for lung cancer? Which patients should be screened?

Previously, routine screening with CXR or sputum cytology had not been shown to reduce mortality. The National Lung Screening Trial was paradigm-changing and led to the revision of NCCN and USPSTF guidelines.

National Lung Screening Trial (*NEJM* 2011, PMID 21714641): PRT of 54,454 patients at high risk for lung cancer randomized to three annual screenings with either low-dose CT or single-view PA CXR. Results: There were 247 vs. 309 deaths from lung cancer per 100,000 person-years in the low-dose CT group vs. the CXR group, representing a relative reduction in mortality from lung cancer of 20% with the use of low-dose CT ($p = .004$). Rate of death from any cause was also reduced by 7% ($p = .02$) in the low-dose CT group compared with the CXR group. Number needed to screen with low-dose CT to prevent one lung cancer death was 320. **Conclusion: CT screening reduces mortality from lung cancer.**

What defines "early-stage" lung cancer? Why is it important to investigate the mediastinum?

Early stage is typically defined as stage I or II, but treatment decision-making is based on the presence or absence of nodal involvement. Therefore, careful staging of the mediastinum is necessary. PET/CT has sensitivity of 79% (CT staging 60%),[21] but investigation of the mediastinum via either mediastinoscopy or EBUS can improve this.

What is the difference between mediastinoscopy and EBUS? What is the sensitivity and NPV of either approach or a combination?

Mediastinoscopy is the historical standard for evaluation of regional LNs, but EBUS has the advantage of being less invasive and providing access to station 10 (hilar nodes). Accurate clinical staging is important to avoid unnecessary thoracotomies, that is, those who will need CHT and/or RT anyway and would not benefit from surgery. Historically, 25% to 30% of thoracotomies were unnecessary due to incomplete clinical staging.

Annema, ASTER Trial (*JAMA* 2010, PMID 21098770): PRT of 241 patients with resectable NSCLC randomized to mediastinoscopy or combined EUS-FNA/EBUS followed by mediastinoscopy if no nodes found. All patients without evidence of mediastinal tumor spread then underwent thoracotomy with LND. Primary outcome was sensitivity for N2/N3 metastases. Results: Sensitivity of mediastinoscopy: 79% (NPV 86%); EUS-FNA/EBUS: 85% (NPV 85%); EUS-FNA/EBUS followed by mediastinoscopy: 94% (NPV 93%). Unnecessary thoracotomies: 18% (mediastinoscopy) vs. 7% (EUS-FNA/EBUS). **Conclusion: EUS-FNA/EBUS followed with mediastinoscopy resulted in fewer unnecessary thoracotomies and increased sensitivity for nodal metastases compared with mediastinoscopy or EUS-FNA/EBUS alone.**

MEDICALLY OPERABLE PATIENTS

What is the surgery of choice? Is wedge resection sufficient?

Ginsberg[22] reported historically that wedge resection is an inferior local therapy to lobectomy, and lobectomy should be considered the surgical procedure of choice. However, recent randomized trials suggest that sub-lobar resection (wedge or segment) is not inferior and may be superior to lobectomy with similar toxicity in patients with small peripheral tumors.[10,11] It is useful to note that "modern" wedge resection is better than wedge resection in the era of Ginsberg.[23]

Which patients with early-stage lung cancer may benefit from postoperative RT (PORT)?

PORT is not indicated in completely resected stage I to II patients. The PORT meta-analysis showed a detriment to routine PORT for patients without pN2 disease.[24,25] In patients with positive margins, re-resection is preferred (NCCN 2024), but PORT is another option.[19] For patients who are surgically upstaged to pN2, PORT is controversial given the results of Lung ART[2] (see Chapter 29). The Trodella study discussed below is notable because it did show a benefit of PORT in completely resected stage I, but this is not routine practice, as it has not been reproduced.

Trodella, Italian Trial (*Radiother Oncol* 2002, PMID 11830308): PRT of adjuvant RT vs. observation in 104 patients with completely resected (R0) pathologic stage I NSCLC. RT was 50.4 Gy/28 fx. Target volume included the bronchial stump and ipsilateral hilum. Results: There were no treatment-related deaths. The 5-year DFS and OS favored the RT arm (71% vs. 60%, p = .039, and 67% vs. 58%, p = .048, respectively). **Conclusion: Adjuvant RT may be safe and beneficial in terms of DFS and OS in select stage I patients.**

Which patients benefit from adjuvant CHT?

Adjuvant CHT should be considered for stage II patients based on the LACE meta-analysis. Stage IB is debatable; the CALGB study (included in the LACE analysis, see below) suggested a benefit for tumors ≥4 cm. A Japanese study showed a benefit to uracil-tegafur, but it is not used in the United States.[26]

Pignon, LACE Pooled Analysis (*JCO* 2008, PMID 18506026): Pooled individual data from 4,584 patients included on five PRTs of adjuvant CHT in NSCLC. MFU 5.2 years. Results: Overall HR of death was 0.89 (p = .005), corresponding to 5-year absolute benefit of 5.4%. Benefit varied with stage: detrimental for stage IA (HR 1.4, 95% CI 0.95–2.06), nonsignificant for IB (HR 0.93, 0.78–1.10), and beneficial for stage II (HR 0.83, 0.73–0.95) and III (HR 0.8, 0.72–0.94). Benefit was higher in patients with better performance status. Type of CHT, sex, age, histology, type of surgery, planned RT, and dose of cisplatin were not associated with outcome. **Conclusion: CHT confers a survival advantage in stage II/III NSCLC.**

Strauss, CALGB 9633 (*JCO* 2008, PMID 18809614): PRT of adjuvant paclitaxel (200 mg/m^2) and carboplatin (AUC 6) day 1 every 3 weeks × 4 cycles vs. observation in completely resected stage IB NSCLC. 384 patients randomized. Results: The 3-year OS was 79% vs. 70% favoring CHT (p = .045). No difference in 5-year OS (60% vs. 57%, p = .32). Subgroup analysis showed that for tumors ≥4 cm, there was improved DFS (mDFS 96 vs. 63 months, p = .035) and OS (MS 99 vs. 77 months, p = .043) with CHT. **Conclusion: Although trial initially closed early after planned interim analysis, 5-year data showed no significant OS benefit. However, for patients with tumors ≥4 cm, CHT may improve OS.**

What is the role of adjuvant targeted therapy?

Adjuvant targeted therapies in early-stage NSCLC are reshaping postsurgical management by leveraging molecular insights and personalized approaches for patients with targetable mutations. The ADAURA trial[13] showed significant improvement in 4-year DFS (73% vs. 38%) and 5-year OS (88% vs. 78%) with adjuvant osimertinib compared with placebo for completely resected stage IB to IIIA EGFR mutated NSCLC. Also, the ALINA trial[14] showed significant improvement in 3-year DFS (89% vs. 54%) with adjuvant alectinib vs. platinum-based CHT for completely resected stage IB to IIIA ALK-positive NSCLC.

MEDICALLY INOPERABLE

What are the outcomes with conventional RT for early NSCLC?

Historically, medically inoperable patients received conventionally fractionated definitive RT to 50 to 60 Gy or supportive care only. Conventional RT provided LC in the range of 40% to 60%, with 30% to 40% of patients dying of lung cancer within 2 years. There was some evidence supporting dose escalation to 70.2 Gy and hypofractionation (60 Gy/15 fx), but ultimately, as technology improved, SBRT has rendered previous forms of definitive RT obsolete in most cases.[27]

Cheung, NCIC CTG BR.25 (*JNCI* 2014, PMID 25074417): Multi-institution phase II trial of 80 patients with T1–T3N0 NSCLC treated to 60 Gy/15 fx using 3D-CRT (no IMRT). GTV was tumor only; PTV was 1.5-cm margin (could be decreased to 1.0 cm in transverse plane if close to critical structures). Primary endpoint was 2-year tumor control. MFU 49 months. Results: The 2-year primary tumor control rate was 87%, and the 2-year OS was 69%; the 2-year regional relapse rate was 9% and the distant relapse rate was 22%. The most common grade 3+ toxicities were fatigue (6%), cough (7.5%), dyspnea (14%), and pneumonitis (10%). **Conclusion: Conformal RT to 60 Gy/15 fx using 3D-CRT results in favorable LC and OS without severe toxicities.**

Nyman, SPACE Trial (*Radiother Oncol* 2016, PMID 27600155): Randomized phase II trial of 102 medically inoperable patients with stage I NSCLC comparing SBRT (66 Gy/3 fx over 1 week) and 3D-CRT (70 Gy/35 fx over 7 weeks). MFU 37 months. Results: No difference between 1-, 2-, and 3-year PFS with SBRT (76%, 53%, and 42%) and 3D-CRT (87%, 54%, 42%). By end of study, 70% of SBRT patients had not progressed compared with 59% of 3D-CRT ($p = .26$). Toxicity was lower in SBRT patients (pneumonitis: 19% vs. 34% [$p = .26$]; esophagitis: 8% vs. 30% [$p = .006$]). **Conclusion: No difference in PFS or OS, but trend toward improved control rate in SBRT group with better quality of life and lower toxicity, so SBRT should be standard.**

Ball, TROG 09.02 CHISEL (*Lancet Oncol* 2019, PMID 30770291): International multicenter PRT of 101 medically inoperable patients with PET-diagnosed, biopsy-confirmed, peripheral T1–T2aN0 NSCLC randomized 2:1 to SBRT (54 Gy/3 fx or 48 Gy/4 fx if <2 cm from chest wall) or conventional fractionation (CF; 66 Gy/33 fx or 50 Gy/20 fx per institutional preference). Primary endpoint: time to local treatment failure. MFU 2.6 years for SBRT, 2.1 years for CF. Results (Table 28.3): 14% of SBRT patients progressed locally vs. 31% of CF patients; 39% in the SBRT group died vs. 62% of CF patients. Freedom from local failure (HR 0.32, 95% CI 0.13–0.77) improved in the SBRT group. No significant differences in patient-reported symptoms or functioning. **Conclusion: In inoperable patients with peripheral stage I NSCLC, SBRT yields better LC compared with conventional fractionation with mildly increased toxicities at ~2 years and improves OS.**

Table 28.3 Results of TROG 09.02 CHISEL Randomized Trial			
	SBRT	**Conventional Fractionation**	**Measure of Significance**
Median OS (yrs)	5.0	3.0	HR 0.53, 95% CI 0.30–0.94
2-yr LC	89%	65%	Not provided
2-yr OS	77%	59%	Not provided
Number of grade 3+ AEs (*n*)	8	2	Not provided

Swaminath, LUSTRE (*JAMA Oncology* 2024, PMID 39298144): Phase III PRT of 233 medically inoperable patients with cT1–T2a allocated 2:1 to receive SBRT 48 Gy/4 fx (peripheral tumors) or 60 Gy/8 fx (central tumors) vs. hypofractionated RT 60 Gy/15 fx. The 3-year LC with SBRT was 88% vs. 81% for hypofractionated RT ($p = .15$). The 3-year EFS was 49% with SBRT and 48% with hypofractionated RT ($p = .87$), and the 3-year OS with SBRT was 64% vs. 68% with hypofractionated RT ($p = .4$). One patient in each arm developed grade 3 acute toxic effects (SBRT: fatigue/pneumonia; hypofractionated RT: dyspnea), while late grades 3 to 4 toxicities were reported in 5% of patients in the SBRT group vs. 3% in the hypofractionated RT group. **Conclusion: SBRT showed improvement (not statistically significant) of LC compared with hypofractionated RT.**

What trials defined the role of SBRT?

SBRT, formally defined as high dose per fraction delivered in ≤5 fractions, was first developed in Sweden. Dr. Timmerman at Indiana University led a dose-escalation trial in 2003, which then led to a phase II trial discovering high rates of central toxicity for 60 Gy/3 fx. In 2002, RTOG 0236 opened, which defined the role of SBRT for early-stage peripheral lesions. Since there is debate regarding the value of surgery, RTOG 0618 investigated SBRT for operable patients, reserving surgery for salvage if needed. Since central tumors are considered high risk using 60 Gy/3 fx (but not with 50 Gy/5 fx), RTOG 0813 studied safety and dose escalation for central tumors starting at 50 Gy/5 fx and going to 60 Gy/5 fx. More recently, HILUS and SUNSET studies established the safety of SBRT for ultracentral tumors using 54 Gy/8 fx and 60 Gy/8 fx, respectively (see below).

Timmerman, Indiana (*Chest* 2003, PMID 14605072): Phase I dose-escalation trial of extracranial stereotactic radioablation (ESR) in 37 patients with T1–2N0 biopsy-confirmed NSCLC. Initial dose was 24 Gy/3 fx and increased to tolerated dose of 60 Gy/3 fx. Abdominal compression was used to decrease respiratory motion. MFU 15.2 months. Results: 87% response rate (27% CR). Six patients experienced LF, all receiving doses <18 Gy/fx. One patient (treated at 14 Gy/fx) developed symptomatic pneumonitis. **Conclusion: Extracranial stereotactic radioablation is feasible and results in good response rates**.

Timmerman, Central Toxicity (*JCO* 2006, PMID 17050868; Update *IJROBP* 2009, PMID 19251380): Phase II trial of 70 medically inoperable patients with cT1–2N0 NSCLC treated with SBRT 60 to 66 Gy/3 fx over 1 to 2 weeks. MFU 50.2 months. Results: 3-year LC 88%. Nodal and distant recurrence rates were 9% and 13%, respectively. MS 32.4 months. The 3-year CSS was 82% and the 3-year OS was 43%. MS for T1 vs. T2 tumors was 39 vs. 24.5 months, respectively ($p = .019$). Tumor size or location did not impact control outcomes. Grade 3+ toxicity occurred in 10% of patients with peripheral tumors and 27% of patients with central tumors. **Conclusion: High LC rates with this regimen, but high toxicity for central tumors.**

Onishi, Japan (*JTO* 2007, PMID 17603311): RR of 257 patients (either medically inoperable or refusing surgery) from 14 institutions treated with SBRT. 164 T1N0, 93 T2N0, all tumors <6 cm, all tumor locations included. MFU 38 months. Median BED_{10} was 111 Gy; 5.4% of patients had grade 3+ pulmonary toxicity; 14% of patients had local progression. LR 8% vs. 43% for BED ≥100 Gy and <100 Gy ($p < .001$), respectively; 5-year OS for medically operable patients refusing surgery was 71% for BED ≥100 Gy and 30% for BED <100 Gy ($p < .05$). **Conclusion: SBRT is safe and effective for stage I lung cancer. With BED ≥100 Gy, LC is excellent and the 5-year OS for medically operable patients is similar to surgical series (compared with 70% OS in Ginsburg for lobectomy of only stage IA patients).**

All of the preceding trials come from single institutions. Are there any cooperative group data?

RTOG 0236 is the most notable cooperative SBRT trial.

Timmerman, RTOG 0236 (*JAMA* 2010, PMID 20233825; Update *JAMA Oncol* 2018, PMID 29852036): Phase II multi-institutional study of SBRT for medically inoperable stage I/II NSCLC (peripheral location, T1/T2 N0, tumors <5 cm). EBUS not required. Fifty-five evaluable patients, MFU 48 months. Prescription was 60 Gy/3 fx, although later analysis showed dose was actually 54 Gy/3 fx (with significant variation depending on lung density and tumor size and location) after accounting for heterogeneity. Treatment duration was ≥8 and <14 days. Results: Grade 3 and 4 adverse events 27% and 3.6%. No grade 5 adverse events at 5 years. See Table 28.4 for oncologic outcomes. **Conclusion: Patients with medically inoperable NSCLC treated with SBRT had a modest survival, high rates of local tumor control, and moderate treatment-related morbidity. Longer term follow-up has shown increased lobar and regional failures.** *Note: No EBUS was required in RTOG 0236.*

Table 28.4 Outcomes From RTOG 0236		
	Initial Results (3-Yr)	**Long-Term Results (5-Yr)**
OS	56%	40%
DFS	48%	26%
MS	48 months	48 months

(continued)

Table 28.4 Outcomes from RTOG 0236 (*continued*)

	Initial Results (3-Yr)	Long-Term Results (5-Yr)
LC	98%	93%
Lobar control	91%	80%
LRC	87%	75%
Distant Failure	22%	24%

Is SBRT an appropriate option for medically operable patients?

SBRT is not standard. Multiple trials investigating this question have closed early due to poor accrual. Several analyses attempt to answer this question while we await additional randomized data including ongoing STABLE-MATES[28] and VALOR[29] trials.

Chang, Pooled Analysis of STARS and ROSEL (*Lancet Oncol* 2015, PMID 25981812): Pooled analysis of two independent phase III PRTs of SBRT vs. lobectomy and mediastinal LND, which closed early due to slow accrual. Total of 58 patients. Six surgery patients died compared with one SBRT patient. The 3-year OS was 95% in the SBRT group vs. 79% in the surgery group (HR 0.14, 95% CI 0.017–1.190, p = .037). RFS was similar: 86% SBRT vs. 80% surgery (p = .54). Grade 3+ events were 10% for SBRT compared with 44% for surgery, with one postoperative death. **Conclusion: SBRT appears viable in medically operable patients, but additional PRTs are warranted.** *Note: 2021 STARS update: Single-arm SBRT protocol was compared via propensity score matching with historical cohort of stage IA NSCLC patients treated with VATS + LND. No significant difference in OS, PFS, CSS, or recurrence (local, regional, distant) between SBRT and VATS + LND.*

Onishi, Japan (*IJROBP* 2011, PMID 20638194): Review of outcomes in medically operable patients with stage I NSCLC. MFU 55 months. Cumulative LC rates for T1 and T2 tumors at 5 years after SBRT were 92% and 73%, respectively. Pulmonary complications grade >2 in one patient (1.1%, grade 3). The 5-year OS for stage IA and IB was 72% and 62%, respectively. One patient who developed LR safely underwent salvage surgery. **Conclusion: SBRT is safe and promising for operable stage I NSCLC, with survival rate approximating that for surgery.**

Zheng, Meta-Analysis (*IJROBP* 2014, PMID 25052562): Study-level meta-analysis of 7,071 patients treated with surgery or SBRT (BED ≥100). Median age for SBRT and surgery was 74 and 66 years. MFU 28 months for SBRT and 37 months for surgery. OS rates at 1, 3, and 5 years for SBRT vs. lobectomy were 83% vs. 92%, 56% vs. 77%, and 41% vs. 66%. After adjustment for proportion of operable patients and age, SBRT and surgery have comparable DFS and OS. **Conclusion: SBRT appears comparable to surgery for medically operable patients.**

Timmerman, RTOG 0618 (*JAMA* 2018, PMID 29852037): Single-arm phase II study of SBRT for patients with operable stage I/II NSCLC (peripheral location, T1–3N0, <5 cm). Treatment was 54 Gy/3 fx. Primary endpoint was tumor control. Early surgical salvage was planned per protocol in the event of an LR. Secondary endpoints: survival, AEs, incidence, and outcome of surgical salvage. Results: 33 patients with MFU 48.1 months. The 4-year LRC rate was 88% and distant failure 12%; 4-year DFS 57% and OS 56%. Median DFS and OS were both 55.2 months. **Conclusion: SBRT appears to be associated with high tumor control and infrequent need for surgical salvage.**

Henschke, Pooled Analysis of I-ELCAP and IELCART (*JTO* 2023, PMID 37806384): Pooled analysis of two prospective cohorts: International Early Lung Cancer Action Program (I-ELCAP) and Initiative for Early Lung Cancer Research on Treatment (IELCART). Total of 1,115 patients with first primary cT1a–bN0M0 NSCLC treated by surgery (n = 1,003) or SBRT (n = 112). There was no difference in lung cancer-specific mortality at 10 years (90% vs. 88%, p = .55). Overall survival at 10 years for 110 propensity-matched pairs was not significantly different (p = .74). **Conclusion: SBRT is an appropriate alternative treatment option for small, early-stage NSCLCs.**

Can SBRT be delivered safely in a single fraction?

Yes. Mature phase II data demonstrate durable safety and efficacy.

Videtic, RTOG 0915 (*IJROBP* 2015, PMID 26530743; Update *IJROBP* 2019, PMID 30513377): Randomized phase II study of 94 (84 evaluable) medically inoperable, biopsy-proven, peripheral, T1–2N0 by PET comparing 34 Gy/1 fx (Arm 1) with 48 Gy/4 fx (Arm 2). Primary outcome: rate of grade 3+ AEs. Secondary endpoints: LC, OS, and PFS. MFU 4 years (6 years for those still living). Three percent of patients in Arm 1 vs. 11% in Arm 2 with grade 3+ AEs (see Table 28.5 for oncologic outcomes). **Conclusion: For medically inoperable peripheral T1–2N0 NSCLC, 34 Gy/1 fx and 48 Gy/4 fx offer comparable toxicities and primary tumor control rates. MS of ~4 years in each arm is comparable to RTOG 0236. OS was lower in Arm 1, although the study was not powered for OS. Both regimens may be appropriate in this population.**

Table 28.5 Outcomes of RTOG 0915		
	Arm 1 (34 Gy/1 fx)	Arm 2 (48 Gy/4 fx)
Grade 3+ AE	3%	11%
Median survival (yrs)	4.1	4.6
5-yr LF	11%	7%
5-yr OS	30%	41%
5-yr PFS	19%	33%
5-yr distant failure	38%	41%

Singh, Roswell Park 1509 (*IJROBP* 2019, PMID 31445956): A total of 98 medically inoperable peripheral cT1–T2N0 NSCLC by PET comparing 30 Gy/1 fx (Arm 1) with 60 Gy/3 fx (Arm 2). Primary endpoint: frequency of AEs grade ≥3. Secondary endpoints: LC, OS, PFS, QOL. MFU 54 months. Incidence of thoracic grade 3 AEs 17% in Arm 1 and 15% in Arm 2 ($p = .77$). No grades 4 to 5 AEs. No SS difference in 2-year OS (73% vs. 62%), 2-year PFS (65% vs. 50%), or 2-year LC (95% vs. 97%), although T2a had poorer OS on MVA. Regarding QOL, no significant differences in overall global health or PFTs; Arm 1 had better dyspnea and social functioning. **Conclusion: No differences between single- vs. 3-fx regimens in OS, LC, PFS, or lung function. QOL measures of social functioning and dyspnea improved in single-fx regimen.**

What data exist regarding the safety of SBRT for central and ultracentral lung tumors?

Central location was originally defined as within 2 cm of the proximal bronchial tree by Timmerman et al.,[30] although other definitions of centrality and "ultracentrality" exist (see the following studies), which historically found significant toxicity associated with the treatment of central or ultracentral tumors. However, more recently, multiple mostly phase II trials have been published evaluating SBRT to central and ultracentral tumors (LungTech,[31] HILUS,[17] SUNSET[18]) utilizing different fractionation regimens than previous, such as 60 Gy/8 fx, which have shown favorable acute and late toxicity as well as good LC. 60 Gy/8 fx appears to be emerging as an acceptable fractionation regimen for central and ultracentral tumors.

Bezjak, RTOG 0813 (*JCO* 2019, PMID 30943123): Phase I/II study of maximum tolerated dose (MTD) and efficacy of SBRT for cT1–2 (<5 cm) N0 NSCLC in medically inoperable patients. Centrality defined as tumors within 2 cm of the tracheal–bronchial tree or immediately adjacent to the mediastinal or pericardial pleura (where PTV would touch the pleura). Dose started at 50 Gy/5 fx and was escalated by 0.5 Gy/fx increments to 60 Gy/5 fx QOD over 1.5 to 2 weeks. MTD defined as dose at which probability of dose-limiting toxicity (DLT; any treatment-related grade 3+ AE within the first year) is closest to 20% without exceeding it. Results: 120 patients; MFU 37.9 months. MTD was 12 Gy/fx, and DLT in this group was 7.2%. No patients receiving ≤11 Gy/fx had DLTs; 12% of patients in both 11.5 and 12 Gy groups had DLTs; 2-year LC, PFS, and OS rates with 11.5 Gy/fx were 89%, 52%, and 68% vs. 88%, 55%, and 73% with 12 Gy/fx (all NS). **Conclusion: For SBRT, 60 Gy/5 fx is associated with clinically significant incidence of DLT, but also with excellent LC at 2 years.** *Note: This trial used a broader definition of centrality than the original Timmerman definition.*

Lindberg, Nordic HILUS (*JTO* 2021, PMID 33823286): Phase II trial of 65 patients treated with SBRT for central (≤1 cm from proximal bronchial tree, but not eroding the wall of mainstem bronchi) tumors ≤5 cm, either NSCLC or metastasis from extrapulmonary primary. Subclassified by tumor location: Group A (*n* = 39): tumors <1 cm from the main bronchi and trachea; Group B

($n = 26$): all other tumors. Treatment was 56 Gy/8 fx prescribed to 67% IDL. Primary outcome: LC; secondary endpoints: toxicity and OS. Results: The 2-year LC was 83%. Grades 3 to 5 toxicities noted in 34%, including 10 cases of treatment-related death (bronchopulmonary hemorrhage, $n = 8$; pneumonitis, $n = 1$; fistula, $n = 1$). Greater grade 5 toxicity was reported in Group A ($n = 8$, 21%) than Group B ($n = 2$, 7%). **Conclusion: Risk of serious or fatal toxicity with SBRT for central tumors, particularly with targets near the main bronchi, is significant.**

Levy, LungTech (*JTO* 2024, PMID 38788924): Phase II single-arm trial of 31 patients with inoperable central NSCLC (T1–T3, ≤7 cm). The trial closed early due to poor accrual. Central tumors were defined as those within 2 cm or abutting the proximal bronchial tree or tumors adjacent to the mediastinal or pericardial pleura (of note, the study included ~20% ultracentral tumors on review). The trial utilized 60 Gy/8 fx, with care taken to respect the bronchial dose constraints. Results: At 3 years, freedom from local progression and OS were 82% and 61%, respectively. The rates of local, regional, and distant progression were 7%, 3%, and 30% respectively. SBRT-related acute and late grade 3+ adverse events were reported in 7% (including one acute grade 5 pneumonitis) and 19% (included one grade 5 hemoptysis), respectively. **Conclusion: Outcomes are similar to those of RTOG 0813 with good LC and less reported AEs than those reported on ultracentral HILUS trial.**

Giuliani, SUNSET (*IJROBP* 2024, PMID 38614279): Safety and efficacy trial included 30 patients with T1–3 (≤6 cm) NSCLC and evaluated SBRT 60 Gy/8 fx to ultracentral tumors defined as PTV overlapping with the central bronchial tree, esophagus, or pulmonary vessels. The primary endpoint was the MTD (defined as the dose associated with a ≤30% grade 3+ toxicity). Results: Grade 3+ toxicity rate was 7% (one patient with grade 3 dyspnea and one patient with grade 5 pneumonia). At 3 years, LC 90%, PFS 66%, and OS 73%. **Conclusion: 60 Gy/8 fx for management of ultracentral tumors has a favorable disease control and acceptable AE rate.**

What data exist regarding the safety of SBRT for early-stage NSCLC in patients with interstitial lung disease (ILD)?

Palma, ASPIRE-ILD (*JAMA Oncology* 2024, PMID 38451491): Phase II single-arm study of patients with fibrotic ILD and a diagnosis of T1–2 NSCLC who were not candidates for surgery and treated with SBRT 50 Gy/5 fx QOD. The study prespecified that SBRT would be considered worthwhile if the median OS was longer than 1 year, with a grade 3 to 4 toxicity risk <35% and a grade 5 risk <15%. Results: Of the 39 patients, 70% reported baseline dyspnea; median FEV1 was 80% predicted and median DLCO was 49% predicted. The 1-year OS was 79% ($p < .001$ vs. the unacceptable rate). Median OS 25 months, median PFS 19 months, and 2-year LC 92%. AEs grades 1 to 2 were reported in 31%, grade 3 in 10%, grade 4 in 0%, and grade 5 in 8% (all due to respiratory deterioration). **Conclusion: Despite the efficacy and toxicity rates meeting the prespecified acceptable threshold, about 8% of patients with ILD died secondary to respiratory deterioration after SBRT, which highlights the importance of patient selection and toxicity discussion for this patient population.**

Is there a benefit with the addition of immunotherapy to SBRT?

Regional and distant failures remain the biggest patterns of failure after SBRT. Phase I/II studies evaluated the role of IO with promising results.[32,33] Several ongoing phase III trials will provide further clarity on this topic.[34–36]

REFERENCES

1. Pignon JP, Tribodet H, Scagliotti GV, et al. Lung adjuvant cisplatin evaluation: a pooled analysis by the LACE Collaborative Group. *J Clin Oncol*. 2008;26(21):3552–3559. doi:10.1200/JCO.2007.13.9030
2. Le Pechoux C, Pourel N, Barlesi F, et al. Postoperative radiotherapy versus no postoperative radiotherapy in patients with completely resected non-small-cell lung cancer and proven mediastinal N2 involvement (Lung ART): an open-label, randomised, phase 3 trial. *Lancet Oncol*. 2022;23(1):104–114. doi:10.1016/S1470-2045(21)00606-9
3. Siegel RL, Giaquinto AN, Jemal A. Cancer statistics, 2024. *CA Cancer J Clin*. 2024;74(1):12–49. doi:10.3322/caac.21820

4. Lynch R, Pitson G, Ball D, Claude L, Sarrut D. Computed tomographic atlas for the new international lymph node map for lung cancer: a radiation oncologist perspective. *Pract Radiat Oncol.* 2013;3(1):54–66. doi:10.1016/j.prro.2012.01.007

5. Tammemagi MC, Ruparel M, Tremblay A, et al. USPSTF2013 versus PLCOm2012 lung cancer screening eligibility criteria (International Lung Screening Trial): interim analysis of a prospective cohort study. *Lancet Oncol.* 2022;23(1):138–148. doi:10.1016/S1470-2045(21)00590-8

6. Brunelli A, Kim AW, Berger KI, Addrizzo-Harris DJ. Physiologic evaluation of the patient with lung cancer being considered for resectional surgery: diagnosis and management of lung cancer, 3rd ed: American College of Chest Physicians evidence-based clinical practice guidelines. *Chest.* 2013;143(5 suppl):e166S–e190S. doi:10.1378/chest.12-2395

7. Yokoi K, Kamiya N, Matsuguma H, et al. Detection of brain metastasis in potentially operable non-small cell lung cancer: a comparison of CT and MRI. *Chest.* 1999;115(3):714–719. doi:10.1378/chest.115.3.714

8. McGarry RC, Song G, des Rosiers P, Timmerman R. Observation-only management of early stage, medically inoperable lung cancer: poor outcome. *Chest.* 2002;121(4):1155–1158. doi:10.1378/chest.121.4.1155

9. Christensen J, Prosper AE, Wu CC, et al. ACR Lung-RADS v2022: assessment categories and management recommendations. *J Am Coll Radiol.* 2024;21(3):473–488. doi:10.1016/j.jacr.2023.09.009

10. Altorki N, Wang X, Kozono D, et al. Lobar or sublobar resection for peripheral stage IA non-small-cell lung cancer. *N Engl J Med.* 2023;388(6):489–498. doi:10.1056/NEJMoa2212083

11. Saji H, Okada M, Tsuboi M, et al. Segmentectomy versus lobectomy in small-sized peripheral non-small-cell lung cancer (JCOG0802/WJOG4607L): a multicentre, open-label, phase 3, randomised, controlled, non-inferiority trial. *Lancet.* 2022;399(10335):1607–1617. doi:10.1016/S0140-6736(21)02333-3

12. Yan TD, Black D, Bannon PG, McCaughan BC. Systematic review and meta-analysis of randomized and nonrandomized trials on safety and efficacy of video-assisted thoracic surgery lobectomy for early-stage non-small-cell lung cancer. *J Clin Oncol.* 2009;27(15):2553–2562. doi:10.1200/JCO.2008.18.2733

13. Herbst RS, Wu YL, John T, et al. Adjuvant osimertinib for resected EGFR-mutated stage IB-IIIA non-small-cell lung cancer: updated results from the phase III randomized ADAURA trial. *J Clin Oncol.* 2023;41(10):1830–1840. doi:10.1200/JCO.22.02186

14. Wu YL, Dziadziuszko R, Ahn JS, et al. Alectinib in resected ALK-positive non-small-cell lung cancer. *N Engl J Med.* 2024;390(14):1265–1276. doi:10.1056/NEJMoa2310532

15. Trodella L, Granone P, Valente S, et al. Adjuvant radiotherapy in non-small cell lung cancer with pathological stage I: definitive results of a phase III randomized trial. *Radiother Oncol.* 2002;62(1):11–19. doi:10.1016/s0167-8140(01)00478-9

16. Bezjak A, Paulus R, Gaspar LE, et al. Safety and efficacy of a five-fraction stereotactic body radiotherapy schedule for centrally located non-small-cell lung cancer: NRG Oncology/RTOG 0813 trial. *J Clin Oncol.* 2019;37(15):1316–1325. doi:10.1200/JCO.18.00622

17. Lindberg K, Grozman V, Karlsson K, et al. The HILUS-trial-a prospective nordic multicenter phase 2 study of ultracentral lung tumors treated with stereotactic body radiotherapy. *J Thorac Oncol.* 2021;16(7):1200–1210. doi:10.1016/j.jtho.2021.03.019

18. Giuliani ME, Filion E, Faria S, et al. Stereotactic radiation for ultra-central non-small cell lung cancer: a safety and efficacy trial (SUNSET). *Int J Radiat Oncol Biol Phys.* 2024;120(3):669–677. doi:10.1016/j.ijrobp.2024.03.050

19. Serrano J, Crespo PC, Taboada B, et al. Postoperative radiotherapy in resected non-small cell lung cancer: the never-ending story. *World J Clin Oncol.* 2021;12(10):833–844. doi:10.5306/wjco.v12.i10.833

20. Vassil AD, Mossolly LM, Woody NM, et al. *Handbook of Treatment Planning in Radiation Oncology.* 3rd ed. Springer Publishing Company.

21. Fischer B, Lassen U, Mortensen J, et al. Preoperative staging of lung cancer with combined PET-CT. *N Engl J Med.* 2009;361(1):32–39. doi:10.1056/NEJMoa0900043

22. Ginsberg RJ, Rubinstein LV. Randomized trial of lobectomy versus limited resection for T1 N0 non-small cell lung cancer. Lung Cancer Study Group. *Ann Thorac Surg.* 1995;60(3):615–622. doi:10.1016/0003-4975(95)00537-u

23. Fernando HC, Landreneau RJ, Mandrekar SJ, et al. Impact of brachytherapy on local recurrence rates after sublobar resection: results from ACOSOG Z4032 (Alliance), a phase III randomized trial for high-risk operable non-small-cell lung cancer. *J Clin Oncol.* 2014;32(23):2456–2462. doi:10.1200/JCO.2013.53.4115

24. Postoperative radiotherapy in non-small-cell lung cancer: systematic review and meta-analysis of individual patient data from nine randomised controlled trials. PORT Meta-analysis Trialists Group. *Lancet.* 1998;352(9124):257–2563. PMID:9690404

25. Burdett S, Stewart L, Group PM-analysis Group. Postoperative radiotherapy in non-small-cell lung cancer: update of an individual patient data meta-analysis. *Lung Cancer.* 2005;47(1):81–83. doi:10.1016/j.lungcan.2004.09.010

26. Kato H, Ichinose Y, Ohta M, et al. A randomized trial of adjuvant chemotherapy with uracil-tegafur for adenocarcinoma of the lung. *N Engl J Med.* 2004;350(17):1713–1721. doi:10.1056/NEJMoa032792

27. Buchberger DS, Videtic GMM. Stereotactic body radiotherapy for the management of early-stage non-small-cell lung cancer: a clinical overview. *JCO Oncol Pract*. 2023;19(5):239–249. doi:10.1200/OP.22.00475

28. Sublobar Resection or Stereotactic Ablative Radiotherapy in Treating Patients with Stage I Non-small Cell Lung Cancer, The STABLE-MATES Trial. https://www.cancer.gov/research/participate/clinical-trials -search/v?id=NCI-2015-01676

29. Ritter TA, Timmerman RD, Hanfi HI, et al. Centralized quality assurance of stereotactic body radiation therapy for the veterans affairs cooperative studies program study number 2005: a phase 3 randomized trial of lung cancer surgery or stereotactic radiotherapy for operable early-stage non-small cell lung cancer (VALOR). *Pract Radiat Oncol*. 2025;15(1):e29–e39. doi:10.1016/j.prro.2024.07.010

30. Timmerman R, McGarry R, Yiannoutsos C, et al. Excessive toxicity when treating central tumors in a phase II study of stereotactic body radiation therapy for medically inoperable early-stage lung cancer. *J Clin Oncol*. 2006;24(30):4833–4839. doi:10.1200/JCO.2006.07.5937

31. Levy A, Adebahr S, Hurkmans C, et al. Stereotactic body radiotherapy for centrally located inoperable early-stage NSCLC: EORTC 22113-08113 lungtech phase II trial results. *J Thorac Oncol*. 2024;19(9):1297–1309. doi:10.1016/j.jtho.2024.05.366

32. Wu TC, Stube A, Felix C, et al. Safety and efficacy results from iSABR, a phase 1 study of stereotactic ablative radiotherapy in combination with durvalumab for early-stage medically inoperable non-small cell lung cancer. *Int J Radiat Oncol Biol Phys*. 2023;117(1):118–122. doi:10.1016/j.ijrobp.2023.03.069

33. Chang JY, Lin SH, Dong W, et al. Stereotactic ablative radiotherapy with or without immunotherapy for early-stage or isolated lung parenchymal recurrent node-negative non-small-cell lung cancer: an open-label, randomised, phase 2 trial. *Lancet*. 2023;402(10405):871–881. doi:10.1016/S0140-6736(23)01384-3

34. Robinson C, Hu C, Machtay M, et al. P1.18-12 PACIFIC-4/RTOG 3515: phase III study of durvalumab following SBRT for unresected stage I/II, lymph-node negative NSCLC. *J Thorac Oncol*. 2019;14(10):S630–S631. doi:10.1016/j.jtho.2019.08.1328

35. Daly ME, Redman M, Simone CB, et al. SWOG/NRG S1914: a randomized phase III trial of Induction/Consolidation Atezolizumab + SBRT vs. SBRT alone in high risk, early-stage NSCLC (NCT#04214262). *Int J Radiat Oncol Biol Phys*. 2022;114(3 suppl):e414. doi:10.1016/j.ijrobp.2022.07.1600

36. Jabbour SK, Houghton B, Robinson AG, et al. Phase 3, randomized, placebo-controlled study of Stereotactic Body Radiotherapy (SBRT) with or without pembrolizumab in patients with unresected stage I or II Non–Small Cell Lung Cancer (NSCLC): KEYNOTE-867. *J Clin Oncol*. 2022;40(16_suppl):TPS8597. doi:10.1200/JCO.2022.40.16_suppl.TPS8597

Jenna E. Kocsis, Aditya Juloori, Kevin L. Stephans, and Gregory M. M. Videtic

QUICK HIT Treatment of stage III NSCLC is heterogeneous due to a wide range of local and nodal presentations (see Table 29.1). Treatment is frequently impacted by patient performance and medical comorbidities. Treatment options involve appropriate selection and possible combination of CHT, RT, immunotherapy (IO), and surgery.

Table 29.1 General Treatment Paradigm for Stage III Lung Cancer[1]		
Treatment Option	**Appropriate Candidate**	**Treatment Details**
Neoadjuvant CRT followed by resection (trimodality)	Good performance, lobectomy-appropriate, nonbulky nonmultistation mediastinal nodes	45 Gy/25 fx with concurrent CHT
Neoadjuvant systemic therapy (immune checkpoint inhibitor [ICI] + CHT) followed by resection*	Resectable disease at diagnosis with no contraindication to ICI[†]	ICI + platinum-doublet CHT × 4 cycles
Initial surgery	Good performance, cT1–3N0–1	Adjuvant CHT for stage ≥II Consider adjuvant CRT for occult N2 or positive margins (54–60 Gy, CHT sequential or concurrent)
Definitive concurrent CRT followed by adjuvant IO	Good performance status, stage III, acceptable baseline pulmonary function Adjuvant IO if PD-L1 >0, no targetable mutations and no contraindications to ICI[†]	60 Gy/30 fx with concurrent cisplatin/etoposide (EP) or carboplatin AUC 2/paclitaxel 45 mg/m² followed by 1 yr of durvalumab
Sequential CRT	Impaired performance status OR stage III (any T/N) with impaired baseline pulmonary function (see Workup section)	CHT ± IO followed by 60 Gy/30 fx or 60 Gy/15 fx (or as determined by clinician)
RT alone	Marginal performance status	60 Gy/30 fx, 60 Gy/15 fx, 45 Gy/15 fx, 30 Gy/10 fx, 17 Gy/2 fx
Palliative care alone	Poor performance, poor risk IIIB NSCLC	

*NCCN recommends that all patients with potentially resectable disease be evaluated for neoadjuvant therapy. Strong consideration should be given to those with tumors ≥4 cm or positive nodes. Evaluation includes testing for PD-L1 status. Should also test for EGFR mutations and ALK rearrangements, as these patients are less likely to benefit from PD-1/PD-L1 inhibitors.
[†]Contraindications to checkpoint inhibitors include active/prior autoimmune disease or current immunosuppressive agents.
Source: NCCN Clinical Practice Guidelines in Oncology: Non-Small Cell Lung Cancer. https://www.nccn.org/professionals/physician_gls/pdf/nscl.pdf.

EPIDEMIOLOGY, RISK FACTORS, ANATOMY, PATHOLOGY, GENETICS, SCREENING: See Chapter 28.

CLINICAL PRESENTATION: Cough, dyspnea, wheeze, stridor, hemoptysis, anorexia, weight loss, decline in performance status, paraneoplastic syndromes such as hypercalcemia from PTHrP (SCC), or hypertrophic pulmonary osteoarthropathy. Hoarseness from recurrent laryngeal (left-sided more common), Horner syndrome (ptosis, miosis, anhidrosis). Pancoast syndrome (Horner, brachial plexopathy, shoulder pain). SVC syndrome.

WORKUP: H&P. ACCP guidelines define the standard for PFT evaluation and recommend FEV1 and DLCO be measured in all patients who are being considered for surgery.[2] For any surgery (including pneumonectomy), predicted postoperative FEV1 and DLCO >60% may not require further pulmonary testing as the risk for perioperative death and cardiopulmonary complications is low. If predicted FEV1 or DLCO is <60% but >30%, a low-technology exercise test (stair climb or shuttle walk) is recommended. If predicted FEV1 or DLCO is <30% or poor performance on the low-technology exercise test, a formal cardiopulmonary exercise test with measurement of maximal oxygen consumption is recommended. If O2 max <10 mL/kg/min or <35% predicted, patients should be counseled on minimally invasive surgeries, sublobar resections, or nonoperative treatments. In patients undergoing neoadjuvant therapy, repeat PFTs should be performed after completion of neoadjuvant therapy. For definitive CRT, pretreatment FEV1 ≥1 to 1.2 L has been used as criteria for clinical trials.[3,4] Note that these are different from the criteria for early-stage lung undergoing lobectomy (see Chapter 28).

Labs: CBC, CMP.

Imaging: CT chest and upper abdomen (with contrast if evaluating nodes; review liver and adrenals) and PET/CT (upstages ~20%, prevents unnecessary thoracotomies but no improvement in survival).[5] "Pathologic" LNs defined as short-axis diameter >1 cm and "bulky" lymphadenopathy as short-axis diameter >3 cm, multiple matted nodes, radiographic ECE, or ≥3 stations involved. MRI brain for stage ≥II.[1] CT brain with contrast sufficient if MRI contraindicated.[6] For T4 and/or superior sulcus tumors, consider MRI to investigate the degree of local invasion, and consider octreotide scan for carcinoid.

Procedures: Biopsy indicated (EBUS, CT-guided, or thoracentesis depending on location/presence of effusion; sputum pathology is unreliable but at least three needed to be negative). EBUS/mediastinoscopy to confirm positive LNs on CT or PET and for all T3 or central T1–2 tumors (EBUS/mediastinoscopy reaches stations 2, 4, 7; EBUS also reaches station 10). Chamberlain procedure (anterior mediastinotomy) or VATS is required to reach stations 5 and 6, and EUS for stations 8 and 9.

PROGNOSTIC FACTORS[7]: Stage, weight loss >5% in 3 months,[8] KPS <90, age >70, marital status. Females and never smokers with improved OS.[9]

STAGING: See Chapter 28 for AJCC 8th edition staging.

TREATMENT PARADIGM

Surgery: Surgery is the standard local therapy modality for medically operable disease.[1] Sublobar resections are not recommended for stage III disease due to the need for mediastinal lymphadenectomy. Surgical plan should be decided prior to initiation of any treatment. Role of surgery in N2 disease is controversial (see the following). N3 disease, bulky N2 disease (>3 cm), and multiple N2 nodes are relative contraindications to surgery. Pneumonectomy carries increased risk of operative mortality.

Chemotherapy[1,10]: CHT is indicated in essentially all stage III patients who are fit enough to tolerate treatment. CHT can be delivered preoperatively, postoperatively, or sequenced along with RT either concurrently or sequentially. For those with operable stage IIIA disease, induction therapy followed by surgery may be offered and options include neoadjuvant CHT-IO, neoadjuvant CHT, or neoadjuvant concurrent CRT. Patients with resected stage III disease who did not receive neoadjuvant systemic therapy should be offered adjuvant platinum-based CHT. Platinum-based doublet CHT is preferred for definitive concurrent CRT, and preferred regimens include cisplatin + etoposide (EP), carboplatin + paclitaxel, cisplatin + pemetrexed (nonsquamous only), and cisplatin + vinorelbine. Cisplatin 50 mg/m² on days 1, 8, 29, and 36 and etoposide 50 mg/m² days 1 to 5 and 29 to 33 or carboplatin AUC 2 and paclitaxel 50 mg/m² weekly are two regimens most commonly used. For definitive sequential CRT, give carboplatin AUC 6 and paclitaxel 200 mg/m² q3 weeks for two cycles followed by RT.

Immunotherapy: As the role for IO in metastatic NSCLC has become first line, its role in the definitive management of locally advanced NSCLC is increasing. The standard of care in patients undergoing nonoperative management is definitive CRT followed by 1 year of durvalumab, per the PACIFIC trial.[11] Stage III patients who are planned for surgical resection can be considered for neoadjuvant CHT-IO given the EFS benefits seen on CheckMate 816 and Keynote-671.[12–15]

Targeted Therapy: Patients with resected or unresectable stage III NSCLC with an EGFR exon 19 deletion or exon 21 L858R mutation should be offered adjuvant osimertinib based off the results of the ADAURA and LAURA trials given a significant PFS and OS benefit.[12,16–18] Patients with completely resected ALK-positive NSCLC should be offered adjuvant alectinib given the results of the ALINA trial showing a DFS benefit over adjuvant CHT.[19]

Radiation

Indications: RT is an option for definitive local therapy when surgery is not recommended or as an adjunct delivered either before or after surgery. In the neoadjuvant setting, CRT is delivered to 45 Gy/25 followed by resection. Postoperatively, for microscopic positive margins give 54 to 60 Gy and for gross residual give 60 Gy. For definitive CRT, concurrent RT provides survival benefit compared with sequential CRT. RT dose escalation for definitive CRT does not improve outcomes. Definitive CRT dose is 60 Gy/30 fx. For poor-performance patients who are not candidates for combined CRT, options include 60 Gy/30 fx, 60 Gy/15 fx, 45 Gy/15 fx, or palliative treatment alone. Historically, RT was commonly utilized in the adjuvant setting (PORT) for resected N2 disease to improve LC. Although this was not shown to provide an OS benefit in the Lung ART RCT, LC remains statistically significantly improved with PORT.[20]

Toxicity: Acute: fatigue, cough, shortness of breath, pneumonitis, esophagitis. Late: pneumonitis, cardiac toxicity, brachial plexopathy.

Procedure: See *Handbook of Treatment Planning in Radiation Oncology*, Chapter 6.[21]

EVIDENCE-BASED Q&A

MEDICALLY OPERABLE STAGE III

Which stage III patients are optimal candidates for initial surgery?

Surgery is the optimal LC method for patients with locally advanced NSCLC. The role of surgery in N2 patients remains controversial as the presence of N2 LNs substantially increases the likelihood of N3 LNs. Induction therapy is also considered in all stage III patients to facilitate surgery and can include neoadjuvant systemic therapy ± RT. Patients felt not to be good candidates for surgery should be treated with definitive CRT as follows if tolerable.

After surgical resection, what is the role of adjuvant systemic therapy?

Adjuvant CHT following surgery consistently provides 5% to 8% absolute benefit to 5-year OS. Many trials exist, but a few to be familiar with include IALT (cisplatin doublet vs. observation, 4% OS benefit at 5 years), ANITA (vinorelbine + cisplatin vs. observation, 8% OS benefit at 5 years for stage II and IIIA),[22] and LACE meta-analysis (see Chapter 28).[23] Distant failure continues to be the predominant mode of failure, and interest in the role of IO and targeted agents continues to increase. In patients who receive upfront surgery, consider adjuvant CHT followed by IO per Impower010, which demonstrated a DFS benefit with adjuvant atezolizumab after platinum-based CHT.[24] In those with EGFR or ALK mutations, consider adjuvant osimertinib or alectinib based on the ADAURA (improves 5-year DFS and OS)[16,25] and ALINA[19] (improves 2-year DFS) trials, respectively.

Which patients should be offered PORT?

Historically, pN2 disease and positive margins were considered indications for PORT. With older RT techniques, in pN2 patients, the PORT meta-analysis showed an LC benefit and the ANITA secondary analysis showed an OS benefit with the addition of PORT.[26–28] However, given the more recent findings from Lung ART and PORT-C showing no PFS or OS improvement with the addition of PORT to pN2 patients, ASCO guidelines state that PORT should not be routinely offered for completely resected NSCLC patients with mediastinal N2 involvement without ECE who have received neoadjuvant or adjuvant platinum-based CHT.[29] This recommendation nonetheless is controversial given the significant LC improvements with PORT.[29]

Pechoux, Lung ART (*Lancet Oncol* 2022, PMID 34919827): Phase III trial of 501 patients with completely resected stage IIIA N2 NSCLC followed by mediastinal PORT (54 Gy in 27–30 fx; 252 patients) vs. no PORT (249 patients). The primary endpoint was 3-year DFS with rates of 47% (with

PORT) and 44% (without), NS. Mediastinal relapse was less common with PORT (25% vs. 46%), although death as a first event was more common (15% vs. 5%) and possibly attributed to a higher rate of cardiopulmonary toxicity (16% of deaths in the PORT arm vs. 2% of deaths in the control arm). Late G3–4 cardiopulmonary toxicity in 11% of PORT vs. 5% without. Patients receiving PORT died less frequently of progression or recurrence (69% vs. 86%). **Conclusion: PORT is not associated with an overall improvement in DFS, which may be associated with cardiopulmonary toxicity. LC remains significantly improved with PORT.**

Hui, PORT-C (*JAMA Oncol* 2021, PMID 34165501): Phase III RCT of 394 patients with pathologic stage IIIA to N2 NSCLC s/p complete resection and adjuvant platinum-based CHT (× 4 cycles) randomized to PORT vs. observation. PORT delivered with a dose up to 50 Gy/25 fx within 6 weeks of CHT. Primary endpoint DFS and MFU 46.0 months. See Table 29.2 for results. PORT significantly improved the 3-year LRFS and LR rates but not the 3-year DFS or OS. An improvement in 3-year DFS was significant in the per-protocol analysis (43% vs. 31%; HR 0.75, 95% CI 0.57–1.00). No grades 4 to 5 adverse events related to RT. **Conclusion: PORT does not offer a DFS or OS benefit in an unselected population.** *Of note: ~24% of patients in the PORT arm refused RT.*

Table 29.2 Results From PORT-C Trial				
Arm	3-Yr DFS	3-Yr OS	3-Yr LRFS	3-Yr LR
PORT	41%	78%	67%	10%
Observation	33%	83%	60%	18%
p value	.20	.93	.03	.04

Is there a role for induction therapy?

Neoadjuvant therapy can be considered to facilitate surgery and improve R0 rates. This is especially true in those with N2 disease where definitive CRT has historically been the standard. Neoadjuvant therapy began with CHT alone (EORTC 08941) and evolved into CRT to improve pathologic response rates (German LCCG and INT0139), and now includes CHT-IO to improve both pCR and EFS. Table 29.3 describes multiple recent trials utilizing induction CHT-IO.

Van Meerbeeck, EORTC 08941 (*JNCI* 2007, PMID 17374834): PRT of 579 patients with N2 NSCLC treated with three cycles of platinum-doublet induction CHT and then randomized to surgery vs. RT 60 to 62.5 Gy. PORT (56 Gy) only delivered for positive margins. Sixty-one percent responded to CHT and were randomized. In the surgery arm, 42% showed nodal downstaging, 25% nodal clearance, and 5% pCR. Only 50% achieved R0 resection. MS was no different: 16.4 months in the surgery arm vs. 17.5 months for RT. **Conclusion: For N2 disease, induction CHT followed by surgery did not improve OS or PFS compared with sequential CRT, and RT should be considered the preferred locoregional treatment.**

Thomas, German Lung Cancer Cooperative Group (*Lancet Oncol* 2008, PMID 18583190): Phase III PRT randomizing 524 patients with stage IIIA to B NSCLC after invasive mediastinal staging to either EP × 3 cycles, then surgery, then RT (54 Gy) or EP × 3 cycles, then concurrent CRT (45 Gy/30 fx BID), and then surgery. Primary endpoint PFS. CRT improved mediastinal downstaging (46% vs. 29%, *p* = .02) and pathologic response (60% vs. 20%, *p* < .0001) but no difference in PFS (9.5 vs. 10 months). Pneumonectomy required in 35% for both groups, but mortality after CRT was higher (14% vs. 6%, NS). **Conclusion: Neoadjuvant CRT improved the response rates but not OS.**

Albain, INT 0139 (*Lancet* 2009, PMID 19632716): PRT of 429 potentially resectable NSCLC patients with biopsy-proven N2 disease randomized to either induction CRT followed by surgery 3 to 5 weeks later or to definitive CRT. Induction therapy for both arms was cisplatin 50 mg/m² and etoposide 50 mg/m² for two cycles (weeks 1 and 5) concurrent with 45 Gy/25 fx; those on definitive arm continued RT to 61 Gy without interruption; two cycles of consolidation EP were given after local therapy. No significant difference in MS between groups (23.6 vs. 22.2 months); 5-year OS 27% for surgery and 20% for CRT. PFS improved in the surgery arm (median 12.8 vs. 10.5 months, *p* = .017). Treatment-related death rate was 8% for surgery and 2% for CRT. Exploratory analysis demonstrated improved OS for lobectomy patients compared with CRT (not true for pneumonectomy).

Conclusion: Given no OS difference, definitive CRT is often favored. However, for healthy lobectomy patients, trimodality may be considered. *Comment: Pneumonectomy mortality rate was higher than expected at 26%.*

Forde, CheckMate 816 (*NEJM* 2022, PMID 35403841): Phase III study of 358 patients with stage IB to IIIA resectable NSCLC treated with neoadjuvant platinum doublet CHT ± nivolumab followed by surgery. EFS and pCR rates were co-primary endpoints. The pCR rate was 24% vs. 2% in favor of the IO group (*p* < .001). The median EFS was 31.6 vs. 28 months in favor of the IO group (*p* = .005). Grade 3/4 toxicities were similar between groups at ~35%. Three-year update from ESMO: 3-year EFS 57% in the CHT-IO arm vs. 43% in the CHT alone arm (HR 0.68, 95% CI 0.49–0.93).[30] **Conclusion: Neoadjuvant CHT-IO is associated with improved pCR rates and EFS compared with neoadjuvant CHT alone.**

Table 29.3 Summary of Neoadjuvant CHT-IO Trials in Locally Advanced NSCLC				
	Population	*N*	**Randomization**	**Results***
CheckMate 816 (2022)[13,30]	IB–IIIA	358	Neoadjuvant CHT ± nivolumab	mEFS 32 vs. 21 months; pCR 24% vs. 2%
Keynote 671 (2023)[14,15]	IIA–IIIB	797	Neoadjuvant CHT + neoadjuvant and adjuvant pembrolizumab vs. neoadjuvant CHT + placebo	3-yr OS: 71% vs. 64% mEFS: 47.2 vs. 18.3 months 2-yr pCR: 30% vs. 11%
AEGEAN (2023)[31]	IIA–IIIB	802	Neoadjuvant CHT + neoadjuvant and adjuvant durvalumab vs. neoadjuvant CHT + placebo	1-yr EFS 73% vs. 65% pCR 17% vs. 4%
NADIM II (2023)[32]	IIIA–IIIB	86	Neoadjuvant CHT ± nivolumab; those in nivolumab arm with R0 resection received adjuvant nivolumab	pCR 37% vs. 7% 2-yr PFS 67% vs. 41% 2-yr OS 85% vs. 64%

*All statistically significant.

NONOPERATIVE MANAGEMENT

Is RT alone an optimal strategy for stage III NSCLC?

RT alone is an option for patients unable to tolerate multimodality therapy given poor performance status. RTOG 7301 was a dose-escalation study that determined the standard dose of 60 Gy/30 fx for definitive RT. Hypofractionation is often considered in poor-performing stage III patients as UTSW demonstrated similar outcomes in patients receiving 60 Gy/15 fx vs. 60 Gy/30 fx.

Perez, RTOG 7301 (*IJROBP* 1980, PMID 6998937): Four-arm PRT of definitive RT dose escalation for stage III NSCLC: 40 Gy split course (20 Gy/5 fx, 2-week break, then another 20 Gy/5 fx) or 40 Gy, 50 Gy, or 60 Gy given 5 fx/week. OS at 2 years was 10% for split course compared with 14% to 18% with the other groups. Response was better in the 50 and 60 Gy arms. **Conclusion: 60 Gy is standard dose.**

Iyengar, UTSW (*JAMA Oncol* 2021, PMID 34383006): Phase III PRT of RT alone with hypofractionation (60 Gy/15 fx) vs. conventionally fractionated RT (60 Gy/30 fx) in patients with stage II/III NSCLC, ECOG ≥2, ≥10% weight loss in 6 months, and/or ineligible for concurrent CRT. Results: Closed early due to interim analysis suggesting futility of demonstrating an OS benefit. There was no SS difference in 1-year OS, mOS, PFS, LF, DM, or G3+ AE. **Conclusion: Hypofractionated RT alone at 60 Gy/15 fx is not superior to standard RT in patients with poor performance status not eligible for concurrent CRT.**

Does CHT followed by RT improve survival? Is concurrent CRT better than sequential CRT?

Multiple studies, including CALGB 8433 and RTOG 8808/ECOG 4588, show that the addition of CHT to RT improves OS.[33–35] In well-performing patients, consider concurrent CRT rather than sequential CRT given OS benefit was seen on RTOG 0914 and confirmed on the Auperin meta-analysis.

Dillman, CALGB 8433 (*NEJM* 1990, PMID 2169587; Update *JNCI* 1996, PMID 8780630): PRT of 155 patients with stage III NSCLC randomized to cisplatin with vinblastine followed by 60 Gy/30 fx vs. immediate identical RT. Long-term results reported 5-year OS rate of 17% vs. 6% (*p* = .012) in favor of CHT arm and confirmed the initial results. **Conclusion: Sequential CRT is superior to RT alone.**

Sause, RTOG 8808/ECOG 4588 (*JNCI* 1995, PMID 7707407): Three-arm PRT of 452 patients with stage II to IIIB unresectable NSCLC randomized to either 60 Gy/30 fx alone, induction cisplatin/vinblastine followed by 60 Gy/30 fx, or hyperfractionated RT alone 69.6 Gy/58 fx at 1.2 Gy/fx BID. MS in each arm was 11.4, 13.8, and 12.3 months, respectively, with statistically significant improvement in the CHT arm. **Conclusion: Sequential CRT is superior to standard and hyperfractionated RT alone.**

Curran, RTOG 9410 (*JNCI* 2011, PMID 21903745): Three-arm PRT of 610 patients with unresectable stage III NSCLC. See Table 29.4 for randomization and results. Statistical significance was demonstrated between sequential and concurrent daily arms (*p* = .046). **Conclusion: Concurrent CHT is superior to sequential.**

Table 29.4 RTOG 9410 Stage III Lung Trial		
Arm	5-Yr OS	MS (Months)
Sequential cisplatin/vinblastine × 2C, then 63 Gy/34 fx	10%	14.6
Concurrent cisplatin/vinblastine × 2C with 63 Gy/34 fx	16%	17
Concurrent cisplatin/etoposide with 69.6 Gy at 1.2 Gy/fx BID	13%	15.6

Note: 63 Gy total was delivered: 45 Gy/25 fx followed by 18 Gy/9 fx boost. Without heterogeneity corrections, this is comparable to 60 Gy/30 fx.

Aupérin, NSCLC Collaborative Group Meta-Analysis (*JCO* 2010, PMID 20351327): Individual patient data meta-analysis of six of seven eligible trials, 1,205 patients. Concurrent CRT demonstrated 4.5% absolute survival benefit at 5 years compared with sequential CRT. Concurrent therapy decreased locoregional but not distant progression and increased esophageal but not pulmonary toxicity. **Conclusion: Concurrent CRT improves survival at the cost of manageable but increased esophageal toxicity.**

What is the optimal CHT regimen when given concurrently with RT?

Many regimens have been used, but cisplatin/etoposide (EP) and carboplatin/paclitaxel are the most common regimens used in the United States. Carboplatin/paclitaxel and cisplatin/pemetrexed (for nonsquamous cancers) may have similar efficacy with reduced toxicity. Retrospective data suggest that carboplatin/paclitaxel is associated with increased radiation pneumonitis, which was confirmed by Liang as follows.[36] However, others feel EP is more difficult to tolerate.[37]

Liang, China (*Ann Oncol* 2017, PMID 28137739): PRT comparing EP with carboplatin/paclitaxel both with concurrent RT to 60 to 66 Gy. Primary endpoint OS, powered for 17% improvement in 3-year OS. 200 patients, MFU 73 months. The 3-year OS improved in the EP arm by 15% (*p* = .024); MS 23.3 vs. 20.7 months. Grade ≥2 pneumonitis increased in the carboplatin/paclitaxel arm (33% vs. 19%, *p* = .036), but esophagitis increased in the EP arm (20% vs. 6%, *p* = .009). **Conclusion: Cisplatin/etoposide may be superior to carboplatin/paclitaxel.**

Senan, PROCLAIM (*JCO* 2016, PMID 26811519): PRT of 555 patients with unresectable stage IIIA/B nonsquamous NSCLC randomized to receive either (a) pemetrexed 500 mg/m² and cisplatin 75 mg/m² q3 weeks for 3 cycles + 60 to 66 Gy followed by consolidation pemetrexed q3 weeks for four cycles or (b) cisplatin 50 mg/m² with etoposide 50 mg/m² q4 weeks for two cycles + same RT with consolidation platinum doublet. Trial stopped early due to futility. Pemetrexed was not superior but was associated with fewer grades 3 to 4 AEs. **Conclusion: Pemetrexed is not superior but may be associated with fewer adverse events.**

Does RT dose escalation improve outcomes when given with concurrent CHT?

Dating back to the 1970s, RTOG 7301 demonstrated 60 Gy/30 fx to be the standard regimen. RTOG 9311 was a phase I/II dose-escalation trial that delivered escalated dose based on achieved V20, with doses ranging from 70.9 to 90.3 Gy without concurrent CHT. This led to RTOG 0617, in which dose escalation to 74 Gy had worse OS outcomes compared with 60 Gy with concurrent CHT (47% treated with IMRT). RTOG 1106 attempted dose escalation with a boost to residual avid disease on midtreatment PET; however, this again did not improve outcomes.

Bradley, RTOG 0617 (*Lancet Oncol* 2015, PMID 25601342): 2×2 PRT of 544 patients randomized to either 60 Gy/30 fx or 74 Gy/37 fx both with concurrent carboplatin AUC 2/paclitaxel 45 mg/ m^2 weekly. Adjuvant CHT given 2 weeks after RT with carboplatin AUC 6/paclitaxel 200 mg/m^2 with second randomization ± cetuximab during adjuvant phase; 47% treated with IMRT. Dose escalation led to worse OS. See Table 29.5 for the results. Overall, no difference in toxicity rates between 60 and 74 Gy, but grade ≥3 esophagitis was increased in the 74 Gy arm. Noncompliance was higher in the 74 Gy arm. Cetuximab increased grade ≥3 toxicity but did not improve OS, PFS, or DM. **Conclusion: 60 Gy is standard of care as escalation to 74 Gy is harmful and not superior. No benefit to cetuximab.** *Comment: Hypotheses as to why 74 Gy survival was inferior: treatment-related deaths were highest in the 74 Gy + cetuximab arm, effect of RT on heart, PTV coverage was sacrificed in the 74 Gy arm for safety thus leading to failures. Second analysis demonstrated dosimetric benefits to IMRT, reduced lung dosimetry, and correlation of heart V40 with survival.*[38]

Table 29.5 Results of RTOG 0617 for Stage III NSCLC						
Arms	MS (Months)	1-Yr OS	mPFS (Months)	1-Yr PFS	1-Yr LF	1-Yr DM
60 Gy/30 fx	28.7	80%	11.8	49%	16%	32%
74 Gy/37 fx	20.3	70%	9.8	41%	25%	35%
p value	.004	.004	.12	.12	.13	.48

Chun, RTOG 0617 IMRT Second Analysis (*JCO* 2016, PMID 28034064): Secondary analysis comparing IMRT with 3D-CRT planning. Results: The IMRT group had larger PTVs (median, 427 vs. 486 mL, $p = .005$), larger PTV/volume of lung ratio (median, 0.13 vs. 0.15, $p = .013$), and more stage IIIB disease (30% vs. 39%, $p = .056$). The 2-year OS, PFS, LF, and DMFS were not different between IMRT and 3D-CRT. IMRT associated with less grade ≥3 pneumonitis (8% vs. 4%, $p = .039$) and a reduced risk in adjusted analyses (OR 0.41, 95% CI 0.17–0.99). IMRT also produced lower heart doses ($p < .05$), and the V40 of the heart was significantly associated with OS on adjusted analysis ($p < .05$). Lung V5 was not associated with any grade ≥3 toxicity, whereas lung V20 was associated with increased grade ≥3 pneumonitis risk on MVA ($p = .026$). **Conclusion: Although with no OS benefit, IMRT was associated with lower cardiac dose and rates of severe pneumonitis, which supports consideration of IMRT for locally advanced NSCLC.**

Kong, RTOG 1106/ECOG-ACRIN 6697 (*JCO* 2024, PMID 39365957): Phase II PRT of 127 patients receiving CRT randomized to either standard RT (60 Gy/30 fx) or adaptive RT with boost delivered to residual avid disease on midtreatment FDG PET/CT. Primary endpoint: freedom from locoregional progression (FFLP) at 2 years. With the boost, patients in the adaptive RT arm received a mean dose of 71 Gy/30 fx. Results: No difference in 2-year FFLP in standard vs. adaptive (60% vs. 55%, $p = .66$). No statistically significant difference in grade 3 toxicity, OS, or PFS. **Conclusion: Adaptive dose escalation RT to residual PET-avid disease does not improve LC.**

Can the addition of IO to concurrent CRT improve OS in locally advanced lung cancer?

The seminal PACIFIC trial has established a new standard of care for management of nonoperative stage III NSCLC given its finding on the benefits of adjuvant IO. PACIFIC-2 and EA5181 are two ongoing trials investigating the role of concurrent IO with CRT.

Antonia, PACIFIC (*NEJM* 2018, PMID 30280658; Update *JCO* 2020, PMID 31622733): PRT of stage IIIA/B NSCLC s/p definitive CRT randomized to consolidation durvalumab for up to 12 months vs. placebo. Co-primary endpoints were PFS and OS. Results: 712 patients, MFU 25.5 months. Durvalumab significantly prolonged OS (HR 0.68, 99% CI 0.47–0.997). Median time to death or DM (28.3 vs. 16.2 months; HR 0.53, 95% CI 0.41–0.68), overall response rate (30% vs. 18, $p < .001$), and median duration of response (NR vs. 18.4 months) favored durvalumab (see Table 29.6); 15% vs. 10% discontinued drug due to AE in durvalumab and placebo, respectively. Although both subsets benefitted, patients with higher PD-L1 seemed to derive the most benefit. **Conclusion: Adjuvant durvalumab is the new standard of care following CRT for stage III NSCLC.**

Table 29.6 Results of PACIFIC Trial

Arm	Median PFS	2-Yr OS	3-Yr OS	Grade 3/4 AE
Durvalumab	17.2 months	66%	57%	31%
Placebo	5.6 months	56%	44%	26%
p value	SS	.005	SS	

Is there benefit to adding induction CHT prior to concurrent CRT or additional consolidation CHT after concurrent CRT?

Consolidation CHT after definitive CRT was given in RTOG 0617, but its current use is diminishing given its lack of definitive benefit with increased toxicity along with the increasing role of IO.[39–41] Induction CHT provides no OS benefit but in selected cases may help in downsizing tumors to meet OAR constraints prior to definitive RT.

Ahn, Korean KCSG-LU05-04 (*JCO* 2015, PMID 26150444): PRT of 437 patients with stage III NSCLC treated to 66 Gy with cisplatin/docetaxel, then randomized to receive either three additional cycles of docetaxel/cisplatin or no further treatment; 62% in consolidation arm completed the treatment. PFS 8.1 months in observation vs. 9.1 months in consolidation arm (*p* = .36). MS was also not different (20.6 vs. 21.8 months, *p* = .44). **Conclusion: Additional CHT did not improve outcomes after CRT.**

Hanna, Hoosier Oncology Group (*JCO* 2008, PMID 19001323; Update *Ann Oncol* 2012, PMID 22156624): Phase III PRT of 203 patients with stage IIIA/B NSCLC treated with EP concurrent with RT to 59.4 Gy, then randomized to adjuvant docetaxel vs. observation. Closed early due to futility. MS not significantly different (initial publication 21.7 vs. 21.2 months, no difference on update). Toxicity increased in docetaxel arm. **Conclusion: Consolidation docetaxel increases toxicity and does not improve OS.**

Vokes, CALGB 39801 (*JCO* 2007, PMID 17404369): PRT of 366 patients randomized to induction CHT followed by CRT vs. CRT alone. No statistically significant difference in OS. **Conclusion: No benefit to induction CHT prior to CRT.**

Are there targeted agents available to patients with nonoperable locally advanced lung cancer?

Similar to the ADAURA trial in operable patients, LAURA is a phase III PRT of patients with unresectable EGFR-mutated stage III NSCLC treated with definitive CRT who were randomized to adjuvant osimertinib vs. placebo and found that osimertinib significantly improved PFS (39.1 vs. 5.6 months, p < .001).[18]

SUPERIOR SULCUS TUMORS

Superior sulcus tumors were classically associated with poor rates of complete resection. SWOG 9416 changed the paradigm, and these tumors are now recommended to undergo induction CRT to facilitate resection.

Rusch, SWOG 9416/INT 0160 (*J Thorac Cardiovasc Surg* 2001, PMID 11241082; Update *JCO* 2007, PMID 17235046): Single-arm phase II trial of 111 patients with mediastinoscopy-negative and supraclavicular node-negative T3–4N0–1 superior sulcus tumor treated with two cycles of EP with concurrent RT 45 Gy/25 fx. If disease was stable or responding on reassessment, thoracotomy was performed 3 to 5 weeks later. Thereafter, two more cycles of CHT were delivered. 111 enrolled, 95 eligible for surgery and 83 underwent thoracotomy, 72 had complete resection (92%). Sixty-five percent of thoracotomy specimens demonstrated CR. On update, the 5-year OS was 44% overall and 56% after complete resection. **Conclusion: Combined-modality induction therapy is the standard for superior sulcus tumors.**

REFERENCES

1.   NCCN Clinical Practice Guidelines in Oncology: Non-Small Cell Lung Cancer. Accessed March 2025. https://www.nccn.org/professionals/physician_gls/pdf/nscl.pdf

2. Brunelli A, Kim AW, Berger KI, Addrizzo-Harris DJ. Physiologic evaluation of the patient with lung cancer being considered for resectional surgery: Diagnosis and management of lung cancer, 3rd ed: American College of Chest Physicians evidence-based clinical practice guidelines. *Chest*. 2013;143(5 Suppl):e166S–e190S. doi:10.1378/chest.12-2395

3. Bradley JD, Bae K, Graham MV, et al. Primary analysis of the phase II component of a phase I/II dose intensification study using three-dimensional conformal radiation therapy and concurrent chemotherapy for patients with inoperable non-small-cell lung cancer: RTOG 0117. *J Clin Oncol*. 2010;28(14):2475–2480. doi:10.1200/JCO.2009.27.1205

4. Bradley JD, Paulus R, Komaki R, et al. Standard-dose versus high-dose conformal radiotherapy with concurrent and consolidation carboplatin plus paclitaxel with or without cetuximab for patients with stage IIIA or IIIB non-small-cell lung cancer (RTOG 0617): a randomised, two-by-two factorial phase 3 study. *Lancet Oncol*. 2015;16(2):187–199. doi:10.1016/S1470-2045(14)71207-0

5. Fischer B, Lassen U, Mortensen J, et al. Preoperative staging of lung cancer with combined PET-CT. *N Engl J Med*. 2009;361(1):32–39. doi:10.1056/NEJMoa0900043

6. Yokoi K, Kamiya N, Matsuguma H, et al. Detection of brain metastasis in potentially operable non-small cell lung cancer: a comparison of CT and MRI. *Chest*. 1999;115(3):714–719. doi:10.1378/chest.115.3.714

7. Garinet S, Wang P, Mansuet-Lupo A, Fournel L, Wislez M, Blons H. Updated prognostic factors in localized NSCLC. *Cancers (Basel)*. 2022;14(6):1400. doi:10.3390/cancers14061400

8. Simmons CP, Koinis F, Fallon MT, et al. Prognosis in advanced lung cancer–a prospective study examining key clinicopathological factors. *Lung Cancer*. 2015;88(3):304–309. doi:10.1016/j.lungcan.2015.03.020

9. Kawaguchi T, Takada M, Kubo A, et al. Performance status and smoking status are independent favorable prognostic factors for survival in non-small cell lung cancer: a comprehensive analysis of 26,957 patients with NSCLC. *J Thorac Oncol*. 2010;5(5):620–630. doi:10.1097/JTO.0b013e3181d2dcd9

10. Daly ME, Singh N, Ismaila N, et al. Management of stage III non-small-cell lung cancer: ASCO guideline. *J Clin Oncol*. 2022;40(12):1356–1384. doi:10.1200/JCO.21.02528

11. Antonia SJ, Villegas A, Daniel D, et al. Overall survival with durvalumab after chemoradiotherapy in stage III NSCLC. *N Engl J Med*. 2018;379(24):2342–2350. doi:10.1056/NEJMoa1809697

12. Singh N, Daly ME, Ismaila N, Management of Stage IIINGEP. Management of stage III non-small-cell lung cancer: ASCO guideline rapid recommendation update. *J Clin Oncol*. 2023;41(27):4430–4432. doi:10.1200/JCO.23.01261

13. Forde PM, Spicer J, Lu S, et al. Neoadjuvant nivolumab plus chemotherapy in resectable lung cancer. *N Engl J Med*. 2022;386(21):1973–1985. doi:10.1056/NEJMoa2202170

14. Wakelee H, Liberman M, Kato T, et al. Perioperative pembrolizumab for early-stage non-small-cell lung cancer. *N Engl J Med*. 2023;389(6):491–503. doi:10.1056/NEJMoa2302983

15. Spicer JD, Garassino MC, Wakelee H, et al. Neoadjuvant pembrolizumab plus chemotherapy followed by adjuvant pembrolizumab compared with neoadjuvant chemotherapy alone in patients with early-stage non-small-cell lung cancer (KEYNOTE-671): a randomised, double-blind, placebo-controlled, phase 3 trial. *Lancet*. 2024;404(10459):1240–1252. doi:10.1016/S0140-6736(24)01756-2

16. Wu YL, Tsuboi M, He J, et al. Osimertinib in resected EGFR-mutated non-small-cell lung cancer. *N Engl J Med*. 2020;383(18):1711–1723. doi:10.1056/NEJMoa2027071

17. Daly ME, Singh N, Ismaila N, Management of Stage IIINGEP. Management of stage III non-small cell lung cancer: ASCO guideline rapid recommendation update. *J Clin Oncol*. 2024;42(25):3058–3060. doi:10.1200/JCO-24-01324

18. Lu S, Kato T, Dong X, et al. Osimertinib after chemoradiotherapy in stage III *EGFR*-mutated NSCLC. *N Engl J Med*. 2024;391(7):585–597. doi:10.1056/NEJMoa2402614

19. Wu YL, Dziadziuszko R, Ahn JS, et al. Alectinib in resected *ALK*-positive non-small-cell lung cancer. *N Engl J Med*. 2024;390(14):1265–1276. doi:10.1056/NEJMoa2310532

20. Le Pechoux C, Pourel N, Barlesi F, et al. Postoperative radiotherapy versus no postoperative radiotherapy in patients with completely resected non-small-cell lung cancer and proven mediastinal N2 involvement (Lung ART): an open-label, randomised, phase 3 trial. *Lancet Oncol*. 2022;23(1):104–114. doi:10.1016/S1470-2045(21)00606-9

21. Videtic GNM, Vassil AD, Woody NM. *Handbook of Treatment Planning in Radiation Oncology*. 3rd ed. Demos Medical; 2020.

22. Douillard JY, Rosell R, De Lena M, et al. Adjuvant vinorelbine plus cisplatin versus observation in patients with completely resected stage IB-IIIA non-small-cell lung cancer (Adjuvant Navelbine International Trialist Association [ANITA]): a randomised controlled trial. *Lancet Oncol*. 2006;7(9):719–727. doi:10.1016/S1470-2045(06)70804-X

23. Arriagada R, Bergman B, Dunant A, et al. Cisplatin-based adjuvant chemotherapy in patients with completely resected non-small-cell lung cancer. *N Engl J Med*. 2004;350(4):351–360. doi:10.1056/NEJMoa031644

24. Felip E, Altorki N, Zhou C, et al. Adjuvant atezolizumab after adjuvant chemotherapy in resected stage IB-IIIA non-small-cell lung cancer (IMpower010): a randomised, multicentre, open-label, phase 3 trial. *Lancet*. 2021;398(10308):1344–1357. doi:10.1016/S0140-6736(21)02098-5

25. Tsuboi M, Herbst RS, John T, et al. Overall survival with osimertinib in resected *EGFR*-mutated NSCLC. *N Engl J Med*. 2023;389(2):137–147. doi:10.1056/NEJMoa2304594

26. Douillard JY, Rosell R, De Lena M, et al. Impact of postoperative radiation therapy on survival in patients with complete resection and stage I, II, or IIIA non-small-cell lung cancer treated with adjuvant chemotherapy: the adjuvant Navelbine International Trialist Association (ANITA) randomized trial. *Int J Radiat Oncol Biol Phys*. 2008;72(3):695–701. doi:10.1016/j.ijrobp.2008.01.044

27. Postoperative radiotherapy in non-small-cell lung cancer: systematic review and meta-analysis of individual patient data from nine randomised controlled trials. PORT Meta-analysis Trialists Group. *Lancet*. 1998;352(9124):257–263.

28. Burdett S, Stewart L, PORT Meta-analysis Group. Postoperative radiotherapy in non-small-cell lung cancer: update of an individual patient data meta-analysis. *Lung Cancer*. 2005;47(1):81–83. doi:10.1016/j.lungcan.2004.09.010

29. Simone CB 2nd, Bradley J, Chen AB, et al. ASTRO radiation therapy summary of the ASCO guideline on management of stage III non-small cell lung cancer. *Pract Radiat Oncol*. 2023;13(3):195–202. doi:10.1016/j.prro.2023.01.005

30. Forde PM, et al. 84O Neoadjuvant nivolumab (N) + platinum-doublet chemotherapy (C) for resectable NSCLC: 3-y update from CheckMate 816. *J Thorac Oncol*. 2023;18(4):S89–S90. doi:10.1016/S1556-0864(23)00338-6

31. Heymach JV, Harpole D, Mitsudomi T, et al. Perioperative durvalumab for resectable non-small-cell lung cancer. *N Engl J Med*. 2023;389(18):1672–1684. doi:10.1056/NEJMoa2304875

32. Provencio M, Nadal E, Gonzalez-Larriba JL, et al. Perioperative nivolumab and chemotherapy in stage III non-small-cell lung cancer. *N Engl J Med*. 2023;389(6):504–513. doi:10.1056/NEJMoa2215530

33. Dillman RO, Herndon J, Seagren SL, Eaton WL Jr, Green MR. Improved survival in stage III non-small-cell lung cancer: seven-year follow-up of Cancer and leukemia group B (CALGB) 8433 trial. *J Natl Cancer Inst*. 1996;88(17):1210–1215. doi:10.1093/jnci/88.17.1210

34. Dillman RO, Seagren SL, Propert KJ, et al. A randomized trial of induction chemotherapy plus high-dose radiation versus radiation alone in stage III non-small-cell lung cancer. *N Engl J Med*. 1990;323(14):940–945. doi:10.1056/NEJM199010043231403

35. Sause WT, Scott C, Taylor S, et al. Radiation Therapy Oncology Group (RTOG) 88-08 and Eastern Cooperative Oncology Group (ECOG) 4588: preliminary results of a phase III trial in regionally advanced, unresectable non-small-cell lung cancer. *J Natl Cancer Inst*. 1995;87(3):198–205. doi:10.1093/jnci/87.3.198

36. Palma DA, Senan S, Tsujino K, et al. Predicting radiation pneumonitis after chemoradiation therapy for lung cancer: an international individual patient data meta-analysis. *Int J Radiat Oncol Biol Phys*. 2013;85(2):444–450. doi:10.1016/j.ijrobp.2012.04.043

37. Santana-Davila R, Devisetty K, Szabo A, et al. Cisplatin and etoposide versus carboplatin and paclitaxel with concurrent radiotherapy for stage III non-small-cell lung cancer: an analysis of Veterans Health Administration data. *J Clin Oncol*. 2015;33(6):567–574. doi:10.1200/JCO.2014.56.2587

38. Chun SG, Hu C, Choy H, et al. Impact of intensity-modulated radiation therapy technique for locally advanced non-small-cell lung cancer: a secondary analysis of the NRG Oncology RTOG 0617 randomized clinical trial. *J Clin Oncol*. 2017;35(1):56–62. doi:10.1200/JCO.2016.69.1378

39. Belani CP, Choy H, Bonomi P, et al. Combined chemoradiotherapy regimens of paclitaxel and carboplatin for locally advanced non-small-cell lung cancer: a randomized phase II locally advanced multi-modality protocol. *J Clin Oncol*. 2005;23(25):5883–5891. doi:10.1200/JCO.2005.55.405

40. Hanna N, Neubauer M, Yiannoutsos C, et al. Phase III study of cisplatin, etoposide, and concurrent chest radiation with or without consolidation docetaxel in patients with inoperable stage III non-small-cell lung cancer: the Hoosier Oncology Group and U.S. Oncology. *J Clin Oncol*. 2008;26(35):5755–5760. doi:10.1200/JCO.2008.17.7840

41. Jalal SI, Riggs HD, Melnyk A, et al. Updated survival and outcomes for older adults with inoperable stage III non-small-cell lung cancer treated with cisplatin, etoposide, and concurrent chest radiation with or without consolidation docetaxel: analysis of a phase III trial from the Hoosier Oncology Group (HOG) and US Oncology. *Ann Oncol*. 2012;23(7):1730–1738. doi:10.1093/annonc/mdr565

30 SMALL-CELL LUNG CANCER

Anirudh Bommireddy and Gregory M. M. Videtic

QUICK HIT Small-cell lung cancer (SCLC) is classically described as either limited-stage (fits within one radiation portal; LS-SCLC) or extensive-stage (metastatic; ES-SCLC). Treatment for LS-SCLC consists of concurrent CRT with four cycles of platinum-based regimens and RT starting with cycle 1 or 2 of CHT followed by adjuvant immunotherapy (IO), with prophylactic cranial irradiation (PCI) offered for those with response to therapy. Treatment for ES-SCLC consists of four cycles of CHT with concurrent IO followed by IO maintenance (Table 30.1). In the IO era, the role and timing of post-CHT/IO thoracic RT and PCI for ES-SCLC are controversial. Outcomes are generally modest, with MS 20 to 30 months for LS-SCLC and 9 to 12 months for ES-SCLC.

Table 30.1 General Treatment Paradigm for Small-Cell Lung Carcinoma	
Disease Extent	**General Treatment Paradigm**
Limited stage (30% of SCLC)	• Concurrent CRT with EP CHT × 4C, RT to start with either C1 or C2 followed by adjuvant durvalumab • CHT: cisplatin 60 mg/m^2 d1 and etoposide 120 mg/m^2 d1–3 q3 weeks × 4C • RT standard: 45 Gy/30 fx in 3 weeks at 1.5 Gy/fx BID; consider dose escalation to 54–60 Gy BID • Durvalumab: 1,500 mg q4 weeks for up to 24 months • PCI: 25 Gy/10 fx for responders • T1–T2N0M0 disease (5% of cases): primary resection with adjuvant CHT + consideration of PCI; if pN+ then consider postoperative RT; medically inoperable cases: consider SBRT as surgical surrogate

Extensive stage (70% SCLC)	• Cisplatin-based CHT (4C) with concurrent and maintenance IO
	• Palliative RT to symptomatic sites
	• Areas of controversy:
	  1. In patients without brain metastases and *any* response to CHT, consider PCI (25 Gy/10 fx).
	  2. In selected patients, consider post-CHT/IO consolidative thoracic RT 30 Gy/10 fx.

EPIDEMIOLOGY: SCLC represents ~14% of all lung cancer diagnoses with decreasing incidence.[1] Approximately 30,000 people are diagnosed in the United States each year.[2] More common in men, although gender difference is narrowing.[1]

RISK FACTORS: Occurs almost exclusively in smokers (>98%)—typically heavy smokers. Uranium mining is another risk factor (radon exposure from uranium decay).[3]

ANATOMY: See Chapter 28.

PATHOLOGY: SCLC is of neuroendocrine origin and lies along a spectrum of other lung neuroendocrine tumors including low-grade neuroendocrine carcinoma (typical carcinoid), intermediate-grade (atypical carcinoid), and high-grade (large-cell neuroendocrine carcinoma [LCNEC] and SCLC). Light microscopy classically reveals clusters or sheets of small round blue cells, twice the size of normal lymphocytes. "Crush artifact" is a classic descriptor on cytology and is considered diagnostic. Cytoplasm is sparse, and the nucleus manifests finely dispersed chromatin without distinct nucleoli. Mitotic rates are high, and necrosis is common. Up to 30% of SCLC autopsy specimens have areas of differentiation into NSCLC, suggestive that carcinogenesis occurs in pluripotent stem cells capable of varied differentiation.[4–6] Three groups of antigen clusters have been identified: neural, epithelial, and neuroendocrine. Epithelial markers include keratin, epithelial membrane antigen, and TTF1. Nearly all SCLCs are immunoreactive for keratin and epithelial membrane antigen, and a majority express TTF1. Neuroendocrine and neural markers include DOPA decarboxylase, calcitonin, NSE, synaptophysin, chromogranin A, CD56 (NCAM), gastrin releasing peptide, and IGF-1. Although these are common in SCLC, they are not specific, with about 10% of NSCLCs being positive for these classic neuroendocrine markers.[7] Seventy-five percent of SCLC will manifest at least one neural/neuroendocrine marker.

GENETICS: In contrast to NSCLC, driving alterations in EGFR, K-ras, ALK, and p16 are rarely seen.

CLINICAL PRESENTATION: SCLC arises submucosally in the central airways, often obstructing the bronchial lumen. Commonly appears on imaging as a large hilar mass with bulky mediastinal adenopathy.[8] Two-thirds of patients present with extensive-stage disease, one-third with limited-stage disease. Common symptoms include new or worsening cough, dyspnea, chest pain, hoarseness, hemoptysis, malaise, anorexia, and weight loss. If other thoracic structures are compromised by the enlarging mass, dysphagia or SVC syndrome (facial edema/plethora, distension of superficial veins, laryngeal edema, altered mental status) may be present. The most common sites of distant spread are the liver, adrenals, bone, and brain. Brain metastasis incidence: 10% to 20% at diagnosis, 50% to 80% at 2 years.[9,10] As detailed in Table 30.2, patients may present with paraneoplastic syndromes (SCLC is the most common solid tumor associated with paraneoplastic syndromes).[11] Fundamentally, treatment of the underlying malignancy is necessary to manage these syndromes, but temporizing management steps are described as follows.

Table 30.2 Paraneoplastic Syndromes Commonly Diagnosed in SCLC	
SIADH	Overproduction of ADH with euvolemic hyponatremia. May present with altered mental status or seizures. Treat with water restriction, hypertonic saline, demeclocycline, vasopressin inhibitors, and/or lithium.
Cushing syndrome	Ectopic production of ACTH. Treat with ketoconazole.
Lambert–Eaton	Autoantibodies to presynaptic calcium channels. Proximal muscle weakness that improves later in the day. Treat with pyridostigmine, prednisone, IVIG, and by treating cancer.
Others (rare)	Subacute cerebellar degeneration, subacute sensory neuropathy, limbic encephalopathy, encephalomyelitis (anti-Hu antibodies).

WORKUP: H&P. Encourage smoking cessation.[12]

Labs: CBC, BMP, LFTs, LDH, alkaline phosphatase, PFTs.

Imaging: CT chest with contrast (including liver and adrenals) and PET/CT (nearly 100% sensitive for SCLC; note that PET upstages 19% of patients initially diagnosed with LS disease).[13] Forego bone scan if PET obtained. Contrast-enhanced MRI brain (preferred) or CT brain (CT brain positive in 10%; MRI brain positive in 20%).[10]

Biopsy: For tissue diagnosis: sputum, bronchoscopy with biopsy/FNA (although note that FNA may not always adequately differentiate SCLC from carcinoid tumors), CT-guided biopsy, or thoracentesis for pleural effusion. Consider bone marrow biopsy if neutropenia/thrombocytopenia/nucleated RBCs on peripheral smear. About 5% of patients present with cT1–2N0 disease. In this setting, mediastinal staging is important (see Chapter 28 for details of mediastinal staging techniques). If LNs are uninvolved, upfront resection (or SBRT in medically inoperable patients) can be considered.

PROGNOSTIC FACTORS: Favorable: LS, female gender, performance status (ECOG 0–1), absence of weight loss, absence of paraneoplastic syndromes, normal labs (LDH, sodium, albumin), smoking cessation.[12,14,15] Hyponatremia (MS 9 months if Na <135, 13 months if Na ≥135, $p < .001$).[16] LDH has been shown to correspond with disease burden, can raise concern for bone marrow involvement, and may be a risk factor for early death.[17] More than 5% weight loss over 6 months is a poor prognostic factor.[18]

NATURAL HISTORY: Distant failure is common with brain metastases in up to 80%.[9,10] Although distant failure is the predominant driver of mortality, LF is also common. If untreated, the MS for LS-SCLC is 12 weeks and is 6 weeks for ES-SCLC.[19]

STAGING: The VA Lung Study Group staging system (Table 30.3) is relevant historically, but AJCC staging is now standard; see Chapter 28.[20]

Table 30.3 VA Lung Cancer Study Group				
Limited stage	Tumor confined to one hemithorax (including both ipsilateral and contralateral mediastinum) and ipsilateral SCV nodes	MS: 20–30 months	2-yr OS: 40%	5-yr OS: 20%–30%
Extensive stage	Tumor beyond boundaries of limited disease, including distant metastases, malignant pericardial/pleural effusions, and contralateral SCV/hilar LN involvement	MS: 12 months	2-yr OS: 5%	5-yr OS: <5%

Source: Adapted from Fox W, Scadding JG. Medical Research Council comparative trial of surgery and radiotherapy for primary treatment of small-celled or oat-celled carcinoma of bronchus. Ten-year follow-up. *Lancet*. 1973;2(7820):63–65. doi:10.1016/s0140-6736(73)93260-1.

TREATMENT PARADIGM

Surgery: Surgery is not standard for most LS-SCLC based on the historical MRC trial published in 1973, which randomized patients to either surgery or RT and showed a survival benefit in those who received RT (mean OS improved from 7 to 10 months, $p = .04$).[21] However, ~5% of SCLC diagnoses present as a solitary pulmonary nodule (SPN). For T1–2 SPN SCLC tumors with negative mediastinal sampling, lobectomy with mediastinal LN dissection is recommended, followed by CHT and/or mediastinal RT depending on pathologic nodal status. Note that adjuvant CHT is indicated, even if pN0.[6] A 2017 NCDB analysis showed an increasing use of definitive surgical management in clinical stage I disease from 15% in 2004 to almost 30% in 2013; the use of SBRT also increased from 0.4% to 6% in this time frame.[22]

Systemic Therapy: Compared with no therapy, CHT improves MS fivefold. Cisplatin and etoposide (EP) are standard and found to be equally effective and less toxic than older regimens.[23,24] Current standard is four cycles of EP with concurrent RT followed by adjuvant durvalumab. Dose of cisplatin is 60 to 100 mg/m^2 on day 1, and etoposide 120 mg/m^2 on days 1 to 3, q3 weeks. Dose of durvalumab is 1,500 mg q4 weeks for up to 24 months. Japanese data showed improved survival with irinotecan + cisplatin vs. EP for ES-SCLC (2-year OS: 20% vs. 5%); however, this was not reproduced by randomized studies in the United States, Canada, or Australia, potentially due to biological differences in the Japanese study population.[25,26] Additional CHT strategies such as dose intensification, triplet therapy, high-dose consolidation, alternating/sequential regimens, and maintenance therapy all have not demonstrated improvements in OS. Some substitute cisplatin with carboplatin for a more favorable side effect profile; the 2012 COCIS meta-analysis of four randomized trials (including both LS and ES disease) showed no difference in response rate (~70%), PFS (~5 months), or OS (~9 months) between the two platinum-based regimens.[27] Several phase III randomized trials now support the addition of concurrent and maintenance IO to platinum-based regimens for ES-SCLC.[28–32] For LS-SCLC, adjuvant therapy with durvalumab after CRT showed improved OS and PFS compared with placebo; however, the addition of concurrent and consolidation atezolizumab to CRT did not improve survival.[33,34]

Radiation

Indications: When added to CHT, RT for LS-SCLC reduces intrathoracic failures by 50% (from 75%–90% to 30%–60%). RT also improves survival by 5% at 2 to 3 years.[35,36] For regimens using EP, concurrent CRT appears superior to sequential. Advantages of concurrent CRT: early use of both treatment modalities, more accurate RT planning, high-intensity treatment in a short time, and radiosensitization of the tumor. Main disadvantage: higher tissue toxicity (esophagitis, pneumonitis, myelosuppression) potentially leading to treatment breaks or discontinuation. Most studies have demonstrated benefit to early RT starting with cycle 1 or 2 of CHT. LS-SCLC patients who have CR or good PR to primary therapy should be treated with PCI to 25 Gy/10 fx, as this reduces the incidence of brain metastases and improves OS.[37] Of note, SBRT may have a role similar to surgery in inoperable early-stage patients. A 2017 multi-institution RR demonstrated excellent 3-year LC (≥95%) for 74 T1–2N0 patients treated with SBRT.[38] This series also showed improved OS in those who received subsequent CHT (31 vs. 14 months, $p = .02$). The role of PCI in those with ES-SCLC without brain metastases at diagnosis who respond to initial CHT remains controversial, particularly in the new IO era.

Dose: Standard accelerated dose is 45 Gy/30 fx at 1.5 Gy/fx BID in 3 weeks with concurrent EP CHT based on results from the landmark Turrisi trial.[39] This schedule has been confirmed by the CONVERT trial. Dose escalation to 70 Gy QD did not improve OS compared with 45 Gy BID on the RTOG 0538/CALGB 30610 trial.[40] Dose escalation to 54 to 60 Gy BID can be considered as improved OS has been demonstrated when compared with 45 Gy BID.[41,42] The results of dose-escalated trials are controversial because of the magnitude of survival improvement without significant differences in failure patterns and toxicity between the two arms. Dose escalation remains an area of investigation. Proposed radiobiological advantages of BID fractionation in SCLC include high growth fraction, short cell cycle time, and small/absent shoulder on cell survival curve. Notwithstanding trial results, a 2019 practice patterns survey found that 76% of clinicians employ a daily fractionation regimen more commonly in their practice.[43] NCCN states that if daily fractionation is used, 60 to 70 Gy should be given (not based on level 1 evidence). Hypofractionated regimens such as 40 Gy/15 fx at 2.67 Gy/fx as employed by Murray et al. are not included in the most recent guidelines.[6,44] If utilizing a hypofractionated regimen, recommend starting RT at cycle 2 of CHT.[45]

Toxicity: Acute: fatigue, esophagitis, pneumonitis, nausea. Chronic: pneumonitis, cardiac injury, dysphagia.

EVIDENCE-BASED Q&A

LIMITED-STAGE SMALL-CELL LUNG CANCER

Is there a benefit to RT in addition to CHT?

Multiple RCTs compared CHT alone with CRT and formed the basis of the seminal Warde and Pignon meta-analyses. Both showed a 5% benefit in OS with the addition of thoracic RT to CHT.

Warde, Ontario Meta-Analysis (*JCO* 1992, PMID 1316951): Meta-analysis of 11 randomized trials of LS-SCLC patients treated with CHT alone vs. CRT. Demonstrated significant ~25% improvement in LC (47% vs. 24%) and 5% improvement in 2-year OS (20% vs. 15%) with the addition of RT. Patients <60 years derived the greatest benefit. There was no significant difference in treatment-related death. **Conclusion: OS and LC in the thorax improve with the addition of RT to CHT.**

Pignon, French Meta-Analysis (*NEJM* 1992, PMID 1331787): Meta-analysis of 13 randomized trials of 2,140 patients with LS-SCLC treated with CHT alone vs. CRT. Addition of thoracic RT improved the 3-year OS by 5% (14% vs. 9%) over CHT alone, with 14% relative reduction in mortality rate. Younger patients (age <55) had greater benefit with the addition of RT compared with patients >70 years. **Conclusion: Thoracic RT improves OS when added to CHT in patients with LS-SCLC.**

What is the ideal dose and fractionation schedule for LS-SCLC?

A schedule of 45 Gy with BID fractionation as initially defined by Turrisi's Intergroup trial is the current standard of care, with the results of the CONVERT and RTOG 0538/CALGB 30610 trials confirming this schedule. Dose escalation to 54 to 60 Gy BID can be considered, as two randomized trials have demonstrated improved OS.[41,42] However, given the magnitude of the survival difference on these trials without significant differences in failure patterns and toxicity between the two arms, the results are controversial.

Turrisi, RTOG 88-15/INT 0096 (*NEJM* 1999, PMID 9920950): Phase III PRT of 417 patients treated with concurrent CHT and either daily or BID RT. CHT was 60 mg/m² cisplatin on day 1 and 120 mg/m² etoposide on days 1 to 3 q3 weeks for 4C. RT was started on day 1 of CHT and was based on the University of Pennsylvania RT technique reported in 1988.[33] RT dose was 45 Gy/25 fx in 5 weeks at 1.8 Gy/fx daily vs. 45 Gy/30 fx in 3 weeks at 1.5 Gy/fx BID. Fields taken off spinal cord at 36 Gy. Patients with CR received PCI 25 Gy/10 fx. BID fractionation improved OS (see Table 30.4). Note that there was 60% to 70% risk of esophagitis in the subgroup of patients aged >70, so altering dose for elderly patients may be important. **Conclusion: BID fractionation significantly improved OS but with higher acute grade 3 esophageal toxicity. No increase in late toxicity.** *Comment: Employing 45 Gy/25 fx as the standard arm may represent suboptimal dose given that this represents low BED for patients with gross disease. Also, the experimental arm tested two additional variables: (a) decreased time between doses and (b) finishing treatment in a shorter period of time—both of which may have independently improved outcomes.*

Table 30.4 Results of Turrisi RTOG 8815/INT 0096, Hyperfractionation for SCLC

Turrisi	MS (Months)	5-Yr OS	LF (Thoracic Relapse)	Acute Grade 3 Esophagitis
45 Gy QD	19	16%	52%	11%
45 Gy BID	23	26%	36%	27%
p value	.04	.04	.06	<.001

Faivre-Finn, CONVERT (*Lancet Oncol* 2017, PMID 28642008): Randomized 547 patients with LS-SCLC to CHT with either BID RT (45 Gy/30 fx BID over 3 weeks) or daily RT (66 Gy/33 fx over 6.5 weeks), both with RT starting on day 1 of C2 of EP CHT, followed by PCI if indicated. Primary endpoint: 2-year OS. MFU 45 months. The 2-year OS and MS were 56% and 30 months for BID and 51% and 25 months for daily RT (p = .14). Toxicities were comparable except for grade 4 neutropenia (increased from 38% in daily RT group to 49% in BID group, p = .05). In each arm, grade 3 esophagitis was 19%. Grade 3 to 4 pneumonitis was rare (~2% in each arm). **Conclusion: The superiority design of the trial suggests the standard arm (BID) remains standard as equivalence was not demonstrated.**

Bogart, RTOG 0538/CALGB 30610 (*JCO* 2023, PMID 36623230): Phase III RCT of 638 patients with LS-SCLC treated with EP CHT and randomized to the following concurrent RT arms: (A) 45 Gy/30 fx in 3 weeks at 1.5 Gy BID, (B) 70 Gy/35 fx in 7 weeks at 2 Gy QD, and (C) 61.2 Gy/34 fx in 5 weeks with 1.8 Gy QD for the first 16 days and 1.8 Gy BID for the last 9 days (Arm C closed at interim analysis due to increased toxicity vs. Arm B). Cycle 1 or 2 start for RT. PCI offered to all patients with a complete or near-CR. The primary endpoint was OS. At MFU of 2.84 years for surviving patients, there was no significant difference in OS for QD vs. BID arms, 30.5 vs. 28.7 months, respectively (HR 0.94, 95% CI 0.76–1.2). No significant differences in PFS. Toxicity was similar between Arms A and B. **Conclusion: Dose escalation to 70 Gy QD did not improve OS vs. 45 Gy BID.**

Yu, China (*Lancet Respir Med* 2024, PMID 39146944): Phase III PRT of 224 Chinese patients ages 18 to 70, ECOG 0 to 1, with LS-SCLC randomized to SOC 45 Gy/30 fx BID vs. dose-escalated 54 Gy/30 fx BID with SIB to primary tumor and nodal sites. Both arms with concurrent platinum-based CHT and PCI in patients who showed response. MFU 45 months. The primary endpoint was OS with a secondary toxicity analysis. mOS was significantly improved in the 54 Gy arm as compared with SOC (62.4 vs. 43.1 months, p = .001). mPFS also improved with dose escalation (30.5 vs. 16.7 months, p = .04). Grades 3 to 4 toxicities were comparable between the arms; notably, esophagitis was minimal in both arms (1% vs. 3%). One grade 5 toxicity in the dose-escalation arm (myocardial infarction). **Conclusion: Compared with SOC with 45 Gy/30 fx BID, dose escalation to 54 Gy/30 fx improved mOS and mPFS with no increase in grades 3 to 4 toxicities.** *Comments: Results remain controversial due to characteristics of treatment population, degree of survival improvement, and absence of toxicity differences.*

What is the optimal timing of CRT?

In an appropriately fit patient, CRT should be given concurrently, and the time from start of any treatment until the end of RT should be <30 days as per De Ruysscher's meta-analysis.[46] There has historically been some controversy as to whether early vs. delayed start is optimal. There are three trials (Murray, Jeremic, Takada) suggesting benefit to early RT, but three other trials (CALGB, Spiro, and Sun) suggesting no benefit.[45,47–51] However, given the findings of De Ruysscher's meta-analysis (with particular attention on start of treatment until end of RT <30 days) as well as the theoretical radiobiological advantages to early treatment in SCLC (rapid cell turnover makes this disease prone to repopulation, which can be more vulnerable to accelerated treatment), most clinicians prefer a cycle 1 or 2 start.

De Ruysscher, Netherlands Meta-Analysis (*Ann Oncol* 2006, PMID 16344277): Meta-analysis of seven trials to determine whether the timing of thoracic RT may influence survival of patients with LS-SCLC. When including all seven trials, the 2- and 5-year OS were not improved between early and late RT. However, looking at only trials using concurrent platinum CHT with RT, the 5-year OS was significantly improved with early RT (OR 0.64, 95% CI 0.44–0.92). In studies with short RT (<30 days treatment time), there was no difference in 2-year survival, but an improvement in 5-year OS was noted (OR 0.56, 0.37–0.85). **Conclusion: In patients who receive platinum CHT, overall treatment time of chest RT <30 days is associated with an increase in 5-year survival.**

De Ruysscher, RTT-SCLC Collaborative Group (*Ann Oncol* 2016, PMID 27436850): Individual patient-level analysis of nine trials comprising 2,305 patients with MFU of 10 years. The authors rationalized this patient-level update based on Spiro's combined RCT/meta-analysis, which showed that early delivery of thoracic RT may contribute to improved survival if patients received CHT regimen as prescribed.[35] When all trials were analyzed together, "earlier or shorter" vs. "later or longer," thoracic RT did not affect OS. However, when limiting analysis to those who were compliant with planned CHT, a benefit to those receiving "earlier or shorter" thoracic RT was observed compared with those who received "later or longer" RT regimens (HR for survival: 0.79, 95% CI 0.69–0.91). Grades 3 to 5 toxicities were greater in the "earlier or shorter" group: Neutropenia increased from 59% to 69% ($p = .001$), and esophagitis increased from 8% to 14% ($p < .001$). Interestingly, the reverse was shown in those unable to complete their planned CHT regimen (better OS with "later or longer": HR 1.19, 1.05–1.34). **Conclusion: "Earlier or shorter" delivery of thoracic RT in those who complete planned CHT significantly improves 5-year OS at the cost of increased toxicity.**

What is the ideal field size? Should the pre- or post-CHT volume be targeted?

Nearly four decades ago, SWOG 7924 suggested use of post-CHT imaging rather than pre-CHT imaging to define RT targets given equivalent LC and OS.[52] Hu et al. have confirmed this in the modern era.[53]

Hu, China (*Cancer* 2020, PMID 31714592): PRT of 309 patients randomized after two cycles of EP and cisplatin to receive RT to the post-CHT tumor volume vs. pre-CHT tumor volume. RT was 45 Gy/30 fx BID. PCI given to responders. LN regions originally involved before induction CHT were included as a nodal CTV for both arms even if the LN disappeared after induction CHT. Study halted early because of slow accrual. Between 2002 and 2017, 159 and 150 patients were randomized to the study arm or the control arm, respectively; 21% and 19% of patients were staged using PET ($p = .31$). MFU was 19.6 months for all patients and 54.1 months for surviving patients. The 3-year local/regional progression-free probability was 58% and 66% in the study and control arms, respectively ($p = .44$). The 5-year OS was 23% and 28% for post- and pre-CHT arms, respectively ($p = .26$). **Conclusion: The use of post-CHT target volumes is valid for RT planning.**

Should elective nodal volumes be included in the CTV?

Designing SCLC targets without elective nodal irradiation had once been controversial, but it is now considered accepted practice in most clinical centers as long as PET imaging is used as a planning tool.[54]

Van Loon, Netherlands (*IJROBP* 2010, PMID 19782478): Single-arm prospective trial of 60 patients with LS-SCLC, RT dose 45 Gy/30 fx BID with EP. Only PET-avid primary and LN stations were irradiated (selective nodal irradiation: SNI). PET altered nodal involvement in 30% of patients. Isolated nodal relapse occurred in only 3% ($n = 2$). Acute grade 3 esophagitis occurred in 12% (lower than on Turrisi trial). MS was 19 months. **Conclusion: PET appears to help in the selection of nodal stations for RT, which may reduce toxicity and keep regional failures low.** *Note: Only prospective study to show value of PET for SNI in LS-SCLC.*

Does the addition of IO to CHT improve outcomes for LS-SCLC?

The ADRIATIC trial evaluated the addition of adjuvant durvalumab or durvalumab/tremelimumab to standard-of-care CRT, and the first planned interim analysis comparing adjuvant durvalumab with placebo showed improved OS and PFS.[33] Adjuvant durvalumab is now an NCCN Category 1 recommendation for those with LS-SCLC who have CR, PR, or stable disease after CRT. LU005 evaluated the addition of concurrent and adjuvant atezolizumab to standard CRT, but showed no improvement in survival.[34]

Cheng, Adriatic (*NEJM* 2024, PMID 39268857): Phase III RCT of patients with LS-SCLC randomized to durvalumab, durvalumab + tremelimumab, or placebo q4 weeks for up to 24 months. Primary endpoints OS and PFS. Durvalumab group had improved mOS compared with placebo, 55.9 vs. 33.4 months ($p = .01$), respectively, and improved mPFS, 16.6 vs. 9.2 months ($p = .02$), respectively. Incidence of grades 3 to 4 adverse events was 24% in both groups. **Conclusion: Adjuvant durvalumab improves OS and PFS in patients with LS-SCLC.**

Higgins, LU005 (ASTRO 2024): Phase III RCT of patients with LS-SCLC randomized to standard CRT ± concurrent and adjuvant atezolizumab. The primary endpoint was OS. PCI was recommended but not required. 544 patients with MFU of 21.0 months. The 3-year OS was 50% for CRT vs. 45% for atezo + CRT. There was no difference in median OS (39.5 vs. 33.1 months), PFS (11.5 vs. 12.0 months), DMFS (13.2 vs. 16.8 months), cumulative incidence of LF at 2 years (14% vs. 13%), and complete or partial response (58.5% vs. 59.1%). Grade 3+ pneumonitis was 3% and 6% on CRT and atezo + CRT. Patients treated with BID RT had higher mOS compared with daily RT (35.4 vs. 28.3 months), regardless of receipt of atezolizumab. **Conclusion: CRT with concurrent and consolidation atezolizumab did not improve survival in LS-SCLC.**

EXTENSIVE-STAGE SMALL-CELL LUNG CANCER

Does the addition of IO to CHT improve the outcomes for first-line treatment of ES-SCLC?

Several randomized trials have demonstrated improved OS and PFS with the incorporation of IO as summarized in Table 30.5.[28–32]

Table 30.5 Summary of Immunotherapy Trials for ES-SCLC					
Trial Name	**IMpower133**	**CASPIAN**	**CAPSTONE-1**	**KEYNOTE-604**	**ASTRUM-005**
N	201 vs. 202	268 vs. 269	230 vs. 232	228 vs. 225	389 vs. 196
Primary Outcome	OS, PFS	OS	OS	PFS, OS	OS
Treatment Arms	Atezolizumab + EC vs. placebo + EC	Durvalumab + EC/EP vs. EC/EP	Adebrelimab + EC vs. placebo + EC	Pembrolizumab + EC/EP vs. placebo + EC/EP	Serplulimab + EC vs. placebo + EC
OS (months; HR, 95% CI)	12.3 vs. 10.3; 0.70, 0.54–0.91	13.0 vs. 10.3; 0.73, 0.59–0.91	15.3 vs. 12.8; 0.72, 0.58–0.90	10.8 vs. 9.7; 0.80, 0.64–0.98 *Significance threshold not met*	15.4 vs. 10.9; 0.63, 0.49–0.82
PFS (months; HR, 95% CI)	5.2 vs. 4.3; 0.77, 0.62–0.96	5.1 vs. 5.4; 0.78, 0.65–0.94	5.8 vs. 5.6; 0.67, 0.54–0.83	4.5 vs. 4.3; 0.75, 0.61–0.91	5.7 vs. 4.3; 0.48, 0.38–0.59

EC, etoposide/carboplatin; EP, etoposide/cisplatin.

Should consolidative thoracic RT be delivered to ES-SCLC patients with response to CHT?

With the addition of IO to standard-of-care CHT for ES-SCLC, the role, if any, and timing of thoracic RT are now highly controversial. Thoracic RT had been considered in favorable patients who had demonstrated response when only CHT was used. As per 2020 guidelines, if thoracic RT is given, it is advised to start after CHT is complete and to deliver it simultaneously with PCI (if given; more in the following).[44] NRG-LU007 (RAPTOR trial) will be evaluating if adding RT to atezolizumab for patients with ES-SCLC improves PFS and OS compared with atezolizumab alone.

Jeremic, Yugoslavia (*JCO* 1999, PMID 10561263): PRT of 210 patients with ES-SCLC treated with EP × 3C. Patients with distant level CR and either local CR or PR received either (Group 1) hyperfractionated (HFX) RT to 54 Gy/36 fx over 18 days with concurrent carboplatin/etoposide (EC) followed by EP × 2C or (Group 2) EP × 4C. All patients with CR at distant level received PCI (25 Gy/10 fx). RT fields included gross disease and ipsilateral hilum with 2-cm margin, mediastinum with 1-cm margin, and bilateral SCV. Patients with PR at distant level were treated nonrandomly with CHT and/or later HFX CRT, and patients with progressive disease received supportive care or oral etoposide. Among all patients, MS was 9 months and the 5-year OS was 3%. MS and 5-year OS superior in Group 1: 17 vs. 11 months and 9% vs. 4% (p = .04). LC nonsignificantly better in Group 1 (p = .06). No difference in DM. Acute grade 3/4 toxicity higher in Group 2 (see Table 30.6). **Conclusion: Addition of HFX RT for most favorable subset of patients leads to improved OS over CHT alone.**

Table 30.6 Results of Jeremic Trial for Consolidative Chest RT in ES-SCLC					
210 ES-SCLC patients treated with 3C of EP, 109 patients with CR or PR, all received PCI and randomized to CHT alone vs. CRT		**5-Yr LRFS**	**5-Yr DMFS**	**MS (Months)**	**Nausea and Vomiting**
	CRT (RT + EC CHT; 54 Gy/36 fx BID) + EP × 2C	20%	27%	17	4%
	CHT alone (EP × 4C)	8%	14%	11	20%
		p = .06	p = .35	p = .04	p = .004

Slotman, Netherlands (*Lancet* 2015, PMID 25230595): Phase III RCT of 498 patients with WHO performance status 0 to 2 and ES-SCLC who responded to CHT, all of whom received PCI and then randomized to thoracic RT (30 Gy/10 fx) or observation. Primary endpoint was 1-year OS; PFS was secondary endpoint. MFU 24 months. OS at 1 year was not significantly different between groups: 33% for the thoracic RT arm vs. 28% for the control group (HR 0.84, 95% CI 0.69–1.01). However, in secondary analysis, 2-year OS was 13% vs. 3% (*p* = .004). At 6 months, PFS was 24% in the thoracic RT group vs. 7% in the control group (*p* = .001). No significant difference in toxicity between groups. **Conclusion: Thoracic RT + PCI should be considered for patients with ES-SCLC who respond to CHT.**

Gore, RTOG 0937 (*J Thorac Oncol* 2017, PMID 28648948): Randomized phase II study of 97 patients with ES-SCLC with one to four extracranial metastases randomized to either PCI alone vs. PCI with consolidative RT to the intrathoracic disease and extracranial metastases, 45 Gy/15 fx (acceptable alternative: 30–40 Gy in 10 fx). MFU 9 months. The 1-year OS was 60% (PCI) vs. 51% (PCI + consolidation, *p* = .21); 12-month progression was 80% vs. 75%, favoring consolidation (HR 0.53, 95% CI 0.32–0.87). **Conclusion: OS analysis was underpowered due to high rate of survival. Consolidation may reduce progression but did not alter OS.**

PROPHYLACTIC CRANIAL IRRADIATION

Who should be treated with PCI?

Historically, patients with LS-SCLC with CR or good PR after CRT have received PCI per the Auperin meta-analysis. In ES-SCLC, some have relied on findings of Slotman's 2007 study to justify PCI for any responders to CHT, but this remains controversial as this study did not require pre-randomization brain MRI to confirm absence of brain metastases prior to PCI. In contrast, the 2017 Takahashi study incorporated pre-randomization brain MRI. The PCILESS prospective trial is a single-arm study of LS-SCLC after definitive treatment with at least a good response, utilizing watchful observation rather than PCI, with results awaited.[55] Per 2020 consensus guidelines, PCI is strongly recommended for stage II or III patients who respond to CRT, with a caveat that this should be a shared decision for those at higher risk of neurocognitive toxicities; PCI is "conditionally not recommended" for stage I patients; for ES-SCLC, the authors recommend consideration of PCI vs. MRI surveillance.[44]

Auperin, French Meta-Analysis (*NEJM* 1999, PMID 10441603): Meta-analysis of 987 SCLC patients from seven RCTs conducted between 1965 and 1995 comparing PCI vs. no PCI. Most patients on this meta-analysis were LS but ~15% were ES. PCI was performed in varied doses and fractionations. An analysis of four dose groups was performed: 8 Gy/1 fx vs. 24–25 Gy/8–12 fx vs. 30 Gy/10 fx vs. 36–40 Gy/18–20 fx. PCI improved the 3-year OS and reduced the incidence of brain mets (see Table 30.7). Effect of PCI on OS did not differ significantly according to total dose. However, there was a trend toward lower risk of brain mets as RT dose increased. There was also a trend toward greater effect of PCI on incidence of brain mets in patients randomized sooner (<6 months) after CHT. **Conclusion: PCI improves OS and incidence of brain mets in SCLC patients.** *However, pre-randomization brain MRI was not required.*

Table 30.7 Results of Auperin Meta-Analysis of PCI		
	Incidence of Brain Mets	3-Yr OS
PCI	33%	21%
No PCI	59%	15%
	p < .001	*p* = .01

Slotman, EORTC 08993-22993 (*NEJM* 2007, PMID 17699816): Phase III RCT of PCI in ES-SCLC, including patients age 18 to 75, PS 0 to 2, any response to CHT, no previous RT, no clinical suggestion of brain mets (imaging not required), *n* = 286. Dose ranged from 20 to 30 Gy with fractionation that was variable but consistent within an institution. Median interval between diagnosis and randomization was 4.2 months. Primary endpoint was reduction in symptomatic brain mets. There was no difference in extracranial disease progression between groups. There was no difference in cognitive and emotional function with PCI (see Table 30.8). **Conclusion: PCI reduces the incidence of symptomatic brain metastases and prolongs DFS and OS.** *Comment: Brain imaging was not required prior to randomization.*

Table 30.8 Results of Slotman PCI for ES-SCLC

	Symptomatic Brain Mets at 1 Yr	Median DFS (Weeks)	MS (Months)	1-Yr OS
No PCI	40%	12	5.4	13%
PCI	15%	14.7	6.7	27%
	p < .001	p = .02	p = .03	p = .003

Takahashi, Japan (*Lancet Oncol* 2017, PMID 28343976): Phase III RCT of PCI in ES-SCLC including patients aged ≥20, PS 0 to 2, any response to platinum-based doublet CHT, and no brain mets on MRI obtained within 4 weeks of PCI, randomized to 25 Gy/10 fx vs. no PCI. Post-PCI brain MRI was obtained at 3-month intervals up to 12 months, then at 18 and 24 months. Primary endpoint was OS. The trial was terminated early due to likely futility (see Table 30.9). **Conclusion: PCI does not improve OS in ES-SCLC in this prescreened population, although it does reduce the incidence of MRI-detected brain mets at all timepoints.** *Comment: Close MRI surveillance was performed and should be considered necessary to replicate the results if PCI is omitted.*

Table 30.9 Results of Takahashi PCI for ES-SCLC

	MS (Months)	Incidence of Brain Mets at 12 Months	Overall Grade 3–4 Toxicity
PCI	11.6	33%	3%
No PCI	13.7	59%	4%
	p = .094	p < .0001	NS

What dose of PCI should be delivered?

25 Gy/10 fx is standard. This was investigated in the EORTC/RTOG 0212 prospective randomized trial composed of three treatment arms: 25 Gy/10 fx, 36 Gy/18 fx QD, and 36 Gy/24 fx BID. Incidence of brain mets at 2 years was ~25% in all arms with no statistical difference; rates of chronic neurotoxicity were greater in the 36 Gy cohort (p = .02).[56–58]

Is there a role for hippocampal avoidance in PCI?

The role of HA-PCI is currently evolving. The PREMER phase III study demonstrated better cognitive preservation with hippocampal avoidance. A phase III RCT from the Netherlands demonstrated no difference in HVLT at 4 months following PCI vs. HA-PCI. NRG CC003 showed improved prevention of first failure in any neurocognitive test with HA-PCI.

Rodriguez de Dios, PREMER (*JCO* 2012, PMID 34379442): Phase III RCT of 150 patients with SCLC randomized to PCI vs. HA-PCI. Seventy-one percent of patients had LS disease. The primary endpoint was delayed free recall (DFR) at 3 months. At MFU of 40.4 months, decline on DFR from baseline was lower in the HA-PCI arm vs. PCI, 6% vs. 24%, respectively (OR 5.0, 95% CI 1.57–15.86). The incidence of brain mets, OS, and QOL were not significantly different. **Conclusion: HA-PCI preserves cognitive function vs. standard PCI in patients with SCLC, with no difference in OS, brain failure, or QOL.**

Belderbos, NCT01780675 (*JTO* 2021, PMID 33545387): Phase III RCT of 168 patients with SCLC randomized to PCI vs. HA-PCI. Seventy percent of patients had LS-SCLC. Primary endpoint: 4-month HVLT total recall. At MFU of 26.6 months, decline on HVLT total recall score at 4 months was not different between arms (29% PCI vs. 28% HA-PCI, p = 1.000). No difference in performance on other cognitive tests. No difference in OS or 2-year incidence of brain mets between groups. **Conclusion: HA-PCI did not offer a lower probability of cognitive decline than standard PCI in patients with SCLC. No difference in OS or rate of brain mets.**

Gondi, NRG CC003 (ASTRO 2023): Phase II/III PRT of 392 patients with LS or ES-SCLC randomized to PCI or HA-PCI. Seventy percent with LS-SCLC. Primary endpoint of phase II portion was 12-month intracranial relapse (ICR) and phase III was 6-month HVLT-R failure. Other neurocognitive tests including trailmaking test (TMT) and Controlled Oral Word Association (COWA) were recorded with time to first neurocognitive test failure (NCF) as a secondary endpoint. MFU

14.9 months. ICR at 12 months was noninferior with HA-PCI (PCI 15% vs. HA-PCI 14%). Primary endpoint of 6-month HVLT-R failure was not significantly different (PCI 30% vs. HA-PCI 26%, p = .31). HA-PCI prevented first failure in any neurocognitive test (HR 0.77, 95% CI 0.61–0.98). **Conclusion: HA-PCI failed to improve HVLT but appears to prevent first failure in any neuro-cognitive tests over PCI with noninferior intracranial control.**

REFERENCES

1. Govindan R, Page N, Morgensztern D, et al. Changing epidemiology of small-cell lung cancer in the United States over the last 30 years: analysis of the surveillance, epidemiologic, and end results database. *J Clin Oncol*. 2006;24(28):4539–4544. doi:10.1200/JCO.2005.04.4859
2. Siegel RL, Giaquinto AN, Jemal A. Cancer statistics, 2024. *CA Cancer J Clin*. 2024;74(1):12–49. doi:10.3322/caac.21820
3. Pesch B, Kendzia B, Gustavsson P, et al. Cigarette smoking and lung cancer–relative risk estimates for the major histological types from a pooled analysis of case-control studies. *Int J Cancer*. 2012;131(5):1210–1219. doi:10.1002/ijc.27339
4. Kreuzer M, Muller KM, Brachner A, et al. Histopathologic findings of lung carcinoma in German uranium miners. *Cancer*. 2000;89(12):2613–2621. doi:10.1002/1097-0142(20001215)89:12<2613::aid-cncr14>3.0.co;2-y
5. Travis WD, Brambilla E, Noguchi M, et al. International association for the study of lung cancer/american thoracic society/european respiratory society international multidisciplinary classification of lung adeno-carcinoma. *J Thorac Oncol*. 2011;6(2):244–285. doi:10.1097/JTO.0b013e318206a221
6. National Comprehensive Cancer Network. Small Cell Lung Cancer (Version 2.2025). Accessed October 15, 2024. https://www.nccn.org/professionals/physician_gls/pdf/sclc.pdf
7. Travis WD. Advances in neuroendocrine lung tumors. *Ann Oncol*. 2010;21(Suppl 7):vii65–vii71. doi:10.1093/annonc/mdq380
8. Rivera MP, Mehta AC, Wahidi MM. Establishing the diagnosis of lung cancer: diagnosis and management of lung cancer, 3rd ed: American College of Chest Physicians evidence-based clinical practice guidelines. *Chest*. 2013;143(5 Suppl):e142S–e165S. doi:10.1378/chest.12-2353
9. Nugent JL, Bunn PA Jr, Matthews MJ, et al. CNS metastases in small cell bronchogenic carcinoma: increasing frequency and changing pattern with lengthening survival. *Cancer*. 1979;44(5):1885–1893. doi:10.1002/1097-0142(197911)44:5<1885::aid-cncr2820440550>3.0.co;2-f
10. Seute T, Leffers P, ten Velde GP, Twijnstra A. Detection of brain metastases from small cell lung cancer: consequences of changing imaging techniques (CT versus MRI). *Cancer*. 2008;112(8):1827–1834. doi:10.1002/cncr.23361
11. Castillo JJ, Vincent M, Justice E. Diagnosis and management of hyponatremia in cancer patients. *Oncologist*. 2012;17(6):756–765. doi:10.1634/theoncologist.2011-0400
12. Videtic GM, Stitt LW, Dar AR, et al. Continued cigarette smoking by patients receiving concurrent chemo-radiotherapy for limited-stage small-cell lung cancer is associated with decreased survival. *J Clin Oncol*. 2003;21(8):1544–1549. doi:10.1200/JCO.2003.10.089
13. Kalemkerian GP. Staging and imaging of small cell lung cancer. *Cancer Imaging*. 2012;11(1):253–258. doi:10.1102/1470-7330.2011.0036
14. Foster NR, Mandrekar SJ, Schild SE, et al. Prognostic factors differ by tumor stage for small cell lung cancer: a pooled analysis of North Central Cancer Treatment Group trials. *Cancer*. 2009;115(12):2721–2731. doi:10.1002/cncr.24314
15. Albain KS, Crowley JJ, LeBlanc M, Livingston RB. Determinants of improved outcome in small-cell lung cancer: an analysis of the 2,580-patient Southwest Oncology Group data base. *J Clin Oncol*. 1990;8(9):1563–1574. doi:10.1200/JCO.1990.8.9.1563
16. Hermes A, Waschki B, Reck M. Hyponatremia as prognostic factor in small cell lung cancer–a retrospective single institution analysis. *Respir Med*. 2012;106(6):900–904. doi:10.1016/j.rmed.2012.02.010
17. Lassen UN, Osterlind K, Hirsch FR, Bergman B, Dombernowsky P, Hansen HH. Early death during chemotherapy in patients with small-cell lung cancer: derivation of a prognostic index for toxic death and progression. *Br J Cancer*. 1999;79(3–4):515–519. doi:10.1038/sj.bjc.6690080
18. Fearon K, Strasser F, Anker SD, et al. Definition and classification of cancer cachexia: an international consensus. *Lancet Oncol*. 2011;12(5):489–495. doi:10.1016/S1470-2045(10)70218-7
19. National Institute for Health and Care Excellence (NICE). The Diagnosis and Treatment of Lung Cancer (Update). Cardiff (UK). National Collaborating Centre for Cancer. NICE Clinical Guidelines NC, Treatment of SCLC. Accessed October 15, 2024. www.ncbi.nlm.nih.gov/books/NBK99023.
20. Kalemkerian GP, Gadgeel SM. Modern staging of small cell lung cancer. *J Natl Compr Canc Netw*. 2013; 11(1):99–104. doi:10.6004/jnccn.2013.0012
21. Fox W, Scadding JG. Medical Research Council comparative trial of surgery and radiotherapy for primary treatment of small-celled or oat-celled carcinoma of bronchus. Ten-year follow-up. *Lancet*. 1973;2(7820): 63–65. doi:10.1016/s0140-6736(73)93260-1

22. Stahl JM, Corso CD, Verma V, et al. Trends in stereotactic body radiation therapy for stage I small cell lung cancer. *Lung Cancer*. 2017;103:11–16. doi:10.1016/j.lungcan.2016.11.009

23. Roth BJ, Johnson DH, Einhorn LH, et al. Randomized study of cyclophosphamide, doxorubicin, and vincristine versus etoposide and cisplatin versus alternation of these two regimens in extensive small-cell lung cancer: a phase III trial of the Southeastern Cancer Study Group. *J Clin Oncol*. 1992;10(2):282–291. doi:10.1200/JCO.1992.10.2.282

24. Sundstrom S, Bremnes RM, Kaasa S, et al. Cisplatin and etoposide regimen is superior to cyclophosphamide, epirubicin, and vincristine regimen in small-cell lung cancer: results from a randomized phase III trial with 5 years' follow-up. *J Clin Oncol*. 2002;20(24):4665–4672. doi:10.1200/JCO.2002.12.111

25. Noda K, Nishiwaki Y, Kawahara M, et al. Irinotecan plus cisplatin compared with etoposide plus cisplatin for extensive small-cell lung cancer. *N Engl J Med*. 2002;346(2):85–91. doi:10.1056/NEJMoa003034

26. Lara PN Jr, Natale R, Crowley J, et al. Phase III trial of irinotecan/cisplatin compared with etoposide/cisplatin in extensive-stage small-cell lung cancer: clinical and pharmacogenomic results from SWOG S0124. *J Clin Oncol*. 2009;27(15):2530–2535. doi:10.1200/JCO.2008.20.1061

27. Rossi A, Di Maio M, Chiodini P, et al. Carboplatin- or cisplatin-based chemotherapy in first-line treatment of small-cell lung cancer: the COCIS meta-analysis of individual patient data. *J Clin Oncol*. 2012;30(14): 1692–1698. doi:10.1200/JCO.2011.40.4905

28. Liu SV, Reck M, Mansfield AS, et al. Updated overall survival and pd-l1 subgroup analysis of patients with extensive-stage small-cell lung cancer treated with atezolizumab, carboplatin, and etoposide (IMpower133). *J Clin Oncol*. 2021;39(6):619–630. doi:10.1200/JCO.20.01055

29. Paz-Ares L, Dvorkin M, Chen Y, et al. Durvalumab plus platinum-etoposide versus platinum-etoposide in first-line treatment of extensive-stage small-cell lung cancer (CASPIAN): a randomised, controlled, open-label, phase 3 trial. *Lancet*. 2019;394(10212):1929–1939. doi:10.1016/S0140-6736(19)32222-6

30. Cheng Y, Han L, Wu L, et al. Effect of first-line serplulimab vs placebo added to chemotherapy on survival in patients with extensive-stage small cell lung cancer: the ASTRUM-005 randomized clinical trial. *JAMA*. 2022;328(12):1223–1232. doi:10.1001/jama.2022.16464

31. Wang J, Zhou C, Yao W, et al. Adebrelimab or placebo plus carboplatin and etoposide as first-line treatment for extensive-stage small-cell lung cancer (CAPSTONE-1): a multicentre, randomised, double-blind, placebo-controlled, phase 3 trial. *Lancet Oncol*. 2022;23(6):739–747. doi:10.1016/S1470-2045(22)00224-8

32. Rudin CM, Awad MM, Navarro A, et al. Pembrolizumab or placebo plus etoposide and platinum as first-line therapy for extensive-stage small-cell lung cancer: randomized, double-blind, phase III KEYNOTE-604 study. *J Clin Oncol*. 2020;38(21):2369–2379. doi:10.1200/JCO.20.00793

33. Cheng Y, Spigel DR, Cho BC, et al. Durvalumab after chemoradiotherapy in limited-stage small-cell lung cancer. *N Engl J Med*. 2024;391(14):1313–1327. doi:10.1056/NEJMoa2404873

34. Higgins K, Hu C, Ross HJ, et al. Concurrent chemoradiation ± atezolizumab (atezo) in Limited-Stage Small Cell Lung Cancer (LS-SCLC): results of NRG oncology/alliance LU005. *Int J Radiat Oncol Biol Phys*. 2024;120(2):S2. doi:10.1016/j.ijrobp.2024.08.013

35. Warde P, Payne D. Does thoracic irradiation improve survival and local control in limited-stage small-cell carcinoma of the lung? A meta-analysis. *J Clin Oncol*. 1992;10(6):890–895. doi:10.1200/JCO.1992.10.6.890

36. Pignon JP, Arriagada R, Ihde DC, et al. A meta-analysis of thoracic radiotherapy for small-cell lung cancer. *N Engl J Med*. 1992;327(23):1618–1624. doi:10.1056/NEJM199212033272302

37. Auperin A, Arriagada R, Pignon JP, et al. Prophylactic cranial irradiation for patients with small-cell lung cancer in complete remission. Prophylactic cranial irradiation overview collaborative group. *N Engl J Med*. 1999;341(7):476–484. doi:10.1056/NEJM199908123410703

38. Verma V, Simone CB 2nd, Allen PK, et al. Multi-institutional experience of stereotactic ablative radiation therapy for stage i small cell lung cancer. *Int J Radiat Oncol Biol Phys*. 2017;97(2):362–371. doi:10.1016/j .ijrobp.2016.10.041

39. Turrisi AT 3rd, Kim K, Blum R, et al. Twice-daily compared with once-daily thoracic radiotherapy in limited small-cell lung cancer treated concurrently with cisplatin and etoposide. *N Engl J Med*. 1999;340(4):265–271. doi:10.1056/NEJM199901283400403

40. Bogart J, Wang X, Masters G, et al. High-dose once-daily thoracic radiotherapy in limited-stage small-cell lung cancer: CALGB 30610 (Alliance)/RTOG 0538. *J Clin Oncol*. 2023;41(13):2394–2402. doi:10.1200/JCO.22.01359

41. Yu J, Jiang L, Zhao L, et al. High-dose hyperfractionated simultaneous integrated boost radiotherapy versus standard-dose radiotherapy for limited-stage small-cell lung cancer in China: a multicentre, open-label, randomised, phase 3 trial. *Lancet Respir Med*. 2024;12(10):799–809. doi:10.1016/S2213-2600(24)00189-9

42. Gronberg BH, Killingberg KT, Flotten O, et al. High-dose versus standard-dose twice-daily thoracic radiotherapy for patients with limited stage small-cell lung cancer: an open-label, randomised, phase 2 trial. *Lancet Oncol*. 2021;22(3):321–331. doi:10.1016/S1470-2045(20)30742-7

43. Farrell MJ, Yahya JB, Degnin C, et al. Radiation dose and fractionation for limited-stage small-cell lung cancer: survey of US radiation oncologists on practice patterns. *Clin Lung Cancer*. 2019;20(1):13–19. doi:10.1016/j.cllc.2018.08.015

44. Simone CB 2nd, Bogart JA, Cabrera AR, et al. Radiation therapy for small cell lung cancer: an ASTRO clinical practice guideline. *Pract Radiat Oncol*. 2020;10(3):158–173. doi:10.1016/j.prro.2020.02.009

45. Murray N, Coy P, Pater JL, et al. Importance of timing for thoracic irradiation in the combined modality treatment of limited-stage small-cell lung cancer. The National Cancer Institute of Canada clinical trials group. *J Clin Oncol*. 1993;11(2):336–344. doi:10.1200/JCO.1993.11.2.336

46. De Ruysscher D, Pijls-Johannesma M, Bentzen SM, et al. Time between the first day of chemotherapy and the last day of chest radiation is the most important predictor of survival in limited-disease small-cell lung cancer. *J Clin Oncol*. 2006;24(7):1057–1063. doi:10.1200/JCO.2005.02.9793

47. Jeremic B, Shibamoto Y, Acimovic L, Milisavljevic S. Initial versus delayed accelerated hyperfractionated radiation therapy and concurrent chemotherapy in limited small-cell lung cancer: a randomized study. *J Clin Oncol*. 1997;15(3):893–900. doi:10.1200/JCO.1997.15.3.893

48. Takada M, Fukuoka M, Kawahara M, et al. Phase III study of concurrent versus sequential thoracic radiotherapy in combination with cisplatin and etoposide for limited-stage small-cell lung cancer: results of the Japan Clinical Oncology Group Study 9104. *J Clin Oncol*. 2002;20(14):3054–3060. doi:10.1200/JCO.2002.12.071

49. Perry MC, Eaton WL, Propert KJ, et al. Chemotherapy with or without radiation therapy in limited small-cell carcinoma of the lung. *N Engl J Med*. 1987;316(15):912–918. doi:10.1056/NEJM198704093161504

50. Spiro SG, James LE, Rudd RM, et al. Early compared with late radiotherapy in combined modality treatment for limited disease small-cell lung cancer: a London Lung Cancer Group multicenter randomized clinical trial and meta-analysis. *J Clin Oncol*. 2006;24(24):3823–3830. doi:10.1200/JCO.2005.05.3181

51. Sun JM, Ahn YC, Choi EK, et al. Phase III trial of concurrent thoracic radiotherapy with either first- or third-cycle chemotherapy for limited-disease small-cell lung cancer. *Ann Oncol*. 2013;24(8):2088–2092. doi:10.1093/annonc/mdt140

52. Kies MS, Mira JG, Crowley JJ, et al. Multimodal therapy for limited small-cell lung cancer: a randomized study of induction combination chemotherapy with or without thoracic radiation in complete responders; and with wide-field versus reduced-field radiation in partial responders: a Southwest Oncology Group Study. *J Clin Oncol*. 1987;5(4):592–600. doi:10.1200/JCO.1987.5.4.592

53. Hu X, Bao Y, Xu YJ, et al. Final report of a prospective randomized study on thoracic radiotherapy target volume for limited-stage small cell lung cancer with radiation dosimetric analyses. *Cancer*. 2020;126(4):840–849. doi:10.1002/cncr.32586

54. Videtic GM, Belderbos JS, Spring Kong FM, Kepka L, Martel MK, Jeremic B. Report from the International Atomic Energy Agency (IAEA) consultants' meeting on elective nodal irradiation in lung cancer: Small-Cell Lung Cancer (SCLC). *Int J Radiat Oncol Biol Phys*. 2008;72(2):327–334. doi:10.1016/j.ijrobp.2008.03.075

55. U.S. National Library of Medicine. Watchful Observation of Patients With LD-SCLC Instead of the PCI (PCILESS); 2019. Accessed October 15, 2024. https://www.clinicaltrials.gov/ct2/show/NCT04168281

56. Le Pechoux C, Dunant A, Senan S, et al. Standard-dose versus higher-dose prophylactic cranial irradiation (PCI) in patients with limited-stage small-cell lung cancer in complete remission after chemotherapy and thoracic radiotherapy (PCI 99-01, EORTC 22003-08004, RTOG 0212, and IFCT 99-01): a randomised clinical trial. *Lancet Oncol*. 2009;10(5):467–474. doi:10.1016/S1470-2045(09)70101-9

57. Le Pechoux C, Laplanche A, Faivre-Finn C, et al. Clinical neurological outcome and quality of life among patients with limited small-cell cancer treated with two different doses of prophylactic cranial irradiation in the intergroup phase III trial (PCI99-01, EORTC 22003-08004, RTOG 0212 and IFCT 99-01). *Ann Oncol*. 2011;22(5):1154–1163. doi:10.1093/annonc/mdq576

58. Wolfson AH, Bae K, Komaki R, et al. Primary analysis of a phase II randomized trial Radiation Therapy Oncology Group (RTOG) 0212: impact of different total doses and schedules of prophylactic cranial irradiation on chronic neurotoxicity and quality of life for patients with limited-disease small-cell lung cancer. *Int J Radiat Oncol Biol Phys*. 2011;81(1):77–84. doi:10.1016/j.ijrobp.2010.05.013

31 MESOTHELIOMA

David S. Buchberger and Gregory M. M. Videtic

QUICK HIT Mesothelioma is a rare thoracic malignancy associated with progressive morbidity. Patients are rarely curable due to disease extent and comorbidity at diagnosis. Historically, extrapleural pneumonectomy (EPP) and pleurectomy and decortication (P/D) were surgical options for nonmetastatic, medically operable patients with epithelioid histology. Recent management trends favor non-operative approaches (Table 31.1). CHT and RT are used mainly for palliation, although can be considered in the perioperative setting. Immunotherapy (IO) plays an increasing role in both the upfront and progressive settings.

Table 31.1 General Treatment Paradigm for Mesothelioma[1]	
Patient	**Treatment Options**
Clinical stage I **Epithelioid histology** **Medically operable** **Resectable disease**	• Induction CHT (cisplatin/pemetrexed) or IO, reassessment, P/D followed by observation or pleural IMRT • Induction CHT (cisplatin/pemetrexed) or IO, reassessment, consider pleural IMRT
Clinical stage II–IV **Epithelioid, biphasic, or** **sarcomatoid histology** **Medically inoperable** **Unresectable**	• Various systemic therapy combinations (most commonly: CHT, IO, CHT/IO) • Consider palliative RT

Source: Data from NCCN Clinical Practice Guidelines in Oncology: Mesothelioma: Pleural https://www.nccn.org/professionals/physician_gls/pdf/meso_pleural.pdf.

EPIDEMIOLOGY: U.S. incidence of mesothelioma is 3,000 cases per year. Incidence peaked around 2000 and has been steadily declining secondary to OSHA limitations on acceptable asbestos exposure initiated in the 1970s.[2]

RISK FACTORS: Exposure to asbestos is the most significant risk factor with 90% of cases related to asbestos. Exposure is most commonly occupational (used as a flame retardant in automobile brakes, shipbuilding, ceiling tiles, pool tiles) and more rarely environmental. Occult transmission of asbestos fibers may occur from workers to family members. Lifetime risk of an asbestos worker developing mesothelioma is as high as 10%. Dose–response relationship and latency period of 20 to 40 years exist between exposure and development of disease. Known synergistic effect of asbestos and smoking. Other risk factors include ionizing RT, carbon nanotubes, and potentially viral oncogenes and genetic susceptibility (BAP1 mutation).[2]

ANATOMY: Arises from any mesothelial surface including the pleura (80%), and less commonly the peritoneum, tunica vaginalis, or pericardium. Two areas of pleura that are particularly challenging to identify and adequately cover after EPP are the ipsilateral diaphragmatic crura and the lowest posterior point of the diaphragm. The right crus extends to L3 and the left crus extends to L2. The lowest point of pleural space can extend as low as L4. Distribution of pleural mesothelioma: 60% right-sided, 35% left-sided, and 5% bilateral.[3]

PATHOLOGY: Three histologic variants: epithelioid (most common, 60% of cases), sarcomatoid, and **biphasic** (combination of the latter two), although several variations exist. Histology is more prognostic than stage. IHC is crucial for diagnosis (mesothelin glycoprotein is 67% sensitive and 98% specific); osteopontin and gene expression assays may be helpful.[2]

CLINICAL PRESENTATION: The majority of patients affected are over age 60 and present 20 to 40 years after asbestos exposure. Symptoms include weight loss, fatigue, chest pain, dyspnea, cough, hoarseness, and dysphagia. Physical exam findings are usually indicative of pleural effusion, with unilateral dullness to percussion or decreased air exchange. Features on CXR suggestive of mesothelioma include unilateral pleural density or thickening, persistent pleural effusion, mediastinal shift, lung volume loss, and asbestosis demonstrated as bibasilar interstitial fibrosis.

WORKUP: H&P with risk factor assessment.

Tests: Assess operability with PFTs including DLCO, perfusion scanning (if FEV1 <80%), cardiac stress test.[4]

Imaging: CT chest with contrast. PET/CT. MRI chest is optional but may be helpful in determining resectability.

Biopsy: Historically, thoracentesis was used for histologic diagnosis, although it was only diagnostic in 26% of cases. In contrast, VATS biopsy is diagnostic in 98% of cases and provides evidence of stromal, fibroadipose, or lung parenchymal invasion that is needed to differentiate between reactive hyperplasia, fibrous pleurisy, and malignancy; 10% risk of seeding biopsy tract, and tract should be excised at surgery. For patients who are potentially resectable, mediastinal staging with mediastinoscopy or EBUS is recommended.

PROGNOSTIC FACTORS: Stage and histology are the most significant prognostic factors. Sarcomatoid and biphasic histologies have worse prognosis compared with epithelioid histology. Poor performance status, age >75, elevated LDH, and hematologic abnormalities (thrombocytosis, leukocytosis, anemia) are associated with worse prognosis.[4]

NATURAL HISTORY: Prognosis is poor, with OS of 9 to 17 months. Distant metastatic disease is less common but can involve the bone, liver, and the CNS. Most patients succumb to local progression of disease with respiratory failure, arrhythmia, heart failure, or stroke.

STAGING: See Table 31.2.

T/M \ N		cN0	cN1	cN2
T1	• Ipsilateral parietal pleura with extension to visceral, mediastinal, or diaphragmatic pleura	IA	II	IIIB
T2	• Involving all ipsilateral pleural surfaces (parietal, mediastinal, diaphragmatic, and visceral) with at least one of the following: • Diaphragmatic muscle • Underlying pulmonary parenchyma	IB	II	IIIB
T3	• Involving all ipsilateral pleural surfaces with involvement of at least one of the following: • Endothoracic fascia • Mediastinal fat • Solitary, resectable focus of tumor extending into chest wall soft tissue • Nontransmural pericardium	IB	IIIA	IIIB
T4	• Involving all ipsilateral pleural surfaces with involvement of at least one of the following: • Multifocal chest wall mass • Transdiaphragmatic extension to peritoneum • Direct extension to contralateral pleura • Direct extension to mediastinal organs • Direct extension into spine • Direct extension to inner surface of pericardium • Direct extension to myocardium	IIIB	IIIB	IIIB
M1	• Distant metastasis	IV	IV	IV

Table 31.2 AJCC 8th Edition (2017): Staging for Malignant Pleural Mesothelioma

cN1: ipsilateral bronchopulmonary, hilar, mediastinal (including internal mammary, peridiaphragmatic, pericardial fat pad, or intercostal) LNs; cN2: contralateral mediastinal or any supraclavicular LNs.

TREATMENT PARADIGM

Surgery: Increasingly, non-operative approaches are preferred. If performed, radical surgery should be limited to carefully selected patients as it is associated with significant morbidity and mortality (early series demonstrate 31% mortality with EPP). Surgical candidates are those with resectable disease, limited to one hemithorax (clinical stages I–III), adequate cardiopulmonary function, and ECOG PS <2. Nearly all surgical series demonstrate OS benefit to surgery when limited to pure epithelioid subtype. Patients with biphasic or sarcomatoid subtypes often have an OS similar to or shorter than expected with nonoperative management.

Historically, definitive surgical procedures included EPP and P/D. P/D provides an opportunity to preserve lung parenchyma. The decision is based on surgeon's judgment on obtaining an R0 resection. RRs suggest P/D may have less morbidity and mortality compared with EPP with comparable OS (see Flores data in the Evidence-Based Q&A section).

- EPP: En bloc resection of parietal and visceral pleura, ipsilateral lung, pericardium, and diaphragm. If there is no involvement of pericardium or diaphragm, these structures can remain intact.
- P/D: Parietal and visceral pleurectomy with removal of all gross tumor without diaphragm and pericardial resection.
- Extended P/D: Parietal and visceral pleurectomy with removal of all gross tumor and resection of diaphragm and pericardium.

Pleurodesis is a surgical option used to palliate symptoms from pleural effusion, and it involves obliteration of the pleural space through injection of sterile, asbestos-free talc to cause adhesion of the visceral and parietal pleura. Complete drainage of the pleural effusion by tube thoracostomy or video thoracoscopy usually precedes this procedure.

Systemic Therapy: CHT has a role in the neoadjuvant, adjuvant, and palliative settings. Cisplatin and pemetrexed demonstrate prolonged OS in patients with unresectable disease. A phase II multicenter study by Krug et al. used neoadjuvant pemetrexed and cisplatin for four cycles, followed by EPP in those patients who did not have disease progression, followed by adjuvant RT (54 Gy), and demonstrated an MS of 16.8 months.[5] The patients who were able to complete all therapy had an MS of 29.1 months. Alternative CHT regimens include cisplatin + gemcitabine and carboplatin + pemetrexed. A survival benefit with the addition of bevacizumab to CHT has also been shown in a randomized setting, although with increased toxicity.[11] IO has shown promise in both the upfront and progressive settings compared with standard CHT.[6] The use of IO as a preferred first-line agent was adopted by the 2024 NCCN guidelines supporting the use of nivolumab/ipilimumab.[1]

Radiation

Indications: Adjuvant after EPP, consolidation after P/D, and palliative.

Dose: After EPP: if negative margins, use 50 to 54 Gy; if positive margins, boost to 54 to 60 Gy. After P/D: total dose (maximum 50.4 Gy) is limited by mean lung dose of 20 Gy to residual lungs; mandates use of IMRT.

Toxicity: Fatigue, esophagitis, pneumonitis (caution with contralateral lung in postpneumonectomy patients).[7]

EVIDENCE-BASED Q&A

What is the benefit of EPP? What is the benefit of P/D?

LC is the main goal of EPP. There is high rate of mortality with EPP; however, with careful selection of patients, there may be a survival benefit. The MARS study in 2011 showed P/D to be the less morbid option; however, recent data from MARS2 suggest that proper patient selection is still paramount to improving outcomes even with less extensive surgery.

Treasure, MARS Study (*Lancet Oncol* 2011, PMID 21723781): PRT of 50 patients from 12 UK hospitals who received neoadjuvant CHT, randomized to ± EPP, followed by RT. Of the 24 patients randomized to EPP, 16 underwent EPP, and 30-day mortality rate was 13%. HR for OS with EPP was 1.90 (95% CI 0.92–3.93). After adjustment for sex, histologic subtype, stage, and age, HR for EPP was 2.75 (1.21–6.26). **Conclusion: Despite study deficiencies, EPP had worse OS compared with no EPP, suggesting the importance of choosing EPP candidates carefully.**

Lim, MARS 2 Study (*Lancet Respir Med* 2024, PMID 38740044): PRT of 335 patients from 26 UK hospitals. After two cycles of CHT, patients were randomized to surgery with P/D followed by further CHT or continued CHT alone; 86% epithelioid histology. MFU 22.4 months. Median survival was 19.3 months in the surgery arm vs. 24.8 months in the CHT-alone arm (*p* = .019). In the first 42 months, the HR for death in the surgery/CHT arm vs. the CHT-alone arm was 1.28, suggesting a 28% increase in the risk of death in the surgery group. 318 serious AEs in the surgery arm vs. 169 in the CHT-alone arm (*p* < .0001), including cardiac, respiratory, and infectious complications. QOL scores favored the CHT-alone group. **Conclusion: Even with P/D, surgical resection combined with CHT has a high rate of morbidity and mortality, underscoring the importance of patient selection and expertise regardless of surgical approach.**

What are the outcomes after EPP compared with P/D?

Data are conflicting with some showing improved LC and OS with EPP, while others demonstrate improved outcomes with P/D. EPP is shown to have higher perioperative morbidity and mortality.

Flores, MSKCC (*J Thorac Cardiovasc Surg* 2008, PMID 18329481): RR of 663 patients from three institutions treated between 1990 and 2006 with EPP or P/D. EPP had perioperative mortality rate of 7% vs. 4% with P/D. Stage (*p* < .001), epithelioid histology (*p* < .001), EPP (*p* < .001), and multimodality therapy (*p* < .001) were all significantly associated with improved survival. MVA demonstrated an HR of 1.4 for EPP (*p* < .001), controlling for stage, histology, gender, and multimodality therapy. **Conclusion: Although subject to selection bias, P/D is associated with improved OS. EPP is associated with a higher risk of perioperative mortality.**

Lang-Lazdunski, UK (*J Thorac Oncol* 2012, PMID 22425923): Nonrandomized prospective study of 22 patients receiving neoadjuvant CHT, EPP, with adjuvant RT and 54 patients receiving neoadjuvant CHT, P/D, and adjuvant CHT. The 30-day mortality rate was 5% in the EPP arm and 0% for P/D. Complications observed in 68% of the EPP group vs. 28% in the P/D group. Trimodality therapy completed by 68% in EPP and 100% in P/D. Survival was significantly better in P/D compared with EPP (2-year OS 49% vs. 18% and 5-year OS 30% vs. 9%, *p* = .004). Epithelioid histology, P/D, and R0 resection were all associated with improved survival on MVA. **Conclusion: Compared with EPP with multimodality therapy, P/D with perioperative CHT improved survival in this nonrandomized study.**

Is trimodality therapy safe and effective? Which patients are the best candidates?

Trimodality therapy is generally safe and effective in very carefully selected patients. Epithelioid histology, R0 resection, and N0 patients have been shown to have 5-year OS as high as 50% with trimodality therapy.

Sugarbaker (*J Thorac Cardiovasc Surg* 1999, PMID 9869758): RR of 183 patients treated with EPP followed by adjuvant CHT and RT. MFU 13 months. Perioperative mortality rate was 4% at 2 years, with 50% morbidity. Survival was 37% at 1 year and 15% at 5 years. MS 19 months. Three variables significantly associated with improved survival: (a) epithelial type (52% 2-year OS, 21% 5-year OS, 26-month MS); (b) negative resection margins (44% 2-year OS, 25% 5-year OS, 23-month MS); and (c) negative LNs (42% 2-year OS, 17% 5-year OS, 21-month MS). Patients with all three variables had 62% 2-year OS, 46% 5-year OS, and MS of 51 months. **Conclusion: Trimodality therapy is feasible and mediastinal LN evaluation is important in selecting optimal patients. Epithelioid type, R0 resection, and extrapleural node-negative patients have extended survival.**

Pagan (*J Thorac Cardiovasc Surg* 2006, PMID 17033611): Prospective nonrandomized trial of EPP followed by carboplatin/paclitaxel and RT (50 Gy). The 30-day mortality rate was 5% and overall complication rate was 50%. No major complications observed. MS was 20 months and the 5-year OS was 19%. Patients with epithelioid histology, R0 resection, and N0–1 had 5-year OS of 50%. **Conclusion: Trimodality therapy is associated with prolonged survival in carefully selected patients.**

What is the benefit of postoperative RT after EPP? Is there a role for IMRT?

LR rates following EPP are reported up to 50% to 70%.[8,9] The addition of postoperative RT has been shown to decrease locoregional failure rates by ~50%. Various studies have employed IMRT showing that it can be safely used when appropriate mean lung dose constraints are met for the remaining lung.

Rusch (*J Thorac Cardiovasc Surgery* **2001, PMID 11581615):** Phase II trial of 55 patients who underwent EPP or P/D followed by postoperative hemithoracic RT (54 Gy/30 fx). RT was AP/PA with photons and electron boost to areas requiring shielding. LRF in 13%, grade 4 pneumonitis in 9%. MS was 33.8 months for stage I and II and 10 months for stage III and IV tumors (*p* = .04). **Conclusion: Hemithoracic RT after surgery is feasible and reduces LR risk.**

Allen (*IJROBP* **2006, PMID 16751058):** RR of 13 patients treated with hemithoracic IMRT (54 Gy/30 fx) after EPP and adjuvant CHT with cisplatin or cisplatin/pemetrexed. Fatal pneumonitis rate was 46%. Patients with fatal pneumonitis had V20 of 15% to 22%, V5 81% to 100%, and mean lung dose 13.3 to 17 Gy. **Conclusion: IMRT after EPP requires close attention to lung constraints given high risk of fatal pneumonitis.**

Rice (*Ann Thorac Surg* **2007, PMID 17954086):** RR of 100 patients who underwent EPP and of whom 63 received IMRT (median dose 45 Gy); CHT not routinely administered. Nonepithelioid histology in 33%, stage III in 72%, and ipsilateral nodal metastases in 54%. Perioperative mortality was 8%. MS for the entire cohort was 10.2 months, and it was 14.2 months for those who received IMRT. In the IMRT group, node-negative patients with epithelioid histology had MS of 28 months. LRR was 13% and only 5% had in-field recurrence. Distant recurrences in 54% of patients. Rate of fatal lung events was 10% and V20 predicted for pulmonary-related death on MVA. **Conclusion: IMRT after EPP results in excellent LC, but distant metastases remain the main driver of OS.**

Is there a role for postoperative RT after P/D?

There are series evaluating its use, initially using 3D-CRT, which observed residual gross disease could not be eradicated. More recent studies employing IMRT have been done showing improvement in survival as compared with palliative approaches, although at the cost of increased toxicity, and thus its use is generally limited to centers of expertise.

Chance (*IJROPB* **2015, PMID 25442335):** Matched-pair analysis of 24 patients who underwent P/D followed by adjuvant CHT and hemithoracic IMRT to 45 Gy. Outcomes were compared with a matched cohort of 24 patients who received EPP followed by IMRT. MFU 12.2 months. There was statistically significant decrease in FVC, FEV1, and DLCO both after P/D and then further after IMRT. MS was 28.4 vs. 14.2 months (*p* = .04) and median PFS was 16.4 vs. 8.2 months (*p* = .01) for PD/IMRT vs. EPP/IMRT, respectively. There was no significant difference in grades 4 to 5 toxicities between the two groups (0% vs. 13%, *p* = .23). **Conclusion: Hemithoracic IMRT after P/D leads to a decline in pulmonary function. However, OS and PFS improved in P/D-IMRT vs. EPP-IMRT.**

Rimner, IMPRINT (*JCO* **2016, PMID 27325859):** Phase II study of 27 patients who received neoadjuvant platinum CHT and pemetrexed, P/D, followed by adjuvant hemithoracic IMRT (median dose 46.8 Gy). MFU 21.6 months. Grade 2 pneumonitis was 22% and grade 3 pneumonitis was 7%; all resolved with steroids. Median PFS and OS were 12.4 and 23.7 months, respectively. The 2-year OS was 59%. **Conclusion: Hemithoracic IMRT after P/D is safe and should be considered in the treatment paradigm.**

Trovo (*IJROBP* **2020, PMID 33259933):** Phase III study of 108 patients undergoing lung-sparing surgery with gross residual disease randomized to adjuvant hemithoracic IMRT (50 Gy/25 fx + 60 Gy SIB to gross disease) vs. palliative RT (most commonly 30–35 Gy/10 fx). All patients received CHT. MFU 14.6 months. Hemithoracic IMRT improved LC with 2-year cumulative LRR of 27% vs. 83% for palliative RT. Median OS was 35.6 months for hemithoracic RT vs. 12.4 months with palliative RT (*p* ≤ .001). No grade 3 toxicity with palliative RT, while 20% with hemithoracic RT had grade ≥3 acute toxicities and 31% had grades 3 to 4 late toxicities, including 16% grade ≥2 pneumonitis including one possible fatal event. **Conclusion: Adjuvant hemithoracic IMRT with SIB to gross residual disease is feasible and improves LC and OS as compared with palliative RT with increased rates of both acute and late toxicities.**

Which CHT regimens are most effective? What is the role of IO?

Platinum-doublet CHT has shown good outcomes in both the neoadjuvant and palliative settings with improvements in PFS, response rates, and a trend toward improved OS.[5,10] *The addition of bevacizumab to platinum doublet in the palliative setting showed a potential survival benefit.*[11] *Recent studies have shown improvements in survival and toxicity with IO compared with traditional platinum-doublet CHT, and IO (nivolumab/ipilimumab) remains a preferred first-line therapy option in the 2025 NCCN guidelines.*

Zalcman, MAPS (*Lancet* 2016, PMID 26719230): PRT of 448 patients with unresectable disease randomized to cisplatin/pemetrexed ± bevacizumab in 21-day cycles for up to six cycles. OS was significantly longer with the addition of bevacizumab (18.8 vs. 16.1 months, p = .0167). There were more grade 3 hypertension (23% vs. 0%) and thrombotic events (6% vs. 1%) with bevacizumab. **Conclusion: The addition of bevacizumab to cisplatin/pemetrexed improves OS but with an increase in toxicity.**

Fennell, CONFIRM (*Lancet Oncol* 2021, PMID 34656227): Prospective RCT at 24 hospitals in the UK. 332 patients with ECOG 0 or 1 with progression after platinum-doublet CHT randomized to placebo vs. nivolumab in a 2:1 fashion. Stratified by histology (epithelioid vs. nonepithelioid). MFU 11.6 months. Median PFS 3 months in the nivolumab group vs. 1.8 months in the placebo group (p = .0012). Median OS 10.2 months in the nivolumab arm vs. 6.9 months for placebo (p = .009). Epithelioid histology benefitted most; however, the trial was not powered to differentiate between histologies. **Conclusion: Nivolumab after progression on platinum-doublet CHT improves PFS and OS.**

Baas, CHECKMATE 743 (*Lancet* 2021, PMID 33485464): International PRT randomizing 605 patients with unresectable malignant pleural mesothelioma (MPM) to nivolumab/ipilimumab or CHT as first-line treatment. At interim analysis (MFU 29.7 months), median OS in the nivolumab/ipilimumab arm was 18.1 vs. 14.1 months in the CHT group (p = .002). No significant difference in G3–4 adverse events (30% vs. 32%). OS benefit observed in nonepithelioid but not epithelioid histologies. **Conclusion: IO as first-line treatment in unresectable MPM has an OS benefit for nonepithelioid histologies.**

If the biopsy tract is not surgically excised, can RT reduce the risk of tract recurrence?

Small PRTs show no difference in rates of tract recurrences with the addition of RT; recurrence rates ~10%.[12,13] Currently, the role of tract RT depends on the clinical setting and primary form of treatment.

Clive, SMART Trial (*Lancet Oncol* 2016, PMID 27345639): PRT of 203 patients from 22 UK hospitals who underwent large-bore pleural intervention randomized to prophylactic RT (21 Gy/3 fx within 42 days of pleural intervention) vs. salvage RT (21 Gy/3 fx upon procedure tract metastasis [PTM]). Primary outcome was incidence of PTM within 7 cm of the site of pleural intervention within 12 months of randomization, and no difference was found with the addition of prophylactic RT (9% vs. 16%, p = .14). **Conclusion: There is no role for prophylactic RT after large-bore thoracic interventions.**

Is there benefit to dose-escalated RT in mesothelioma?

Historically, typical mesothelioma doses were ~30 Gy given planning limitations and toxicity. Allen et al. found that dose escalation to 54 Gy resulted in improved LC.[14] With the advent of IMRT and improved planning techniques, 54 Gy has become standard. Currently, there is no evidence to increase the dose beyond 54 Gy in the adjuvant setting.

Is RT useful for treating pain in mesothelioma?

RT can be used in mesothelioma for palliation of symptoms. Multiple studies have shown improvement in pain with RT, especially with doses ≥4 Gy/fx.[15,16]

McLeod (*J Thorac Oncol* 2015, PMID 25654216): Phase II trial of 40 patients, with assessments of pain and other symptoms at baseline, who received 20 Gy/5 fx to areas of pain. Primary endpoint was assessment of pain at the site of RT at 5 weeks. Forty-seven percent of patients alive at week 5 had an improvement in pain. **Conclusion: RT is an effective palliative treatment in patients with mesothelioma.**

de Graaf-Strukowska (*IJROBP* 1999, PMID 10078630): RR of 189 patients; higher local response rate for patients treated with 4 Gy/fx compared with <4 Gy/fx (50% vs. 39%). Duration of response was short, with pain recurring predominantly in the RT field after a median of 69 days (range 32–363). **Conclusion: Use fraction sizes of ≥4 Gy when palliating mesothelioma.**

Are there alternative therapies available for unresectable mesothelioma?

There is evidence to support the addition of tumor treating fields (TTF), but further study is warranted. TTF is a noninvasive cancer treatment that uses low-intensity electric fields to disrupt the division of cancer cells. To date, its role in the setting of IO use remains unknown for malignant pleural mesothelioma.

Ceresoli, STELLAR (*Lancet Oncol 2019*, PMID 31628016): Prospective single-arm trial of 80 patients with unresectable disease receiving platinum-doublet CHT + Novo-TTF-100L. MS was 18.2 months and 21.2 months in the epithelioid histology subset. No increase in serious toxicity. **Conclusion: Novo-TTF when added to standard CHT is safe with encouraging survival results, and future study is warranted.**

REFERENCES

1. NCCN Clinical Practice Guidelines in Oncology: Mesothelioma: Pleural, 2025. Accessed June 8, 2025. https://www.nccn.org/professionals/physician_gls/pdf/meso_pleural.pdf

2. Ai J, Stevenson JP. Current issues in malignant pleural mesothelioma evaluation and management. *Oncologist*. 2014;19(9):975–984. doi:10.1634/theoncologist.2014-0122

3. Rosenzweig KE, Giraud P. Radiation therapy for malignant pleural mesothelioma. *Cancer Radiother*. 2017;21(1):73–76. doi:10.1016/j.canrad.2016.09.009

4. Patel SC, Dowell JE. Modern management of malignant pleural mesothelioma. *Lung Cancer (Auckl)*. 2016;7:63–72. doi:10.2147/LCTT.S83338

5. Krug LM, Pass HI, Rusch VW, et al. Multicenter phase II trial of neoadjuvant pemetrexed plus cisplatin followed by extrapleural pneumonectomy and radiation for malignant pleural mesothelioma. *J Clin Oncol*. 2009;27(18):3007–3013. doi:10.1200/JCO.2008.20.3943

6. Reuss JE, Forde PM. Immunotherapy for mesothelioma: rationale and new approaches. *Clin Adv Hematol Oncol*. 2020;18(9):562–572.

7. Allen AM, Czerminska M, Janne PA, et al. Fatal pneumonitis associated with intensity-modulated radiation therapy for mesothelioma. *Int J Radiat Oncol Biol Phys*. 2006;65(3):640–645. doi:10.1016/j.ijrobp.2006.03.012

8. Pass HI, Kranda K, Temeck BK, Feuerstein I, Steinberg SM. Surgically debulked malignant pleural mesothelioma: results and prognostic factors. *Ann Surg Oncol*. 1997;4(3):215–222. doi:10.1007/BF02306613

9. Rusch VW, Rosenzweig K, Venkatraman E, et al. A phase II trial of surgical resection and adjuvant high-dose hemithoracic radiation for malignant pleural mesothelioma. *J Thorac Cardiovasc Surg*. 2001;122(4):788–795. doi:10.1067/mtc.2001.116560

10. Vogelzang NJ, Rusthoven JJ, Symanowski J, et al. Phase III study of pemetrexed in combination with cisplatin versus cisplatin alone in patients with malignant pleural mesothelioma. *J Clin Oncol*. 2003;21(14):2636–2644. doi:10.1200/JCO.2003.11.136

11. Zalcman G, Mazieres J, Margery J, et al. Bevacizumab for newly diagnosed pleural mesothelioma in the Mesothelioma Avastin Cisplatin Pemetrexed Study (MAPS): a randomised, controlled, open-label, phase 3 trial. *Lancet*. 2016;387(10026):1405–1414. doi:10.1016/S0140-6736(15)01238-6

12. Bydder S, Phillips M, Joseph DJ, et al. A randomised trial of single-dose radiotherapy to prevent procedure tract metastasis by malignant mesothelioma. *Br J Cancer*. 2004;91(1):9–10. doi:10.1038/sj.bjc.6601957

13. O'Rourke N, Garcia JC, Paul J, Lawless C, McMenemin R, Hill J. A randomised controlled trial of intervention site radiotherapy in malignant pleural mesothelioma. *Radiother Oncol*. 2007;84(1):18–22. doi:10.1016/j.radonc.2007.05.022

14. Allen AM, Den R, Wong JS, et al. Influence of radiotherapy technique and dose on patterns of failure for mesothelioma patients after extrapleural pneumonectomy. *Int J Radiat Oncol Biol Phys*. 2007;68(5):1366–1374. doi:10.1016/j.ijrobp.2007.02.047

15. MacLeod N, Chalmers A, O'Rourke N, et al. Is radiotherapy useful for treating pain in mesothelioma?: a phase II trial. *J Thorac Oncol*. 2015;10(6):944–950. doi:10.1097/JTO.0000000000000499

16. de Graaf-Strukowska L, van der Zee J, van Putten W, Senan S. Factors influencing the outcome of radiotherapy in malignant mesothelioma of the pleura–a single-institution experience with 189 patients. *Int J Radiat Oncol Biol Phys*. 1999;43(3):511–516. doi:10.1016/s0360-3016(98)00409-x

32 THYMOMA

Cole Billena, Christopher W. Fleming, and Gregory M. M. Videtic

QUICK HIT Thymoma is a rare tumor of the anterior mediastinum associated with myasthenia gravis (MG) and managed primarily with surgery. Postoperative RT (PORT) is indicated for Masaoka–Koga stage III disease or incomplete resection, and CHT is usually employed for potentially resectable tumors to facilitate surgery (Table 32.1). Metastatic thymoma may have a very long natural history; systemic therapy has limited benefits, and local therapies (surgery, RT) may be appropriate as indicated by patient and tumor presentations. Thymic carcinoma is a more aggressive entity and generally warrants PORT for all stages.

Table 32.1 General Treatment Paradigm for Thymoma			
Thymic neoplasm suspected and resection possible?	Yes → proceed to total thymectomy (biopsy may be omitted in selected cases)	Stage I	No adjuvant therapy
		Stage II	No adjuvant therapy (PORT controversial)
		Stage III–IVA, +margin, or thymic carcinoma	PORT 45–50 Gy (negative/close margins), 54 Gy (microscopic +margins), 60–70 Gy (gross residual); CHT controversial, may be considered for gross residual or thymic carcinomas
	No (locally advanced, solitary or potentially resectable metastases)	Core needle biopsy followed by induction CHT	Individualized by disease burden and performance status, including CHT +/– local therapy (surgery/RT) as indicated

EPIDEMIOLOGY: 1.5 cases per million person-years in the United States.[1] Typically occurs in adults aged 40 to 60. Comprises ~20% of all mediastinal tumors but half of all anterior mediastinal tumors. Thymic carcinomas represent <1% of thymic tumors.

RISK FACTORS: No known etiologic factors.

ANATOMY: The thymus is an anterior mediastinal structure responsible for the maturation of T-cells. Lymphatic drainage is to the lower cervical, internal mammary, and hilar nodes. Structurally, the thymus consists of the capsule, cortex, and medulla. Histologically, it includes epithelial cells, epithelioreticular cells (form Hassall's corpuscles), myoid cells, early T lymphocytes ("thymocytes"), and B lymphocytes.

PATHOLOGY: See Table 32.2.

Table 32.2 2021 WHO Thymoma Grading	
WHO Type[2,3]	Histology
A	Medullary thymoma
AB	Mixed thymoma
B1	Predominantly cortical thymoma
B2	Cortical thymoma
B3	Well-differentiated thymic carcinoma
C	Thymic carcinoma

CLINICAL PRESENTATION: Often an incidental finding on imaging. Local symptoms due to mass effect may include chest pain, dyspnea, cough, phrenic nerve palsy, and SVC syndrome. Paraneoplastic syndromes may be present prior to or after diagnosis. Up to 50% of patients will present with MG; it is less common for MG patients to have associated thymoma. Other less common paraneoplastic syndromes include red cell aplasia, immunodeficiency, and multiorgan autoimmunity.

WORKUP: H&P. If thymoma suspected and considered resectable, biopsy may be omitted and resection performed. If unresectable/medically inoperable, obtain core needle biopsy to confirm diagnosis (open biopsy also possible; biopsy should not violate pleural space). Multidisciplinary evaluation indicated. Perform PFTs.

Labs: As indicated by clinical and radiographic findings. Serum β-hCG and AFP (rule out germ cell tumor), CBC, CMP, serum level of anti-ACh antibodies to assess for MG.

Imaging: Chest CT with contrast, PET/CT (optional).

PROGNOSTIC FACTORS: Masaoka stage, histology, degree of resection (R0 vs. R1 vs. R2).[4] Thymoma is an indolent but locally aggressive disease with a long natural history even in the setting of metastases. Thymic carcinoma is a more aggressive disease, with poorer outcomes due to early metastatic spread.

STAGING: Historically, Masaoka Staging System and Koga Modification of Masaoka Staging System have been utilized (see Table 32.3). TNM staging system was first implemented in 2017 with the AJCC 8th edition (see Table 32.4).

Table 32.3 Masaoka–Koga Staging System for Thymoma[5]	
Stage	**Definition**
I	Grossly and microscopically completely encapsulated tumor
IIA	Microscopic transcapsular invasion
IIB	Macroscopic invasion into surrounding fatty tissue or grossly adherent to but not breaking through mediastinal pleura or pericardium
III	Macroscopic invasion into neighboring organ (e.g., pericardium, great vessels, or lung)
IVA	Pleural or pericardial dissemination
IVB	Distant metastasis

Source: Masaoka A, Monden Y, Nakahara K, Tanioka T. Follow-up study of thymomas with special reference to their clinical stages. *Cancer.* 1981;48(11):2485–2492. doi:10.1002/1097-0142(19811201)48:11<2485::aid-cncr2820481123>3.0.co;2-r.

Table 32.4 AJCC 8th Edition (2017): Staging for Thymic Tumors					
T/M		N	N0	N1	N2
T1	**T1a:** No mediastinal pleura involvement		I		
	T1b: Direct invasion of mediastinal pleura				
T2	• Direct invasion of the pericardium (either partial or full thickness)		II	IVA	IVB
T3	• Direct invasion into lung, brachiocephalic vein, SVC, phrenic nerve, chest wall, or extrapericardial pulmonary artery or veins		IIIA		
T4	• Invasion into aorta, arch vessels, intrapericardial pulmonary artery, myocardium, trachea, esophagus		IIIB		
M1	**M1a:** Separate pleural or pericardial nodule(s)				
	M1b: Pulmonary intraparenchymal nodule or distant organ metastasis				

N1: metastasis in anterior (perithymic) LNs; N2: metastasis in deep intrathoracic or cervical LNs.

TREATMENT PARADIGM

Surgery: Total thymectomy with negative margins is the mainstay of therapy in resectable cases. This is typically performed with median sternotomy. Resection of both phrenic nerves should be avoided to prevent severe respiratory compromise. Signs and symptoms of MG should be controlled medically with anticholinesterase inhibitors prior to surgery.

Chemotherapy: Platinum-based CHT is indicated for locally advanced, medically inoperable/unresectable thymoma or thymic carcinoma. CHT can also be used for downstaging preoperatively or given postoperatively based on the degree of resection. For diffuse metastases, consider CHT alone. No randomized trials have identified a superior regimen. Common regimens include cyclophosphamide (CYC)/adriamycin/cisplatin, cisplatin/etoposide (EP), or carboplatin/paclitaxel.

Radiation

Indications: PORT should be offered for positive surgical margins or stage III disease, and it should be considered for any thymic carcinoma.

Dose: RT dosing is based on degree of resection, with 45 to 50 Gy, 54 Gy, and 60 to 70 Gy given for R0, R1, and R2, respectively. Definitive RT indicated for medically inoperable disease, with the addition of CHT and its sequencing empirically based.

Toxicity: Acute: fatigue, cough, skin erythema. Late: cardiac morbidity, hypothyroidism, second malignancy.

EVIDENCE-BASED Q&A

What are the outcomes for completely resected thymoma by stage and when should PORT be considered?

Surgery is the mainstay of therapy for operable patients with locoregional disease given excellent LC and survival for R0 resections. PORT is always indicated for residual disease if repeat resection is not feasible. Conventionally, stage III/IVA disease has been managed by surgery followed by PORT, independent of margins. Some authors have recommended PORT for stage II/III disease with positive or close margin (<1 mm), gross fibrous adhesion to pleura, or WHO high grade (B3), but otherwise PORT is not recommended for R0 resected thymoma.[6] However, a meta-analysis by Tateishi et al. found the use of PORT in completely resected stage II/III thymoma to be associated with improved OS. There are challenges reconciling these results with some data from large Japanese institutional series. At present, PORT for stage III would be generally recommended.[7]

Kondo, Japan (*Ann Thorac Surg* 2003, PMID 12963221): RR of 1,320 patients with thymic epithelial tumors from 115 special thoracic surgery institutes across Japan. Patients with stage I thymoma received surgery alone, and patients with stage II/III thymoma and thymic carcinoid underwent surgery + PORT. Patients with stage IV thymoma and thymic carcinoma were treated with RT or CHT. In stage III and IV thymoma, 5-year survival rates of GTR, STR, and inoperable groups were 93%, 64%, and 36%, respectively. In thymic carcinoma, 5-year survival rates of GTR, STR, and inoperable groups were 67%, 30%, and 24%, respectively. PORT did not change LR rates in patients with totally resected stage II and III thymoma. Adjuvant therapy (RT or CHT) did not improve prognosis in patients with totally resected III and IV thymoma and thymic carcinoma (see Table 32.5). **Conclusion: Total resection is the most important factor in the treatment of thymic epithelial tumors. Adjuvant therapy may not improve outcomes for totally resected invasive thymoma and thymic carcinoma.**

Table 32.5 Results of Japanese Retrospective Study for Thymoma by Kondo et al.				
Masaoka Stage	**I**	**II**	**III**	**IVA**
Complete resection	100%	100%	85%	42%
Recurrence	1%	4%	28%	34%
5-yr OS	100%	98%	89%	71%

Omasa, Japan (*Cancer* 2015, PMID 25565590): Database study including 1,265 patients with stage II/III thymoma or thymic carcinoma (12%). Majority (71%) were stage II. PORT delivered to 403 (32%) patients; those receiving PORT had significantly higher rates of incomplete surgery. For stage II/III thymoma, PORT was not associated with improved RFS or OS (*p* = .350). PORT for stage II/III thymic carcinoma was associated with improved RFS ($p = .003$) but not OS ($p = .536$). **Conclusion: PORT did not increase RFS or OS for stage II or III thymoma but did increase RFS for stage II or III thymic carcinoma.** *Comment: Higher rates of incomplete resection without worse outcomes suggest potential benefit to PORT for stage II to III thymoma.*

Rimner, ITMIG group (*J Thorac Oncol* **2016, PMID 27346413):** Database study including 1,263 patients with completely resected stage II/III thymoma; 870 (69%) had stage II thymoma and 827 (70%) had grade B1, B2, or B3. The 5- and 10-year OS rates for patients receiving PORT were 95% and 86%, respectively, compared with 90% and 79% for patients receiving resection alone ($p = .002$). OS benefit remained significant when stage II ($p = .02$) and III ($p = .0005$) patients were analyzed separately. On MVA, younger age, female gender, absence of paraneoplastic syndromes, stage II disease, and use of PORT were significantly associated with longer OS. **Conclusion: OS benefit was observed with the use of PORT in completely resected stage II and III thymoma.**

Jackson, NCDB (*J Thorac Oncol* **2017, PMID 28126540):** NCDB study including 4,056 patients who underwent surgery for thymoma or thymic carcinoma. PORT delivered to 49%. MVA and propensity score-matched analyses found survival advantage associated with PORT. Subset analysis indicated longer OS in association with PORT for patients with positive margins or stage IIB to III thymoma ($p < .05$), but not for stage I to IIA patients ($p = .156$). **Conclusions: PORT was associated with longer OS, with the greatest relative benefits observed for stage IIB to III disease and positive margins.**

Tateishi, Japan (*J Thorac Oncol* **2021, PMID 33515812):** Meta-analysis of five studies (including the above Omasa, Rimner, and Jackson studies) involving 4,746 patients comparing surgery alone vs. surgery + PORT for completely resected Masaoka/Masaoka–Koga (M/MK) stage II/III thymoma. PORT was not associated with improved DFS (HR 0.96, 95% CI 0.70–1.33) but was associated with improved OS (HR 0.68, 0.57–0.83), which was similar on subgroup analysis of M/MK stage II disease (HR 0.63, 0.44–0.91) and stage III disease (HR 0.72, 0.55–0.95). **Conclusion: PORT was associated with OS improvement in stage II/III thymomas after R0.**

What are the reported outcomes for thymic carcinoma?

Ahmad, ITMIG Group (*J Thorac Cardiovasc Surg* **2015, PMID 25524678):** ITMIG database study of 1,042 patients with thymic carcinoma; 370 patients (45%) were stage III and 274 (33%) stage IV. 166 patients (22%) underwent induction CHT, and 48 (6%) underwent preoperative RT. R0 resection in 447 (61%), R1 in 102 (14%), and R2 in 184 (25%). SCC was the predominant histologic subtype ($n = 560$; 79%). RT was utilized for the majority of patients (72%), with the exception of stage I patients (45% underwent RT). Likewise, CHT was utilized for most (65%), with the exception of stage I and II patients (42% and 34%, respectively). Median OS 6.6 years, and the cumulative incidence of recurrence at 5 years was 35%. On MVA, R0 resection and use of RT were associated with prolonged OS. **Conclusion: R0 resection and RT are associated with improved OS for thymic carcinomas.**

Rimner, ITMIG Group (*J Thorac Oncol* **2024, PMID 38070599):** Retrospective analysis of 462 patients with thymic carcinoma from the ITMIG database. Overall, receipt of PORT was associated with improved OS (5-year OS 68% with PORT vs. 53% without). When stratified by resection margins, PORT was associated with increased OS in both R0 and R1/2 resection for stage III to IV disease. On MVA, PORT, R0 resection, and pathologic stage were associated with OS. **Conclusion: PORT is associated with an OS benefit in advanced thymic carcinoma following resection.**

What are the management options for unresectable/inoperable thymic tumors?

In the unresectable setting, downstaging with neoadjuvant therapy may be attempted with induction CHT ± RT. With good response to CHT, RT is often deferred in favor of resection, allowing pathologic stage to dictate necessity for PORT. In those who are medically inoperable or remain unresectable, completion of definitive treatment using combined-modality therapy may be appropriate. Data for definitive RT are modest given this rare clinical scenario. Diffuse systemic metastatic disease is typically treated with CHT alone, and palliative RT considered for symptomatic progression.

Loehrer, SWOG/SECSG/ECOG (*JCO* **1997, PMID 9294472):** Prospective single-arm study conducted from 1983 to 1995 involving 26 patients with limited-stage unresectable thymoma or thymic carcinoma. Patients received two to four cycles q3 weeks of cisplatin, doxorubicin, and CYC (PAC) followed by RT with 54 Gy to primary tumor and regional LNs for patients without progressive disease. Twenty-three patients were evaluable. Toxicity was mild. There were 5 CR and 11 PR to CHT (overall response rate, 70%). Median time to treatment failure was 93.2 months, and MS was 93 months. The 5-year OS was 53%. **Conclusion: PAC combination CHT produces response rates in management of patients with unresectable thymoma. Combined-modality therapy is feasible and associated with prolonged PFS. Benefit of combined-modality therapy over RT alone is suggested for patients with unresectable thymoma.**

Shin, MD Anderson (*Ann Intern Med* 1998, PMID 9669967): Prospective cohort study from 1990 to 1996 of 13 patients with newly diagnosed, histologically proven, unresectable malignant thymoma. Patients treated with induction CHT (three cycles of CYC, doxorubicin, cisplatin, and prednisone), surgical resection, PORT, and consolidation CHT with three more cycles of the same regimen. Twelve patients were evaluable. CR to CHT in three patients (25%), PR in eight patients (67%), and one patient had minor response (8%). Eleven patients underwent surgical resection, with one refusing surgery. R0 resection in 9 (82%) and incompletely in 2 (18%) of 11 patients who had been receiving RT and consolidation CHT. All 12 patients were alive at 7 years, with MFU of 43 months, while 10 of 12 were disease-free (7-year DFS 73%). **Conclusion: Aggressive multimodal treatment may be appropriate for locally advanced, unresectable malignant thymoma.**

When is concurrent CRT recommended?

There are very little data on concurrent CHT for thymic neoplasms. The following phase II trial from China found 60 Gy with concurrent cisplatin/etoposide (EP) to be well-tolerated and efficacious. There are no prospective data comparing definitive RT alone with concurrent or sequential CHT regimens.

Fan, China (*IJROBP* 2020, PMID 31987968): Phase II trial of 56 patients with unresectable thymic malignancies (22 thymoma, 34 thymic carcinoma) undergoing 60 Gy IMRT with concurrent and adjuvant EP. Seventy-five percent were stage IVB. Objective response rate was 86%. The 1-, 2-, and 5-year PFS rates were 66%, 48%, and 30%, and the 1-, 2-, and 5-year OS rates were 91%, 76%, and 56%, respectively. The most common grade 3 to 4 adverse event was leukopenia (43%). G3 esophagitis rate 5%, no radiation pneumonitis. G3 pulmonary fibrosis in 5%. **Conclusion: Concurrent RT and CHT with EP may be a suitable treatment option for patients with unresectable thymic neoplasms.**

REFERENCES

1. Engels EA. Epidemiology of thymoma and associated malignancies. *J Thorac Oncol.* 2010;5(10 suppl 4):S260–S265. doi:10.1097/JTO.0b013e3181f1f62d
2. Falkson CB, Bezjak A, Darling G, et al. The management of thymoma: a systematic review and practice guideline. *J Thorac Oncol.* 2009;4(7):911–919. doi:10.1097/jto.0b013e3181a4b8e0
3. Kondo K, Yoshizawa K, Tsuyuguchi M, et al. WHO histologic classification is a prognostic indicator in thymoma. *Ann Thorac Surg.* 2004;77(4):1183–1188. doi:10.1016/j.athoracsur.2003.07.042
4. Safieddine N, Liu G, Cuningham K, et al. Prognostic factors for cure, recurrence and long-term survival after surgical resection of thymoma. *J Thorac Oncol.* 2014;9(7):1018–1022. doi:10.1097/JTO.0000000000000215
5. Masaoka A, Monden Y, Nakahara K, Tanioka T. Follow-up study of thymomas with special reference to their clinical stages. *Cancer.* 1981;48(11):2485–2492. doi:10.1002/1097-0142(19811201)48:11<2485::aid-cncr2820481123>3.0.co;2-r
6. Wright CD. Management of thymomas. *Crit Rev Oncol Hematol.* 2008;65(2):109–120. doi:10.1016/j.critrevonc.2007.04.005
7. Tateishi Y, Horita N, Namkoong H, Enomoto T, Takeda A, Kaneko T. Postoperative radiotherapy for completely resected masaoka/masaoka-koga stage II/III thymoma improves overall survival: an updated meta-analysis of 4746 patients. *J Thorac Oncol.* 2021;16(4):677–685. doi:10.1016/j.jtho.2020.12.023

PART VI: Gastrointestinal

33 ESOPHAGEAL CANCER

Sean M. Parker, Ehsan H. Balagamwala, and Gregory M. M. Videtic

QUICK HIT Most esophageal cancer patients present with either locally advanced or metastatic disease. Palliative RT is therefore commonly used to relieve pain or obstruction. In potentially curable patients, EBRT may be employed in the definitive, neoadjuvant, or adjuvant settings, as the individual roles and sequencing of surgery, CHT, and RT in contributing to cure remain controversial. Brachytherapy may be an option in select curative cases as a boost treatment or in advanced cases for palliation (Table 33.1).

Table 33.1 General Treatment Paradigm for Esophageal Cancer[1]	
Stage I	Tis/T1a (SCC or ACA): endoscopic resection/ablation (preferred) vs. esophagectomy T1b (SCC): endoscopic resection/ablation T1b (ACA): esophagectomy
Stage II–IVA (T4a only)	1. Preoperative CRT for SCC (41.4–50.4 Gy with concurrent CHT) followed by postoperative nivolumab if R0 without pCR <div align="center">or</div>2. Definitive CRT 50.4 Gy with concurrent CHT (60–66 Gy historically delivered for cervical location) <div align="center">or</div>3. Perioperative FLOT CHT for ACA (4 preoperative and 4 postoperative cycles) with surgery <div align="center">or</div>4. Postoperative CRT for pathologic stages IIA(T3N0)–IVA; any stage with R1/R2 resection Can consider esophagectomy for T1b–T2 low risk lesions, <3 cm, well-differentiated
Stage IVA (T4b)	Definitive CRT, 50.4 Gy; can consider CHT alone if invasion to trachea, great vessels, or heart
Stage IVB	Palliation with EBRT, brachytherapy, CHT, and/or best supportive care

Source: Data from Ajani JA, D'Amico TA, Bentrem DJ, et al. Esophageal and esophagogastric junction cancers, version 4.2024, NCCN clinical practice guidelines in oncology. *J Natl Compr Canc Netw.* 2024;21(4):393–422. doi:10.6004/jnccn.2023.0019.

EPIDEMIOLOGY: Approximately 22,000 new esophageal cancers diagnosed with nearly 16,000 deaths per year in the United States.[2] Incidence peaks in the sixth and seventh decades. Globally, squamous cell carcinoma (SCC) accounts for 90% of cases, with the majority of these cases arising in endemic regions of Eastern Europe and Asia.[3] However, adenocarcinoma (ACA) is more common in North America and Western European countries, comprising ~70% of cases.[3,4] Both histologic subtypes are more common in men, but the relative increased incidence in males is more pronounced for ACA.

RISK FACTORS: For SCC (mnemonic: ABCDEF)[3,4]: **a**chalasia, **b**ad diet (nutritional deficiency, high fat, low fruit/vegetables, drinking beverages at high temperatures causing thermal injury to mucosa), **c**austic stricture (lye ingestion), **c**igarette smoking, **d**ysplasia/**d**iverticuli, **e**sophageal webs (Plummer–Vinson syndrome: iron-deficiency anemia, atrophic glossitis, webs), **e**thanol (alcohol), **f**amilial. For ACA (mnemonic: BOG)[3,4]: **B**arrett esophagus (squamocolumnar metaplasia; risk ~0.5% per year for nondysplastic lesions; ranges from 1% to 5% for dysplastic lesions),[5,6] **o**besity, **G**ERD (weekly symptoms increase risk by factor of 5, daily symptoms increase risk by factor of 7)[7] cigarette smoking (less so than SCC); also associated with hiatal hernia and EGFR polymorphisms. Rarely, hereditary predisposition syndromes may be implicated, including tylosis, Bloom syndrome, Fanconi anemia for SCC, and familial Barrett syndrome for ACA.[1]

ANATOMY: Anatomic key features of the esophagus include no true serosa, nonkeratinized squamous epithelium superiorly that transitions to glandular epithelium inferiorly, and extensive submucosal lymphatic plexus that often results in skip metastases. Approximately 25 cm long, it begins at the cricopharyngeus muscle at about 15 cm from the incisors to gastroesophageal junction (GEJ), about 40 cm from the incisors (Table 33.2). The esophagus extends from the vertebral levels C6 to T10. GEJ tumors are defined as within 5 cm from the true GEJ (epithelial change) and are classified according to the modified Siewert system, with class I tumors originating from 1 to 5 cm superior to the true GEJ, class II tumors originating from 1 cm above to 2 cm below, and class III tumors from 2 to 5 cm below the GEJ.[8,9]

Table 33.2 Anatomic and Endoscopic Landmarks of the Esophagus		
Anatomic Site	**Description**	**Approximate Distance From the Incisors**
Cervical	Upper esophageal sphincter (UES) to thoracic inlet (sternal notch)	15–20 cm
Upper thoracic	Sternal notch to azygos vein	20–25 cm
Middle thoracic	Azygos vein to inferior pulmonary vein	25–30 cm
Lower thoracic	Inferior pulmonary vein to GEJ	30–40 cm
Lower abdominal/GEJ/cardia	GEJ to 5 cm below GEJ (see Chapter 34)	40–45 cm

PATHOLOGY: As noted earlier, SCC accounts for 90% of cases globally, but ACA comprises 70% of cases in North America and Western Europe. "Mixed adenosquamous" and "carcinomas, NOS" are categorized as SCC for purposes of staging. Rare histologies include small-cell carcinoma and sarcoma.

CLINICAL PRESENTATION[4]: Common symptoms include progressive dysphagia, weight loss, heartburn that does not respond to medical therapy, melena, and/or symptoms of asymptomatic blood loss. Less commonly, patients may present with symptoms of laryngeal nerve paralysis such as hoarseness, cough, and pneumonia. Note that asymptomatic cases may be detected due to Barrett esophagus screening. Given association with other aerodigestive malignancies, it is important to evaluate for symptoms related to H&N SCC.

WORKUP[1]: H&P with careful neck and abdominal exam.

Labs: CBC, CMP, MSI/MMR. HER2-neu and PD-L1 testing for unresectable, recurrent, or metastatic ACA (~25% of esophageal cancers are HER2-neu positive).[10,11]

Imaging: Barium swallow, CT chest/abdomen/pelvis with oral and IV contrast; PET/CT for distant metastases (has poor sensitivity and specificity for nodal metastases: ~50% and 80%, respectively).[12] Endoscopic ultrasound (EUS) more accurate than CT and PET-CT for local/nodal staging (Table 33.3).[13]

Procedures: Upper GI endoscopy with biopsy. EUS permits biopsy of suspicious nodes. Lesions at or above the carina need bronchoscopy to rule out tracheoesophageal fistula.

PROGNOSTIC FACTORS: Age, KPS, stage, grade, weight loss, pretreatment and postinduction dysphagia.[14] RPA of esophageal patients showed only weight loss, specifically loss of ≥10% in the preceding 6 months, as prognostic.[15]

NATURAL HISTORY: The 5-year OS is ~40% if confined to primary site, 20% if spread to regional LNs, and 4% if DMs present.

STAGING

Table 33.3 AJCC 8th Edition (2017): Staging for Esophageal Cancer					
Tumor		**Node**		**Distant Metastasis**	
T1	a. Invades lamina propria or muscularis mucosa	N0	• No regional LNs	M0	• No distant metastasis
	b. Invades submucosa				
T2	• Invades muscularis propria	N1	• 1–2 regional LNs	M1	• Distant metastasis
T3	• Invades adventitia	N2	• 3–6 regional LNs		
T4	a. Resectable[1]	N3	• ≥7 regional LNs		
	b. Unresectable[2]				

Notes: Resectable[1] = invades pleura, pericardium, diaphragm, azygos vein, or peritoneum. Unresectable[2] = invades aorta, vertebral body, or airway. AJCC suggests ≥10 nodes be removed and examined for pT1 tumors, ≥20 for pT2, and ≥30 for pT3–4.

(continued)

Table 33.3 AJCC 8th Edition (2017): Staging for Esophageal Cancer (*continued*)			
Stage Grouping (AJCC 8th Edition) *Note that the AJCC 8th Edition includes a pathologic TNM and a post-neoadjuvant pathologic TNM, which are not displayed here.*			
Squamous Cell Carcinoma		**Adenocarcinoma**	
Clinical Stage	**Clinical TNM**	**Clinical Stage**	**Clinical TNM**
0	TisN0	0	TisN0
I	T1N0–1	I	T1N0
II	T2N0–1 T3N0	IIA	T1N1
		IIB	T2N0
III	T3N1 T1–3N2	III	T2N1 T3N0–1 T4aN0–1
IVA	T4N0–2 Any T, N3	IVA	T1–4aN2 T4bN0–2 Any T, N3
IVB	Any T, Any N, M1	IVB	Any T, Any N, M1

Source: Adapted from AJCC Cancer Staging Manual, 8th edition, 2017.

TREATMENT PARADIGM

Surgery: Surgery is a commonly utilized modality for locoregionally confined disease and options are based on the patient's medical condition, tumor location, and stage. Cervical tumors are typically treated nonoperatively because these lesions may also need laryngopharyngectomy with permanent stoma. For upper and middle thoracic tumors (>5 cm below cricopharyngeus), total esophagectomy with gastric pull-through is standard. Distal esophagogastrectomy is standard for lesions of the GEJ and lower thoracic esophagus. Contraindications to surgery include DMs, T4b lesions (involvement of the heart, great vessels, trachea, or other surrounding organs), bulky multistation adenopathy, and medical comorbidity.

Three techniques are commonly employed in North America for total esophagectomy: Ivor Lewis, McKeown (tri-incisional), and transhiatal. Both Ivor Lewis esophagogastrectomy and McKeown esophagogastrectomy require right thoracotomy incisions, with the latter permitting access to more superiorly located tumors. Transhiatal esophagogastrectomy can be used for cervical, thoracic, and GEJ lesions and requires abdominal and left cervical incisions; thoracotomy is not performed (often resulting in shorter operative times). There is some evidence of lower postoperative morbidity with a transhiatal approach[16]; however, several disadvantages are associated with this technique and include difficulty in resecting large, midesophageal and/or paratracheal tumors and an inability to perform a full thoracic lymphadenectomy. Postoperative mortality at high-volume centers is typically <5%[17–19] but can be ≥10% after neoadjuvant CRT.[20–22]

For most distal lesions, mediastinal and upper abdominal lymphadenectomy is performed. Minimum number of LNs to optimize staging and survival is controversial, with recommendations varying from 6 to 23 LNs.[23–26] Retrospective evidence exists for improved OS with increased number of LNs resected.[24]

Minimally invasive surgery (thoracoscopy with upper abdominal laparoscopy) is an acceptable approach, with two randomized trials reporting reduction in complications compared with open esophagectomy.[27,28] Furthermore, robot-assisted minimally invasive surgery offers reduced complications compared with open esophagectomy and improves LN dissection yield compared with minimally invasive surgery alone.[29,30]

Chemotherapy: CHT is commonly utilized for T2–T4 or N+ tumors in neoadjuvant, perioperative, adjuvant, or definitive settings.[1]

In both preoperative and definitive settings, common regimens concurrent with RT include cisplatin + infusional 5-FU or carboplatin + paclitaxel. Infusional 5-FU is thought to be superior to bolus 5-FU based on data from gastric cancer.[1,31] Oral capecitabine can be substituted for infusional 5-FU.[1] Addition of cetuximab to standard cytotoxic therapy has shown no benefit.[32,33] There is no benefit to the addition of trastuzumab to definitive CRT in HER2+ esophageal ACA.[34] Trastuzumab can be considered for HER2+ metastatic ACAs of GEJ based on a survival benefit demonstrated by the TOGA trial.[35] If perioperative CHT alone is being considered in the management of GEJ or esophageal ACA, FLOT (5-FU, leucovorin, oxaliplatin, and docetaxel) should be regarded as the recommended regimen.[36,37] Perioperative FLOT recently demonstrated a superior OS compared with neoadjuvant CRT for esophageal ACA.[37] For esophageal SCC, triplet therapy with docetaxel, cisplatin, and 5-FU may be favored.[38]

Immunotherapy: The role of immune checkpoint inhibitors in esophageal cancer continues to evolve. In patients without a pCR following neoadjuvant CRT with R0 resection, adjuvant immunotherapy (IO) with nivolumab is recommended.[1,39] The addition of IO failed to improve survival outcomes when added to perioperative CHT in two trials for GEJ/gastric cancer.[40,41] However, for patients with ACA that is MSI-H/dMMR, neoadjuvant or perioperative immune checkpoint inhibitors should be considered per NCCN.[1,42]

Radiation

Indications: Typically delivered with concurrent CHT in the preoperative or definitive setting for T2–T4 or N+ tumors.

Dose: With concurrent CHT, 50–50.4 Gy/25–28 fx is standard. Without CHT, 64 Gy/32 fx is standard (see Herskovic). Randomized trials show benefit to concurrent CHT and no benefit to dose escalation beyond 50.4 Gy.[43–46] In the preoperative setting, 41.4 Gy is the appropriate dose based on the CROSS trial. Brachytherapy boost can be selectively employed, although it does not improve survival and may be associated with morbidity.[47,48]

Palliation: EBRT and brachytherapy can be used. Other options include dilation, laser therapy, endoscopic injection therapies, endoscopic mucosal resection (EMR), photodynamic therapy (PDT), and stenting (preferable in those with malignant fistula). Safe to treat with palliative RT post-stenting.

Toxicity: Acute: esophagitis, fatigue, weight loss, subacute pneumonitis. Late: strictures, pulmonary fibrosis, pericarditis, coronary artery disease.

Procedure: See *Handbook of Treatment Planning in Radiation Oncology*, Chapter 6.[49]

Endoscopic Therapy: Endoscopic management of early esophageal cancer may be performed using EMR or endoscopic submucosal dissection (ESD). Both techniques allow resection of mucosa (and possibly a portion of the submucosa) containing early tumor without interruption of deeper layers. EMR can remove lesions <2 cm in size en bloc. Larger lesions may require resection in a piecemeal fashion, limiting assessment of margins. ESD offers en bloc dissection of tumor regardless of size. ESD is performed with specialized needle knives, which allow incision followed by careful dissection of the lesion within the submucosal layer. ESD is labor-intensive and has an increased risk of perforation. Esophageal stenosis remains a concern after extensive EMR or ESD.

Locally Ablative Modalities: Include thermal destruction by laser, multipolar electrocoagulation (MPEC), argon plasma coagulation (APC), or radiofrequency ablation; cryotherapy; and PDT. PDT may eradicate high-grade dysplasia and Barrett's.

EVIDENCE-BASED Q&A

UNRESECTABLE/INOPERABLE ESOPHAGEAL CANCER

Is RT alone sufficient for esophageal cancer or should concurrent CHT be added?

RT alone is insufficient since OS is improved with the addition of CHT to RT.

Herskovic, RTOG 8501 (*NEJM* 1992, PMID 1584260; Update Al-Sarraf, *JCO* 1997, PMID 8996153; Update Cooper, *JAMA* 1999, PMID 10235156): Phase III PRT of 129 patients with ACA (12%) or SCC (88%) cT1–3N0–1 randomized to RT alone (64 Gy/32 fx) vs. CRT (concurrent cisplatin/5-FU + 50 Gy/25 fx). CHT was cisplatin 75 mg/m^2 and 5-FU 1,000 mg/m^2 on weeks 1, 5, 8, and 11. Initial

RT field extended from SCV fossa to GEJ (except SCV was optional for distal one-third tumors). For the CRT arm, extended field was taken to 30 Gy followed by 20 Gy boost to tumor + 5 cm. For the RT-alone arm, extended field was taken to 50 Gy followed by 14 Gy boost to tumor + 5 cm. Trial stopped early due to survival difference. The 5-year OS was 26% vs. 0% favoring CRT. Persistent disease was the most common mode of failure: 26% in the CRT arm and 37% in the RT-alone arm. Severe/life-threatening acute toxicities were 44%/20% with CRT and 25%/3% with RT alone. No differences in late toxicity. **Conclusion: When treating nonoperatively, concurrent CRT is superior to RT alone for T1–3N0–1 esophageal cancer.**

Does RT dose escalation improve survival in the setting of CHT?

There is no evidence that dose escalation improves outcomes. An NCDB analysis evaluating dose escalation (≥50 Gy) with modern techniques found no benefit, consistent with the results of the Minsky trial.[50] Using a less toxic CHT regimen with more modern RT techniques, the phase III ARTDECO trial attempted dose escalation, but again failed to demonstrate a benefit. Additionally, the phase III CONCORDE/PRODIGE-26 trial (only presented in abstract form) found no benefit to dose escalation from 50 Gy to 66 Gy with concurrent FOLFOX-4 adding to the growing collection of data showing no benefit to dose escalation in this population.[43]

Minsky, RTOG 94-05/INT 0123 (*JCO* 2002, PMID 11870157): Phase III PRT of 218 patients with T1–4N0–1 ACA (15%) or SCC (85%) treated with low-dose (50.4 Gy) vs. high-dose (64.8 Gy) RT with both arms receiving concurrent CHT (cisplatin + 5-FU). For the high-dose arm, RT was 50.4 Gy/28 fx to tumor + 5 cm sup–inf (and 2 cm laterally), with 14.4 Gy boost to tumor + 2 cm. CHT was cisplatin 75 mg/m^2 and 5-FU 1,000 mg/m^2 on weeks 1, 5, 9, and 13 in the low-dose arm, and weeks 1, 5, 11, and 15 in the high-dose arm. Closed early because no benefit seen in the high-dose arm. See Table 33.4. **Conclusion: No benefit to high-dose RT with concurrent CHT, with higher incidence of treatment-related death in this trial.** *Note: Some authors have commented that the higher mortality observed in the high-dose arm may not be related to RT dose given 7 of 11 deaths occurred at ≤50.4 Gy.*

Table 33.4 RTOG 9405 Minsky: RT Dose Escalation for Esophageal Cancer				
	MS (Months)	**2-Yr OS**	**2-Yr LR**	**Treatment-Related Deaths**
High-dose CRT (64.8 Gy)	13.0	31%	56%	10% (7/11 deaths at ≤50.4 Gy)
Low-dose CRT (50.4 Gy)	18.1	40%	52%	2%
p value	NS	NS	.71	

Hulshof, ARTDECO (*JCO* 2021, PMID 34101496): Phase III PRT of 260 patients with medically inoperable esophageal cancer (61% SCC, 39% ACA) undergoing definitive CRT randomly assigned to receive 50.4 Gy or 61.6 Gy. CTV consisted of GTV + regional LN area up to 3 cm superior and inferior to the GTV, with a margin of at least 0.5 cm; PTV was a 1-cm expansion on CTV. CHT in both arms was concurrent weekly carboplatin (AUC 2)/paclitaxel (50 mg/m^2) for 6 weeks. Primary endpoint was local progression-free survival (LPFS). MFU 50 months. The 3-year LPFS was 70% in the 50.4 Gy arm vs. 73% in the 61.6 Gy arm (NS). No significant difference in grades 4 to 5 toxicities. **Conclusion: For definitive CRT for inoperable esophageal cancer, dose escalation to 61.6 Gy did not result in improved LC over 50.4 Gy for both ACA and SCC subtypes.**

Should elective nodal stations be targeted when treating patients definitively?

There is no strong evidence to suggest that elective nodal stations should not be included, and current NCCN guidelines suggest that the CTV should include elective nodes respective to the primary tumor location.[1] Of note, the randomized study from China below suggests nonelective treatment is safe.

Lyu (*Cancer Med* 2020, PMID 32841543): PRT of 228 stage II to III thoracic SCC esophageal patients randomized to involved field irradiation (IFI) or elective nodal irradiation (ENI). RT was delivered daily in 1.8 to 2 Gy/fx to a total dose of 60 to 66 Gy to the GTV and 50 to 54 Gy to the CTV. Initial results in 2018 revealed significant decreases in treatment-related esophagitis and pneumonitis in the IFI arm. In this current report, for ENI and IFI groups, respectively, PFS (20 vs. 21 months) and OS (33 vs 35 months) were similar. **Conclusion: IFI was associated with similar survival as ENI and is an acceptable treatment method for patients with thoracic esophageal SCC.**

RESECTABLE/OPERABLE ESOPHAGEAL CANCER

Is there benefit to trimodality therapy as compared with definitive CRT?

To date, there is no phase III evidence to suggest that surgery improves OS, although PFS appears to improve by reducing locoregional failure. Note that the Stahl trial limited the inclusion criteria to SCC only and that 90% of patients in the Bedenne trial had SCC.

Stahl, "Stahl I" (*JCO* 2005, PMID 15800321): Phase III PRT of 172 patients with locally advanced upper–mid SCC esophageal cancer, uT3–4N0–1M0, age ≥70, randomized to either (A) induction CHT, preop CRT (40 Gy/20 fx), then surgery; or (B) induction CHT, then definitive CRT (≥65 Gy) without surgery. Induction CHT was bolus 5-FU, leucovorin, etoposide, and cisplatin q3 weeks for three cycles. Concurrent CHT was cisplatin/etoposide (EP). In Arm B, T4 and obstructing T3 tumors received 50 Gy/25 fx, with EBRT boost to 65 Gy with 15 Gy/10 fx BID over the last week. For nonobstructing T3 tumors, patients received 60 Gy/30 fx with HDR brachytherapy boost of 4 Gy × 2 fx to 5 mm depth. MFU 6 years. No difference in 2-year OS (40% vs. 35%) or MS (16 vs. 15 months). The surgery arm had better 2-year PFS (64% vs. 41%, *p* = .003) due to improved LC, but also higher treatment-related mortality (13% vs. 4%, *p* = .03). In Arm A, only 66% proceeded to surgery, but complete resection was possible in 82% of those who did. Seventy percent of surgery patients had at least one severe complication; 11% postop hospital mortality; 35% had pCR. Response to induction CHT was associated with improved survival. **Conclusion: Adding surgery to CRT improves LC but does not improve OS. Patients who respond to induction treatment may be treated definitively with CRT, while poor responders may benefit from surgery.**

Bedenne, French FFCD 9102 (*JCO* 2007, PMID 17401004): Phase III PRT of operable T3N0–1M0 thoracic esophageal cancer patients comparing (A) neoadjuvant CRT followed by surgery vs. (B) higher dose definitive CRT in those with response to upfront CRT. Patients received two cycles of 5-FU and cisplatin (days 1–5 and 22–26) and either conventional (46 Gy in 4.5 weeks) or split-course (15 Gy, days 1–5 and 22–26) concomitant RT (investigator choice). Patients with response and no contraindication to either treatment were randomly assigned to surgery (Arm A) or continuation of CRT (Arm B; three additional cycles of 5-FU/cisplatin and either conventional [20 Gy] or split-course [15 Gy] RT). CRT was considered equivalent to surgery if difference in 2-year survival rate was <10%. Histologic composition: 90% SCC, 10% ACA. No difference in MS between Arm A and Arm B (17.7 vs. 19.3 months, *p* = .44). The 2-year LC improved with surgery (66% vs. 57%, *p* = .03). Fewer stents were required in the surgery arm (5% vs. 32%, *p* < .001). **Conclusion: LC is improved with surgery but no difference in OS.**

Does CHT with surgery improve OS compared with surgery alone?

Yes. Multiple trials studied neoadjuvant and perioperative regimens, with most demonstrating an OS benefit.[51,52] However, local response was often inadequate (pCR rates typically <5%). The MAGIC trial, investigating perioperative ECF (epirubicin, cisplatin, and fluorouracil) for gastric/GEJ cancers, showed improved OS for ECF + surgery compared with surgery alone.[53] FLOT-4, which compared perioperative FLOT with ECF, established FLOT as the perioperative CHT standard since it is superior to ECF.[36]

Does preoperative CRT improve OS compared with surgery alone?

Yes. The CROSS PRT found that trimodality therapy doubled OS compared with surgery alone.

Van Hagen, CROSS (*NEJM* 2012, PMID 22646630; Update Shapiro, *Lancet Oncol* 2015, PMID 26254683; Update Eyck, *JCO* 2021, PMID 33891478): Phase III PRT of neoadjuvant CRT + surgery vs. surgery alone. 366 potentially resectable patients randomized to carboplatin (AUC 2 mg/mm/min)/paclitaxel (50 mg/m^2) and concurrent RT (41.4 Gy/23 fx) followed by surgery (transthoracic or transhiatal approach) vs. surgery alone. Surgery was performed within 4 to 6 weeks of completion of CRT; 75% ACA, 23% SCC, and 2% had large-cell undifferentiated carcinoma. Initial publication showed that MS improved from 24 to 49.4 months with the addition of preop CRT (*p* = .003). Update with MFU 147 months. Complete resection (R0) rate was higher with CRT, 92% vs. 69% (*p* < .001). pCR in 29% overall (49% in SCC subgroup) of those treated with CRT. MS improved in CRT + surgery group vs. surgery alone (see Table 33.5); absolute 10-year OS benefit was 13%. Locoregional control remained strong at 10 years with CRT, but isolated distant relapse was comparable across arms. **Conclusion: Preoperative CRT improved MS among patients with potentially curable esophageal or GEJ cancer.**

Table 33.5 CROSS Trial of Neoadjuvant CRT for Esophageal Cancer			
	Neoadjuvant CRT + Surgery	Surgery Alone	p value
MS, all	48.6 months	24 months	.003
MS, SCC	81.6 months	21.1 months	.008
MS, ACA	43.2 months	27.1 months	.038

Does neoadjuvant CRT improve OS as compared with neoadjuvant/perioperative CHT?

Multiple trials and meta-analyses demonstrate conflicting results. The Stahl II trial supports benefit to CRT as compared with CHT alone, although it was underpowered. Furthermore, two large meta-analyses demonstrated among multiple treatment approaches that neoadjuvant CRT had the largest OS benefit.[54,55] More recently, NeoAEGIS demonstrated equipoise between modern perioperative CHT with modified MAGIC regimen (amended to include FLOT) and CROSS approach, although pCR/R0 resections were more likely with CRT. A more modern meta-analysis of RCTs directly comparing pre/perioperative CHT with neoadjuvant CRT for esophageal ACA demonstrated similar OS with either approach.[56] The ESOPEC trial directly compared perioperative FLOT with neoadjuvant CRT for esophageal ACA demonstrating improved OS with similar pCR rates for perioperative FLOT. In the setting of esophageal SCC, the JCOG 1109 NeXT trial showed similar OS between neoadjuvant triplet CHT and neoadjuvant CRT.

Stahl, "Stahl II" POET Trial (*JCO* 2009, PMID 19139439): Phase III PRT of neoadjuvant CHT vs. neoadjuvant CRT in patients with locally advanced (T3–4NxM0) resectable ACA of the GEJ; 126 patients (goal 394; closed due to poor accrual) randomized to (A) PLF (cisplatin/leucovorin/fluorouracil) × 2.5 cycles vs. (B) PLF × 2 cycles, then 3 weeks of CRT, 30 Gy/15 fx with EP. Both arms followed by tumor resection 3 to 4 weeks after induction. Comparing Arm A with Arm B, R0 resection: 70% vs. 72%; pCR: 2% vs. 16% ($p = .03$); 3-year OS: 28% vs. 47% ($p = .07$). **Conclusion: Preoperative CRT trends to improved OS compared with preoperative CHT alone.** *Comment: Trial closed early and is underpowered.*

Ronellenfitsch, Network Meta-Analysis (*JAMA Netw Open* 2024, PMID 39093560): Meta-analysis of 2,549 patients with esophageal ACA (gastric/SCC excluded) from 17 trials (conducted 1989–2016) comparing preoperative CRT + surgery with preoperative/perioperative CHT + surgery, one intervention with surgery alone, or all three treatments. Both preoperative CRT + surgery (HR 0.75, 95% CI 0.62–0.90) and pre/perioperative CHT (HR 0.78, 0.64–0.91) improved OS compared with surgery alone. Similar OS (HR 1.04, 0.83–1.28) was observed between CRT and pre/perioperative CHT. **Conclusion: For patients with esophageal ACA, both neoadjuvant CRT and pre/perioperative CHT approaches demonstrate similar efficacy.** *Comment: Few patients received FLOT, ESOPEC not included.*

Reynolds, Neo-AEGIS (*Lancet Gastroenter Hepatol* 2023, PMID 37734399): Phase III PRT of 377 patients with locally advanced esophageal ACA (T2–3N0–3) randomized to CROSS (carbo/taxol, 41.4 Gy RT) vs. perioperative CHT (MAGIC or FLOT) administered pre- and postsurgery. Eighty-four percent of patients were cT3; 58% cN1. MFU 39 months. No difference in median OS (48 months CHT vs. 49 months CRT) or median DFS (32 months CHT vs. 24 months CRT). Trimodality therapy improved pCR (OR 0.33, 95% CI 0.14–0.81), major pathologic response (0.21, 0.12–0.38), and R0 rates (0.21, 0.08–0.53). No differences in operative mortality (5 [3%] deaths in the perioperative CHT group vs. 4 [2%] in the trimodality group), major morbidity, or in global health status at 1 and 3 years. **Conclusion: Compared with CRT (CROSS regimen), perioperative CHT (FLOT or MAGIC) demonstrated similar OS and perioperative mortality with worse R0 rates and pathologic major/complete response.** *Comment: Trial was underpowered and incomplete (70% accrual) with multiple amendments.*

Hoeppner, ESOPEC (*NEJM* 2025, PMID 39842010): Phase III PRT of 438 patients with resectable locally advanced esophageal ACA (cT1–4aN1-3) randomized to CROSS regimen vs. perioperative FLOT. Primary endpoint OS. MFU 55 months. Median OS improved in FLOT arm (66 vs. 37 months). The 3-year OS rates were 57% for FLOT and 51% for CROSS (HR 0.70, 95% CI 0.53–0.92). pCR was achieved in 19% in FLOT and 14% in CROSS. **Conclusion: Perioperative FLOT improves OS in resectable esophageal ACA compared with CROSS. Grade 3 or higher toxicity was 47% in of FLOT and 42% in CROSS cohorts.** *Comment: pCR rate in the CROSS arm was lower than expected; adjuvant nivolumab not included in trial design.*

Kato, JCOG 1109 NExT (*Lancet* 2024, PMID 38876133): Phase III PRT of 601 patients with potentially resectable locally advanced esophageal SCC randomized to (a) preop cisplatin/5FU (CF), (b) preoperative docetaxel + cisplatin/5FU (DCF), or (c) RT (41.4 Gy) + cisplatin/5FU (CF-RT) followed by surgery. Primary endpoint OS. MFU 51 months. Compared with the CF group, the 3-year OS was significantly higher in the DCF group (72% vs. 63%; HR 0.68, 95% CI 0.50–0.92) but not in the CF-RT group (68%; HR 0.84, 0.63–1.12). Treatment-related adverse events leading to termination of neoadjuvant therapy were more common in the DCF group than in the CF-RT group (9% vs. 6%). **Conclusion: For esophageal SCC, neoadjuvant triplet CHT improves OS compared with doublet therapy but not compared with neoadjuvant CRT.**

Is there a role for adding neoadjuvant CRT to perioperative CHT?

In two trials, neoadjuvant CRT has demonstrated superior pCR over peri/preoperative CHT alone, but this has not translated to improved survival outcomes.[57,58] However, according to the results of ESOPEC, perioperative FLOT and CROSS appear to demonstrate similar pCR rates. Theoretically, combining perioperative CHT and neoadjuvant CRT approaches may improve pCR and survival outcomes. The TOPGEAR trial evaluated the addition of CRT to perioperative CHT (FLOT accounted for 33%) for gastric/GEJ ACA and found improved pCR but no difference in OS or PFS. Paradigms involving organ preservation for patients with pCR following this approach are currently under investigation.[59,60]

Leong, TOPGEAR (*NEJM* 2024, PMID 39282905): Phase III PRT of 574 patients with resectable ACA of the stomach or GEJ randomized to perioperative CHT (either ECX/ECF or FLOT) ± preoperative CRT (45 Gy/25 fx + continuous 5-FU). One less cycle of preoperative CHT delivered in those receiving CRT. GEJ accounted for one-third of patients. FLOT was received by 33% of patients. MFU 67 months. No differences observed in median OS or PFS between cohorts. More patients in the CRT group had a pCR (17% vs. 8%) and greater tumor downstaging. Toxicity was similar. **Conclusion: Addition of neoadjuvant CRT to perioperative CHT did not improve PFS or OS but did improve pCR.**

Is there a role for neoadjuvant or adjuvant immunotherapy?

CheckMate 577 supports the addition of adjuvant nivolumab following preoperative CRT for those patients achieving R0 resection but with an incomplete pathologic response. In the setting of gastric/GEJ ACA, KEYNOTE-585 demonstrated improved pCR but no benefit to EFS or OS with the addition of IO to neoadjuvant CHT. Similarly, ATTRACTION-5 found no improvement in RFS among gastric/GEJ cancer treated with adjuvant nivolumab following upfront surgery.[41] The DANTE trial evaluating the addition of atezolizumab to perioperative FLOT has demonstrated improved pCR at interim analysis, with phase III endpoints awaited.[61] For patients with ACA that is MSI-H/dMMR, the NEONIPIGA phase II trial demonstrated an impressive pCR rate of 58% with perioperative nivolumab/ipilimumab, and thus addition of IO should be considered for this population.[1,42]

Kelly, CheckMate 577 (*NEJM* 2021, PMID 33789008): Phase III PRT of 794 patients with resected (R0) stage II to III esophageal/GEJ cancer without a pCR who had received neoadjuvant CRT randomized to adjuvant nivolumab (240 mg every 2 weeks for 16 weeks, then 480 mg every 4 weeks for 1 year) vs. observation. MFU 24.4 months. Median DFS was significantly better in the nivolumab group (HR 0.69, 95% CI 0.56–0.86). **Conclusion: DFS was improved with adjuvant nivolumab among patients with resected esophageal/GEJ cancer that received neoadjuvant CRT and achieved R0 resection with incomplete pathologic response.**

If a patient gets initial surgery, what is the role of adjuvant therapy?

The McDonald trial (INT 0116) evaluated the role of adjuvant CRT in patients with GEJ or gastric cancer and demonstrated an improvement in 3-year OS (from 41% to 50%, p = .005) in those who received adjuvant CRT (bolus 5-FU + leucovorin with concurrent RT, 45 Gy/25 fx).[62] A meta-analysis of over 6,000 patients from 33 RCTs with resectable esophageal carcinoma found no significant advantage in OS in patients who received surgery + adjuvant therapy (HR 0.87, 95% CI 0.67–1.14), whereas neoadjuvant therapies followed by surgery were associated with a survival advantage (HR 0.83, 0.76–0.90).[63]

Is there benefit to IMRT for esophageal cancer?

3D-conformal RT via three or four fields is the standard technique for esophageal cancer, with NCCN suggesting IMRT in cases when OAR constraints cannot be met.[1] Retrospective data suggest IMRT benefit with respect to cardiac toxicity, but selection and follow-up bias remains the issue and further study is necessary. Guidelines for IMRT planning are available.[64]

Lin, MDACC (*IJROBP* 2012, PMID 22867894): RR of 676 patients (413 3D-CRT, 263 IMRT) with stage IB to IVA esophageal cancer treated with CRT (46% also received surgery) from 1998 to 2008 at MDACC. Inverse probability-weighted adjusted Cox model used to compare OS. OS was independently associated with stage, performance status, PET staging, induction CHT, and treatment modality (IMRT vs. 3D-CRT, HR 0.72, $p < .001$). Compared with IMRT, 3D-CRT patients had significantly greater risk of dying (73% vs. 53%, $p < .0001$) and of LRR ($p = .004$). No difference seen in cancer-specific mortality ($p = .86$) or DM ($p = .99$). Increased cumulative incidence of cardiac death in 3D-CRT group ($p = .049$), as well as undocumented deaths (5-year estimate: 12% in 3D-CRT vs. 5% in IMRT, $p = .003$). **Conclusion: IMRT should be considered for the treatment of esophageal cancer.**

PROTON THERAPY

Proton therapy (PBT) in the setting of thoracic tumors, including esophageal cancer, remains investigational. However, the study by Lin et al. is the first published randomized study of proton vs. photon RT and bears knowing, even for its unusual endpoint.

Lin (*JCO* 2020, PMID 32160096): Phase IIB randomized trial of PBT vs. IMRT (50.4 Gy) in stage II to III unresectable and potentially resectable esophageal cancer patients eligible to receive concurrent CHT; 145 patients randomly assigned (72 IMRT, 73 PBT) and 107 patients (61 IMRT, 46 PBT) evaluable. Primary endpoints were total toxicity burden (TTB) and PFS. TTB synthesizes the cumulative severity of multiple AEs that patients may experience after CHT-RT with or without surgery. The posterior mean TTB was 2.3 times higher for IMRT (40; 95% highest posterior density interval, 26–55) than PBT (17; 11–25). The mean postoperative complication score was 7.6× higher for IMRT (19; 7–32) vs. PBT (3; 0.3–5). The posterior probability that mean TTB was lower for PBT compared with IMRT was 0.9989, which exceeded the trial's stopping boundary of 0.9942 at the 67% interim analysis. The 3-year PFS (~51%) and OS (~45%) rates were similar in both arms. **Conclusion: PBT for neoadjuvant or definitive treatment of locally advanced esophageal cancer produced a lower toxicity profile, but with similar PFS and OS compared with IMRT.**

ESOPHAGEAL BRACHYTHERAPY

What is the role for esophageal brachytherapy in the modern era?

Classically, brachytherapy was developed as a boost to EBRT and for palliation of dysphagia related to esophageal cancer. ABS consensus guidelines have been established for brachytherapy.[46] Brachytherapy is less utilized in the modern era, likely due to availability of other advanced RT techniques, limited indications, and potential complications.

Does brachytherapy boost improve outcomes when added to definitive CRT?

This was investigated in RTOG 9207, a phase I/II study of definitive CRT to 50 Gy/25 fx with cisplatin/5-FU followed by brachytherapy boost (if HDR: initially 15 Gy/3 fx, then reduced to 10 Gy/2 fx prescribed to 1 cm depth; if LDR: 20 Gy in 1 fx).[48] Results showed a 12% fistula rate that was lethal in 50% of patients, and outcomes were no better than prior trials looking at CRT alone. Of note, CHT was given concurrently with brachytherapy in this trial and may have contributed to high toxicity rates.

Which is the most effective method of palliation: metal stent or brachytherapy?

Homs, Dutch SIREC (*Lancet* 2004, PMID 15500894): Phase III PRT of 209 patients with either metastatic disease or medically inoperable esophageal/GEJ cancer randomized to stent or brachytherapy 12 Gy/fx (10 mm diameter applicator, prescribed to 1 cm from source axis, sucralfate × 4 weeks, lifelong omeprazole). Excluded tumors >12 cm, fistula, tumor within 3 cm of UES, previous RT, or stent. Primary endpoint was physician-reported dysphagia; patient-reported outcomes recorded as well. Stenting demonstrated more rapid relief; brachytherapy demonstrated more long-term relief. Late hemorrhage occurred more with stenting (33% vs. 22%, $p = .02$); QOL scores favored brachytherapy, and medical costs were similar; fistula formation occurred in three patients in each group. **Conclusion: Brachytherapy has more durable dysphagia relief and fewer complications than stenting.**

REFERENCES

1.   Ajani JA, D'Amico TA, Bentrem DJ, et al. Esophageal and esophagogastric junction cancers, version 4.2024, NCCN clinical practice guidelines in oncology. *J Natl Compr Canc Netw.* 2024;21(4):393–422. doi:10.6004/jnccn.2023.0019

2.   Siegel RL, Giaquinto AN, Jemal A. Cancer statistics, 2024. *CA Cancer J Clin.* 2024;74(1):12–49. doi:10.3322/caac.21820

3.   Uhlenhopp DJ, Then EO, Sunkara T, Gaduputi V. Epidemiology of esophageal cancer: update in global trends, etiology and risk factors. *Clin J Gastroenterol.* 2020;13(6):1010–1021. doi:10.1007/s12328-020-01237-x

4.   Rustgi AK, El-Serag HB. Esophageal carcinoma. *N Engl J Med.* 2014;371(26):2499–2509. doi:10.1056/nejmra1314530

5.   Hvid-Jensen F, Pedersen L, Drewes AM, Sørensen HT, Funch-Jensen P. Incidence of adenocarcinoma among patients with barrett's esophagus. *N Engl J Med.* 2011;365(15):1375–1383. doi:10.1056/nejmoa1103042

6.   de Jonge PJ, van Blankenstein M, Looman CWN, Casparie MK, Meijer GA, Kuipers EJ. Risk of malignant progression in patients with Barrett's oesophagus: a Dutch nationwide cohort study. *Gut.* 2010;59(8):1030–1036. doi:10.1136/gut.2009.176701

7.   Rubenstein JH, Taylor JB. Meta-analysis: the association of oesophageal adenocarcinoma with symptoms of gastro-oesophageal reflux. *Aliment Pharmacol Ther.* 2010;32(10):1222–1227. doi:10.1111/j.1365-2036.2010.04471.x

8.   Rüdiger Siewert J, Feith M, Werner M, Stein HJ. Adenocarcinoma of the esophagogastric junction: results of surgical therapy based on anatomical/topographic classification in 1,002 consecutive patients. *Ann Surg.* 2000;232(3):353–361. doi:10.1097/00000658-200009000-00007

9.   Siewert JR, Stein HJ. Classification of adenocarcinoma of the oesophagogastric junction. *Br J Surg.* 1998;85(11):1457–1459. doi:10.1046/j.1365-2168.1998.00940.x

10.   Gowryshankar A, Nagaraja V, Eslick GD. HER2 status in Barrett's esophagus & esophageal cancer: a meta analysis. *J Gastrointest Oncol.* 2014;5(1):25–35. doi:10.3978/j.issn.2078-6891.2013.039

11.   Bartley AN, Washington MK, Ismaila N, Ajani JA. HER2 testing and clinical decision making in gastroesophageal adenocarcinoma: guideline summary from the college of American pathologists, American society for clinical pathology, and American society of clinical oncology. *J Oncol Pract.* 2017;13(1):53–57. doi:10.1200/jop.2016.018929

12.   van Westreenen HL, Westerterp M, Bossuyt PMM, et al. Systematic review of the staging performance of 18F-fluorodeoxyglucose positron emission tomography in esophageal cancer. *J Clin Oncol.* 2004;22(18):3805–3812. doi:10.1200/jco.2004.01.083

13.   Lightdale CJ, Kulkarni KG. Role of endoscopic ultrasonography in the staging and follow-up of esophageal cancer. *J Clin Oncol.* 2005;23(20):4483–4489. doi:10.1200/jco.2005.20.644

14.   McNamara MJ, Adelstein DJ, Allende DS, et al. Persistent dysphagia after induction chemotherapy in patients with esophageal adenocarcinoma predicts poor post-operative outcomes. *J Gastrointest Cancer.* 2017;48(2):181–189. doi:10.1007/s12029-016-9881-x

15.   Thomas CR Jr, Berkey BA, Minsky BD, et al. Recursive partitioning analysis of pretreatment variables of 416 patients with locoregional esophageal cancer treated with definitive concomitant chemoradiotherapy on Intergroup and Radiation Therapy Oncology Group trials. *Int J Radiat Oncol Biol Phys.* 2004;58(5):1405–1410. doi:10.1016/j.ijrobp.2003.09.022

16.   Hulscher JB, van Sandick JW, de Boer AG, et al. Extended transthoracic resection compared with limited transhiatal resection for adenocarcinoma of the esophagus. *N Engl J Med.* 2002;347(21):1662–1669. doi:10.1056/nejmoa022343

17.   Karl RC, Schreiber R, Boulware D, Baker S, Coppola D. Factors affecting morbidity, mortality, and survival in patients undergoing Ivor Lewis esophagogastrectomy. *Ann Surg.* 2000;231(5):635–643. doi:10.1097/00000658-200005000-00003

18.   Orringer MB, Marshall B, Chang AC, Lee J, Pickens A, Lau CL. Two thousand transhiatal esophagectomies: changing trends, lessons learned. *Ann Surg.* 2007;246(3):363–374. doi:10.1097/sla.0b013e31814697f2

19.   Orringer MB, Marshall B, Iannettoni MD. Transhiatal esophagectomy: clinical experience and refinements. *Ann Surg.* 1999;230(3):392. doi:10.1097/00000658-199909000-00012

20.   Bedenne L, Michel P, Bouché O, et al. Chemoradiation followed by surgery compared with chemoradiation alone in squamous cancer of the esophagus: FFCD 9102. *J Clin Oncol.* 2007;25(10):1160–1168. doi:10.1200/jco.2005.04.7118

21.   Bosset JF, Gignoux M, Triboulet JP, et al. Chemoradiotherapy followed by surgery compared with surgery alone in squamous-cell cancer of the esophagus. *N Engl J Med.* 1997;337(3):161–167. doi:10.1056/nejm199707173370304

22. Stahl M, Stuschke M, Lehmann N, et al. Chemoradiation with and without surgery in patients with locally advanced squamous cell carcinoma of the esophagus. *J Clin Oncol.* 2005;23(10):2310–2317. doi:10.1200/jco.2005.00.034

23. Bogoevski D, Onken F, Koenig A, et al. Is it time for a new TNM classification in esophageal carcinoma? *Ann Surg.* 2008;247(4):633–641. doi:10.1097/sla.0b013e3181656d07

24. Greenstein AJ, Litle VR, Swanson SJ, Divino CM, Packer S, Wisnivesky JP. Effect of the number of lymph nodes sampled on postoperative survival of lymph node-negative esophageal cancer. *Cancer.* 2008;112(6):1239–1246. doi:10.1002/cncr.23309

25. Hu Y, Hu C, Zhang H, Ping Y, Chen LQ. How does the number of resected lymph nodes influence TNM staging and prognosis for esophageal carcinoma? *Ann Surg Oncol.* 2010;17(3):784–790. doi:10.1245/s10434-009-0818-5

26. Peyre CG, Hagen JA, DeMeester SR, et al. The number of lymph nodes removed predicts survival in esophageal cancer: an international study on the impact of extent of surgical resection. *Ann Surg.* 2008;248(4):549–556. doi:10.1097/sla.0b013e318188c474

27. Biere SS, van Berge Henegouwen MI, Maas KW, et al. Minimally invasive versus open oesophagectomy for patients with oesophageal cancer: a multicentre, open-label, randomised controlled trial. *Lancet.* 2012;379(9829):1887–1892. doi:10.1016/s0140-6736(12)60516-9

28. Mariette C, Markar S, Dabakuyo-Yonli TS, et al. Health-related quality of life following hybrid minimally invasive versus open esophagectomy for patients with esophageal cancer, analysis of a multicenter, open-label, randomized phase III controlled trial: the MIRO trial. *Ann Surg.* 2019;271(6):1023–1029. doi:10.1097/sla.0000000000003559

29. van der Sluis PC, van der Horst S, May AM, et al. Robot-assisted minimally invasive thoracolaparoscopic esophagectomy versus open transthoracic esophagectomy for resectable esophageal cancer. *Ann Surg.* 2019;269(4):621–630. doi:10.1097/sla.0000000000003031

30. Yang Y, Li B, Yi J, et al. Robot-assisted versus conventional minimally invasive esophagectomy for resectable esophageal squamous cell carcinoma: early results of a multicenter randomized controlled trial: the RAMIE trial. *Ann Surg.* 2022;275(4):646–653. doi:10.1097/SLA.0000000000005023

31. Wagner AD, Grothe W, Haerting J, Kleber G, Grothey A, Fleig WE. Chemotherapy in advanced gastric cancer: a systematic review and meta-analysis based on aggregate data. *J Clin Oncol.* 2006;24(18):2903–2909. doi:10.1200/jco.2005.05.0245

32. Crosby T, Hurt CN, Falk S, et al. Chemoradiotherapy with or without cetuximab in patients with oesophageal cancer (SCOPE1): a multicentre, phase 2/3 randomised trial. *Lancet Oncol.* 2013;14(7):627–637. doi:10.1016/s1470-2045(13)70136-0

33. Suntharalingam M, Winter K, Ilson D, et al. Effect of the addition of cetuximab to paclitaxel, cisplatin, and radiation therapy for patients with esophageal cancer: the NRG Oncology RTOG 0436 Phase 3 randomized clinical trial. *JAMA Oncol.* 2017;3(11):1520–1528. doi:10.1001/jamaoncol.2017.1598

34. Safran HP, Winter K, Ilson DH, et al. Trastuzumab with trimodality treatment for oesophageal adenocarcinoma with HER2 overexpression (NRG Oncology/RTOG 1010): a multicentre, randomised, phase 3 trial. *Lancet Oncol.* 2022;23(2):259–269. doi:10.1016/s1470-2045(21)00718-x

35. Bang YJ, Van Cutsem E, Feyereislova A, et al. Trastuzumab in combination with chemotherapy versus chemotherapy alone for treatment of HER2-positive advanced gastric or gastro-oesophageal junction cancer (ToGA): a phase 3, open-label, randomised controlled trial. *Lancet.* 2010;376(9742):687–697. doi:10.1016/s0140-6736(10)61121-x

36. Al-Batran SE, Homann N, Pauligk C, et al. Perioperative chemotherapy with fluorouracil plus leucovorin, oxaliplatin, and docetaxel versus fluorouracil or capecitabine plus cisplatin and epirubicin for locally advanced, resectable gastric or gastro-oesophageal junction adenocarcinoma (FLOT4): a randomised, phase 2/3 trial. *Lancet.* 2019;393(10184):1948–1957. doi:10.1016/s0140-6736(18)32557-1

37. Hoeppner J, Brunner T, Lordick F, et al. Prospective randomized multicenter phase III trial comparing perioperative chemotherapy (FLOT protocol) to neoadjuvant chemoradiation (CROSS protocol) in patients with adenocarcinoma of the esophagus (ESOPEC trial). *J Clin Oncol.* 2024;42(17_suppl):LBA1. doi:10.1200/JCO.2024.42.17_suppl.LBA1

38. Kato K, Machida R, Ito Y, et al. Doublet chemotherapy, triplet chemotherapy, or doublet chemotherapy combined with radiotherapy as neoadjuvant treatment for locally advanced oesophageal cancer (JCOG1109 NExT): a randomised, controlled, open-label, phase 3 trial. *Lancet.* 2024;404(10447):55–66. doi:10.1016/S0140-6736(24)00745-1

39. Kelly RJ, Ajani JA, Kuzdzal J, et al. Adjuvant nivolumab in resected esophageal or gastroesophageal junction cancer. *N Engl J Med.* 2021;384(13):1191–1203. doi:10.1056/NEJMoa2032125

40. Shitara K, Rha SY, Wyrwicz LS, et al. Neoadjuvant and adjuvant pembrolizumab plus chemotherapy in locally advanced gastric or gastro-oesophageal cancer (KEYNOTE-585): an interim analysis of the multicentre, double-blind, randomised phase 3 study. *Lancet Oncol.* 2024;25(2):212–224. doi:10.1016/S1470-2045(23)00541-7

41. Terashima M, Kang YK, Kim YW, et al. ATTRACTION-5: a phase 3 study of nivolumab plus chemotherapy as postoperative adjuvant treatment for pathological stage III (pStage III) Gastric or Gastroesophageal Junction (G/GEJ) cancer. *J Clin Oncol.* 2023;41(16_suppl):4000. doi:10.1200/JCO.2023.41.16_suppl.4000

42. André T, Tougeron D, Piessen G, et al. Neoadjuvant nivolumab plus ipilimumab and adjuvant nivolumab in localized deficient mismatch repair/microsatellite instability–high gastric or esophagogastric junction adenocarcinoma: the GERCOR NEONIPIGA phase II study. *J Clin Oncol.* 2023;41(2):255–265. doi:10.1200/JCO.22.00686

43. Crehange G, M'Vondo C, Bertaut A, et al. Exclusive chemoradiotherapy with or without radiation dose escalation in esophageal cancer: multicenter phase 2/3 randomized trial CONCORDE (PRODIGE-26). *Int J Radiat Oncol Biol Phys.* 2021;111(3):S5. doi:10.1016/j.ijrobp.2021.07.045

44. Herskovic A, Martz K, Al-Sarraf M, et al. Combined chemotherapy and radiotherapy compared with radiotherapy alone in patients with cancer of the esophagus. *N Engl J Med.* 1992;326(24):1593–1598. doi:10.1056/nejm199206113262403

45. Hulshof MCCM, Geijsen ED, Rozema T, et al. Randomized study on dose escalation in definitive chemoradiation for patients with locally advanced esophageal cancer (ARTDECO Study). *J Clin Oncol.* 2021;39(25):2816–2824. doi:10.1200/jco.20.03697

46. Minsky BD, Pajak TF, Ginsberg RJ, et al. INT 0123 (Radiation Therapy Oncology Group 94-05) phase III trial of combined-modality therapy for esophageal cancer: high-dose versus standard-dose radiation therapy. *J Clin Oncol.* 2002;20(5):1167–1174. doi:10.1200/jco.2002.20.5.1167

47. Gaspar LE, Nag S, Herskovic A, Mantravadi R, Speiser B, Committee ABSPPATCR. American Brachytherapy Society (ABS) consensus guidelines for brachytherapy of esophageal cancer. *Int J Radiat Oncol Biol Phys.* 1997;38(1):127–132. doi:10.1016/s0360-3016(97)00231-9

48. Gaspar LE, Winter K, Kocha WI, Coia LR, Herskovic A, Graham M. A phase I/II study of external beam radiation, brachytherapy, and concurrent chemotherapy for patients with localized carcinoma of the esophagus (Radiation Therapy Oncology Group Study 9207): final report. *Cancer.* 2000;88(5):988–995. PMID:10699886

49. Videtic GMM, Woody NM, Vassil AD. *Handbook of Treatment Planning in Radiation Oncology.* 3rd ed. Demos Medical; 2020.

50. Brower JV, Chen S, Bassetti MF, et al. Radiation dose escalation in esophageal cancer revisited: a contemporary analysis of the national cancer data base, 2004 to 2012. *Int J Radiat Oncol Biol Phys.* 2016;96(5):985–993. doi:10.1016/j.ijrobp.2016.08.016

51. Ychou M, Boige V, Pignon JP, et al. Perioperative chemotherapy compared with surgery alone for resectable gastroesophageal adenocarcinoma: an FNCLCC and FFCD multicenter phase III trial. *J Clin Oncol.* 2011;29(13):1715–1721. doi:10.1200/jco.2010.33.0597

52. Medical Research Council Oesophageal Cancer Working Group. Surgical resection with or without preoperative chemotherapy in oesophageal cancer: a randomised controlled trial. *Lancet.* 2002;359(9319):1727–1733. doi:10.1016/s0140-6736(02)08651-8

53. Cunningham D, Allum WH, Stenning SP, et al. Perioperative chemotherapy versus surgery alone for resectable gastroesophageal cancer. *N Engl J Med.* 2006;355(1):11–20. doi:10.1056/NEJMoa055531

54. Gebski V, Burmeister B, Smithers BM, et al. Survival benefits from neoadjuvant chemoradiotherapy or chemotherapy in oesophageal carcinoma: a meta-analysis. *Lancet Oncol.* 2007;8(3):226–234. doi:10.1016/S1470-2045(07)70039-6

55. Pasquali S, Yim G, Vohra RS, et al. Survival after neoadjuvant and adjuvant treatments compared to surgery alone for resectable esophageal carcinoma: a network meta-analysis. *Ann Surg.* 2017;265(3):481–491. doi:10.1097/SLA.0000000000001905

56. Ronellenfitsch U, Friedrichs J, Barbier E, et al. Preoperative chemoradiotherapy vs chemotherapy for adenocarcinoma of the esophagogastric junction: a network meta-analysis. *JAMA Netw Open.* 2024;7(8):e2425581. doi:10.1001/jamanetworkopen.2024.25581

57. Klevebro F, Alexandersson von Döbeln G, Wang N, et al. A randomized clinical trial of neoadjuvant chemotherapy versus neoadjuvant chemoradiotherapy for cancer of the oesophagus or gastro-oesophageal junction. *Ann Oncol.* 2016;27(4):660–667. doi:10.1093/annonc/mdw010

58. Reynolds JV, Preston SR, O'Neill B, et al. Trimodality therapy versus perioperative chemotherapy in the management of locally advanced adenocarcinoma of the oesophagus and oesophagogastric junction (Neo-AEGIS): an open-label, randomised, phase 3 trial. *Lancet Gastroenterol Hepatol.* 2023;8(11):1015–1027. doi:10.1016/S2468-1253(23)00243-1

59. Lorenzen S, Biederstädt A, Ronellenfitsch U, et al. RACE-trial: neoadjuvant radiochemotherapy versus chemotherapy for patients with locally advanced, potentially resectable adenocarcinoma of the gastroesophageal junction-a randomized phase III joint study of the AIO, ARO and DGAV. *BMC Cancer.* 2020;20(1):886. doi:10.1186/s12885-020-07388-x

60. van der Wilk BJ, Eyck BM, Wijnhoven BPL, et al. LBA75 Neoadjuvant chemoradiotherapy followed by surgery versus active surveillance for oesophageal cancer (SANO-trial): a phase-III stepped-wedge cluster randomised trial. *Ann Oncol.* 2023;34(2):S1317. doi:10.1016/j.annonc.2023.10.076

61. Lorenzen S, Götze TO, Thuss-Patience P, et al. Perioperative atezolizumab plus fluorouracil, leucovorin, oxaliplatin, and docetaxel for resectable esophagogastric cancer: interim results from the randomized, multicenter, phase II/III DANTE/IKF-s633 trial. *J Clin Oncol.* 2024;42(4):410–420. doi:10.1200/JCO.23.00975

62. Macdonald JS, Smalley SR, Benedetti J, et al. Chemoradiotherapy after surgery compared with surgery alone for adenocarcinoma of the stomach or gastroesophageal junction. *N Engl J Med.* 2001;345(10):725–730. doi:10.1056/nejmoa010187

63. Pasquali S, Yim G, Vohra RS, et al. Survival after neoadjuvant and adjuvant treatments compared to surgery alone for resectable esophageal carcinoma. *Ann Surg.* 2017;265(3):481–491. doi:10.1097/sla.0000000000001905

64. Wu AJ, Bosch WR, Chang DT, et al. Expert consensus contouring guidelines for intensity modulated radiation therapy in esophageal and gastroesophageal junction cancer. *Int J Radiat Oncol Biol Phys.* 2015;92(4):911–920. doi:10.1016/j.ijrobp.2015.03.030

34 GASTRIC CANCER

Ahmed Halima, Kevin L. Stephans, and Gregory M. M. Videtic

QUICK HIT Most gastric patients present with locoregionally advanced or metastatic disease. For cT2–4 or N+ locoregionally confined disease, management involves surgery, perioperative CHT, preoperative CRT, or postoperative CRT (Table 34.1). Surgery can be either partial or total gastrectomy depending on disease location and extent, with regional lymph node dissection (D2 dissection recommended including ≥15 LNs).

Table 34.1 General Treatment Paradigm for Gastric Cancer[1]	
Tis/T1a (≤3 cm, nonulcerated, well-differentiated)	• Endoscopic mucosal resection or endoscopic submucosal dissection or surgery
T1a–bN0	• Gastrectomy and regional lymph node dissection (LND) • No adjuvant therapy indicated
T2–4N0-3 or T1N+	• Gastrectomy and regional LND • Perioperative CHT (category 1) or preoperative CRT (category 2B) • For pT2N0, who have not received preoperative CHT or CRT: observation or adjuvant CHT and RT for patients with high-risk features (poorly differentiated or higher grade cancer, LVI, neural invasion, or <50 years of age, or patients who did not undergo D2 LND) • Consider neoadjuvant or perioperative immunotherapy (IO) if tumor is MSI-H/dMMR • Adjuvant CHT and RT indicated for T2–T4 or LN+ disease • Adjuvant RT (per INT 0116): 45 Gy/25 fx starting on day 29 of CHT (5 cycles of bolus 5-FU/LCV) • Adjuvant CRT for R1 or R2 who have not received preoperative CHT ± RT
M1	• Palliative CHT and/or RT

Source: NCCN. NCCN Clinical Practice Guidelines in Oncology. Gastric Cancer. 5.2024.

EPIDEMIOLOGY: Gastric cancer has an estimated incidence of 26,890 cases and estimated deaths of 10,880 in the United States in 2024.[2] Gastric cancer is the 15th leading cause of cancer death in the United States and the fourth leading cause of cancer death worldwide. It is most common in East Asia (China, Japan, Korea, and Taiwan), with the lowest incidence in the United States and Canada. In the United States, the most common location is within the proximal stomach (GEJ and cardia).[3]

RISK FACTORS: Increased salt intake, salt-preserved foods (salted fish, cured meat, and salted vegetables), nitrates, smoked and processed meats, fried food, low consumption of fruits and vegetables, and low vitamin A and C.[4–6] Obesity (BMI ≥25, OR 1.22),[7] smoking,[8] and pathogens such as *Helicobacter pylori* and Epstein–Barr virus.[9,10] Hereditary syndromes due to HDGC, GAPPS, and FIGC represent about 1% to 3% of cases.[11]

ANATOMY

Stomach: Starts at GEJ (40–45 cm from incisions) and ends at pylorus. There are three main parts: fundus/cardia, body, and antrum/pylorus. There are five layers of stomach (starting from luminal surface): mucosa, submucosa, muscularis (outer longitudinal, middle circular, inner oblique), subserosa, and serosa. Gastric submucosal plexus is rich, and carcinoma can spread superficially along the stomach to the esophagus, which also has rich submucosal plexus. Access to subserosal channels allows distal tumor spread to duodenum via subserosal lymphatic plexus.

Vascular: Vascular supply is derived from celiac axis, which is composed of three branches (Table 34.2).

Table 34.2 Vascular Supply of Stomach		
Celiac axis	Branches	Supply
Left gastric	Esophageal and gastric	Lesser curvature/right portion of stomach
Common hepatic	Right gastric	Lesser curvature/inferior right stomach
	Right gastroepiploic	Greater curvature
Splenic	Left gastroepiploic	Upper portion of greater curvature
	Short gastrics	Fundus/proximal stomach

Lymphatics: JRSGC proposed 16 regional LN stations for stomach in 1963. See Table 34.3. N1/2 LN stations are considered regional and N3/4 are considered distant.[12]

Table 34.3 JRSGC Nodal Stations		
N1	1	Right cardia
	2	Left cardia
	3	Lesser curvature
	4	Greater curvature
	5	Suprapyloric
	6	Infrapyloric
N2	7	Left gastric artery
	8	Common hepatic artery
	9	Celiac axis
	10	Splenic hila
	11	Splenic artery
N3	12	Hepatoduodenal ligament
	13	Post. pancreatic head
	14	Mesenteric root
N4	15	Transverse mesocolon
	16	Para-aortic

PATHOLOGY: Adenocarcinoma (ACA) is the most common histology (90%–95%), followed by MALT lymphoma. Rare histologies include leiomyosarcoma (2%), carcinoid (1%), adenoacanthoma (1%), and squamous cell carcinoma (1%).

Lauren Histologic Classification: There are two distinct types of ACA (intestinal and diffuse types). Intestinal type is more likely to be associated with environmental exposures (*H. pylori*, chronic gastritis, tobacco, diet), is more prevalent in high-incidence areas, and has better prognosis. Diffuse type (also known as "linitis plastica") tends to present as diffuse involvement of the gastric mucosa, is characterized by organized clusters of signet ring (mucin-rich) cells, is more predominant in younger women, and is associated with poorer prognosis.[14]

Siewert Classification of GEJ Tumors (Based on Location): Class I: arises from metaplasia of the distal esophagus and invades distally into the stomach; Class II: arises from gastric cardia; Class III: arises from subcardia and invades proximally into the esophagus.[15]

Bormann Classification: Class I: polypoid/fungating; Class II: ulcerative with raised borders; Class III: ulceration with invasion into gastric wall; Class IV: diffuse infiltration (linitis plastic).[16]

GENETICS: Her2 positivity was seen in 22% of patients screened for ToGA trial.[17]

SCREENING: Observational studies suggest that screening in high-incidence areas may reduce gastric cancer mortality; however, there are no randomized data to support this finding.[18,19] Population-based screening has been implemented in Japan, Korea, Venezuela, and Chile, although screening intervals and modalities vary and randomized data have not established an optimal program.[18,20,21] In Japan, universal screening is recommended for all individuals >50 years of age, with upper endoscopy every 2 to 3 years or double-contrast barium study every year. Alternatively, in Korea, upper endoscopy is recommended every 2 years for those 40 to 75 years of age.[22] In the United States, screening can be considered for patients with atrophic gastritis, pernicious anemia, gastric adenomas, Barrett esophagus, and familial gastric cancer syndromes.

CLINICAL PRESENTATION: Symptoms include weight loss, epigastric pain, nausea, vomiting, anorexia, dysphagia, early satiety, melena, and weakness. Characteristic physical exam findings include palpable stomach, succussion splash, palpable lymphadenopathy: Virchow's node (left supraclavicular), Irish's node (left axillary node), Sister Mary Joseph node (periumbilical node), Blumer's shelf (rectal shelf), and Krukenberg tumor (metastatic deposit to ovary).

WORKUP: H&P.

Labs: CBC, CMP.

Imaging: Includes CT chest, abdomen, pelvis with IV and oral contrast. Consider PET/CT in the absence of M1 disease on CT scans.

Pathology: EGD with biopsies (six to eight biopsies should be obtained), and endoscopic ultrasound to assess for tumor invasion and LN staging. Diagnostic laparoscopy to assess peritoneal cavity prior to surgery is indicated for clinical stage T1b and higher.[1] Obtain Her2-Neu status if metastatic.[1]

PROGNOSTIC FACTORS: Poor KPS, advanced T and N stage, subtotal resection or gross residual disease (R2 > R1 > R0), and diffuse-type histology are all poor prognostic features.[21] Retrospective multicenter study from Italy demonstrated that patients with 0, 1 to 3, 4 to 6, and >6 LNs involved had 10-year OS after surgery of 92%, 82%, 73%, and 27%, respectively.[23] Metabolic response (≥35% decrease in PET SUV max) after neoadjuvant CHT is associated with improved MS.[24]

NATURAL HISTORY: Majority of patients (90%) present with locally advanced or metastatic disease, with 80% presenting with nodal metastases, 40% peritoneal metastases, and 30% liver metastases, for which prognosis is poor. Patients with early-stage gastric cancer (≤T1bN0) have excellent outcomes: 5-year OS of 100% with mucosal invasion and 80% to 90% with submucosal involvement.[25]

STAGING: Cancers with midpoint in lower thoracic esophagus, GEJ, or within the proximal 5 cm of the stomach *and* extending to the GE junction or esophagus are staged as *esophageal neoplasms*. Cancers with midpoint in stomach >5 cm distal to GEJ or within 5 cm of GEJ but *not* involving GEJ or esophagus are staged as gastric cancer. AJCC is based on number of nodes, whereas JRSGC is based on anatomic location. Positive peritoneal cytology is defined as pM1. See Table 34.4.

T/M	N	cN0	cN1	cN2	cN3a	cN3b
Table 34.4 AJCC 8th Edition (2017): Gastric Cancer Staging[13]						
T1	a. Lamina propria or muscularis mucosae	I	IIA			
	b. Submucosa					
T2	• Muscularis propria					
T3	• Subserosal connective tissue	IIB	III			
T4	a. Visceral peritoneum					
	b. Adjacent organs	IVA				
M1	• Distant metastasis	IVB				

cN1: 1–2 regional LNs; cN2: 3–6 regional LNs; cN3a: 7–15 regional LNs; cN3b: ≥16 regional LNs.

TREATMENT PARADIGM

Surgery: Surgery is the mainstay of therapy, which includes endoscopic resection (small subset of patients) and partial or total gastrectomy. Endoscopic resection includes endoscopic mucosal resection and endoscopic submucosal dissection, both shown in retrospective data to have high rate of LC in appropriately selected patients.[26] Optimal selection criteria for endoscopic resection are evolving, with routine features being high likelihood of en bloc resection, intestinal type histology, tumor limited to mucosa, no LVSI, and tumor size <2 cm without ulceration.[27-29]

Survival is similar between partial and total gastrectomy in the setting of satisfactory margins, with partial gastrectomy associated with improved nutritional status and quality of life, except in proximal lesions, in which partial gastrectomy was associated with higher rates of reflux and anastomotic stenosis compared with total gastrectomy.[30,31] Therefore, total gastrectomy is typically utilized for lesions in the upper one-third of the stomach, and partial gastrectomy is utilized for lesions in the lower two-thirds.[31] Total gastrectomy involves esophagojejunostomy with Roux-en-Y anastomosis to prevent reflux of bile and pancreatic fluid. Billroth I is end-to-end gastrojejunal anastomosis using gastric resection margin. Billroth II is end-to-side gastrojejunal anastomosis, with closure of duodenal stump and lesser curvature (gastric resection margin not used for anastomosis). Complications include anastomotic failure, bleeding, ileus, B_{12} deficiency, dumping syndrome, and reflux.

LND: Extent of LND is controversial, but it is recommended that at least 15 LNs be removed for adequate staging. See Table 34.5 for data regarding extent of LND. Gastrectomy with D2 LND is standard of care in Eastern Asia.[32]

Table 34.5 Definition of Extent of Lymph Node Dissection for Gastric Cancer	
D0	No LND
D1	JRSGC N1 nodes
D2	D1 dissection + JRSGC N2 nodes with distal pancreatectomy and splenectomy
D3	D2 dissection + JRSGC N3 nodes
D4	D3 dissection + JRSGC N4 nodes

Chemotherapy: GASTRIC meta-analysis demonstrated OS benefit of ~6% with use of 5-FU-based CHT in adjuvant setting compared with surgery alone.[33] Historical option in the United States was perioperative epirubicin, cisplatin, and 5-FU (ECF) per MAGIC trial, which has now been replaced with perioperative FLOT per FLOT4-AIO trial showing an OS benefit to FLOT over ECF.[34] Alternatively, adjuvant CHT with bolus 5-FU and LCV concurrent with RT per INT 0116 may be used.[35] ToGA trial demonstrated OS benefit to trastuzumab in addition to standard CHT (5-FU or capecitabine with cisplatin, 13.8 vs. 11.1 months, p = .0046) for locally advanced, recurrent, or metastatic and inoperable Her-2 Neu-amplified cancers of the GEJ and stomach.[17] The CheckMate-649 and the Keynote-859 trials established an OS benefit to the addition of IO (nivolumab and pembrolizumab, respectively) to CHT as first-line treatment in patients with metastatic or locally advanced unresectable HER2-negative gastric cancer.[36,37] The addition of pembrolizumab to trastuzumab + fluoropyrimidine and platinum-based CHT has been shown to improve PFS and OS in patients with advanced or metastatic HER2-positive gastric or gastroesophageal junction ACA.[38,39] Furthermore, zolbetuximab, a novel antibody against claudin 18.2 (a tight junction protein that is typically expressed in normal gastric epithelia and is retained during malignant transformation),[40] was shown to improve PFS and OS over FOLFOX/CAPOX in advanced or metastatic claudin 18.2-positive gastric or gastroesophageal junction ACA.[41,42] Nivolumab and ipilimumab-based neoadjuvant therapy was feasible and associated with a high pCR rate (59%) in patients with deficient mismatch repair/microsatellite instability-high gastric or gastroesophageal cancer in a prospective phase II trial.[43]

Radiation

Indications: Indications for adjuvant RT include T2–4, N+, or positive margins. Preoperative RT is an option for borderline resectable or definitive RT for unresectable disease. RT can also be used in patients with positive margins (R1/R2 resection).[1]

Dose: Dosing for adjuvant RT is 45 Gy/25 fx. Consider 5.4 to 5.9 Gy boost for positive margins or gross residual disease.[1] Tumor bed is covered and coverage of gastric remnant is dependent on risk and organs at risk. LN coverage in adjuvant setting is dependent on anatomic site of primary (see the following). Can consider omission of nodal coverage in patients with T2–3N0 and >15 LNs removed.[44-46]

Perigastric LNs: Always covered, except for proximal T1–2aN0 patients with negative margins >5 cm and 10 to 15 LNs removed.

Celiac and suprapancreatic LNs: Cover for T4, N+, or T3N0 with <15 LNs resected.

Portahepatic LN: Cover all T4 or N+, except proximal lesions with only 1 to 2 involved LNs and >15 LNs resected.

Splenic LN: Cover for all T4 or N+, except distal lesions with only 1 to 2 involved LNs and >15 LNs resected.

Distal paraesophageal LN: Lesions with esophageal extension.

Toxicity: Acute: fatigue, nausea, vomiting, diarrhea, gastritis, esophagitis. Late: stricture, renal insufficiency, second malignancy.

Procedure: See *Handbook of Treatment Planning in Radiation Oncology*, Chapter 7.[47]

EVIDENCE-BASED Q&A

What is the optimal extent of LND?

It is recommended that at least 15 LNs be dissected for satisfactory staging, with NCCN recommending D2 dissection. However, extent of LND is controversial. There are four randomized clinical trials and meta-analysis demonstrating no survival advantage and higher postoperative morbidity and mortality with extensive LND.[48–51] On the other hand, several nonrandomized clinical trials have suggested improvement in survival with more radical LND.[30,52]

Bonenkamp, Dutch Gastric Cancer Group (*NEJM* 1999, PMID 10089184): PRT of 711 patients with gastric cancer undergoing curative resection randomized to D1 LND (*n* = 380) or D2 LND (*n* = 331). Patients with D2 LND had significantly higher rates of postoperative complications compared with D1 LND (43% vs. 25%, *p* < .001) and postoperative deaths (10% vs. 4%, *p* = .004). The 5-year OS was similar between groups (45% vs. 47%), for D1 and D2 LND, respectively. **Conclusion: D2 LND resulted in significantly higher toxicity and no survival benefit compared with D1 LND.**

Is there benefit to neoadjuvant CHT compared with surgery alone and what is the optimal CHT regimen?

There are two PRTs (MAGIC/FFCD) that demonstrate significant survival benefit with use of neoadjuvant CHT compared with surgery alone, while EORTC 40954 demonstrated no survival benefit.[34,53] A meta-analysis of 12 RCTs[54] showed that neoadjuvant CHT was associated with significantly improved OS, 3-year PFS, and R0 resection rate with no significant increase in operative complications, perioperative morality, or grade 3 or 4 adverse effects. Neoadjuvant CHT may be particularly beneficial in patients at high risk of developing distant metastases (T3/T4 tumors, high clinical nodal burden, diffuse histology). The FLOT4-AIO trial compared FLOT with ECF, with FLOT having improved OS and now is the recommended standard-of-care perioperative CHT in gastric cancer. A summary of neoadjuvant CHT trials is provided in Table 34.6.

Table 34.6 Neoadjuvant/Perioperative CHT Phase III Trials in Gastric Cancer						
Trial	N	CHT	R0 Resection	LR	DM	OS
MAGIC[34] (2006) Perioperative CHT vs. surgery alone	250 253	Epirubicin/ cisplatin/5-FU	69% vs. 66%	14% vs. 21%	24% vs. 37%	**5-yr** 36%* vs. 23%*
FFCD/FNCLCC[55] (2011) Perioperative CHT vs. surgery	113 111	Cisplatin/5-FU	87%* vs. 74%*	24% vs. 26%	42% vs. 56%	**5-yr** 38%* vs. 24%*
EORTC 40954[53] (2010) Neoadjuvant CHT vs. surgery	72 72	Cisplatin/5-FU/ LCV	82%* vs. 67%*	–	–	**2-yr** 73% vs. 70%
FLOT4-AIO[56] (2019) perioperative CHT	360 356	ECF/ECX vs. FLOT	78%* vs. 85%*	–	–	**5-yr** 36%* vs. 45%*

*Statistically significant.

Is there benefit to the addition of CRT to neoadjuvant CHT?

The impact of RT, in addition to neoadjuvant CHT, is unclear, but Stahl and RTOG 9904 suggest some benefit. The TOPGEAR trial assessed neoadjuvant CHT (ECF/FLOT) with RT + adjuvant ECF/FLOT vs. neoadjuvant and adjuvant ECF/FLOT alone and showed no OS or PFS benefit to addition of preoperative RT despite showing increased pCR and downstaging.[57]

Stahl, Germany (*JCO* 2009, PMID 19139439): PRT of 354 patients with locally advanced ACA of the lower third of the esophagus or gastric cardia undergoing surgery randomized to induction CHT for 15 weeks (cisplatin, 5-FU, LCV) followed by surgery or induction CHT for 13 weeks followed by concurrent CHT (cisplatin and etoposide) and RT (30 Gy/15 fx) followed by surgery. Neoadjuvant CRT demonstrated higher rate of pCR (16% vs. 2%) and N0 status (65% vs. 38%), compared with neoadjuvant CHT alone. The 3-year OS was 48% vs. 28% (*p* = .07) for neoadjuvant CRT and neoadjuvant CHT, respectively. **Conclusion: Neoadjuvant CRT had higher pCR and trended toward improved survival, although not statistically significant compared with neoadjuvant CHT alone.**

Ajani, RTOG 9904 (*JCO* 2006, PMID 16921048): Phase II trial of 49 patients with potentially resectable T2–3NxM0 gastric ACA treated with induction CHT (cisplatin, 5-FU, LCV) for two cycles, followed by concurrent CHT (5-FU, paclitaxel) and RT (45 Gy/25 fx) and then surgery (D2 LND recommended). pCR was 26% and R0 resection was obtained in 77% of patients. The 1-year OS was 82% for patients who had pCR and 69% for patients who had less than pCR. **Conclusion: Neoadjuvant CRT had 26% pCR rate, which may be associated with higher OS.**

Leong, TOPGEAR (*NEJM* 2024, PMID 39282905): Phase III randomized trial of 574 patients randomized to perioperative CHT (ECF or FLOT) vs. perioperative CHT in addition to preoperative CRT (45 Gy in 25 fractions with concurrent 5-FU). The primary endpoint was OS. Secondary endpoints were PFS, pCR, toxic effects, and QOL. One-third of the cohort had GEJ tumors. A higher pCR rate was seen in the preoperative CRT arms (17% vs. 8%) as well as greater downstaging after resection. However, at MFU of 67 months, there were no significant differences in OS (median 46 vs. 49 months) and PFS (31 vs. 32 months). **Conclusion: Addition of preoperative CRT did not provide an OS or a PFS benefit over perioperative CHT alone, although it improved tumor downstaging and pCR rates.**

Is there benefit to adjuvant CHT compared with surgery alone?

The role of adjuvant CHT is unclear for Western patients, as trials performed in European populations have not shown survival benefit (GOIRC/GOIM). Only one trial (ACTS-GC) has demonstrated OS benefit in Japanese population, while the CLASSIC trial demonstrated a DFS benefit in patients from South Korea, China, and Taiwan. A meta-analysis of 17 PRTs[58] found that adjuvant RT is associated with significant PFS and 5-year OS benefit compared with surgery alone. A summary of adjuvant CHT trials is provided in Table 34.7.

Table 34.7 Summary of Adjuvant CHT Trials in Gastric Cancer					
Trial	**N**	**CHT**	**LRR**	**DM**	**OS**
ACTS-GC[59] (2007) Adjuvant CHT vs. surgery alone	529 530	Tegafur/gimeracil/ oteracil (S1)	8% vs. 13%	26% vs. 32%	**5-yr** 72%* vs. 61%*
GOIM[60] (2007) Adjuvant CHT vs. surgery alone	112 113	Epirubicin/LCV/5-FU/etoposide	–	–	**5-yr** 41% vs. 34%
GOIRC[61] (2008) Adjuvant CHT vs. surgery alone	130 128	Epirubicin/LCV/5-FU/cisplatin	–	–	**5-yr** 48% vs. 49%
CLASSIC[62] (2012) Adjuvant CHT vs. surgery alone	520 515	Oxaliplatin/ capecitabine	–	–	3-yr DFS 74%* vs. 60%*

*Statistically significant.

Is there benefit to adjuvant CRT compared with surgery alone?

In the United States, for patients undergoing surgery first, adjuvant CRT is preferred.

MacDonald, INT0116 (*NEJM* 2001, PMID 11547741; Update Smalley, *JCO* 2012, PMID 22585691): PRT of 556 patients with stage IB to IV (M0) gastric cancer or GEJ ACA with R0 resection randomized to surgery alone vs. surgery followed by adjuvant CRT. CHT was bolus 5-FU 425 mg/m^2 and LCV 20 mg/m^2/day on days 1 to 5 for two cycles. RT was 45 Gy/25 fx and was started on day 1 of cycle 2 with 5-FU dose reduced to 400 mg/m^2 during RT and cycle 3 as 5-FU alone. After completion of RT, bolus 5-FU and LCV was given for two more cycles. MFU 5 years. D0 LND 54%, D1 LND 36%, and D2 LND 10%. Sixty-nine percent were T3–4 and 85% N+. See Table 34.8 for the results. With MFU >10 years, OS remained significantly improved with CRT (HR 1.32, p = .0046) and there was benefit in all subsets except diffuse histology. **Conclusion: Postop CRT should be considered for resected gastric cancer given RFs, DFS, and OS benefit.**

Table 34.8 Results of INT0116 Adjuvant CRT for Gastric Cancer[35]						
	3-Yr RFS	Median DFS	DM	LRR	MS	3-Yr OS
Surgery	31%	19 months	18%	29%	27 months	41%
Surgery + adjuvant CRT	48%	30 months	33%	19%	36 months	50%
p value	<.001	<.001	NS		.006	.005

Source: Data from Macdonald JS, Smalley SR, Benedetti J, et al. Chemoradiotherapy after surgery compared with surgery alone for adenocarcinoma of the stomach or gastroesophageal junction. *N Engl J Med.* 2001;345(10):725–730. doi:10.1056/NEJMoa010187.

Is there benefit to adjuvant CRT compared with adjuvant CHT alone?

The CRITICS trial did not demonstrate a benefit to adjuvant CRT compared with adjuvant CHT alone.[63] The ARTIST trial demonstrated a trend to DFS benefit for adjuvant CRT in patients who had R0 resection with D2 LND. Subset analysis demonstrated DFS benefit in N+ or intestinal-type histology patients.[64] The ARTIST II trial randomized patients with D2-resected gastric cancer to S1, S1 + oxaliplatin, and S1 + oxaliplatin + RT. It showed benefit to SOX and SOXRT over S1 alone, but no added benefit to addition of RT to SOX.[65]

Lee, ARTIST Trial (*JCO* 2015, PMID 25559811): PRT of 458 patients with R0 resection and D2 LND randomized to adjuvant capecitabine and cisplatin (XP) for six cycles or XP for two cycles followed by RT (45 Gy/25 fx) with capecitabine, followed by XP for two cycles. OS was similar between the two groups. Subgroup analysis demonstrated that addition of RT to XP significantly improved 3-year DFS for patients with N+ disease (76% vs. 72%, p = .04) and intestinal histology (94% vs. 83%, p = .01). **Conclusion: Adjuvant CRT did not significantly improve DFS and OS compared with adjuvant CHT alone.** *Comment: There may be a subset of patients with N+ and intestinal type histology who have DFS benefit from adjuvant CRT.*

Park, ARTIST II Trial (*Ann of Onc* 2021, PMID 33278599): PRT of 546 patients with stage II to III gastric ACA (AJCC 7th ed.) who underwent curative gastrectomy and D2 LND randomized 1:1:1 to adjuvant S1, S1 + oxaliplatin (SOX), or S1 + oxaliplatin + RT (SOXRT; 45 Gy/25 fx with concurrent S1). Primary endpoint was DFS. Secondary endpoints were OS, pattern of recurrence, and QOL. The 3-year DFS was 65%, 74%, and 73% in the S1, SOX, and SOXRT arms, respectively. HR for DFS in the control arm (S1) was shorter than that in the SOX and SOXRT arms: S1 vs. SOX (0.692; p = .042) and S1 vs. SOXRT (0.724; p = .074). No difference in DFS was found between SOX and SOXRT (HR 0.971, p = .879). Adverse events were generally well-tolerated and manageable. **Conclusion: Adjuvant SOX and SOXRT prolonged DFS compared with adjuvant S1 alone in stage II to III, D2-resected, N+, gastric cancer. The addition of RT to SOX did not significantly reduce the rate of recurrence after D2 gastrectomy.**

Cats, CRITICS (*Lancet* 2018, PMID 29650363): PRT of 788 patients from Netherlands, Denmark, and Sweden with stage IB to IV (M0) gastric cancer who received neoadjuvant CHT (epirubicin, capecitabine, and cisplatin or oxaliplatin: ECX or EOX) for three cycles and resection with D2 dissection, then randomized to three cycles of ECX/EOX or CRT (45 Gy/25 fx with weekly XP). Eighty-seven percent of patients had ≥D1 LND and removal of a median of 20 LNs. Only 47% of patients completed adjuvant CHT and 55% completed adjuvant CRT. See Table 34.9 for the results. **Conclusion: Adjuvant CRT did not significantly improve OS compared with adjuvant CHT alone after preoperative CHT and surgery.**

Table 34.9 Results of CRITICS Gastric Cancer Trial[63]		
	Median OS	**Grade 3+ GI Toxicity**
CHT + surgery + adjuvant CHT	43 months	37%
CHT + surgery + adjuvant CRT	37 months	42%
p value	.90	.14

Source: Cats A, Jansen EPM, van Grieken NCT, et al. Chemotherapy versus chemoradiotherapy after surgery and preoperative chemotherapy for resectable gastric cancer (CRITICS): an international, open-label, randomised phase 3 trial. *Lancet Oncol.* 2018;19(5):616–628. doi:10.1016/S1470-2045(18)30132-3.

Is there a role for neoadjuvant or adjuvant immunotherapy?

KEYNOTE-585[66] demonstrated improved pCR but no benefit to EFS or OS with the addition of IO to neoadjuvant CHT. Similarly, ATTRACTION-5 found no improvement in RFS among gastric/GEJ cancer treated with adjuvant nivolumab following upfront surgery.[67] The DANTE trial evaluating the addition of atezolizumab to perioperative FLOT has demonstrated improved pCR at interim analysis with phase III endpoints awaited.[68] For patients with gastric ACA that is MSI-H/dMMR, the NEONIPIGA phase II trial demonstrated an impressive pCR rate of 58% with perioperative nivolumab/ipilimumab, and thus the addition of IO should be considered for this population.[43,69]

REFERENCES

1. NCCN. NCCN Clinical Practice Guidelines in Oncology. Gastric Cancer. 5.2024.
2. Siegel RL, Giaquinto AN, Jemal A. Cancer statistics, 2024. *CA Cancer J Clin.* 2024;74(1):12–49. doi:10.3322/caac.21820
3. Siegel RL, Miller KD, Jemal A. Cancer statistics, 2020. *CA Cancer J Clin.* 2020;70(1):7–30. doi:10.3322/caac.21590
4. Kono S, Hirohata T. Nutrition and stomach cancer. *Cancer Causes Control.* 1996;7(1):41–55. doi:10.1007/bf00115637
5. González CA, Jakszyn P, Pera G, et al. Meat intake and risk of stomach and esophageal adenocarcinoma within the European Prospective Investigation Into Cancer and Nutrition (EPIC). *J Natl Cancer Inst.* 2006;98(5):345–354. doi:10.1093/jnci/djj071
6. Zhu H, Yang X, Zhang C, et al. Red and processed meat intake is associated with higher gastric cancer risk: a meta-analysis of epidemiological observational studies. *PLoS One.* 2013;8(8):e70955. doi:10.1371/journal.pone.0070955
7. Yang P, Zhou Y, Chen B, et al. Overweight, obesity and gastric cancer risk: results from a meta-analysis of cohort studies. *Eur J Cancer.* 2009;45(16):2867–2873. doi:10.1016/j.ejca.2009.04.019
8. Ladeiras-Lopes R, Pereira AK, Nogueira A, et al. Smoking and gastric cancer: systematic review and meta-analysis of cohort studies. *Cancer Causes Control.* 2008;19(7):689–701. doi:10.1007/s10552-008-9132-y
9. Fox JG, Dangler CA, Taylor NS, King A, Koh TJ, Wang TC. High-salt diet induces gastric epithelial hyperplasia and parietal cell loss, and enhances Helicobacter pylori colonization in C57BL/6 mice. *Cancer Res.* 1999;59(19):4823–4828. PMID:10519391
10. Boysen T, Mohammadi M, Melbye M, et al. EBV-associated gastric carcinoma in high-and low-incidence areas for nasopharyngeal carcinoma. *Br J Cancer.* 2009;101(3):530–533. doi:10.1038/sj.bjc.6605168
11. Oliveira C, Pinheiro H, Figueiredo J, Seruca R, Carneiro F. Familial gastric cancer: genetic susceptibility, pathology, and implications for management. *Lancet Oncol.* 2015;16(2):e60–e70. doi:10.1016/s1470-2045(14)71016-2
12. Morón FE, Szklaruk J. Learning the nodal stations in the abdomen. *Br J Radiol.* 2007;80(958):841–848. doi:10.1259/bjr/64292252
13. Amin MB, Edge SB, Greene FL, et al, eds. . *AJCC Cancer Staging Manual.* Springer. 2017.
14. Correa P. Human gastric carcinogenesis: a multistep and multifactorial process–First American Cancer Society Award Lecture on Cancer Epidemiology and Prevention. *Cancer Res.* 1992;52(24):6735–6740.
15. Siewert J, Hölscher A, Becker K, Gössner W. Cardia cancer: attempt at a therapeutically relevant classification. *Chirurg.* 1987;58(1):25–32. PMID:3829805

16. Hu B, El Hajj N, Sittler S, Lammert N, Barnes R, Meloni-Ehrig A. Gastric cancer: Classification, histology and application of molecular pathology. *J Gastrointest Oncol.* 2012;3(3):251–261. doi:10.3978/j.issn.2078-6891.2012.021

17. Bang YJ, Van Cutsem E, Feyereislova A, et al. Trastuzumab in combination with chemotherapy versus chemotherapy alone for treatment of HER2-positive advanced gastric or gastro-oesophageal junction cancer (ToGA): a phase 3, open-label, randomised controlled trial. *Lancet.* 2010;376(9742):687–697. doi:10.1016/S0140-6736(10)61121-X

18. Mizoue T, Yoshimura T, Tokui N, et al. Prospective study of screening for stomach cancer in Japan. *Int J Cancer.* 2003;106(1):103–107. doi:10.1002/ijc.11183

19. Kunisaki C, Ishino J, Nakajima S, et al. Outcomes of mass screening for gastric carcinoma. *Ann Surg Oncol.* 2006;13(2):221–228. doi:10.1245/ASO.2006.04.028

20. Llorens P. Gastric cancer mass survey in Chile. *Semin Surg Oncol.* 1991;7(6):339–343. doi:10.1002/ssu.2980070604

21. Pisani P, Oliver WE, Parkin DM, Alvarez N, Vivas J. Case-control study of gastric cancer screening in Venezuela. *Br J Cancer.* 1994;69(6):1102–1105. doi:10.1038/bjc.1994.216

22. Choi KS, Suh M. Screening for gastric cancer: the usefulness of endoscopy. *Clin Endosc.* 2014;47(6):490–496. doi:10.5946/ce.2014.47.6.490

23. Roviello F, Rossi S, Marrelli D, et al. Number of lymph node metastases and its prognostic significance in early gastric cancer: a multicenter Italian study. *J Surg Oncol.* 2006;94(4):275–280. doi:10.1002/jso.20566

24. Lordick F, Ott K, Krause BJ, et al. PET to assess early metabolic response and to guide treatment of adenocarcinoma of the oesophagogastric junction: the MUNICON phase II trial. *Lancet Oncol.* 2007;8(9):797–805. doi:10.1016/S1470-2045(07)70244-9

25. Okada K, Fujisaki J, Yoshida T, et al. Long-term outcomes of endoscopic submucosal dissection for undifferentiated-type early gastric cancer. *Endoscopy.* 2012;44(2):122–127. doi:10.1055/s-0031-1291486

26. Takekoshi T, Baba Y, Ota H, et al. Endoscopic resection of early gastric carcinoma: results of a retrospective analysis of 308 cases. *Endoscopy.* 1994;26(4):352–358. doi:10.1055/s-2007-1008990

27. Soetikno R, Kaltenbach T, Yeh R, Gotoda T. Endoscopic mucosal resection for early cancers of the upper gastrointestinal tract. *J Clin Oncol.* 2005;23(20):4490–4498. doi:10.1200/JCO.2005.19.935

28. Min YW, Min BH, Lee JH, Kim JJ. Endoscopic treatment for early gastric cancer. *World J Gastroenterol.* 2014;20(16):4566–4573. doi:10.3748/wjg.v20.i16.4566

29. Gotoda T. Endoscopic resection of early gastric cancer: the Japanese perspective. *Curr Opin Gastroenterol.* 2006;22(5):561–569. doi:10.1097/01.mog.0000239873.06243.00

30. Bozzetti F, Marubini E, Bonfanti G, Miceli R, Piano C, Gennari L. Subtotal versus total gastrectomy for gastric cancer: five-year survival rates in a multicenter randomized Italian trial. Italian Gastrointestinal Tumor Study Group. *Ann Surg.* 1999;230(2):170–178. doi:10.1097/00000658-199908000-00006

31. Pu YW, Gong W, Wu YY, Chen Q, He TF, Xing CG. Proximal gastrectomy versus total gastrectomy for proximal gastric carcinoma. A meta-analysis on postoperative complications, 5-year survival, and recurrence rate. *Saudi Med J.* 2013;34(12):1223–1228. PMID:24343461

32. Degiuli M, De Manzoni G, Di Leo A, et al. Gastric cancer: current status of lymph node dissection. *World J Gastroenterol.* 2016;22(10):2875–2893. doi:10.3748/wjg.v22.i10.2875

33. Paoletti X, Oba K, Burzykowski T, et al. Benefit of adjuvant chemotherapy for resectable gastric cancer a meta-analysis. *JAMA.* 2010;303(17):1729–1737. doi:10.1001/jama.2010.534

34. Cunningham D, Allum WH, Stenning SP, et al. Perioperative chemotherapy versus surgery alone for resectable gastroesophageal cancer. *N Engl J Med.* 2006;355(1):11–20. doi:10.1056/NEJMoa055531

35. Macdonald JS, Smalley SR, Benedetti J, et al. Chemoradiotherapy after surgery compared with surgery alone for adenocarcinoma of the stomach or gastroesophageal junction. *N Engl J Med.* 2001;345(10):725–730. doi:10.1056/NEJMoa010187

36. Janjigian YY, Shitara K, Moehler M, et al. First-line nivolumab plus chemotherapy versus chemotherapy alone for advanced gastric, gastro-oesophageal junction, and oesophageal adenocarcinoma (CheckMate 649): a randomised, open-label, phase 3 trial. *Lancet.* 2021;398(10294):27–40. doi:10.1016/S0140-6736(21)00797-2

37. Rha SY, Oh DY, Yañez P, et al. Pembrolizumab plus chemotherapy versus placebo plus chemotherapy for HER2-negative advanced gastric cancer (KEYNOTE-859): a multicentre, randomised, double-blind, phase 3 trial. *Lancet Oncol.* 2023;24(11):1181–1195. doi:10.1016/S1470-2045(23)00515-6

38. Janjigian YY, Kawazoe A, Bai Y, et al. Pembrolizumab plus trastuzumab and chemotherapy for HER2-positive gastric or gastro-oesophageal junction adenocarcinoma: interim analyses from the phase 3 KEYNOTE-811 randomised placebo-controlled trial. *Lancet.* 2023;402(10418):2197–2208. doi:10.1016/S0140-6736(23)02033-0

39. Janjigian Y, Kawazoe A, Bai Y, et al. 1400O Final overall survival for the phase III, KEYNOTE-811 study of pembrolizumab plus trastuzumab and chemotherapy for HER2+ advanced, unresectable or metastatic G/GEJ adenocarcinoma. *Ann Oncol.* 2024;35(2):S877–S878. doi:10.1016/j.annonc.2024.08.1466

40. Angerilli V, Ghelardi F, Nappo F, et al. Claudin-18.2 testing and its impact in the therapeutic management of patients with gastric and gastroesophageal adenocarcinomas: a literature review with expert opinion. *Pathol Res Pract*. 2024;254:155145. doi:10.1016/j.prp.2024.155145

41. Shitara K, Lordick F, Bang YJ, et al. Zolbetuximab plus mFOLFOX6 in patients with CLDN18. 2-positive, HER2-negative, untreated, locally advanced unresectable or metastatic gastric or gastro-oesophageal junction adenocarcinoma (SPOTLIGHT): a multicentre, randomised, double-blind, phase 3 trial. *Lancet*. 2023;401(10389):1655–1668. doi:10.1016/S0140-6736(23)00620-7

42. Shah MA, Shitara K, Ajani JA, et al. Zolbetuximab plus CAPOX in CLDN18. 2-positive gastric or gastroesophageal junction adenocarcinoma: the randomized, phase 3 GLOW trial. *Nat Med*. 2023;29(8):2133–2141. doi:10.1038/s41591-023-02465-7

43. André T, Tougeron D, Piessen G, et al. Neoadjuvant nivolumab plus ipilimumab and adjuvant nivolumab in localized deficient mismatch repair/microsatellite instability–high gastric or esophagogastric junction adenocarcinoma: the GERCOR NEONIPIGA phase II study. *J Clin Oncol*. 2023 ;41(2):255–265. doi:10.1200/JCO.22.00686

44. Tepper JE, Gunderson LL. Radiation treatment parameters in the adjuvant postoperative therapy of gastric cancer. *Semin Radiat Oncol*. 2002;12(2):187–195. doi:10.1053/srao.2002.30827

45. Smalley SR, Gunderson L, Tepper J, et al. Gastric surgical adjuvant radiotherapy consensus report: rationale and treatment implementation. *Int J Radiat Oncol Biol Phys*. 2002;52(2):283–293. doi:10.1016/s0360-3016(01)02646-3

46. Wo JY, Yoon SS, Guimaraes AR, Wolfgang J, Mamon HJ, Hong TS. Gastric lymph node contouring atlas: a tool to aid in clinical target volume definition in 3-dimensional treatment planning for gastric cancer. *Pract Radiat Oncol*. 2013;3(1):e11–e19. doi:10.1016/j.prro.2012.03.007

47. Videtic GM, Vassil AD, Woody NM. *Handbook of Treatment Planning in Radiation Oncology*. Springer Publishing Company; 2020.

48. Bonenkamp J, Hermans J, Sasako M, et al. Extended lymph-node dissection for gastric cancer. *N Eng J Med*. 1999;340(12):908–914. doi:10.1056/NEJM199903253401202

49. Cuschieri A, Weeden S, Fielding J, et al. Patient survival after D1 and D2 resections for gastric cancer: long-term results of the MRC randomized surgical trial. *Br J Cancer*. 1999;79(9–10):1522–1530. doi:10.1038/sj.bjc.6690243

50. Sasako M, Sano T, Yamamoto S, et al. D2 lymphadenectomy alone or with para-aortic nodal dissection for gastric cancer. *N Eng J Med*. 2008;359(5):453–462. doi:10.1056/NEJMoa0707035

51. Seevaratnam R, Bocicariu A, Cardoso R, et al. A meta-analysis of D1 versus D2 lymph node dissection. *Gastric Cancer*. 2012;15(suppl 1):60–69. doi:10.1007/s10120-011-0110-9

52. Schwarz RE, Smith DD. Clinical impact of lymphadenectomy extent in resectable gastric cancer of advanced stage. *Ann Surg Oncol*. 2007;14(2):317–328. doi:10.1245/s10434-006-9218-2

53. Schuhmacher C, Gretschel S, Lordick F, et al. Neoadjuvant chemotherapy compared with surgery alone for locally advanced cancer of the stomach and cardia: European Organisation for Research and Treatment of Cancer randomized trial 40954. *J Clin Oncol*. 2010;28(35):5210–5218. doi:10.1200/JCO.2009.26.6114

54. Xiong BH, Cheng Y, Ma L, Zhang CQ. An updated meta-analysis of randomized controlled trial assessing the effect of neoadjuvant chemotherapy in advanced gastric cancer. *Cancer Invest*. 2014;32(6):272–284. doi:10.3109/07357907.2014.911877

55. Ychou M, Boige V, Pignon JP, et al. Perioperative chemotherapy compared with surgery alone for resectable gastroesophageal adenocarcinoma: an FNCLCC and FFCD multicenter phase III trial. *J Clin Oncol*. 2011;29(13):1715–1721. doi:10.1200/jco.2010.33.0597

56. Al-Batran SE, Homann N, Pauligk C, et al. Perioperative chemotherapy with fluorouracil plus leucovorin, oxaliplatin, and docetaxel versus fluorouracil or capecitabine plus cisplatin and epirubicin for locally advanced, resectable gastric or gastro-oesophageal junction adenocarcinoma (FLOT4): a randomised, phase 2/3 trial. *Lancet*. 2019;393(10184):1948–1957. doi:10.1016/S0140-6736(18)32557-1

57. Stahl M, Walz MK, Stuschke M, et al. Phase III comparison of preoperative chemotherapy compared with chemoradiotherapy in patients with locally advanced adenocarcinoma of the esophagogastric junction. *J Clin Oncol*. 2009;27(6):851–856. doi:10.1200/jco.2008.17.0506

58. Paoletti X, Oba K, Burzykowski T, et al. Benefit of adjuvant chemotherapy for resectable gastric cancer: a meta-analysis. *JAMA*. 2010;303(17):1729–1737. doi:10.1001/jama.2010.534

59. Sakuramoto S, Sasako M, Yamaguchi T, et al. Adjuvant chemotherapy for gastric cancer with S-1, an oral fluoropyrimidine. *N Engl J Med*. 2007;357(18):1810–1820. doi:10.1056/NEJMoa072252

60. De Vita F, Giuliani F, Orditura M, et al. Adjuvant chemotherapy with epirubicin, leucovorin, 5-fluorouracil and etoposide regimen in resected gastric cancer patients: a randomized phase III trial by the Gruppo Oncologico Italia Meridionale (GOIM 9602 Study). *Ann Oncol*. 2007;18(8):1354–1358. doi:10.1093/annonc/mdm128

61. Di Costanzo F, Gasperoni S, Manzione L, et al. Adjuvant chemotherapy in completely resected gastric cancer: a randomized phase III trial conducted by GOIRC. *J Natl Cancer Inst*. 2008;100(6):388–398. doi:10.1093/jnci/djn054

62. Bang YJ, Kim YW, Yang HK, et al. Adjuvant capecitabine and oxaliplatin for gastric cancer after D2 gastrectomy (CLASSIC): a phase 3 open-label, randomised controlled trial. *Lancet*. 2012;379(9813):315–321. doi:10.1016/s0140-6736(11)61873-4

63. Cats A, Jansen EPM, van Grieken NCT, et al. Chemotherapy versus chemoradiotherapy after surgery and preoperative chemotherapy for resectable gastric cancer (CRITICS): an international, open-label, randomised phase 3 trial. *Lancet Oncol*. 2018;19(5):616–628. doi:10.1016/S1470-2045(18)30132-3

64. Park SH, Sohn TS, Lee J, et al. Phase III trial to compare adjuvant chemotherapy with capecitabine and cisplatin versus concurrent chemoradiotherapy in gastric cancer: final report of the adjuvant chemoradiotherapy in stomach tumors trial, including survival and subset analyses. *J Clin Oncol*. 2015;33(28):3130–3136. doi:10.1200/jco.2014.58.3930

65. Park SH, Lim DH, Sohn TS, et al. A randomized phase III trial comparing adjuvant single-agent S1, S-1 with oxaliplatin, and postoperative chemoradiation with S-1 and oxaliplatin in patients with node-positive gastric cancer after D2 resection: the ARTIST 2 trial. *Ann Oncol*. 2021;32(3):368–374. doi:10.1016/j.annonc.2020.11.017

66. Shitara K, Rha SY, Wyrwicz LS, et al. Neoadjuvant and adjuvant pembrolizumab plus chemotherapy in locally advanced gastric or gastro-oesophageal cancer (KEYNOTE-585): an interim analysis of the multicentre, double-blind, randomised phase 3 study. *Lancet Oncol*. 2024;25(2):212–224. doi:10.1016/S1470-2045(23)00541-7

67. Terashima M, Kang YK, Kim YW, et al. ATTRACTION-5: A phase 3 study of nivolumab plus chemotherapy as postoperative adjuvant treatment for pathological stage III (pStage III) gastric or gastroesophageal junction (G/GEJ) cancer. *J Clin Oncol*. 2023;41(16_suppl):4000. doi:10.1200/JCO.2023.41.16_suppl.4000

68. Lorenzen S, Götze TO, Thuss-Patience P, et al. Perioperative atezolizumab plus fluorouracil, leucovorin, oxaliplatin, and docetaxel for resectable esophagogastric cancer: interim results from the randomized, multicenter, Phase II/III DANTE/IKF-s633 trial. *J Clin Oncol*. 2024 ;42(4):410–420. doi:10.1200/JCO.23.00975

69. Ajani JA, D'Amico TA, Bentrem DJ, et al. Esophageal and Esophagogastric Junction Cancers, Version 4.2024, NCCN Clinical Practice Guidelines in Oncology. *J Nat Compr Canc Netw*. 2024;21(4):393–422. doi:10.6004/jnccn.2023.0019

35 HEPATOCELLULAR CARCINOMA

Erik M. Davies and Kevin L. Stephans

QUICK HIT Hepatocellular carcinoma (HCC) is associated with liver disease, particularly cirrhosis and hepatitis B and C. Screening of patients with chronic hepatitis infection and those with cirrhosis may result in early detection and improved outcomes. Diagnosis is commonly clinical, based on AFP and imaging characteristics. Patients are staged according to the BCLC staging system, and early tumors are treated with surgical resection (if liver function allows), or liver transplantation if within Milan criteria (1 tumor ≤5 cm or 2–3 tumors each ≤3 cm; no extrahepatic disease or vascular invasion). Patients with multiple tumors, larger tumors, or reduced functional status may be treated with focal therapies including RFA, TACE, radioembolization (Y^{90}), or RT (proton or SBRT). Patients who respond to first-line locoregional therapy may be downstaged within Milan criteria and become eligible for transplant. Patients with advanced disease may be candidates for atezolizumab/bevacizumab, durvalumab/tremelimumab, or other systemic agents, which have been shown to improve OS in advanced disease.

EPIDEMIOLOGY: Second leading cause of cancer death worldwide in men and sixth leading cause of cancer death in women. In the United States, incidence of primary liver cancer (HCC and intrahepatic bile duct) is 8.8 cases per 100,000 and is the fifth leading cause of cancer death among men as of 2021.[1] HCC is more common in areas with high rates of hepatitis B (HBV) and hepatitis C (HCV) infection. Incidence has been increasing in the United States due to the prevalence of HCV infection and NASH contributing to cirrhosis.

RISK FACTORS: Most strongly associated with cirrhosis and primarily related to HBV and HCV infections, which are present in ~80% of cases. Treatment of viral infection has been shown to reduce future cancer risk in HBV by 50% to 60% and in HCV by 70%.[2] Other risk factors include male gender (relative risk 2–3), diabetes (relative risk 2), smoking, hereditary hemochromatosis, alcohol use, chemical exposure, obesity, and exposure to environmental toxins including aflatoxin and microcystin.

ANATOMY: The liver is the largest solid organ in the body, surrounded by the peritoneal membrane (Glisson's capsule), and can be divided based on vasculature into eight segments. On the left numbering begins with the caudate lobe (segment 1), followed by the lateral (segments 2 and 3), and medial portion (segment 4). On the right, numbering starts with the anterior inferior segment (5) and moves in clockwise direction; posterior inferior, posterior superior, and anterior superior segments are numbered 6, 7, and 8, respectively. There are no anatomic borders between segments and thus no barriers to intrahepatic spread of disease. The liver receives a dual blood supply; the portal vein (75%) supplies the normal hepatic parenchyma, and the hepatic artery (25%) supplies the normal hepatic parenchyma, but also preferentially supplies malignant tumors. Increased portal venous pressure potentiates the development of varices.

PATHOLOGY: HCC can be diagnosed clinically based on AFP and radiographic criteria (see Workup section) or less commonly with biopsy. HCC can be conventional type, which is graded from I to IV, based on the presence of trabecular organization and nuclear appearance. Molecular markers including HepPar1, albumin, fibrinogen, α1-antitrypsin, AFP, and GPC-3 can help confirm the diagnosis.

SCREENING: AASLD has developed screening guidelines (updated 2018) for patients with chronic HBV infection and/or cirrhosis.[3] All patients with cirrhosis (except Child–Pugh C not on transplant list) and high-risk HBV should undergo surveillance with AFP and ultrasound (US) q6 months. Patients on the transplant waiting list should continue to be screened to ensure they do not develop HCC while awaiting transplant. Patients found to have a lesion <1 cm on US should have a repeat US in 3 months, and patients with lesions ≥1 cm or AFP ≥20 ng/mL should receive diagnostic imaging with a four-phase CT or MRI. A randomized trial of 18,816 patients in China using AFP and US showed low compliance rate of 58% but achieved a 37% reduction in HCC mortality (no equivalent U.S.-based study).[4] NCCN guidelines recommend screening with AFP and US q6 months.[5]

CLINICAL PRESENTATION: Most commonly asymptomatic, and symptoms related to the predisposing chronic liver disease are most evident. Patients may have mild to moderate abdominal pain, weight loss, early satiety, diarrhea, fever, and fatigue. Signs and symptoms of decompensated cirrhosis include ascites, encephalopathy, jaundice, and variceal bleeding. May present with paraneoplastic syndrome including erythrocytosis, hypercalcemia, hypoglycemia, and watery diarrhea. Paraneoplastic symptoms, except erythrocytosis, are associated with worse prognosis. HCC can be associated with cutaneous features including dermatomyositis, pemphigus foliaceus, sign of Leser–Trelat, pityriasis rotunda, and porphyria cutanea tarda, although these are not specific to HCC.

WORKUP: Detailed H&P including evaluation of prior liver disease and treatment history.

Labs: HBV and HCV serology, AFP, CMP, CBC, and PT/INR.

Imaging: Diagnostic four-phase CT or MRI to evaluate lesions ≥1 cm on US with or without an elevated AFP. Imaging must include hepatic arterial phase, portal venous phase, and delayed phase, and may include a precontrast phase as well. For cirrhotic (or other high-risk) patients, multiple imaging criteria have been suggested by AASLD, OPTN, EASL, and LI-RADS for lesions ≥1 cm (lesions <1 cm are indeterminate),[6–9] including arterial hyperenhancement, venous washout, pseudocapsule, and growth. These criteria do not apply to patients without cirrhosis. Larger tumor volumes, rim enhancement on arterial phase, peritumoral hypointensity on hepatobiliary phase, nonsmooth margin, multifocal lesions, and T1 hypointensity are predictive of microvascular invasion on MRI.[10] Systemic staging includes CT of chest, abdomen, pelvis, and bone scan if symptoms are present. PET/CT is not recommended.

Biopsy: Can be done for lesions that are not diagnostic based on imaging criteria. Biopsy may be associated with a small risk of tract seeding, and in cases where an indeterminate lesion is resectable, it may be preferable to resect for simultaneous diagnosis and treatment.

PROGNOSTIC FACTORS: Tumor stage, functional status, Child–Pugh score (Table 35.1), and presence of metastatic disease are all prognostic of survival, which in some cases is more determined by cirrhosis than HCC. Child–Pugh is a validated assessment of underlying liver function and is incorporated into many clinical decision schemas for treating HCC. The primary criticism of the Child–Pugh classification concerns the subjective grading of the extent of ascites and encephalopathy. A more recent alternative is the albumin-bilirubin (ALBI) grade, which has been prospectively validated in patients with or without cirrhosis.[11]

Table 35.1 Child–Pugh Classification for Chronic Liver Disease			
Measure	1 Point	2 Points	3 Points
Total bilirubin (mg/dL)	<2	2–3	>3
Serum albumin (g/dL)	>3.5	2.8–3.5	<2.8
Prothrombin time or INR	<4.0 <1.7	4.0–6.0 1.7–2.3	>6.0 >2.3
Ascites	None	Moderate	Severe
Encephalopathy	None	Grades 1–2 or controlled with medication	Grades 3–4 or refractory

Sum of all points: 5–6 (Class A), 7–9 (Class B), 10–15 (Class C).
2-yr OS for Child–Pugh Class A, B, and C is 85%, 57%, and 35%, respectively.

STAGING: Although AJCC TNM staging system exists for HCC, patients are typically staged according to BCLC (Tables 35.2 and 35.3). BCLC staging includes patient performance status, liver function, and tumor characteristics, and each stage is accompanied by a recommended treatment strategy.[12] BCLC-B (intermediate stage) is a heterogeneous group that can be considered for a range of therapies per the BCLC 2022 treatment strategy update.[13] Following initial local therapy, BCLC-B patients with well-defined nodules and lower AFP (≤1,000 ng/dL) can be considered for transplant even with limited progression exceeding Milan criteria. No consensus guidelines exist regarding cutoffs for transplant eligibility, however. By contrast, some patients with BCLC-B disease harbor tumors with diffuse liver infiltration ineligible for transplant, and in these instances systemic therapy should be prioritized over local therapies.[13]

Table 35.2 BCLC Staging System for HCC		
	Stage Characteristics	Suggested Treatment
Very early stage (0)	ECOG PS 0, Child–Pugh A, single tumor ≤2 cm	Resection if candidate for transplant, otherwise ablation
Early stage (A)	ECOG PS 0, Child–Pugh A–B, 1–3 tumors, each ≤3 cm	Single nodule with normal portal pressure and bilirubin → resection. Multiple nodules or increased portal pressure/bilirubin → transplant or ablation
Intermediate stage (B)	ECOG PS 0, Child–Pugh A–B, multiple tumors not meeting stage A	Well-defined tumors → consider transplant or TACE. Diffuse disease → systemic therapy (as below)
Advanced stage (C)	ECOG PS 0-2, Child–Pugh A–B, portal invasion, nodal or distant metastasis	Atezolizumab/bevacizumab or durvalumab/tremelimumab (sorafenib or lenvatinib if ineligible)
Terminal stage (D)	ECOG PS >2 or Child–Pugh C	Supportive care

Table 35.3 AJCC 8th Edition (2017): Staging System for HCC				
T/M	N		cN0	cN1
T1	a. Solitary tumor ≤2 cm		IA	IVA
	b. Solitary tumor >2 cm without vascular invasion		IB	
T2	• Solitary tumor >2 cm with vascular invasion • Multiple tumors ≤5 cm		II	
T3	• Multiple tumors, at least one >5 cm		IIIA	
T4	• Involvement of major branch of portal or hepatic vein • Direct invasion of adjacent organs (other than gallbladder) • Perforation of visceral peritoneum		IIIB	
M1	• Distant metastasis		IVB	

cN1: regional LN metastasis.

TREATMENT PARADIGM: As per BCLC staging system, treatment is based on tumor, patient, and liver function. Surgical resection or transplantation is preferred as the curative option for early-stage patients, while nonsurgical options including radiofrequency ablation (RFA), Y^{90}, transcatheter arterial chemoembolization (TACE), and RT may be used for definitive treatment, downstaging, or as bridge to liver transplantation.[14–17] Systemic therapy is reserved for advanced disease.

Prevention: Vaccination of infants reduces rates of HBV infection and reduces incidence of HCC. Studies of universal vaccination in Taiwan beginning in 1984 revealed 50% decline in pediatric cases of HCC.[18] Similarly, treatment of HBV and HCV should be undertaken in affected patients, and precautions should be taken to avoid transmission.[5]

Surgery: For early-stage patients, surgical resection is the mainstay of cure, and for very small early lesions, partial hepatectomy can provide high rates of cure.[19] However, many patients are not candidates for partial hepatectomy based on tumor features or liver function. In such cases, orthotopic liver transplantation (OLT) may be an alternative surgical approach. For patients without cirrhosis, partial hepatectomy has equivalent cure rates to liver transplantation.[20] Since OLT is also used for benign indications, patients are carefully selected for transplantation based on Milan criteria defined as single tumor ≤5 cm or ≤3 tumors each ≤3 cm, with no extrahepatic spread or macrovascular involvement. The Milan criteria resulted in 5-year OS of ~70% and recurrence rates <15%.[21] UCSF validated expanded transplant criteria for HCC: single lesion ≤6.5 cm in diameter or two lesions ≤4.5 cm each with total tumor diameter ≤8 cm, which has also demonstrated low rates of recurrence.[22] Patients listed for OLT are stratified based on risk of death using the MELD scoring system, which is the sum of an equation using creatinine, bilirubin, and INR and serves similar purpose to the older Child–Pugh score.[23] In addition, patients with HCC can be listed based on exception points, reflecting the risk that their tumor could progress and make them ineligible for transplantation. The number of points granted has changed over time to balance access to organs for cancer and noncancer transplant candidates.

Systemic Therapy: CHT is difficult to administer in patients with HCC who often have associated poor liver function. Multiple agents have been studied with small benefits at the cost of significant toxicity, but newer agents are promising. Until recently, sorafenib was the first-line agent in unresectable HCC in patients with Child–Pugh A cirrhosis with only modest survival outcomes.[24,25] Current first-line agents include atezolizumab/bevacizumab and durvalumab/tremelimumab with improved OS compared with sorafenib in separate phase III RCTs.[22,26,27] Subsequent-line therapy includes sorafenib, lenvatinib, regorafenib, and cabozantinib.[5,13]

Radiation

Indications: Historically, RT played a minor role in treatment due to intrinsic sensitivity of the liver and large treatment volumes. However, conformal techniques including SBRT and proton therapy permit adequate liver sparing, and RT is now a more favorable local therapy. In some patients, RT may be preferable to other ablative or invasive techniques, particularly in tumors exhibiting vascular invasion, tumor thrombosis, inaccessible lesions, or those with vascular shunting. Caution is necessary for Child–Pugh B and C patients as decompensation after RT can pose significant risk.

Dose: Dose varies by technique, and 3- and 5-fx regimens have been deployed up to 54–60 Gy/3 fx or 50 Gy/5 fx, with dose reduction based on dose limits to normal liver. For patients requiring palliation, 8 Gy/1 fx to the involved liver or the whole liver can provide symptomatic improvement in 50% to 70% of patients.[28,29]

Toxicity: Radiation-induced liver disease (RILD) may occur 1 to 2 months after RT (range 0.5–8 months). Two types: classic (fatigue, pain, hepatomegaly, anicteric ascites, elevated ALP but not AST/ALT) and nonclassic (jaundice, elevated ALT/AST). No effective treatment for RILD exists.[30] With more conformal modern RT techniques, RILD is less common; however, 10% to 30% of patients may still suffer worsening Child–Pugh score with definitive intent RT.

Procedure: See *Handbook of Treatment Planning in Radiation Oncology*, Chapter 7.[31]

RFA: Percutaneous or laparoscopic technique; involves thermal ablation of lesion with one or more probes. Larger lesions and difficult locations such as subcapsular, hepatic dome, caudate lobe, central biliary tree, proximal to major blood vessels, and those abutting the gallbladder, small bowel, kidney, and stomach can be problematic. Advantages include single-day treatment and high control rates, particularly for small tumors.[32,33]

TACE: Combines arterial embolization of tumor vasculature with infusion of chemotherapeutic agents, increasing transit time of chemotherapeutic agents, and thus increasing apoptosis and necrosis. Generally considered for patients with preserved liver function and lesions without vascular invasion or extrahepatic spread. There are limited data on the safety and efficacy of TACE in the setting of portal vein thrombus. A RCT of 112 patients comparing TACE with bland embolization and conservative treatment showed an OS advantage to TACE (HR 0.47, $p = .025$), and the 2-year OS was 63% with TACE vs. 50% with bland embolization.[34] There is controversy regarding the survival benefit of TACE as other randomized studies have not shown a survival benefit over conservative management.[34] TACE can be given using either CHT mixed with lipiodol or on drug-eluting beads (DEB). Studies have not shown a significant difference between conventional (lipiodol) and DEB-TACE. Chemotherapeutic agents employed include cisplatin, doxorubicin, and MMC. Postembolization syndrome is seen in 80% of patients and symptoms include RUQ pain, nausea, ileus, fatigue, fever, and transaminitis. It typically lasts 3 to 4 days, and as such many patients are observed in the hospital for 24 hours following treatment. As many as 9% of procedures may result in irreversible hepatotoxicity.[35]

Radioembolization: Yttrium-90 microspheres: Y^{90} is a pure β emitter, with average energy ~1 MeV delivered via the hepatic artery. Prior to radioembolization, patients undergo pretreatment ^{99}mTc macro-aggregated albumin scan, which facilitates prediction of distribution of radioactive beads. If anticipated lung exposure is ≥30 Gy, lung shunt fraction exceeds 20%, or significant GI tract dose is observed, then the distribution catheter needs to be repositioned. If the target cannot be isolated without significant shunting, the procedure is contraindicated. Encephalopathy, Child–Pugh C status, and biliary obstruction are other contraindications. A longitudinal cohort study of Y^{90} in 291 patients receiving 526 treatments revealed overall time to progression of 7.9 months. Child–Pugh A patients had a median survival of 17 months vs. 8 months for Child–Pugh B patients, and Child–Pugh B patients with portal vein thrombus had a median survival of 6 months.[36] Y^{90} may be particularly useful in the setting of portal vein thrombus, and a prospective study of 30 patients found an MS of 13 months.[37] Alternatively, iodine 131-labeled lipiodol has also been employed for radioembolization.

EVIDENCE-BASED Q&A

What are the key studies defining the current role of SBRT for HCC?

Prospective and retrospective studies demonstrate high rates of LC and favorable OS for patients treated with SBRT, often after prior liver-directed therapy.

Bujold, PMH Phase I and II (*JCO* 2013, PMID 23547075): Combined analysis of prospective phase I and II studies of liver SBRT in Canada; 102 patients with HCC unsuitable for TACE, RFA, and surgery enrolled and treated to doses of 24–54 Gy/6 fx; 52% of patients had prior liver-directed therapy and 55% had tumor vascular thrombus. The 1-year LC was 87% and MS was 17 months. Grade 3+ toxicity was seen in 30% of patients, and seven patients experienced possible grade 5 toxicity. Tumor vascular thrombosis significant for worse OS on UVA and MVA. **Conclusion: SBRT is effective in the treatment of HCC, with 1-year LC of 87%.**

Yoon, South Korea (*Clin Mol Hepatol* 2020, PMID 32646200): Phase II single-arm trial of 50 patients receiving SBRT 45 Gy/3 fx for inoperable, untreated single-lesion HCC. MFU 48 months. Median tumor size 1.3 cm (range 0.7–3.1 cm). The 2-year and 5-year LC were 100% and 97%, respectively. The 5-year OS was 78%. Following SBRT, radiologic response was noted in 49 of 53 lesions (92%) per modified RECIST criteria. No patients experienced grade 3+ adverse events. **Conclusion: LC and OS following SBRT for untreated solitary HCC were excellent despite candidates being unfit for other curative treatment modalities.**

Dawson, RTOG 1112 (*JAMA Oncol* 2024, PMID 39699905): Phase III PRT of 193 Child–Pugh A patients with locally advanced HCC not eligible for other local therapy (82% BCLC stage C, 74% macrovascular invasion, 4% with metastatic disease [<3 cm lesions], 60% multifocal) randomized to sorafenib alone vs. sorafenib with SBRT (27.5–50 Gy/5 fx). Trial accrual was closed early secondary to atezolizumab/bevacizumab becoming standard of care, limiting statistical power of analysis. With MFU of 13.2 months, 33.7 months for alive patients, the addition of SBRT improved the median OS (15.8 vs. 12.3 months, $p = .06$) and PFS (9.2 vs. 5.5 months, $p < .001$). OS difference was statistically significant on MVA after adjusting for performance status, degree of macrovascular invasion, M stage, and liver function. No significant difference in grade 3+ AEs between the two groups. Strong suggestion for QOL improvement in SBRT cohort at 6 months (35% vs. 10%). **Conclusion: Despite closing early to accrual, compared with sorafenib alone, the addition of SBRT improved PFS with a strong trend toward improvement in OS in patients with locally advanced HCC, without a significant increase in toxicity.**

Is SBRT safe in Child–Pugh B and C patients?

Original reports of SBRT in Child–Pugh B to C patients demonstrated high rates of toxicity, but newer series demonstrate that, in carefully selected Child–Pugh B to C patients, SBRT is feasible. In one small retrospective series, almost two-thirds of Child–Pugh B and C patients had a decline in Child–Pugh by at least 2 index points at 3 months.[38] A small prospective cohort of 23 Child–Pugh B and C patients demonstrated LC of 92% at 1 year and MS of 14.5 months with no RILD; one of seven deaths in this cohort were attributed to SBRT.[39]

Can SBRT be used as a bridge to liver transplantation?

In small RRs, SBRT as a bridge to transplantation appears to be associated with favorable outcomes. In one review of 60 patients at Indiana University, 2-year LC was 90% and 23 patients (38%) eventually proceeded to OLT.[40] In a similar review of 27 patients from Mount Sinai, 17 patients proceeded to OLT following SBRT.[41]

What data are available to compare the efficacy of ablative treatments for HCC?

Data comparing the efficacy of liver-directed therapies are limited, but in most studies SBRT demonstrates very favorable LC.

Xi (*JCO* 2024, PMID 39693584): RCT of patients with solitary recurrent HCC (≤5 cm) randomized to SBRT vs. RFA. The primary endpoint was LPFS. 166 patients randomized with MFU of 43 months. The 2-year LPFS was 93% in the SBRT arm vs. 76% in the RFA arm (SS). The effect was most pronounced among lesions ≤2 cm. mPFS was 38 months with SBRT and 28 months with RFA (NS). The 2-year OS was 98% in the SBRT arm vs. 94% in the RFA arm (NS). Acute and late AEs were similar in both arms. **Conclusion: In the setting of solitary recurrent HCC ≤5 cm, SBRT shows superior LPFS compared with RFA, with no difference in 2-year OS or incidence of adverse effects.**

Wahl, Michigan (*JCO* 2016, PMID 26628466): RR of 224 patients treated with RFA (161 patients with 250 tumors) or SBRT (63 patients with 83 tumors). Patients treated with SBRT had lower Child–Pugh scores, higher pretreatment AFP, and more prior treatments. The 1-year FFLP was increased with SBRT 97% vs. 84% for RFA. Increasing size was associated with reduced control for RFA but not for SBRT. For tumors >2 cm, SBRT has significantly higher FFLP (HR 3.35, SS). No differences in 1- or 2-year OS. **Conclusion: For tumors >2 cm, SBRT is superior to RFA in terms of FFLP.**

Bush, Loma Linda (*Cancer* 2023, PMID 37503907): PRT of 76 patients with new diagnosis of HCC meeting either Milan or UCSF criteria for transplantation randomized to TACE vs. proton therapy (PBT) 70.2 Gy/15 fx. Median tumor size 3.2 cm. At MFU of 30 months, 2-year LC and PFS higher in PBT, and 2-year OS not significantly different. Total hospitalization days within 30 days of treatment was significantly higher with TACE (166 vs. 24 days, SS), and PBT was associated with numerically higher CR rate among patients proceeding to transplantation (25% vs. 10%, NS). **Conclusion: PBT may have better efficacy and lower toxicity than TACE as a bridge to transplantation.**

Méndez Romero, TRENDY (*IJROBP* 2023, PMID 37037359): Multicenter, randomized, phase II study of 30 TACE- or transplant-eligible patients with inoperable HCC comparing TACE-DEB with SBRT. Closed early due to slow accrual. MFU 28 months. Primary endpoint was time to progression (TTP). Secondary endpoints included LC and OS. TTP was 12 months for TACE-DEB vs. 19 months for SBRT (NS). Post-hoc analysis showed significantly superior LC in the SBRT arm at 1 and 2 years. mOS was 37 months for TACE-DEB and 33 months for SBRT (NS). Response rate of >80% and similar quality of life scores in both arms. **Conclusion: Time to progression is not significantly improved by SBRT when compared with standard TACE-DEB. SBRT can be administered without detriment to OS or response rate. Superior LC with SBRT compared with TACE-DEB.**

Comito, Italy (*Curr Oncol* 2022, PMID 36421345): Single-institution RCT of SBRT vs. TAE/TACE rechallenge among 40 patients with incomplete response to prior TAE/TACE. Median tumor size 2.5 cm. Primary endpoint was 1-year LC. Closed early due to accrual. SBRT resulted in superior LC compared with TAE/TACE (median not reached vs. 8 months, SS). No significant improvement in OS in the SBRT arm. **Conclusion: SBRT following failure of TAE/TACE is associated with significantly superior LC when compared with TAE/TACE rechallenge.**

Kim, Korea (*Hepatology* 2020, PMID 33031846): Phase III randomized noninferiority trial of RFA vs. PBT for recurrent/residual one to two HCC lesions, each <3 cm. 144 patients total, 72 each arm. PBT was 66 GyE/10 fx. The per-protocol noninferiority analysis was set at 15% for the primary endpoint 2-year LPFS. The 2-year LPFS for PBT was 95% compared with 84% for RFA (SS). Median PFS for PBT was 13.4 months and 13.7 months in RFA. The 2-year OS was 89% in PBT and 93% in RFA (NS). CR was seen in 84% of PBT and 97% of RFA cases. Median time to best tumor response was 4.4 months for PBT and 1 month for RFA. There was a higher incidence of LFT increase and pain with RFA, but higher pneumonitis with PBT (all grade 1; SS). **Conclusion: PBT is noninferior to RFA in terms of LPFS. PBT is safe and tolerable.**

Can SBRT be combined with TACE to improve outcomes?

It appears safe and effective to give SBRT either combined with TACE or as salvage treatment after TACE.

Hardy-Abeloos, Mt. Sinai (*IJROBP* 2019, PMID 31536781): RR of 99 patients with MFU 9.8 months who received SBRT after TACE or TARE. Thirty-one had SBRT after segmental TARE and 68 post-TACE. There was a significant increase in post-SBRT Child–Pugh and ALBI scores (SS) for both groups; however, the increase was comparable for both. There was no significant increase in grade 3+ toxicity post-segmental TARE. There was also no significant difference in LC and OS between cohorts. **Conclusion: SBRT after segmental TARE appears to have acceptable tolerability and is effective compared with SBRT after TACE.**

Su, China (*BMC Cancer* 2016, PMID 27809890): RR of 127 patients with unresectable HCC who received SBRT followed by TAE or TACE (*n* = 77) compared with SBRT alone (*n* = 50). SBRT was 30–50 Gy/3–5 fx. Eligibility criteria included tumor >5 cm (median 8.5 cm) and Child–Pugh A to B. The PFS and LRFS were not significantly different between the groups. In the entire cohort, BED_{10} ≥100 Gy and EQD2 ≥74 Gy were significant prognostic factors for OS, PFS, LRFS, and DMFS. **Conclusion: SBRT combined with TAE/TACE may be an effective complementary treatment approach for HCC >5 cm. Treat to BED_{10} ≥100 Gy if feasible.**

Can hypofractionated RT or SBRT improve outcomes in the setting of portal vein tumor thrombus and can it be safely combined with other treatments?

Patient series out of Asia demonstrate improved outcomes with SBRT, with or without other therapies, in patients with portal vein tumor thrombus (PVT). Retrospective analyses suggest OS and PFS benefit to TACE + SBRT vs. TACE + sorafenib among patients with macroscopic vascular invasion.[42] SBRT is also superior to conventionally fractionated RT and is the preferred RT modality.[43]

Kang, Beijing (*Mol Clin Oncol* 2014, PMID 24649306): PRT of 101 patients with HCC and PVT randomized to SBRT followed by TACE, TACE followed by SBRT, or SBRT alone. SBRT ranged from 21 to 60 Gy/6 fx with median dose of 40 Gy. The 1-year LC trended toward improvement in SBRT followed by TACE (56%) vs. TACE followed by SBRT (49%) and SBRT alone (43%). CR of tumor thrombus to SBRT was achieved in 18% and PR in 53%. TACE followed by SBRT was associated with a slightly higher rate of increase in Child–Pugh score of 41% vs. 30% in other arms. **Conclusion: SBRT improves outcomes in HCC with PVT and can be safely combined with TACE. It may be most advantageous to sequence SBRT followed by TACE to preserve liver function.**

Yoon, Korea (*JAMA Oncol* 2018, PMID 29543938): PRT comparing TACE + RT vs. sorafenib in 90 treatment-naïve Child–Pugh A HCC patients with macroscopic vascular invasion. TACE given q6 weeks, RT was 45 Gy/15–18 fx, and sorafenib was 400 mg BID. At 12 weeks, PFS significantly higher with TACE + RT than sorafenib (87% vs. 34%, SS). OS significantly improved with TACE + RT vs. sorafenib (55 vs. 43 weeks, SS). Eleven percent of TACE + RT patients underwent curative surgical resection due to downstaging. **Conclusion: TACE + RT significantly improved PFS and OS compared with sorafenib alone in HCC patients with vascular invasion.**

Zhang, China (*PLoS One* 2022, PMID 35594278): Meta-analysis of nine studies (including Kang, above) comprising 938 patients examining clinical outcomes of patients with known PVT treated with SBRT + TACE vs. SBRT or TACE alone. Although multimodality therapy did not produce superior response rate on follow-up imaging, survival at 1 and 2 years was significantly improved with the combination of TACE and SBRT. This survival benefit did not hold among patients in whom the SBRT-TACE interval was ≥28 days. **Conclusion: Combined SBRT and TACE is safe in patients with PVT and extends survival relative to TACE or SBRT alone. Minimize the interval between SBRT and TACE to <28 days.**

Is RT safe and effective in the setting of IVC and/or right atrium involvement?

Data are limited; however, a recently published multicenter trial suggests RT is safe and effective.

Rim, KROG 17-10 (*IJROBP* 2020, PMID 31977276): From 2009 to 2016, 49 HCC patients with IVC and/or right atrium involvement received RT with a median dose of 46.7 Gy (range 35.4–71.5 Gy). MFU 9.3 months with MS 10 months. LC 89% and 75% at 1 and 2 years, respectively. The 1- and

2-year OS rates were 44% and 30%, respectively. Factors affecting OS were AFP ≥300 ng/mL, tumor multiplicity, and patient volume at institution (all *SS*). One case of possible RILD noted. **Conclusion: RT can yield favorable LC in HCC with extensive vascular involvement.**

Are there data to support pre- or postoperative RT for resectable HCC with portal vein tumor thrombus?

Recently published RCTs from China showed improved recurrence and survival outcomes for RT combined with surgery; however, this is primarily in HBV patients where surgery is more common. One study evaluated neoadjuvant 3D-CRT (18 Gy/6 fx) prior to hepatectomy and demonstrated statistically significant improvements in OS; on MVA, RT reduced HCC-related mortality and recurrence rates.[44] Similarly, in an RCT, postoperative IMRT (50 Gy/25 fx) demonstrated improved DFS and OS with the addition to RT after hepatectomy ± thrombectomy.[45]

Is there an advantage to proton therapy for HCC?

Given the dosimetric characteristics of protons, there may be an advantage to spare normal liver and reduce the risk of RILD. However, prospective studies have been limited to single-arm investigations.[46,47]

Sanford, MGH (*IJROBP* 2019, PMID 30684667): RR of 113 unresectable patients treated with RT; 37% treated with PBT. RT was 45 Gy/15 fx or 30 Gy/5–6 fx. In the photon arm, there were more Child–Pugh B/C patients (28% vs. 8%, SS) and more patients received prior liver-directed treatment (45% vs. 24%, NS). PBT was associated with improved OS; median OS 31 months compared with 14 months for photon patients. PBT was associated with significantly decreased risk of nonclassic RILD (seen in 4 PBT and 17 photon patients, *p* = .03). There was no difference in LC (2-year 93% PBT and 90% photon, *p* = .67). **Conclusion: Receipt of PBT was associated with better OS; however, selection bias and imbalance in the photon and proton arms may have contributed to this difference.**

Mizumoto, Japan (*IJROBP* 2024, PMID 37778422): Prospective registry of 576 patients treated with PBT, MFU 39 months. mOS was 49 months and 2-year OS was 69%. LR noted in 45 (8%) patients. Median PFS 15 months and 2-year was PFS 38%. Smaller tumors (<5 cm) and Child–Pugh A/B tumors had significantly superior OS to large tumors and Child–Pugh C patients. Twenty-seven patients (5%) with grade 3+ late adverse events. **Conclusion: Proton therapy for HCC results in excellent LC with an acceptable late toxicity profile.**

Bush, Loma Linda (*Cancer* 2011, PMID 21264826): Phase II study of PBT for 67 Child–Pugh A to C HCC patients with 63 GyE/15 fx. MS for Child–Pugh A, B, and C patients was 34, 13, and 12 months, respectively. In all patients, the median PFS was 36 months, and 19 patients underwent liver transplantation with 33% pCR. For transplanted patients, the 3-year OS was 70%, with average time from RT to transplantation of 13.2 months. No significant change in liver function seen within 6 months posttreatment. **Conclusion: PBT is a safe and effective treatment for inoperable HCC.**

REFERENCES

1. Siegel RL, Giaquinto AN, Jemal A. Cancer statistics, 2024. *CA Cancer J Clin.* 2024;74(1):12–49. doi:10.3322/caac.21820
2. Ioannou GN, Green PK, Berry K. HCV eradication induced by direct-acting antiviral agents reduces the risk of hepatocellular carcinoma. *J Hepatol.* 2018;68(1):25–32. doi:10.1016/j.jhep.2017.08.030
3. Marrero JA, Kulik LM, Sirlin CB, et al. Diagnosis, staging, and management of hepatocellular carcinoma: 2018 practice guidance by the American association for the study of liver diseases. *Hepatology.* 2018;68(2):723–750. doi:10.1002/hep.29913
4. Zhang BH, Yang BH, Tang ZY. Randomized controlled trial of screening for hepatocellular carcinoma. *J Cancer Res Clin Oncol.* 2004;130(7):417–422. doi:10.1007/s00432-004-0552-0
5. Network NCC. Hepatocellular Carcinoma (Version 2.2024). Accessed September 23, 2024, https://www.nccn.org/professionals/physician_gls/pdf/hcc.pdf
6. Pomfret EA, Washburn K, Wald C, et al. Report of a national conference on liver allocation in patients with hepatocellular carcinoma in the United States. *Liver Transpl.* 2010;16(3):262–278. doi:10.1002/lt.21999
7. Chernyak V, Fowler KJ, Kamaya A, et al. Liver Imaging Reporting and Data System (LI-RADS) version 2018: imaging of hepatocellular carcinoma in at-risk patients. *Radiology.* 2018;289(3):816–830. doi:10.1148/radiol.2018181494

8. Bruix J, Sherman M, American Association for the Study of Liver Diseases. Management of hepatocellular carcinoma: an update. *Hepatology*. 2011;53(3):1020–1022. doi:10.1002/hep.24199
9. European Association for the Study of the Liver. EASL clinical practice guidelines: management of hepatocellular carcinoma. *J Hepatol*. 2018;69(1):182–236. doi:10.1016/j.jhep.2018.03.019
10. Hong SB, Choi SH, Kim SY, et al. MRI features for predicting microvascular invasion of hepatocellular carcinoma: a systematic review and meta-analysis. *Liver Cancer*. 2021;10(2):94–106. doi:10.1159/000513704
11. Johnson PJ, Berhane S, Kagebayashi C, et al. Assessment of liver function in patients with hepatocellular carcinoma: a new evidence-based approach-the ALBI grade. *J Clin Oncol*. 2015;33(6):550–558. doi:10.1200/JCO.2014.57.9151
12. Forner A, Reig ME, de Lope CR, Bruix J. Current strategy for staging and treatment: the BCLC update and future prospects. *Semin Liver Dis*. 2010;30(1):61–74. doi:10.1055/s-0030-1247133
13. Reig M, Forner A, Rimola J, et al. BCLC strategy for prognosis prediction and treatment recommendation: the 2022 update. *J Hepatol*. 2022;76(3):681–693. doi:10.1016/j.jhep.2021.11.018
14. O'Connor JK, Trotter J, Davis GL, Dempster J, Klintmalm GB, Goldstein RM. Long-term outcomes of stereotactic body radiation therapy in the treatment of hepatocellular cancer as a bridge to transplantation. *Liver Transpl*. 2012;18(8):949–954. doi:10.1002/lt.23439
15. Kulik LM, Atassi B, van Holsbeeck L, et al. Yttrium-90 microspheres (TheraSphere) treatment of unresectable hepatocellular carcinoma: downstaging to resection, RFA and bridge to transplantation. *J Surg Oncol*. 2006;94(7):572–586. doi:10.1002/jso.20609
16. Llovet JM, Fuster J, Bruix J. Intention-to-treat analysis of surgical treatment for early hepatocellular carcinoma: resection versus transplantation. *Hepatology*. 1999;30(6):1434–1440. doi:10.1002/hep.510300629
17. Graziadei IW, Sandmueller H, Waldenberger P, et al. Chemoembolization followed by liver transplantation for hepatocellular carcinoma impedes tumor progression while on the waiting list and leads to excellent outcome. *Liver Transpl*. 2003;9(6):557–563. doi:10.1053/jlts.2003.50106
18. Amin J, O'Connell D, Bartlett M, et al. Liver cancer and hepatitis B and C in New South Wales, 1990-2002: a linkage study. *Aust N Z J Public Health*. 2007;31(5):475–482. doi:10.1111/j.1753-6405.2007.00121.x
19. Poon RT, Fan ST, Lo CM, Liu CL, Wong J. Long-term survival and pattern of recurrence after resection of small hepatocellular carcinoma in patients with preserved liver function: implications for a strategy of salvage transplantation. *Ann Surg*. 2002;235(3):373–382. doi:10.1097/00000658-200203000-00009
20. Iwatsuki S, Starzl TE, Sheahan DG, et al. Hepatic resection versus transplantation for hepatocellular carcinoma. *Ann Surg*. 1991;214(3):221–229. doi:10.1097/00000658-199109000-00005
21. Mazzaferro V, Regalia E, Doci R, et al. Liver transplantation for the treatment of small hepatocellular carcinomas in patients with cirrhosis. *N Engl J Med*. 1996;334(11):693–699. doi:10.1056/NEJM199603143341104
22. Yao FY, Xiao L, Bass NM, Kerlan R, Ascher NL, Roberts JP. Liver transplantation for hepatocellular carcinoma: validation of the UCSF-expanded criteria based on preoperative imaging. *Am J Transplant*. 2007;7(11):2587–2596. doi:10.1111/j.1600-6143.2007.01965.x
23. Wiesner R, Edwards E, Freeman R, et al. Model for end-stage liver disease (MELD) and allocation of donor livers. *Gastroenterology*. 2003;124(1):91–96. doi:10.1053/gast.2003.50016
24. Vilgrain V, Pereira H, Assenat E, et al. Efficacy and safety of selective internal radiotherapy with yttrium-90 resin microspheres compared with sorafenib in locally advanced and inoperable hepatocellular carcinoma (SARAH): an open-label randomised controlled phase 3 trial. *Lancet Oncol*. 2017;18(12):1624–1636. doi:10.1016/S1470-2045(17)30683-6
25. Kudo M, Finn RS, Qin S, et al. Lenvatinib versus sorafenib in first-line treatment of patients with unresectable hepatocellular carcinoma: a randomised phase 3 non-inferiority trial. *Lancet*. 2018;391(10126):1163–1173. doi:10.1016/S0140-6736(18)30207-1
26. Hack SP, Spahn J, Chen M, et al. IMbrave 050: a Phase III trial of atezolizumab plus bevacizumab in high-risk hepatocellular carcinoma after curative resection or ablation. *Future Oncol*. 2020;16(15):975–989. doi:10.2217/fon-2020-0162
27. Abou-Alfa GK, Lau G, Kudo M, et al. Tremelimumab plus durvalumab in unresectable hepatocellular carcinoma. *NEJM Evid*. 2022;1(8):EVIDoa2100070. doi:10.1056/EVIDoa2100070
28. Soliman H, Ringash J, Jiang H, et al. Phase II trial of palliative radiotherapy for hepatocellular carcinoma and liver metastases. *J Clin Oncol*. 2013;31(31):3980–3986. doi:10.1200/JCO.2013.49.9202
29. Dawson LA, Ringash J, Fairchild A, et al. Palliative radiotherapy versus best supportive care in patients with painful hepatic cancer (CCTG HE1): a multicentre, open-label, randomised, controlled, phase 3 study. *Lancet Oncol*. 2024;25(10):1337–1346. doi:10.1016/S1470-2045(24)00438-8
30. Benson R, Madan R, Kilambi R, Chander S. Radiation induced liver disease: a clinical update. *J Egypt Natl Canc Inst*. 2016;28(1):7–11. doi:10.1016/j.jnci.2015.08.001
31. Videtic GMM, Vassil AD, Woody NM. *Handbook of Treatment Planning in Radiation Oncology*. 3rd ed. Springer Publishing Company; 2020.
32. Tateishi R, Shiina S, Teratani T, et al. Percutaneous radiofrequency ablation for hepatocellular carcinoma. An analysis of 1000 cases. *Cancer*. 2005;103(6):1201–1209. doi:10.1002/cncr.20892

33. Tanabe KK, Curley SA, Dodd GD, Siperstein AE, Goldberg SN. Radiofrequency ablation: the experts weigh in. *Cancer*. 2004;100(3):641–650. doi:10.1002/cncr.11919

34. Llovet JM, Real MI, Montana X, et al. Arterial embolisation or chemoembolisation versus symptomatic treatment in patients with unresectable hepatocellular carcinoma: a randomised controlled trial. *Lancet*. 2002;359(9319):1734–1739. doi:10.1016/S0140-6736(02)08649-X

35. Garwood ER, Fidelman N, Hoch SE, Kerlan RK Jr, Yao FY. Morbidity and mortality following transarterial liver chemoembolization in patients with hepatocellular carcinoma and synthetic hepatic dysfunction. *Liver Transpl*. 2013;19(2):164–173. doi:10.1002/lt.23552

36. Salem R, Lewandowski RJ, Mulcahy MF, et al. Radioembolization for hepatocellular carcinoma using Yttrium-90 microspheres: a comprehensive report of long-term outcomes. *Gastroenterology*. 2010;138(1): 52–64. doi:10.1053/j.gastro.2009.09.006

37. Kokabi N, Camacho JC, Xing M, et al. Open-label prospective study of the safety and efficacy of glass-based yttrium 90 radioembolization for infiltrative hepatocellular carcinoma with portal vein thrombosis. *Cancer*. 2015;121(13):2164–2174. doi:10.1002/cncr.29275

38. Culleton S, Jiang H, Haddad CR, et al. Outcomes following definitive stereotactic body radiotherapy for patients with Child-Pugh B or C hepatocellular carcinoma. *Radiother Oncol*. 2014;111(3):412–417. doi:10.1016/j.radonc.2014.05.002

39. Lee P, Ma Y, Zacharias I, et al. Stereotactic body radiation therapy for hepatocellular carcinoma in patients with Child-Pugh B or C cirrhosis. *Adv Radiat Oncol*. 2020;5(5):889–896. doi:10.1016/j.adro.2020.01.009

40. Andolino DL, Johnson CS, Maluccio M, et al. Stereotactic body radiotherapy for primary hepatocellular carcinoma. *Int J Radiat Oncol Biol Phys*. 2011;81(4):e447–e453. doi:10.1016/j.ijrobp.2011.04.011

41. Facciuto ME, Singh MK, Rochon C, et al. Stereotactic body radiation therapy in hepatocellular carcinoma and cirrhosis: evaluation of radiological and pathological response. *J Surg Oncol*. 2012;105(7):692–698. doi:10.1002/jso.22104

42. Shen L, Xi M, Zhao L, et al. Combination therapy after TACE for hepatocellular carcinoma with macroscopic vascular invasion: stereotactic body radiotherapy versus sorafenib. *Cancers (Basel)*. 2018;10(12):516. doi:10.3390/cancers10120516

43. Yang JF, Lo CH, Lee MS, et al. Stereotactic ablative radiotherapy versus conventionally fractionated radiotherapy in the treatment of hepatocellular carcinoma with portal vein invasion: a retrospective analysis. *Radiat Oncol*. 2019;14(1):180. doi:10.1186/s13014-019-1382-1

44. Wei X, Jiang Y, Zhang X, et al. Neoadjuvant three-dimensional conformal radiotherapy for resectable hepatocellular carcinoma with portal vein tumor thrombus: a randomized, open-label, multicenter controlled study. *J Clin Oncol*. 2019;37(24):2141–2151. doi:10.1200/JCO.18.02184

45. Sun J, Yang L, Shi J, et al. Postoperative adjuvant IMRT for patients with HCC and portal vein tumor thrombus: an open-label randomized controlled trial. *Radiother Oncol*. 2019;140:20–25. doi:10.1016/j.radonc.2019.05.006

46. Cheng JY, Liu CM, Wang YM, et al. Proton versus photon radiotherapy for primary hepatocellular carcinoma: a propensity-matched analysis. *Radiat Oncol*. 2020;15(1):159. doi:10.1186/s13014-020-01605-4

47. Sanford NN, Pursley J, Noe B, et al. Protons versus photons for unresectable hepatocellular carcinoma: liver decompensation and overall survival. *Int J Radiat Oncol Biol Phys*. 2019;105(1):64–72. doi:10.1016/j.ijrobp.2019.01.076

36 PANCREATIC ADENOCARCINOMA

Ahmed Halima, James R. Broughman, Jacob A. Miller, and Ehsan H. Balagamwala

QUICK HIT   Pancreatic adenocarcinoma is the fourth leading cause of cancer death in the United States. Although it is prone to wide dissemination, up to a third of patients die of complications from local progression. For the 15% of patients with resectable disease at presentation, upfront surgery ± neoadjuvant CHT is standard and represents the only means of cure. Adjuvant treatment consists of CHT ± RT. Twenty percent present with borderline-resectable disease; however, only ~60% of these patients will undergo surgery with a clear margin. Patients with borderline-resectable disease may undergo downstaging with CHT ± RT to increase the likelihood of a R0 resection (see Table 36.1). Combined-agent CHT regimens such as FOLFIRINOX/gemcitabine + abraxane are preferred over single-agent regimens in fit patients. Pancreatic cancer is intrinsically radioresistant, so there is growing interest in utilizing SBRT to improve LC, although this is technically challenging due to the proximity of tumors to the duodenum, jejunum, and stomach.

Table 36.1 General Treatment Paradigm for Pancreatic Cancer

Setting	Initial Option	Additional Treatment(s)
Resectable disease	Neoadjuvant CHT	Surgery followed by adjuvant CHT ± RT (for positive margins)
	Surgery	CHT alone[1] • 5-FU-based multiagent regimen (e.g., FOLFIRINOX) • Gemcitabine ± capecitabine • 5-FU
		CHT followed by CRT to 45–54 Gy with concurrent 5-FU or gemcitabine for positive margins and/or LN+
Borderline resectable	Neoadjuvant CHT followed by CRT (45–54 Gy), reassessment, then surgery	
	Neoadjuvant CHT followed by surgery; adjuvant CRT for positive margins and/or LN+	
Locally advanced/ unresectable	Initial CHT	SBRT (preferred) or in select cases CRT
	SBRT (if symptomatic)	CHT
	CHT alone	
Metastatic	Treated with multiagent or single-agent systemic therapy ± palliative surgery/biliary stent/RT	

EPIDEMIOLOGY: Estimated 66,440 new cases in 2024 in the United States, with 51,750 deaths; fourth leading cause of cancer mortality in men and third most common cause of cancer mortality in females.[1] Higher incidence in males vs. females (1.3:1), higher incidence in Black individuals vs. Caucasians, and more common in developed nations.[2,3] Rare under 40 years of age with a median age of 60 at diagnosis. Peak incidence sixth to seventh decade, which makes aggressive treatment challenging.[3]

RISK FACTORS: Chronic pancreatitis (relative risk [RR] 16–69), cigarette smoking (RR 1–3), high BMI (RR 1–2), chronic diabetes (RR 1–3), heavy alcohol consumption (RR 2–4), red meat (RR 1–1.5), exposure to hydrocarbon compounds/pesticides/heavy metals, and cystic fibrosis.[4-7] There is emerging evidence for increased risk in those previously infected with *Helicobacter pylori*, HBV, and HCV.[4,8] Hereditary conditions include familial predisposition, hereditary pancreatitis (*PRSS1/SPINK1*; RR 50–67), Peutz–Jeghers (*STK11/LKB1*; RR 132), FAMMM syndrome (*CDKN2A/TP16*; RR 48), mutations in *BRCA1/BRCA2* (RR 2–7), Lynch syndrome (*MLH1/MSH2/MSH6/PMS2*), or ataxia telangiectasia.[4,9-14] Of the cases, 5% to 10% have an inherited component, although if one first-degree relative RR 1.5–13, if two relatives RR 18, and if three relatives RR 57.[15-18] Other risk factors include non-O blood type (RR 1–2) and partial gastrectomy/cholecystectomy/appendectomy[19,20]

ANATOMY: Pancreas: retroperitoneal and located anterior to L1/L2. It extends from the concavity of the duodenum to the hilum of the spleen. Divided into head (including uncinate process), neck, body, and tail. The superior mesenteric vessels pass anterior to the uncinate process. The pancreatic duct and accessory duct combine with the common bile duct, which courses posterior to the head of the pancreas and enter the duodenum via the sphincter of Oddi at the ampulla of Vater. The splenic vein and the superior mesenteric vein (SMV) join posterior to the neck of the pancreas to form the portal vein. The inferior mesenteric vein drains into the splenic vein. Peritoneal involvement is more common with body and tail tumors. Arterial supply of the pancreas is through derivatives of the celiac artery except for the inferior half of the head and the uncinate process, which is supplied by the inferior pancreaticoduodenal artery, a branch of the SMA. Venous drainage is via portal system. Celiac axis is at the level of T11/T12, and SMA is at the level of L1. Nerve supply follows the distribution of the arterial supply. Tumor invasion posteriorly can lead to lung/pleural metastasis via vena cava drainage. The pancreas is directly adjacent to or in close proximity to the stomach, duodenum, jejunum, kidneys, spleen, and several blood vessels (celiac axis, superior mesenteric artery, splenic artery, and associated veins as well as portal vein), and common bile duct.

Lymphatics/Patterns of Spread: Regional drainage is to peripancreatic, celiac, superior mesenteric, porta hepatic, and para-aortic LNs. Frequently metastasizes hematogenously to the liver via portal venous network. Tumors of the head and neck drain along the common bile duct, common hepatic artery, portal vein, posterior/anterior pancreaticoduodenal arcades, SMV, and right lateral wall of SMA. Tumors of body and tail drain along common hepatic artery, celiac axis, splenic artery, and splenic hilum.

PATHOLOGY: Greater than 80% are ductal adenocarcinoma (ACA).[21] Approximately 60% arise from head, 15% in body or tail, and 20% diffusely involve the pancreas.[21] Periampullary tumors can originate from the head of the pancreas, distal common bile duct, ampulla of Vater, or adjacent duodenum. Acinar cell tumors are associated with fat necrosis, elevated lipase, rash, eosinophilia, polyarthralgia, and poor prognosis. Others include mucinous cystadenoma and adenosquamous carcinoma.[22] Other histologies include signet ring, medullary, adenosquamous, serous, and mixed acinar/ductal/neuroendocrine carcinoma. Approximately 5% of all pancreatic tumors are indolent endocrine tumors with long natural history and circulating polypeptides.[23]

GENETICS: *KRAS* and *P53* oncogene mutation in >90%.[21,24] Overexpression of *MMP* or *EGFR* in 60% to 70%. *TP53* mutation in 60%. *SMAD4* tumor suppressor mutated/deleted in ~30% and is a poor prognostic marker linked to higher predisposition for metastatic disease and shortened survival.[21,24]

SCREENING: The International Cancer of the Pancreas Screening (CAPS) consortium[25] recommends annual screening with endoscopic ultrasound (EUS), MRI/MRCP, and fasting blood glucose or HbA1C at baseline and with alternating MRI/MRCP and EUS thereafter for high-risk individuals defined as patients with:

1. Peutz–Jeghers (carriers of a germline *LKB1/STK11* gene mutation)
2. All carriers of a germline *CDKN2A* mutation
3. Carriers of a germline *BRCA2*, *BRCA1*, *PALB2*, *ATM*, *MLH1*, *MSH2*, or *MSH6* gene mutation with at least one affected first-degree blood relative
4. Individuals who have at least one first-degree relative with pancreatic cancer who in turn also has a first-degree relative with pancreatic cancer (familial pancreatic cancer kindred)

Age to initiate surveillance depends on an individual's gene mutation status and family history. No consensus exists on age to initiate or terminate screening/surveillance, but generally starts at age 40 for Peutz–Jeghers and CDKN2A mutations and at age 45 to 50 or 10 years younger than the youngest affected blood relative in carriers of other listed mutations. Higher detection rate when screened with EUS over MRI or CT imaging.[25-28]

CLINICAL PRESENTATION: Due to gross or microscopic involvement of the celiac plexus, ~40% to 60% of patients present with pain particularly in the upper abdomen radiating to the back, which is intermittent and can be exacerbated by eating and/or alleviated by specific positions such as leaning forward or lying on the left side or in fetal position. Other symptoms include weight loss (80%–85%); fatigue (85%); nausea (~25%); diarrhea/steatorrhea; jaundice (~55%), often with acholic stools and/or dark urine; and hepatomegaly.[29-31] Classically, painless jaundice in resectable patients associated with a pancreatic head mass has a more favorable prognosis than those with symptomatic jaundice. Patients may suddenly develop diabetes 2 to 3 years prior to presentation with malignancy.

Eponyms: Enlarged nontender gallbladder (Courvoisier's sign), migratory thrombophlebitis (Trousseau's sign), left SCV LN (Virchow's node), left axillary node (Irish's node), periumbilical node (Sister Mary Joseph node), rectal shelf (Blumer's shelf), periumbilical ecchymosis (Cullen's sign), or flank ecchymosis (Grey Turner sign).

WORKUP: H&P.

Labs: CBC, CMP (including LFTs), CA 19–9 (may be undetectable in Lewis antigen-negative patients).

Imaging: Multidetector pancreatic protocol CT (early arterial, late arterial, and venous phases) obtaining thin (0.5–1 mm) slices is recommended even if a standard CT of the abdomen is available. MRI (abdomen and pelvis) can also be performed. Imaging should be before stent placement if possible.[32] Systemic staging with CT CAP. PET/CT can be considered in patients at high risk of extrapancreatic metastasis but is not a substitute to high-quality contrast-enhanced pancreatic protocol CT.[32] PET/CT detects unsuspected CT-occult DM in 33% of patients.[32]

Biopsy: Via EUS, ERCP, or CT guidance. EUS-guided biopsy is associated with better diagnostic yield, potentially lower risk of peritoneal seeding, and safety compared with CT-guided biopsy in nonmetastatic disease.[33-35] Biopsy is not necessarily required before surgery in patients with resectable disease, however is necessary before administration of neoadjuvant therapy, in patients with unresectable or metastatic disease (biopsy of metastatic site may be preferable), or enrollment in a clinical trial. ERCP (with brushing/biopsy) may be useful in symptomatic obstructive jaundice requiring stent placement. MRCP is useful when looking for occult primary (benefits are no contrast and no increased risk of post-ERCP pancreatitis).[36] Diagnostic staging laparoscopy (especially for body and tail lesions) can be utilized to rule out unresectable disease and peritoneal metastases not seen on imaging. Imaging-guided biopsy is preferred for potentially metastatic lesions in the liver.[37-39]

PROGNOSTIC FACTORS: Age, stage, grade, KPS, histology, location (head lesions are more favorable and present earlier), visceral artery involvement, extent of resection, response to neoadjuvant therapy, perineural invasion, LN status/ratio, and both pre- and postoperative serum CA 19–9 levels.[40-44]

STAGING: See Table 36.2.

Table 36.2 AJCC 8th Edition (2017) Staging for Exocrine Pancreatic Cancer					
T/M	N	cN0	cN1	cN2
T1	a. ≤0.5 cm	IA	IIB	III
	b. >0.5 and <1 cm			
	c. 1–2 cm			
T2	• 2.1–4 cm	IB		
T3	• >4 cm	IIA		
T4	• Involvement[1] regardless of size			
M1	• Distant metastasis	IV		

Notes: Involvement[1] = celiac axis, SMA, and/or common hepatic artery.
cN1: 1–3 LNs; cN2: ≥4 LNs.

TREATMENT PARADIGM

Surgery: Surgery is currently the only potentially curative option for pancreatic cancer (Table 36.3). Twenty percent present with apparently resectable disease; however, ~20% of patients thought to have resectable disease do not have resectable disease at the time of surgery (e.g., peritoneal involvement, etc.). Approximately 50% of patients present with disseminated disease (commonly liver, peritoneum, and lungs). The remainder have borderline resectable disease (i.e., tumor is neither clearly resectable nor clearly unresectable) or locally advanced unresectable disease. Ultimately, ~15% of patients with newly diagnosed pancreatic cancer have upfront resectable disease. If neoadjuvant therapy is pursued, restaging after completion of neoadjuvant therapy is necessary before proceeding with surgery. Whipple procedure (pancreaticoduodenectomy) is the standard therapeutic operation for pancreatic head tumors and involves en bloc resection of pancreatic head/body, distal stomach, duodenum, proximal jejunum, gallbladder, and distal common bile duct. Four PRTs have shown no difference in survival between variations on pancreaticoduodenectomy including pylorus-preserving, subtotal stomach-preserving, and minimally invasive techniques.[45–48] In addition, more extensive surgery, including extended lymphadenectomy and arterial en bloc resection, does not improve outcomes.[48,49] Operative mortality at high-volume centers is <5%.[50] After Whipple, remnant organs are attached to the jejunum (pancreaticojejunostomy, gastrojejunostomy, and choledochojejunostomy) with vagotomy. The most common site of positive margin is retroperitoneal margin. This margin is also referred to as "uncinate margin," "posterior margin," and "SMA margin." It represents soft tissue directly adjacent to the proximal 3 to 4 cm of the SMA. Tail lesions can be considered for distal pancreatectomy depending on disease involvement. For highly selected patients with body/tail lesions with celiac artery involvement, Appleby procedure may be an option (includes splenectomy, distal pancreatectomy and celiac artery resection, relies on collateral circulation for hepatic perfusion). Postoperative complications include anastomotic leaks, which can lead to peritonitis, abscess, autodigestion, hemorrhage, and delayed gastric emptying.

Table 36.3 NCCN Criteria for Resectability at Diagnosis[32]		
Resectability Status	**Arterial**	**Venous**
Resectable	No arterial tumor contact (celiac axis, SMA, and common hepatic artery)	No radiographic evidence of SMV or portal vein contact or ≤180° contact without vein contour irregularity
Borderline resectable	1. Head/uncinate process tumor 　a. Involvement of common hepatic artery without celiac axis or hepatic bifurcation involved 　b. Abutment of SMA of ≤180° 　c. Contact with anatomic arterial variant (e.g., replaced or accessory artery) 2. Body/tail tumors: involvement of ≤180° of celiac axis	3. Involvement of SMV/portal vein of >180° OR ≤180° with contour irregularity of vein 4. SMV/portal impingement (distortion/narrowing/occlusion/thrombosis), which can be resected/reconstructed 5. Solid tumor contact with the inferior vena cava
Unresectable	1. DM, including LN beyond field of resection 2. Head/uncinate process tumor: abutment >180° with SMA or celiac axis 3. Body/tail tumors 　a. Abutment of >180° with the SMA or celiac axis 　b. Aortic invasion or encasement	4. Unreconstructable SMV/portal vein occlusion due to tumor involvement or occlusion (even bland thrombus)

Source: NCCN Clinical Practice Guidelines in Oncology: Pancreatic Adenocarcinoma. https://www.nccn.org/professionals/physician_gls/pdf/pancreatic.pdf.

Systemic Therapy: Systemic therapy is used in all stages of pancreatic cancer. Historically, 5-FU was used in both the metastatic and adjuvant settings. Gemcitabine was the first agent to show a modest advantage over 5-FU in patients with advanced pancreatic cancer.[51] In both the adjuvant and metastatic settings, FOLFIRINOX was shown to be superior to single-agent gemcitabine.[52,53] Separately, the addition of nab-paclitaxel (Abraxane) to gemcitabine showed a survival advantage over gemcitabine alone in both the metastatic and nonmetastatic setting.[54,55] Gemcitabine/nab-paclitaxel and FOLFIRINOX were never compared head-to-head in a trial. However, ASCO/NCCN guidelines recommend FOLFIRINOX as first line in patients with an ECOG performance status of 0 to 1 who are able to tolerate it.[56] NALIRINOX (liposomal irinotecan, oxaliplatin, leucovorin, and 5FU) has recently shown to improve survival compared with gemcitabine/nab-paclitaxel in the metastatic setting in the NAPOLI-3 trial.[57] Single-agent gemcitabine and 5-FU are reserved for patients with a poor performance status. PARP inhibitors are approved for BRCA- and PALB2-mutated pancreatic cancer after at least 16 weeks of platinum-based combination CHT based on the POLO trial.[58] Immunotherapy can be utilized in a small subset of patients with MSI-high and high tumor mutational burden (TMB).[59]

Radiation

Indications: RT can be delivered in neoadjuvant, postoperative, definitive, or palliative setting. Neoadjuvant RT has been utilized for borderline resectable patients in an attempt to optimize downstaging and provide LC in the event resection does not occur. However, this continues to be controversial in the setting of multiagent neoadjuvant CHT. Adjuvant RT should be considered in patients with positive margins and/or positive LNs.[60] Definitive RT for unresectable/locally advanced cases improves LC and reduces pain. However, survival benefit has not been shown in modern trials (see below). For locally advanced tumors, ASCO Guidelines recommend initial CHT followed by SBRT or CRT in the setting of local progression or stable disease to avoid progression to second- or third-line CHT.[61] Contouring guidelines per RTOG 1102 for locally advanced disease and RTOG 0848 for adjuvant therapy.[62–64]

Dose: Conventional RT: 50.4 Gy/28 fx. SBRT: 25 to 50 Gy/5 fx delivered every other day.

Toxicity: Acute: fatigue, dermatitis, nausea, vomiting, diarrhea, appetite loss, weight loss, stomach ulcers. Late: fatigue, skin discoloration, liver/renal dysfunction, bowel obstruction, stomach/bowel ulcers, dry/hyperpigmented skin.

Procedure: See *Handbook of Treatment Planning in Radiation Oncology,* Chapter 7.[65]

Palliation: Celiac plexus and intrapleural nerve blocks and neurolysis can provide effective pain relief for select patients; however, relief can be transient in those who respond and others derive minimal relief after procedure.[66,67] In patients who do not respond to celiac plexus block, palliative SBRT can be utilized for pain and tumor control. SBRT has been shown to help achieve pain relief in >85% of patients and is the preferred palliative option when appropriate.[68] In a single-arm, phase II trial, palliative SBRT to the celiac plexus (25 Gy/1 fx with lower dose to areas close to OARs) was shown to improve QOL, decrease pain at 3 and 6 weeks, and decrease opioid use.[69] A nonrandomized phase II trial of 24 Gy in 3 weekly fractions also showed improved pain and QOL.[70] Alternative palliative SBRT regimens includes 25 to 50 Gy in 5 fx. In patients who are not SBRT candidates, palliative RT with 30 Gy/10 fx can improve pain in ~50% to 65% of patients.[71] Roux-En-Y gastric bypass and biliary bypass or Whipple procedure can offer palliation for duodenal obstruction and jaundice. Endoscopic stent placement (frequently plastic for resectable disease and expandable metal stent for unresectable disease) is preferred method (compared with percutaneous stents).

EVIDENCE-BASED Q&A

RESECTABLE PANCREATIC CANCER

Is surgery necessary in the management of pancreatic cancer?

Surgery, if possible, carries a significant survival benefit. Retroperitoneal lymphadenectomy is not necessary as it provides no OS advantage, and pylorus preservation carries a higher risk of positive margins (21% vs. 5%).[51]

Doi, Japan (*Surg Today* 2008, PMID 18958561): Japanese multi-institution RCT of resectable pancreatic ACA (no involvement of SMA/common hepatic artery, no PA LN+) randomized to surgery (pancreaticoduodenectomy or distal pancreatectomy + regional LN dissection) vs. CRT (continuous infusion 5-FU at 200 mg/m²/day with 50.4 Gy/28 fx, four-field technique, tumor + 1–3 cm margin covering regional LN). Closed early due to survival benefit (42/150 enrolled) favoring surgical resection. MS 12.1 vs. 8.9 months, 3-year OS 20% vs. 0% (*p* < .03), 5-year OS 10% vs. 0% (NS). LC not reported. **Conclusion: Surgery significantly improves OS in resectable pancreatic cancer.**

Is there a benefit to neoadjuvant systemic therapy in resectable patients?

Neoadjuvant CHT (4–6 months) is preferred for resectable patients. While NORPACT-1 did not show a survival benefit to neoadjuvant compared with adjuvant CHT, neoadjuvant is favored, *allowing for maximum control of systemic disease and an increased rate of R0 resections.*

Labori, NORPACT-1 (*Lancet Gastroenterol Hepatol* 2024, PMID 38237621): Phase II trial of 140 patients with resectable pancreatic cancer randomized to neoadjuvant FOLFIRINOX for four cycles followed by surgery and adjuvant CHT (77 patients) or immediate surgery followed by adjuvant CHT (63 patients). Adjuvant CHT was initially gemcitabine + capecitabine; however, this was addended to allow adjuvant FOLFIRINOX. Primary endpoint was OS at 18 months. Of 77 patients, 61 (79%) in the neoadjuvant FOLFIRINOX received the neoadjuvant therapy and 8 patients were excluded from the upfront surgery group. Eighty-two percent of the neoadjuvant group and 89% of patients in the upfront surgery group had resection ($p = .24$). OS at 18 months by intention to treat was 60% in the neoadjuvant FOLFIRINOX arm and 73% in the upfront surgery group ($p = .032$). OS at 18 months by per-protocol analysis was 57% in neoadjuvant group and 70% in the upfront surgery group ($p = .14$). Fifty-eight percent of the neoadjuvant FOLFIRINOX group vs. 40% of the upfront surgery group experienced a grade 3+ adverse event. **Conclusion: This phase II trial did not show a survival benefit to neoadjuvant FOLFIRINOX in resectable pancreatic ductal ACA.**

Is there a benefit to adjuvant CRT compared with surgery alone?

The benefit to adjuvant CRT compared with surgery alone is controversial given the results of the following two trials. Latest ASCO guidelines suggest consideration of adjuvant CRT to patients who did not receive preoperative therapy and present postresection with microscopic positive margins and/or positive LNs. CRT should be given after completion of 4 to 6 months of adjuvant CHT.[60]

Kalser, GITSG 91-73 (*Arch Surg* 1985, PMID 4015380; Confirmation Arm, *Cancer* 1987, PMID 3567862): PRT of 43 patients with negative margins following resection without peritoneal mets randomized to postop CRT vs. observation. Treatment was split-course 40 Gy with 2-week break + 5-FU 500 mg/m² d1–3, with each 20 Gy course, then weekly 5-FU for 2 years or until recurrence. RT covered pancreas, pancreatic bed, and regional LNs. Subtotal Whipple in 68%, total Whipple in 32%; 25% did not start adjuvant treatment for >10 weeks postop. CRT significantly increased MS and 2-year OS (Table 36.4). **Conclusion: Combined use of CRT as adjuvant therapy after curative resection is effective and is preferred to no adjuvant therapy.** *Comment: Terminated early after 8 years due to poor accrual and early benefit to CRT presented in 1985. Additional 30 patients were accrued to receive adjuvant CRT after closure were presented in 1987 to demonstrate replication of results ("confirmation arm").*

Table 36.4 Results of GITSG 91-73 Adjuvant Pancreas Trial			
GITSG	**MS**	**2-Yr OS**	**5-Yr OS**
Surgery alone	11 months	15%	5%
Adjuvant CRT	20 months	42%	15%
Confirmation arm	18 months	46%	17%

Klinkenbijl, EORTC 40891 (*Ann Surg* 1999, PMID 10615932; Reanalysis Garofalo, *Ann Surg* 2006, PMID 16858208; Update Smeenk, *Ann Surg* 2007, PMID 17968163): PRT of 218 patients with T1–2N0–1a pancreatic head ACA ($n = 114$) or T1–3N0–1a periampullary ACA ($n = 104$) s/p resection. N1a was defined as LNs within resection specimen. Positive margins were included. Randomized to adjuvant concurrent CRT (40 Gy split course, with 5-FU 25 mg/kg on d1–5 and 29–34) vs. no adjuvant therapy. CHT was similar to GITSG 9173 with no maintenance CHT. Adjuvant treatment arm had more pancreatic head tumors than observation arm and fewer periampullary tumors. Overall, no difference in OS, but study was underpowered (Table 36.5). Trend of benefit to adjuvant CRT for pancreatic head tumors (excluding periampullary). **Conclusion: Routine use of postop CRT is not recommended; 12-year update confirmed no benefit.** *Comment: Study limitations included patients with positive margins, no maintenance CHT, split-course RT, low RT dose, no RT QA, and inclusion of periampullary and N1a patients. Twenty percent of patients randomized to CRT did not receive it.*

Table 36.5 Results of EORTC 40891 Adjuvant CRT for Pancreas Cancer							
EORTC 40891 (12-Yr Update)	**MS (Yrs)**	**5-Yr OS**	**10-Yr OS**	**Median PFS (Yrs)**	**5-Yr PFS**	**10-Yr PFS**	**MS Pancreatic Head (Yrs)**
Surgery alone	1.6	22%	18%	1.2	20%	17%	1
Adjuvant CRT	1.8	25%	17%	1.5	21%	16%	1.3
p value	NS	NS	NS	NS	NS	NS	NS

Is there benefit to postoperative CRT compared with postoperative CHT?

On the basis of ESPAC-1, postoperative CRT is not beneficial and possibly detrimental compared with post-operative CHT.[67] However, both ESPAC-1 and EORTC 40891 had numerous flaws and thus results do not preclude CRT as an acceptable choice in adjuvant setting based on GITSG 91-73. Systemic therapy has greatly improved since these trials were conducted. Phase III RTOG 0848 trial investigated the role of adjuvant RT in the setting of modern systemic therapy and showed no OS in the overall cohort, but showed an OS and DFS benefit in node-negative patients. Current guidelines support consideration of adjuvant CRT in the setting of positive margins and/or positive LNs after completion of adjuvant systemic thearpy.[60] However, RTOG 0848 reported no DFS or OS benefit in node-positive patients.[72]

Neoptolemos, ESPAC-1 (*Lancet* 2001, PMID 11716884; Update *NEJM* 2004, PMID 15028824): PRT of 541 patients with grossly resected pancreatic ductal carcinoma randomized to 2×2 factorial design to surgery followed by observation vs. CHT alone vs. CRT vs. CRT + consolidative CHT. Altered to boost accrual with randomization into one of main treatment comparisons (CRT vs. no CRT or CHT vs. no CHT). CHT was 5-FU 425 mg/m^2 d1–5 + LCV 20 mg/m^2 q28d × 6 cycles. CRT regimen was 40 Gy split course (20 Gy/10 fx + bolus 5-FU 500 mg/m^2 followed by 2-week break followed by 20 Gy/10 fx + bolus 5-FU 500 mg/m^2); 285 patients randomized to 2×2 design: 68 to ± CRT and 188 to ± CHT. MFU 47 months. Eighty-one percent with R0 resection, 19% had positive margins. Median time from resection to treatment was 46 days in CHT arm and 61 days in CRT arm. Prognostic factors were higher grade, LN+ and tumor >2 cm. QOL parameters were equivalent between groups. Overall results are in Table 36.6. After adjusting for prognostic factors, there was no benefit for adjuvant CRT, but there was a survival benefit for adjuvant CHT. **Conclusion: CHT alone improved survival compared with observation. Adjuvant 5-FU-based CRT did not improve survival and may have had deleterious effect.** *Comment: Study limitations included no central RT QA, selection bias (physician allowed to select which randomization), background treatment allowed by clinician choice (CHT or CRT), nearly one-third of observation arm and one-third of CHT arm received RT, and RT dose was inconsistent—designed at 40 Gy, but choice of up to 60 Gy allowed.*

Table 36.6 Results of ESPAC 1 for Pancreas Cancer

ESPAC 1: 2 × 2 Subset Only (2004)	MS	Time to Recurrence	5-Yr OS
CRT	15.9 months	10.7 months	10%
No CRT	17.9 months	15.2 months	20%
p value (± CRT)		.04	.05
CHT	20.1 months	15.3 months	21%
No CHT	15.5 months	10.5 months	8%
p value (± CHT)		.02	.009

Stocken, Pancreatic Cancer Meta-Analysis Group (*Br J Cancer* 2005, PMID 15812554): Systematic review and meta-analysis of five RCTs (GITSG, Norway, EORTC, Japan, ESPAC-1) of adjuvant CHT and CRT for 1,136 patients. CHT showed reduction in risk of death by 25% (HR 0.75, 95% CI 0.64–0.90) and improved MS. No significant difference in risk of death with CRT (HR 1.09, CI 0.89–1.32; Table 36.7). Subgroup analysis showed CRT more effective with positive margins and CHT alone less effective. **Conclusion: CHT is an effective adjuvant therapy, while CRT is not unless patient has margin-positive disease.**

Table 36.7 Results of Stocken Meta-Analysis

Stocken Meta-Analysis	MS	2-Yr OS	5-Yr OS
CHT alone	19.0 months	38%	19%
Observation (vs. CHT)	13.5 months	28%	12%
CRT	15.8 months	30%	12%
Observation (vs. CRT)	15.2 months	34%	17%

Abrams, RTOG 0848 (ASCO 2024 Abstract): Part 2 of RTOG 0848; 354 patients without progression after five cycles of adjuvant CHT (± erlotinib) further randomized to concurrent CRT (50.4 Gy/28 fx) vs. no additional treatment. MFU for all and alive patients was 2 and 7 years, respectively.

Eighty-three percent of patients had negative margins, 26% were node-negative. Thirteen percent of patients randomized to CRT did not receive RT. Overall, OS was not improved. However, in pN0 patients, there was an improvement in OS (5-year OS 48% vs. 29%, p = .0063) and DFS (5-year DFS 47% vs. 19%, p = .014) in patients who received CHT followed by CRT. There was an overall DFS benefit (5-year DFS 21% vs. 15%, p = .045) driven by the benefit seen in node-negative patients. **Conclusion: Adjuvant CHT + CRT did not improve OS, but it did improve DFS. In node-negative patients, both OS and DFS were improved with adjuvant CHT + CRT without an increase in grades 4 to 5 AEs.**

What is the optimal adjuvant CHT regimen?

ESPAC-1[68] and German CONKO-001[69,70] demonstrated a survival benefit to adjuvant CHT as compared with surgery alone and used 5-FU and gemcitabine monotherapy, respectively. In the modern era, mFOLFIRINOX and gemcitabine/capecitabine are preferred regimens based on the results of PRODIGE-24[71] and ESPAC-4,[72] respectively, which both demonstrated an OS advantage to multiagent CHT as compared with gemcitabine alone. Gemcitabine/nab-paclitaxel as well as gemcitabine and 5-FU/LCV are acceptable alternatives.

What is the optimal adjuvant CRT regimen?

Regine, RTOG 97-04 (*JAMA* 2008, PMID 18319412; Update *Ann Surg Oncol* 2011, PMID 21499862): PRT of 451 patients s/p GTR of T1–4N0–1M0 pancreatic ACA (excluded ampullary cancers) with KPS >60 randomized to PVI 5-FU × 3 weeks → CRT → PVI 5-FU × 2 months or weekly gemcitabine × 3 → CRT → gemcitabine × 2 months. CRT was 50.4 Gy/28 fx (cone-down after 45 Gy) with concurrent PVI 5-FU. Primary endpoint OS. MFU 1.5 years overall and 7 years for alive patients; 67% were N1, 75% were T3–4 (more in gemcitabine arm), 34% had positive margins (25% had unknown margin status), and 86% pancreatic head tumors. Overall, no difference in OS or DFS (Table 36.8). **Conclusion: No difference in OS of patients with gemcitabine or 5-FU given before/after CRT. Gemcitabine was associated with greater heme toxicity.** *Comment: Second analysis demonstrated effect between RT QA and protocol compliance on OS.[73] Furthermore, significantly worse OS reported in patients with postresection CA 19–9 >90 U/mL (HR 3.1, p < .0001).[74]*

Table 36.8 Results of RTOG 97-04				
RTOG 97-04 (All Patients)	**LR**	**3-Yr OS**	**5-Yr OS**	**Grade 4 Heme Toxicity**
5-FU arm	28%	22%	18%	1%
Gemcitabine arm	23%	31%	22%	14%
p value	NS		.12	<.001

BORDERLINE RESECTABLE

What is the rationale for neoadjuvant CRT?

Neoadjuvant CRT may help downstage patients, reduce nodal burden, reduce rate of positive margins, and improve resectability in borderline patients.[40,75,76] CHT regimens include concurrent 5-FU or gemcitabine. Recently, attention is being paid to neoadjuvant regimens incorporating more aggressive CHT with or without RT, such as FOLFIRINOX, mFOLFIRINOX, gemcitabine/docetaxel/capecitabine, or gemcitabine/capecitabine, and continues to be evaluated on trials.[77–79] The Alliance A021501 trial[80] showed no OS benefit to the addition of neoadjuvant SBRT or hypofractionated RT to mFOLFIRINOX in an unselected population, while a single-arm phase II trial of FOLFIRINOX followed by individualized hypofractionated/conventional CRT followed by surgery showed favorable outcome in terms of R0 resection rates and survival.[81]

Versteijne, PREOPANC-1 (*JCO* 2020, PMID 32105518): Phase III RCT of 246 patients with resectable or borderline resectable pancreatic cancer randomized to immediate surgery (Arm A) vs. preop CRT (Arm B; three cycles gemcitabine with 36 Gy/15 fx during cycle 2). Both arms received adjuvant gemcitabine (six cycles in arm A; four cycles in arm B). No difference in the primary endpoint of OS (Arm A: 14.3 months vs. Arm B: 16 months, p = .096). However, on subset analysis of borderline resectable patients, there was an OS benefit for preop CRT (13.2 vs. 17.6 months, p = .029). Preop

CRT also improved R0 resection rate (40% vs. 71%, $p < .001$). No difference in serious adverse events. **Conclusion: CRT improves OS among borderline resectable pancreatic cancer patients.**

Koerkamp, PREOPANC-2 (*ESMO* 2023, Abstract): Phase III RCT of 375 patients with resectable or borderline resectable pancreatic cancer randomized to eight cycles of FOLFIRINOX (q2 weeks) followed by surgery vs. neoadjuvant hypofractionated CRT (three cycles of gemcitabine with 36 Gy/15 fx initiated during cycle 2) followed by surgery and four cycles of adjuvant gemcitabine. Primary endpoint OS. At MFU of 41.7 months with 254 events, median OS was 21.9 months in the CHT arm and 21.3 months in the CRT arm (HR 0.87, 95% CI 0.68–1.12). Resection rates: 77% with CHT vs. 75% with CRT ($p = .69$). Serious AE rates: 49% with CHT vs. 43% with CRT arm ($p = .26$). **Conclusion: Neoadjuvant CHT with FOLFIRINOX did not improve OS compared with neoadjuvant gemcitabine-based CRT in patients with borderline-resectable and resectable pancreatic cancer.**

Katz, Alliance A021501 (*JAMA Onc* 2022, PMID 35834226): Randomized multicenter phase II trial in borderline resectable pancreatic ACA. Seventy patients (54 randomized, 16 following closure of Arm 2 at interim analysis) randomized to Arm 1, preoperative eight cycles of mFOLFIRINOX, and 56 patients randomized to Arm 2, seven cycles of mFOLFIRINOX + SBRT (33–40 Gy/5 fx) or hypofractionated RT (25 Gy/5 fx). Patients in both arms without disease progression underwent pancreatectomy followed by four cycles of FOLFOX. A planned interim analysis mandated closure of either arm for which 11 or fewer of the first 30 accrued patients underwent margin-negative (R0) resection. Among the first 30 evaluable patients enrolled to each arm, 17 patients in Arm 1 (57%) and 10 patients in Arm 2 (33%) had undergone R0 resection, leading to closure of Arm 2 but continuation to full enrollment in Arm 1. mFOLFIRINOX with SBRT/hypofractionated RT did not improve OS. The 18-month OS rate was 68% with mFOLFIRINOX and 47% in mFOLFIRINOX + RT. Notably, only 20 patients in the mFOLFIRINOX arm completed all treatments compared with 10 patients in the mFOLFIRINOX + RT arm. **Conclusion: Addition of SBRT or hypofractionated RT to neoadjuvant mFOLFIRINOX did not improve OS at 18 months.**

Murphy (*JAMA Onc* 2018, PMID 29800971): Single-arm, phase II trial of 48 borderline resectable pancreatic cancer patients treated with eight cycles of FOLFIRINOX. Patients with resolution of vascular involvement received short-course CRT (25 Gy/5 fx with protons or 30 Gy/10 fx with photons) with capecitabine. Patients with persistent vascular involvement received long-course CRT with 50.4 Gy/28 fx with IMRT with an SIB to 58.8 Gy/28 fx with concurrent 5-FU/capecitabine. Surgery was performed 1 to 3 weeks after short-course RT or 4 to 8 weeks after long-course RT. Primary endpoint was rate of R0 resection. Five patients received CHT and CRT but did not have surgery due to disease progression. Seven patients had an attempt at surgery but were found to be unresectable. Thirty-two patients underwent surgical resection, of whom 31 had an R0 resection (97% R0 resection rate). No pCR was seen. Median PFS for the whole group was 14.7 months (2-year PFS 43%) and 48.6 months (2-year PFS 55%) for patients who underwent surgery. **Conclusion: FOLFIRINOX followed by individualized CRT shows a high rate of R0 resection and prolonged survival.**

LOCALLY ADVANCED/UNRESECTABLE PANCREATIC CANCER

What is the optimal CHT to palliate symptoms from advanced pancreatic cancer?

Multiagent CHT is preferred over single-agent CHT in patients who are candidates given the results of the PRODIGE trial[82] showing improved OS with FOLFIRINOX over gemcitabine (11.1 vs. 6.8 months, $p < .001$). Regimens such as FOLFIRINOX, gemcitabine/abraxane, or NALIRINOX are recommended. Single-agent options include 5-FU or gemcitabine.[51–59,83] A multi-institution PRT showed gemcitabine improved time to clinical benefit over 5-FU.[51]

What is the rationale for definitive CRT in locally advanced unresectable pancreatic cancer?

As with resectable pancreatic cancer, use of CRT as part of standard management of locally advanced or unresectable disease is controversial due to conflicting results of randomized studies. In general, biliary stent (if jaundice) can be performed first followed by induction CHT with restaging, followed by CRT or continued CHT alone (see ASCO guidelines).[58] The following trials (Table 36.9) support the use of CRT, whereas later trials (Chauffert, Krishnan, and Hammel) do not support CRT. SBRT/hypofractionated RT has become an important consideration in this setting (see next section).

Table 36.9 Trials Supporting Use of CRT for Locally Advanced/Unresectable Pancreatic Cancer			
Trial	Arms	Results	Notes
Mayo Clinic[84] (1969)	RT alone vs. CRT (35–40 Gy ± 5-FU)	MS 6.3 months vs. 10.4 months	
GITSG 9273[85] (1981)	RT alone (60 Gy) vs. CRT (40 Gy) vs. CRT (60 Gy)	MS 22.9 weeks vs. 42.2 weeks vs. 40.3 weeks	RT given with 2-week break every 20 Gy, CHT 5-FU concurrent and maintenance RT-alone arm with worse OS (SS)
GITSG 9283[86] (1988)	CHT alone vs. CRT	1-yr OS 19% vs. 41%	CHT alone: SMF (streptozocin, MMC, and 5-FU) CRT: 54 Gy + 5-FU
ECOG E4201[87] (2008)	CHT alone vs. CRT	MS 9.2 vs. 11.1 ($p = .017$)	CHT alone: gemcitabine CRT: gemcitabine + 50.4 Gy/28 fx Closed early due to poor accrual
CONKO-007[88] (2022)	CHT → CRT vs. CHT	2-yr OS 35% vs. 33% (NS), R0 resection (25% vs. 18%, NS); R0 circumferential resection margin negative (20% vs. 9%, SS)	CHT alone: mostly FOLFIRINOX, some gemcitabine CRT: 50.4 Gy with concurrent gemcitabine Initial primary endpoint was OS, changed to R0 resection due to poor accrual Primary endpoint negative, but more negative circumferential resection margins (CRM−) with CRT; patients with CRM− had better OS (2-year OS 67% vs. 41%)

Chauffert, French FFCD-SFRO (*Ann Oncol* 2008, PMID 18467316; Update *Cancer Radiother* 2011, PMID 21315644): PRT of 119 patients with locally advanced pancreatic cancer and WHO PS 0 randomized to induction CRT (60 Gy/30 fx with PVI 5-FU, 300 mg/m², d1–5 ×6 weeks and cisplatin 20 mg/m², d1–5 during weeks 1 and 5) or induction gemcitabine alone (1,000 mg/m² weekly ×7 weeks). Maintenance gemcitabine (1,000 mg/m² weekly, 3/4 weeks) given in both arms until disease progression or toxicity. Stopped early due to lower MS with CRT (8.6 vs. 13 months, $p = .03$) and higher toxicity (grades 3–4 toxicities 36% vs. 22% during induction and 32% vs. 18% during maintenance). **Conclusion: Induction CRT showed increased toxicity and decreased effectiveness than gemcitabine alone.** *Comment: Updated results published in 2011 confirmed the original results.89 CRT regimen in this trial was nonstandard and toxic.*

Hammel, LAP07 (*JAMA* 2016, PMID 27139057): PRT of 442 patients. Two randomizations: first to either gemcitabine (1,000 mg/m² weekly ×3 weeks) or gemcitabine with erlotinib (100 mg/day for 4 months). Those with no progression after 4 months ($n = 269$) were randomized again to further CHT ± RT (54 Gy and capecitabine 1,600 mg/m²/day). Patients receiving erlotinib received maintenance erlotinib after completion. MFU 36.7 months. MS was 16.5 with CHT and 15.2 months with CHT + RT ($p = .83$). MS was 13.6 months in those undergoing gemcitabine and 11.9 months for gemcitabine + erlotinib ($p = .09$). Reduced LR was noted with CRT (32% vs. 46%, $p = .03$) with no increased grades 3 to 4 toxicities except nausea. **Conclusion: No significant difference in OS with CRT vs. CHT or with addition of gemcitabine in conjunction with erlotinib used as maintenance CHT. However, CRT did improve LC.** *Comment: After formal RT QA, only 32% of patients in CRT arm were treated per protocol, while 50% had minor deviations and 18% had major deviations.*

What is the role of SBRT/dose-escalated hypofractionated RT in locally advanced pancreatic cancer?

Although there are no randomized trials comparing SBRT with CRT, there is growing interest in SBRT or dose-escalated hypofractionated RT as a means to improve LC while minimizing interruption of systemic therapy.

Chang, Stanford (*Cancer* 2009, PMID 19117351): RR of 77 patients with unresectable pancreatic cancer (58% locally advanced, 14% medically inoperable, 8% locally recurrent, 19% metastatic) treated with 25 Gy/1 fx with CyberKnife®. Twenty-one percent also received 45 to 54 Gy of fractionated EBRT. Various gemcitabine-based regimens in 96% of patients. Isolated LF at 6 and 12 months was 5%. PFS at 6 and 12 months was 26% and 9%, respectively. OS at 6 and 12 months was 56% and 21%. Grade ≥2 acute toxicity was 5%. Grade ≥3 late toxicity was 9%. **Conclusion: 25 Gy/1 fx provides effective LC, although concerns about late toxicity, most commonly ulceration. A subsequent dose–volume analysis of duodenal toxicity (*n* = 73) showed the 12-month risk of duodenal toxicity was 29%.**[90]

Pollom, Stanford (*IJROBP* 2014, PMID 25585785): RR of 167 patients treated with SBRT with either single fx (46%) or 5 fx (55%) regimens. MFU 7.9 months. No difference in recurrence by fractionation scheme with 6/12-month rates of LR 5%/10% for single fraction and 3%/12% for 5 fx, respectively. No difference in OS by fractionation scheme with 6/12-month rates of OS 67%/31% for single fraction and 76%/35% for 5 fx, respectively. Significantly less grade ≥2 toxicity with 5 fx regimen. In single fx group, 6- and 12-month rates of GI toxicity grade ≥3 were 8% and 12%, respectively, while both were 6% in 5 fx group (NS). **Conclusion: Multifraction SBRT reduces GI toxicity without detriment in LC.**

Moningi, Johns Hopkins (*Ann Surg Oncol* 2015, PMID 25564157): RR of 88 patients with pancreatic ACA receiving SBRT (25–33 Gy/5 fx) from 2010 to 2014. Seventy-four locally advanced (MFU 14.5 months) and 14 borderline resectable (MFU 10.3 months). Most patients received pre-SBRT CHT. MS 18.4 months and median PFS 9.8 months. Only three patients had grade 3+ toxicity and five patients had late grade 2+ GI toxicity; 19 patients underwent resection, of whom 15 (79%) had locally advanced disease and 16 (84%) had R0 resection. **Conclusion: SBRT after CHT for either locally advanced or borderline resectable pancreatic cancer results in low acute and late toxicity. Majority of patients completed resection without significant radiographic response.**

What is the role of SBRT for palliation of pain?

Palliative SBRT has been shown to improve QOL and pain control and decrease opioid use.[69,70]

Lawrence (*Lancet Onc* 2024, PMID 39029483): International single-arm phase II trial that included patients with an average pain level of ≥5/11 on the Brief Pain Inventory (BPI), ECOG 0 to 2, and anatomic involvement of the celiac axis from pancreatic and other upper GI malignancies. The trial accrued 145 patients, of whom 125 received RT and 90 were evaluable. SBRT was a single fraction of 25 Gy delivered to the celiac plexus. The primary endpoint was "complete or partial (≥2 points) pain response" based on the BPI "average pain" 11-point scale. Secondary endpoint was changes in health-related QOL at 3 and 6 weeks compared with baseline. At 3 weeks, 48 (53%) had at least a partial pain response. Opioid usage decrease at 3 weeks was not significant, but it was significant at 6 weeks (*p* = .005). QOL outcomes were also improved at 3 and 6 weeks. **Conclusions: Celiac plexus SBRT decreases pain and opioid use among patients with pancreatic cancer and other tumors invading the celiac axis. The treatment appears to improve QOL.**

PAINPANC Trial (*IJROBP* 2024, PMID 37647972): Prospective, phase II, single-center nonrandomized trial of 29 patients who received palliative RT (24 Gy in 3 weekly fx) for pancreatic cancer-related pain. Primary endpoint of the study was defined as clinically relevant average decrease in ≥2 points in pain severity within 7 weeks after the start of RT. Secondary endpoint was improvement in global QOL by 5 to 10 points (on a 0–100 scale). Acute toxicity and OS were also assessed. The study showed a clinically relevant mean pain severity reduction (3.15-point average decrease at 7 weeks, *p* = .045), improvement in the global QOL (50.5 to 60.8 improvement, *p* = .001), and reduction in the median oral morphine equivalent dose used. Grade 3 acute toxicity occurred in three patients and no grades 4 to 5 toxicities were observed. Median OS was 11.8 weeks. **Conclusion: Short-course palliative RT for pancreatic cancer-related pain was associated with clinically relevant reduction in pain severity and improvement in global QOL with mostly mild toxicity.**

REFERENCES

1. Siegel RL, Giaquinto AN, Jemal A. Cancer statistics, 2024. *CA Cancer J Clin.* 2024;74(1):12–49. doi:10.3322/caac.21820
2. Rawla P, Sunkara T, Gaduputi V. Epidemiology of pancreatic cancer: global trends, etiology and risk factors. *World J Oncol.* 2019;10(1):10–27. doi:10.14740/wjon1166
3. Ma J, Siegel R, Jemal A. Pancreatic cancer death rates by race among US men and women, 1970–2009. *J Natl Cancer Inst.* 2013;105(22):1694–700. doi:10.1093/jnci/djt292

4.   Barone E, Corrado A, Gemignani F, Landi S. Environmental risk factors for pancreatic cancer: an update. *Arch Toxicol.* 2016;90(11):2617–2642. doi:10.1007/s00204-016-1821-9

5.   Fuchs CS, Colditz GA, Stampfer MJ, et al. A prospective study of cigarette smoking and the risk of pancreatic cancer. *Arch Intern Med.* 1996;156(19):2255–2260. PMID:8885826

6.   Michaud DS, Giovannucci E, Willett WC, Colditz GA, Stampfer MJ, Fuchs CS. Physical activity, obesity, height, and the risk of pancreatic cancer. *JAMA.* 2001;286(8):921–929. doi:10.1001/jama.286.8.921

7.   Yamada A, Komaki Y, Komaki F, Micic D, Zullow S, Sakuraba A. Risk of gastrointestinal cancers in patients with cystic fibrosis: a systematic review and meta-analysis. *Lancet Oncol.* 2018;19(6):758–767. doi:10.1016/s1470-2045(18)30188-8

8.   Hassan MM, Li D, El-Deeb AS, et al. Association between hepatitis B virus and pancreatic cancer. *J Clin Oncol.* 2008;26(28):4557–4562. doi:10.1200/jco.2008.17.3526

9.   Giardiello FM, Brensinger JD, Tersmette AC, et al. Very high risk of cancer in familial Peutz-Jeghers syndrome. *Gastroenterology.* 2000;119(6):1447–1453. doi:10.1053/gast.2000.20228

10. van Lier MG, Wagner A, Mathus-Vliegen EM, Kuipers EJ, Steyerberg EW, van Leerdam ME. High cancer risk in Peutz-Jeghers syndrome: a systematic review and surveillance recommendations. *Am J Gastroenterol.* 2010;105(6):1258–1264. doi:10.1038/ajg.2009.725

11. Lim W, Olschwang S, Keller JJ, et al. Relative frequency and morphology of cancers in STK11 mutation carriers. *Gastroenterology.* 2004;126(7):1788–1794. doi:10.1053/j.gastro.2004.03.014

12. de Snoo FA, Bishop DT, Bergman W, et al. Increased risk of cancer other than melanoma in CDKN2A founder mutation (p16-Leiden)-positive melanoma families. *Clin Cancer Res.* 2008;14(21):7151–7157. doi:10.1158/1078-0432.Ccr-08-0403

13. Roberts NJ, Jiao Y, Yu J, et al. ATM mutations in patients with hereditary pancreatic cancer. *Cancer Discov.* 2012;2(1):41–46. doi:10.1158/2159-8290.Cd-11-0194

14. Iqbal J, Ragone A, Lubinski J, et al. The incidence of pancreatic cancer in BRCA1 and BRCA2 mutation carriers. *Br J Cancer.* 2012;107(12):2005–2009. doi:10.1038/bjc.2012.483

15. Olson SH, Kurtz RC. Epidemiology of pancreatic cancer and the role of family history. *J Surg Oncol.* 2013;107(1):1–7. doi:10.1002/jso.23149

16. Klein AP. Genetic susceptibility to pancreatic cancer. *Mol Carcinog.* 2012;51(1):14–24. doi:10.1002/mc.20855

17. Klein AP, Hruban RH, Brune KA, Petersen GM, Goggins M. Familial pancreatic cancer. *Cancer J.* 2001; 7(4):266–273. PMID:11561603

18. Solomon S, Das S, Brand R, Whitcomb DC. Inherited pancreatic cancer syndromes. *Cancer J.* 2012;18(6): 485–491. doi:10.1097/PPO.0b013e318278c4a6

19. Amundadottir L, Kraft P, Stolzenberg-Solomon RZ, et al. Genome-wide association study identifies variants in the ABO locus associated with susceptibility to pancreatic cancer. *Nat Genet.* 2009;41(9):986–990. doi:10.1038/ng.429

20. Wolpin BM, Chan AT, Hartge P, et al. ABO blood group and the risk of pancreatic cancer. *J Natl Cancer Inst.* 2009;101(6):424–431. doi:10.1093/jnci/djp020

21. Esposito I, Konukiewitz B, Schlitter AM, Klöppel G. Pathology of pancreatic ductal adenocarcinoma: facts, challenges and future developments. *World J Gastroenterol.* 2014;20(38):13833–13841. doi:10.3748/wjg.v20.i38.13833

22. La Rosa S, Sessa F, Capella C. Acinar cell carcinoma of the pancreas: overview of clinicopathologic features and insights into the molecular pathology. *Front Med (Lausanne).* 2015;2:41. doi:10.3389/fmed.2015.00041

23. Klimstra DS. Nonductal neoplasms of the pancreas. *Mod Pathol.* 2007;20(suppl 1):S94–S112. doi:10.1038/modpathol.3800686

24. Winter JM, Maitra A, Yeo CJ. Genetics and pathology of pancreatic cancer. *HPB (Oxford).* 2006;8(5):324–336. doi:10.1080/13651820600804203

25. Goggins M, Overbeek KA, Brand R, et al. Management of patients with increased risk for familial pancreatic cancer: updated recommendations from the International Cancer of the Pancreas Screening (CAPS) Consortium. *Gut.* 2020;69(1):7–17. doi:10.1136/gutjnl-2019-319352

26. Canto MI, Goggins M, Hruban RH, et al. Screening for early pancreatic neoplasia in high-risk individuals: a prospective controlled study. *Clin Gastroenterol Hepatol.* 2006;4(6):766–781. doi:10.1016/j.cgh.2006.02.005

27. Stoffel EM, Brand RE, Goggins M. Pancreatic cancer: changing epidemiology and new approaches to risk assessment, early detection, and prevention. *Gastroenterology.* 2023;164(5):752–765. doi:10.1053/j.gastro.2023.02.012

28. Canto MI, Harinck F, Hruban RH, et al. International Cancer of the Pancreas Screening (CAPS) consortium summit on the management of patients with increased risk for familial pancreatic cancer. *Gut.* 2013;62(3):339–347. doi:10.1136/gutjnl-2012-303108

29. Porta M, Fabregat X, Malats N, et al. Exocrine pancreatic cancer: symptoms at presentation and their relation to tumour site and stage. *Clin Transl Oncol.* 2005;7(5):189–197. doi:10.1007/bf02712816

30. Kalser MH, Barkin J, MacIntyre JM. Pancreatic cancer. Assessment of prognosis by clinical presentation. *Cancer.* 1985;56(2):397–402. doi:10.1002/1097-0142(19850715)56:2<397::aid-cncr2820560232>3.0.co;2-i

31. Bakkevold KE, Arnesjø B, Kambestad B. Carcinoma of the pancreas and papilla of Vater: presenting symptoms, signs, and diagnosis related to stage and tumour site. A prospective multicentre trial in 472 patients. Norwegian Pancreatic Cancer Trial. *Scand J Gastroenterol*. 1992;27(4):317–325. doi:10.3109/00365529209000081

32. NCCN Clinical Practice Guidelines in Oncology: Pancreatic Adenocarcinoma. Accessed January 15, 2025. https://www.nccn.org/professionals/physician_gls/pdf/pancreatic.pdf

33. Canto MI, Hruban RH, Fishman EK, et al. Frequent detection of pancreatic lesions in asymptomatic high-risk individuals. *Gastroenterology*. 2012;142(4):796–804. doi:10.1053/j.gastro.2012.01.005

34. Poley JW, Kluijt I, Gouma DJ, et al. The yield of first-time endoscopic ultrasonography in screening individuals at a high risk of developing pancreatic cancer. *Am J Gastroenterol*. 2009;104(9):2175–2181. doi:10.1038/ajg.2009.276

35. Kandel P, Wallace MB. Recent advancement in EUS-guided fine needle sampling. *J Gastroenterol*. 2019;54(5):377–387. doi:10.1007/s00535-019-01552-2

36. Lee ES, Lee JM. Imaging diagnosis of pancreatic cancer: a state-of-the-art review. *World J Gastroenterol*. 2014;20(24):7864–7877. doi:10.3748/wjg.v20.i24.7864

37. Ahmed SI, Bochkarev V, Oleynikov D, Sasson AR. Patients with pancreatic adenocarcinoma benefit from staging laparoscopy. *J Laparoendosc Adv Surg Tech A*. 2006;16(5):458–463. doi:10.1089/lap.2006.16.458

38. Allen VB, Gurusamy KS, Takwoingi Y, Kalia A, Davidson BR. Diagnostic accuracy of laparoscopy following Computed Tomography (CT) scanning for assessing the resectability with curative intent in pancreatic and periampullary cancer. *Cochrane Database Syst Rev*. 2013;11:Cd009323. doi:10.1002/14651858.CD009323.pub2

39. Warshaw AL, Gu ZY, Wittenberg J, Waltman AC. Preoperative staging and assessment of resectability of pancreatic cancer. *Arch Surg*. 1990;125(2):230–233. doi:10.1001/archsurg.1990.01410140108018

40. Gillen S, Schuster T, Meyer Zum Buschenfelde C, Friess H, Kleeff J. Preoperative/neoadjuvant therapy in pancreatic cancer: a systematic review and meta-analysis of response and resection percentages. *PLoS Med*. 2010;7(4):e1000267. doi:10.1371/journal.pmed.1000267

41. Andrén-Sandberg A. Prognostic factors in pancreatic cancer. *N Am J Med Sci*. 2012;4(1):9–12. doi:10.4103/1947-2714.92893

42. Bilici A. Prognostic factors related with survival in patients with pancreatic adenocarcinoma. *World J Gastroenterol*. 2014;20(31):10802–10812. doi:10.3748/wjg.v20.i31.10802

43. Tas F, Sen F, Keskin S, Kilic L, Yildiz I. Prognostic factors in metastatic pancreatic cancer: older patients are associated with reduced overall survival. *Mol Clin Oncol*. 2013;1(4):788–792. doi:10.3892/mco.2013.131

44. Eloubeidi MA, Desmond RA, Wilcox CM, et al. Prognostic factors for survival in pancreatic cancer: a population-based study. *Am J Surg*. 2006;192(3):322–329. doi:10.1016/j.amjsurg.2006.02.017

45. Tran KT, Smeenk HG, van Eijck CH, et al. Pylorus preserving pancreaticoduodenectomy versus standard Whipple procedure: a prospective, randomized, multicenter analysis of 170 patients with pancreatic and periampullary tumors. *Ann Surg*. 2004;240(5):738–745. doi:10.1097/01.sla.0000143248.71964.29

46. Lin PW, Shan YS, Lin YJ, Hung CJ. Pancreaticoduodenectomy for pancreatic head cancer: PPPD versus Whipple procedure. *Hepatogastroenterology*. 2005;52(65):1601–1604. PMID:16201125

47. Seiler CA, Wagner M, Bachmann T, et al. Randomized clinical trial of pylorus-preserving duodenopancreatectomy versus classical Whipple resection-long term results. *Br J Surg*. 2005;92(5):547–556. doi:10.1002/bjs.4881

48. Riall TS, Cameron JL, Lillemoe KD, et al. Pancreaticoduodenectomy with or without distal gastrectomy and extended retroperitoneal lymphadenectomy for periampullary adenocarcinoma–part 3: update on 5-year survival. *J Gastrointest Surg*. 2005;9(9):1191–1206. doi:10.1016/j.gassur.2005.08.034

49. Yeo CJ, Cameron JL, Sohn TA, et al. Pancreaticoduodenectomy with or without extended retroperitoneal lymphadenectomy for periampullary adenocarcinoma: comparison of morbidity and mortality and short-term outcome. *Ann Surg*. 1999;229(5):613–622. doi:10.1097/00000658-199905000-00003

50. Langer B. Role of volume outcome data in assuring quality in HPB surgery. *HPB (Oxford)*. 2007;9(5):330–334. doi:10.1080/13651820701611234

51. Burris HA 3rd, Moore MJ, Andersen J, et al. Improvements in survival and clinical benefit with gemcitabine as first-line therapy for patients with advanced pancreas cancer: a randomized trial. *J Clin Oncol*. 1997;15(6):2403–2413. doi:10.1200/jco.1997.15.6.2403

52. Conroy T, Desseigne F, Ychou M, et al. FOLFIRINOX versus gemcitabine for metastatic pancreatic cancer. *N Engl J Med*. 2011;364(19):1817–1825. doi:10.1056/NEJMoa1011923

53. Conroy T, Hammel P, Hebbar M, et al. FOLFIRINOX or Gemcitabine as adjuvant therapy for pancreatic cancer. *N Engl J Med*. 2018;379(25):2395–2406. doi:10.1056/NEJMoa1809775

54. Von Hoff DD, Ervin T, Arena FP, et al. Increased survival in pancreatic cancer with nab-paclitaxel plus gemcitabine. *N Engl J Med*. 2013;369(18):1691–1703. doi:10.1056/NEJMoa1304369

55. Tempero MA, Pelzer U, O'Reilly EM, et al. Adjuvant nab-Paclitaxel + Gemcitabine in resected pancreatic ductal adenocarcinoma: results from a randomized, open-label, phase III trial. *J Clin Oncol*. 2023;41(11):2007–2019. doi:10.1200/jco.22.01134

56. Sohal DPS, Kennedy EB, Cinar P, et al. Metastatic pancreatic cancer: ASCO guideline update. *J Clin Oncol.* 2020;38(27):3217–3230. doi:10.1200/jco.20.01364

57. Wainberg ZA, Melisi D, Macarulla T, et al. NALIRIFOX versus nab-paclitaxel and gemcitabine in treatment-naive patients with metastatic pancreatic ductal adenocarcinoma (NAPOLI 3): a randomised, open-label, phase 3 trial. *Lancet.* 2023;402(10409):1272–1281. doi:10.1016/s0140-6736(23)01366-1

58. Golan T, Hammel P, Reni M, et al. Maintenance olaparib for Germline BRCA-mutated metastatic pancreatic cancer. *N Engl J Med.* 2019;381(4):317–327. doi:10.1056/NEJMoa1903387

59. Brown TJ, Reiss KA, O'Hara MH. Advancements in systemic therapy for pancreatic cancer. *Am Soc Clin Oncol Educ Book.* 2023;43:e397082. doi:10.1200/edbk_397082

60. Khorana AA, McKernin SE, Berlin J, et al. Potentially curable pancreatic adenocarcinoma: ASCO clinical practice guideline update. *J Clin Oncol.* 2019;37(23):2082–2088. doi:10.1200/jco.19.00946

61. Balaban EP, Mangu PB, Yee NS. Locally advanced unresectable pancreatic cancer: American Society of Clinical Oncology clinical practice guideline summary. *J Oncol Pract.* 2017;13(4):265–269. doi:10.1200/jop.2016.017376

62. Brunner TB, Haustermans K, Huguet F, et al. ESTRO ACROP guidelines for target volume definition in pancreatic cancer. *Radiother Oncol.* 2021;154:60–69. doi:10.1016/j.radonc.2020.07.052

63. Sanford NN, Narang AK, Aguilera TA, et al. NRG oncology international consensus contouring atlas on target volumes and dosing strategies for dose-escalated pancreatic cancer radiation therapy. *Int J Radiat Oncol Biol Phys.* 2025;121(4):918–929. doi:10.1016/j.ijrobp.2024.10.026

64. Goodman KA, Regine WF, Dawson LA, et al. Radiation Therapy Oncology Group consensus panel guidelines for the delineation of the clinical target volume in the postoperative treatment of pancreatic head cancer. *Int J Radiat Oncol Biol Phys.* 2012;83(3):901–908. doi:10.1016/j.ijrobp.2012.01.022

65. Videtic GM, Vassil AD, Woody NM. *Handbook of Treatment Planning in Radiation Oncology.* Springer Publishing Company; 2020.

66. Arcidiacono PG, Calori G, Carrara S, McNicol ED, Testoni PA. Celiac plexus block for pancreatic cancer pain in adults. *Cochrane Database Syst Rev.* 2011;2011(3):CD007519. doi:10.1002/14651858.CD007519.pub2

67. Eisenberg E, Carr DB, Chalmers TC. Neurolytic celiac plexus block for treatment of cancer pain: a meta-analysis. *Anesth Analg.* 1995;80(2):290–295. doi:10.1097/00000539-199502000-00015

68. Buwenge M, Arcelli A, Cellini F, et al. Pain relief after stereotactic radiotherapy of pancreatic adenocarcinoma: an updated systematic review. *Curr Oncol.* 2022;29(4):2616–2629. doi:10.3390/curroncol29040214

69. Lawrence YR, Miszczyk M, Dawson LA, et al. Celiac plexus radiosurgery for pain management in advanced cancer: a multicentre, single-arm, phase 2 trial. *Lancet Oncol.* 2024;25(8):1070–1079. doi:10.1016/s1470-2045(24)00223-7

70. Tello Valverde CP, Ebrahimi G, Sprangers MA, et al. Impact of short-course palliative radiation therapy on pancreatic cancer-related pain: prospective phase 2 nonrandomized PAINPANC trial. *Int J Radiat Oncol Biol Phys.* 2024;118(2):352–361. doi:10.1016/j.ijrobp.2023.08.055

71. Morganti AG, Trodella L, Valentini V, et al. Pain relief with short-term irradiation in locally advanced carcinoma of the pancreas. *J Palliat Care.* 2003;19(4):258–262. PMID:14959596

72. Abrams RA, Winter KA, Goodman KA, et al. NRG Oncology/RTOG 0848: results after adjuvant chemotherapy +/– chemoradiation for patients with resected periampullary Pancreatic Adenocarcinoma (PA). *J Clin Oncol.* 2024;42(16_suppl):4005. doi:10.1200/JCO.2024.42.16_suppl.4005

73. Abrams RA, Winter KA, Regine WF, et al. Failure to adhere to protocol specified radiation therapy guidelines was associated with decreased survival in RTOG 9704–a phase III trial of adjuvant chemotherapy and chemoradiotherapy for patients with resected adenocarcinoma of the pancreas. *Int J Radiat Oncol Biol Phys.* 2012;82(2):809–816. doi:10.1016/j.ijrobp.2010.11.039

74. Berger AC, Winter K, Hoffman JP, et al. Five year results of US intergroup/RTOG 9704 with postoperative CA 19-9 ≤90 U/mL and comparison to the CONKO-001 trial. *Int J Radiat Oncol Biol Phys.* 2012;84(3):e291–e297. doi:10.1016/j.ijrobp.2012.04.035

75. Laurence JM, Tran PD, Morarji K, Eslick GD, Lam VW, Sandroussi C. A systematic review and meta-analysis of survival and surgical outcomes following neoadjuvant chemoradiotherapy for pancreatic cancer. *J Gastrointest Surg.* 2011;15(11):2059–2069. doi:10.1007/s11605-011-1659-7

76. Jang JY, Han Y, Lee H, et al. Oncological benefits of neoadjuvant chemoradiation with gemcitabine versus upfront surgery in patients with borderline resectable pancreatic cancer: a prospective, randomized, open-label, multicenter phase 2/3 trial. *Ann Surg.* 2018;268(2):215–222. doi:10.1097/SLA.0000000000002705

77. Paniccia A, Edil BH, Schulick RD, et al. Neoadjuvant FOLFIRINOX application in borderline resectable pancreatic adenocarcinoma: a retrospective cohort study. *Medicine (Baltimore).* 2014;93(27):e198. doi:10.1097/md.0000000000000198

78. Blazer M, Wu C, Goldberg RM, et al. Neoadjuvant modified (m) FOLFIRINOX for locally advanced unresectable (LAPC) and borderline resectable (BRPC) adenocarcinoma of the pancreas. *Ann Surg Oncol.* 2015;22(4):1153–1159. doi:10.1245/s10434-014-4225-1

79. Sherman WH, Chu K, Chabot J, et al. Neoadjuvant gemcitabine, docetaxel, and capecitabine followed by gemcitabine and capecitabine/radiation therapy and surgery in locally advanced, unresectable pancreatic adenocarcinoma. *Cancer*. 2015;121(5):673–680. doi:10.1002/cncr.29112

80. Katz MHG, Shi Q, Meyers J, et al. Efficacy of preoperative mFOLFIRINOX vs mFOLFIRINOX plus hypofractionated radiotherapy for borderline resectable adenocarcinoma of the pancreas: the A021501 phase 2 randomized clinical trial. *JAMA Oncol*. 2022;8(9):1263–1270. doi:10.1001/jamaoncol.2022.2319

81. Murphy JE, Wo JY, Ryan DP, et al. Total neoadjuvant therapy with FOLFIRINOX followed by individualized chemoradiotherapy for borderline resectable pancreatic adenocarcinoma: a phase 2 clinical trial. *JAMA Oncol*. 2018;4(7):963–969. doi:10.1001/jamaoncol.2018.0329

82. Conroy T, Desseigne F, Ychou M, et al. FOLFIRINOX versus gemcitabine for metastatic pancreatic cancer. *N Engl J Med*. 2011;364(19):1817–1825. doi:10.1056/NEJMoa1011923

83. Maeda A, Boku N, Fukutomi A, et al. Randomized phase III trial of adjuvant chemotherapy with gemcitabine versus S-1 in patients with resected pancreatic cancer: Japan Adjuvant Study Group of Pancreatic Cancer (JASPAC-01). *Jpn J Clin Oncol*. 2008;38(3):227–229. doi:10.1093/jjco/hym178

84. Moertel CG, Childs DS Jr, Reitemeier RJ, Colby MY Jr, Holbrook MA. Combined 5-fluorouracil and supervoltage radiation therapy of locally unresectable gastrointestinal cancer. *Lancet*. 1969;2(7626):865–867. doi:10.1016/s0140-6736(69)92326-5

85. Moertel CG, Frytak S, Hahn RG, et al. Therapy of locally unresectable pancreatic carcinoma: a randomized comparison of high dose (6000 rads) radiation alone, moderate dose radiation (4000 rads + 5-fluorouracil), and high dose radiation + 5-fluorouracil: The Gastrointestinal Tumor Study Group. *Cancer*. 1981;48(8):1705–1710. doi:10.1002/1097-0142(19811015)48:8<1705::aid-cncr2820480803>3.0.co;2-4

86. Treatment of locally unresectable carcinoma of the pancreas: comparison of combined-modality therapy (chemotherapy plus radiotherapy) to chemotherapy alone. Gastrointestinal Tumor Study Group. *J Natl Cancer Inst*. 1988;80(10):751–755. PMID:2898536

87. Loehrer PJ Sr, Feng Y, Cardenes H, et al. Gemcitabine alone versus gemcitabine plus radiotherapy in patients with locally advanced pancreatic cancer: an Eastern Cooperative Oncology Group trial. *J Clin Oncol*. 2011;29(31):4105–4112. doi:10.1200/jco.2011.34.8904

88. Fietkau R, Ghadimi M, Grützmann R, et al. Randomized phase III trial of induction chemotherapy followed by chemoradiotherapy or chemotherapy alone for nonresectable locally advanced pancreatic cancer: first results of the CONKO-007 trial. *J Clin Oncol*. 2022;40(16_suppl):4008. doi:10.1200/JCO.2022.40.16_suppl.4008

89. Barhoumi M, Mornex F, Bonnetain F, et al. Locally advanced unresectable pancreatic cancer: Induction chemoradiotherapy followed by maintenance gemcitabine versus gemcitabine alone: Definitive results of the 2000-2001 FFCD/SFRO phase III trial. *Cancer Radiother*. 2011;15(3):182–191. doi:10.1016/j.canrad.2010.10.001

90. Murphy JD, Christman-Skieller C, Kim J, Dieterich S, Chang DT, Koong AC. A dosimetric model of duodenal toxicity after stereotactic body radiotherapy for pancreatic cancer. *Int J Radiat Oncol Biol Phys*. 2010;78(5):1420–1426. doi:10.1016/j.ijrobp.2009.09.075

37 RECTAL CANCER

David S. Buchberger, Ian W. Winter, Jacob A. Miller, and Sudha R. Amarnath

QUICK HIT   Colorectal cancer (CRC) is the third most common cancer in the United States, with increasing incidence in younger adults.[1,2] Several new treatment paradigms have emerged. While surgical resection remains standard and typically involves TME by either LAR (sphincter-sparing) or APR (not sphincter-sparing), increasing evidence supports nonoperative management (NOM) with total neoadjuvant therapy (TNT) for patients with clinical complete responses (cCR), as well as the potential omission of RT/use of less invasive surgeries in low-risk populations (Table 37.1).

Table 37.1 General Treatment Paradigm for Rectal Cancer	
	Treatment Options
Stage I	cT1N0: consider endoscopic or local excision alone followed by observation for low-risk lesions (pT1 lesion <3 cm, <30% circumference, within 8 cm of anal verge, grades 1–2, margin >3 mm, no LVSI).[3] If pT1 with high-risk features (piecemeal excision, +margins, LVSI, PNI, poorly differentiated, submucosal depth >1 mm) or pT2, proceed with APR/LAR with TME followed by adjuvant therapy as indicated. cT2N0: APR/LAR as indicated with TME (can consider neoadjuvant CRT to improve chances for sphincter-sparing procedure). No adjuvant treatment if pT1–2N0. If pT3N0 or pT1–3N1–2, adjuvant CHT ± adjuvant CRT.
Stage II/III	cT3a/bN0, EMVI absent, MRF clear, mid/upper rectum: TME or neoadjuvant CHT with response-guided CRT prior to TME. cT4, N2, EMVI, threatened MRF, or low rectum: TNT, typically with long-course CRT* (LC-CRT) followed by CHT, then TME vs. watch-and-wait (W&W) NOM for cCR. cT3c/dN0 or cT2–3N1, MRF clear, mid/upper rectum: TNT with LC-CRT or short-course RT (SC-RT) followed by CHT, then TME vs. W&W NOM for cCR. Alternatively, neoadjuvant CHT with response-guided CRT prior to surgery for patients not desiring W&W.
Stage IVA (resectable metastasis)	Individualize therapy based on presentation and multidisciplinary discussion. General options include: SC-RT followed by combination CHT, then staged or synchronous resection (primary and metastasis) and adjuvant CHT *OR* Combination CHT followed by RT (short or long course), then staged or synchronous resection (primary with metastasis) and adjuvant CHT *OR* CRT followed by staged or synchronous resection (primary and metastasis) and adjuvant CHT
Isolated pelvic or anastomotic recurrence	Resectable: preoperative CRT → resection ± IORT Unresectable: CHT ± RT If prior pelvic RT, consider BID re-RT. May also consider SBRT in the unresectable setting.
dMMR	For locally advanced dMMR disease, initial treatment with immunotherapy (IO) monotherapy is recommended with surveillance for cCR.

*LC-CRT preferred to SC-RT secondary to possible decrease in LR rates among advanced tumors. If obstructed, may need diverting colostomy prior to neoadjuvant therapy.

EPIDEMIOLOGY: CRC is the third most common cancer and the third leading cause of cancer-related deaths in the United States in both males and females. In 2024, the estimated incidence of CRC was 152,810, of which 46,220 were rectal cancers.[4] Incidence of CRC is higher in men and in Black individuals compared with women and Caucasians. Incidence is declining in both genders but has risen sharply in young patients.[1,2] In the United States, the average lifetime risk of developing CRC is 4% to 5%.[4]

RISK FACTORS: Age, male sex, IBD (especially UC[5]), high fat, low fiber, alcohol use, tobacco, family history, genetic syndromes (Table 37.2), diabetes, red meat, cholecystectomy. Protective factors: NSAIDs, fiber, vitamin B[6].

Table 37.2 Familial Colorectal Cancer Syndromes	
FAP	Autosomal dominant germline mutation in *APC* gene located on chr 5. CRC occurs at younger age than in the general population and usually does not arise from an adenoma. Variants include Gardner's (sarcomas, osteomas, desmoid tumors) and Turcot's (GBM, medulloblastoma).
HNPCC (Lynch)	Due to microsatellite instability as a result of mutations in mismatch repair genes, most commonly *hMLH1*, *hMSH2*, *hMSH6*, or *PMS2*. Synchronous and metachronous tumors are possible. Patients with HNPCC also have increased risk of endometrial, ovarian, stomach, small bowel, hepatobiliary system, brain, renal pelvis, and ureteral cancers.

ANATOMY: Rectal cancer defined as a lesion straddling or inferior to the peritoneal reflection (landmark is middle transverse fold at ~11 cm from anal verge) OR lesion within 12 cm of verge. If lesion is completely above this level, it is treated as colon cancer (note: trials have used anywhere up to 16 cm from verge). Layers of rectum: mucosa, muscularis mucosa, submucosa, muscularis propria, serosa, fat. Rectum is ~12 to 15 cm in length, beginning proximally at rectosigmoid junction (~S3) and extending to anorectal ring, just proximal to the dentate line. Proximal third is peritonealized anteriorly and laterally and is supplied by the superior rectal artery (from IMA). Middle third is peritonealized anteriorly and is supplied by the middle rectal artery (from internal iliac). Lower rectum is not peritonealized and is supplied by the inferior rectal artery (from internal pudendal artery). Anorectal ring is composed of the internal and external sphincters and levator ani muscles. Mesorectum is not true mesentery but rather loose connective tissue that is thicker posteriorly. It contains the terminal branches of IMA and needs to be removed for adequate surgery (see TME in the following). Anorectal ring: (a) represents internal anal sphincter muscle and is necessary for anal continence, (b) represents inferior limit for functional sphincter preservation surgery, and (c) defines lymphatic watershed for rectal cancer spread. *Nodal drainage*: Superior half of the rectum drains along the superior rectal artery to pararectal, presacral, sigmoidal, and inferior mesenteric nodes. Inferior half of the rectum drains along the middle rectal artery to the internal iliac nodes. Tumors extending to the anal canal (below dentate line) may drain to the superficial inguinal nodes. Tumors that invade anteriorly (into pelvic organs) can drain to the external iliac nodes. *Pattern of metastasis*: Liver is the most common site of metastatic disease in both colon and rectal cancers. However, rectal cancer has increased propensity for lung as compared with colon cancer. Upper rectal tumors spread along the superior rectal vein to the portal system and into the liver. Middle and inferior rectal tumors spread along the middle and inferior rectal veins, into the internal iliac LNs, into systemic circulation, and into the lung.

PATHOLOGY: More than 90% of rectal cancers are adenocarcinomas (ACA). Approximately 15% to 20% of ACAs have colloid (extracellular mucin); however, there is no prognostic significance. Tumors with signet ring (intracellular mucin) compose 1% to 2% of ACAs and have worse prognosis. Other histologies: small cell, carcinoid, leiomyosarcoma, lymphoma.

SCREENING[6,7]: For average-risk patients, NCCN suggests at 45 years of age and every 10 years if negative. If polyps are identified, repeat colonoscopy every 3 or 5 years depending on risk of polyp. Other options include stool-based testing, imaging with CT colonoscopy, or combination of flexible sigmoidoscopy with stool guaiac. Stool-based tests include stool guaiac, fecal immunochemical test (FIT), or fecal DNA; if positive, proceed to colonoscopy. In patients with family history of CRC, start screening at 40 years of age or 10 years before diagnosis in affected first-degree relative, then repeat colonoscopy every 5 years. If IBD, annual colonoscopy starting 8 years after symptom onset. If FAP, elective colectomy or proctocolectomy after onset of polyposis. If HNPCC, colonoscopy every 1 to 2 years starting at 20 to 25 years of age.

CLINICAL PRESENTATION: Hematochezia is the most common presenting symptom in rectal and lower sigmoid cancers. Abdominal pain is more common in colon cancer. Other symptoms are constipation, diarrhea, reduced stool caliber, and in locally advanced disease tenesmus, rectal urgency, inadequate emptying, urinary symptoms, and buttock and perineal pain.

WORKUP: H&P, including DRE (size, location, mobility, sphincter function); pelvic exam in women.

Labs: CBC, LFTs, CEA.

Procedures: Colonoscopy with biopsies.

Imaging: CT chest, abdomen, pelvis. MRI rectum with IV and rectal contrast is standard for clinical staging. Rectal ultrasound can be utilized if MRI is not available. PET/CT is not routine, but it is utilized in many practices.

PROGNOSTIC FACTORS: Stage (both T and N classifications; Table 37.3), circumferential resection margin (CRM), extramural venous invasion (EMVI), depth of extramural invasion, and lymphovascular space invasion (LVSI) are the most important factors. Performance status, grade (G3 worse), surgery, administration of CHT, and hemoglobin levels before (<12 vs. ≥12 g/dL) and during RT also predict outcomes.[8] Preoperative CEA >5 ng/mL has been associated with inferior RFS and OS. Distance from anal verge is associated with positive margins and bowel function. ESMO clinical practice guidelines further stratify T3 tumors on the basis of depth of invasion. See Tables 37.3 and 37.4 for staging.

STAGING

Table 37.3 AJCC 8th Edition (2017): Staging for Rectal Cancer[9]								
T/M	N	cN0	cN1a	cN1b	cN1c	cN2a	cN2b
T1	Invades submucosa	I	IIIA				
T2	Invades muscularis propria						
T3	Invades into pericolorectal soft tissue	IIA	IIIB				
T4	Invades into visceral peritoneum[1]	IIB					
	Invades or adherent to adjacent organs/structures	IIC	IIIC				
M1a	Distant metastasis to 1 site or organ without peritoneal metastasis	IVA					
M1b	Distant metastasis to ≥2 sites or organs without peritoneal metastasis	IVB					
M1c	Metastasis to peritoneal surface with or without other organ or site	IVC					

Notes: Peritoneum[1] = includes gross perforation of bowel through tumor and continuous invasion of tumor through areas of inflammation to surface of visceral peritoneum.
cN1a: 1 regional LN; cN1b: 2–3 regional LNs; cN1c: no positive regional LNs, but subserosal, mesenteric, nonperitoneal pericolic or perirectal tumor deposits; cN2a: 4–6 regional LNs; cN2b: ≥7 regional LNs.

Table 37.4 ESMO Subclassification of T3 Rectal Cancer[10,11]	
T Stage	Depth of Invasion Beyond Muscularis Propria (mm)
T3a	<1
T3b	1–5
T3c	6–15
T3d	>15

Source: Glynne-Jones R, Wyrwicz L, Tiret E, et al. Rectal cancer: ESMO Clinical Practice Guidelines for diagnosis, treatment and follow-up. *Ann Oncol.* 2018;29(suppl 4):iv263. doi:10.1093/annonc/mdy161; Glynne-Jones R, Wyrwicz L, Tiret E, et al. Rectal cancer: ESMO Clinical Practice Guidelines for diagnosis, treatment and follow-up. *Ann Oncol.* 2017;28(suppl 4):iv22–iv40. doi:10.1093/annonc/mdx224.

TREATMENT PARADIGM

Surgery: Surgery is the mainstay of treatment, although a W&W approach for cCR is emerging as an option for patients who desire NOM. T1 tumors can be initially managed with transanal excision. All other tumors should undergo transabdominal resection (LAR or APR) with sharp TME and at least 12 LNs resected for staging.

Local Excision (Transanal Excision, Transanal Endoscopic Microsurgery, or Transanal Minimally Invasive Surgery): Possible for T1 tumors <3 cm in greatest diameter, <30% of rectal circumference, within 8 cm of dentate line or below middle rectal valve, low-grade histology, and no LVSI.[3]

Low Anterior Resection (LAR): Sphincter-sparing surgery with coloanal anastomosis (or alternatively colonic J-pouch or coloplasty). With modern surgical techniques, distal margin of 2 cm or even less is adequate and crucial margin is CRM.

Abdominoperineal Resection (APR): Historically used for tumors <5 cm from anal verge where sphincter-sparing surgery was not thought possible. Rectosigmoid is oversewn via abdominal incision and pulled out with anal canal via perineal incision. Requires permanent colostomy. NSABP R-04 did not show worse QOL at 1 year between APR compared with sphincter-sparing surgery, but profiles of QOL were different.[12]

Total Mesorectal Excision (TME): Standard of care regardless of APR or LAR. Involves sharp en bloc removal of mesorectum including associated vascular and lymphatic structures, fatty tissue, and mesorectal fascia as "package" through sharp dissection, designed to spare autonomic nerves. TME improves LC and reduces autonomic nerve damage (impotence, retrograde ejaculation, and urinary incontinence) compared with standard blunt dissection of conventional surgery but with higher rate of anastomotic leaks.

Chemotherapy: Utilization of CHT leads to improved LC and OS as well as decreased risk of developing DM.[13]

Indications: Historically, CHT is used in pre/postop setting for T3/T4, N1/N2 disease, adjuvantly for positive margins or those at high risk for LR (high-grade positive or close margin). Concurrent and induction/consolidative regimens are a standard part of the TNT approach.

Concurrent CHT:

1. PVI 5-FU: With concurrent RT improves LC, DFS, and OS (per Mayo Clinic/NCCTG study, in the following); PVI 5-FU compared with bolus 5-FU has lower rate of recurrence and DM, with improvement in 4-year OS from 60% to 70%.[14] PVI 5-FU dose is 225 mg/m² throughout RT (7 days/week).

2. Capecitabine: Several trials suggest noninferiority relative to PVI 5-FU.[15] German phase III trial (included pre- and postop CRT) showed significant reduction in DM and trend toward OS and DFS benefit.[16] Associated with more hand foot syndrome, fatigue, proctitis, and less leukopenia compared with 5-FU. Concurrent dose is 825 mg/m² BID 5 days/week. Without RT, dose is 1,000 to 1,250 mg/m² BID days 1 to 14, q3 weekly cycle.

3. Oxaliplatin: Not recommended concurrent with RT as no benefit was observed on multiple trials despite increased toxicity.[15,17-19]

Adjuvant CHT: Historical role for adjuvant CHT was controversial but often performed given German Rectal Trial.[20] Common adjuvant regimens included FOLFOX, CAPOX, 5-FU, or 5-FU+leucovorin. The ADORE trial showed improved 3-year DFS (72% vs. 63%, *p* = .047) with adjuvant FOLFOX compared with 5-FU + leucovorin.[21] Similarly, the CAO/ARO/AIO-04 trial comparing preoperative CRT with 5-FU ± oxaliplatin followed by surgery and adjuvant 5-FU + LCV ± oxaliplatin showed improved DFS with oxaliplatin.[22] In contrast, a meta-analysis shows no benefit to adjuvant CHT in patients who underwent concurrent preop CRT followed by surgery.[23,24] Use of adjuvant CHT is now decreasing in favor of neoadjuvant or TNT regimens.[25]

Neoadjuvant (TNT): The most commonly used regimens include CAPOX, FOLFOX, and mFOLFIRINOX, all of which have shown efficacy in multiple recently published clinical trials (see below).

Immunotherapy: PD-1 monotherapy (dostarlimab) for the treatment of dMMR rectal ACA demonstrated a 100% cCR rate at short-term follow-up (6 months) in a small cohort.[26] PD-1 monotherapy for dMMR rectal cancer is now an accepted standard of care. Trials investigating the use of IO in pMMR disease have been published with impressive initial results.[27-29] Further investigation is underway.

Radiation: RT improves LC, reduces deaths from rectal cancer, and possibly improves OS.[30,31]

Preoperative RT: cT3-4, cN1–2, EMVI, threatened mesorectal fascia (MRF), or cT1–2N0 requiring APR. Options include short course (25 Gy/5 fx with surgery within 7–10 days and adjuvant CHT if N+) or long course (50.4 Gy/28 fx with concurrent CHT followed by surgery 7–8 weeks later). After SC-RT, postoperative complications increase after 5 days and substantially increase after 10 days (between surgery and RT). Although waiting 4 to 5 weeks after short course leads to improved downstaging (44% vs. 13%), there is no improvement in sphincter-sparing surgery.[32] Consider colostomy prior to RT in select patients including patients with severe obstruction.

Postoperative RT (PORT): Indications include pT4, pN2, positive margins, or poor differentiation. Select pT3 or pN1 tumors with no other risk factors may be spared PORT, although guidelines differ.[33] Consider boost to 55 to 60 Gy for gross residual disease.

RT Boost, Dose Escalation: With the emergence of TNT and W&W strategies, the benefit of boosting and/or dose escalating to facilitate optimized organ preservation has been investigated.[31,34] The OPERA and MORPHEUS trials showed an LC benefit with contact brachytherapy boosts (90 Gy/3 fx or 30 Gy/3 fx) in relatively low-risk populations.[35,36] Other trials such as WW2 (primary tumor treated with SIB to 62 Gy) and OPRA (primary tumor treated to 50–56 Gy, median 54 Gy) showed dose escalation above historical standards is safe and feasible, perhaps resulting in better complete response rates.[37–39]

Procedure: See *Handbook of Treatment Planning in Radiation Oncology,* Chapter 7.[40]

Other Modalities: Other options for small T1 tumors include thermal electrocoagulation, endocavitary RT, or HDR brachytherapy.

EVIDENCE-BASED Q&A

HISTORIC RT TRIALS

What historical studies established the addition of CRT to surgery as a standard for rectal cancer?

GITSG 7175 was a PRT of surgery alone, postop CHT, PORT, or postop CRT for locally advanced rectal cancer. It closed early due to the significant benefits in LR and OS observed with CRT.[41] NSABP-R01 compared surgery alone vs. postop CHT vs. PORT and found that CHT improved OS while RT improved LC.[42] NCCTG 794751 compared PORT alone with postop CRT and showed that all oncologic outcomes, including OS, were improved with CRT.[43] NSABP R-02 found that CRT improved LC but not OS.[44]

What is the benefit of preoperative CRT over postoperative CRT? Is CHT needed?

After establishing the benefit of CRT in the treatment of rectal cancer, the German Rectal Study demonstrated that neoadjuvant CRT with adjuvant CHT was preferred to postop CRT alone. NSABP R-03 similarly found a benefit to preoperative CRT over postop treatment.[45] Additional studies showed increased LC with CRT vs. RT alone.[46,47]

Sauer, German Rectal Study (*NEJM* 2004, PMID 15496622; Update *JCO* 2012, PMID 22529255): PRT of 823 patients ≤75 years with cT3–4 or cN+ rectal ACA with inferior margin ≤16 cm from anal verge randomized to (a) preop CRT 50.4 Gy/28 fx and concurrent continuous infusion 5-FU followed by TME in 6 weeks or (b) postop CRT 50.4 Gy/28 fx with 5.4 Gy boost to tumor bed 4 weeks following surgery. All patients had TME, and adjuvant CHT started 4 weeks after surgery or after completion of postop CRT composed of four cycles of 5-FU 500 mg/m^2 IV bolus. Compliance higher in preop arm at 90% vs. ~50% in postop arm. Overall, sphincter-preserving surgery was not more common in the preop group, although preop therapy improved the likelihood of sphincter-sparing operation via downstaging (39% vs. 19%, *p* = .004). Preop CRT improved acute and late toxicity as well as 10-year LR. pCR was 8%, and nodal involvement decreased (40% vs. 25%). No improvement in distant recurrence, OS, or DFS (Table 37.5); 18% of patients in the postop arm were clinically overstaged. **Conclusion: Preoperative CRT improves LC and tumor downstaging, reduces late effects, and is preferred to postoperative CRT.**

Table 37.5 Long-Term Results of German Rectal Study

	10-Yr LR	10-Yr DM	10-Yr OS	10-Yr DFS	Acute Grades 3–4 AEs	Late Grades 3–4 AEs
Preop CRT	7%	30%	60%	68%	27%	14%
Postop CRT	10%	30%	60%	68%	40%	24%
p value	.048	.9	.85	.65	.001	.01

Can additional CHT after preop long-course CRT (LC-CRT) increase pCR rates?

Phase II nonrandomized data[48] showed that LC-CRT followed by CHT with mFOLFOX6 before TME significantly increased rates of pCR. Rates increased with the number of cycles delivered. Results suggest investigation of nonoperative management of rectal cancer.

Is short-course preoperative RT effective compared with surgery alone? What about with TME?

The Swedish Rectal Cancer Trial found that preop short-course RT (SC-RT) improved LC and OS with non-TME surgery. SC-RT in the setting of TME was validated by a Dutch study showing improved LC. A British PRT confirmed that neoadjuvant SC-RT was superior to selective postop CRT for LC and DFS.[49] Subsequent comparisons to LC-CRT did not show significant differences between the two approaches. In the setting of TNT, LC-CRT is preferred (below), but studies are ongoing to further elucidate the role of SC-RT in TNT.

Folkesson, Swedish Rectal Cancer Trial (*NEJM* 1997, PMID 9091798; Update *JCO* 2005, PMID 16110023): PRT of 1,168 patients with resectable rectal ACA, age <80, planned abdominal surgery, and no mets randomized to (a) 25 Gy/5 fx followed by surgery within 1 week or (b) surgery alone. Primary endpoints were LR and postoperative mortality. See Table 37.6 for the results. **Conclusion: Preop SC-RT is associated with significantly improved LC and OS compared with surgery alone.** *Comment: Study criticized because it was unclear how many T1 patients were included, non-TME surgery was used, and there was an increased risk of late small bowel obstruction in the RT group.*

Table 37.6 Results of Short-Course RT Swedish Rectal Trial

	13-Yr LR	13-Yr OS	13-Yr CSS
Preop SC-RT 25 Gy/5 fx	9%	38%	72%
Surgery alone	26%	30%	62%
p value	<.001	.004	<.001

Kapiteijn, Dutch CKVO 9504 (*NEJM* 2001, PMID 11547717; Update *Ann Surg* 2007, PMID 17968156; *Lancet Oncol* 2011, PMID 21596621): PRT of 1,861 patients with clinically resectable ACA of the rectum, inferior tumor margin <15 cm from anal verge randomized to (a) 25 Gy/5 fx followed by TME or (b) TME alone. The 10-year LR was reduced from 11% to 5% with the addition of RT (*p* < .0001) with no change in OS or DM. Of note, there was a significant OS benefit in stage III patients who had negative CRM (50% vs. 40%, *p* = .03). **Conclusion: Preoperative SC-RT with 25 Gy/5 fx significantly improves LC, even with good surgery (TME), but does not improve OS.**

How does preop long-course CRT compare to short-course preop RT?

Bujko, Polish Study (*Br J Surg* 2006, PMID 16983741): PRT of 312 patients with cT3–4 and no sphincter involvement randomized to (a) 25 Gy/5 fx followed by TME within 7 days or (b) 50.4 Gy/28 fx with concurrent bolus 5-FU + LCV followed by TME 4 to 6 weeks later. Primary endpoint was sphincter preservation, and no difference was seen. The 4-year LC (11% vs. 16%), OS (67% vs. 66%), and DFS (58% vs. 56%) rates were similar between SC-RT and LC-CRT. **Conclusion: LC-CRT did not improve OS, LC, or late toxicity compared with SC-RT.** *Comment: Limitations to this study include clinical staging (no US or MRI), no standard postop CHT, not all TME, and no RT QA.*

Ngan, TROG Intergroup Trial (*JCO* 2012, PMID 23008301): PRT of 326 patients with cT3N0–2M0 rectal ACA within 12 cm of verge (US or MRI staged) randomized to (1) 25 Gy/5 fx, surgery in 3 to 7 days, six cycles 5-FU with folinic acid; or (2) 50.4 Gy/28 fx + continuous infusion 5-FU (225 mg/m²), surgery in 4 to 6 weeks, four cycles of 5-FU with folinic acid. No differences in LR, DR, OS, or late grades 3 to 4 toxicities (Table 37.7). For distally located tumors, LR was 13% in Arm 1 vs. 3% in Arm 2 (p = .21). **Conclusion: Preop SC-RT is equivalent to preop LC-CRT without increased late toxicity. Unclear if short course is equivalent to long course for distally located tumors.**

Table 37.7 Results of TROG Short vs. Long-Course Rectal Trial				
TROG 01.04	**3-Yr LR**	**5-Yr DR**	**5-Yr OS**	**Late Grades 3–4 Toxicity**
LC-CRT	4%	30%	70%	8%
SC-RT	8%	27%	74%	6%
p value	.24	.92	.62	NS

Bujko, Polish II Trial (*Ann Oncol* 2016, PMID 26884592; Update Cisel, *Ann Oncol* 2019, PMID 31192355): Phase III PRT of 515 patients with either fixed cT3 or cT4 rectal cancer randomized to 25 Gy/5 fx followed by three cycles of FOLFOX4 (Group A, n = 261) or 50.4 Gy/28 fx combined with two 5-day cycles of bolus 5-FU 325 mg/m²/day and LCV 20 mg/m²/day during the first and fifth weeks of RT along with five infusions of oxaliplatin 50 mg/m² once weekly (Group B, n = 254). Protocol amended to allow optional oxaliplatin in both groups. At MFU of 35 months, preop treatment acute toxicity was lower in Group A than Group B (p = .006), any toxicity being 75% vs. 83%, grades 3 to 4 23% vs. 21%, and toxic deaths 1% vs. 3%, respectively. R0 resection rates (primary endpoint) and pCR rates in Group A and Group B were, respectively, 77% vs. 71% (p = .07), and 16% vs. 12% (p = .17). The 3- and 8-year results are shown in Table 37.8. The 3-year OS improvement with SC-RT disappeared with longer follow-up. There was no difference in postop complications (29% vs. 25%, p = .18) or grade ≥3 late complications (11% vs. 9%, p = .66). **Conclusion: With long-term follow-up, 25 Gy/5 fx with consolidation CHT is not superior to LC-CRT.**

Table 37.8 Results of Polish II Trial Short vs. Long-Course Rectal Trial								
	3-Yr				**8-Yr**			
	OS	**DFS**	**LF**	**DM**	**OS**	**DFS**	**LF**	**DM**
SC-RT	73%	53%	22%	30%	49%	43%	35%	36%
LC-CRT	65%	52%	21%	27%	49%	41%	32%	34%
p value	.046	.85	.82	.26	.38	.65	.60	.54

OMISSION OF THERAPIES

In the modern era, when can neoadjuvant RT be omitted?

FOWARC,[50] a phase III RCT from China, found no difference in 3-year DFS or OS between neoadjuvant CRT vs. neoadjuvant CHT alone, but neoadjuvant CRT had higher pCR rates. This led to the CONVERT phase III noninferiority trial in China. The PROSPECT trial also found that preop FOLFOX is noninferior to preop CRT in patients with favorable-risk upper rectal cancer amenable to LAR.

Mei, CONVERT (*Ann Surg* 2022, PMID 36538627): Phase III noninferiority trial from China of 589 patients with locally advanced rectal ACA defined as tumors within 12 cm of the anal verge with uninvolved MRF (included cT2N+ or cT3–T4aN+; excluded T4b). Patients randomized to receive either neoadjuvant CHT with four cycles of CAPOX or neoadjuvant CRT (50 Gy/25 fx with concurrent capecitabine) followed by surgery. The pCR rate was 11% vs. 14% in the CHT vs. CRT arms, respectively (p = .33). Neoadjuvant CHT was associated with lower rates of periop DM (0.7% vs. 3%, p = .03) and preventive ileostomy rate (52% vs. 64%, p = .008). Two patients in the neoadjuvant CHT group and five in the CRT group achieved a cCR and proceeded with a W&W approach. **Conclusion: Neoadjuvant CAPOX (with omission of RT) results in similar pCR and downstaging rates with improved periop DM and ileostomy rates.**

Schrag, PROSPECT (*NEJM* 2023, PMID 37272534): Phase III PRT of 1,128 patients with cT2N+, cT3N0, or cT3N+ rectal ACA who are candidates for sphincter-sparing surgery randomized to six cycles of neoadjuvant FOLFOX vs. LC-CRT (50.4 Gy/28 fx with concurrent 5-FU or capecitabine followed by adjuvant FOLFOX). Patients with low tumors, T4 tumors, ≥4 nodes >1 cm, and tumors within 3 mm of the radial margin were excluded. In the FOLFOX arm, patients whose primary tumor decreased by <20% received additional neoadjuvant CRT (9% of FOLFOX patients required this). FOLFOX was noninferior to CRT for DFS (81% vs. 79%, $p = .005$). No difference in 5-year OS (90% vs. 90%) or LR (<2% in each group). Preoperative G3+ adverse event rate higher in the FOLFOX arm (41% vs. 23%). **Conclusion: Preop FOLFOX is noninferior to preop LC-CRT with respect to oncologic outcomes for relatively low-risk rectal cancer patients.** *Comment: How neoadjuvant FOLFOX compares to TNT remains an active question.*

Basch, PROSPECT QOL (*J Clin Oncol* 2023, PMID 37270691): Patient-reported QOL outcomes from the PROSPECT trial. Presurgery, the FOLFOX arm had higher rates of anxiety, appetite loss, constipation, depression, dysphagia, dyspnea, edema, fatigue, mucositis, nausea, neuropathy, and vomiting ($p < .05$), with patients in the CRT arm having worse rates of diarrhea and bowel function. One year after surgery, the FOLFOX arm reported improved rates of fatigue, neuropathy, and sexual function relative to the CRT arm ($p < .05$). **Conclusion: In the PROSPECT trial, both arms have distinct side effect profiles that can help inform patient decision-making.**

Which patients can be treated with upfront surgery alone?

Advances in MRI and the ability to detect involvement of the MRF have led to investigations into whether TME alone is appropriate for certain low-risk patients. The OCUM study[51] classified rectal cancer patients (cT2–4, any cN, M0) into low- and high-risk groups and found low rates of 5-year LR (3%) and DM (16%) in low-risk patients treated with upfront surgery. High-risk patients (MRF+, cT4, and cT3 in the lower third of the rectum) had 5-year LR of 6% and DM of 35%, suggesting a need for intensified therapy. A Dutch cohort study[52] further validated the use of MRI in determining a low-risk patient population based on MRF involvement that can avoid neoadjuvant CRT and proceed directly to TME. However, a Chinese noninferiority RCT showed greater LR rates in those who proceeded directly to surgery, and the trial was terminated (see below).

Li, MRI for Adjuvant CRT (*IJROBP* 2024, PMID 38185388): Noninferiority RCT from China investigating the omission of neoadjuvant CRT in 275 patients with locally advanced rectal cancer with tumors within 6 to 12 cm of the anal verge and no MRF involvement per MRI. Patients were randomized to either primary surgery and risk-adapted adjuvant therapy (CRT for positive margins, CHT for negative margins) or preoperative CRT followed by surgery and adjuvant CHT. Six patients (4%) had an LR in the primary surgery arm vs. none in the standard arm, which led to the early termination of the trial. **Conclusion: In this trial of patients with locally advanced rectal cancer and no MRF involvement per MRI, the omission of neoadjuvant CRT resulted in higher LF rates and is not a recommended strategy.**

What are the data on surgical de-escalation?

The LASRE RCT[53] compared laparoscopic vs. open surgery for the resection of low rectal tumors and found no difference in complete mesorectal excision, negative CRM or distal resection margins, number of LN removed, or postop complication rate. Laparoscopic surgery was associated with higher rates of preserved sphincter function and shorter hospital duration. The NEO phase II trial[54] showed that in patients with cT1–T3abN0 low or mid-rectal ACA that respond to neoadjuvant CHT, TES (rather than TME) may be sufficient. The TAU-TEM study[55] is a RCT aiming to demonstrate noninferiority of LC and an improvement in morbidity with CRT followed by transanal endoscopic microsurgery rather than TME. Early results show high pCR rates (44%) with reduced postop morbidity (21% vs. 51%, $p < .001$). Outcomes data are maturing.

TOTAL NEOADJUVANT THERAPY

What are the data assessing the utility and outcomes of total neoadjuvant therapy (TNT)?

The TNT paradigm involves administering all CHT upfront (although variations exist), either prior to or following LC-CRT/SC-RT, but prior to surgery. The phase II Spanish GCR-3 trial[56] found no difference in oncologic outcomes between induction CAPOX and adjuvant CAPOX after surgery, but induction CAPOX increased compliance along with reducing acute toxicity. Recently published data have shown this to be a safe and efficacious strategy, and TNT has emerged as the preferred treatment strategy for high-risk/locally advanced disease.

Conroy, PRODIGE 23 (*Ann Oncol*** 2024, PMID 38986769):** Phase III PRT in France randomizing locally advanced (mostly cT3–4, N1–2) rectal cancer patients to two different schedules, including TNT with neoadjuvant mFOLFIRINOX followed by CRT, surgery, and additional adjuvant CHT (6 cycles) vs. standard therapy with CRT, surgery, and adjuvant CHT (12 cycles). The 7-year DFS, MFS, and OS all favored the group receiving neoadjuvant mFOLFIRINOX (Table 37.9). Previously reported data (ASCO 2020) also showed a higher pCR in the TNT arm (28% vs. 12%, $p < .001$). Treatment was well-tolerated, with no differences in compliance or surgical morbidity. **Conclusion: TNT with neoadjuvant mFOLFIRINOX and LC-CRT was associated with improved 7-year DFS, MFS, and OS rates vs. standard therapy.**

Table 37.9 Results of the PRODIGE 23 Study

	7-Yr DFS	7-Yr MFS	7-Yr OS
TNT arm (CHT → CRT → TME → CHT)	68%	79%	82%
Standard arm (CRT → TME → CHT)	63%	72%	76%
p value	.048	.021	.033

Jin, STELLAR (*JCO*** 2022, PMID 35263150):** Phase III noninferiority trial of 599 patients with cT3–4 and/or N+ mid- to distal rectal ACA randomized to standard neoadjuvant CRT (50 Gy/25 fx with concurrent capecitabine) vs. neoadjuvant TNT. TNT arm was SC-RT (25 Gy/5 fx) followed by four cycles of CAPOX. Following surgery, patients in the standard arm received six cycles of CAPOX and the TNT arm received two additional cycles. There were no significant differences in 3-year DFS (65% vs. 62%), MFS (77% vs. 75%), or LRR (8% vs. 11%) for TNT vs. standard CRT, respectively. However, the 3-year OS was improved in the TNT arm (87% vs. 75%, $p = .033$). Complete clinical response (11% vs. 4%) and pCR (22% vs. 12%, $p = .002$) were improved with TNT. **Conclusion: TNT with SC-RT followed by CHT showed an improvement in OS without improvement in DFS or DMFS.**

Is SC-RT or LC-CRT the preferred TNT strategy?

Both SC-RT and LC-CRT are accepted historical standards in the neoadjuvant paradigm. While emerging data suggest LC-CRT may be the best choice in a TNT approach,[31,57] SCRT is more cost-effective with attractive QOL outcomes, and institutional practices vary.[58,59]

Bahadoer, RAPIDO (*Lancet Oncol*** 2020, PMID 33301740; Update ***Ann Surg*** 2023, PMID 36661037):** Phase III PRT of 912 patients in Europe and United States with primary locally advanced rectal cancer with high-risk features on MRI (cT4a/b, EMVI, cN2, MRF involvement, or enlarged lateral LNs) randomized to TNT vs. standard therapy. TNT arm: SC-RT (25 Gy/5 fx) followed by either six cycles of CAPOX or nine cycles of FOLFOX4, followed by TME. Standard arm: CRT, 50–50.4 Gy/25–28 fx, with concurrent capecitabine, followed by TME and adjuvant CHT (if stipulated by hospital policy), either 8 cycles of CAPOX or 12 cycles of FOLFOX4. Primary endpoint was 3-year disease-related treatment failure (DRTF) defined as first occurrence of LRF, DM, new primary CRC tumor, or treatment-related death. At MFU of 4.6 years, the 3-year cumulative probability of DRTF and rates of DM favored the TNT arm (Table 37.10). No difference in LRF or OS. pCR achieved in 28% of TNT arm vs. 14% for standard (OR 2.37, 95% CI 1.67–3.37). Serious adverse events were similar, 38% for TNT vs. 34% for standard arm, with four treatment-related deaths in each arm. At 5-year follow-up, LRR was higher in the TNT arm. **Conclusion: TNT with SC-RT followed by CHT and delayed surgery is associated with decreased 3-year disease-related treatment failure vs. standard therapy, but at 5 years there is an increased risk of LRR with SC-RT. LC-CRT may be the preferred TNT strategy, but further investigation is needed.** *Comment: Fifty-two percent of patients in the standard arm did not receive adjuvant CHT; however, on subset analysis, there was no difference in DM or LRF with and without CHT in the standard arm.*

Table 37.10 3- and 5-Year Results of RAPIDO

	3-Yr DRTF	3-Yr DM	3-Yr LRF	3-Yr OS	5-Yr LRF	5-Yr LRR
TNT (SC-RT → CHT → TME)	24%	20%	8%	89%	12%	10%
CRT → TME → ±CHT	30%	27%	6%	89%	8%	6%
p value	.019	.0048	.12	.59	.07	.027

Francois, PRODIGE 42/GERICO 12 (*Eur J Cancer* 2023, PMID 36535196): RCT from France evaluating SC-RT vs. LC-CRT followed by surgery in the elderly. 103 patients ≥75 years of age with resectable T3–T4 rectal ACA within 12 cm of the anal verge or T2 tumors of the low rectum were randomized between neoadjuvant SC-RT (25 Gy/5 fx) followed by surgery vs. neoadjuvant LC-CRT (50 Gy/25 fx with concurrent capecitabine) with surgery 7 to 8 weeks later. R0 resection rate was 84% in the SC-RT group vs. 88% in LC-RT (noninferiority *p* = .28). There was no difference in the activities of daily living score between the two groups preop or at 12 months postop (although it was worse in the LC-RT group at the 3-month postop time point). No difference in postop serious adverse events between groups. **Conclusion: Both short-course neoadjuvant RT and long-course neoadjuvant CRT are viable options in the elderly. LC-CRT has a higher R0 resection rate with no detriment in postop activities of daily living at 1 year.**

Francois, PRODIGE 42/GERICO 12 QOL Assessment (*Radiother Oncol* 2024, PMID 38341097): Secondary analysis of QOL for the above trial with mixed results. No overall difference in global EORTC QLQ-C30 score between the SC-RT and LC-CRT groups, but SC-RT did outperform LC-CRT at 3 months in the domains of cognitive function, fatigue, and appetite. The ELD14 score, which quantifies perception of disease burden, also favored the SC-RT group at 3, 6, and 12 months. The GDS15 depression score was significantly improved in the SC-RT group. No difference between groups in scores of ADLs, walking speed, nutritional status, and MMSE. **Conclusion: SC-RT outperforms preoperative LC-CRT in some QOL and functionality domains in the elderly, with no difference in others.**

What is the preferred TNT sequencing?

The phase II CAO/ARO/AIO-12 study[60] found no difference in DFS, LRR, DM, chronic toxicity, or QOL between induction CHT and consolidation CHT after CRT, but the rate of pCR was higher in the CRT first arm (25% vs. 17%, p = .04). The phase II OPRA trial (below) found that sequencing CRT first increases the chance of organ preservation.

Garcia-Aguilar, OPRA (*JCO* 2022 PMID 35483010; Update *JCO* 2024, PMID 37883738): Phase II PRT of 324 patients with stage II/III (mostly cT3–4N+) rectal ACA randomized to induction CHT (FOLFOX or CAPEOX) followed by CRT or CRT followed by consolidation CHT. CRT was 5-FU or capecitabine based with 50 to 56 Gy. Response was assessed 8 to 12 weeks after TNT with DRE, flexible sigmoidoscopy, and MRI. Patients with CR and near-CR were offered W&W, while those with incomplete response received TME. No difference in compliance between the arms. No differences in LRFS, DMFS, or OS. The 5-year updated outcomes are shown in Table 37.11. **Conclusion: There were no differences in DFS or DMFS with timing of CRT and CHT components of TNT, but improved organ preservation rates were demonstrated with CRT → CHT → TME.**

Table 37.11 Results of the OPRA study

	5-Yr DFS	5-Yr DMFS	5-Yr TME-Free Survival
Induction CHT arm (CHT → CRT → TME)	71%	80%	39%
Consolidation CHT arm (CRT → CHT → TME)	69%	78%	54%
p value	.68	.64	.012

For patients undergoing TNT who have a clinical complete response (cCR), is W&W a viable option?

This is an active area of investigation and not standard. However, accumulating evidence suggests this is a feasible strategy when strict surveillance occurs. Promising results from Brazil led to the idea of organ preservation in rectal cancer. In the OPRA study (above), over half of the patients treated on the consolidative CHT arm were TME-free at 5 years. Additionally, improvements in QOL have been reported in multiple studies.[61] A 2024 NCDB analysis[62] shows a 10% increase in the absolute annual proportion of organ preservation from 2006 to 2020 in the United States.

Habr-Gama, Brazil (*Semin Radiat Oncol* 2011, PMID 21645869): RR of 173 patients (63% cT3/ T4, 21% cTxN1–2) from 1991 to 2009 treated with neoadjuvant CRT 50.4 to 54 Gy with concurrent 5-FU. MFU 65 months. Sixty-seven patients (39%) developed cCR. Of these 67 patients, 13% underwent rectal biopsy and 87% were managed without surgical procedures. Recurrence occurred in 15 patients (21%): 8 patients developed local-only recurrence and 7 developed DM. Of eight patients who recurred locally, seven were successfully salvaged; 5-year OS 96% and 5-year DFS 72%. **Conclusion: Early retrospective data suggest it may be feasible to reserve surgery for salvage after cCR to CRT.**

Renehan, OnCoRe (*Lancet Oncol* 2016, PMID 26705854): Propensity-matched cohort study from UK evaluating W&W strategy in patients who achieve cCR after preop CRT. A total of 259 patients were included, of whom 228 underwent surgery and 31 (12%) had cCR and underwent W&W. An additional 98 patients with cCR were included via national registry for a total of 129 patients managed by W&W. MFU 33 months. Of 129 W&W patients, 44 (34%) had LR and 36 of 41 patients were salvaged. In matched analysis, there was no significant difference in nonregrowth DFS between W&W and immediate post-CRT surgery (88% vs. 78%) or 3-year OS (96% vs. 87%). Significantly improved 3-year colostomy-free survival in W&W cohort (74% vs. 47%). **Conclusion: Watch and wait can be considered in many patients without detriment in 3-year OS.**

Smith, MSKCC (*JAMA Oncol* 2019, PMID 30629084): Retrospective series of 113 patients with stage II/III rectal cancer who underwent neoadjuvant therapy (various regimens, most commonly RT 45–54 Gy/25–28 fx with concurrent 5-FU or capecitabine) who achieved cCR and were followed by W&W, compared with patients who underwent neoadjuvant therapy followed by TME found to have pCR. Twenty-two (19%) local regrowths occurred in the W&W group, of which 20 (91%) were controlled with salvage surgery; the 5-year OS was 73% in the W&W group vs. 94% in the surgery group and DFS 75% vs. 92%. Rate of DM was 36% in W&W patients with local regrowth vs. 1% in WW patients without local failure ($p < .001$). **Conclusion: Excellent rectal preservation and pelvic tumor control with W&W for patients who achieved cCR after neoadjuvant therapy, but with worse OS and higher risk of DM in those with local regrowth.**

Chin, WashU (*IJROBP* 2021, PMID 34653579): RR of 86 patients with stage I to III (95% locally advanced) rectal ACA undergoing SC-RT followed by consolidation CHT with W&W in those with cCR. With an MFU of 30 months, 50% of patients had an initial cCR. Local regrowth-free survival was 81% in those with initial cCR, and all patients with a recurrence were salvaged successfully. The 2-year regional control (98% vs. 85%), DMFS (100% vs. 80%), DFS (98% vs. 71%), and OS (100% vs. 88%) rates were significantly improved in those with a cCR compared with a non-cCR. **Conclusion: SC-RT followed by consolidation CHT is a feasible organ preservation strategy in patients with rectal ACA.**

What about dose and dose-escalation?

In the era of NOM, dose escalation has been considered as a way to maximize LC. OPRA treated from 50 to 56 Gy with a median of 54 Gy/30 fx.[38,39] The WW2 study dose-escalated to 62 Gy with impressive rates of LC and pCR.[37] More recent international retrospective data (ATLANTIS) suggest that patients with T3/T4 tumors treated to 56 to 60 Gy have higher pCR rates (27% vs. 17%, SS) with minimal increases in G3+ GI toxicity (6% vs. 2%, SS).[63] Other studies such as OPERA (below) and MORPHEUS[35] have investigated the use of contact brachytherapy for ultra-dose escalation with promising results, although the generalizability of this method remains uncertain.

Gerard, OPERA (*Lancet Gastroenterol Hepatol* 2023, PMID 36801007): Phase III European RCT assessing the role of contact brachytherapy boost in the setting of organ preservation. 141 patients with cT2, cT3a, cT3b ACA of the low to mid-rectum <5 cm in diameter with cN0 or cN1 disease (<8 mm) were included. All patients received CRT with 45 Gy/25 fx and concurrent capecitabine. Patients were then randomized to Group A (EBRT boost; 9 Gy/5 fx) vs. Group B (contact brachytherapy boost; 90 Gy/3 fx). MFU of 38.2 months. The 3-year organ preservation rate was 59% in Group A vs. 81% in Group B ($p = .0026$). For tumors <3 cm, the 3-year organ preservation rates were 63% vs. 97% in favor of Group B ($p = .012$). For tumors ≥3 cm, the 3-year organ preservation rates were 55% vs. 68% ($p = .11$). Late G1–2 bleeding was more common in Group B (12% vs. 63%, $p = .0001$). **Conclusion: CRT followed by a contact brachytherapy boost improved 3-year organ preservation rates (notably for tumors <3 cm) with higher rates of late rectal bleeding.**

What is the role of immunotherapy (IO) in TNT?

IO has an increasing role in the treatment of rectal cancer, particularly for MMRd tumors, with early data showing impressive CR rates with IO monotherapy in this population.[26,64] Efforts are underway to incorporate IO into TNT paradigms for pMMR patients.[27,28]

Cercek, Dostarlimab for MMRd Disease (*NEJM* 2022, PMID 35660797): Phase II study investigating single-agent dostarlimab in the treatment of MMRd stage II or III rectal ACA. Twelve patients were evaluated, and at a minimum of 6 months of follow-up (range 6–25 months) all 12 patients had a cCR with none requiring any additional therapy (no CRT or surgery). There were no G3+ adverse events. **Conclusion: MMRd rectal ACA is highly sensitive to dostarlimab monotherapy; longer follow-up is needed.**

Lin, UNION (*Ann Oncol* 2024, PMID 38964714): Phase III randomized multicenter Chinese trial investigating the adoption of IO into a TNT paradigm. 231 patients were assigned to either SC-RT followed by two cycles of CHT-IO (capecitabine/oxaliplatin with camrelizumab) then surgery and an additional six cycles of CHT-IO or LC-CRT followed by two cycles of capecitabine/oxaliplatin then surgery and an additional six cycles of capecitabine/oxaliplatin. pCR was 40% in the IO arm vs. 15% in the control arm. There was no difference in surgical complication rates or G3 AEs. **Conclusion: TNT with SC-RT and neoadjuvant CHT-IO is an evolving paradigm with notable pCR rates; additional outcomes data are maturing.**

OTHER CONSIDERATIONS

Does increased time interval between preop CRT and surgery impact pCR rates?

Data are conflicting. Historically, prior to TNT, the German Rectal Cancer Study used a time interval of ~6 weeks from completion of neoadjuvant LC-CRT to surgery.[20] The GRECCAR-6 trial randomized patients undergoing LC-CRT to surgery at 7 weeks or 11 weeks, and there was no difference in pCR rate between surgery at 7 vs. 11 weeks (15% vs. 17%, p = .598). Morbidity was significantly increased in the 11-week surgery group (45% vs. 32%, p = .04) and quality of TME was worse.[65] Contrarily, a Polish study randomizing patients after SC-RT to early (7–10 days) vs. delayed (4–5 weeks) surgery showed a significantly higher rate of downstaging was achieved (44% vs. 13%) for the delayed group.[32] Additionally, a separate Swedish study found no difference in pathologic response between early and delayed surgery with worse complications in patients who underwent early surgery (within 1 week).[66] For patients not receiving TNT, guidelines recommend an interval of 6 to 11 weeks.[31] The optimal timing of surgery following TNT is unknown—on the RAPIDO and STELLAR studies, the median time from the end of RT to surgery was 23 and 20 weeks.

Is tumor response after preop CRT predictive of outcomes?

Patel, Mercury Study (*JCO* 2011, PMID 21876084): Prospective cohort study of 111 patients treated with preop LC-RT alone or LC-CRT who underwent preop MRI 4 to 6 weeks following preop treatment. All patients had to have at least 5 mm of initial tumor extension beyond the muscularis propria. Tumor regression on MRI was significantly predictive of OS (HR 4.4) and DFS (HR 3.3). If CRM was involved based on posttreatment MRI, there was significantly increased risk of LR (28% vs. 12%, *p* < .05). The 5-year OS for patients with pathologic involved CRM vs. clear CRM was 30% vs. 63% (*p* = .001), DFS was 34% vs. 63% (*p* < .001), and LR was 26% vs. 7% (*p* < .001). **Conclusion: Tumor regression as documented by MRI predicts DFS and OS, and MRI-predicted CRM involvement is associated with increased risk of LR.**

Fokas, German Rectal Trial Posthoc Analysis (*JCO* 2014, PMID 24752056): See trial details previously. The authors evaluated pathologic response based on viable tumor vs. fibrosis—Tumor Regression Grading (TRG): grade 0, no regression; grade 1, minor regression (dominant tumor mass with obvious fibrosis in ≤25% of tumor mass); grade 2, moderate regression (dominant tumor mass with obvious fibrosis in 26%–50% of tumor mass); grade 3, good regression (dominant fibrosis outgrowing tumor mass; i.e., >50% tumor regression); and grade 4, total regression (no viable tumor cells; fibrotic mass only). MFU 132 months. MVA showed that ypN+ and TRG were the only independent prognosticators for DM and DFS. ypN+ and LVSI were predictive of LR. Cienfuegos et al. also showed that in patients with PNI/LVSI, TRG had no impact on OS. However, in patients without PNI/LVSI, TRG was predictive of OS and DFS.[67] Finally, pathologic response correlated with DFS, LR, and DM (Table 37.12).

Table 37.12 German Rectal Trial Secondary Analysis on Tumor Regression Grade		
10-Yr results	**DM**	**DFS**
TRG 4	11%	90%
TRG 2/3	29%	74%
TRG 0/1	40%	63%
p value	.005	.008

Is IMRT for rectal cancer safe and effective?

Hong, RTOG 0822 (*IJROBP* 2015, PMID 26163334): Phase II study of cT3–4, N0–2 low to mid-rectal cancers treated with IMRT 45 Gy/25 fx followed by 3D-CRT boost of 5.4 Gy/3 fx with concurrent capecitabine and oxaliplatin. Of 68 analyzable patients, 51% developed grade 2+ GI toxicity, which was not improved relative to historical controls (RTOG 0247); 15% of patients developed pCR and the 4-year LRF was 7%. **Conclusion: IMRT is feasible, but it did not demonstrate significant toxicity improvement relative to historical controls.**

RECURRENT RECTAL CANCER

Is re-irradiation of recurrent rectal cancer feasible?

Despite improved outcomes with TNT and TME, 5% to 10% of patients will experience LR after curative intent therapy.[68] Re-RT is commonly required in this scenario, and early studies including a phase II trial from Italy (see below) showed efficacy and acceptable toxicity with an accelerated hyperfractionated approach delivering BID treatment.[69–71] IORT is commonly used in this setting, especially for patients at risk for close or positive surgical margins.[72,73] For nonsurgical patients, SBRT and particle therapy are emerging options for dose escalation.[74–76]

Valentini, STORM (*IJROBP* 2006, PMID 16414206): Phase II trial of pelvic recurrences in patients with previous RT <55 Gy and KPS ≥60. Preop RT: PTV2 (GTV + 4 cm) 30 Gy/25 fx at 1.2 Gy/fx BID followed by boost to PTV1 (GTV + 2 cm) to 10.8 Gy/9 fx at 1.2 Gy/fx BID with concurrent PVI 5-FU. Patients who were resectable underwent surgery 6 to 8 weeks later. Fifty-nine patients were enrolled. Median time to re-RT was 27 months (minimum 9 months). Majority (86%) completed therapy; 8.5% of patients developed pCR. Grade 3 GI toxicity was 5%. Overall response rate was 44%. **Conclusion: Hyperfractionated re-RT with CHT is safe and effective for locally recurrent rectal cancer.**

Lee, Systematic Review (*Radiother Oncol* 2019, PMID 31176204): Included 17 studies and 744 patients with locally recurrent rectal cancer undergoing re-RT, with a variety of techniques and heterogeneity between studies. The 3-year OS for the entire group, surgical patients, and nonsurgical patients was 38%, 52%, and 24%, respectively. The 3-year LC for the surgical and nonsurgical groups was 47% and 45%, respectively. The rate of pooled G3+ acute and late complications was 12% for surgical group and 25% for nonsurgical patients, with more late complications in the surgery group. Overall palliation rate was 75%. **Conclusion: Mindful of heterogeneity, pooled data from numerous studies continue to suggest that re-RT is a reasonable option for recurrent rectal cancer; surgical patients have better survival, with the potential for more late complications.**

REFERENCES

1. Stoffel EM, Murphy CC. Epidemiology and mechanisms of the increasing incidence of colon and rectal cancers in young adults. *Gastroenterology*. 2020;158(2):341–353. doi:10.1053/j.gastro.2019.07.055
2. Siegel RL, Fedewa SA, Anderson WF, et al. Colorectal cancer incidence patterns in the United States, 1974-2013. *J Natl Cancer Inst*. 2017;109(8):djw322. doi:10.1093/jnci/djw322
3. National Comprehensive Cancer Network. *Clinical Practice Guidelines in Oncology: Rectal Cancer*. 2024.
4. Siegel RL, Giaquinto AN, Jemal A. Cancer statistics, 2024. *CA Cancer J Clin*. 2024;74(1):12–49. doi:10.3322/caac.21820
5. Ekbom A, Helmick C, Zack M, Adami HO. Ulcerative colitis and colorectal cancer. A population-based study. *N Engl J Med*. 1990;323(18):1228–1233. doi:10.1056/NEJM199011013231802
6. National Comprehensive Cancer Network. *Clinical Practice Guidelines in Oncology: Colorectal Cancer Screening*. 2024. Accessed February 2025. https://www.nccn.org/patients/guidelines/content/PDF/colorectal-screening-patient.pdf

7.   National Comprehensive Cancer Network. *Clinical Practice Guidelines in Oncology: Genetic/Familial High-Risk Assessment: Colorectal.* 2025. https://www.nccn.org/professionals/physician_gls/pdf/genetics_ceg.pdf

8.   Rades D, Kuhn H, Schultze J, et al. Prognostic factors affecting locally recurrent rectal cancer and clinical significance of hemoglobin. *Int J Radiat Oncol Biol Phys.* 2008;70(4):1087–1093. doi:10.1016/j.ijrobp.2007.07.2364

9.   Amin MB, Edge SB, Greene FL, et al, eds. *AJCC Cancer Staging Manual.* 8th ed. Springer International Publishing; 2017.

10. Glynne-Jones R, Wyrwicz L, Tiret E, et al. Rectal cancer: ESMO Clinical Practice Guidelines for diagnosis, treatment and follow-up. *Ann Oncol.* 2018;29(suppl 4):iv263. doi:10.1093/annonc/mdy161

11. Glynne-Jones R, Wyrwicz L, Tiret E, et al. Rectal cancer: ESMO Clinical Practice Guidelines for diagnosis, treatment and follow-up. *Ann Oncol.* 2017;28(suppl 4):iv22–iv40. doi:10.1093/annonc/mdx224

12. Russell MM, Ganz PA, Lopa S, et al. Comparative effectiveness of sphincter-sparing surgery versus abdominoperineal resection in rectal cancer: patient-reported outcomes in National Surgical Adjuvant Breast and Bowel Project randomized trial R-04. *Ann Surg.* 2015;261(1):144–148. doi:10.1097/SLA.0000000000000594

13. Buyse M, Zeleniuch-Jacquotte A, Chalmers TC. Adjuvant therapy of colorectal cancer. Why we still don't know. *JAMA.* 1988;259(24):3571–3578. doi:10.1001/jama.1988.03720240033028

14. O'Connell MJ, Martenson JA, Wieand HS, et al. Improving adjuvant therapy for rectal cancer by combining protracted-infusion fluorouracil with radiation therapy after curative surgery. *N Engl J Med.* 1994;331(8):502–507. doi:10.1056/NEJM199408253310803

15. Allegra CJ, Yothers G, O'Connell MJ, et al. Neoadjuvant 5-FU or capecitabine plus radiation with or without oxaliplatin in rectal cancer patients: a phase III randomized clinical trial. *J Natl Cancer Inst.* 2015;107(11):djv248. doi:10.1093/jnci/djv248

16. Hofheinz RD, Wenz F, Post S, et al. Chemoradiotherapy with capecitabine versus fluorouracil for locally advanced rectal cancer: a randomised, multicentre, non-inferiority, phase 3 trial. *Lancet Oncol.* 2012;13(6):579–588. doi:10.1016/S1470-2045(12)70116-X

17. Aschele C, Cionini L, Lonardi S, et al. Primary tumor response to preoperative chemoradiation with or without oxaliplatin in locally advanced rectal cancer: pathologic results of the STAR-01 randomized phase III trial. *J Clin Oncol.* 2011;29(20):2773–2780. doi:10.1200/JCO.2010.34.4911

18. Gerard JP, Azria D, Gourgou-Bourgade S, et al. Comparison of two neoadjuvant chemoradiotherapy regimens for locally advanced rectal cancer: results of the phase III trial ACCORD 12/0405-Prodige 2. *J Clin Oncol.* 2010;28(10):1638–1644. doi:10.1200/JCO.2009.25.8376

19. Hong TS, Moughan J, Garofalo MC, et al. NRG Oncology Radiation Therapy Oncology Group 0822: a phase 2 study of preoperative chemoradiation therapy using intensity modulated radiation therapy in combination with capecitabine and oxaliplatin for patients with locally advanced rectal cancer. *Int J Radiat Oncol Biol Phys.* 2015;93(1):29–36. doi:10.1016/j.ijrobp.2015.05.005

20. Sauer R, Liersch T, Merkel S, et al. Preoperative versus postoperative chemoradiotherapy for locally advanced rectal cancer: results of the German CAO/ARO/AIO-94 randomized phase III trial after a median follow-up of 11 years. *J Clin Oncol.* 2012;30(16):1926–1933. doi:10.1200/JCO.2011.40.1836

21. Hong YS, Nam BH, Kim KP, et al. Oxaliplatin, fluorouracil, and leucovorin versus fluorouracil and leucovorin as adjuvant chemotherapy for locally advanced rectal cancer after preoperative chemoradiotherapy (ADORE): an open-label, multicentre, phase 2, randomised controlled trial. *Lancet Oncol.* 2014;15(11):1245–1253. doi:10.1016/S1470-2045(14)70377-8

22. Rödel C, Liersch T, Becker H, et al. Preoperative chemoradiotherapy and postoperative chemotherapy with fluorouracil and oxaliplatin versus fluorouracil alone in locally advanced rectal cancer: initial results of the German CAO/ARO/AIO-04 randomised phase 3 trial. *Lancet Oncol.* 2012;13(7):679–687. doi:10.1016/S1470-2045(12)70187-0

23. Breugom AJ, Swets M, Bosset JF, et al. Adjuvant chemotherapy after preoperative (chemo)radiotherapy and surgery for patients with rectal cancer: a systematic review and meta-analysis of individual patient data. *Lancet Oncol.* 2015;16(2):200–207. doi:10.1016/S1470-2045(14)71199-4

24. Colorectal Cancer Collaborative Group. Adjuvant radiotherapy for rectal cancer: a systematic overview of 8,507 patients from 22 randomised trials. *Lancet.* 2001;358(9290):1291–1304. doi:10.1016/S0140-6736(01)06409-1

25. Bahadoer RR, Dijkstra EA, van Etten B, et al. Short-course radiotherapy followed by chemotherapy before total mesorectal excision (TME) versus preoperative chemoradiotherapy, TME, and optional adjuvant chemotherapy in locally advanced rectal cancer (RAPIDO): a randomised, open-label, phase 3 trial. *Lancet Oncol.* 2021;22(1):29–42. doi:10.1016/S1470-2045(20)30555-6

26. Cercek A, Lumish M, Sinopoli J, et al. PD-1 blockade in mismatch repair-deficient, locally advanced rectal cancer. *N Engl J Med.* 2022;386(25):2363–2376. doi:10.1056/NEJMoa2201445

27. Li Y, Pan C, Gao Y, et al. Total neoadjuvant therapy with PD-1 blockade for high-risk proficient mismatch repair rectal cancer. *JAMA Surg.* 2024;159(5):529–537. doi:10.1001/jamasurg.2023.7996

28. Xia F, Wang Y, Wang H, et al. Randomized phase II trial of immunotherapy-based total neoadjuvant therapy for proficient mismatch repair or microsatellite stable locally advanced rectal cancer (TORCH). *J Clin Oncol.* 2024;42(28):3308–3318. doi:10.1200/JCO.23.02261

29. Lin ZY, Zhang P, Chi P, et al. Neoadjuvant short-course radiotherapy followed by camrelizumab and chemotherapy in locally advanced rectal cancer (UNION): early outcomes of a multicenter randomized phase III trial. *Ann Oncol.* 2024;35(10):882–891. doi:10.1016/j.annonc.2024.06.015

30. Camma C, Giunta M, Fiorica F, Pagliaro L, Craxi A, Cottone M. Preoperative radiotherapy for resectable rectal cancer: a meta-analysis. *JAMA.* 2000;284(8):1008–1015. doi:10.1001/jama.284.8.1008

31. Wo JY, Ashman JB, Bhadkamkar NA, et al. Radiation therapy for rectal cancer: an ASTRO Clinical Practice Guideline Focused Update. *Pract Radiat Oncol.* 2024. doi:10.1016/j.prro.2024.11.003

32. Pach R, Kulig J, Richter P, Gach T, Szura M, Kowalska T. Randomized clinical trial on preoperative radiotherapy 25 Gy in rectal cancer--treatment results at 5-year follow-up. *Langenbecks Arch Surg.* 2012;397(5): 801–807. doi:10.1007/s00423-011-0890-8

33. Song C, Song S, Kim JS, et al. Impact of postoperative chemoradiotherapy versus chemotherapy alone on recurrence and survival in patients with stage II and III upper rectal cancer: a propensity score-matched analysis. *PLoS One.* 2015;10(4):e0123657. doi:10.1371/journal.pone.0123657

34. Wojcieszynski AP, Chuong MD, Hawkins M, et al. Rectal cancer update: which treatment effects are the least "brutal"? *Int J Radiat Oncol Biol Phys.* 2024;118(1):1–7. doi:10.1016/j.ijrobp.2023.08.012

35. Garant A, Vasilevsky CA, Boutros M, et al. MORPHEUS phase II–III study: a pre-planned interim safety analysis and preliminary results. *Cancers (Basel).* 2022;14(15):3665. doi:10.3390/cancers14153665

36. Gerard JP, Barbet N, Schiappa R, et al. Neoadjuvant chemoradiotherapy with radiation dose escalation with contact x-ray brachytherapy boost or external beam radiotherapy boost for organ preservation in early cT2-cT3 rectal adenocarcinoma (OPERA): a phase 3, randomised controlled trial. *Lancet Gastroenterol Hepatol.* 2023;8(4):356–367. doi:10.1016/S2468-1253(22)00392-2

37. Jensen LH, Risum S, Nielsen JD. Curative chemoradiation for low rectal cancer: primary clinical outcomes from a multicenter phase II trial. *J Clin Oncol.* 2022;40(17):LBA3514.

38. Garcia-Aguilar J, Patil S, Gollub MJ, et al. Organ preservation in patients with rectal adenocarcinoma treated with total neoadjuvant therapy. *J Clin Oncol.* 2022;40(23):2546–2556. doi:10.1200/JCO.22.00032

39. Verheij FS, Omer DM, Williams H, et al. Long-term results of organ preservation in patients with rectal adenocarcinoma treated with total neoadjuvant therapy: the randomized phase II OPRA trial. *J Clin Oncol.* 2024;42(5):500–506. doi:10.1200/JCO.23.01208

40. Videtic GMM, Woody NM, Vassil AD. *Handbook of Treatment Planning in Radiation Oncology.* 3rd ed. Demos Medical; 2020.

41. Gastrointestinal Tumor Study Group. Prolongation of the disease-free interval in surgically treated rectal carcinoma. *N Engl J Med.* 1985;312(23):1465–1472. doi:10.1056/NEJM198506063122301

42. Fisher B, Wolmark N, Rockette H, et al. Postoperative adjuvant chemotherapy or radiation therapy for rectal cancer: results from NSABP protocol R-01. *J Natl Cancer Inst.* 1988;80(1):21–29. doi:10.1093/jnci/80.1.21

43. Krook JE, Moertel CG, Gunderson LL, et al. Effective surgical adjuvant therapy for high-risk rectal carcinoma. *N Engl J Med.* 1991;324(11):709–715. doi:10.1056/NEJM199103143241101

44. Wolmark N, Wieand HS, Hyams DM, et al. Randomized trial of postoperative adjuvant chemotherapy with or without radiotherapy for carcinoma of the rectum: National Surgical Adjuvant Breast and Bowel Project Protocol R-02. *J Natl Cancer Inst.* 2000;92(5):388–396. doi:10.1093/jnci/92.5.388

45. Roh MS, Colangelo LH, O'Connell MJ, et al. Preoperative multimodality therapy improves disease-free survival in patients with carcinoma of the rectum: NSABP R-03. *J Clin Oncol.* 2009;27(31):5124–5130. doi:10.1200/JCO.2009.22.0467

46. Bosset JF, Collette L, Calais G, et al. Chemotherapy with preoperative radiotherapy in rectal cancer. *N Engl J Med.* 2006;355(11):1114–1123. doi:10.1056/NEJMoa060829

47. Gerard JP, Conroy T, Bonnetain F, et al. Preoperative radiotherapy with or without concurrent fluorouracil and leucovorin in T3-4 rectal cancers: results of FFCD 9203. *J Clin Oncol.* 2006;24(28):4620–4625. doi:10.1200/JCO.2006.06.7629

48. Garcia-Aguilar J, Chow OS, Smith DD, et al. Effect of adding mFOLFOX6 after neoadjuvant chemoradiation in locally advanced rectal cancer: a multicentre, phase 2 trial. *Lancet Oncol.* 2015;16(8):957–966. doi:10.1016/S1470-2045(15)00004-2

49. Sebag-Montefiore D, Stephens RJ, Steele R, et al. Preoperative radiotherapy versus selective postoperative chemoradiotherapy in patients with rectal cancer (MRC CR07 and NCIC-CTG C016): a multicentre, randomised trial. *Lancet.* 2009;373(9666):811–820. doi:10.1016/S0140-6736(09)60484-0

50. Deng Y, Chi P, Lan P, et al. Neoadjuvant modified FOLFOX6 with or without radiation versus fluorouracil plus radiation for locally advanced rectal cancer: final results of the Chinese FOWARC trial. *J Clin Oncol.* 2019;37(34):3223–3233. doi:10.1200/JCO.18.02309

51. Ruppert R, Junginger T, Kube R, et al. Risk-adapted neoadjuvant chemoradiotherapy in rectal cancer: final report of the OCUM study. *J Clin Oncol.* 2023;41(24):4025–4034. doi:10.1200/JCO.22.02166

52. Hazen SJA, Sluckin TC, Intven MPW, et al. Abandonment of routine radiotherapy for nonlocally advanced rectal cancer and oncological outcomes. *JAMA Oncol.* 2024;10(2):202–211. doi:10.1001/jamaoncol.2023.5444

53. Jiang WZ, Xu JM, Xing JD, et al. Short-term outcomes of laparoscopy-assisted vs open surgery for patients with low rectal cancer: the LASRE randomized clinical trial. *JAMA Oncol.* 2022;8(11):1607–1615. doi:10.1001/jamaoncol.2022.4079

54. Kennecke HF, O'Callaghan CJ, Loree JM, et al. Neoadjuvant chemotherapy, excision, and observation for early rectal cancer: the phase II NEO trial (CCTG CO.28) primary end point results. *J Clin Oncol.* 2023;41(2):233–242. doi:10.1200/JCO.22.00184

55. Serra-Aracil X, Pericay C, Badia-Closa J, et al. Short-term outcomes of chemoradiotherapy and local excision versus total mesorectal excision in T2-T3ab,N0,M0 rectal cancer: a multicentre randomised, controlled, phase III trial (the TAU-TEM study). *Ann Oncol.* 2023;34(1):78–90. doi:10.1016/j.annonc.2022.09.160

56. Fernandez-Martos C, Garcia-Albeniz X, Pericay C, et al. Chemoradiation, surgery and adjuvant chemotherapy versus induction chemotherapy followed by chemoradiation and surgery: long-term results of the Spanish GCR-3 phase II randomized trial. *Ann Oncol.* 2015;26(8):1722–1728. doi:10.1093/annonc/mdv223

57. Bercz A, Park BK, Pappou E, et al. Organ preservation after neoadjuvant long-course chemoradiotherapy versus short-course radiotherapy. *Ann Oncol.* 2024;35(11):1003–1014. doi:10.1016/j.annonc.2024.07.729

58. Chin RI, Otegbeye EE, Kang KH, et al. Cost-effectiveness of total neoadjuvant therapy with short-course radiotherapy for resectable locally advanced rectal cancer. *JAMA Netw Open.* 2022;5(2):e2146312. doi:10.1001/jamanetworkopen.2021.46312

59. Ma H, Li H, Xu T, et al. Quality of life and functional outcomes in patients with locally advanced rectal cancer receiving total neoadjuvant therapy versus concurrent chemoradiotherapy: an analysis of the XXX trial. *Int J Radiat Oncol Biol Phys.* 2025. doi:10.1016/j.ijrobp.2024.12.035

60. Fokas E, Schlenska-Lange A, Polat B, et al. Chemoradiotherapy plus induction or consolidation chemotherapy as total neoadjuvant therapy for patients with locally advanced rectal cancer: long-term results of the CAO/ARO/AIO-12 randomized clinical trial. *JAMA Oncol.* 2022;8(1):e215445. doi:10.1001/jamaoncol.2021.5445

61. Custers PA, van der Sande ME, Grotenhuis BA, et al. Long-term quality of life and functional outcome of patients with rectal cancer following a watch-and-wait approach. *JAMA Surg.* 2023;158(5):e230146. doi:10.1001/jamasurg.2023.0146

62. Loria A, Tejani MA, Temple LK, et al. Practice patterns for organ preservation in US patients with rectal cancer, 2006–2020. *JAMA Oncol.* 2024;10(1):79–86. doi:10.1001/jamaoncol.2023.4845

63. Nicosia L, Bonu ML, Angelicone I, et al. Analysis of patients with locally advanced rectal cancer given neoadjuvant radiochemotherapy with or without RT dose intensification: a multicenter retrospective study - ATLANTIS part I. *Radiother Oncol.* 2025;204:110701. doi:10.1016/j.radonc.2024.110701

64. Andre T, Berton D, Curigliano G, et al. Antitumor activity and safety of dostarlimab monotherapy in patients with mismatch repair deficient solid tumors: a nonrandomized controlled trial. *JAMA Netw Open.* 2023;6(11):e2341165. doi:10.1001/jamanetworkopen.2023.41165

65. Lefevre JH, Mineur L, Cachanado M, et al. Does a longer waiting period after neoadjuvant radio-chemotherapy improve the oncological prognosis of rectal cancer?: three years' follow-up results of the Greccar-6 randomized multicenter trial. *Ann Surg.* 2019;270(5):747–754. doi:10.1097/SLA.0000000000003530

66. Erlandsson J, Holm T, Pettersson D, et al. Optimal fractionation of preoperative radiotherapy and timing to surgery for rectal cancer (Stockholm III): a multicentre, randomised, non-blinded, phase 3, non-inferiority trial. *Lancet Oncol.* 2017;18(3):336–346. doi:10.1016/S1470-2045(17)30086-4

67. Cienfuegos JA, Rotellar F, Baixauli J, et al. Impact of perineural and lymphovascular invasion on oncological outcomes in rectal cancer treated with neoadjuvant chemoradiotherapy and surgery. *Ann Surg Oncol.* 2015;22(3):916–923. doi:10.1245/s10434-014-4051-5

68. Regan SN, Hendren S, Krauss JC, Crysler OV, Cuneo KC. Treatment of locally recurrent rectal cancer: a review. *Cancer J.* 2024;30(4):264–271. doi:10.1097/PPO.0000000000000728

69. Mohiuddin M, Marks G, Marks J. Long-term results of reirradiation for patients with recurrent rectal carcinoma. *Cancer.* 2002;95(5):1144–1150. doi:10.1002/cncr.10799

70. Valentini V, Morganti AG, Gambacorta MA, et al. Preoperative hyperfractionated chemoradiation for locally recurrent rectal cancer in patients previously irradiated to the pelvis: a multicentric phase II study. *Int J Radiat Oncol Biol Phys.* 2006;64(4):1129–1139. doi:10.1016/j.ijrobp.2005.09.017

71. Tao R, Tsai CJ, Jensen G, et al. Hyperfractionated accelerated reirradiation for rectal cancer: an analysis of outcomes and toxicity. *Radiother Oncol.* 2017;122(1):146–151. doi:10.1016/j.radonc.2016.12.015

72. Haddock MG. Intraoperative radiation therapy for colon and rectal cancers: a clinical review. *Radiat Oncol.* 2017;12(1):11. doi:10.1186/s13014-016-0752-1

73. Amarnath SR. The role of intraoperative radiotherapy treatment of locally advanced rectal cancer. *Clin Colon Rectal Surg.* 2024;37(4):239–247. doi:10.1055/s-0043-1770718

74. Johnstone P, Okonta L, Aitken K, et al. A multicentre retrospective review of SABR reirradiation in rectal cancer recurrence. *Radiother Oncol.* 2021;162:1–6. doi:10.1016/j.radonc.2021.06.030

75. Koroulakis A, Molitoris J, Kaiser A, et al. Reirradiation for rectal cancer using pencil beam scanning proton therapy: a single institutional experience. *Adv Radiat Oncol.* 2021;6(1):100595. doi:10.1016/j.adro.2020.10.008

76. Jeans EB, Ebner DK, Takiyama H, et al. Comparing oncologic outcomes and toxicity for combined modality therapy vs. carbon-ion radiotherapy for previously irradiated locally recurrent rectal cancer. *Cancers (Basel).* 2023;15(11):3057. doi:10.3390/cancers15113057

Katherine R. Amarell, Jacob A. Miller, and Sudha R. Amarnath

QUICK HIT   Squamous cell carcinoma (SCC) of the anal canal is a relatively rare but often curable cancer (Table 38.1). Standard of care is concurrent CRT with 5-FU and mitomycin C (MMC). Select T1N0 patients with well-differentiated anal margin cancers may be treated with wide local excision (WLE) with 1-cm margins. Acute treatment-related toxicities are often severe, but treatment breaks should be avoided as prolonged treatment time has been associated with increased failure rates. IMRT has been shown to reduce hematologic, GI, and skin toxicities, but expertise is required with this approach.

Table 38.1 General Treatment Paradigm for Anal Cancer	
Stage	**Treatment Recommendations***
T1N0 (anal margin, well-differentiated)	WLE ± CRT if inadequate margins
T1–T2N0 (anal canal)	50.4 Gy/28 fx to primary, 42 Gy/28 fx to elective LNs Per NCCN, can consider excision alone if the tumor meets criteria for "superficial SCC," i.e., <3 mm invasion past basement membrane and <7 mm horizontal spread
T3/T4N0	54 Gy/30 fx to primary, 45 Gy/30 fx to elective LNs
Node-positive	54 Gy/30 fx to primary Involved nodes: ≤3 cm: 50.4 Gy/28 fx; >3 cm: 54 Gy/30 fx

*IMRT doses per RTOG 0529.[1]

EPIDEMIOLOGY: Approximately 10,540 new diagnoses with 2,190 anal cancer-related deaths in the United States in 2024.[2] Lifetime risk is 1 in 500.[3] Comprises 2.6% of GI malignancies[2] (rectal cancer is 5× as common). Incidence in men and women has increased over the past 30 years. Average age at diagnosis is early 60s.[3] Incidence of anal cancer is more than twice as high in females as it is in males.[2] Incidence has not decreased in the era of HAART.[4]

RISK FACTORS: HPV (most commonly HPV 16, but also 18, 31, 33, and 45).[3] High-risk HPV DNA has been detected in up to 84% of specimens in large-scale anal cancer studies.[5] Other risk factors include HIV infection; history of cervical, vulvar, or vaginal cancer (HPV-related); immunosuppression after organ transplant; smoking; and history of receptive anal intercourse.

ANATOMY: The anal canal is 4 cm long and extends proximally from the anal verge (palpable junction between non–hair-bearing and hair-bearing squamous epithelium) to the dentate line (line between simple columnar epithelium proximally to stratified squamous epithelium distally). The anal margin is the skin within 5 cm of the anal verge. The canal is surrounded by the internal and external anal sphincters.

Histology: Three zones: *cutaneous zone* is the anal margin; *transition zone* is in the canal and ends at the dentate line, contains squamous epithelium without hair; *true mucosa* starts at the dentate line and contains columns of Morgagni and holds transitional epithelium for about 2 cm before the true mucosa of the rectum begins.

Lymphatics: For tumors that arise below the dentate line, the drainage pattern is to the inguinal and femoral nodes that arise from the external iliacs. Above the dentate line, the nodal drainage pattern is similar to that of rectal cancer: perirectal and internal iliacs.

PATHOLOGY: About 75% to 80% are SCC. Other, more rare anal cancers include adenocarcinoma (treated like rectal cancer), melanoma, neuroendocrine, carcinoid, Kaposi's, leiomyosarcoma, and lymphoma. Perianal skin tumors (SCC, BCC, melanoma, Bowen's, Paget's) should be treated as skin cancer.

CLINICAL PRESENTATION: About 45% of patients present with rectal bleeding; 30% will experience either pain or sensation of a rectal mass.[6] Patients with more proximally located tumors can also present with alteration in bowel movements. At presentation, ~50% will present with localized disease, 30% with regional LN involvement, and 10% with DMs (most commonly liver and lung).[7] Risk of nodal involvement is higher in patients with sphincter involvement or poorly differentiated tumors.

WORKUP: H&P (with careful attention to inguinal nodes and digital rectal exam to determine extent of tumor and sphincter function). GYN exam/cervical screening for females.

Labs: CBC, BMP, LFTs, CEA, HIV if there are risk factors (and CD4 if HIV+).

Procedures: Anoscopy with biopsy of primary, excisional biopsy or FNA of suspicious inguinal LNs, and HPV status. Sigmoidoscopy/colonoscopy often performed as well.

Imaging: CT chest, abdomen, and pelvis; MRI of pelvis with contrast; PET/CT.

PROGNOSTIC FACTORS: Male sex, N+, and tumor size >5 cm were independently prognostic of worse OS on RTOG 98–11.

STAGING: See Table 38.2.

Table 38.2 AJCC 9th Edition (2022): Staging for Anal Cancer					
T/M		cN0	cN1a	cN1b	cN1c
T1	≤2 cm	I		IIB	
T2	>2 cm but ≤5 cm	IIA			
T3	>5 cm		IIIA		
T4	Invasion into adjacent organs[1]	IIIB		IIIC	
M1	Distant metastasis		IV		

Notes: Organs[1] = invasion of vagina, urethra, or bladder. Invasion of rectal wall, perirectal skin, subcutaneous tissue, or sphincter muscle are not always T4.
cN1a: metastasis in inguinal, mesorectal, superior rectal, obturator, or internal iliac nodes; cN1b: metastasis in external iliac nodes; cN1c: metastasis in external iliac node as well as any N1a nodal involvement.

TREATMENT PARADIGM

Surgery: Before the 1970s, anal cancer was treated with abdominoperineal resection (APR) and permanent colostomy with historical 5-year OS rates of 60% for T1/2 disease, 40% for T3 disease, and 20% for LN+ disease. In the 1970s, the Nigro regimen was established after high CR rates to neoadjuvant CRT were noted. Concurrent CRT is now standard but has never been prospectively compared with surgery. Local excision is a treatment option per NCCN for those with T1N0 well-differentiated tumors of the anal margin.[8] Patients with adequate margins (>1 cm) can be observed. Those resected with positive margins require re-excision, adjuvant RT, or CRT.

Chemotherapy: Definitive CRT, as established by Nigro, is indicated for T2+ or any N+ disease. Standard of care is two cycles of 5-FU/MMC concurrent with RT; 5-FU dose is 1,000 mg/m^2 on days 1 to 4 and 29 to 32 (start of week 5). MMC is often given concurrently with 5-FU, two cycles on days 1 and 29, 10 mg/m^2 IV bolus. Some providers are currently using single-dose MMC (12 mg/m^2) on week 1 with 5-FU given on weeks 1 and 5 per the ACT I trial or replacing 5-FU with daily Xeloda during RT, which is similar to rectal cancer CHT administration, but with the addition of MMC. Major limiting toxicity of MMC is neutropenia. Cisplatin is used at some institutions in place of MMC given the equivalent response rates seen on the ACT II trial. However, no trials to date have demonstrated an oncologic benefit to the use of cisplatin.

Radiation

Indications: RT is indicated in all cases except T1N0 tumors of the anal margin treated with WLE, although RT alone may be appropriate for T1N0 (controversial). For others (cT2–4 or N+), organ preservation therapy is standard with concurrent CRT.

Dose: No prospective data exist to guide RT dosing strategies. One common standard is defined by RTOG 0529 (see Table 38.1 for dosing). IMRT is standard of care. Ongoing clinical trials (DECREASE study) are investigating deintensified CRT in the early-stage setting.

Toxicity: Acute: skin desquamation, fatigue, nausea, vomiting, diarrhea, urethritis, cystitis, pain, neutropenia. Late: cystitis, proctitis, sexual dysfunction (females), infertility, sacral insufficiency fracture, second malignancy, bowel stricture, fistula, hyperpigmentation, bowel incontinence.

Procedure: See *Handbook of Treatment Planning in Radiation Oncology*, Chapter 7.[9]

EVIDENCE-BASED Q&A

What is the basis for nonsurgical management of anal cancer?

Historically, primary treatment was APR. Use of preoperative CRT in the Wayne State study demonstrated excellent rates of CR and thus established that CRT alone was adequate. There has not been a direct phase III comparison with surgery, although definitive CRT compares favorably in RRs with the benefit of allowing for sphincter preservation. T1 patients were not included in the original Nigro studies.

Leichman, Wayne State "Nigro Regimen" (*Am J Med* 1985, PMID 3918441): RR of 45 patients (T2+) treated with continuous infusion 5-FU (1,000 mg/m²) for 96 hours × 2 cycles days 1 to 4 and 29 to 32, as well as one cycle bolus of MMC (15 mg/m²) on day 1. RT was 30 Gy/15 fx over 3 weeks using AP/PA technique to pelvis and inguinal nodes. Posttreatment biopsy was taken 4 to 6 weeks after completion of CRT. Originally, APR was required for all patients, but the first five out of six patients had pCR. Thus, in the remainder of the study, APR was required only for those with positive posttreatment biopsy. Eighty-four percent of patients had negative biopsy after CRT, and there were no recurrences observed in this population, with an OS rate of 89% at 50 months. Overall, the 5-year OS was 67% and the 5-year CFS 59%. **Conclusion: Definitive treatment with CRT alone is an effective treatment for anal cancer.**

Is concurrent CRT superior to RT alone?

Two major RCTs have been performed to answer this question. Both trials included more locally advanced patients and demonstrated that the addition of CHT to RT improves pCR rates, LC, colostomy-free survival (CFS), and DSS, although no noted improvement in OS. Addition of CHT did not significantly increase late toxicity. Update of ACT I shows that the benefit provided by adjuvant CRT persists at 13 years.

UK ACT I (*Lancet* 1996, PMID 8874455; Update Northover, *Br J Cancer* 2010, PMID 20354531): PRT of 577 patients with stage II to IV anal SCC randomized to RT alone vs. CRT. The RT regimen was either 45 Gy/20 fx or 45 Gy/25 fx depending on institutional preference. In the CRT arm, the regimen was two cycles of continuous infusion 5-FU (1,000 mg/m² days 1–4 or 750 mg/m² days 1–5) during the first and last week of RT. One cycle of bolus MMC was given on day 1 (12 mg/m²). Clinical response was assessed at 6 weeks and those with response received additional 15 Gy boost with EBRT or 25 Gy boost with Ir-192 brachytherapy. Those without response had salvage surgery. Primary endpoint was LF. See Table 38.3. Addition of concurrent CHT to RT significantly improved LC and CSS. Acute toxicity was worse with CHT, but there was no observed increase in late toxicity. The 13-year update demonstrated that for every 100 patients treated with CRT, there were 25 fewer locoregional relapses and 12.5 fewer anal cancer deaths, with no difference in late toxicity. The CRT arm had an initial increase in nonanal cancer-related deaths in the first 5 years, but this was not seen in long-term follow-up. **Conclusion: CHT in addition to RT improves LC and CSS without increasing late toxicity.**

Table 38.3 Initial Results of ACT I Concurrent CRT for Anal Cancer					
	3-Yr LF	**3-Yr OS**	**3-Yr CSS**	**Acute Morbidity**	**Late Morbidity**
RT	61%	58%	61%	39%	38%
RT + 5-FU/MMC	39%	65%	72%	48%	42%
p value	<.0001	.25	.02	.03	.39

Bartelink, EORTC 22861 (*JCO* 1997, PMID 9164216): PRT of 103 patients with T3/T4 or N+ disease randomized to RT vs. CRT. RT was 45 Gy/25 fx, with assessment at 6 weeks followed by 20 Gy boost for PR and 15 Gy boost for CR. APR was used if there was no response. CHT was continuous infusion 5-FU 750 mg/m² on days 1 to 5 and days 29 to 33 and a single dose of MMC 15 mg/m² on day 1. See Table 38.4. Addition of concurrent CHT improves LC, CFS, and CR rates, but not OS.

No significant difference in severe toxicities. **Conclusion: CRT improves oncologic outcomes over definitive RT alone.**

Table 38.4 Results of EORTC CRT for Anal Cancer				
	5-Yr CR	5-Yr LC	5-Yr CFS	5-Yr OS
RT (*n* = 52)	54%	50%	40%	56%
RT + 5-FU/MMC (*n* = 51)	80%	68%	72%	56%
p value	.02	.02	.002	.17

Is concurrent 5-FU alone sufficient in comparison to 5-FU/MMC?

Multiple studies have shown that the addition of MMC to 5-FU-based CRT improves outcomes of LC, CFS, and OS despite greater toxicity. Most notable is RTOG 8704 as follows, but the Princess Margaret study also confirmed the importance of adding MMC.[10]

Flam, ECOG 1289/RTOG 8704 (*JCO* 1996, PMID 8823332): PRT of 291 patients with anal cancer of any T/N stage treated with definitive CRT and randomized to either concurrent 5-FU and MMC or 5-FU alone. Regimen was 5-FU 1,000 mg/m^2 continuous infusion on days 1 to 4 and 28 to 33 and MMC 10 mg/m^2 bolus on days 1 and 28. RT was 45 Gy/25 fx to the pelvis with 5.4 Gy boost if palpable disease present at the end of the initial RT course. Biopsy was performed 4 to 6 weeks after CRT. If biopsy was positive, further 9 Gy was given with concurrent 5-FU and cisplatin. Patients with residual tumor underwent APR. With concurrent MMC, rates of colostomy were lower (9% vs. 22%, *p* = .002), CFS was higher (71% vs. 59%, *p* = .014), and DFS was higher (73% vs. 51%, *p* = .003) at 4 years. No significant differences in OS. Grades 4 to 5 toxicities were higher with MMC (23% vs. 7%, *p* ≤ .001). Of 24 patients who underwent salvage CRT after the initial course of CRT, 50% were cured. **Conclusion: Although it is associated with greater toxicity, use of MMC improves DFS and CFS. Salvage CRT may be reasonable for patients with residual disease as opposed to salvage APR.**

Can MMC be replaced with cisplatin?

RTOG 98–11 showed that replacing MMC with cisplatin along with the addition of induction CHT significantly decreased hematologic toxicities but also increased colostomy rates and reduced DFS and OS. However, the ACT II trial established that replacement of MMC with cisplatin does not affect the rate of CR. Due to ACT II showing that CHT regimens are equal in terms of response rate, some have suggested that the results of RTOG 98–11 are indicative that induction CHT may be detrimental.

Ajani, RTOG 98–11 (*JAMA* 2008, PMID 18430910; Update Gunderson, *JCO* 2012, PMID 23150707): PRT of 649 patients with T2–T4, N0–N3 disease randomized to (a) RT + concurrent 5-FU/MMC or (b) RT + induction/concurrent 5-FU/cisplatin. RT was 45 Gy/25 fx with 55 to 59 Gy boost to primary tumor and involved nodes for those with T3–T4, N+, or T2 patients with residual disease after 45 Gy. Elective nodal sites were treated to 30.6–36 Gy/17–20 fx. CHT in Arm A was 5-FU 1,000 mg/m^2 continuous infusion on days 1 to 4 and 29 to 32 and MMC 10 mg/m^2 bolus on days 1 and 29. In Arm B, two cycles of induction 5-FU and cisplatin were given, and RT started on day 57 with the third cycle of CHT and was continued through the end of the fourth cycle. Cisplatin given in four bolus administrations: 75 mg/m^2 on days 1, 29, 57, and 85, with two cycles prior to the start of RT. See Table 38.5. OS and DFS were superior in Arm A. **Conclusion: Use of concurrent 5-FU/MMC without induction CHT should remain standard of care.**

Table 38.5 Results of RTOG 98–11					
	5-Yr OS	5-Yr CFS	5-Yr DFS	Grades 3–4 Heme Toxicity	Grades 3–4 Nonheme Toxicity
RT + concurrent 5-FU/MMC	78%	72%	68%	61%	74%
RT + induction/concurrent 5-FU/cisplatin	71%	65%	58%	42%	74%
p value	.026	.05	.006	.0013	NS

James, UK ACT II (*Lancet Oncol* 2013, PMID 23578724): PRT of 940 T1–T4 patients randomized in 2 × 2 fashion to either concurrent 5-FU/cisplatin or concurrent 5-FU/MMC, followed by second randomization to 5-FU × 2 cycles after completion of CRT (maintenance) or observation. RT dose was 50.4 Gy/28 fx. MFU 5.1 years. CR was ~90% with either concurrent CHT regimen; 3-year PFS was 74% with maintenance CHT vs. 73% with observation (NS). **Conclusion: MMC/5-FU + RT remains standard. There was no benefit to the addition of maintenance CHT after completion of standard therapy.**

Are there any advantages to dose escalation?

RTOG 9208 demonstrated that there is no role for dose escalation, although the study was limited due to a mandatory treatment break.[11] Patients were treated to 59.4 Gy with concurrent 5-FU/MMC with mandatory 2-week break (then amended to be continuous without break). Higher dose in this study was associated with increased colostomy rate and no significant difference in OS or LC compared with historical standards (RTOG 8704). These findings are supported by the ACCORD 03 trial, which also showed no improvement in oncologic outcomes with high-dose boost (see the following).

Should we add induction CHT or high-dose boost?

The results of ACCORD 03 are in line with the findings of RTOG 98–11—there is no benefit to induction CHT. One retrospective study has suggested there may be a benefit in CFS with use of induction CHT in T4 patients, although this has not been validated prospectively.[12] There is no role for high-dose boost at this time.

Peiffert, ACCORD 03 (*JCO* 2012, PMID 22529257): PRT of 307 patients with anal SCC (either ≥4 cm or N+) randomized in 2 × 2 fashion: ± induction CHT and either standard or high-dose boost in addition to concurrent CRT (45 Gy/25 fx with concurrent 5-FU/cisplatin). Standard boost was 15 Gy. High-dose boost was 20 Gy for CR or ≥80% reduction and 25 Gy for PR (<80% reduction). Primary endpoint CFS. See Table 38.6. At MFU of 50 months, there was no statistically significant difference between the four arms. Considering the 2 × 2 analysis, the 5-year CFS was 77% vs. 75% (*p* = .37) in Arms A and B vs. C and D, respectively, and 74% vs. 78% (*p* = .067) in Arms A and C vs. C and D, respectively. **Conclusion: No benefit to induction CHT or high-dose boost. Further evaluation of dose intensification is needed given the trend in improved CFS.**

Table 38.6 Results of ACCORD 03 for Anal Cancer			
Arm	5-Yr CFS	5-Yr LC	5-Yr DSS
A. Induction + CRT + standard boost	70%	72%	77%
B. Induction + CRT + high-dose boost	82%	88%	89%
C. CRT + standard boost	77%	84%	81%
D. CRT + high-dose boost	73%	78%	76%

Is there benefit to IMRT?

RTOG 0529[1] was a phase II trial evaluating the use of IMRT for anal cancer and demonstrated significant reduction in hematologic, GI, and skin toxicity, compared with historical 3D-CRT standards. NCCN consensus is that IMRT is preferred over 3D-CRT; however, IMRT requires expertise in its application as 81% of patients on study required replanning on central review. RTOG 0529 is an appropriate guideline for use of IMRT in anal cancer.

What salvage options are available for recurrence after definitive CRT?

APR is used for salvage in the setting of LF after definitive CRT. Salvage surgery results vary widely in the literature due to small patient populations and selection bias. One study performed in the Netherlands of 47 patients undergoing salvage APR demonstrated negative margin resections in 81% with a 5-year OS rate of 42%. However, 45% of the cohort ultimately recurred.[13]

For incomplete posttreatment response, when should biopsy be performed?

Initial guidelines recommended response assessment at 6 to 12 weeks after treatment; however, post-hoc analysis of ACT II showed that there can be a delayed clinical response up to 26 weeks without a negative impact on survival.

Glynne-Jones (*Lancet* 2017, PMID 28209296): Post-hoc analysis of ACT II to determine an optimal response assessment time point. Complete clinical response (cCR) was evaluated at three time points measured from start of CRT: 11 weeks, 18 weeks, and 26 weeks. cCR was defined as no evidence of residual tumor or nodal disease by clinical exam. At 11, 18, and 26 weeks, cCR rates were 52%, 71%, and 78%, respectively. The 5-year OS for cCR at each time point was 83%, 84%, and 87% vs. 72%, 59%, and 46% for those who did not have a cCR at each time point. **Conclusion: Many patients without cCR at 11 weeks will respond by 26 weeks, and any salvage interventions should be delayed until after this time point to avoid unnecessary surgeries.**

What is the recommendation for T1N0 patients?

This patient subset was not included in the original Nigro studies, and they were also excluded from RTOG 98–11, ACT I, ACT II, and EORTC 22861. NCCN recommends local excision with adequate margins (defined as 1 cm) for anal margin cancers and CRT for anal canal lesions. Options for inadequate margins include re-excision (preferred) or local RT ± concurrent CHT. Retrospective series have suggested good outcomes with definitive RT in this patient subset.

What are the outcomes with nonregional LN metastasis (PA LNs) treated definitively?

There may be a small subset of patients who have good outcomes with extended DFS when treated definitively with extended field RT and CHT.

Holliday (*IJROPB* 2018, PMID 29907489): RR of 30 patients with de novo SCC of the anal canal metastatic to PA LNs, treated with extended field CRT (median dose 51 Gy) and cisplatin/5-FU/Xeloda, 5-FU/MMC, or daily Xeloda. The 3-year OS and DFS rates were 67% and 42%; the 3-year rate of DM was 50%. **Conclusion: In patients presenting with SCC of the anal canal with metastases limited to the PA LNs, extended-field CRT is a viable treatment option.**

REFERENCES

1. Kachnic LA, Winter K, Myerson RJ, et al. RTOG 0529: a phase 2 evaluation of dose-painted intensity modulated radiation therapy in combination with 5-fluorouracil and mitomycin-C for the reduction of acute morbidity in carcinoma of the anal canal. *Int J Radiat Oncol Biol Phys*. 2013;86(1):27–33. doi:10.1016/j.ijrobp.2012.09.023

2. Siegel RL, Giaquinto AN, Jemal A. Cancer statistics, 2024. *CA Cancer J Clin*. 2024;74(1):12–49. doi:10.3322/caac.21820

3. American Cancer Society - Anal Cancer. *Key Statistics for Anal Cancer*. 2020. Accessed November 5, 2025. https://www.cancer.org/cancer/anal-cancer/about/what-is-key-statistics.html

4. Crum-Cianflone NF, Hullsiek KH, Marconi VC, et al. Anal cancers among HIV-infected persons: HAART is not slowing rising incidence. *AIDS*. 2010;24(4):535–543. doi:10.1097/QAD.0b013e328331f6e2

5. Frisch M, Glimelius B, van den Brule AJ, et al. Sexually transmitted infection as a cause of anal cancer. *N Engl J Med*. 1997;337(19):1350–1358. doi:10.1056/NEJM199711063371904

6. Ryan DP, Compton CC, Mayer RJ. Carcinoma of the anal canal. *N Engl J Med*. 2000;342(11):792–800. doi:10.1056/NEJM200003163421107

7. Altekruse S, Kosary CL, Krapcho M, et al, eds. SEER Cancer Statistics Review, 1975–2007. National Cancer Institute; 2010. Accessed November 5, 2025. https://seer.cancer.gov/explorer/application.html?site=34&data_type=1&graph_type=4&compareBy=sex&chk_sex_3=3&chk_sex_2=2&race=1&age_range=1&advopt_precision=1

8. National Comprehensive Cancer Network. NCCN Clinical Practice Guidelines in Oncology: Anal Carcinoma. *Version 1.2025*. National Comprehensive Cancer Network; 2025. Accessed November 5, 2025. https://www.nccn.org

9. Gregory M. M. Videtic MDCMF, Vassil AD, Woody NM. *Handbook of Treatment Planning in Radiation Oncology*. Springer Publishing Company; 2020.

10. Cummings BJ, Keane TJ, O'Sullivan B, Wong CS, Catton CN. Epidermoid anal cancer: treatment by radiation alone or by radiation and 5-fluorouracil with and without mitomycin C. *Int J Radiat Oncol Biol Phys*. 1991;21(5):1115–1125. doi:10.1016/0360-3016(91)90265-6

11. Konski A, Garcia M Jr, John M, et al. Evaluation of planned treatment breaks during radiation therapy for anal cancer: update of RTOG 92-08. *Int J Radiat Oncol Biol Phys*. 2008;72(1):114–118. doi:10.1016/j.ijrobp.2007.12.027

12. Moureau-Zabotto L, Viret F, Giovaninni M, et al. Is neoadjuvant chemotherapy prior to radio-chemotherapy beneficial in T4 anal carcinoma? *J Surg Oncol*. 2011;104(1):66–71. doi:10.1002/jso.21866

13. Hagemans JAW, Blinde SE, Nuyttens JJ, et al. Salvage abdominoperineal resection for squamous cell anal cancer: a 30-year single-institution experience. *Ann Surg Oncol*. 2018;25(7):1970–1979. doi:10.1245/s10434-018-6483-9

Winston Vuong, Christopher W. Fleming, and Kevin L. Stephans

QUICK HIT Cholangiocarcinoma (CC) is a rare and highly lethal cancer, with a propensity for both local and distant recurrence. Surgery is the ideal local approach; however, the majority of patients present with advanced, unresectable disease. CC is categorized based on three sites of origin: intrahepatic, perihilar, and distal extrahepatic. The general treatment paradigm for resectable CC consists of surgery, followed by adjuvant CHT, with RT reserved for positive margins or positive LNs. Unresectable patients receive CHT and can be considered for dose-escalated hypofractionated RT. Transplant protocols, consisting of neoadjuvant CRT, brachytherapy boost, and orthotopic liver transplant (OLT), have shown excellent outcomes for patients with perihilar CC with unresectable disease or arising in the setting of primary sclerosing cholangitis (PSC).

EPIDEMIOLOGY: Incidence in the United States is 2 to 4 per 100,000 people annually and appears to be increasing due to a rise in intrahepatic CC.[1,2] Worldwide, the highest incidence is found in Thailand and Southeast Asia, with nearly 20× higher incidence than Western countries.[3] Patients are typically diagnosed between ages 50 and 70, although patients with PSC often present at a younger age.

RISK FACTORS: PSC is the strongest risk factor, with an estimated lifetime risk of 5% to 20%.[4] Other established risk factors include hepatobiliary lithiasis, congenital biliary duct cysts (seen in Caroli disease), infection with the liver flukes *Opisthorchis viverrini* and *Clonorchis sinensis* (most commonly found in Southeast Asia and Thailand), and exposure to Thorotrast, a radiologic contrast agent banned in the 1960s. Other risk factors include genetic disorders such as Lynch syndrome and cystic fibrosis, smoking, diabetes, obesity, nitrosamine intake, inflammatory bowel disease (IBD), cirrhosis, and hepatitis B and C.[5] Although CC is separated into fluke-associated vs. non–fluke-associated, management remains the same.

ANATOMY: CC originates from the bile duct epithelium and is classified based on site of origin: intrahepatic, perihilar, and distal extrahepatic. Perihilar tumors have been further classified based on extent of ductal involvement using the Bismuth–Corlette system; those involving the common hepatic duct bifurcation are referred to as Klatskin tumors.

PATHOLOGY: The vast majority are adenocarcinoma and often marked by significant peritumoral desmoplasia, lowering the diagnostic yield of biopsy and cytology. The cell of origin is the cholangiocyte, and a subset of intrahepatic CC can originate from hepatocytes that transdifferentiate into biliary lineages, leading to a subtype referred to as hepatocholangiocarcinoma or primary liver carcinoma with biphenotypic differentiation. CC is often multifocal and has a strong propensity for perineural invasion.[6] Intrahepatic CCs are associated with characteristic growth patterns including mass-forming (65%), which originates in the small intrahepatic bile ducts and forms a mass lesion; periductal-infiltrating (6%), which grows along the walls of the larger biliary ducts and is associated with progressive wall thickening/strictures; and intraductal-growing (4%), which presents as a polypoid or papillary tumor, or a mixed pattern. Periductal infiltrating can often adopt features of mass-forming (~25%).[7] Perihilar and extrahepatic CCs tend to grow as flat or poorly defined nodular sclerosing lesions that diffusely infiltrate adjacent structures. Perihilar tumors are particularly challenging to diagnose, as only half of the patients will have a diagnostic biopsy. The need for tissue diagnosis has been questioned, as patients diagnosed using clinical criteria alone (see Workup section) have similar likelihood of malignancy found on explanted livers. CK7 is generally positive by IHC, although not specific to biliary cancers. FISH testing for chromosomal abnormalities may aid in diagnosis when cytology is inconclusive for malignancy, increasing the diagnostic yield.

GENETICS: Lynch syndrome and PSC-associated with IBD are the primary genetic syndromes associated with CC. CC is associated with various somatic mutations that may influence systemic therapy options. Molecular testing (for unresectable/metastatic cases) includes *FGFR2* fusion or rearrangement, *IDH1* mutation, *HER2* overexpression or amplification, *RET* gene fusion, *KRAS G12C* mutation, *BRAF V600E* mutation, *NTRK* gene fusion, TMB-H, or MSI-H/dMMR.

SCREENING: PSC patients are generally recommended at least annual surveillance with CA 19–9 and US, CT, or MRI.

CLINICAL PRESENTATION: Perihilar and distal extrahepatic CCs often present with obstructive symptoms of jaundice, pruritus, malabsorption, and dark urine. Intrahepatic CC is less likely to cause obstruction unless very advanced, due to unaffected contralateral or nearby biliary branch drainage, and generally presents with RUQ pain, weight loss, and fever.

WORKUP: H&P, with attention to symptoms as previously noted.

Labs: CBC, CMP, CA 19–9, CEA, AFP (elevated in HCC and mixed hepatocholangiocarcinoma). Patients presenting with cholangitis should have tumor markers redrawn after infection and obstruction have resolved, as these can spuriously elevate marker levels. Check serum IgG4 in cases of extrahepatic CC to rule out IgG4-cholangitis that may mimic CC.

Imaging: Patients often have undergone CT and US of the liver during workup but should undergo MRI or MRCP for assessment of local tumor extent and resectability. If stent placement is required for obstruction, MRI is ideally performed prior to avoid artifact. CT chest or PET/CT to evaluate for DM, most commonly to the liver, peritoneum, bone, and lungs.

Procedures: ERCP and PTHC (percutaneous transhepatic cholangiography) allow for visualization of the biliary tree as well as therapeutic drainage. Staging laparoscopy should be performed prior to surgery to assess for resectability as well as peritoneal metastases.

Biopsy: EUS with FNA (for distal lesions) only after surgical consultation due to risk of peritoneal seeding and/or ERCP with brush cytology for pathologic confirmation. Because of the dense peritumoral desmoplasia, potential background PSC, and often poorly visualized tumors, the diagnostic yield of a biopsy or brushing is low (50% of patients with perihilar tumors have pathologic confirmation). Because of this, clinical criteria have been developed that signal for a similar likelihood of malignancy on explanted livers.[8]

Criteria for Diagnosis of Perihilar CC: Presence of a malignant-appearing stricture on percutaneous or endoscopic cholangiography and one of the following: malignant cytology or histology on transluminal brushings or biopsy, polysomy on FISH, CA 19–9 >100 U/mL, or mass on cross-sectional imaging at the site of the malignant-appearing stricture.[8]

PROGNOSTIC FACTORS: Age, stage, grade, margin status, tumor markers.[9] Overall, the 5-year OS is estimated between 2% and 30%.[10] CC is marked by a high rate of local and distant failure. At presentation, one-third of patients will have regional LN metastases.[11–13] An additional one-third to two-thirds present with DM.[14] In unresected CC, there is a 1-year OS of <20% in those who do not pursue additional therapy or are treated medically alone without modern CHT.[15] For those who receive adjuvant CRT, ~25% will recur locoregionally, 63% of those with LRF will require biliary intervention, and one-third of those patients will die from biliary complications.[16]

STAGING: AJCCs 8th edition has separate TNM and group staging for each site of origin (Table 39.1).

Table 39.1 AJCC 8th Edition: Staging for Cholangiocarcinoma			
	Intrahepatic	**Perihilar**	**Distal**
T1	**a.** ≤5 cm, no vascular invasion	Confined to bile duct, extension up to muscle layer or fibrous tissue	Invades bile duct wall, depth <5 mm
	b. >5 cm, no vascular invasion		
T2	Single tumor with vascular invasion, or multiple tumors	**a.** Invasion into surrounding fat	Invades bile duct wall, depth 5–12 mm
		b. Invasion into adjacent liver	
T3	Perforates visceral peritoneum	Invades unilateral branches of portal vein or hepatic artery	Invades bile duct wall, depth >12 mm

(continued)

Table 39.1 AJCC 8th Edition: Staging for Cholangiocarcinoma (*continued*)			
	Intrahepatic	Perihilar	Distal
T4	Invasion[1]	Invasion[2]	Invasion[3]
N0	No regional lymph node metastases		
N1	Involves regional nodes	1–3 regional nodes	
N2	N/A	4+ regional nodes	
M0	No distant metastases		
M1	Distant metastases present		

Notes: Invasion[1] = invasion into local extrahepatic structures. Invasion[2] = invasion into main portal vein or its bilateral branches, common hepatic artery, or unilateral second-order biliary radicals with contralateral portal vein or hepatic artery involvement. Invasion[3] = invasion of celiac axis, SMA, or common hepatic artery.
Group staging also varies for each location; see AJCC Staging Manual.[17]
Source: Adapted from AJCC Cancer Staging Manual. 8th ed. Springer International Publishing; 2017.

TREATMENT PARADIGM

Surgery: Surgery is performed for all resectable patients. Patients considered for resection are those without DM, in whom margin-negative resection would maintain adequate hepatic function postoperatively; this unfortunately represents the minority of patients. Variable degrees of vascular, biliary tree, and diaphragmatic involvement are considered resectable based on center experience. Contraindications to surgery include DM, nodal metastases beyond the porta hepatis, and multifocal hepatic disease, although resection can be considered in highly selected situations. Preoperative portal vein embolization may be used to induce hypertrophy of the future liver remnant to allow for more extensive resections.

Intrahepatic Tumors: Resected via partial hepatectomy. At least 1-cm margins are preferred, as smaller margins are associated with higher risk of recurrence, although this remains an area of controversy.[18]

Distal Extrahepatic Tumors: Resected via pancreaticoduodenectomy (Whipple procedure) and are more likely to be resectable at diagnosis.[19]

Perihilar Tumors: Often unresectable due to the degree of bile duct involvement. Some may be amenable to bile duct excision and partial hepatectomy, although recurrence rates after local excision are high,[20] as is perioperative mortality.[21] These factors have led to increasing adoption of OLT for early-stage perihilar CC, as well as for CC arising in the setting of PSC (see Transplant Protocol below).

Chemotherapy

Adjuvant: CHT (or enrollment on a clinical trial) is the preferred option for all patients after R0/R1 resection or pN+ disease. Capecitabine (1,250 mg/m^2 BID on days 1–14 of a 21-day cycle for 8 cycles) is the only Category 1 recommendation, although alternatives can include gemcitabine ± (capecitabine or cisplatin) or single-agent 5-FU.

Concurrent: Capecitabine (1,330 mg/m^2 daily with RT per SWOG 0809) or alternatively 825 mg/m^2 BID or 5-FU 225 mg/m^2 daily.

R2 Resection/Unresectable/Metastatic: Gemcitabine + cisplatin + (durvalumab per TOPAZ-1 or pembrolizumab per KN-966) is the preferred regimen.[22,23] Cisplatin (25 mg/m^2) and gemcitabine (1,000 mg/m^2) are given on days 1 and 8 q3 weeks for up to eight cycles. Durvalumab (1,500 mg) is given on day 1 of each 3-week cycle then once monthly after completion of gemcitabine/cisplatin until progression. Pembrolizumab (200 mg) is given once q3 weeks for up to 35 cycles until progression. Alternatives include gemcitabine + cisplatin (Category 1 alternative)[24]; gemcitabine monotherapy or with either nab-paclitaxel or capecitabine or oxaliplatin; capecitabine single-agent or combined with oxaliplatin; FOLFOX; or single-agent 5-FU. The ACTICCA-1 trial is an ongoing phase III trial comparing combination gemcitabine/cisplatin to capecitabine in the adjuvant setting.[25]

Radiation Therapy

Adjuvant: Traditional indications include positive margins and consideration for positive LN. Adjuvant CRT can be considered in select cases of R0 resected extrahepatic CC. For extrahepatic biliary cancers with R1 resection, ASCO guidelines recommend consideration of adjuvant CRT with capecitabine based on the results of the SWOG 0809 trial.[10] Patients received four cycles of gemcitabine (1,000 mg/m² on days 1 and 8) and capecitabine (1,500 mg/m² per day on days 1–14) q21 days followed by concurrent capecitabine (1,330 mg/m² per day) and RT, consisting of 45 Gy to the regional lymphatics with a boost to 54 to 59.4 Gy to the resection bed. Note: *Intrahepatic CC was not included due to the challenge of identifying the positive margin.*

Unresectable: Unresectable patients will often start treatment with CHT alone, with locoregional therapy considered for those who do not progress distantly. Dose-escalated hypofractionated RT ± concurrent CHT has shown promising results in single-institution studies for unresectable intrahepatic CC.[26,27] NRG GI-001 was investigating the benefit of RT following three cycles of gemcitabine/ cisplatin, with doses up to 67.5 Gy/15 fx, with dose reductions based on mean liver dose (MLD) and proximity to the porta hepatis, although this was terminated due to poor accrual. SBRT has also been used in this setting; common prescriptions include 40–60 Gy/5 fx and 30–60 Gy/3 fx.[28] A small proportion of patients will convert to resectable disease after RT.

Mayo Clinic Transplant Protocol for Perihilar CC: Mayo Clinic has pioneered the use of OLT for perihilar tumors and CC arising in the setting of PSC. This protocol consists of neoadjuvant CRT, brachytherapy boost, maintenance CHT, followed by OLT. Staging laparoscopy is required prior to transplant.[29]

Inclusion criteria:

- Diagnosis of CC either pathologically or with clinical criteria as noted previously
- Perihilar CC arising in the setting of PSC or anatomically unresectable
- Radial tumor diameter ≤3 cm
- Absence of intra- and extrahepatic metastases, including regional LNs
- Candidate for OLT

CRT: 45 Gy/30 fx BID with concurrent 5-FU or capecitabine.

Brachytherapy: 15 Gy/3 fx or 9.3 Gy/1 fx HDR or 20–30 Gy/3 fx LDR. In patients who are not candidates for brachytherapy (e.g., unable to place biliary catheters), SBRT has been used to replace brachytherapy[30] and the external RT component.[31,32] Another option includes an EBRT sequential boost to 54 to 60 Gy for non-brachy candidates.[33]

Maintenance CHT: 5-FU or capecitabine until transplant.

EVIDENCE-BASED Q&A

What is the benefit of adjuvant CHT?

Adjuvant CHT is indicated for all patients with positive margins or positive regional LNs. There is controversy regarding its use in N0 patients after R0 resection. The long-term follow-up of BILCAP demonstrates persisting OS benefit in the per-protocol analysis but not in the intention-to-treat analysis.[34]

Primrose, BILCAP (*Lancet Oncol* 2019, PMID 30922733): Multicenter phase III trial randomizing 447 patients with CC or gallbladder carcinoma after macroscopically complete resection to adjuvant capecitabine vs. observation; 62% had R0 resection and 53% were pN0. By intention to treat, the median OS was 51 vs. 36 months in favor of adjuvant capecitabine (*p* = .097). Per-protocol analysis showed OS of 53 vs. 36 months (*p* = .028). **Conclusion: Adjuvant capecitabine can improve OS in resected biliary tract cancer.**

What are the indications for adjuvant RT?

General indications include positive margins and positive LNs. Controversy exists regarding the use of adjuvant RT for intrahepatic CC due to difficulty in identifying the positive margin. SWOG 0809 enrolled extrahepatic-only CC and showed favorable outcomes compared with historical reports, with no difference in OS or LR between R0 and R1 resection after high-dose postoperative CHT and RT, providing an evidence-based adjuvant regimen for clinicians. A meta-analysis of extrahepatic CC/gallbladder cancers suggests an OS benefit to adjuvant RT.

Ben-Josef, SWOG 0809 (*JCO*** 2015, PMID 25964250):** Prospective, single-arm, phase II trial including 79 patients with extrahepatic CC or gallbladder carcinoma, surgically resected with pT2–T4, positive nodes, or positive margins. Patients received four cycles of adjuvant gemcitabine/capecitabine, followed by RT (45 Gy to regional lymphatics; 54–59.4 Gy to tumor bed) with concurrent capecitabine. Eighty-six percent completed treatment per protocol; the 2-year OS was 65% and the 2-year LR was 11%, neither of which was different between R0/R1 patients, suggesting potential efficacy of the treatment regimen. **Conclusion: This combination was well-tolerated, has promising efficacy, and provides a well-supported adjuvant regimen for clinical use.**

Ren, EHCC/GBC Meta-Analysis (*Radiat Oncol*** 2020, PMID 31941520):** Meta-analysis from 21 clinical trials involving 1,465 patients with extrahepatic CC or gallbladder cancer examining OS and LR in those who received adjuvant RT (PORT) or not. PORT was associated with significantly improved 5-year OS particularly from those with positive margins or N+ disease and numerically but not significantly improved 5-year OS in those with negative margins. LR was significantly lower in the PORT group and there was no difference in DM between the groups. **Conclusion: PORT is an effective therapy particularly in those with positive margins or N+ disease.**

How should RT be delivered for unresectable CC?

For patients who remain free of metastatic disease after initial CHT, RT can be added to prolong LC and potentially OS. The best evidence exists for dose-escalated hypofractionated RT, which was being investigated on NRG GI-001, randomizing patients with intrahepatic CC to observation vs. hypofractionated RT after initial gemcitabine/cisplatin; this was terminated due to poor accrual. Outcomes after SBRT have been reported as well.[32,35]

Tao, MD Anderson (*JCO*** 2016, PMID 26503201):** RR of 79 patients with inoperable intrahepatic CC treated with definitive RT between 2002 and 2014. Doses ranged from 35 to 100 Gy in 3 to 30 fx, with a median BED of 80.5 Gy. Eighty-nine percent received CHT prior to RT. Median OS 30 months, 3-year OS 44%. For patients receiving BED >80.5 Gy, the 3-year OS was 73% vs. 38% (*p* = .017) and the 3-year LC 78% vs. 45% (*p* = .04). No significant RT-related toxicities. **Conclusion: Higher BED is associated with improved LC and OS.**

Hong, Multi-Institutional (*JCO*** 2016, PMID 26668346).** Phase II study of 92 patients with unresectable HCC or intrahepatic CC (*n* = 41) undergoing high-dose hypofractionated proton beam therapy. Median RT dose 58 GyE (range 15.1–67.5) in 15 fx; 2-year LC 94% for both HCC and CC; 2-year OS 63% for HCC and 47% CC; 5% rate of grade 3 adverse effects. **Conclusion: High-dose hypofractionated proton therapy demonstrated high LC with low rates of toxicity.**

What studies have led to the adoption of OLT for unresectable hilar CC?

Early experiences with transplantation alone were disappointing, with 5-year OS <30%.[36] The University of Nebraska then pioneered a neoadjuvant regimen with CRT, followed by OLT, showing 45% long-term survival.[37] This approach was later adopted by the Mayo Clinic, which published excellent initial outcomes, with 5-year OS of 82% for those completing the protocol.[38] Several other institutions adopted this protocol, with reproducible results. Due to the success of this paradigm, some have suggested implementation of OLT for resectable hilar and intrahepatic CC.[39–41]

Rosen, Mayo Clinic (*HPB*** 2008, PMID 18773052):** Review of 148 patients enrolled on prospective institutional protocol; 61% underwent OLT; 5-year OS for all patients 55%, 71% for those who proceeded to transplant. **Conclusion: Transplant protocol achieves significantly lower recurrence and higher long-term survival rates than resection, OLT alone, or medical treatment in hilar CC.**

Darwish Murad, Multi-Institutional (*Gastroenterology*** 2012, PMID 22504095):** RR of 287 patients from 12 U.S. transplant centers (67% from Mayo Clinic) enrolled on OLT protocols. In the 75% who underwent OLT, the 5-year RFS was 65%. The 5-year OS was 53% in all patients. No difference in outcomes between centers. **Conclusion: Transplant protocol proved to be reproducible across multiple transplant centers.**

Ethun, Multi-Institutional (*Ann Surg*** 2018, PMID 29064885):** RR of 304 patients with hilar CC treated at 10 U.S. institutions; 234 underwent attempted resection, and 70 enrolled on transplant protocols. Patients who underwent transplant had improved OS, compared with resection (3-year 72% vs. 33%; 5-year 64% vs. 18%; *p* < .001). Among patients who underwent resection for tumors

<3 cm with LN-negative disease and excluding PSC patients, transplant was still associated with improved OS (3-year 54% vs. 44%; 5-year 54% vs. 29%; p = .03). Transplant remained associated with improved OS on intention-to-treat analysis, even after accounting for tumor size, LN status, and PSC (p = .049). **Conclusion: Resection for hilar CC meeting the criteria for transplantation (<3 cm, LN-negative) is associated with substantially decreased OS compared with transplant for unresectable disease.**

REFERENCES

1. Patel N, Benipal B. Incidence of cholangiocarcinoma in the USA from 2001 to 2015: a US cancer statistics analysis of 50 states. *Cureus*. 2019;11(1):e3962–e3962. doi:10.7759/cureus.3962
2. Javle M, Lee S, Azad NS, et al. Temporal changes in cholangiocarcinoma incidence and mortality in the United States from 2001 to 2017. *The Oncologist*. 2022;27(10):874–883. doi:10.1093/oncolo/oyac150
3. Sripa B, Pairojkul C. Cholangiocarcinoma: lessons from Thailand. *Curr Opin Gastroenterol*. 2008;24(3): 349–356. doi:10.1097/MOG.0b013e3282fbf9b3
4. Fung BM, Lindor KD, Tabibian JH. Cancer risk in primary sclerosing cholangitis: epidemiology, prevention, and surveillance strategies. *World J Gastroenterol*. 2019;25(6):659–671. doi:10.3748/wjg.v25.i6.659
5. Tyson GL, El-Serag HB. Risk factors for cholangiocarcinoma. *Hepatology*. 2011;54(1):173–184. doi:10.1002/hep.24351
6. Li CG, Zhou ZP, Tan XL, Zhao ZM. Perineural invasion of hilar cholangiocarcinoma in Chinese population: one center's experience. *World J Gastrointest Oncol*. 2020;12(4):457–466. doi:10.4251/wjgo.v12.i4.457
7. Rodrigues PM, Olaizola P, Paiva NA, et al. Pathogenesis of cholangiocarcinoma. *Annu Rev Pathol Mech Dis*. 2021;16(1):433–463. doi:10.1146/annurev-pathol-030220-020455
8. Rosen CB, Murad SD, Heimbach JK, Nyberg SL, Nagorney DM, Gores GJ. Neoadjuvant therapy and liver transplantation for hilar cholangiocarcinoma: is pretreatment pathological confirmation of diagnosis necessary? *J Am Coll Surg*. 2012;215(1):31–38. doi:10.1016/j.jamcollsurg.2012.03.014
9. Mavros MN, Economopoulos KP, Alexiou VG, Pawlik TM. Treatment and prognosis for patients with intrahepatic cholangiocarcinoma. *JAMA Surgery*. 2014;149(6):565. doi:10.1001/jamasurg.2013.5137
10. Shroff RT, Kennedy EB, Bachini M, et al. Adjuvant Therapy for Resected Biliary Tract Cancer: ASCO Clinical Practice Guideline. *J Clin Oncol*. 2019;37(12):1015–1027. doi:10.1200/jco.18.02178
11. Kiriyama M, Ebata T, Aoba T, et al. Prognostic impact of lymph node metastasis in distal cholangiocarcinoma. *Br J Surg*. 2015;102(4):399–406. doi:10.1002/bjs.9752
12. Bagante F, Tran T, Spolverato G, et al. Perihilar cholangiocarcinoma: number of nodes examined and optimal lymph node prognostic scheme. *J Am Coll Surg*. 2016;222(5):750–759.e2. doi:10.1016/j.jamcollsurg.2016.02.012
13. Jutric Z, Johnston WC, Hoen HM, et al. Impact of lymph node status in patients with intrahepatic cholangiocarcinoma treated by major hepatectomy: a review of the National Cancer Database. *HPB (Oxford)*. 2016;18(1):79–87. doi:10.1016/j.hpb.2015.07.006
14. Ellington TD, Momin B, Wilson RJ, Henley SJ, Wu M, Ryerson AB. Incidence and mortality of cancers of the biliary tract, gallbladder, and liver by sex, age, race/ethnicity, and stage at diagnosis: United States, 2013 to 2017. *Cancer Epidemiol Biomarkers Prev*. 2021;30(9):1607–1614. doi:10.1158/1055-9965.EPI-21-0265
15. Farley DR, Weaver AL, Nagorney DM. "Natural history" of unresected cholangiocarcinoma: patient outcome after noncurative intervention. *Mayo Clin Proc*. 1995;70(5):425–429. doi:10.4065/70.5.425
16. Dee EC, Freret ME, Horick N, et al. Patterns of failure and the need for biliary intervention in resected biliary tract cancers after chemoradiation. *Ann Surg Oncol*. 2020;27(13):5161–5172. doi:10.1245/s10434-020-08967-9
17. Amin MB, Edge SB, Greene FL, et al , eds. *AJCC Cancer Staging Manual*. 8th ed. Springer Publishing Company; 2017.
18. Spolverato G, Yakoob MY, Kim Y, et al. The impact of surgical margin status on long-term outcome after resection for intrahepatic cholangiocarcinoma. *Ann Surg Oncol*. 2015;22(12):4020–4028. doi:10.1245/s10434-015-4472-9
19. Nakeeb A, Pitt HA, Sohn TA, et al. Cholangiocarcinoma: a spectrum of intrahepatic, perihilar, and distal tumors. *Ann Surg*. 1996;224(4):463–475. doi:10.1097/00000658-199610000-00005
20. Groot Koerkamp B, Wiggers JK, Coelen RJ, et al. Recurrence rate and pattern of perihilar cholangiocarcinoma after curative intent resection. *HPB (Oxford)*. 2016;18:e868. doi:10.1016/j.hpb.2016.01.503
21. Loehrer AP, House MG, Nakeeb A, Kilbane ME, Pitt HA. Cholangiocarcinoma: are North American surgical outcomes optimal? *J Am Coll Surg*. 2013;216(2):192–200. doi:10.1016/j.jamcollsurg.2012.11.002
22. Oh DY, He AR, Qin S, et al. Durvalumab plus gemcitabine and cisplatin in advanced biliary tract cancer. *NEJM Evid*. 2022;1(8):EVIDoa2200015. doi:10.1056/EVIDoa2200015

23. Kelley RK, Ueno M, Yoo C, et al. Pembrolizumab in combination with gemcitabine and cisplatin compared with gemcitabine and cisplatin alone for patients with advanced biliary tract cancer (KEYNOTE-966): a randomized, double-blind, placebo-controlled, phase 3 trial. *Lancet.* 2023;401(10391):1853–1865. doi:10.1016/S0140-6736(23)00727-4

24. Valle J, Wasan H, Palmer DH, et al. Cisplatin plus gemcitabine versus gemcitabine for biliary tract cancer. *N Engl J Med.* 2010;362(14):1273–1281. doi:10.1056/NEJMoa0908721

25. Stein A, Arnold D, Bridgewater J, et al. Adjuvant chemotherapy with gemcitabine and cisplatin compared to observation after curative intent resection of cholangiocarcinoma and muscle invasive gallbladder carcinoma (ACTICCA-1 trial) - a randomized, multidisciplinary, multinational phase III trial. *BMC Cancer.* 2015;15:564. doi:10.1186/s12885-015-1498-0

26. Hong TS, Wo JY, Yeap BY, et al. Multi-institutional phase II study of high-dose hypofractionated proton beam therapy in patients with localized, unresectable hepatocellular carcinoma and intrahepatic cholangiocarcinoma. *J Clin Oncol.* 2016;34(5):460–468. doi:10.1200/JCO.2015.64.2710

27. Tao R, Krishnan S, Bhosale PR, et al. Ablative radiotherapy doses lead to a substantial prolongation of survival in patients with inoperable intrahepatic cholangiocarcinoma: a retrospective dose response analysis. *J Clin Oncol.* 2016;34(3):219–226. doi:10.1200/JCO.2015.61.3778

28. Lee J, Yoon WS, Koom WS, Rim CH. Efficacy of stereotactic body radiotherapy for unresectable or recurrent cholangiocarcinoma: a meta-analysis and systematic review. *Strahlenther Onkol.* 2018;195(2):93–102. doi:10.1007/s00066-018-1367-2

29. Rosen CB, Heimbach JK, Gores GJ. Liver transplantation for cholangiocarcinoma. *Transpl Int.* 2010;23(7):692–697. doi:10.1111/j.1432-2277.2010.01108.x

30. Broughman J, Sittenfeld S, Bauer-Nilsen K, Stephans K. Substituting stereotactic body radiation therapy boost for brachytherapy using Mayo protocol for peri-hilar cholangiocarcinoma. *Appl Radiat Oncol.* 2019:43–45. doi:10.37549/aro1205

31. Welling TH, Feng M, Wan S, et al. Neoadjuvant stereotactic body radiation therapy, capecitabine, and liver transplantation for unresectable hilar cholangiocarcinoma. *Liver Transpl.* 2014;20(1):81–88. doi:10.1002/lt.23757

32. Sandler KA, Veruttipong D, Agopian VG, et al. Stereotactic Body Radiotherapy (SBRT) for locally advanced extrahepatic and intrahepatic cholangiocarcinoma. *Adv Radiat Oncol.* 2016;1(4):237–243. doi:10.1016/j.adro.2016.10.008

33. Keltner SJ, Hallemeier C, Wang K, et al. Neoadjuvant therapy regimens for hilar cholangiocarcinoma before liver transplant. *Am J Clin Oncol.* 2023;46(6):276–278. doi:10.1097/COC.0000000000001002

34. Bridgewater J, Fletcher P, Palmer DH, et al. Long-term outcomes and exploratory analyses of the randomized phase III BILCAP study. *J Clin Oncol.* 2022;40(18):2048–2057. doi:10.1200/JCO.21.02568

35. Frakulli R, Buwenge M, Macchia G, et al. Stereotactic body radiation therapy in cholangiocarcinoma: a systematic review. *Br J Radiol.* 2019;92(1097):20180688. doi:10.1259/bjr.20180688

36. Iwatsuki S, Todo S, Marsh JW, et al. Treatment of hilar cholangiocarcinoma (Klatskin tumors) with hepatic resection or transplantation. *J Am Coll Surg.* 1998;187(4):358–364. doi:10.1016/s1072-7515(98)00207-5

37. Sudan D, DeRoover A, Chinnakotla S, et al. Radiochemotherapy and transplantation allow long-term survival for nonresectable hilar cholangiocarcinoma. *Am J Transplant.* 2002;2(8):774–779. doi:10.1034/j.1600-6143.2002.20812.x

38. Rea DJ, Heimbach JK, Rosen CB, et al. Liver transplantation with neoadjuvant chemoradiation is more effective than resection for hilar cholangiocarcinoma. *Ann Surg.* 2005;242(3):451–461. doi:10.1097/01.sla.0000179678.13285.fa

39. Ethun CG, Lopez-Aguiar AG, Anderson DJ, et al. Transplantation versus resection for hilar cholangiocarcinoma: an argument for shifting treatment paradigms for resectable disease. *Ann Surg.* 2018;267(5):797–805. doi:10.1097/SLA.0000000000002574

40. Goldaracena N, Gorgen A, Sapisochin G. Current status of liver transplantation for cholangiocarcinoma. *Liver Transpl.* 2018;24(2):294–303. doi:10.1002/lt.24955

41. Lunsford KE, Javle M, Heyne K, et al. Liver transplantation for locally advanced intrahepatic cholangiocarcinoma treated with neoadjuvant therapy: a prospective case-series. *Lancet Gastroenterol Hepatol.* 2018;3(5):337–348. doi:10.1016/S2468-1253(18)30045-1

PART VII: Genitourinary

40 LOW-RISK PROSTATE CANCER

Zachary S. Mayo, Timothy D. Smile, Omar Y. Mian, and Rahul D. Tendulkar

QUICK HIT Low-risk prostate cancer includes organ-confined disease typically detected by a screening PSA or DRE (T1–T2a), with a PSA <10 ng/mL and Gleason score (GS) ≤6. Standard treatment options include active surveillance, prostatectomy, EBRT, or brachytherapy (see Table 40.1). Prostate cancer-specific survival (PCSS) is >95% for each. Therefore, treatment selection is guided by side effect profiles and patient preference, with national guidelines recommending active surveillance for very-low and low-risk patients. Definitive treatment is offered only if life expectancy is >10 years. Dose-escalated RT improves biochemical control compared with "conventional" doses, and concurrent ADT is not indicated. The PROST-QA and ProtecT trials included patient-reported outcomes and are helpful to inform patient decisions.

Table 40.1 General Overview of Treatment Options for Low-Risk Prostate Cancer

Treatment Option	General Overview/ Example	Pros	Cons	Patient Selection
Watchful waiting (WW)	No further testing, treatment only when symptoms develop	Avoids overtreatment, reduces cost	Risk of disease progression	Patients with severe comorbidity and/or limited lifespan
Active surveillance (AS)	Regimented follow-up with PSA testing and repeat biopsies +/– MRI; consider genomic testing and MRI-guided biopsy	Avoids immediate side effects and cost of treatment; delays or eliminates need for definitive treatment	Patient anxiety; risk of disease progression; costs increase over time	Compliant patients with low-risk or favorable intermediate-risk disease motivated toward deferring treatment
Radical prostatectomy (RP)	Robotic, laparoscopic, or open, usually with pelvic LN dissection	Removes all tumor/prostate, relieves obstructive symptoms; obtains pathologic staging; avoids RT exposure	Operative risk; higher risk of ED and incontinence than nonoperative options	Younger, healthier patients motivated toward avoiding RT; concerns of urinary or bowel effects of RT; significant obstructive symptoms
IMRT (standard fractionation)	74–80 Gy over 7–9 weeks	RT regimen with long-term follow-up	Protracted course is inconvenient; potential late effects include cystitis, proctitis, ED, second malignancy	Patients motivated toward nonoperative intervention or specific concerns of ED or incontinence from RP
IMRT (moderate hypofractionation)	60–70 Gy over 4–5.5 weeks	Reduces treatment time, large randomized trials, reduced cost over conventional IMRT	Treatment time still moderately protracted; potential late effects include cystitis, proctitis, ED, second malignancy	

(continued)

Treatment Option	General Overview/ Example	Pros	Cons	Patient Selection
Table 40.1 General Overview of Treatment Options for Low-Risk Prostate Cancer (*continued*)				
SBRT (extreme hypofractionation)	35–40 Gy/5 fx QOD	Significantly reduces treatment time; late effects appear favorable compared with more protracted courses	Long-term follow-up data not available; potential late effects include cystitis, proctitis, ED, second malignancy	
Brachytherapy	LDR with I-125/P-103 OR HDR with Ir-192	Single-day procedure (LDR); long-term follow-up available	Pronounced acute LUTS; potential late effects include urinary retention, cystitis, ED, second malignancy	

EPIDEMIOLOGY: Estimated 299,010 new cases and ~35,250 deaths in 2024.[1] Prostate cancer is the most common noncutaneous malignancy in men in the United States (lifetime risk is approximately 1 in 7) and the second most common cause of cancer death in men (behind lung cancer). The median age of diagnosis is 67 years.[2] The incidence is highest in Scandinavia and lowest in Asia. In the United States, the incidence is higher in Black men compared with White men (1.7:1).[2]

RISK FACTORS: Age and family history are the strongest known factors.[3] Black men have had worse outcomes than White men, although the contribution of biological vs. nonbiological factors is unclear.[3–7] Mutations in genes responsible for DNA repair (e.g. germline BRCA2 mutation) may be associated with higher GS and worse prognosis.[8,9] Other general syndromes associated with increased risk of prostate cancer are Lynch syndrome, BRCA2, Fanconi anemia, and HOXB13.[10–12]

ANATOMY: The prostate is composed of two-thirds glandular elements and one-third fibromuscular stroma. The glandular part is divided into three zones: peripheral zone (comprises 70% of prostate volume, majority of prostate cancers arising from this zone), central zone (comprises 25% of prostate volume, 5% of prostate cancers arising from this zone), and transition zone (comprises 5% of the prostate volume, site of benign prostatic hyperplasia). The neurovascular bundles are located posterolaterally. The fibromuscular stroma (or anterior zone) extends superiorly from the smooth muscle of the bladder neck and inferiorly to the urethra, prostate apex, and external sphincter. The seminal vesicles (SVs) are coaxial with the gland and adjacent to the posterolateral aspect of the prostate, joining the vas deferens to the ejaculatory duct and entering the prostatic urethra at the verumontanum. The position of the prostate and SVs varies with filling of the rectum and bladder. Typical prostate variability is as follows (standard deviation): Ant-Post—2.4 mm, Inf-Sup—2.1 mm, and Med-Lat—0.4 mm; SV displacement: Ant-Post—3.5 mm, Inf-Sup—2.1 mm, and Med-Lat—0.8 mm.[13] Lymphatic drainage of the prostate includes internal iliac, external iliac, obturator, and presacral LNs, with occasional drainage directly to the common iliac nodes. The SVs typically drain to the external iliac nodes.

PATHOLOGY: Ninety-five percent of prostate cancers are adenocarcinomas. Other histologies such as small cell (neuroendocrine) carcinoma, ductal adenocarcinoma, transitional cell carcinoma, sarcomatoid carcinoma, and sarcoma are associated with a worse prognosis.[14–17] The Gleason score (GS) is based on the architectural structure of the malignant cells and is determined by summing the two most prevalent grades seen on biopsied tissue (primary grade + secondary grade). Tertiary grades are given only in RP specimens if there is a component (<5%) of higher grade tumor than the two predominant patterns.[18] Extracapsular extension (ECE) is seen in ~45% of patients with clinically localized disease and is within 2.5 mm in 96% of cases.[19] SV involvement increases with risk group: low-risk ~1%, intermediate risk ~15%, and high risk ~30%. The median length of involvement is 1 cm, with ~1% risk of SV involvement beyond 2 cm.[20] A grade grouping system was developed by the International Society of Urological Pathology (ISUP) based on GS, which demonstrated an increased risk of biochemical recurrence with increasing grade group (Table 40.2).[21]

Table 40.2 ISUP Consensus Grouping[21]		
Grade Group	**Gleason Score(s)**	**HR of Biochemical Recurrence**
1	≤6	Reference
2	3 + 4 = 7	1.9
3	4 + 3 = 7	5.4
4	8	8.0
5	9 or 10	11.7

Source: Data from Kestin L, Goldstein N, Vicini F, Yan D, Korman H, Martinez A. Treatment of prostate cancer with radiotherapy: should the entire seminal vesicles be included in the clinical target volume? *Int J Radiat Oncol Biol Phys.* 2002;54(3):686–697. doi:10.1016/S0360-3016(02)02968-3.

GENETICS: Several tissue-based tests have been developed to determine prognosis, including Oncotype DX Genomic Prostate Score (Genomic Health, Redwood City, California), which is a 17-gene expression panel that predicts the risk of recurrence, prostate cancer death, and aggressive features on pathology (GS ≥4 + 3 or pT3) after RP.[22] Decipher Prostate is a 22-gene genomic classifier (GC) derived from biopsy specimens and has been shown to correlate with risk of metastasis, PCSM, and OS.[23,24] A Decipher GC score ≥0.6 is associated with a shorter time on AS and shorter time to treatment failure for those undergoing radical therapy.[25] NCCN states that genomic biomarkers should be considered for low-risk, localized prostate cancer to guide decision-making for AS.[26] AUA/ASTRO 2022 guidelines state that tissue-based genomic biomarkers should not be routinely used for clinical decision-making.[27] Combining a GC test with clinical factors can accurately predict 10-year DM rates.[28]

SCREENING: The updated 2023 American Urological Association (AUA) guidelines recommend PSA screening every 2 to 4 years for men ages 50 to 69 (Grade A evidence). Baseline PSA screening should also be offered to men ages 45 to 50 (Grade B) as well as men ages 40 to 45 at increased risk (Grade B).[29] The 2018 USPSTF guidelines state that screening for men ages 55 to 69 is an individual one (Grade C) and recommend against screening for patients 70 years or older (Grade D).[30] SEER data suggest that the 2012 USPSTF recommendation against PSA screening for all men increased the incidence of metastatic prostate cancer.[31] Free PSA (ratio of free PSA/total PSA, with lower free PSA predicting higher risk of cancer) and PSA velocity (>0.75 ng/mL/yr) can increase the PPV of screening.[32] PSA velocity of >2 ng/mL in the year previous to diagnosis has been associated with increased risk of death due to prostate cancer.[33] The half-life of PSA is ~2.2 days. PSA levels can be increased by prostatitis, urinary retention, DRE, ejaculation, TRUS biopsy, TURP, and BPH. Medical treatment for BPH with 5α-reductase inhibitors such as finasteride decreases PSA by ~50% within 6 months of use, and thus correct PSA by multiplying by 2 in the first 2 years and by 2.3 for longer term use.[34,35] National screening guidelines do not recommend DRE alone for screening (poor PPV of 4%–11%).[36] Combined DRE and PSA screening is left to the discretion of physicians, and DRE is recommended in any patient with suspicious PSA.[37] DRE palpates only the posterior and lateral aspects of the prostate gland, which inherently limits its screening utility, but 85% of prostate cancers arise from these locations. DRE has a sensitivity of 53% and specificity of 86% in one study.[38] A multicenter screening study demonstrated that PSA detected significantly more prostate cancer than DRE (82% vs. 55%, $p = .001$).[39] Prostate cancer antigen 3 (PCA3) is an RNA biomarker overexpressed by malignant cells and can be found in urine after an "attentive" DRE with a "minimum of 6 pressed strokes on the prostate from lateral to medial." This test may be a useful surrogate to repeat biopsies in the detection of cancer with a high NPV (88%), but its use is not routine.[40] The 4K score is a blood test that measures prostate-specific kallikrein used to determine patient-specific probability of finding GS ≥7 on biopsy.[41] Serum levels are combined with an algorithm including patient age, presence of palpable nodule on DRE, and prior negative biopsy to give a percent risk score (1%–95%) of having aggressive cancer on biopsy.

CLINICAL PRESENTATION: Prostate cancer is usually asymptomatic, with the majority diagnosed by PSA or as an incidental finding on TURP. Suspicious DRE findings include areas of nodularity, asymmetry, or induration. Some patients with locally advanced disease may present with obstructive urinary symptoms, polyuria, and less frequently dysuria and hematuria. Unexplained bony pain may suggest metastatic disease, but this is rare in patients with otherwise low-risk prostate cancer.

WORKUP: H&P, including DRE and assessment of baseline urinary, bowel, and sexual function. The AUA score (a.k.a. International Prostate Symptom Score [IPSS]) can be used to assess urinary function (range 0–5 points for seven questions; total score 35, with higher score implying worse symptoms) based on incomplete emptying, frequency, intermittency, urgency, weak stream, straining, and nocturia. The Sexual Health Inventory for Men (SHIM) is commonly used to assess baseline erectile function (range 0/1–5 points for five questions; total score 25, with higher score signifying better erectile function).

Labs: PSA, preoperative workup if surgery is indicated.

Biopsy: TRUS-guided random biopsy involving removal of 8 to 12 cores of tissue is the most common approach for diagnosis. A systematic review suggested that MRI-targeted biopsy may detect clinically significant cancers with less core samples compared with conventional prostate biopsy techniques.[42] Many low-risk prostate cancers will not be identified on MRI.

Imaging: No role for routine staging scans in low-risk prostate cancer. Multiparametric MRI may be used in patients considering AS as it may detect lesions concerning for GS ≥7 cancer or ECE.

PROGNOSTIC FACTORS: Risk stratification of prostate cancer is based primarily on clinical staging by DRE, pretreatment PSA, GS/grade group on biopsy, and the number of biopsy cores involved with cancer. Several risk classifications exist, including the NCCN, D'Amico, and American Joint Committee on Cancer (AJCC) risk categories (Tables 40.3 and 40.4). Other prognostic factors also exist, including cancer volume (>4 cm^3 demonstrated shorter time to PSA failure),[43] PNI on biopsy (associated with higher rate of positive margin, but has not been shown to be an independent predictor of PSA recurrence),[44] and the presence of disseminated cancer cells (>5 disseminated cancer cells per 7.5 mL associated with shorter OS in three randomized trials).[45] The UCSF-CAPRA nomogram includes age (≥50 vs. <50 years), PSA, GS, clinical stage (T1/T2 vs. T3a), and percentage of biopsy core involved (<34% vs. ≥34%) to predict the likelihood of disease recurrence or progression.[46] Refer to the Genetics section for the prognostic role of genomic classifiers.

NATURAL HISTORY: In the modern era, the risk of death from early-stage, low-risk disease is 1% at 10 years and 3% at 15 years (per active monitoring arm of the ProtecT trial).[47] As per the Pound study of patients with biochemical failure (bF) after prostatectomy, metastases developed at a median of 8 years after bF and death occurred at a median of 5 years from the development of DM.[48]

STAGING

Table 40.3 AJCC 8th Edition (2017) Prostate Cancer Staging							
cT		pT		N		M	
T1	a. Incidental finding in ≤5% of tissue resected			N0	• No regional LNs	M1a	• Nonregional LNs
	b. Incidental finding in >5% of tissue resected						
	c. Identified by needle biopsy (e.g., PSA), but not palpable						
T2	a. Palpable ≤½ of one lobe or less	T2	• Organ confined disease	N1	• Metastasis in regional LNs	M1b	• Metastasis to bone
	b. Palpable >½ of one lobe, but not both lobes						
	c. Palpable both lobes						
T3	a. EPE	T3	a. EPE or microscopic bladder neck invasion			M1c	• Metastasis to other sites with or without bone disease
	b. SV invasion		b. SV invasion				
T4	Invasion[1]	T4	• Invasion[1]				

Notes: Invasion[1] = invasion into bladder, external sphincter, rectum, levator muscles, and pelvic wall.

(continued)

Table 40.3 AJCC 8th Edition (2017) Prostate Cancer Staging (*continued*)	
AJCC 8th Edition 2017, Prognostic Stage Groups	
I	cT1a–c, cT2a or pT2 + PSA <10 ng/mL + grade group 1
IIA	cT1a–c or cT2a + PSA ≥10 and <20 ng/mL + grade group 1 cT2b–c + PSA <20 ng/mL + grade group 1
IIB	T1–T2, PSA <20 ng/mL, grade group 2
IIC	T1–T2, PSA <20 ng/mL, grade group 3 T1–T2, PSA <20 ng/mL, grade group 4
IIIA	T1–T2, PSA ≥20, grade groups 1–4
IIIB	T3–T4, any PSA, grade groups 1–4
IIIC	Any T, any PSA, grade group 5
IVA	Any T, N1, any PSA, any grade group
IVB	Any T, M1, any PSA, any grade group

Source: Adapted from AJCC Cancer Staging Manual. 8th ed. Springer International Publishing; 2017.

Table 40.4 Other Risk Stratifications for Prostate Cancer		
NCCN Risk Classification[26]		**D'Amico Risk Categories**[49]
Very low risk	T1 GS ≤6 PSA <10 ng/mL <3 positive biopsy cores ≤50% cancer in any core PSA density <0.15 ng/mL/gram	**Low risk** T1–2a, and GS ≤6, and PSA <10 ng/mL
Low risk	T1–T2a, and GS ≤6/grade group 1, and PSA <10 ng/mL	
Favorable intermediate risk (FIR)	T2b–T2c, or GS 3 + 4 = 7/grade group 2, or PSA 10–20 ng/mL, and % of positive biopsy cores <50%	**Intermediate risk** T2b, or GS 7, or PSA 10–20 ng/mL
Unfavorable intermediate risk (UIR)	2 or 3 intermediate risk factors (above), and/or Grade group 3, and/or ≥50% cores positive	
High risk	T3a–cT4, or GS 8/grade group 4, or GS 9–10/grade group 5, or PSA >20 ng/mL	**High risk** ≥T2c, or GS 8–10, or PSA >20 ng/mL
Very high risk	At least 2 of the following: – cT3 or cT4 – Grade group 4 or 5 (GS 8–10) – PSA >40 ng/mL	

TREATMENT PARADIGM

AS and WW: AS involves regular monitoring of patients with PSA, DRE, and biopsy, and evidence of progression will prompt conversion to potentially curative treatment. This is different from WW in which monitoring continues, but treatment is typically initiated only when symptoms develop. NCCN recommends AS for very low-risk and low-risk disease (GS ≤6) with life expectancy >10 years.[26] Genomic profiling helps identify patients appropriate for AS. WW recommendations also vary and can be considered for patients with low-risk cancer and limited life expectancy (<10 years).[26,50]

Prevention: The role of 5α-reductase inhibitors in preventing cancer progression in the setting of AS is debatable among consensus guidelines, but the REDEEM trial revealed lower 3-year rates of prostate cancer progression with dutasteride compared with placebo (38% vs. 48%, $p = .009$).[51]

Neither dutasteride nor finasteride is currently approved by the FDA for the prevention of prostate cancer.

Surgery: RP approaches include retropubic or laparoscopic/robotic approach. Robotic surgery has been compared with open surgery in one single-institution RCT, which reported early outcomes at 6 and 12 weeks and demonstrated similar rates of positive surgical margins, postoperative complications, intraoperative adverse events, and similar patient-reported urinary and sexual function scores for both techniques.[52] A perineal approach omits lymphadenectomy and SV removal and has been shown to be associated with higher rates of bF, positive margins, capsular incisions, and rectal injury.[53] The positive margin rate for open, laparoscopic, and robotic techniques are estimated to be 23%, 15%, and 14%, respectively.[54] Perioperative complications are rare and include mortality (<1%), rectal injury (<1%), thromboembolism (1%–3%), myocardial infarction (1%–8%), wound infection (<1%), blood loss, and pelvic pain.[55,56] Impotence and incontinence are the most common postoperative adverse effects. Bilateral nerve-sparing procedure is associated with an estimated 50% rate of impotence, and unilateral nerve-sparing is associated with an impotence rate of ~75%. In one study, an estimated 32% of patients reported total urinary control, 40% occasional leakage, 7% frequent leakage, and 1% to 2% no urinary control.[57] A standard LN dissection involves sampling of the obturator and external iliac LN. It is uncertain whether an extended LN dissection improves outcomes.

Radiation

Indications: Definitive RT is an option for low-risk prostate cancer without contraindications such as prior pelvic RT or inflammatory bowel disease.

Dose: Dose escalation with conventional EBRT has been shown to improve biochemical outcomes in several randomized trials but without an improvement in OS. Dose and fractionation vary widely in practice. Common conventionally fractionated regimens include 78 Gy/39 fx or 79.2 Gy/44 fx. Moderately hypofractionated options such as 70 Gy/28 fx or 60 Gy/20 fx have been tested in large prospective trials. For SBRT, 36.25 to 40 Gy in 5 fx delivered QOD is a commonly utilized regimen. The phase III PACE-B prospective randomized trial showed similar rates of RTOG grade ≥2 GI and GU toxicity between SBRT and conventionally fractionated RT with similar rates of biochemical control.[58,59] Brachytherapy is frequently used for low-risk prostate cancer with comparable outcomes to surgery and EBRT, but no randomized trial has compared these modalities directly for assessment of clinical outcomes. Dose for LDR brachytherapy is 145 Gy for I-125 or 125 Gy for Pd-103. For low-risk and FIR prostate cancer, there is no role for combining EBRT with brachytherapy boost or with ADT; monotherapy is sufficient. Recent evidence suggests HDR brachytherapy monotherapy delivered in two fractions is well-tolerated with favorable 5-year outcomes and is superior to single-fraction HDR brachytherapy.[60] After RT, PSA surveillance should occur every 6 months. Per RTOG-ASTRO Phoenix Consensus, the definition of bF is a rise of 2 ng/mL above the posttreatment nadir PSA.[61] A PSA "bounce" phenomenon may occur in some patients, particularly after brachytherapy, and is not associated with worse outcomes.

Toxicity: Acute: fatigue, dysuria, urgency, frequency, retention, rectal urgency, diarrhea. Late: stricture, cystitis, proctitis, sexual dysfunction, second malignancy. QOL outcomes have been compared between these therapies, and each modality is associated with distinct patterns of change in terms of urinary, bowel, and sexual function (see the ProtecT and PROST-QA trials).

Procedure: See *Handbook of Treatment Planning in Radiation Oncology*, Chapter 8.[62]

Other: Other treatments such as high-frequency ultrasound (HIFU) and cryotherapy are emerging techniques but are not recommended as first-line options per NCCN guidelines.

EVIDENCE-BASED Q&A

SCREENING AND PREVENTION

What is the value of PSA screening? Why did the U.S. Preventive Services Task Force (USPSTF) previously recommend against PSA screening?

In 2012, the USPSTF recommended against PSA screening given the risk of harm from screening (i.e., false-positive test results leading to more testing and possible side effects) as well as the likelihood that the cancer itself would not have caused symptoms or death. Unfortunately, this led to a significant increase in the incidence of metastatic prostate cancer across races and age groups. The updated 2018 USPSTF guidelines recommended against routine PSA for men over 70 years old, but recommended screening for men ages 55 to 69 years be "an individual one."[30] The ERSPC, Swedish Trial, and CAP showed a PCSM benefit for PSA screening, while the PLCO did not. CAP evaluated a single invitation for PSA screening (with subsequent PSA screening if PSA ≥3) vs. no PSA screening and found a small but significant PCSM benefit at 15 years (0.69% vs. 0.78%, p = .03).[63] Notably, it is difficult to keep people in the "observation" arm from being screened, which is one of the criticisms of the PLCO trial.

Schröder, ERSPC (*NEJM* 2009, PMID 19297566; Update *Lancet* 2014, PMID 25108889; Update *Eur Urol* 2019, PMID 30824296): 162,388 men (55–69 years of age) randomized to PSA q4 years (on average) vs. no screening. PSA ≥3 ng/mL was an indication for biopsy in most centers; 1° endpoint PCM. Incidence of prostate cancer was 9.55/1,000 person-years for screening vs. 6.23/1,000 person-years for control group. At 13 years, 355 men in the screening group and 545 men in the control died of prostate cancer, yielding a PCM rate ratio of 0.79 (*p* = .001), corresponding to a number needed to screen (NNS) of 781 and a number needed to detect (NND) of 27 to prevent one death. At 16 years, the NNS was reduced to 570 and NND to 18. No difference in ACM. **Conclusion: Reduction in PCM was observed in the cohort randomized to PSA screening.** *Comment: Did not report treatment type, assumed arms were balanced, and overall rate of screening in the control group was not reported; there was variance among European centers for recruiting, use of DRE, TRUS, and screening intervals. There is increased survival and decreased progression but at a cost of overdetection and overtreatment.*

Hugosson, Swedish Trial (*Lancet Oncol* 2010, PMID 20598634; Update *J Urol* 2022, PMID 35422134): 20,000 men 50 to 64 years of age living in Göteborg, Sweden, randomly selected by computer to be screened by PSA every other year or not (no informed consent). PSA >3 ng/mL was an indication for DRE and biopsies; 1° endpoint was PCM. Seventy-eight percent reached max follow-up of 14 years, with 76% compliance with screening. Incidence and metastatic burden decreased by screening. Prostate cancer incidence of 13% in the screening group vs. 8% in the control group (HR 1.64, 95% CI 1.50–1.80). Rate ratio for PCM was 0.56 (95% CI 0.39–0.82) for screening vs. control group. Forty-six screened men vs. 87 controls were diagnosed with metastatic disease (*p* = .003). NNS = 293, NNT = 12 to prevent one prostate cancer death. Risk of prostate cancer was only 2.6% if the first PSA was <1. In the 22-year update, the rate ratio for PCM was 0.71 (95% CI 0.55–0.91). The NNS was 221 and NND was 9 to prevent one prostate cancer death. **Conclusion: PSA screening reduces the risk of death from prostate cancer.** *Comment: This is the "purest" trial because of the randomization and lack of informed consent with good follow-up, and it also had the lowest NNS.*

Andriole, PLCO Cancer Screening Trial (*NEJM* 2009, PMID 19297565; Update *J Natl Cancer Inst* 2012, PMID 22228146; Update Pinsky, *Cancer* 2017, PMID 27911486): 76,693 men 55 to 74 years of age randomized to annual screening with PSA + DRE vs. usual care. PSA >4 ng/mL or abnormal DRE was an indication for biopsy. Ninety-two percent of participants were followed to 10 years. Incidence of prostate cancer was 108 vs. 97 per 10,000 person-years for the screening arm vs. the control arm, which is a 12% relative increase in incidence rates (RR 1.12), but there was no statistical difference in PCM in the screening vs. the control arm (3.7 vs. 3.4 deaths per 10,000 person-years). The 15-year update again showed no benefit to screening on PCM with a rate ratio of 1.04 (95% CI 0.87–1.24). **Conclusion: No evidence of PCM benefit from annual screening.** *Comment: 45% of men had PSA in the 3 years preceding randomization, eliminating prostate cancer prior to randomization; 52% (86% at the update) of men in the control arm underwent PSA testing. Because of the crossover contamination and prescreening PSA, many feel these data are insufficient to conclude PSA screening is not useful.*

How does the incorporation of MRI-directed prostate biopsy compare to standard TRUS biopsy?

Eklund, STHLM3-MRI (*NEJM* 2021, PMID 34237810): Population-based, noninferiority trial of prostate cancer screening in 12,750 men aged 50 to 74. Those with PSA >3 were randomized in a 2:3 ratio to standard 12 core biopsy vs. MRI, with targeted and standard biopsy if the MRI suggested prostate cancer (PI-RADS score 3). 1,532 men with PSA >3. Seventy-three percent of men in the standard group underwent biopsy compared with 36% in the MRI group. In the intention-to-treat analysis, clinically significant prostate cancer (GS ≥7) was diagnosed in 21% of the experimental group vs. 18% of the standard biopsy group. MRI-guided biopsy resulted in fewer clinically insignificant (GS 6) prostate cancer (4% vs. 12%) and fewer benign biopsies (11% vs. 43%). **Conclusion: Among men with an indication for prostate biopsy (PSA >3), the use of MRI halved the number of men undergoing biopsy and was noninferior at diagnosing clinically significant prostate cancer when MRI-targeted and standard biopsies are performed.**

Klotz (*JAMA Oncol* 2021, PMID 33538782): Phase III RCT comparing MRI with targeted only biopsy vs. standard 12-core TRUS biopsy in the detection of clinically significant prostate cancer (at least GG2 histology). 453 patients. Clinically significant cancer was found in 35% in the MRI arm and 30% in the standard biopsy arm, demonstrating noninferiority. In the MRI arm, 37% of patients avoided biopsy and diagnosis of GG1 was reduced by 50%. **Conclusion: MRI-guided targeted biopsy is noninferior to standard TRUS biopsy in detecting clinically significant cancers.**

Can prostate cancer be prevented with 5α-reductase inhibitors (5-ARIs)?

Yes, although 5-ARIs primarily reduce the risk of low-grade cancer. The PCPT trial randomized ~19,000 men to finasteride vs. placebo and found that, compared with placebo, the finasteride group had a significant relative risk reduction in low-grade cancers (GS 2–6; RR 0.57, 95% CI 0.52–0.63), but an increased risk in high-grade cancers, with no difference in 15-year OS.[35,64] The REDUCE trial had similar findings when randomizing ~7,000 men to dutasteride vs. placebo. There was a reduction in GS 5–6 cancers in the dutasteride group (13% vs. 18%, p < .001), with an increase in GS 8–10 tumors in years 3 and 4. There was no difference in OS.[65] The increase in high GS tumors may be due to gland shrinkage and increased biopsy yield.

ACTIVE SURVEILLANCE

Compared with upfront local therapy, is AS an appropriate management strategy for low-risk prostate cancer? How do the outcomes of AS compare with RP or RT?

The 15-year follow-up data from both the phase III ProtecT trial and the single-arm prospective data by Klotz show excellent PCSS rates of >95%. Notably, two older surgical phase III RCTs (PIVOT and SPCG-4) comparing RP vs. WW/AS showed OS rates that are worse than those reported on ProtecT. The PIVOT trial reported no difference in cumulative incidence of death from prostate cancer (7% RP vs. 11% AS, p = .06) with an MFU of 12.7 years. However, the 22-year follow-up showed a small all-cause mortality benefit to RP (13.6 years mean survival vs. 12.6 years), although this benefit was lost when restricted to only low-risk patients.[66] The SPCG-4 trial demonstrated a reduction in cumulative incidence of death from prostate cancer at 18 years, with a rate of 18% for RP vs. 29% in the WW group. The 23-year update reported a mean of 2.9 extra life-years gained with surgery.[67]

Klotz (*JCO* 2010, PMID 19917860; Update *JCO* 2015, PMID 25512465): Single-arm cohort of 993 patients followed under AS. Between 1995 and 1999, this trial included all GS ≤6 and PSA ≤10 ng/mL. If >70 years of age, PSA ≤15 ng/mL or GS ≤3+4. Starting in 2000, inclusion was restricted to GS ≤6 and PSA ≤10 ng/mL or patients with FIR disease (PSA 10–20 ng/mL and/or GS 3+4) with significant comorbidities and life expectancy <10 years. The 10- and 15-year actuarial prostate cancer survival rates were 98% and 94%, respectively. Only 15 of 933 (1.5%) died of prostate cancer and 3% developed metastatic disease. The 10- and 15-year OS rates were 80% and 62%, respectively. At 5, 10, and 15 years, 76%, 64%, and 55% of patients remained untreated and on AS. Patients were 9.2× more likely to die of causes other than prostate cancer. **Conclusion: AS for low-risk and select FIR patients is safe.**

Hamdy, UK ProtecT (*NEJM* 2016, PMID 27626136; QOL Donovan, *NEJM* 2016, PMID 27626365; Update *Eur Urol* 2020, PMID 31771797; *NEJM* 2023, PMID 36912538): 1,643 patients aged 50 to 69 with localized prostate cancer randomized to "active monitoring" (AM, PSA monitoring only), surgery (RP), or RT with ADT. Median age was 62 years and median PSA was 4.6 ng/mL (range 3–19.9). Seventy-seven percent had GS 6 and 76% had T1c. Contemporary risk stratification reveals 24% had intermediate-risk disease and 10% had high-risk. AM group had PSA q3 months the first year and q6–12 months thereafter; increase in 50% PSA in the previous 12 months triggered a review to continue monitoring or pursue treatment. RT arm had ADT for 3 to 6 months before and concurrent with 3D-CRT to 74 Gy/37 fx. RP arm had postop PSA q3 months for the first year then q6–12 months. Primary outcome was death from prostate cancer. MFU 15 years, see Table 40.5 for results. PCSM for AM, RP, and RT groups was 3.1%, 2.2%, and 2.9%, respectively, without any significant difference among groups (*p* = .53). Metastases developed in 9.4%, 4.7%, and 5.0% in the AM, RP, and RT groups, respectively. Upfront treatment with RP or RT reduced the risk of distant disease by 0.47 and 0.48, respectively. In the AM arm (*n* = 545), 61% received a radical treatment at 15 years. RP NNT = 27 and RT NNT = 33 to avoid one patient having metastatic disease. NNT = 9 with either RP or RT to avoid one patient having clinical progression. **Conclusion: Irrespective of treatment arm, PCM remained low at <5% at 15 years. Rates of disease progression and metastatic disease were significantly lower for RP or RT compared with AM.**

Table 40.5 Results of ProtecT Randomized Trial						
	5-Yr PCSS	10-Yr PCSS	15-Yr PCSS	Clinical Progression Rate Per 1,000 Person-Years (Hazard Ratio)	Metastatic Disease Rate Per 1,000 Person-Years (HR)	All-Cause Deaths Per 1,000 Person-Years (HR)
Active monitoring	99%	98%	97%	21.4 (ref)	7.1 (ref)	16.2 (ref)
Surgery	100%	99%	97%	8 (0.36)	3.5 (0.47)	15 (0.89)
Radiation	100%	99%	98%	8.4 (0.35)	3.7 (0.48)	15 (0.88)
p value	.48	.48	.51			

How does the side effect profile compare between RP, EBRT, and brachytherapy?

Generally, RP has worse incontinence and impotence, EBRT has worse bowel/rectal irritation (without rectal spacer use), and brachytherapy has worse urinary irritation/obstruction. Placement of a rectal spacer can significantly reduce rectal dose and side effects from EBRT.[68]

Sanda, PROST-QA (NEJM 2008, PMID 18354103): First major prospective study (nonrandomized) to document patient- and partner-reported QOL outcomes. Prospective questionnaire of 1,201 patients and 625 spouses given pre- and post- (up to 24 months) definitive RP, brachytherapy, and EBRT for localized T1–T2 cancer. Patients who received EBRT had the greatest number of baseline comorbidities followed by brachytherapy and RP. RP was associated with worse sexual and urinary incontinence scores despite higher baseline function. Nerve-sparing surgical procedures had better recovery of sexual QOL. EBRT was associated with more irritative and obstructive side effects, as well as bowel toxicity. Large prostates had greater urinary irritation with brachytherapy and greater relief with RP. The use of ADT decreased vitality scores. On MVA, the most important factors associated with overall patient satisfaction were sexual function, vitality, and urinary function, in descending order. Patient-related factors that diminished health-related QOL included obesity, large prostate size, elevated initial PSA, older age, and African American race. **Conclusion: RP is associated with higher rates of urinary incontinence and sexual dysfunction, while RT is associated with increased bowel and bladder side effects.**

Donovan, ProtecT Trial QOL (NEJM 2016, PMID 27626365; Update NEJM Evid, PMID 38320051): Same trial as noted previously (Hamdy et al.). Patient-reported outcomes through questionnaires given before diagnosis, 6 and 12 months, then annually, and reported through 6 years. RP had the greatest negative effect on sexual function (erections firm enough for intercourse at 6 months: 52% AM, 22% RT, 12% surgery) and urinary incontinence. RT had a peak negative effect on sexual function at 6 months but recovered and stabilized (note: all patients received short-term ADT). RT had little effect on urinary continence, but urinary voiding and nocturia problems peaked at 6 months, then recovered by 12 months to be similar to other groups. RT had worse bowel function at 6 months compared with other arms but then recovered (except for frequency of bloody stools, which remained ~5%), while other groups had stable bowel function. Sexual function gradually declined in the AM group (erections firm enough for intercourse: 41% at year 3 and 30% at year 6), as well as urinary function. No differences in anxiety, depression, and general health-related or cancer-related QOL among groups. The 7- to 12-year update showed that urinary leakage requiring pads was worse in the RP group (18%–24% RP vs. 9%–11% AM vs. 3%–8% RT), erections sufficient for intercourse at 7 years was worse in the RP group (18% RP, 30% AM, 27% RT), nocturia was better in the RP group (34% RP vs. 47% AM vs. 48% RT), and fecal leakage was worse in the RT group (12% RT vs. 6% AM vs. 6% RP). **Conclusion: RP is associated with higher rates of urinary incontinence and sexual dysfunction but lower rates of urinary voiding/nocturia. In contrast, RT (in the pre-spacer era) can increase the risk of bloody stools and fecal leakage.**

Can a 5α-reductase inhibitor (dutasteride) or an androgen receptor inhibitor (enzalutamide) reduce the rates of progression for patients undergoing AS?

Yes. However, enzalutamide is technically an intervention with associated side effects.

Fleshner, REDEEM Trial (Lancet 2012, PMID 22277570): 302 men with Gleason 5 to 6 and PSA ≤11 placed on AS randomized to dutasteride 0.5 mg daily vs. placebo. Patients followed q3 months for 1 year, then q6 months with a PSA and DRE at each visit q18 months. All patients had repeat biopsy at 18 months and 3 years or if concerning PSA/DRE. Progression defined as ≥4 cores involved, ≥50% of one core, or Gleason pattern of 4. At 3 years, prostate cancer progression decreased from 48% to 38% with dutasteride (HR 0.62, 95% CI 0.43–0.89). **Conclusion: Dutasteride may be beneficial in reducing progression in AS patients.**

Shore, ENACT Trial (*JAMA Onc 2022, PMID 35980389*): Phase II clinical trial enrolling 277 men with low- to intermediate-risk localized prostate cancer diagnosed by screening who opted for AS randomized to AS + enzalutamide or AS alone. Enzalutamide reduced the risk of prostate cancer progression by 46% and increased the odds of a negative biopsy result by 3.5. The most common toxicities were fatigue (55%) and gynecomastia (37%). **Conclusion: Enzalutamide added to AS was well-tolerated and reduced the rates of disease progression.**

EXTERNAL BEAM RADIATION THERAPY

With conventional EBRT, does dose escalation improve outcomes?

There have been at least five major randomized trials investigating "dose escalation," with each one showing a biochemical control benefit (but no difference in OS) for higher doses compared with "conventional" lower doses (~70 Gy at 1.8–2.0 Gy/fx), but also higher rates of rectal bleeding. The current standard dose is 78 to 80 Gy with conventional fractionation (see Table 40.6).

Table 40.6 Summary of Phase III Dose Escalation Trials for Prostate Cancer

	Pasalic, MDACC[69]	Zietman, MGH[70]	Heemsbergen, Dutch[68]	Dearnaley, MRC[71]	Michalski, RTOG 0126[72]
Doses	70 vs. 78 Gy	70.2 vs. 79.2 Gy	68 vs. 78 Gy	64 vs. 74 Gy	70.2 vs. 79.2 Gy
N	301	393	669	843	1,499
Technique	Four-field box and 3D-CRT	Four-field box and proton boost	3D	3D	3D or IMRT
MFU (yrs)	14.3	8.9	9.1	10	8.4
Biochemical control	81% vs. 88%, $p = .042$	68% vs. 83%, $p < .0001$	49% vs. 43%, $p = .046$	43% vs. 55%, $p = .0003$	65% vs. 80%, $p < .001$

Is moderate hypofractionation safe and effective?

There have been several randomized trials examining moderate hypofractionation (2.4–4 Gy/fx to 60–70 Gy) compared with conventional fractionation (Table 40.7). The potential advantages include improved convenience for patients, lower cost, and potentially improved outcomes (due to hypothesized low α/β ratio). Follow-up is moderate, with MFU ranging from 5 to 10 years. Updated results of RTOG 0415 comparing conventionally fractionated vs. moderately hypofractionated RT in the management of low-risk prostate cancer demonstrated noninferiority of moderate hypofractionation. The 12-year DFS rate was 56% for conventional fractionation vs. 62% for moderate hypofractionation, and the 12-year biochemical recurrence rate was 17% vs. 10%, respectively, meeting protocol-specified noninferiority criteria. Late grade ≥3 GI and ≥3 GU toxicity were also noninferior, with rates <5% for both hypofractionated and conventional fractionation.[73] Moderate hypofractionation is endorsed across all risk groups by NCCN guidelines.

Table 40.7 Summary of Moderate Hypofractionation Trials in Prostate Cancer

Author, Institution	MFU	Eligibility	Hypofx Arm	Conventional Arm	Outcome
Hoffman, MDACC[74]	8.5 yrs	LR-IR	72 Gy at 2.4 Gy/fx	75.6 at 1.8 Gy/fx	8-yr bRFS 89% vs. 85%, 10-yr 89% vs. 76%, $p = .04$ favoring hypofx arm. No diff in OS or late GI or GU toxicity (but hypofx arm had nonsignificantly more rectal bleeding after treatment). Better control emerged after 5 yrs.

(continued)

Table 40.7 Summary of Moderate Hypofractionation Trials in Prostate Cancer (*continued*)

Author, Institution	MFU	Eligibility	Hypofx Arm	Conventional Arm	Outcome
Avkshtol, Fox Chase[75]	10.2 yrs	IR-HR	70.2 Gy at 2.7 Gy/fx	76 Gy at 2 Gy/fx	10-yr biochemical/clinical disease failure: 31% vs. 26% (*p* = NS). No diff in late toxicity (except those with poor urinary function IPSS >12 had higher toxicity in hypofx arm). No diff in bF, PCSM, or OS, but trend toward higher DM in hypofx arm.
Lee, RTOG 0415[73,76]	12.8 yrs	LR	70 Gy at 2.5 Gy/fx	73.8 at 1.8 Gy/fx	Noninferior 12-yr DFS (56% CF vs. 62% HF) and 12-yr BR (17% CF vs. 10% HF). Noninferior late grade ≥3 GI (3% CF vs. 4% HF) and ≥3 GU (3% CF vs. 4% HF). Publication at MFU 5.8 yrs showed more late grade 2 GI (18.3% vs. 11.4%, *p* = .002) and GU toxicity (26.2% vs. 20.5%, *p* = .06) with hypofx, but this was not clinically significant in patient-reported outcomes.
Dearnaley, CHHiP[77]	5.2 yrs	All (most IR)	60 or 57 Gy at 3 Gy/fx	74 at 2 Gy/fx	5-yr bRFS: 88% (74 Gy) vs. 91% (60 Gy) vs. 86% (57 Gy). 60 Gy not inferior to 74 Gy but noninferiority could NOT be claimed for 57 Gy vs. 74 Gy. No diff in GI/GU toxicity between arms.

HR, high risk; IR, intermediate risk; LR, low risk.

Is extreme hypofractionation (>4–10 Gy/fx) delivered with SBRT safe and effective?

The Prostate Advances in Comparative Evidence (PACE) has conducted a set of three large randomized trials that demonstrate the safety and efficacy of SBRT in the management of prostate cancer. In each of these trials, SBRT is delivered to a dose of 36.25 Gy in five fractions. PACE-A is an international phase III trial comparing SBRT with RP in patients with localized prostate cancer. The 2-year toxicity results showed lower use of urinary pads (7% vs. 50%, p < .001) and improved sexual subdomain scores for SBRT compared with RP. More SBRT patients did report a reduction from baseline in bowel domain scores at 24 months compared with those with RP (45% vs. 14%, p < .001).[78] PACE-B (discussed below) randomized patients with low- and intermediate-risk prostate cancer to conventional/hypofractionated RT vs. SBRT and demonstrated favorable results.[58] PACE-C (completed accrual, pending results) randomized patients with intermediate- and high-risk disease who are receiving hormone therapy to conventional RT vs. SBRT.

Tree, PACE-B Trial (*Lancet Onc* 2019, PMID 31540791; *Lancet Onc* 2022, PMID 36113498; Update NEJM 2024, PMID 39413377): Phase III RCT conducted in the UK, Ireland, and Canada randomizing 874 men with low- (9%) to intermediate-risk (91%) prostate cancer to either conventionally fx/moderately hypofx EBRT (78 Gy in 39 fx or 62 Gy in 20 fx) or SBRT (36.25 Gy in 5 fx). Per 2019 *Lancet* paper, SBRT and EBRT demonstrated similar rates of acute grade ≥2 GI toxicity (10% and 12%, respectively) and acute grade ≥2 GU toxicity (23% and 27%, respectively), neither of which was significant. Per the 2022 update, there was no difference in the co-primary endpoints of grade ≥2 GI (3% EBRT vs. 2% SBRT) or GU toxicity (2% EBRT vs. 3% SBRT) at 24 months. With an MFU of 74 months, SBRT was noninferior in terms of incidence of freedom from biochemical or clinical failure (96% EBRT vs. 95% SBRT, *p* = .004 for noninferiority). The 5-year RTOG ≥2 GU toxicity was seen in 7% SBRT vs. 5% of EBRT (*p* = .14), but cumulative incidence of RTOG ≥2 GU toxicity was higher in the SBRT arm (27% vs. 18%, *p* < .001). RTOG ≥2 GI toxicity was <1% for both arms, and cumulative incidence was not significantly different between the two arms (11% vs. 10%, *p* = .94). **Conclusion: Prostate SBRT has a safe toxicity profile and is noninferior to conventionally fractionated RT in terms of biochemical failure.**

Widmark, HYPO-RT-PC (*Lancet* 2019, PMID 31227373): PRT of 1,180 men undergoing RT for intermediate- (89%) or high-risk (11%) prostate cancer randomized to conventional fractionation (78 Gy/39 fx) vs. ultra-hypofractionation (42.7 Gy/7 fx QOD). No ADT was allowed, and the primary endpoint was time to biochemical or clinical failure. MFU 5 years. The estimated failure-free survival was 84% in both arms, with adjusted HR of 1.002 ($p = .99$). There was a trend toward higher incidence of >G2 acute urinary toxicity in ultra-hypofractionation arm (28% vs. 23%, $p = .057$), and urinary toxicity was higher in ultra-hypofractionation arm at 1 year (6% vs. 2%, $p = .0037$). **Conclusion: Ultra-hypofractionation is noninferior to conventionally fractionated RT with regard to failure-free survival, although acute toxicity is slightly more pronounced.**

Jackson, Meta-Analysis (*IJROBP* 2020, PMID 30959121): Meta-analysis of 6,116 men receiving prostate SBRT in 38 prospective trials, of which 92% included low-risk, 78% included intermediate-risk, and 38% included high-risk patients. MFU 39 months. Overall, 5- and 7-year bRFS rates were 95% and 94%, respectively. Late grade ≥3 GU and GI toxicities were 2% and 1%, respectively. Increased SBRT dose was associated with improved biochemical control ($p = .018$) but worse late grade ≥3 GU toxicity ($p = .014$). **Conclusion: Prostate SBRT achieves favorable biochemical control and toxicity outcomes.**

Does the fractionation schedule of SBRT affect toxicity outcomes?

The early experience from Stanford found that QOD treatment resulted in less toxicity than once-daily SBRT (nonrandomized), and so most have adopted a QOD schedule.[79] The prospective PATRIOT trial reported decreased patient-reported acute bowel QOL decrement with once-weekly compared with QOD fractionation in men receiving 40 Gy/5 fx.[80] Long-term follow-up, however, revealed similarly low rates of late GI and GU toxicity with either fractionation regimen.[81]

Does placement of SpaceOAR hydrogel improve rectal toxicity in patients undergoing SBRT?

SpaceOAR hydrogel placement was prospectively evaluated in 2:1 randomization with no hydrogel in patients undergoing standard dose-escalated RT with 79.2 Gy/44 fx. The 2-year grade >2 rectal toxicity rate was 0% in the SpaceOAR arm vs. 5.7% in the control arm. Urinary and bowel quality of life scores were significantly higher in the SpaceOAR arm.[82,83]

Is daily image guidance necessary?

There have been many data reporting inter- and intra-fraction prostate motion signifying the importance of image guidance during treatment.

De Crevoisier (*IJROBP* 2018, PMID 30071296): PRT of daily vs. weekly (days 1, 2, and 3, then weekly) IGRT in N0 localized prostate cancer, treating prostate only with IMRT (mean dose 78 Gy). 470 men enrolled; primary endpoint 5-year RFS, secondary outcomes OS and toxicity. No difference in RFS. OS worse in the daily IGRT group compared with weekly group ($p = .042$), with more secondary cancer events (11 vs. 24). Acute rectal bleeding and late rectal toxicity lower in daily IGRT group (6% vs. 11%, $p = .014$). Biochemical progression-free interval and clinical progression-free interval both improved with daily IGRT; risk of biochemical and clinical recurrence reduced by a factor of 2 with daily IGRT. **Conclusion: Daily IGRT improves biochemical control and reduces toxicity compared with weekly IGRT, with potential increase in second malignancies, although too few events to conclude.**

REFERENCES

1. Siegel RL, Giaquinto AN, Jemal A. Cancer statistics, 2024. *CA Cancer J Clin.* 2024;74(1):12–49. doi:10.3322/caac.21820
2. National Cancer Institute Surveillance, Epidemiology, and End Results Program. *Cancer Stat Facts: Prostate Cancer.* Accessed May 15, 2024. https://seer.cancer.gov/statfacts/html/prost.html
3. Hoffman RM, Gilliland FD, Eley JW, et al. Racial and ethnic differences in advanced-stage prostate cancer: the Prostate Cancer Outcomes Study. *J Natl Cancer Inst.* 2001;93(5):388–395. doi:10.1093/jnci/93.5.388
4. Deka R, Courtney PT, Parsons JK, et al. Association between African American race and clinical outcomes in men treated for low-risk prostate cancer with active surveillance. *JAMA.* 2020;324(17):1747–1754. doi:10.1001/jama.2020.17020

5.   Butler S, Muralidhar V, Chavez J, et al. Active surveillance for low-risk prostate cancer in Black patients. *N Engl J Med*. 2019;380(21):2070–2072. doi:10.1056/NEJMc1900333

6.   Dess RT, Hartman HE, Mahal BA, et al. Association of Black race with prostate cancer-specific and other-cause mortality. *JAMA Oncol*. 2019;5(7):975–983. doi:10.1001/jamaoncol.2019.0826

7.   Hamilton RJ, Aronson WJ, Presti JC Jr, et al. Race, biochemical disease recurrence, and prostate-specific antigen doubling time after radical prostatectomy: results from the SEARCH database. *Cancer*. 2007;110(10): 2202–2209. doi:10.1002/cncr.23012

8.   Agalliu I, Gern R, Leanza S, Burk RD. Associations of high-grade prostate cancer with BRCA1 and BRCA2 founder mutations. *Clin Cancer Res*. 2009;15(3):1112–1120. doi:10.1158/1078-0432.CCR-08-1822

9.   Castro E, Goh C, Olmos D, et al. Germline BRCA mutations are associated with higher risk of nodal involvement, distant metastasis, and poor survival outcomes in prostate cancer. *J Clin Oncol*. 2013;31(14):1748–1757. doi:10.1200/JCO.2012.43.1882

10. Raymond VM, Mukherjee B, Wang F, et al. Elevated risk of prostate cancer among men with Lynch syndrome. *J Clin Oncol*. 2013;31(14):1713–1718. doi:10.1200/JCO.2012.44.1238

11. Tischkowitz M, Easton DF, Ball J, Hodgson SV, Mathew CG. Cancer incidence in relatives of British Fanconi anemia patients. *BMC Cancer*. 2008;8:257. doi:10.1186/1471-2407-8-257

12. Ewing CM, Ray AM, Lange EM, et al. Germline mutations in HOXB13 and prostate-cancer risk. *N Engl J Med*. 2012;366(2):141–149. doi:10.1056/NEJMoa1110000

13. Deurloo KE, Steenbakkers RJ, Zijp LJ, et al. Quantification of shape variation of prostate and seminal vesicles during external beam radiotherapy. *Int J Radiat Oncol Biol Phys*. 2005;61(1):228–238. doi:10.1016/j.ijrobp.2004.09.023

14. Epstein JI, Egevad L, Amin MB, et al. The 2014 International Society of Urological Pathology (ISUP) consensus conference on gleason grading of prostatic carcinoma: definition of grading patterns and proposal for a new grading system. *Am J Surg Pathol*. 2016;40(2):244–252. doi:10.1097/PAS.0000000000000530

15. Tetu B, Ro JY, Ayala AG, Johnson DE, Logothetis CJ, Ordonez NG. Small cell carcinoma of the prostate. Part I. A clinicopathologic study of 20 cases. *Cancer*. 1987;59(10):1803–1809. doi:10.1002/1097-0142 (19870515)59:10<1803::AID-CNCR2820591018>3.0.CO;2-7

16. Robinson B, Magi-Galluzzi C, Zhou M. Intraductal carcinoma of the prostate. *Arch Pathol Lab Med*. 2012;136(4):418–425. doi:10.5858/arpa.2011-0519-RA

17. Palou J, Wood D, Bochner BH, et al. ICUD-EAU International Consultation on Bladder Cancer 2012: urothelial carcinoma of the prostate. *Eur Urol*. 2013;63(1):81–87. doi:10.1016/j.eururo.2012.08.011

18. Markowski MC, Eisenberger MA, Zahurak M, Epstein JI, Paller CJ. Sarcomatoid carcinoma of the prostate: retrospective review of a case series from the Johns Hopkins Hospital. *Urology*. 2015;86(3):539–543. doi:10.1016/j.urology.2015.06.011

19. Gordetsky J, Epstein J. Grading of prostatic adenocarcinoma: current state and prognostic implications. *Diagn Pathol*. 2016;11:25. doi:10.1186/s13000-016-0478-2

20. Davis BJ, Pisansky TM, Wilson TM, et al. The radial distance of extraprostatic extension of prostate carcinoma: implications for prostate brachytherapy. *Cancer*. 1999;85(12):2630–2637. doi:10.1002/(SICI)1097 -0142(19990615)85:12<2630::AID-CNCR20>3.0.CO;2-9

21. Kestin L, Goldstein N, Vicini F, Yan D, Korman H, Martinez A. Treatment of prostate cancer with radiotherapy: should the entire seminal vesicles be included in the clinical target volume? *Int J Radiat Oncol Biol Phys*. 2002;54(3):686–697. doi:10.1016/S0360-3016(02)02968-3

22. Cullen J, Rosner IL, Brand TC, et al. A biopsy-based 17-gene genomic prostate score predicts recurrence after radical prostatectomy and adverse surgical pathology in a racially diverse population of men with clinically low- and intermediate-risk prostate cancer. *Eur Urol*. 2015;68(1):123–131. doi:10.1016/j.eururo .2014.11.030

23. Nguyen PL, Haddad Z, Ross AE, et al. Ability of a genomic classifier to predict metastasis and prostate cancer-specific mortality after radiation or surgery based on needle biopsy specimens. *Eur Urol*. 2017;72(5): 845–852. doi:10.1016/j.eururo.2017.05.009

24. Nguyen PL, Huang HR, Spratt DE, et al. Analysis of a biopsy-based genomic classifier in high-risk prostate cancer: meta-analysis of the NRG Oncology/Radiation Therapy Oncology Group 9202, 9413, and 9902 phase 3 randomized trials. *Int J Radiat Oncol Biol Phys*. 2023;116(3):521–529. doi:10.1016/j.ijrobp.2022.12.035

25. Vince RA Jr, Jiang R, Qi J, et al. Impact of Decipher biopsy testing on clinical outcomes in localized prostate cancer in a prospective statewide collaborative. *Prostate Cancer Prostatic Dis*. 2022;25(4):677–683. doi:10 .1038/s41391-021-00428-y

26. National Comprehensive Cancer Network. *NCCN Clinical Practice Guidelines in Oncology: Prostate Cancer* (Version 3.2024). Accessed May 15, 2024. https://www.nccn.org/professionals/physician_gls/pdf/ prostate_blocks.pdf

27. Eastham JA, Auffenberg GB, Barocas DA, et al. Clinically localized prostate cancer: AUA/ASTRO Guideline, Part II: principles of active surveillance, principles of surgery, and follow-up. *J Urol*. 2022;208(1):19–25. doi:10.1097/JU.0000000000002758

28. Spratt DE, Zhang J, Santiago-Jiménez M, et al. Development and validation of a novel integrated clinical-genomic risk group classification for localized prostate cancer. *J Clin Oncol.* 2018;36(6):581–590. doi:10.1200/JCO.2017.74.2940

29. Wei JT, Barocas D, Carlsson S, et al. Early detection of prostate cancer: AUA/SUO Guideline Part I: prostate cancer screening. *J Urol.* 2023;210(1):46–53. doi:10.1097/JU.0000000000003491

30. US Preventive Services Task Force, Grossman DC, Curry SJ, et al. Screening for prostate cancer: US Preventive Services Task Force recommendation statement. *JAMA.* 2018;319(18):1901–1913. doi:10.1001/jama.2018.3710

31. Desai MM, Cacciamani GE, Gill K, et al. Trends in incidence of metastatic prostate cancer in the US. *JAMA Netw Open.* 2022;5(3):e222246. doi:10.1001/jamanetworkopen.2022.2246

32. Catalona WJ, Partin AW, Slawin KM, et al. Use of the percentage of free prostate-specific antigen to enhance differentiation of prostate cancer from benign prostatic disease: a prospective multicenter clinical trial. *JAMA.* 1998;279(19):1542–1547. doi:10.1001/jama.279.19.1542

33. D'Amico AV, Chen MH, Roehl KA, Catalona WJ. Preoperative PSA velocity and the risk of death from prostate cancer after radical prostatectomy. *N Engl J Med.* 2004;351(2):125–135. doi:10.1056/NEJMoa032975

34. Guess HA, Heyse JF, Gormley GJ. The effect of finasteride on prostate-specific antigen in men with benign prostatic hyperplasia. *Prostate.* 1993;22(1):31–37. doi:10.1002/pros.2990220106

35. Thompson IM, Goodman PJ, Tangen CM, et al. The influence of finasteride on the development of prostate cancer. *N Engl J Med.* 2003;349(3):215–224. doi:10.1056/NEJMoa030660

36. Schroder FH, van der Maas P, Beemsterboer P, et al. Evaluation of the digital rectal examination as a screening test for prostate cancer. Rotterdam section of the European Randomized Study of Screening for Prostate Cancer. *J Natl Cancer Inst.* 1998;90(23):1817–1823. doi:10.1093/jnci/90.23.1817

37. Gershman B, Van Houten HK, Herrin J, et al. Impact of Prostate-Specific Antigen (PSA) screening trials and revised PSA screening guidelines on rates of prostate biopsy and postbiopsy complications. *Eur Urol.* 2016;70(1):85–93. doi:10.1016/j.eururo.2016.03.015

38. Mistry K, Cable G. Meta-analysis of prostate-specific antigen and digital rectal examination as screening tests for prostate carcinoma. *J Am Board Fam Pract.* 2003;16(2):95–101. doi:10.3122/jabfm.16.2.95

39. Catalona WJ, Richie JP, Ahmann FR, et al. Comparison of digital rectal examination and serum prostate specific antigen in the early detection of prostate cancer: results of a multicenter clinical trial of 6,630 men. *J Urol.* 1994;151(5):1283–1290. doi:10.1016/S0022-5347(17)35233-3

40. Wei JT, Feng Z, Partin AW, et al. Can urinary PCA3 supplement PSA in the early detection of prostate cancer? *J Clin Oncol.* 2014;32(36):4066–4072. doi:10.1200/JCO.2013.52.8505

41. Parekh DJ, Punnen S, Sjoberg DD, et al. A multi-institutional prospective trial in the USA confirms that the 4Kscore accurately identifies men with high-grade prostate cancer. *Eur Urol.* 2015;68(3):464–470. doi:10.1016/j.eururo.2014.10.021

42. Moore CM, Robertson NL, Arsanious N, et al. Image-guided prostate biopsy using magnetic resonance imaging-derived targets: a systematic review. *Eur Urol.* 2013;63(1):125–140. doi:10.1016/j.eururo.2012.06.004

43. D'Amico AV, Whittington R, Malkowicz SB, et al. Calculated prostate cancer volume greater than 4.0 cm3 identifies patients with localized prostate cancer who have a poor prognosis following radical prostatectomy or external-beam radiation therapy. *J Clin Oncol.* 1998;16(9):3094–3100. doi:10.1200/JCO.1998.16.9.3094

44. D'Amico AV, Wu Y, Chen MH, Nash M, Renshaw AA, Richie JP. Perineural invasion as a predictor of biochemical outcome following radical prostatectomy for select men with clinically localized prostate cancer. *J Urol.* 2001;165(1):126–129. doi:10.1097/00005392-200101000-00031

45. Goldkorn A, Ely B, Quinn DI, et al. Circulating tumor cell counts are prognostic of overall survival in SWOG S0421: a phase III trial of docetaxel with or without atrasentan for metastatic castration-resistant prostate cancer. *J Clin Oncol.* 2014;32(11):1136–1142. doi:10.1200/JCO.2013.51.7417

46. Punnen S, Freedland SJ, Presti JC Jr, et al. Multi-institutional validation of the CAPRA-S score to predict disease recurrence and mortality after radical prostatectomy. *Eur Urol.* 2014;65(6):1171–1177. doi:10.1016/j.eururo.2013.03.058

47. Hamdy FC, Donovan JL, Lane JA, et al. Fifteen-year outcomes after monitoring, surgery, or radiotherapy for prostate cancer. *N Engl J Med.* 2023;388(17):1547–1558. doi:10.1056/NEJMoa2214122

48. Pound CR, Partin AW, Eisenberger MA, Chan DW, Pearson JD, Walsh PC. Natural history of progression after PSA elevation following radical prostatectomy. *JAMA.* 1999;281(17):1591–1597. doi:10.1001/jama.281.17.1591

49. D'Amico AV, Whittington R, Malkowicz SB, et al. Biochemical outcome after radical prostatectomy, external beam radiation therapy, or interstitial radiation therapy for clinically localized prostate cancer. *JAMA.* 1998;280(11):969–974. doi:10.1001/jama.280.11.969

50. Chen RC, Rumble RB, Loblaw DA, et al. Active surveillance for the management of localized prostate cancer (Cancer Care Ontario Guideline): American Society of Clinical Oncology Clinical Practice Guideline Endorsement. *J Clin Oncol.* 2016;34(18):2182–2190. doi:10.1200/JCO.2015.65.7759

51. Fleshner NE, Lucia MS, Egerdie B, et al. Dutasteride in localized prostate cancer management: the REDEEM randomized, double-blind, placebo-controlled trial. *Lancet.* 2012;379(9821):1103–1111. doi:10.1016/S0140 -6736(11)61619-X

52. Yaxley JW, Coughlin GD, Chambers SK, et al. Robot-assisted laparoscopic prostatectomy versus open radical retropubic prostatectomy: early outcomes from a randomized controlled phase 3 study. *Lancet.* 2016;388(10049):1057–1066. doi:10.1016/S0140-6736(16)30592-X

53. Boccon-Gibod L, Ravery V, Vordos D, Toublanc M, Delmas V, Boccon-Gibod L. Radical prostatectomy for prostate cancer: the perineal approach increases the risk of surgically induced positive margins and capsular incisions. *J Urol.* 1998;160(4):1383–1385. doi:10.1016/S0022-5347(01)62543-0

54. Sooriakumaran P, Srivastava A, Shariat SF, et al. A multinational, multi-institutional study comparing positive surgical margin rates among 22,393 open, laparoscopic, and robot-assisted radical prostatectomy patients. *Eur Urol.* 2014;66(3):450–456. doi:10.1016/j.eururo.2013.11.018

55. Alibhai SM, Leach M, Tomlinson G, et al. 30-day mortality and major complications after radical prostatectomy: influence of age and comorbidity. *J Natl Cancer Inst.* 2005;97(20):1525–1532. doi:10.1093/jnci/dji313

56. Van Hemelrijck M, Garmo H, Holmberg L, et al. Thromboembolic events following surgery for prostate cancer. *Eur Urol.* 2013;63(2):354–363. doi:10.1016/j.eururo.2012.09.041

57. Stanford JL, Feng Z, Hamilton AS, et al. Urinary and sexual function after radical prostatectomy for clinically localized prostate cancer: the Prostate Cancer Outcomes Study. *JAMA.* 2000;283(3):354–360. doi:10.1001/jama.283.3.354

58. Tree AC, Ostler P, van der Voet H, et al. Intensity-modulated radiotherapy versus stereotactic body radiotherapy for prostate cancer (PACE-B): 2-year toxicity results from an open-label, randomized, phase 3, non-inferiority trial. *Lancet Oncol.* 2022;23(10):1308–1320. doi:10.1016/S1470-2045(22)00517-4

59. van As N, Griffin C, Tree A, et al. Phase 3 trial of stereotactic body radiotherapy in localized prostate cancer. *N Engl J Med.* 2024;391(15):1413–1425. doi:10.1056/NEJMoa2403365

60. Morton G, McGuffin M, Chung HT, et al. Prostate high dose-rate brachytherapy as monotherapy for low and intermediate risk prostate cancer: efficacy results from a randomized phase II clinical trial of one fraction of 19 Gy or two fractions of 13.5 Gy. *Radiother Oncol.* 2020;146:90–96. doi:10.1016/j.radonc.2020.02.009

61. Roach M 3rd, Hanks G, Thames H Jr, et al. Defining biochemical failure following radiotherapy with or without hormonal therapy in men with clinically localized prostate cancer: recommendations of the RTOG-ASTRO Phoenix Consensus Conference. *Int J Radiat Oncol Biol Phys.* 2006;65(4):965–974. doi:10.1016/j .ijrobp.2006.04.029

62. Videtic GMM, Woody N, Vassil AD. *Handbook of Treatment Planning in Radiation Oncology.* 2nd ed. Demos Medical; 2015.

63. Martin RM, Turner EL, Young GJ, et al. Prostate-specific antigen screening and 15-year prostate cancer mortality: a secondary analysis of the CAP randomized clinical trial. *JAMA.* 2024;331(17):1460–1470. doi:10.1001/jama.2024.4011

64. Thompson IM Jr, Goodman PJ, Tangen CM, et al. Long-term survival of participants in the prostate cancer prevention trial. *N Engl J Med.* 2013;369(7):603–610. doi:10.1056/NEJMoa1215932

65. Andriole GL, Bostwick DG, Brawley OW, et al. Effect of dutasteride on the risk of prostate cancer. *N Engl J Med.* 2010;362(13):1192–1202. doi:10.1056/NEJMoa0908127

66. Wilt TJ, Vo TN, Langsetmo L, et al. Radical prostatectomy or observation for clinically localized prostate cancer: extended follow-up of the Prostate Cancer Intervention Versus Observation Trial (PIVOT). *Eur Urol.* 2020;77(6):713–724. doi:10.1016/j.eururo.2020.02.009

67. Bill-Axelson A, Holmberg L, Garmo H, et al. Radical prostatectomy or watchful waiting in prostate cancer - 29-year follow-up. *N Engl J Med.* 2018;379(24):2319–2329. doi:10.1056/NEJMoa1807801

68. Heemsbergen WD, Al-Mamgani A, Slot A, Dielwart MF, Lebesque JV. Long-term results of the Dutch randomized prostate cancer trial: impact of dose-escalation on local, biochemical, clinical failure, and survival. *Radiother Oncol.* 2014;110(1):104–109. doi:10.1016/j.radonc.2013.09.026

69. Pasalic D, Kuban DA, Allen PK, et al. Dose escalation for prostate adenocarcinoma: a long-term update on the outcomes of a phase 3, single institution randomized clinical trial. *Int J Radiat Oncol Biol Phys.* 2019;104(4):790–797. doi:10.1016/j.ijrobp.2019.02.045

70. Zietman AL, Bae K, Slater JD, et al. Randomized trial comparing conventional-dose with high-dose conformal radiation therapy in early-stage adenocarcinoma of the prostate: long-term results from Proton Radiation Oncology Group/American College of Radiology 95-09. *J Clin Oncol.* 2010;28(7):1106–1111. doi:10.1200/JCO.2009.25.8475

71. Dearnaley DP, Jovic G, Syndikus I, et al. Escalated-dose versus control-dose conformal radiotherapy for prostate cancer: long-term results from the MRC RT01 randomized controlled trial. *Lancet Oncol.* 2014;15(4):464–473. doi:10.1016/S1470-2045(14)70040-3

72. Michalski JM, Moughan J, Purdy J, et al. Effect of standard vs dose-escalated radiation therapy for patients with intermediate-risk prostate cancer: the NRG Oncology RTOG 0126 randomized clinical trial. *JAMA Oncol.* 2018;4(6):e180039. doi:10.1001/jamaoncol.2018.0039

73. Lee WR, Dignam JJ, Amin MB, et al. Long-term analysis of NRG Oncology RTOG 0415: a randomized phase III noninferiority study comparing two fractionation schedules in patients with low-risk prostate cancer. *J Clin Oncol.* 2024;42(16):1875–1883. doi:10.1200/JCO.23.02445

74. Hoffman KE, Voong KR, Levy LB, et al. Randomized trial of hypofractionated, dose-escalated, Intensity-Modulated Radiation Therapy (IMRT) versus conventionally fractionated IMRT for localized prostate cancer. *J Clin Oncol.* 2018;36(17):1681–1689. doi:10.1200/JCO.2018.77.9868

75. Avkshtol V, Ruth KJ, Ross EA, et al. Ten-year update of a randomized, prospective trial of conventional fractionated versus moderate hypofractionated radiation therapy for localized prostate cancer. *J Clin Oncol.* 2020;38(15):1676–1684. doi:10.1200/JCO.19.01485

76. Lee WR, Dignam JJ, Amin MB, et al. Randomized phase III noninferiority study comparing two radiotherapy fractionation schedules in patients with low-risk prostate cancer. *J Clin Oncol.* 2016;34(20):2325–2332. doi:10.1200/JCO.2016.67.0448

77. Dearnaley D, Syndikus I, Mossop H, et al. Conventional versus hypofractionated high-dose intensity-modulated radiotherapy for prostate cancer: 5-year outcomes of the randomized, non-inferiority, phase 3 CHHiP trial. *Lancet Oncol.* 2016;17(8):1047–1060. doi:10.1016/S1470-2045(16)30102-4

78. van As N, Yasar B, Griffin C, et al. Radical prostatectomy versus stereotactic radiotherapy for clinically localised prostate cancer: results of the PACE-A randomized trial. *Eur Urol.* 2024;86(3):267–276. doi:10.1016/j.eururo.2024.08.030

79. King CR, Brooks JD, Gill H, Presti JC Jr. Long-term outcomes from a prospective trial of stereotactic body radiotherapy for low-risk prostate cancer. *Int J Radiat Oncol Biol Phys.* 2012;82(2):877–882. doi:10.1016/j.ijrobp.2010.11.054

80. Quon HC, Ong A, Cheung P, et al. Once-weekly versus every-other-day stereotactic body radiotherapy in patients with prostate cancer (PATRIOT): a phase 2 randomized trial. *Radiother Oncol.* 2018;127(2):206–212. doi:10.1016/j.radonc.2018.02.029

81. Alayed Y, Quon H, Ong A, et al. Accelerating prostate stereotactic ablative body radiotherapy: efficacy and toxicity of a randomized phase II study of 11 versus 29 days overall treatment time (PATRIOT). *Radiother Oncol.* 2020;149:8–13. doi:10.1016/j.radonc.2020.04.039

82. Hamstra DA, Mariados N, Sylvester J, et al. Continued benefit to rectal separation for prostate radiation therapy: final results of a phase III trial. *Int J Radiat Oncol Biol Phys.* 2017;97(5):976–985. doi:10.1016/j.ijrobp.2016.12.024

83. Mariados N, Sylvester J, Shah D, et al. Hydrogel spacer prospective multicenter randomized controlled pivotal trial: dosimetric and clinical effects of perirectal spacer application in men undergoing prostate image guided intensity modulated radiation therapy. *Int J Radiat Oncol Biol Phys.* 2015;92(5):971–977. doi:10.1016/j.ijrobp.2015.04.030

Cole Billena, Omar Y. Mian, and Rahul D. Tendulkar

QUICK HIT Prostate cancer demonstrates highly heterogeneous clinical behavior. Most patients with unfavorable intermediate-risk and nearly all with high-risk disease are treated with local therapy (as opposed to active surveillance). Multimodality therapy is often required, consisting of either prostatectomy ± postoperative RT (depending on pathology findings and PSA kinetics) or definitive RT combined with ADT (4–6 months for intermediate-risk and 18–36 months for high-risk) ± brachytherapy boost (Table 41.1).

Table 41.1 General Treatment Paradigm for Intermediate- and High-Risk Prostate Cancer[1]	
Definitions (NCCN)	**Treatment Options**

Intermediate Risk (IR):
No high or very high-risk features and ≥1 intermediate risk factors (IRF):
  – cT2b–cT2c
  – Grade group 2 or 3
  – PSA 10–20 ng/mL
Favorable Intermediate Risk (FIR)
  – cT2b–cT2c OR
  – GS 3 + 4 = 7 (GG2) OR
  – PSA 10–20
    AND
  – <50% biopsy cores positive
Unfavorable Intermediate Risk (UIR)
  – 2 or 3 IRFs and/or
  – Grade group 3 and/or
  – ≥50% biopsy cores positive
	• Active surveillance (if life expectancy <10 years)
	• EBRT ± short-term ADT (4–6 months; consider ADT based on FIR vs. UIR, or genomic testing)
	• Brachytherapy alone (primarily for FIR)
	• RP; consider postoperative EBRT for adverse features (+ margins, seminal vesicle invasion [SVI], extracapsular extension [ECE], detectable postoperative PSA)

High Risk
≥1 high-risk features but does not meet very high-risk criteria:
  – cT3 or cT4
  – Grade group 4 or 5 (GS 8–10)
  – PSA >20 ng/mL
Very High Risk
Has at least 2 of the following:
  – cT3 or cT4
  – Grade group 4 or 5 (GS 8–10)
  – PSA >40 ng/mL
	• EBRT + long-term ADT (18–36 months)
	• EBRT + brachytherapy boost ± long-term ADT RP (in select patients); consider postoperative EBRT for adverse features (+margins, SVI, ECE, detectable postoperative PSA); if pN1, consider ADT + pelvic EBRT
	• ADT alone in rare patients who are not otherwise candidates for local therapy

Clinically N+	• RT + long-term ADT (2–3 years) + abiraterone • ADT alone in rare patients who are not otherwise candidates for local therapy

Source: Data from Prostate Cancer, NCCN Guidelines Version 1.2025.

EPIDEMIOLOGY: See Chapter 40. About 15% of new prostate cancer diagnoses are composed of high-risk disease.[2]

RISK FACTORS: See Chapter 40. Prostate cancer is more common in Black men, in whom it presents at an earlier age, and many studies have demonstrated higher PSA levels, higher Gleason score (GS), more advanced stage of disease at diagnosis, and significantly higher biochemical disease recurrence (HR 1.28, 95% CI 1.07–1.54), even when adjusting for socioeconomic, clinical, and pathologic confounders.[3,4] Family history, specifically having a father who survived <24 months from prostate cancer, has been associated with higher risk disease.[5] Germline mutations in DNA repair genes occur in ~5% of localized cases, and in particular germline BRCA2 mutations are associated with a higher GS and a worse prognosis.[6–8] Other general syndromes associated with increased risk of prostate cancer are Lynch syndrome, Fanconi anemia, and HOXB13.[9–11]

ANATOMY, PATHOLOGY, SCREENING, CLINICAL PRESENTATION: See Chapter 40. The risk of pelvic nodal involvement has been estimated by both Partin tables and the Roach formula (2/3*PSA+[GS-6]*10), which tends to overestimate risk in the modern era.[12,13]

WORKUP: H&P including DRE and assessment of baseline urinary, bowel, and sexual function.

Labs: PSA, preoperative workup as indicated.

Imaging: Bone and soft tissue imaging is recommended by NCCN guidelines for patients with UIR, high-risk, and very high-risk disease.[1] PSMA-PET scan is now preferred for initial staging of bone and soft tissue disease without prerequisite conventional imaging (as often required by insurance) due to increased sensitivity and specificity. Bony disease is conventionally assessed by technetium-99m bone scan, and soft tissue disease is conventionally evaluated using CT chest/abdomen/pelvis and/or MRI abdomen/pelvis. Multiparametric (mp) MRI pelvis is preferred over CT pelvis. In addition to anatomic T2 imaging, mpMRI includes at least one additional sequence, such as diffusion-weighted imaging (DWI) or dynamic contrast-enhanced (DCE) imaging.

NATURAL HISTORY: The Connecticut Tumor Registry demonstrated the probability of dying from untreated prostate cancer within 15 years in a patient with GS 8–10 disease is 60% to 87%.[14] Most men treated for high-risk prostate cancer live >10 years and remain at risk of death from other causes.[15]

PROGNOSTIC FACTORS, STAGING: See Chapter 40 for prognostic factors, AJCC 8th edition staging, and risk classifications.

TREATMENT PARADIGM

Active Surveillance: Observation is not a standard management option for UIR and high-risk prostate cancer but may have a role in select patients with a limited life expectancy and multiple medical comorbidities.[16]

Surgery: Radical prostatectomy (RP) is an option for IR and high-risk prostate cancer, although some patients will require postoperative RT for a rising PSA. There have been no prospective randomized trials comparing RP with EBRT for high-risk prostate cancer, and retrospective comparisons are difficult to interpret due to significant selection biases. Thus, either operative or nonoperative approaches may be considered. See Chapter 40 for details regarding surgical options.

Androgen Deprivation Therapy (ADT): The decision to use ADT, timing, and sequencing is dependent on disease characteristics and patient factors (Table 41.2). For IR disease, 4 to 6 months of ADT can be added to EBRT given a DFS benefit in most trials, but no OS benefit. Generally, 2 to 3 years of concurrent ADT is recommended for high-risk disease treated with EBRT, with one trial suggesting that 18 months may be sufficient.[17] The most commonly used agents are GnRH agonists alone or with oral antiandrogens (combined androgen blockade). The most common GnRH agonist is leuprolide, administered as a depot injection. Relugolix is an oral GnRH antagonist that achieves suppression of testosterone levels superior to that with leuprolide, with a lower risk of major adverse cardiovascular events and quicker testosterone recovery.[18] ADT alone can be used for select patients who are not otherwise candidates for definitive local therapy. Side effects include impotence, decreased libido, fatigue, weight gain, hot flashes, cognitive changes, depression, osteoporosis and potentially cardiovascular disease.

Table 41.2 Androgen Deprivation Therapy Medications

Method	Mechanism	Examples
Surgical castration	Removes 90%–95% of circulating testosterone and results in prompt decline in testosterone.	Bilateral orchiectomy
Gonadotropin-releasing hormone (GnRH) agonists	Induce initial stimulation of LH and subsequent testosterone release, followed by gradual decline. By days 20–28, testosterone levels are in castration range. Initial transient elevation in testosterone can exacerbate pain in patients with metastatic disease. An antiandrogen is commonly used concurrently for 1 month on initiation of GnRH agonist to avoid this flare reaction.	Leuprolide (7.5 mg/month), goserelin acetate (3.6 mg/month), buserelin, triptorelin

(continued)

Table 41.2 Androgen Deprivation Therapy Medications (*continued*)		
Method	Mechanism	Examples
GnRH antagonists	Suppresses testosterone while avoiding flare reaction.	Degarelix, relugolix
Steroidal antiandrogens	Inhibition of testosterone and dihydrotestosterone (DHT) from binding to the androgen receptor in prostatic nuclei.	Megestrol acetate, cyproterone acetate
Nonsteroidal antiandrogens	Competitive inhibitors of androgen binding to androgen receptors, preventing nuclear translocation of androgen receptors and binding to DNA response elements.	Bicalutamide (50 mg; *gynecomastia*), Flutamide (*hepatotoxicity*), Enzalutamide (*gynecomastia*), apalutamide, darolutamide
Adrenal suppression	Suppresses synthesis of multiple adrenal steroids.	Ketoconazole (most rapid drug for reducing testosterone)
5α-reductase inhibitors	Suppresses the enzyme that catalyzes the conversion of testosterone to DHT.	Finasteride, dutasteride
CYP17A1 inhibitors	Inhibits the formation of DHEA and androstenedione, precursors of testosterone.	Abiraterone (must be given with prednisolone)

Radiation

Indications: Generally, EBRT is an appropriate option for all patients with IR and high-risk prostate cancer. EBRT with brachytherapy boost can be considered in UIR and high-risk patients. IR patients may be candidates for short-term ADT (4–6 months) in combination with EBRT. High-risk patients are candidates for pelvic nodal RT and ADT for a total of 2 to 3 years.[19] When nodal RT is performed, the updated NRG Oncology guidelines recommend including the common iliac (up to L4–L5), external iliac, internal iliac, presacral (S1–S3), and obturator LNs.[20]

Dose: With standard fractionation, dose escalation to 74 to 81 Gy improves biochemical PFS, but does not improve OS (see Chapter 40 for details).[21-24] Moderate hypofractionation options include 70 Gy/28 fx, 70.2 Gy/26 fx, or 60 Gy/20 fx. If brachytherapy boost is planned, EBRT dose is typically 45 to 50 Gy to prostate and SVs followed by 110 Gy if I-125 or 100 Gy if Pd-103 (RTOG 0232, FIR) or 46 Gy/23 fx to whole pelvis followed by 115 Gy I-125 (ASCENDE-RT, IR and high-risk).[25,26] EBRT 77 Gy/25 fx with an SIB up to 95 Gy/35 fx to the macroscopic tumor in the prostate was shown to prolong biochemical DFS in the FLAME trial.[27] Whole pelvis regimens include 45 Gy/25 fx followed by sequential cone down of 34.2 Gy/19 fx boost to prostate (RTOG 0924, high-risk). Whole pelvis RT can also be delivered in 50.4 Gy/28 fx or 44 Gy/20 fx with corresponding simultaneous dose escalation to the prostate. SBRT to the prostate alone is delivered to a dose of 36.25–40 Gy/5 fx. Pathologic analysis of prostatectomy specimens demonstrated the median length of SVI to be 1 cm, with 90% within 2 cm. SVI was found most commonly in patients with PSA ≥10 ng/mL, GS ≥7, or ≥cT2b. Therefore, the proximal 1 to 2 cm of the SVs is included within the CTV for IR and high-risk patients.[28] An analysis of prostatectomy specimens found that ECE extended 4 mm in 90% of cases, which has implications for CTV margins (typically ≥5 mm).[29]

Toxicity: Acute: fatigue, dysuria, urinary frequency, urinary and rectal urgency. If treating pelvic nodes, diarrhea and cramping may occur. Late: radiation cystitis, urethral stricture, radiation proctitis, bowel obstruction, fistula, pelvic insufficiency fracture, secondary malignancies.

Procedure: See *Handbook of Treatment Planning in Radiation Oncology*, Chapter 8.[30]

EVIDENCE-BASED Q&A

For patients with IR prostate cancer, is there a benefit to ADT with EBRT over EBRT alone?

Several studies have demonstrated a DFS benefit without an OS benefit with the addition of short-term ADT (ST-ADT) to EBRT as summarized in Table 41.3. Of note, RTOG 9408 demonstrated an OS benefit with ADT in the subset of IR patients, but the RT dose was relatively low compared with the other trials. The standard duration of ADT for IR disease is 4 to 6 months.

Table 41.3 Summary of Prospective Randomized Trials Evaluating ST-ADT for IR Disease

	ADT (months)	RT Dose	% IR	Conclusion
RTOG 9408 (Jones, *NEJM*, 2011)[31]	4 vs. 0	66.6 Gy	54%	↑OS in IR ↓BF, DM, PCSM
EORTC 22991 (Bolla, *JCO*, 2021)[32]	6 vs. 0	70, 74, or 78 Gy	75%	↑bDFS, cDFS, not DMFS or OS
GETUG 14 (Dubray, *ASCO*, 2016)[33]	4 vs. 0	80 Gy	100%	↑EFS, not OS
RTOG 0815 (Krauss, *JCO*, 2023)[34]	6 vs. 0	79.2 Gy or 45 Gy + brachy boost	100%	↓bF, DM, not OS

Nabid, Canadian PCS III (*Eur J Cancer* 2021, PMID 33279855): PRT of 600 patients with IR prostate cancer (23% FIR, 77% UIR) randomized to ST-ADT (bicalutamide and goserelin for 6 months, with 4 months given neoadjuvantly) with conventional dose EBRT (70 Gy, Arm 1) or ST-ADT with dose-escalated EBRT (76 Gy, Arm 2) or dose-escalated EBRT alone (76 Gy, Arm 3) with 3D-CRT. The primary endpoint of biochemical failure (bF) was higher in Arm 3 (30% at 10 years) than in Arm 1 (16%) or Arm 2 (13%; $p < .001$). Rates of prostate cancer progression (5% vs. 3% vs. 12%, for Arms 1 vs. 2 vs. 3, respectively, $p = .001$) and PCSM (3% vs. 1.5% vs. 6%, $p = .03$) were also worse with dose-escalated RT alone than either arm with ADT. No significant difference in OS between the three arms. Grade ≥2 GI toxicity was higher with 76 Gy than with 70 Gy (16% vs. 5%, $p < .001$). **Conclusion: Combination ST-ADT and EBRT, even with lower RT doses, leads to superior biochemical control and PCSM compared with dose-escalated EBRT alone in IR prostate cancer (77% of whom were UIR).**

Krauss, RTOG 0815 (*JCO* 2023, PMID 37104748): Phase III randomized study of dose-escalated EBRT (79.2 Gy/1.8 Gy) ± ST-ADT (GnRH agonist/antagonist + oral antiandrogen started 8 weeks prior to RT, 6 months total) for IR prostate cancer. Eligibility: ≥1 of the following risk factors: cT2b–T2c, GS 7, PSA 10 to 20 (except for patients with all three RFs and ≥50% cores positive, who were excluded). RT was EBRT alone 79.2 Gy or EBRT 45 Gy followed by LDR or HDR boost; pelvic RT not permitted. Patients stratified by number of RFs, boost modality, and baseline comorbidities, then randomized to EBRT ± ST-ADT. Primary endpoint: OS; secondary endpoints: DM, death due to prostate cancer, bF. Results: 1,492 patients randomized. Sixty-seven percent had a single RF. Majority (88%) got EBRT without brachytherapy boost. MFU 6.3 years. No difference in OS, but significantly improved 8-year bF (10% vs. 21%), DM (1% vs. 4%), and death from prostate cancer (1 vs. 10 deaths) in EBRT + ADT group. More acute toxicity in ADT group, but no difference in late toxicity. **Conclusion: The addition of ADT to dose-escalated RT does not improve OS, but improves death due to prostate cancer, DM rate, and bF, supporting the use of ADT with RT for IR prostate cancer.** *Comment: Unclear which subset of IR patients derive the largest benefit from ADT.*

For IR prostate cancer, does longer term ADT improve outcomes?

For patients with IR prostate cancer receiving ADT, ST-ADT (4 months) has been shown to be equivalent to longer term regimens (9 months on RTOG 9910, 28 months on DART).

Pisansky, RTOG 9910 (*JCO* 2015, PMID 25534388): PRT of 1,579 patients with IR prostate cancer randomized to neoadjuvant ADT for 8 weeks vs. 28 weeks prior to EBRT (70.2 Gy/39 fx) followed by 8 weeks of concurrent ADT (total 4 months vs. 9 months). At 10 years, both 4 months and 9 months of ADT, respectively, yielded similar rates of bF (27% vs. 27%), CSS (95% vs. 96%), and OS (66% vs. 67%). **Conclusion: Longer duration of ADT does not improve outcomes in patients with IR prostate cancer.**

What is the optimal sequencing of short-term ADT and RT?

Historically, ADT has often been given neoadjuvantly for ~2 months prior to starting RT. Recent evidence suggests that when ST-ADT is utilized, it can be given concurrently/adjuvantly with the start of RT.[35,36] There are no such comparative data in the setting of long-term ADT.

Malone, Canadian (*JCO* 2019, PMID 31829912): PRT of 432 patients with primarily IR prostate cancer (GS 6–7, T1b–T3a, and PSA <30) randomized to 6 months of neoadjuvant/concurrent ADT starting 4 months before RT or RT with concurrent/adjuvant ADT (6 months total). Primary endpoint was bRFS, but also measured OS and late grade 3+ toxicity. No SS difference in 10-year bRFS, OS, or grade 3+ toxicity. **Conclusion: Timing of ST-ADT in relation to RT does not impact biochemical control, OS, or toxicity. Neoadjuvant ADT is not necessary—RT and ADT can be started concurrently.**

Is LDR brachytherapy alone sufficient treatment for FIR prostate cancer?

Michalski, RTOG 0232 (*JCO* 2023, PMID 37315297): PRT of 579 patients with IR prostate cancer, defined as T1c–T2b, GS 2 to 6 with PSA 10 to 20 ng/mL, or GS 7 with PSA <10 ng/mL (but not multiple IR features), randomized to EBRT (45 Gy/25 fx to prostate and SVs; LNs optional) followed by LDR brachytherapy with Pd-103 (100 Gy) or I-125 (110 Gy) or brachytherapy alone with Pd-103 (125 Gy) or I-125 (145 Gy). Only 20% of GS 7 were 4+3 (grade group 3). Freedom from progression was not improved at 5 years with the addition of EBRT. Grade ≥2 and grade ≥3 acute toxicities were similar, but late grade ≥2 (43% vs. 26%, $p < .0001$) and late grade ≥3 (8% vs. 4%, $p = .006$) toxicities were higher in the EBRT + brachytherapy arm. **Conclusion: The addition of EBRT to brachytherapy did not significantly improve 5-year freedom from progression and increased late toxicity in patients with mostly favorable IR prostate cancer.**

For high-risk or locally advanced prostate cancer, what is the benefit of combining ADT with EBRT over EBRT alone?

Multiple trials demonstrated a survival benefit to the addition of ADT to EBRT as summarized in Table 41.4. These trials used heterogenous inclusion criteria and sequencing/duration of ADT. They also largely did not utilize dose-escalated EBRT, and all included pelvic nodal RT.

Table 41.4 Summary of Prospective RCTs Evaluating ADT for Locally Advanced or High-Risk Disease				
	Inclusion	ADT (Months)	RT Dose	Conclusion
EORTC 22863 (**Bolla**, *Lancet Oncol*, 2010)[37]	T1–2 grade 3 or T3–4	36 vs. 0 (included antiandrogen)	70 Gy	ADT ↑bPFS, DFS, and OS
RTOG 8531 (**Pilepich**, *IJROBP*, 2005)[38]	T3N0–1	Lifelong/ orchiectomy vs. 0	65–70 Gy	ADT ↑bNED, OS ↓LF, DM
RTOG 8610 (**Roach**, *JCO*, 2008)[39]	T2–4N0–1	4 vs. 0 (included antiandrogen)	65–70 Gy	ADT ↑DFS, PCSM, not OS
DFCI 95-096 (**D'Amico**, *JAMA*, 2008)[40]	PSA 10–40, GS 7–10, or T3	6 vs. 0 (included antiandrogen)	70 Gy	ADT ↑OS in patients with minimal comorbidity
TROG 9601 (Denham, *Lancet Oncol*, 2011)	cT2b–4N0	6 vs. 3 vs. 0	66 Gy	Compared with EBRT alone, 3 months ADT: ↓PSA progression, ↑EFS; 6 months ADT: ↓PSA progression, ↑EFS, ↓DM, PCSM, ACM

What is the optimal duration of hormone therapy for high-risk prostate cancer?

For patients with high-risk prostate cancer, an OS benefit has been demonstrated with long-term ADT (LT-ADT) compared with ST-ADT (Table 41.5), with most recent data demonstrating a 2- to 3-year benefit with ADT even in the dose escalation era (DART trial). Notably, PCS IV found similar oncologic outcomes between 18 months and 36 months of ADT, although it was not powered to demonstrate noninferiority, suggesting a shorter duration of 18 months of ADT may be sufficient for some patients.[17] On the other hand, the DART 01/05 trial initially reported improved DFS, MFS, and OS with 28 months of ADT vs. 4 months, but this improvement did not hold at 10-year follow-up.[19,41]

Table 41.5 Summary Table of Prospective RCTs Comparing Various Durations of ADT in Patients With High-Risk Prostate Cancer

	Inclusion	ADT (Months)	RT Dose	Conclusion
RTOG 9202 (Horwitz, *JCO*, 2008)[42,43]	T2c–T4	4 vs. 28	65–70 Gy	↑DFS, OS with LT-ADT at 20 yrs
EORTC 22961 (Bolla, *NEJM*, 2009)[44]	T2c–T4 or N1	6 vs. 36	70 Gy	↑bPFS, OS with LT-ADT
TROG 9601 (Denham, *Lancet Oncol*, 2011)[45]	T2b–4N0	0 vs. 3 vs. 6	66 Gy	↑EFS with any ADT ↓DM, PCSM, and ACM with 6 months
DART 01/05 (Zapatero, *Lancet Oncol*, 2022)[41]	T1c–T3a (IR or high-risk)	4 vs. 28	76–82 Gy	↑DFS, MFS, and OS with LT-ADT at 5 yrs for high-risk (but not IR); no difference in DFS, MFS, or OS at 10 yrs (even for high-risk)
PCS IV (Nabid, *Eur Urol*, 2018)[17]	T3–4, GS 8–10, PSA >20	18 vs. 36	70 Gy	No difference in OS with IT-ADT and LT-ADT (but not powered)
RADAR (Denham, *Lancet Oncol*, 2019)[46]	T2b–T4 or T2a and GS ≥7 and PSA ≥10	6 vs. 18	66, 70, 74 Gy, or 46 Gy + HDR brachy boost	↓PCSM with LT-ADT
TRIP/TRIGU0907 (Yorozu, *IJROBP*, 2024)[47]	cT2c–3, PSA >20, or GS >7	6 vs. 30	45 Gy + LDR brachy boost	No difference in biochemical control

Nabid, PCS IV (*Eur Urol* 2018, PMID 29980331): PRT of 630 patients with high-risk prostate cancer (cT3–T4, Gl 8–10, PSA >20) who received pelvic (44 Gy) and prostate RT (70 Gy/35 fx) and randomized to ADT for either 36 or 18 months (bicalutamide 50 mg for 1 month, goserelin 10.8 mg q3 months). The 10-year OS with 36 months of ADT was 62% vs. 62% with 18 months of ADT (HR 1.02, 95% CI 0.81–1.29). QOL significantly favored 18 months of ADT ($p < .001$) for hot flashes and enjoyable sex. Only 53% of patients in the 36-month arm received full duration compared with 88% in the 18-month arm. Median time to testosterone recovery from randomization was 3.6 years for 18-month ADT and 6.6 years for 36-month ADT ($p < .001$). **Conclusion: In high-risk prostate cancer treated with RT, 36 months of ADT was not superior to 18 months (study was not designed to evaluate if 18 months was noninferior).**

Denham, TROG 03.04 RADAR (*Lancet Oncol* 2019, PMID 30579763): PRT comparing ST-ADT (6 months) + RT vs. IT-ADT (18 months) + RT with or without zoledronic acid in men with locally advanced prostate cancer. All patients received RT to the prostate and SVs, starting from the end of the fifth month of ADT. Dosing options: 66, 70, and 74 Gy in 2 Gy/fx, or 46 Gy in 2 Gy/fx, followed by an HDR brachytherapy boost dose of 19.5 Gy in 6.5 Gy/fx. Primary endpoint PCSM. The addition of zoledronic acid did not affect PCSM. When analyzed by duration of ADT, PCSM was 13% vs. 10% ($p = .035$), favoring 18 months of ADT. **Conclusion: 18 months of ADT + RT is a more effective treatment option for locally advanced prostate cancer than 6 months of ADT + RT. The addition of zoledronic acid is not beneficial.**

Is there significant cardiovascular toxicity associated with ADT?

Multiple pooled analyses have been performed, with mixed results. Some demonstrated no significant difference in cardiovascular (CV) mortality with the use of ADT, while others demonstrated increased CV death and shorter time to fatal myocardial infarction, particularly in men over 65 years of age.[48–51]

Nguyen, Meta-Analysis (*JAMA* 2011, PMID 22147380): Systematic review of 4,141 patients from eight randomized trials. Demonstrated that CV death was not significantly different between patients who received ADT and those who did not, but PCSM and ACM were improved with ADT. There was no excess risk of CV death in long-term ADT (>3 years) vs. short-term ADT (≤6 months). **Conclusion: In patients with IR and high-risk prostate cancer, use of ADT was not associated with an increased risk of CV death; however, ADT did reduce PCSM and ACM.**

Zapatero, DART 01/05 GICOR (*IJROBP* 2016, PMID 27598804): Late RT and CV toxicity reporting of patients on DART 01/05. There was no difference in grade ≥2 rectal or urinary toxicity between treatment arms. On MVA, only treatment arm correlated with risk of CV event (HR 2.269, p = .009). On MVA including treatment arm, myocardial infarction, and number of CV diseases, it was found that LT-ADT (HR 2.09, 95% CI 1.17–3.72) and history of myocardial infarction (HR 2.08, 1.13–3.81) were the only factors associated with risk of CV event. **Conclusion: LT-ADT use with a history of myocardial infarction is associated with increased risk of CV event.**

Can brachytherapy boost improve outcomes in addition to EBRT?

Brachytherapy boost is associated with increased toxicity but better biochemical control.[52,53]

Morris, ASCENDE-RT (*IJROBP* 2016, PMID 28262473; *IJROBP* 2022, PMID 36528488): PRT of 398 patients with IR (31%) and high-risk (69%) prostate cancer treated with neoadjuvant and concurrent ADT (12 months total) and EBRT (46 Gy/23 fx to the whole pelvis) and then randomized to conformal EBRT boost to prostate (32 Gy/16 fx) or I-125 LDR brachytherapy boost (prescribed to a minimum peripheral dose of 115 Gy). Primary endpoint bPFS (defined as nadir + 2 ng/mL). The 9-year bPFS was significantly higher for the brachytherapy boost arm compared with the EBRT boost arm (83% vs. 62%, p < .001), but also associated with a higher risk of GU toxicity. At updated 10-year follow-up, the time to biochemical progression was higher for the brachytherapy arm compared with the EBRT arm (85% vs. 67%, p < .05), but no difference was noted in time to DM or OS. **Conclusion: LDR brachytherapy boost significantly increased biochemical control compared with EBRT boost in patients with IR and high-risk prostate cancer.**

Rodda, ASCENDE-RT Morbidity and HR-QOL (*IJROBP* 2017, PMID 28433432, 28581398): LDR brachytherapy boost increased the risk of temporary catheterization and/or requirement for incontinence pads. At 5 years, the cumulative incidence of grade 3 GU events was increased in patients receiving brachytherapy boost, but the prevalence was not statistically significant (Table 41.6). IPSS ≥16 predicted for grade 2 GU toxicity. No significant difference in grade 3 GI or erectile function between arms. The patient-reported HR-QOL demonstrated a clinically significant decline in both physical and sexual function scales for both groups. There was a larger drop in mean score for men receiving LDR brachytherapy boost in physical function (−15.3 vs. −6.9, p = .03) and urinary function (−3.6 vs. −0.5, p = .04). **Conclusion: LDR brachytherapy boost increased the incidence of grade 3 GU toxicity, but no difference in GI toxicity or erectile function. It is also associated with a larger drop in HR-QOL measures of physical and urinary function.**

Table 41.6 Toxicity Results of ASCENDE-RT					
5-Yr	**Grade 3 GU**		**Grade 3 GI**		**Adequate Erections at Baseline and After Treatment**
	Cumulative Incidence	**Prevalence**	**Cumulative Incidence**	**Prevalence**	
DE-EBRT boost	5%	2%	3%	2%	37%
LDR brachytherapy boost	18%	9%	8%	1%	45%
p value	<.001	.058	.124	NS	.30

Can EBRT boost improve outcomes in patients with IR and high-risk prostate cancer?

The FLAME trial described below improved biochemical DFS using an SIB to the dominant intraprostatic lesion (DIL) using conventional fractionation, while the phase II Hypo-FLAME trial demonstrated the feasibility of an SIB approach with ultra-hypofractionation.

Kerkmeijer, FLAME (*JCO* 2021, PMID 33471548): Phase III PRT of 571 patients with IR and high-risk prostate cancer treated with 77 Gy/35Fx (2.2 Gy/fx) to the entire prostate. Patients were randomized to no SIB vs. an SIB of up to 95 Gy/35fx (2.7 Gy/fx; 95 Gy achieved in 20% of patients) to the DIL visible on mpMRI. OAR constraints were prioritized over the focal boost dose. The primary endpoint was 5-year bDFS. At 5-year follow-up, bDFS was 92% in the SIB arm vs. 85% in the standard arm (p < .001). No difference in OS or prostate CSS. Late toxicities were not significantly different between the two arms. **Conclusion: Addition of a focal boost to the DIL improved bDFS for patients with localized IR and high-risk prostate cancer without impacting toxicity or QOL.**

Draulans, hypo-FLAME (*Radiother and Oncol* 2024, PMID 39362607): Phase II trial evaluating SBRT (35 Gy in 5 weekly fractions with an iso-toxic SIB up to 50 Gy to mpMRI-defined tumors) in 100 men with IR or high-risk prostate cancer. Dose constraints for OARs were prioritized over focal boost dose. With an MFU of 61 months, the 5-year bDFS was 94% and the prevalence of grade ≥2 GU and GI toxicity was 12% and 4%, respectively. **Conclusion: SBRT with focal boost to MRI-defined tumors over 5 weekly fractions is feasible with acceptable biochemical control and toxicity.**

Is there a benefit to elective pelvic nodal RT, and which patients should be considered?

The data are conflicting regarding the benefit of pelvic elective nodal irradiation (ENI). Because most of the seminal high-risk trials used whole pelvic fields, virtually all high-risk patients can be considered candidates for ENI. RTOG 9413 has been a difficult trial to interpret but demonstrates a small PFS benefit to ENI in patients with ≥15% risk of LN metastasis.[54] The POP-RT trial demonstrated favorable MFS and DFS with hypofractionated IMRT with simultaneous treatment of pelvic nodes compared with prostate-only RT.[55] The question of ENI is being further investigated on RTOG 0924.

Roach, RTOG 9413 (*JCO* 2003, PMID 12743142; Update *IJROBP* 2006, PMID 17011443; Update Lawton, *IJROBP* 2007, PMID 17531401; Update Roach, *Lancet Oncol* 2018, PMID 30507486): PRT of 1,275 patients with clinically localized prostate cancer with PSA ≤100 ng/mL with an estimated ≥15% risk of LN-positive disease according to Roach formula. Primary endpoint PFS. Randomization was 2 × 2 design, testing neoadjuvant/concurrent ADT (NHT) vs. adjuvant ADT (AHT) and prostate-only RT (PORT) vs. whole pelvic RT (WPRT). ADT was goserelin or leuprolide with flutamide for 2 months before EBRT and 2 months during EBRT in the NHT arm. AHT was also 4 months but started at end of EBRT. EBRT dose was 50.4 Gy to the whole pelvis with four-field box and boost of 19.8 Gy to the prostate in the WPRT arm and 70.2 Gy in the PORT arm. Initial publication demonstrated PFS improvement with WPRT (both arms) compared with PORT (both arms). In the 2018 update, the NHT + WPRT arm had improved 10-year PFS (28%) compared with NHT + PORT (24%) and compared with AHT + WPRT (19%), but not compared with AHT + PORT (30%; *p* = .0002). There were no differences in OS (*p* = .07) or DM (*p* = .32) between the arms. Late grade 3 toxicity was also higher in the NHT + WPRT arm. **Conclusion: In patients with ≥15% risk of LN metastasis, NHT + WPRT appears to improve PFS compared with NHT + PORT and AHT + WPRT arms, but not compared with AHT + PORT.** *Comment: This trial is controversial due to the 2 × 2 design, short duration of ADT, and low dose to the primary tumor, which may limit the ability to detect a potential effect of ENI.*

Murthy, POP-RT (*JCO* 2021, PMID 33497252): Phase III PRT of patients with nonmetastatic, node-negative (80% of whom were staged by PSMA PET/CT) prostate cancer who had at least a 20% risk of pelvic node involvement per the Roach formula (cT3b–T3a with any GS or PSA; or cT1–T3a with GS 8–10 with any PSA, GS 7 with PSA >15 ng/mL, and GS 6 with PSA >30 ng/mL) randomized to either prostate only RT (PORT) or whole pelvis RT (WPRT). WPRT improved 5-year DFS (90% vs. 77%, *p* = .002) and DMFS (96% vs. 89%, *p* = .01) compared with PORT; however, no difference in 5-year OS was detected. **Conclusion: WPRT improves DFS and DMFS in node-negative prostate cancer patients at high risk for nodal involvement, the majority of whom were staged with PSMA PET/CT.**

Is ultra-hypofractionation or SBRT safe and effective for IR and high-risk prostate cancer?

The pHART8 (prostate/SVs), SHARP, and SATURN (prostate/SVs + pelvis) single-arm phase II studies are more recently published data on SBRT for high-risk patients, which appears efficacious with the bulk of late toxicity grade ≤2. The HYPO-RT-PC phase III RCT showed noninferiority to ultra-hypofractionated RT in comparison to conventional fractionation (CF), with comparable late toxicity. Please refer to Chapter 40 for further SBRT studies as some also included IR/high-risk patients in their analyses.

Widmark, HYPO-RT-PC (*Lancet* 2019, PMID 31227373): PRT of 1,180 men undergoing RT for IR (89%) or high-risk (11%) prostate cancer randomized to CF (78 Gy/39 fx) vs. ultra-hypofractionation (42.7 Gy/7 fx QOD). No ADT was allowed, and the primary endpoint was time to biochemical or clinical failure. At MFU of 5 years, the estimated FFS was 84% in both arms. There was a trend toward higher incidence of acute grade ≥2 urinary toxicity in ultra-hypofractionation arm (28% vs. 23%, *p* = .057), and urinary toxicity was higher in ultra-hypofractionation arm at 1 year (6% vs.

2%, p = .0037). **Conclusion: Ultra-hypofractionation is noninferior to CF RT with regard to FFS, although acute toxicity is slightly more pronounced.**

Can elective nodal irradiation be delivered with moderate hypofractionation or ultra-hypofractionation?

The pHART2-RCT enrolled 180 patients with high-risk disease to moderate hypofractionation (MH, 48 Gy to pelvis with SIB to 68 Gy to prostate in 25 fx) or conventional fractionation (CF, 46 Gy/23 fx to pelvis followed by sequential boost of 32 Gy/16 fx to prostate) and found more late G3+ GI toxicities in the MH arm, but otherwise no difference in G2+ GI or GU toxicity or clinical outcomes with an MFU of more than 5 years.[56] Another trial, PCS5, in high-risk prostate cancer (T3/T4, GS ≥8, and PSA >20) compared hypofractionated RT (68 Gy to prostate and 45 Gy to pelvis in 25 fx) with conventional (76 Gy/38 fx to prostate and 46 Gy/23 fx to pelvis) with 28 months of ADT and reported no differences in OS, prostate CSS, and DMFS at an MFU of 5 years.[57]

With respect to 5 fx ENI, the SATURN trial[58] was a phase I/II trial that found that prostate SBRT with 40 Gy/5 fx with ENI 25 Gy/5 fx was tolerable. The randomized phase II HOPE trial[59] delivered 15 Gy HDR brachytherapy to the prostate in a single fx followed by whole pelvic RT 45 to 46 Gy in 23 to 25 fx vs. 25 Gy in 5 fx QOD. No difference in acute toxicity was seen. Additionally, the phase II SPORT trial[60] compared toxicity of prostate SBRT alone (36.35 Gy/5 fx once weekly) vs. prostate SBRT with ENI (25 Gy/5 fx once weekly) in 30 patients, reporting numerically higher acute and late GU/GI toxicities with prostate + ENI SBRT at 3 years; acute G2+ GI toxicity (0% prostate alone vs. 7% prostate + ENI), acute G2+ GU toxicity (7% vs. 20%), late G2+ GI (7% vs. 13%), and late G2+ GU (7% vs. 33%).

For high-risk or locally advanced prostate cancer, is there a benefit to combined EBRT and ADT over ADT alone?

Two trials demonstrated an OS benefit to combined EBRT + ADT over ADT alone. One older MRC trial did not demonstrate an advantage to the addition of EBRT to ADT, although there were several limitations in this trial.[61]

Widmark, SPCG-7/SFU0-3 (*Lancet* 2009, PMID 19091394): PRT of 875 patients from 47 centers with T1b–T2 and G2–G3 disease or T3, PSA <70 ng/mL, N0, M0 randomized to ADT (3 months total androgen blockage followed by continuous flutamide 250 mg) or ADT + EBRT (70 Gy) to prostate/SVs. The results are in Table 41.7. **Conclusion: The addition of EBRT to flutamide improved bPFS, CSS, and OS for patients with high-risk prostate cancer.**

Table 41.7 SPCG-7 Trial Results							
10-Yr Data	**bPFS**	**CSS**	**OS**	**Erectile Dysfunction**	**Urethral Stricture**	**Urgency**	**Incontinence**
ADT	25%	76%	61%	81%	0%	8%	3%
ADT + EBRT	74%	88%	70%	89%	2%	14%	7%

All results statistically significant.

Warde, NCIC CTG PR.3/MRC UK PR 07 (*Lancet* 2011, PMID 22056152; Update Mason, *JCO* 2015, PMID 25691677): PRT of 1,205 patients with T3–4N0, or T1–2 and PSA >40 ng/mL, or PSA >20 ng/mL and GS >8 randomized to lifelong ADT (bilateral orchiectomy or GnRH agonist) or ADT + EBRT (64–69 Gy to prostate/SVs and 45 Gy to pelvic nodes). The addition of EBRT to ADT improved OS at 7 years (74% vs. 66%, p = .033). Deaths from prostate cancer were significantly reduced by the addition of RT to ADT (HR 0.46, 95% CI 0.34–0.61). **Conclusion: The addition of EBRT to lifelong ADT improves OS in patients with high-risk prostate cancer.**

Is there a role for CHT in high-risk prostate cancer?

Whether there is an OS benefit with the addition of CHT to LT-ADT and dose-escalated EBRT in the modern era for patients with high-risk prostate cancer is unclear. PRTs currently have limited follow-up. RTOG 9902 was a PRT of patients with high-risk prostate cancer randomized to EBRT + LT-ADT (24 months) ± paclitaxel, estramustine, and oral etoposide, and did not show improved outcomes (BF, LF, DM, DFS, or OS).[62] In RTOG 0521, the addition of six cycles of docetaxel to EBRT + LT-ADT (24 months) in patients with high-risk prostate cancer improved OS from 89% to 93% at 4 years, with improved DFS and decreased DM.[63] GETUG 12 randomized patients with high-risk prostate cancer to LT-ADT (3 years) ± 4 cycles of docetaxel and estramustine followed by RP or EBRT and showed improved RFS (62% vs. 50%, p = .57) with CHT.[64] The decision to use CHT should be individualized.

Rosenthal, RTOG 9902 (*IJROBP* 2015, PMID 26209502): PRT of 397 patients with high-risk prostate cancer randomized to EBRT + LT-ADT (GnRH agonist × 24 months) with adjuvant paclitaxel, estramustine, oral etoposide CHT vs. EBRT + ADT alone. No difference in any outcome (bF, LF, DM, DFS, OS) with the addition of this CHT regimen. **Conclusion: The addition of CHT to standard of care EBRT + LT-ADT did not improve outcomes in patients with high-risk prostate cancer.**

Rosenthal, RTOG 0521 (*JCO* 2019, PMID 30860948): PRT of 612 patients with high-risk prostate cancer randomized to EBRT (75.6 Gy) + LT-ADT (24 months) followed by CHT (docetaxel × 6 cycles) or EBRT + LT-ADT alone. EBRT + ADT + CHT had significantly higher 4-year OS (93% vs. 89%, one-sided *p* = .04) and 6-year DFS (65% vs. 55%, two-sided *p* = .04) compared with EBRT + ADT alone. **Conclusion: Adjuvant docetaxel, in addition to EBRT and LT-ADT, may provide a benefit in patients with high-risk prostate cancer.**

Fizazi, GETUG 12 (*Lancet Oncol* 2015, PMID 26028518): PRT of 207 patients with high-risk or N1 prostate cancer randomized to LT-ADT (GnRH agonist × 3 years) with CHT (docetaxel and estramustine × 4 cycles) or ADT alone. Local therapy with RP or EBRT was performed 3 months after systemic treatment. The 8-year RFS was significantly higher with the addition of CHT (62% vs. 50%, *p* = .017). **Conclusion: Docetaxel and estramustine CHT in combination with LT-ADT and local therapy (RP or EBRT) significantly improved RFS in patients with high-risk prostate cancer.**

Is there a role for the use of abiraterone + prednisolone (AA/P) in addition to other ADT (i.e., GNRH agonist) in high-risk nonmetastatic prostate cancer?

Attard, STAMPEDE (*Lancet Oncol* 2022, PMID 34953525): Pooled analysis of two randomized phase III RCTs on the STAMPEDE multigroup, multistage platform protocol investigating combination therapy (ADT + AA/P or ADT + AA/P + enzalutamide) vs. standard ADT alone in patients with high-risk nonmetastatic prostate cancer (defined as node-positive or at least two of the following: T3–4, GS 8–10, and PSA >40 ng/mL) or high-risk relapsing disease (PSA ≥20 ng/mL, PSA ≥4 ng/mL with PSADT <6 months, ≤12 months of total ADT with an interval of ≥12 months without treatment, or nodal disease). 1,974 patients were enrolled in the two trials, with an MFU of 72 months. Compared with ADT alone, combination therapy statistically significantly improved OS (HR 0.60, 95% CI 0.48–0.73), PCSS (0.49, 0.37–0.65), MFS (0.53, 0.44–0.64), PFS (0.44, 0.36–0.54), and BFFS (0.39, 0.33–0.47). AA/P + enzalutamide did not appear to improve MFS over AA/P alone (interaction HR 1.02, *p* = .91). Adverse G3+ events during the first 2 years were higher in the combination therapy arms (37% ADT + AA/P vs. 29% ADT alone in the AA/P trial, and 58% ADT + AA/P + enzalutamide vs. 32% ADT alone in the AA/P + enzalutamide trial). **Conclusion: Combination therapy improves OS and MFS in patients with very high-risk, nonmetastatic prostate cancer.**

Is there a role for ADT prior to prostatectomy?

Klotz, Canada (*J Urol* 2003, PMID 12913699): PRT of 213 patients randomized to prostatectomy with neoadjuvant ADT (cyproterone × 3 months) or prostatectomy alone. MFU 6 years. The positive margin rate was reduced by 50% with the addition of ADT; however, there was no difference in rates of bF (34% vs. 37%, *p* = .07). **Conclusion: The use of preoperative ADT has not been shown to significantly improve clinical outcomes and its use is not considered standard of care.**

LYMPH NODE-POSITIVE PROSTATE CANCER

What is the management of patients with clinically lymph node-positive disease?

Historically, node-positive disease was treated according to a similar treatment paradigm as DMs, with early trial questions evaluating immediate vs. delayed ADT at the time of progression. Current practice patterns have shifted, as most node-positive patients are now treated with combined ADT and EBRT.

Lin, NCDB (*JNCI* 2015, PMID 25957435): RR of 3,450 patients with clinically N+ prostate cancer without DM. ADT + EBRT was associated with a 50% decreased risk of 5-year ACM (HR 0.50, 95%

CI 0.37–0.67). **Conclusion: The combination of ADT + EBRT may be associated with a significant survival benefit in men with clinically node-positive prostate cancer.**

James, STAMPEDE N+ Cohort (*JAMA Oncol* 2015, PMID 26606329): Cohort study of high-risk, ADT-naïve patients with newly diagnosed M0 prostate cancer. In the N+ cohort, RT was encouraged but not required. 177 N1M0 patients were available for analysis, and 97 patients were planned for RT, of whom 29 did not receive RT, while another 10 patients were not planned to receive RT but reported receipt. FFS was better among those planned for radical RT than those not planned, with a 2-year FFS of 81% vs. 64% (HR 0.48, 95% CI 0.29–0.79). Additionally, those who truly received RT vs. not had improved 2-year FFS (89% vs. 64%; HR 0.35, 0.19–0.65). **Conclusion: These exploratory data support the use of combined ADT and RT in patients with N1M0 prostate cancer.**

LOCALLY RECURRENT PROSTATE CANCER AFTER RADIATION

What are treatment options for LR of prostate cancer after previous RT?

Several salvage options exist after prior EBRT, including RP, cryotherapy, brachytherapy, or SBRT. The MASTER meta-analysis demonstrated that the estimated rates of 5-year bRFS on meta-regression were similar between various local salvage therapies, ranging from 50% to 60% after RP, cryotherapy, SBRT, or brachytherapy, with no significant differences between any modality and RP. Severe GU toxicity was lower after all three forms of RT salvage than with RP (20% for RP, 15% for cryotherapy, 6% for SBRT, 10% for HDR brachytherapy, and 9% for LDR brachytherapy; p < .001). GI toxicity was lower with salvage HDR brachytherapy than with RP, but it was <2% across all modalities.[65]

MASTER Meta-Analysis/Systematic Review (*Eur Urol* 2021, PMID 33309278): Systematic review of 150 studies of patients with locally recurrent prostate cancer after definitive RT who received various modalities of salvage therapy as listed in Table 41.8. The 5-year RFS rates varied between 46% and 57%, without significant difference relative to RP. Rates of severe GU toxicity among RT modalities (5%–10%) were significantly lower than that of RP (20%), which was comparable to HIFU. Cryotherapy had 15% GU toxicity. Rates of severe GI toxicity were low and ranged from 0% to 2%. **Conclusion: The salvage modalities have comparable 5-year RFS albeit with varying rates of severe GU and GI toxicity favoring re-RT.**

Table 41.8 Efficacy and Toxicity by Modality Per the MASTER Meta-Analysis			
Modality	5-Yr RFS	Rate of Severe GU AE	Rate of Severe GI AE
RP	53%	20%	1.5%
SBRT	56%	6%	0.0%
HDR	58%	10%	0.0%
LDR	53%	9%	2.1%
HIFU	46%	23%	0.8%
Cryotherapy	57%	15%	0.9%

RTOG 0526 (*IJROBP* 2022, PMID 34740768): Prospective phase II trial of salvage LDR brachytherapy for biopsy-proven LF after EBRT for initial low-intermediate risk prostate cancer. 100 patients were enrolled, with an MFU of 6.7 years and a median time since EBRT of 85 months. ADT was used in 16% of patients. Late G3 GI/GU AEs were seen in 14% of patients (12/92 evaluable pts). The 10-year OS was 70%, 10-year DFS was 33%, 5-year FFBF was 68%, and most postsalvage failures were biochemical (46% at 10 years). Of the patients, 5% had LF and 19% had distant failure at 10 years. **Conclusion: Salvage LDR brachytherapy is a viable re-RT modality with modest toxicity and promising outcomes.**

REFERENCES

1. National Comprehensive Cancer Network. *Prostate Cancer, NCCN Guidelines* Version 1.2025. Accessed January 12, 2025. https://www.nccn.org/professionals/physician_gls/pdf/prostate.pdf
2. Cooperberg MR, Broering JM, Carroll PR. Time trends and local variation in primary treatment of localized prostate cancer. *J Clin Oncol.* 2010;28(7):1117–1123. doi:10.1200/JCO.2009.26.0133

3. Hoffman RM, Gilliland FD, Eley JW, et al. Racial and ethnic differences in advanced-stage prostate cancer: the Prostate Cancer Outcomes Study. *J Natl Cancer Inst.* 2001;93(5):388–395. doi:10.1093/jnci/93.5.388

4. Hamilton RJ, Aronson WJ, Presti JC Jr, et al. Race, biochemical disease recurrence, and prostate-specific antigen doubling time after radical prostatectomy: results from the SEARCH database. *Cancer.* 2007;110(10):2202–2209. doi:10.1002/cncr.23012

5. Hemminki K, Ji J, Försti A, Sundquist J, Lenner P. Concordance of survival in family members with prostate cancer. *J Clin Oncol.* 2008;26(10):1705–1709. doi:10.1200/JCO.2007.13.3355

6. Agalliu I, Gern R, Leanza S, Burk RD. Associations of high-grade prostate cancer with BRCA1 and BRCA2 founder mutations. *Clin Cancer Res.* 2009;15(3):1112–1120. doi:10.1158/1078-0432.CCR-08-1822

7. Castro E, Goh C, Olmos D, et al. Germline BRCA mutations are associated with higher risk of nodal involvement, distant metastasis, and poor survival outcomes in prostate cancer. *J Clin Oncol.* 2013;31(14):1748–1757. doi:10.1200/JCO.2012.43.1882

8. Pritchard CC, Mateo J, Walsh MF, et al. Inherited DNA-repair gene mutations in men with metastatic prostate cancer. *N Engl J Med.* 2016;375(5):443–453. doi:10.1056/NEJMoa1603144

9. Raymond VM, Mukherjee B, Wang F, et al. Elevated risk of prostate cancer among men with Lynch syndrome. *J Clin Oncol.* 2013;31(14):1713–1718. doi:10.1200/JCO.2012.44.1238

10. Tischkowitz M, Easton DF, Ball J, Hodgson SV, Mathew CG. Cancer incidence in relatives of British Fanconi anemia patients. *BMC Cancer.* 2008;8:257. doi:10.1186/1471-2407-8-257

11. Ewing CM, Ray AM, Lange EM, et al. Germline mutations in HOXB13 and prostate-cancer risk. *N Engl J Med.* 2012;366(2):141–149. doi:10.1056/NEJMoa1110000

12. Eifler JB, Feng Z, Lin BM, et al. An updated prostate cancer staging nomogram (Partin tables) based on cases from 2006 to 2011. *BJU Int.* 2013;111(1):22–29. doi:10.1111/j.1464-410X.2012.11324.x

13. Nguyen PL, Chen MH, Hoffman KE, Katz MS, D'Amico AV. Predicting the risk of pelvic node involvement among men with prostate cancer in the contemporary era. *Int J Radiat Oncol Biol Phys.* 2009;74(1):104–109. doi:10.1016/j.ijrobp.2008.07.053

14. Albertsen PC, Hanley JA, Fine J. 20-year outcomes following conservative management of clinically localized prostate cancer. *JAMA.* 2005;293(17):2095–2101. doi:10.1001/jama.293.17.2095

15. Tendulkar RD, Hunter GK, Reddy CA, et al. Causes of mortality after dose-escalated radiation therapy and androgen deprivation for high-risk prostate cancer. *Int J Radiat Oncol Biol Phys.* 2013;87(1):94–99. doi:10.1016/j.ijrobp.2013.05.044

16. Chen RC, Rumble RB, Loblaw DA, et al. Active surveillance for the management of localized prostate cancer (Cancer Care Ontario Guideline): American Society of Clinical Oncology Clinical Practice Guideline Endorsement. *J Clin Oncol.* 2016;34(18):2182–2190. doi:10.1200/JCO.2015.65.7759

17. Nabid A, Carrier N, Martin AG, et al. Duration of androgen deprivation therapy in high-risk prostate cancer: a randomized phase III trial. *Eur Urol.* 2018;74(4):432–441. doi:10.1016/j.eururo.2018.06.018

18. Shore ND, Saad F, Cookson MS, et al. Oral relugolix for androgen-deprivation therapy in advanced prostate cancer. *N Engl J Med.* 2020;382(23):2187–2196. doi:10.1056/NEJMoa2004325

19. Zapatero A, Guerrero A, Maldonado X, et al. High-dose radiotherapy with short-term or long-term androgen deprivation in localised prostate cancer (DART01/05 GICOR): a randomised, controlled, phase 3 trial. *Lancet Oncol.* 2015;16(3):320–327. doi:10.1016/S1470-2045(15)70045-8

20. Hall WA, Paulson E, Davis BJ, et al. NRG Oncology updated international consensus atlas on pelvic lymph node volumes for intact and postoperative prostate cancer. *Int J Radiat Oncol Biol Phys.* 2021;109(1):174–185. doi:10.1016/j.ijrobp.2020.08.034

21. Pasalic D, Kuban DA, Allen PK, et al. Dose escalation for prostate adenocarcinoma: a long-term update on the outcomes of a phase 3, single institution randomized clinical trial. *Int J Radiat Oncol Biol Phys.* 2019;104(4):790–797. doi:10.1016/j.ijrobp.2019.02.045

22. Zietman AL, Bae K, Slater JD, et al. Randomized trial comparing conventional-dose with high-dose conformal radiation therapy in early-stage adenocarcinoma of the prostate: long-term results from Proton Radiation Oncology Group/American College of Radiology 95-09. *J Clin Oncol.* 2010;28(7):1106–1111. doi:10.1200/JCO.2009.25.8475

23. Dearnaley DP, Jovic G, Syndikus I, et al. Escalated-dose versus control-dose conformal radiotherapy for prostate cancer: long-term results from the MRC RT01 randomised controlled trial. *Lancet Oncol.* 2014;15(4):464–473. doi:10.1016/S1470-2045(14)70040-3

24. Heemsbergen WD, Al-Mamgani A, Slot A, Dielwart MF, Lebesque JV. Long-term results of the Dutch randomized prostate cancer trial: impact of dose-escalation on local, biochemical, clinical failure, and survival. *Radiother Oncol.* 2014;110(1):104–109. doi:10.1016/j.radonc.2013.09.026

25. Orio PF 3rd, Nguyen PL, Buzurovic I, Cail DW, Chen YW. The decreased use of brachytherapy boost for intermediate and high-risk prostate cancer despite evidence supporting its effectiveness. *Brachytherapy.* 2016;15(6):701–706. doi:10.1016/j.brachy.2016.05.001

26. Michalski JM, Winter KA, Prestidge BR, et al. Effect of brachytherapy with external beam radiation therapy versus brachytherapy alone for intermediate-risk prostate cancer: NRG Oncology RTOG 0232 randomized clinical trial. *J Clin Oncol.* 2023;41(24):4035–4044. doi:10.1200/JCO.22.01856

27. Kerkmeijer LGW, Groen VH, Pos FJ, et al. Focal boost to the intraprostatic tumor in external beam radiotherapy for patients with localized prostate cancer: results from the FLAME randomized phase III trial. *J Clin Oncol.* 2021;39(7):787–796. doi:10.1200/JCO.20.02873

28. Kestin L, Goldstein N, Vicini F, Yan D, Korman H, Martinez A. Treatment of prostate cancer with radiotherapy: should the entire seminal vesicles be included in the clinical target volume? *Int J Radiat Oncol Biol Phys.* 2002;54(3):686–697. doi:10.1016/S0360-3016(02)02968-3

29. Sohayda C, Kupelian PA, Levin HS, Klein EA. Extent of extracapsular extension in localized prostate cancer. *Urology.* 2000;55(3):382–386. doi:10.1016/S0090-4295(99)00500-8

30. Videtic GMM, Woody N, Vassil AD. *Handbook of Treatment Planning in Radiation Oncology.* 3rd ed. Demos Medical; 2020.

31. Jones CU, Hunt D, McGowan DG, et al. Radiotherapy and short-term androgen deprivation for localized prostate cancer. *N Engl J Med.* 2011;365(2):107–118. doi:10.1056/NEJMoa1012348

32. Bolla M, Neven A, Maingon P, et al. Short androgen suppression and radiation dose escalation in prostate cancer: 12-year results of EORTC trial 22991 in patients with localized intermediate-risk disease. *J Clin Oncol.* 2021;39(27):3022–3033. doi:10.1200/JCO.21.00855

33. Dubray BM, Salleron J, Guerif SG, et al. Does short-term androgen depletion add to high dose radiotherapy (80 Gy) in localized intermediate risk prostate cancer? Final analysis of GETUG 14 randomized trial (EU-20503/NCT00104741). *J Clin Oncol.* 2016;34(15 suppl):5021. doi:10.1200/JCO.2016.34.15_suppl.5021

34. Krauss DJ, Karrison T, Martinez AA, et al. Dose-escalated radiotherapy alone or in combination with short-term androgen deprivation for intermediate-risk prostate cancer: results of a phase III multi-institutional trial. *J Clin Oncol.* 2023;41(17):3203–3216. doi:10.1200/JCO.22.02390

35. Malone S, Roy S, Eapen L, et al. Sequencing of androgen-deprivation therapy with external-beam radiotherapy in localized prostate cancer: a phase III randomized controlled trial. *J Clin Oncol.* 2020;38(6):593–601. doi:10.1200/JCO.19.01904

36. Spratt DE, Malone S, Roy S, et al. Prostate radiotherapy with adjuvant Androgen Deprivation Therapy (ADT) improves metastasis-free survival compared to neoadjuvant ADT: an individual patient meta-analysis. *J Clin Oncol.* 2021;39(2):136–144. doi:10.1200/JCO.20.02438

37. Bolla M, Van Tienhoven G, Warde P, et al. External irradiation with or without long-term androgen suppression for prostate cancer with high metastatic risk: 10-year results of an EORTC randomised study. *Lancet Oncol.* 2010;11(11):1066–1073. doi:10.1016/S1470-2045(10)70223-0

38. Pilepich MV, Winter K, Lawton CA, et al. Androgen suppression adjuvant to definitive radiotherapy in prostate carcinoma--long-term results of phase III RTOG 85-31. *Int J Radiat Oncol Biol Phys.* 2005;61(5):1285–1290. doi:10.1016/j.ijrobp.2004.08.047

39. Roach M 3rd, Bae K, Speight J, et al. Short-term neoadjuvant androgen deprivation therapy and external-beam radiotherapy for locally advanced prostate cancer: long-term results of RTOG 8610. *J Clin Oncol.* 2008;26(4):585–591. doi:10.1200/JCO.2007.13.9881

40. D'Amico AV, Chen MH, Renshaw AA, Loffredo M, Kantoff PW. Androgen suppression and radiation vs radiation alone for prostate cancer: a randomized trial. *JAMA.* 2008;299(3):289–295. doi:10.1001/jama.299.3.289

41. Zapatero A, Guerrero A, Maldonado X, et al. High-dose radiotherapy and risk-adapted androgen deprivation in localised prostate cancer (DART 01/05): 10-year results of a phase 3 randomised, controlled trial. *Lancet Oncol.* 2022;23(5):671–681. doi:10.1016/S1470-2045(22)00190-5

42. Horwitz EM, Bae K, Hanks GE, et al. Ten-year follow-up of Radiation Therapy Oncology Group protocol 92-02: a phase III trial of the duration of elective androgen deprivation in locally advanced prostate cancer. *J Clin Oncol.* 2008;26(15):2497–2504. doi:10.1200/JCO.2007.14.9021

43. Lawton CAF, Lin X, Hanks GE, et al. Duration of androgen deprivation in locally advanced prostate cancer: long-term update of NRG Oncology RTOG 9202. *Int J Radiat Oncol Biol Phys.* 2017;98(2):296–303. doi:10.1016/j.ijrobp.2017.02.004

44. Bolla M, de Reijke TM, Van Tienhoven G, et al. Duration of androgen suppression in the treatment of prostate cancer. *N Engl J Med.* 2009;360(24):2516–2527. doi:10.1056/NEJMoa0810095

45. Denham JW, Steigler A, Lamb DS, et al. Short-term neoadjuvant androgen deprivation and radiotherapy for locally advanced prostate cancer: 10-year data from the TROG 96.01 randomised trial. *Lancet Oncol.* 2011;12(5):451–459. doi:10.1016/S1470-2045(11)70063-8

46. Denham JW, Joseph D, Lamb DS, et al. Short-term androgen suppression and radiotherapy versus intermediate-term androgen suppression and radiotherapy, with or without zoledronic acid, in men with locally advanced prostate cancer (TROG 03.04 RADAR): 10-year results from a randomised, phase 3, factorial trial. *Lancet Oncol.* 2019;20(2):267–281. doi:10.1016/S1470-2045(18)30757-5

47. Yorozu A, Namiki M, Saito S, et al. Trimodality therapy with iodine-125 brachytherapy, external beam radiation therapy, and short- or long-term androgen deprivation therapy for high-risk localized prostate cancer: results of a multicenter, randomized phase 3 trial (TRIP/TRIGU0907). *Int J Radiat Oncol Biol Phys.* 2024;118(2):390–401. doi:10.1016/j.ijrobp.2023.08.046

48. Nguyen PL, Je Y, Schutz FA, et al. Association of androgen deprivation therapy with cardiovascular death in patients with prostate cancer: a meta-analysis of randomized trials. *JAMA.* 2011;306(21):2359–2366. doi:10.1001/jama.2011.1745

49. D'Amico AV, Denham JW, Crook J, et al. Influence of androgen suppression therapy for prostate cancer on the frequency and timing of fatal myocardial infarctions. *J Clin Oncol.* 2007;25(17):2420–2425. doi:10.1200/JCO.2006.09.3369

50. Tsai HK, D'Amico AV, Sadetsky N, Chen MH, Carroll PR. Androgen deprivation therapy for localized prostate cancer and the risk of cardiovascular mortality. *J Natl Cancer Inst.* 2007;99(20):1516–1524. doi:10.1093/jnci/djm168

51. Zapatero A, Guerrero A, Maldonado X, et al. Late radiation and cardiovascular adverse effects after androgen deprivation and high-dose radiation therapy in prostate cancer: results from the DART 01/05 randomized phase 3 trial. *Int J Radiat Oncol Biol Phys.* 2016;96(2):341–348. doi:10.1016/j.ijrobp.2016.06.2445

52. Hoskin PJ, Rojas AM, Bownes PJ, Lowe GJ, Ostler PJ, Bryant L. Randomised trial of external beam radiotherapy alone or combined with high-dose-rate brachytherapy boost for localised prostate cancer. *Radiother Oncol.* 2012;103(2):217–222. doi:10.1016/j.radonc.2012.01.007

53. Morton G, Loblaw A, Cheung P, et al. Is single fraction 15 Gy the preferred high dose-rate brachytherapy boost dose for prostate cancer? *Radiother Oncol.* 2011;100(3):463–467. doi:10.1016/j.radonc.2011.08.022

54. Roach M, Moughan J, Lawton CAF, et al. Sequence of hormonal therapy and radiotherapy field size in unfavourable, localised prostate cancer (NRG/RTOG 9413): long-term results of a randomised, phase 3 trial. *Lancet Oncol.* 2018;19(11):1504–1515. doi:10.1016/S1470-2045(18)30528-X

55. Murthy V, Maitre P, Kannan S, et al. Prostate-only versus whole-pelvic radiation therapy in high-risk and very high-risk prostate cancer (POP-RT): outcomes from phase III randomized controlled trial. *J Clin Oncol.* 2021;39(11):1234–1242. doi:10.1200/JCO.20.03282

56. Glicksman RM, Loblaw A, Morton G, et al. Randomized trial of concomitant hypofractionated intensity modulated radiation therapy boost versus conventionally fractionated intensity modulated radiation therapy boost for localized high-risk prostate cancer (pHART2-RCT). *Int J Radiat Oncol Biol Phys.* 2024;119(1):100–109. doi:10.1016/j.ijrobp.2023.11.006

57. Niazi T, Nabid A, Malagon T, et al. Hypofractionated dose escalation radiotherapy for high-risk prostate cancer: the survival analysis of the Prostate Cancer Study 5, a Groupe de Radio-oncologie Génito-urinaire du Quebec-led phase 3 trial. *Eur Urol.* 2024. doi:10.1016/j.eururo.2024.08.032

58. Musunuru HB, D'Alimonte L, Davidson M, et al. Phase 1-2 study of stereotactic ablative radiotherapy including regional lymph node irradiation in patients with high-risk prostate cancer (SATURN): early toxicity and quality of life. *Int J Radiat Oncol Biol Phys.* 2018;102(5):1438–1447. doi:10.1016/j.ijrobp.2018.07.2005

59. Mendez LC, Crook J, Martell K, et al. Is ultrahypofractionated Whole Pelvis Radiation Therapy (WPRT) as well tolerated as conventionally fractionated WPRT in patients with prostate cancer? Early results from the HOPE trial. *Int J Radiat Oncol Biol Phys.* 2024;119(3):803–812. doi:10.1016/j.ijrobp.2023.11.058

60. Houlihan OA, Redmond K, Fairmichael C, et al. A randomized feasibility trial of stereotactic prostate radiation therapy with or without elective nodal irradiation in high-risk localized prostate cancer (SPORT trial). *Int J Radiat Oncol Biol Phys.* 2023;117(3):594–609. doi:10.1016/j.ijrobp.2023.02.054

61. Fellows GJ, Clark PB, Beynon LL, et al. Treatment of advanced localised prostatic cancer by orchiectomy, radiotherapy, or combined treatment. A Medical Research Council Study. Urological Cancer Working Party--Subgroup on Prostatic Cancer. *Br J Urol.* 1992;70(3):304–309. doi:10.1111/j.1464-410X.1992.tb15736.x

62. Rosenthal SA, Hunt D, Sartor AO, et al. A phase 3 trial of 2 years of androgen suppression and radiation therapy with or without adjuvant chemotherapy for high-risk prostate cancer: final results of Radiation Therapy Oncology Group phase 3 randomized trial NRG Oncology RTOG 9902. *Int J Radiat Oncol Biol Phys.* 2015;93(2):294–302. doi:10.1016/j.ijrobp.2015.05.024

63. Rosenthal SA, Hu C, Sartor O, et al. Effect of chemotherapy with docetaxel with androgen suppression and radiotherapy for localized high-risk prostate cancer: the randomized phase III NRG Oncology RTOG 0521 trial. *J Clin Oncol.* 2019;37(14):1159–1168. doi:10.1200/JCO.18.02158

64. Fizazi K, Faivre L, Lesaunier F, et al. Androgen deprivation therapy plus docetaxel and estramustine versus androgen deprivation therapy alone for high-risk localised prostate cancer (GETUG 12): a phase 3 randomised controlled trial. *Lancet Oncol.* 2015;16(7):787–794. doi:10.1016/S1470-2045(15)00011-X

65. Valle LF, Lehrer EJ, Markovic D, et al. A systematic review and meta-analysis of local salvage therapies after radiotherapy for prostate cancer (MASTER). *Eur Urol.* 2021;80(3):280–292. doi:10.1016/j.eururo.2020.11.010

42 POST-PROSTATECTOMY RADIATION THERAPY

Sean M. Parker, James R. Broughman, Omar Y. Mian, and Rahul D. Tendulkar

QUICK HIT   After radical prostatectomy (RP) ~25% to 30% of patients will have PSA progression postoperatively (>50% among men with pT3 disease or positive margins). Adjuvant RT improves bRFS among patients with positive margins, ECE (pT3a), or SVI (pT3b). Compared with adjuvant RT, early salvage RT has less toxicity and avoids unnecessary treatment without compromising EFS (Table 42.1). The addition of ADT to RT improves outcomes, although patient selection for treatment intensification remains controversial. Prostate bed RT can be delivered using conventional (64–72 Gy in 1.8–2 Gy/fx) or hypofractionated approaches (52.5–62.5 Gy in 20–25 fx). Addition of nodal RT is indicated in pN1 disease and should be considered in men with pN0 disease with higher risk features at the time of biochemical recurrence. Genomic classifiers (e.g. Decipher) and advanced PET imaging are increasingly utilized to guide RT decision-making following RP.

Table 42.1 General Treatment Paradigm for Prostate Cancer After Prostatectomy		
Initial Treatment	**Pathologic Findings**	**Subsequent Treatment Options**
Radical prostatectomy (RP)	No adverse features or LN metastases, PSA <0.1 ng/mL	Close monitoring*
	Adverse features (positive margin, SVI, ECE, high Decipher), PSA <0.1 ng/mL	Close monitoring*
		Adjuvant RT (select patients only)
	LN metastases	ADT + RT to prostate bed + pelvic LNs
		Close monitoring (select patients only)*
	Detectable postoperative PSA (≥0.1 ng/mL) and no evidence of distant metastases	Salvage RT to prostate bed ± pelvic LNs ± ADT
		Close monitoring* (if low grade with slow PSA doubling time [PSADT] and/or limited life expectancy)

*Close monitoring: PSA q6–12 months + annual DRE. Early-salvage RT indicated if PSA rises to 0.2 ng/mL or >2 consecutive rises above 0.1 ng/mL.

EPIDEMIOLOGY: There are ~300,000 diagnoses of prostate cancer and 35,000 deaths in the United States annually.[1] Over 90% have localized disease and over half undergo RP as initial treatment. Following RP, PSA is highly sensitive and biochemical failure (bF) is not uncommon: for men with intermediate-risk prostate cancer, 5-year bRFS is ~80% and 10-year bRFS is ~65%. For high/very high-risk disease, 5-year bRFS is ~70% and 10-year bRFS is ~55%.[2] Laparoscopic/robotic surgery has become more common, with a vast majority undergoing this approach rather than an open technique.[3] Overall, after RP, 25% to 30% have postop PSA progression (>50% if pT3 or positive margins).

RISK FACTORS, ANATOMY, PATHOLOGY, SCREENING, CLINICAL PRESENTATION: See Chapter 40 for further details.

GENETICS: Role of multigene assays in improving RT decision-making following RP is evolving. Decipher incorporates 22 genes to produce a score (range 0–1) that provides independent prognostic value for post-prostatectomy patients, and it has been verified in prospective cohorts.[4–6]

WORKUP: H&P to rule out distant metastatic disease. Palpation of nodule on DRE is suggestive of anastomotic recurrence.

Labs: PSA should be undetectable following RP. A detectable/rising PSA postoperatively warrants investigation for locoregional or distant metastatic disease. The AUA definition of bF is PSA ≥0.2 ng/mL followed by second confirmatory PSA ≥0.2 ng/mL.[7]

Imaging: For patients with good life expectancy, consider bone and soft tissue imaging via PSMA PET/CT; otherwise can consider fluciclovine (Axumin) PET/CT or Tc-99m bone scan (poor sensitivity at PSA <10 ng/mL)[8] with CT abdomen/pelvis. Multiparametric MRI (3T preferred) can be considered as a substitute for CT abdomen/pelvis, especially to identify postoperative bed recurrences[9,10] and assist with treatment planning.[11] Over the last decade, improved prostate cancer-specific nuclear imaging has dramatically improved sensitivity in detecting recurrent/metastatic disease. Both PSMA and fluciclovine PET impact RT decision-making, and the addition of PET to conventional imaging has been shown to improve EFS.[12,13] PSMA PET has demonstrated improved detection over fluciclovine for PSA ≤2.0 ng/mL.[14] Detection rates for PSMA PET are approximately 38% for PSA <0.5 ng/mL and 91% for PSA >2.0 ng/mL.[15]

PROGNOSTIC FACTORS: Surgical margins (positive margins are favorable for response to salvage RT), Gleason score (GS), PSA level, PSADT (<6 months worse), PSA response (ratio of rate of climb to rate of fall before and after ADT), interval from surgery to bF, lack of SV involvement, and high Decipher score.[6,16,17] Tertiary patterns 4 and 5 in prostatectomy specimens behave as high-risk disease.

NATURAL HISTORY: Most common sites of LR following RP: (a) vesicourethral anastomosis (approximately two-thirds of LR), (b) bladder neck, and (c) retrotrigone.[18] Survival following bF is highly variable, ranging from 4 to 15+ years in various series.[19] Historically, the median time to radiographic metastases after post-prostatectomy bF is 8 years without treatment, and the median time to death after developing macrometastatic disease is another 5 years.[20]

STAGING: See Chapter 40 for AJCC 8th edition's staging and risk classifications.

TREATMENT PARADIGM

Surgery: See Chapter 40 for details on upfront prostatectomy techniques.

Chemotherapy: No current role for adjuvant cytotoxic CHT in the setting of biochemical recurrence. The STAMPEDE trial found an OS benefit to the use of docetaxel administered at the time of first-line ADT in metastatic hormone-sensitive prostate cancer patients, although it is unclear if this applies in the nonmetastatic recurrent setting (evaluated by NRG-GU002).[21]

Androgen Deprivation: Four trials have demonstrated benefit to adding ADT to salvage RT.[22–25] Across these trials, there has been indication that patients with higher PSA at bF benefit more, particularly those with PSA ≥0.5 to 0.6 ng/mL. Treatment intensification for patients with higher risk factors (e.g., higher GS, PSA >0.5–1.0, shorter PSADT, high-risk Decipher) continues to evolve. Addition of enzalutamide improved MFS in patients at high risk for biochemical recurrence on the EMBARK trial.[26] The FORMULA-509 trial evaluated the addition of abiraterone/apalutamide for high-risk patients, with preliminary results indicating an MFS benefit for the subset with PSA >0.5 ng/mL. See below discussion and Chapter 41 for details on ADT including dosing and administration.

Radiation

Indications

Adjuvant Therapy: Treatment in the absence of detectable disease, generally started >3 to 4 months after surgery so that patients are allowed time for recovery. Rationale: RT may prevent recurrence in those at high risk when disease burden is minimal. Classic indications: positive margins, ECE (pT3a), or SVI (pT3b), although observation and early salvage therapy is preferred for most.

Salvage Therapy: Treatment in the presence of detectable disease (elevated/rising PSA and/or nodular recurrence). Rationale: RT may eradicate locally recurrent/residual prostate cancer. Clinical indications: LR, persistently elevated postop PSA, or rising PSA.

Pelvic Nodal RT: Indicated in the pN+ setting (see the following for discussion). RTOG 0534 demonstrated that elective nodal RT for pN0 patients improved outcomes over prostate bed RT alone in the setting of ADT.[24] However, the indications for nodal RT for pN0 remain controversial.

Dose: Conventional (64–72 Gy at 1.8–2 Gy/fx) or hypofractionated (52.5–62.5 Gy in 20–25 fx) regimens are appropriate. Doses of at least 66 Gy appear to be associated with improved outcomes in retrospective series[27]; however, the SAKK 09/10 trial showed that dose escalation to 70 Gy/35 fx did not improve bPFS compared with 64 Gy/32 fx but did increase GI toxicity.[28] NRG-GU003 demonstrated that hypofractionation (62.5 Gy/25 fx) increased acute toxicity immediately following RT, but chronic toxicity and bRFS were noninferior when compared with 66.6 Gy/37 fx.[29]

Procedure: See *Handbook of Treatment Planning in Radiation Oncology*, Chapter 8.[30]

EVIDENCE-BASED Q&A

Does immediate post-prostatectomy RT improve outcomes for patients with high-risk features?

the rate of bF after prostatectomy is >50% in those with pT3 disease, positive margins, and high GS.[31,32] Therefore, three major trials evaluated the role of immediate ("adjuvant") RT to the prostate bed vs. observation for pT3 (all trials) and positive margins (SWOG 8794, EORTC 22911). Of note, ~30% of patients had detectable PSA (≥0.2 ng/mL) on SWOG and EORTC studies, whereas ARO required an undetectable ultrasensitive PSA prior to randomization. In all three trials, immediate RT improved bPFS by about 20% to 30%, but only the SWOG trial detected an improvement in DMFS and OS (Table 42.2). Two meta-analyses (Ontario and Cochrane) were also performed with conflicting results.[33,34] However, none of these trials specified the timing or type of salvage treatment provided to patients who failed observation. This was instead left to the treating physician, and ultimately a wide range of treatments were given, including no salvage therapy for some patients.[35] Adjuvant RT was also shown to improve bPFS in patients with organ-confined (pT2) disease with positive margins, a group that is underrepresented in the three major trials and some argue warrants adjuvant treatment.[36]

Table 42.2 Randomized Trials of Adjuvant RT vs. Observation						
	SWOG 8794 (10-Yr)[37]		**EORTC 22911 (10-Yr)**[38]		**ARO 96–02 (10-Yr)**[39]	
	RT	Observation	RT	Observation	RT	Observation
bPFS	64%	34%*	62%	39%*	56%	35%*
DMFS	71%	61%*	90%	89%	~82%	~85%
OS	74%	66%*	77%	80%	~84%	~87%

*Statistically significant.

Is early salvage RT superior to adjuvant RT?

The ARTISTIC meta-analysis combined the results of RAVES, RADICALS-RT, and GETUG-AFU 17 (Table 42.3) and found that early salvage RT may reduce toxicity and avoid unnecessary treatment without compromising EFS compared with adjuvant RT.[40–43] Data from UCLA show that with every 0.1 ng/mL increase, the likelihood of cure decreases by ~3%, suggesting that earlier intervention may lead to better outcomes.[35] Higher grade/stage accounted for a minority of patients enrolled in these studies; thus, the role of adjuvant RT for certain high-risk subgroups may still be warranted.

Vale, ARTISTIC Meta-Analysis (*Lancet* 2020, PMID 33002431): The ARTISTIC collaboration is a planned series of reviews and meta-analyses for RAVES,[40] RADICALS-RT,[41] and GETUG-AFU 17.[42] This first series analyzed EFS defined as (a) PSA ≥0.4 after RT, (b) any PSA ≥2.0, (c) clinical or radiographic progression, (d) nontrial treatment, or (e) death from prostate cancer. Over 70% of patients had at least one of positive margins, ECE, or SVI. At the time of analysis, 39% of men assigned to early salvage therapy had received RT. Adjuvant RT did not improve EFS (89% vs. 88%) compared with early salvage RT. Outcomes were consistent across all three included trials and across patient subgroups. Only 8% to 17% had GS 8 to 10 and 19% to 21% had SVI, suggesting that most enrolled patients had relatively favorable pathology. **Conclusion: Adjuvant RT does not improve EFS in men with pT3 or margin-positive prostate cancer compared with early salvage RT.**

Table 42.3 Randomized Trials of Adjuvant vs. Early-Salvage RT				
Trial	Postop PSA (ng/mL)	Salvage RT Threshold	RT Dose	bPFS (Adjuvant vs. Salvage)
RAVES (5-yr)	<0.1	0.2 ng/mL	64 Gy/32 fx	86% vs. 87%
RADICALS-RT (10-yr)	<0.2	0.1 ng/mL or three successive increases	66 Gy/33 fx or 52.5 Gy/20 fx	76% vs. 75%
GETUG-AFU 17 (5-yr)	<0.1	0.2 ng/mL	66 Gy/33 fx	92% vs. 90%

What prognostic tools are available to identify good candidates for salvage RT?

The Stephenson nomogram has been utilized to predict outcomes after salvage RT and was updated by Tendulkar to help elucidate the efficacy of salvage therapy in the ultrasensitive PSA era.[16] Another update of this nomogram integrated PSADT (<6 months associated with adverse outcomes).[44]

Tendulkar, Multi-Institution Nomogram (*JCO* 2016, PMID 27528718): Multi-institutional RR of 2,460 LN-negative patients s/p RP with a detectable post-RP PSA treated with salvage RT with or without ADT, including patients whose postop PSA was <0.2 ng/mL. Both bRFS and DM rates were improved when salvage RT was delivered at lower PSA levels, even before meeting the AUA criteria for bF of ≥0.2 ng/mL (see Table 42.4). On MVA, pre-RT PSA, GS, EPE, SVI, surgical margins, ADT use, and RT dose were associated with FFBF.

Table 42.4 Tendulkar Nomogram Results						
PSA at Salvage RT	0.01–0.20 ng/mL	0.21–0.5 ng/mL	0.51–1.0 ng/mL	1.01–2 ng/mL	>2.0 ng/mL	p value
5-yr bRFS	71%	63%	54%	43%	37%	<.001
10-yr DM	9%	15%	19%	20%	37%	<.001

Can genomic classifiers help risk-stratify patients?

There is growing evidence that genomic classifiers such as Decipher may improve selection for postoperative RT and/or ADT following RP. Decipher score independently improves prognostication of patients post-RP and has been validated in the RTOG 9601 and SAKK 09/10 cohorts.[4–6] Decipher is now being incorporated into multiple large prospective clinical trials to further clarify the predictive value of the test and identify optimal cutoffs for clinical decision-making.

Can salvage RT be delivered with hypofractionation? Is there a role for dose escalation?

Studies with short-term follow-up suggest hypofractionation is well-tolerated.[45–47] An exploratory analysis of RADICALS-RT found a modest decrease in grade 1/2 GU toxicity and no increase in severe toxicity with hypofractionation (52.5 Gy/20 fx).[48] NRG GU003 sought to prospectively compare toxicity and oncologic outcomes of conventional vs. hypofractionation, and the 2-year results have been reported (see below). The SAKK 09/10 trial demonstrated dose escalation (from 64 Gy to 70 Gy) did not improve oncologic outcomes and worsened late toxicity.[28]

Buyyounouski, NRG GU003 (*JAMA Oncol* 2024, PMID 38483412): Phase III PRT of 296 patients with either (a) detectable PSA (≥0.1 ng/mL) and pT2/3 pNx/0 disease or (b) undetectable PSA (<0.1 ng/mL) with pT2–3 disease and positive margins randomized to 62.5 Gy/25 fx (HYPORT) or 66.6 Gy/37 fx (COPORT). Primary endpoint was 2-year change in GU and GI toxicity score with non-inferiority margins at −5 and −6, respectively. MFU 2.1 years. At the end of RT, mean GI toxicity score was worse with hypofractionation (−15.52 vs. −7.06, $p < .001$). However, at 6 and 12 months, both fractionation schedules returned to baseline levels. At 24 months, hypofractionation met non-inferiority margins for mean GU (HYPORT, −5.01 and COPORT, −4.07; $p = .005$) and GI (HYPORT, −4.17 and COPORT, −1.41; $p = .02$) score differences. Biochemical failure at 2 years was similar between groups (12% HYPORT vs. 8% COPORT, $p = .28$). **Conclusion: Hypofractionation appears noninferior to conventional fractionation at 2 years, with increased acute toxicity immediately following treatment.**

Should we include pelvic lymph nodes in treatment volumes?

RTOG 0534 suggests that nodal RT improves freedom from progression (FFP) over prostate bed RT in the setting of ADT. However, despite the valuable results of RTOG 0534, it remains controversial how best to incorporate initial risk group into treatment decisions and which specific patient subgroups may warrant the treatment intensification.

Pollack, RTOG 0534/SPPORT (*Lancet* 2022, PMID 35569466): Phase III PRT of 1,716 men with pT2/3 or positive margins and PSA 0.1 to 2.0. Three-arm randomization to (1) RT alone (64.8–70.2 Gy), (2) RT + 4 to 6 months of ADT, and (3) RT + PLNRT (45 Gy) + 4 to 6 months of ADT with a primary endpoint of 5-year FFP. The 5-year FFP was 71%, 81%, and 87% for Arms 1, 2, and 3, respectively (all arms with SS difference). PLNRT + ADT had significantly lower rate of DM and PCSM compared with RT alone (HR 0.52, 95% CI 0.34–0.81 for DM; HR 0.51, 0.27–0.94 for PCSM). The addition of ADT to PLNRT improved outcomes across all clinicopathologic variables over RT alone (Table 42.5). No OS difference between arms. Acute ≥G2 toxicity increased with intensification of therapy, although late toxicity was similar between Arms 2 and 3, except for increased hematologic AE in Arm 3 attributed to the nodal field. **Conclusion: PLNRT + 6 months ADT improves 5-year FFP over prostate bed RT + 6 months ADT or prostate bed RT alone without an impact on OS.** *Comment: Median of six LNs were removed on dissection.*

Table 42.5 Hazard Ratios Between RTOG 0534 Arms			
	Arm 2 vs. 1 (RT ± ADT)	Arm 3 vs. 1 (RT ± ADT and Nodal RT)	Arm 3 vs. 2 (RT + ADT ± Nodal RT)
FFP	0.60*	0.50*	0.82*
RF	0.49*	0.28*	0.57
DM	0.74	0.52*	0.71
PCSM	0.73	0.51*	0.70
OS	0.87	0.93	1.07

*Statistically significant.

What is the benefit of adding ADT to salvage RT?

Four randomized trials comparing salvage RT ± ADT have shown a benefit to addition of ADT, although only RTOG 9601 found an OS benefit of 5% at 12 years. RTOG 9601 utilized 2 years of bicalutamide, whereas GETUG-AFU 16 and RTOG 0534 used 4 to 6 months of ADT. RADICALS-HD, the secondary randomization of the RADICALS trial, compared no ADT vs. 6 months vs. 24 months of ADT with 24 months of ADT demonstrating improved MFS. The DADSPORT meta-analysis of the above trials did not find an OS benefit with the addition of ADT but did show an absolute 5-year MFS benefit of 2% in those that received 6 months vs. none. The optimal indications and timing of ADT remain controversial. The TOAD trial, although underpowered with a heterogenous cohort, demonstrated improved OS with immediate over delayed ADT.[49]

Shipley, RTOG 9601 (*NEJM* 2017, PMID 28146658): PRT of 761 patients with bF (postop PSA 0.2–4.0 ng/mL) and either pT2 with positive margins or pT3N0 who received salvage RT (64.8 Gy/36 fx) then randomized to 24 months of 150 mg daily bicalutamide vs. placebo. Median PSA at entry 0.6 ng/mL. MFU 12.6 years. See Table 42.6 for results. **Conclusion: The addition of ADT to salvage RT improved bF, DM, PCM, and OS with tolerable side effects.** *Comment: Relatively high PSA at entry and low RT dose by modern standards.*

Spratt, Secondary Analysis of RTOG 9601 (*JAMA Oncol* 2020, PMID 32215583): See trial details above. A significant OS benefit for bicalutamide was seen in men with PSA >1.5 ng/mL (HR 0.45, 95% CI 0.25–0.81) but not for PSA 0.2 to 1.5 ng/mL (HR 0.87, 0.66–1.16). In a subset analysis of men with PSA of 0.61 to 1.5 ng/mL, bicalutamide was associated with improved OS (HR 0.61, 0.39–0.94). Men receiving bicalutamide with PSA ≤0.6 ng/mL had increased other-cause mortality (HR 1.94, 1.17–3.20) and grades 3 to 5 cardiac events (OR 3.57, 1.09–15.97). **Conclusion: Long-term ADT did not improve OS in patients receiving early salvage RT (PSA ≤0.6 ng/mL) and may be associated with increased risk of other-cause mortality.**

Table 42.6 RTOG 9601 Clinical Outcome					
	12-Yr bF	12-Yr DM	12-Yr PCM	12-Yr OS	Gynecomastia
RT + placebo	68%	23%	13%	71%	11%
RT + bicalutamide	44%*	14%*	6%*	76%*	70%*

*Statistically significant.

Carrie, GETUG-AFU 16 (*Lancet* 2019, PMID 31629656): PRT of 743 men s/p RP with initially undetectable and subsequently rising postop PSA between 0.2 and 2.0 ng/mL randomized to RT alone vs. RT + 6 months of goserelin. RT was 66 Gy/33 fx via 3D-CRT or IMRT. MFU 112 months. RT + ADT improved 5-year bRFS (49% vs. 64%; SS) and 10-year DMFS (69% vs. 75%; SS). **Conclusion: Salvage RT + short-term ADT improves bRFS and DMFS.** *Comment: Men with PSA >0.5 ng/mL had a greater bRFS benefit compared with those with <0.5 ng/mL.*

Parker, RADICALS-HD (*Lancet* 2024, PMID 38763153; Update *Lancet* 2024, PMID 38763154): *Phase III PRT of patients enrolled in RADICALS trial receiving RT (salvage or adjuvant) following RP with PSA <5 ng/mL at diagnosis that underwent secondary randomization to (a) no ADT vs. 6 months ADT (n = 1,480) and (b) 6 months ADT vs. 24 months ADT (n = 1,523 patients). MFS (primary endpoint) was not improved by the addition of 6 months ADT (HR 0.89, 95% CI 0.69–1.14), but MFS was improved with the extension of ADT from 6 months to 24 months (HR 0.77, 0.61–0.98). Grade ≥3 toxicity was more commonly reported in the 24-month group (p = .025). Among those with PSA >0.5 ng/mL, there was a trend to improved MFS (HR 0.67, 0.45–1.0) that was not significant.* **Conclusion: No MFS benefit with the addition of short-course ADT (6 months), but benefit was seen when extending duration to 24 months.**

Is there a role for systemic therapy intensification for high-risk patients receiving salvage RT?

Treatment intensification may be warranted for certain high-risk cohorts. The EMBARK trial detailed below supports the addition of enzalutamide. The FORMULA-509 trial is evaluating the addition of 6 months of abiraterone/apalutamide for a high-risk cohort (GS 8–10, PSA >0.5, pT3/T4, pN1, PSADT <10 months, negative margins, gross local/regional disease, or Decipher high risk), with early results suggesting an MFS benefit for men with PSA >0.5 ng/mL.[50]

Freedland, EMBARK (*NEJM* 2023, PMID 37851874): Phase III PRT of 1,068 patients with high-risk biochemical recurrence (PSADT <9 months, PSA 2 ng/mL from nadir after RT, or PSA ≥1 ng/mL after RP) randomized to (a) enzalutamide + leuprolide, (b) leuprolide alone, or (c) enzalutamide alone. Primary endpoint was MFS. MFU 60.7 months. MFS at 5 years was 87% in the combination group, 71% in the leuprolide-alone group, and 80% in the enzalutamide group. MFS for enzalutamide + leuprolide was superior to leuprolide alone (HR 0.42, 95% CI 0.30–0.61); enzalutamide monotherapy was also superior to leuprolide alone (HR 0.63, 0.46–0.87). **Conclusion: Enzalutamide + leuprolide improves MFS over leuprolide alone for patients with high-risk biochemical recurrences.**

How should we treat patients with lymph node-positive disease following prostatectomy?

The Messing trial established ADT as standard of care for pN1 disease.[51] The role of RT is controversial, although retrospective data suggest benefit particularly for patients with (a) ≤2 +LNs and GS 7 to 10 with pT3b/pT4 disease or positive margins or (b) 3–4 +LNs.[33,52] There is no published RCT that definitively demonstrates the role of adjuvant vs. salvage RT for pN1 patients; these patients only comprised 3% of the ARTISTIC meta-analysis cohort. Retrospective studies suggest an all-cause mortality benefit for adjuvant RT over salvage RT, with increasing benefit to those with an increasing number of positive LNs.[53] Management of oligorecurrent nodal disease following prior RT or RP is evolving and detailed further in Chapter 73.

Messing (*NEJM* 1999, PMID 10588962; Update *Lancet Oncol* 2006, PMID 16750497): Multi-institutional PRT of 98 men with pT1b–T2 prostate cancer s/p RP found to have LN+ disease randomized to immediate (monthly goserelin or bilateral orchiectomy) vs. delayed ADT (initiated at disease progression). MFU 11.9 years. Immediate ADT improved OS (HR 1.84, 95% CI 1.01–3.35), PCSS (HR 4.09, 1.76–9.49), and PFS (HR 3.42, 1.96–5.98). Seventy-nine percent of those in the delayed ADT arm received an active treatment by 5 years. **Conclusion: Immediate postoperative ADT improves OS for LN+ prostate cancer.** *Comment: Study conducted in the pre-PSA era and PSA was not used to guide decision-making (i.e., only clinically palpable nodules were considered LFs); average pretreatment PSA in the delayed ADT arm was 14 ng/mL at the time of initiating ADT; GS was not available from 14 of 36 institutions; an imbalance may exist accounting for the differences in survival.*

Abdollah (*JCO* 2014, PMID 25245445): RR of 1,107 patients with pN1 prostate cancer treated with RP and PLND between 1988 and 2010 treated with ADT with or without RT. Investigators found four variables that could be used to stratify patients according to PCM risk: the number of involved LNs, pathologic GS, tumor stage, and margin status. Men with either (a) ≤2 +LNs and GS 7 to 10 with pT3b/pT4 disease or positive margins (HR 0.30, 95% CI 0.14–0.64) or (b) 3–4 +LNs (HR 0.21, 0.06–0.79) appeared to benefit from combined ADT + RT. These results were confirmed when OS was examined as an endpoint. **Conclusion: Postoperative RT appears to provide benefit in select men with pN+ prostate cancer.**

How can advanced imaging impact postoperative RT?

Conventional imaging (CT, MRI, bone scan) rarely identifies disease at PSA <1.0 ng/mL, but initiation of salvage RT at lower PSA levels improves outcomes. Advanced imaging, such as fluciclovine or PSMA PET, improves detection at lower PSAs, allowing for more individually tailored salvage treatment plans. The addition of fluciclovine PET to conventional imaging has prospectively demonstrated improved EFS.[13] PSMA PET has prospectively outperformed fluciclovine.[14] A meta-analysis of 20 prospective studies analyzing PSMA PET demonstrated detection rates of 38% for PSA <0.5 ng/mL and 91% for PSA >2.0 ng/mL.[15]

Armstrong, PSMA-SRT (*Eur Urol* 2024, PMID 38290964): Phase III PRT of 193 patients with biochemical recurrence of prostate cancer after RP randomized to immediate salvage RT or PSMA PET/CT prior to salvage RT planning. Any other imaging modalities were allowed in both arms. Primary endpoint was bRFS (data still maturing). Median PSA was 0.3 ng/mL. One-third of patients had a positive PSMA PET, including 13% within the prostate fossa, 16% in pelvic LN, and 9% distantly. PSMA PET led to increased rate of significant treatment changes (45% vs. 22%, p = .002) and more treatment intensification (29% vs. 12%, p = .005). **Conclusion: With oncologic data still maturing, PSMA PET appears to significantly impact treatment decision-making, often leading to treatment intensification.**

REFERENCES

1. Siegel RL, Giaquinto AN, Jemal A. Cancer statistics, 2024. *CA Cancer J Clin*. 2024;74(1):12–49. doi:10.3322/caac.21820
2. Boorjian SA, Karnes RJ, Rangel LJ, Bergstralh EJ, Blute ML. Mayo Clinic validation of the D'Amico risk group classification for predicting survival following radical prostatectomy. *J Urol*. 2008;179(4):1354–1361. doi:10.1016/j.juro.2007.11.061
3. Barry MJ, Gallagher PM, Skinner JS, Fowler FJ Jr. Adverse effects of robotic-assisted laparoscopic versus open retropubic radical prostatectomy among a nationwide random sample of Medicare-age men. *J Clin Oncol*. 2012;30(5):513–518. doi:10.1200/JCO.2011.36.8621
4. Dal Pra A, Ghadjar P, Hayoz S, et al. Validation of the Decipher genomic classifier in patients receiving salvage radiotherapy without hormone therapy after radical prostatectomy: an ancillary study of the SAKK 09/10 randomized clinical trial. *Ann Oncol*. 2022;33(9):950–958. doi:10.1016/j.annonc.2022.05.007
5. Feng FY, Huang HC, Spratt DE, et al. Validation of a 22-gene genomic classifier in patients with recurrent prostate cancer: an ancillary study of the NRG/RTOG 9601 randomized clinical trial. *JAMA Oncol*. 2021;7(4):544–552. doi:10.1001/jamaoncol.2020.7671
6. Spratt DE, Yousefi K, Deheshi S, et al. Individual patient-level meta-analysis of the performance of the Decipher genomic classifier in high-risk men after prostatectomy to predict development of metastatic disease. *J Clin Oncol*. 2017;35(18):1991–1998. doi:10.1200/JCO.2016.70.2811
7. Cookson MS, Aus G, Burnett AL, et al. Variation in the definition of biochemical recurrence in patients treated for localized prostate cancer: the American Urological Association Prostate Guidelines for Localized Prostate Cancer Update Panel report and recommendations for a standard in the reporting of surgical outcomes. *J Urol*. 2007;177(2):540–545. doi:10.1016/j.juro.2006.10.097
8. Dotan ZA, Bianco FJ Jr, Rabbani F, et al. Pattern of Prostate-Specific Antigen (PSA) failure dictates the probability of a positive bone scan in patients with an increasing PSA after radical prostatectomy. *J Clin Oncol*. 2005;23(9):1962–1968. doi:10.1200/JCO.2005.06.058
9. Sella T, Schwartz LH, Swindle PW, et al. Suspected local recurrence after radical prostatectomy: endorectal coil MR imaging. *Radiology*. 2004;231(2):379–385. doi:10.1148/radiol.2312030011
10. Silverman JM, Krebs TL. MR imaging evaluation with a transrectal surface coil of local recurrence of prostatic cancer in men who have undergone radical prostatectomy. *AJR Am J Roentgenol*. 1997;168(2):379–385. doi:10.2214/ajr.168.2.9016212
11. Miralbell R, Vees H, Lozano J, et al. Endorectal MRI assessment of local relapse after surgery for prostate cancer: a model to define treatment field guidelines for adjuvant radiotherapy in patients at high risk for local failure. *Int J Radiat Oncol Biol Phys*. 2007;67(2):356–361. doi:10.1016/j.ijrobp.2006.08.079

12. Armstrong WR, Kishan AU, Booker KM, et al. Impact of prostate-specific membrane antigen positron emission tomography/computed tomography on prostate cancer salvage radiotherapy management: results from a prospective multicenter randomized phase 3 trial (PSMA-SRT NCT03582774). *Eur Urol.* 2024;86(1):52–60. doi:10.1016/j.eururo.2024.01.012

13. Jani AB, Schreibmann E, Goyal S, et al. 18F-fluciclovine-PET/CT imaging versus conventional imaging alone to guide postprostatectomy salvage radiotherapy for prostate cancer (EMPIRE-1): a single centre, open-label, phase 2/3 randomised controlled trial. *Lancet.* 2021;397(10288):1895–1904. doi:10.1016/S0140-6736(21)00581-X

14. Pernthaler B, Kulnik R, Gstettner C, Salamon S, Aigner RM, Kvaternik H. A prospective head-to-head comparison of 18F-fluciclovine with 68Ga-PSMA-11 in biochemical recurrence of prostate cancer in PET/CT. *Clin Nucl Med.* 2019;44(10):e522–e528. doi:10.1097/RLU.0000000000002657

15. Mazrani W, Cook GJR, Bomanji J. Role of 68Ga and 18F PSMA PET/CT and PET/MRI in biochemical recurrence of prostate cancer: a systematic review of prospective studies. *Nucl Med Commun.* 2022;43(6):631–641. doi:10.1097/MNM.0000000000001559

16. Stephenson AJ, Scardino PT, Kattan MW, et al. Predicting the outcome of salvage radiation therapy for recurrent prostate cancer after radical prostatectomy. *J Clin Oncol.* 2007;25(15):2035–2041. doi:10.1200/JCO.2006.08.9607

17. Tendulkar RD, Stephans KL. Contemporary external beam radiotherapy. In: Klein EA, Jones JS, eds. *Management of Prostate Cancer.* 3rd ed. Humana Press; 2012:243–261.

18. Connolly JA, Shinohara K, Presti JC, Carroll PR. Local recurrence after radical prostatectomy: characteristics in size, location, and relationship to prostate-specific antigen and surgical margins. *Urology.* 1996;47(2):225–231. doi:10.1016/S0090-4295(99)80421-X

19. Freedland SJ, Humphreys EB, Mangold LA, et al. Risk of prostate cancer-specific mortality following biochemical recurrence after radical prostatectomy. *J Urol.* 2006;175(2):564–564. doi:10.1016/S0022-5347(05)00388-5

20. Pound CR, Partin AW, Eisenberger MA, et al. Natural history of progression after PSA elevation following radical prostatectomy. *J Urol.* 1999;162(4):1548–1548. doi:10.1016/S0022-5347(05)68359-0

21. Clarke NW, Ali A, Ingleby FC, et al. Addition of docetaxel to hormonal therapy in low- and high-burden metastatic hormone sensitive prostate cancer: long-term survival results from the STAMPEDE trial. *Ann Oncol.* 2019;30(12):1992–2003. doi:10.1093/annonc/mdz396

22. Carrie C, Magné N, Burban-Provost P, et al. Short-term androgen deprivation therapy combined with radiotherapy as salvage treatment after radical prostatectomy for prostate cancer (GETUG-AFU 16): a 112-month follow-up of a phase 3, randomised trial. *Lancet Oncol.* 2019;20(12):1740–1749. doi:10.1016/S1470-2045(19)30486-3

23. Parker CC, Kynaston H, Cook AD, et al. Duration of androgen deprivation therapy with postoperative radiotherapy for prostate cancer: a comparison of long-course versus short-course androgen deprivation therapy in the RADICALS-HD randomised trial. *Lancet.* 2024;403(10442):2416–2425. doi:10.1016/S0140-6736(24)00549-X

24. Pollack A, Karrison TG, Balogh AG, et al. The addition of androgen deprivation therapy and pelvic lymph node treatment to prostate bed salvage radiotherapy (NRG Oncology/RTOG 0534 SPPORT): an international, multicentre, randomised phase 3 trial. *Lancet.* 2022;399(10338):1886–1901. doi:10.1016/S0140-6736(21)01790-6

25. Shipley WU, Seiferheld W, Lukka HR, et al. Radiation with or without antiandrogen therapy in recurrent prostate cancer. *N Engl J Med.* 2017;376(5):417–428. doi:10.1056/NEJMoa1607529

26. Freedland SJ, Luz MA, De Giorgi U, et al. Improved outcomes with enzalutamide in biochemically recurrent prostate cancer. *N Engl J Med.* 2023;389(16):1453–1465. doi:10.1056/NEJMoa2303974

27. Pisansky TM, Agrawal S, Hamstra DA, et al. Salvage radiation therapy dose response for biochemical failure of prostate cancer after prostatectomy: a multi-institutional observational study. *Int J Radiat Oncol Biol Phys.* 2016;96(5):1046–1053. doi:10.1016/j.ijrobp.2016.08.043

28. Ghadjar P, Hayoz S, Bernhard J, et al. Dose-intensified versus conventional-dose salvage radiotherapy for biochemically recurrent prostate cancer after prostatectomy: the SAKK 09/10 randomized phase 3 trial. *Eur Urol.* 2021;80(3):306–315. doi:10.1016/j.eururo.2021.05.033

29. Buyyounouski MK, Pugh SL, Chen RC, et al. Noninferiority of hypofractionated vs conventional postprostatectomy radiotherapy for genitourinary and gastrointestinal symptoms: the NRG-GU003 phase 3 randomized clinical trial. *JAMA Oncol.* 2024;10(5):584–591. doi:10.1001/jamaoncol.2023.7291

30. Videtic GM, Woody N, Vassil AD. *Handbook of Treatment Planning in Radiation Oncology.* 3rd ed. Demos Medical; 2020.

31. Han M, Partin AW, Zahurak M, Piantadosi S, Epstein JI, Walsh PC. Biochemical (prostate specific antigen) recurrence probability following radical prostatectomy for clinically localized prostate cancer. *J Urol.* 2003;169(2):517–523. doi:10.1016/S0022-5347(05)63946-8

32. Nguyen CT, Reuther AM, Stephenson AJ, Klein EA, Jones JS. The specific definition of high risk prostate cancer has minimal impact on biochemical relapse-free survival. *J Urol.* 2009;181(1):75–80. doi:10.1016/j.juro.2008.09.027

33. Briganti A, Karnes RJ, Di Filippo L, et al. Combination of adjuvant hormonal and radiation therapy significantly prolongs survival of patients with pT2-4 pN+ prostate cancer: results of a matched analysis. *Eur Urol.* 2011;59(5):832–840. doi:10.1016/j.eururo.2011.02.024

34. Daly T, Hickey BE, Lehman M, Francis DP, See AM. Adjuvant radiotherapy following radical prostatectomy for prostate cancer. *Cochrane Database Syst Rev.* 2011;(12):CD007234. doi:10.1002/14651858.CD007234.pub2

35. King CR. The timing of salvage radiotherapy after radical prostatectomy: a systematic review. *Int J Radiat Oncol Biol Phys.* 2012;84(1):104–111. doi:10.1016/j.ijrobp.2011.10.069

36. Hackman G, Taari K, Tammela TL, et al. Randomised trial of adjuvant radiotherapy following radical prostatectomy versus radical prostatectomy alone in prostate cancer patients with positive margins or extracapsular extension. *Eur Urol.* 2019;76(5):586–595. doi:10.1016/j.eururo.2019.07.001

37. Thompson IM, Tangen CM, Paradelo J, et al. Adjuvant radiotherapy for pathological T3N0M0 prostate cancer significantly reduces risk of metastases and improves survival: long-term followup of a randomized clinical trial. *J Urol.* 2009;181(3):956–962. doi:10.1016/j.juro.2008.11.032

38. Bolla M, Van Poppel H, Tombal B, et al. Postoperative radiotherapy after radical prostatectomy for high-risk prostate cancer: long-term results of a randomised controlled trial (EORTC trial 22911). *Lancet.* 2012;380(9858):2018–2027. doi:10.1016/S0140-6736(12)61253-7

39. Wiegel T, Bartkowiak D, Bottke D, et al. Adjuvant radiotherapy versus wait-and-see after radical prostatectomy: 10-year follow-up of the ARO 96-02/AUO AP 09/95 trial. *Eur Urol.* 2014;66(2):243–250. doi:10.1016/j.eururo.2014.03.011

40. Kneebone A, Fraser-Browne C, Duchesne GM, et al. Adjuvant radiotherapy versus early salvage radiotherapy following radical prostatectomy (TROG 08.03/ANZUP RAVES): a randomised, controlled, phase 3, non-inferiority trial. *Lancet Oncol.* 2020;21(10):1331–1340. doi:10.1016/S1470-2045(20)30456-3

41. Parker CC, Clarke NW, Cook AD, et al. Timing of radiotherapy after radical prostatectomy (RADICALS-RT): a randomised, controlled phase 3 trial. *Lancet.* 2020;396(10260):1413–1421. doi:10.1016/S0140-6736(20)31553-1

42. Sargos P, Chabaud S, Latorzeff I, et al. Adjuvant radiotherapy versus early salvage radiotherapy plus short-term androgen deprivation therapy in men with localised prostate cancer after radical prostatectomy (GETUG-AFU 17): a randomised, phase 3 trial. *Lancet Oncol.* 2020;21(10):1341–1352. doi:10.1016/S1470-2045(20)30454-X

43. Vale CL, Fisher D, Kneebone A, et al. Adjuvant or early salvage radiotherapy for the treatment of localised and locally advanced prostate cancer: a prospectively planned systematic review and meta-analysis of aggregate data. *Lancet.* 2020;396(10260):1422–1431. doi:10.1016/S0140-6736(20)31952-8

44. Campbell SR, Tom MC, Agrawal S, et al. Integrating prostate-specific antigen kinetics into contemporary predictive nomograms of salvage radiotherapy after radical prostatectomy. *Eur Urol Oncol.* 2022;5(3):304–313. doi:10.1016/j.euo.2021.04.011

45. Gladwish A, Loblaw A, Cheung P, et al. Accelerated hypofractionated postoperative radiotherapy for prostate cancer: a prospective phase I/II study. *Clin Oncol (R Coll Radiol).* 2015;27(3):145–152. doi:10.1016/j.clon.2014.12.003

46. Katayama S, Striecker T, Kessel K, et al. Hypofractionated IMRT of the prostate bed after radical prostatectomy: acute toxicity in the PRIAMOS-1 trial. *Int J Radiat Oncol Biol Phys.* 2014;90(4):926–933. doi:10.1016/j.ijrobp.2014.07.015

47. Kruser TJ, Jarrard DF, Graf AK, et al. Early hypofractionated salvage radiotherapy for postprostatectomy biochemical recurrence. *Cancer.* 2011;117(12):2629–2636. doi:10.1002/cncr.25824

48. Petersen PM, Cook AD, Sydes MR, et al. Salvage radiation therapy after radical prostatectomy: analysis of toxicity by dose-fractionation in the RADICALS-RT trial. *Int J Radiat Oncol Biol Phys.* 2023;117(3):624–629. doi:10.1016/j.ijrobp.2023.04.032

49. Duchesne GM, Woo HH, Bassett JK, et al. Timing of androgen-deprivation therapy in patients with prostate cancer with a rising PSA (TROG 03.06 and VCOG PR 01-03 [TOAD]): a randomised, multicentre, non-blinded, phase 3 trial. *Lancet Oncol.* 2016;17(6):727–737. doi:10.1016/S1470-2045(16)00107-8

50. Nguyen PL, Kollmeier M, Rathkopf DE, et al. FORMULA-509: a multicenter randomized trial of post-operative salvage radiotherapy (SRT) and 6 months of GnRH agonist with or without abiraterone acetate/prednisone (AAP) and apalutamide (Apa) post-radical prostatectomy (RP). *J Clin Oncol.* 2023;41(6 suppl):303. doi:10.1200/JCO.2023.41.6_suppl.303

51. Messing EM, Manola J, Yao J, et al. Immediate versus deferred androgen deprivation treatment in patients with node-positive prostate cancer after radical prostatectomy and pelvic lymphadenectomy. *Lancet Oncol.* 2006;7(6):472–479. doi:10.1016/S1470-2045(06)70700-8

52. Abdollah F, Karnes RJ, Suardi N, et al. Impact of adjuvant radiotherapy on survival of patients with node-positive prostate cancer. *J Clin Oncol.* 2014;32(35):3939–3947. doi:10.1200/JCO.2013.54.7893

53. Tilki D, Chen MH, Wu J, Huland H, Graefen M, D'Amico AV. Adjuvant versus early salvage radiation therapy after radical prostatectomy for pN1 prostate cancer and the risk of death. *J Clin Oncol.* 2022;40(20):2186–2192. doi:10.1200/JCO.21.02800

7. Briganti A, Karnes RJ, Di Filippo L, et al. Combination of adjuvant hormonal and radiation therapy significantly prolongs survival of patients with pT2-4 pN+ prostate cancer: results of a matched analysis. *Eur Urol*. 2009;55(3):922–930. doi:10.1016/j.eururo.2011.02.10

8. Daly T, Hickey BE, Lehman M, Francis DP, See AM. Adjuvant radiotherapy following radical prostatectomy for prostate cancer. *Cochrane Database Syst Rev*. 2011;12(12):CD007234. doi:10.1002/14651858.CD007234.pub2

9. King CR. Adjuvant or salvage radiotherapy after radical prostatectomy: a complex convergence of paths. *Int J Radiat Oncol Biol Phys*. 2011;80(4):1046–1047. doi:10.1016/j.ijrobp.2011.01.005

10. Ghadjar P, Hayoz S, Bernhard J, et al. Acute toxicity and quality of life after dose-intensified salvage radiation therapy for biochemically recurrent prostate cancer after prostatectomy: first results of the randomized trial SAKK 09/10. *J Clin Oncol*. 2015;33(35):4158–4166. doi:10.1200/JCO.2015.63.3529

11. Stephenson AJ, Shariat SF, Zelefsky MJ, et al. Salvage radiotherapy for recurrent prostate cancer after radical prostatectomy. *JAMA*. 2004;291(11):1325–1332. doi:10.1001/jama.291.11.1325

12. Trock BJ, Han M, Freedland SJ, et al. Prostate cancer-specific survival following salvage radiotherapy vs observation in men with biochemical recurrence after radical prostatectomy. *JAMA*. 2008;299(23):2760–2769. doi:10.1001/jama.299.23.2760

43 BLADDER CANCER

Winston Vuong, Erik M. Davies, Omar Y. Mian, and Rahul D. Tendulkar

QUICK HIT Bladder cancer is the second most common GU malignancy, and >90% are urothelial carcinomas. About 70% have superficial disease and are managed with TURBT ± intravesical therapy (Table 43.1). Patients with muscle-invasive disease (MIBC) are most often managed with radical cystectomy and perioperative CHT. Selective bladder preservation (SBP) may be utilized in certain patients. Up to 80% achieve a CR to induction CRT, and 70% to 80% will remain free of local recurrence (LR) and retain their native bladder.

Table 43.1 General Treatment Paradigm for Bladder Cancer[1]	
	Treatment Options
Non–muscle-invasive bladder cancer (NMIBC; Ta, Tis, T1)	TURBT followed by surveillance OR intravesical therapy (BCG vs. mitomycin) OR cystectomy (for high risk); BCG + immunotherapy (IO) is an emerging option for high-risk NMIBC[2]
NMIBC, BCG unresponsive or intolerant	Cystectomy (preferred); alternatives include intravesical CHT, IO (pembrolizumab or nogapendekin alfa inbakicept-pmln with BCG), gene therapy with nadofaragene firadenovec-vncg, or definitive CRT
Stage II/IIIA (cT2–4aN0; cT1–4a N1)	Radical cystectomy + neoadjuvant cisplatin-based CHT (if eligible) OR SBP*: Maximal TURBT + CRT (64 Gy/32 fx or 55 Gy/20 fx); less preferred alternatives include cystectomy alone for patients ineligible for cisplatin, RT alone if neither cystectomy nor CRT candidate, or TURBT
Stage IIIB (cT1–4aN2–3)	Induction systemic therapy with response-adapted consolidation (see below) OR Definitive CRT *Consolidation: If CR/PR, consider cystectomy vs. CRT (surveillance an option for CR); if PR/PD, systemic therapy*
Stage IVA (cT4b or M1a)	Systemic therapy (any stage IVA) OR CRT (for cT4bM0) Consolidation recommended regardless of response with either more systemic therapy, CRT, or cystectomy depending on prior therapy; can consider consolidative local therapy for select M1a after CR to systemic therapy
Metastatic stage IVB	Enfortumab vedotin + pembrolizumab ± palliative RT as needed; alternatives are dependent on cisplatin-eligibility: Cisplatin-eligible: gemcitabine/cisplatin + maintenance avelumab or nivolumab/gemcitabine/cisplatin + maintenance nivolumab Cisplatin-ineligible: gemcitabine/carboplatin + maintenance avelumab
Adjuvant	If no neoadjuvant CHT with pT3–4a/N+, consider adjuvant cisplatin-based regimen or nivolumab If ypT2–4a/ypN+ after neoadjuvant CHT, consider nivolumab If pT3-4/N+ or positive margins, consider adjuvant RT

*With response-adapted management based on surveillance CT CAP with contrast and cystoscopies; if no tumor after 2–3 months, continue surveillance. If recurrent Tis/Ta/T1, consider TURBT ± intravesical therapy. If persistent T2, consider salvage cystectomy. If residual tumor after RT alone or TURBT alone, then consider systemic therapy or TURBT ± intravesical therapy. Optimal candidates for SBP: unifocal tumor <5 cm after complete TURBT, cT2–T3 (and selected T4a), cN0, adequate bladder function, compliant with surveillance protocol, no hydronephrosis, no associated CIS, no IBD, no prior RT.
Source: Data from NCCN Guidelines. Bladder Cancer. v6.2024 - January 17, 2025.

EPIDEMIOLOGY: In 2024, ~83,200 new cases, 3:1 male:female ratio, ~17,000 deaths.[3] Median age 70 years.[4] Highest rates in North America/Western Europe.[5]

RISK FACTORS: Majority of cases are related to environmental exposures. Smoking is the most important, with relative risk of 2 to 5 compared with nonsmokers, and is associated with about 50% of cases. Others include chemical exposures (industrial aromatic amines, polycyclic aromatic hydrocarbons, hair dyes, chlorinated water, arsenic), drugs (phenacetin-containing analgesics, cyclophosphamide), schistosomiasis (associated with squamous cell carcinoma [SCC]), chronic inflammation (chronic UTIs, cystitis, stones), and radiation exposure.[5]

ANATOMY: The bladder is divided into the body (above the ureteral orifices), the trigone (area between the ureteral and urethral orifices), and the bladder neck. Layers from internal to external: urothelium (epithelial lining made up of transitional cells bounded by a thin basement membrane), lamina propria (thick layer of fibroelastic connective tissue), and detrusor muscle (smooth muscle arranged in inner longitudinal, middle circular, and outer longitudinal layers). The bladder is anchored to the anterior abdominal wall by the urachus. It is bounded superiorly by peritoneum, and anteriorly/inferiorly/laterally by perivesical fat. Primary LN drainage includes external iliac, internal iliac, obturator, perivesical, and presacral nodes. The common iliacs are a secondary drainage site.[6]

PATHOLOGY: Urothelial carcinoma (>90% of cases in the United States), SCC (~3%), adenocarcinoma (ACA, ~2%), small cell carcinoma (~1%), all others <1% (sarcomas, lymphomas, melanoma, mets). More aggressive urothelial subtypes include micropapillary, plasmacytoid, nested, and sarcomatoid histologies, which may warrant more aggressive management. In *Schistosoma haematobium* endemic areas, SCCs comprise the majority of cases. Urachal tumors are commonly ACA and have better outcomes than nonurachal ACA.

CLINICAL PRESENTATION: Gross or microscopic hematuria is the most common presenting symptom. If gross hematuria, risk of a bladder tumor is 10% to 20%. Less commonly, patients may note obstructive/irritative bladder symptoms or pain.

WORKUP: H&P.

Labs: Urine cytology. Cytology has poor sensitivity (34%) but high specificity (>98%).[7] CBC, CMP, alkaline phosphatase.

Procedures: Cystoscopy. If a suspicious lesion is noted in the bladder, proceeding to transurethral resection of bladder tumor (TURBT) is the standard of care, although cystoscopic biopsy and mpMRI are emerging as a new diagnostic paradigm.[8] TURBT is diagnostic and often therapeutic for T1 disease. Random or targeted biopsies of sites adjacent to the tumor are performed to assess for field defect/CIS, as well as biopsy of the prostate in men. The bladder biopsy specimen should include muscle to assess for invasion. Patients undergoing orthotopic neobladder reconstruction with urethral anastomosis must have a confirmed negative urethral margin first.[9]

Imaging: If cystoscopic appearance of the tumor is solid, high grade, or MIBC, consider CT or MRI of abdomen and pelvis prior to TURBT. In cases of suspected MIBC, mpMRI after cystoscopic biopsy rather than immediate TURBT potentially shortens time to correct therapy.[8] The entire urinary tract should be imaged (e.g., CT urogram with and without contrast including delayed images or MRI urogram). Obtain chest imaging if muscle-invasive. Bone scan if alkaline phosphatase elevated or bone pain. PET/CT should be reserved for further evaluation of abnormal conventional staging. Neuroimaging only for symptomatic or high-risk patients, such as those with small cell histology.

PROGNOSTIC FACTORS: Stage (Table 43.2), grade, multicentricity, size, recurrence, presence of CIS, LVI, growth pattern, histology.

STAGING

Table 43.2 AJCC 8th Edition (2017): Staging for Urinary Bladder Cancer					
T/M	N	cN0	cN1	cN2	cN3
T1	• Invades lamina propria (subepithelial connective tissue)	I			
T2	a. Invades muscularis propria (inner half)	II			
	b. Invades muscularis propria (outer half)		IIIA		IIIB
T3	a. Invades perivesical tissue (microscopic)				
	b. Invades perivesical tissue (macroscopic)				
T4	a. Invades prostatic stroma, seminal vesicles, uterus, vagina				
	b. Invades pelvic wall or abdominal wall	IVA			
M1a	Nonregional LNs				
M1b	Distant metastasis	IVB			

cN1: single pelvic node (perivesicular, obturator, internal iliac, external iliac, or sacral); cN2: multiple LNs in the true pelvis; cN3: common iliac LNs.

NATURAL HISTORY: DM comprises the primary mode of recurrence for pure urothelial carcinoma (~45% of all CRT patients), while invasive LRR makes up ~15% to 20%.[10] Small cell neuroendocrine carcinomas are also primarily driven by distant recurrence, with up to 10% metastasizing to the CNS.[11] Plasmacytoid subtypes have a propensity to grow along the fascial planes and have a high risk of intraperitoneal metatasis.[12] In contrast, morbidity and mortality for nonmetastatic pure SCC of the bladder are driven by LRR.[13] Micropapillary and sarcomatoid tumors are subtypes in which immediate cystectomy might be considered for non–muscle-invasive disease. Bladder neck involvement is associated with urethral recurrences in men (particularly with prostatic stromal involvement with upwards of 20% urethral recurrence) and women in cystectomy series, and an elective urethral CTV is recommended to encompass the proximal urethra in CRT planning.[14,15] Extensive bladder neck involvement in women potentially increases the risk of poor urinary function following RT.[16]

TREATMENT PARADIGM

Surgery

TURBT: First step in diagnosis and is therapeutic for Ta/Tis/T1 non–muscle-invasive disease. Observation can be considered after TURBT in select patients with Ta or low-grade T1 disease without risk factors. Adjuvant intravesical therapy recommended for Tis, high-grade Ta or T1, positive cytology, recurrent disease, or multifocality. TURBT for maximal debulking is recommended as the initial step in patients considering SBP for MIBC.

Cystectomy: Radical cystectomy with urinary diversion is a standard of care for multiple recurrent superficial tumors, high-grade T1 tumors with CIS, MIBC, and variant histologies. The technique includes en bloc resection of the bladder, peritoneal covering, urachus, perivesical fat, lower ureters, bilateral pelvic LNs, proximal urethra (men), entire urethra (all women, and men with CIS/multicentric tumors/involvement of bladder neck or prostatic urethra), prostate, seminal vesicles, pelvic vas deferens (men), uterus, fallopian tubes, ovaries, cervix, and vaginal cuff (women). A bilateral pelvic lymphadenectomy should be performed and include at a minimum the obturator, external iliac, and internal iliac LNs. SWOG 8710 demonstrated improved survival when at least 10 LNs were removed.[17] SWOG S1011 suggests dissecting beyond the standard template may increase morbidity and mortality without benefit in DFS or OS.[18]

Urinary Diversions: Diversion may be either noncontinent or continent. Historically, noncontinent diversions were standard (e.g., ileal conduit). Advances in technique resulted in continent diversion for most patients in the modern era. Broadly, these techniques are categorized as continent cutaneous diversions (e.g., Kock, Indiana, Miami pouches) that require self-catheterization or (more commonly) orthotopic neobladders that connect directly to the native urethra using the external sphincter for continence.

Intravesical Therapy: Allows for high concentrations of agents to be delivered locally to eradicate viable tumor and prevent recurrences. BCG is a live attenuated *Mycobacterium bovis* that functions via an antitumor immunostimulatory mechanism and is considered the adjuvant treatment of choice for high-risk NMIBC (Ta, Tis, or T1 tumors) after TURBT. BCG is initiated 3 to 4 weeks after resection and given weekly for 6 weeks. Meta-analyses have shown BCG to be superior to mitomycin C in NMIBC.[19,20] Common toxicities of BCG include urinary frequency (71%), cystitis (67%), fever (25%), and hematuria (23%).[10] Note that the frequency and dysuria associated with BCG treatment can be severe and many patients do not complete the full 6-week course due to acute toxicity.

Chemotherapy: Can be used perioperatively before or after cystectomy, concurrent with RT as part of bladder preservation therapy, or in the metastatic setting. Evidence is stronger for neoadjuvant CHT before cystectomy rather than for adjuvant—a meta-analysis demonstrated a 5% survival benefit with neoadjuvant platinum-based CHT compared with surgery alone.[21] Current and future trials are assessing the addition of IO in the nonmetastatic setting.

Perioperative: Cisplatin-based regimens including dose-dense methotrexate (MTX); vinblastine, doxorubicin, and cisplatin (DD-MVAC); gemcitabine/cisplatin; and MTX, cisplatin, and vinblastine (MCV). The different regimens have not been directly compared in randomized trials.

Concurrent With RT: NCCN-preferred regimens for concurrent CHT include cisplatin alone (35–40 mg/m^2 weekly; carboplatin is not an acceptable alternative), low-dose gemcitabine (27 mg/m^2

twice per week of conventional RT[22] or 100 mg/m² once per week for hypofractionated RT[23]), or 5-FU/mitomycin-C (BC2001; 5-FU 500 mg/m² on fx 1–5 and 16–20 with mitomycin C 12 mg/m² on day 1).[24] Carbogen can be considered per BCON using 2% CO_2 and 98% O_2 at 15 L/min via closed face mask 5 minutes before and during each fraction, with nicotinamide given PO 40 to 60 mg/kg 1.5 to 2 hours before each fx.[25]

Adjuvant: CheckMate247 demonstrated a DFS and OS benefit to 1 year of adjuvant nivolumab in patients with high-risk disease (ypT2–T4 or N+ disease, or no NAC and pT3–T4a or N+ disease) following radical cystectomy.[26] Adjuvant pembrolizumab has also shown a DFS benefit in high-risk MIBC with the above criteria including those with positive margins.[27] This stands in contrast to the IMvigor010 trial, which showed no DFS improvement with adjuvant atezolizumab.[28] The role of concurrent and adjuvant IO following bladder preservation is unclear.

Metastatic: Enfortumab vedotin with pembrolizumab is the standard-of-care first-line systemic therapy regardless of cisplatin eligibility.[29]

Radiation

Indications: RT may be given for organ preservation as an alternative to cystectomy (SBP), as definitive management in nonsurgical candidates or those who refuse cystectomy, or palliatively. The role of adjuvant RT after cystectomy is evolving, but it may be considered for select cases of pT3–4/N+, positive margins, or ECE (54–60 Gy to positive margin with tumor bed and pelvic nodes to 45–50.4 Gy).[30]

Selective Bladder Preservation (SBP): Ideal candidates include those with a unifocal tumor <5 cm after complete TURBT, cT2–T3 (and selected T4a), cN0, adequate bladder function, compliant with surveillance protocol, no hydronephrosis, no associated CIS, no IBD, and no prior pelvic RT. SBP can be considered in patients with unilateral hydronephrosis, typically following ureteral stenting.

Historical Schema: Maximal TURBT → CRT 40–45 Gy → cystoscopy → if CR (T0/Tis/Ta) boost to ~64 Gy → surveillance. If → T1 on cystoscopy after induction CRT, proceed to salvage cystectomy. Interim cystoscopy may be avoided in patients who are not surgical candidates.

Dose: Multiple regimens have been used, typically treating the pelvis to 40 to 45 Gy followed by a boost to ~64 Gy at 1.8–2.0 Gy/fx. An alternative fractionation is 55 Gy/20 fx, which was associated with good LRC.[31] Elective nodal irradiation (ENI) was typically utilized in RTOG trials, but not in BC2001. ENI is appropriate in high-risk patients, for example, T3/T4 tumors, variant histology, or clinically N1 patients. For clinical N+ disease, consider boosting the involved node up to prescription dose if safely achievable.

Toxicity: Acute: fatigue, nausea, diarrhea, urinary urgency, frequency. Late: cystitis, fibrosis, proctitis, enteritis.

Procedure: See *Handbook of Treatment Planning in Radiation Oncology*, Chapter 8.[32]

EVIDENCE-BASED Q&A

What is the rationale for selective bladder preservation?

Strategies to preserve the native bladder and avoid the potential complications of radical cystectomy and urinary diversion are appealing, particularly for those who are older adults or with significant comorbidities. A series of phase II trials were conducted by the RTOG in the 1980s to 1990s.[33–39] Pooled analysis of these trials demonstrated low rates of toxicity with survival outcomes similar to historical cystectomy series for clinically staged patients.[40] There have been no randomized trials directly comparing SBP with radical cystectomy. Of note, clinical understaging is common and SBP patients are generally older with more comorbidities; therefore, caution must be taken when comparing retrospective series of SBP vs. cystectomy.

Mak, RTOG Pooled Analysis (*JCO* 2014, PMID 25366678): Pooled analysis of five RTOG prospective phase II trials; 468 patients, clinical T2 (61%), T3 (35%), T4 (4%). Following CRT, CR was observed in 69% of patients; 5-year OS associated with T stage: 62% for T2 vs. 49% for T3–4 (*p* = .002); see Table 43.3 for overall results. **Conclusion: Long-term DSS with SBP is comparable to cystectomy series and can be considered as an alternative to surgery.**

Table 43.3 RTOG Pooled Analysis of Selective Bladder Trials

	OS	DSS	Muscle-Invasive LF	Non–Muscle-Invasive LF	DM
5 yrs	57%	71%	13%	31%	31%
10 yrs	36%	65%	14%	36%	35%

Zlotta (*Lancet Oncol* 2023, PMID 37187202): Multi-institutional RR of 722 patients with cT2–4N0M0 MIBC who would be eligible for either trimodality therapy (TMT) or cystectomy to compare the clinical outcomes associated with each therapy against a propensity-matched cohort. The primary endpoint was MFS, and secondary endpoints were OS, CSS, and DFS. MFU 4.4 years in the cystectomy group and 4.9 years in the TMT group. Age, sex, stage, presence of hydronephrosis, and receipt of neoadjuvant or adjuvant CHT were similar between groups. The 5-year MFS was 74% with cystectomy and 75% with TMT (NS). No difference in 5-year CSS or DFS. OS was superior among the TMT group at 5 years (66% cystectomy vs. 73%; HR 0.70, $p = .1$). **Conclusion: TMT is comparable to cystectomy in terms of 5-year MFS, CSS, and DFS in this matched cohort analysis. There may be a 5-year OS benefit to TMT. Consider TMT in all suitable candidates, not only the medically inoperable population.**

Are the rates of toxicity after SBP prohibitive?

Although survival rates are comparable to cystectomy, there is concern regarding late effects. The RTOG pooled analysis suggests high-grade toxicity is uncommon; late grade 3+ toxicity rates were 6% GU and 2% GI. No late grade 4 events, and no patients required a cystectomy due to treatment-related toxicity.[41] Furthermore, patient-reported QOL outcomes from the BC2001 trial discussed in the following reported similar reductions in QOL between arms immediately following treatment, which improved to pretreatment baseline after 6 months, with no evidence that the addition of CHT impairs QOL long term.[42]

Is there a benefit to neoadjuvant/induction CHT prior to SBP?

Neoadjuvant CHT improves survival when delivered prior to radical cystectomy.[21] The older RTOG 8903 trial tested this concept in the SBP setting, but both this trial and other retrospective series showed no benefit to neoadjuvant CHT prior to definitive CRT.[40] This is being revisited with suggestion of potential benefit in more locally advanced disease and is an NCCN-recommended option for stage IIIB/IVA patients.[43]

Shipley, RTOG 8903 (*JCO* 1998, PMID 9817278): PRT to assess the addition of neoadjuvant CHT to SBP. 123 patients with cT2–4a MIBC received TURBT and then randomized to ± 2 cycles of neoadjuvant MCV (methotrexate, cisplatin, vinblastine). All patients were treated to a dose of 39.6 Gy at 1.8 Gy/fx to pelvic field with cisplatin, then underwent cystoscopy at 4 weeks. If <CR, patients proceeded to cystectomy. If CR, patients received a 25.2 Gy tumor boost with cisplatin. No difference in CR rate (61% vs. 55%), 5-year OS (48% vs. 49%), DM (33% vs. 39%), or survival with intact bladder (36% vs. 40%). **Conclusion: Neoadjuvant CHT prior to SBP increased toxicity without improving outcomes.**

Does the addition of CHT to RT improve outcomes with definitive (nonoperative) management?

LR rates with RT alone are high, and early data suggested a benefit to concurrent CHT.[44] This led to the UK Bladder Cancer 2001 (BC2001) trial.[24]

James, BC2001 (*NEJM* 2012, PMID 22512481): PRT of 360 patients with T2–T4a bladder cancer (ACA, TCC, and SCC included). Allowed but did not require neoadjuvant CHT. Randomized to RT alone vs. RT and concurrent CHT with 5-FU 500 mg/m^2 on days 1 to 5 and 16 to 20 and mitomycin C 12 mg/m^2 on day 1. RT either 55 Gy/20 fx or 64 Gy/32 fx, and the pelvic nodes were not electively targeted. Of note, midtreatment cystoscopy was not performed on this protocol; as a result, all patients were treated definitively. Primary endpoint was LRFS. See Table 43.4 for the results. **Conclusion: The addition of 5-FU/MMC to RT improves LRFS over RT alone without significant difference in OS (but not powered for OS). This benefit persisted at 10-year follow-up.[25]**

Table 43.4 UK BC2001 Trial of Definitive RT for Bladder Cancer

BC2001	2-Yr LRFS	Invasive LR	Noninvasive LR	2-Yr Cystectomy	5-Yr OS
RT	54%	19%	17%	17%	35%
CRT	67%	11%	14%	11%	48%
p value	.03	.01		.03	.16

What are some of the CHT regimens utilized for SBP in the modern era?

Cisplatin-based CHT regimens predominate in North America because these are the regimens that have been evaluated by the RTOG. For patients who may not be candidates for platinum-based CHT due to hearing impairment, renal dysfunction, or poor performance status, there have been recent efforts to establish platinum-free CRT regimens. Per BC2001, 5-FU/MMC is an option. Most recently, the RTOG 0712 trial utilized 5-FU/cisplatin + BID RT vs. low-dose gemcitabine + daily RT.[22]

Coen, NRG/RTOG 0712 (*JCO* 2019, PMID 30433852): Phase II PRT in MIBC randomizing 66 patients to FCT (5-FU/cisplatin) concurrent with RT delivered BID vs. GD (gemcitabine) concurrent with RT delivered once daily. Patients underwent TURBT and induction CRT to 40 Gy. Those achieving CR received consolidation CRT to 64 Gy. Non-CR had cystectomy performed. Patients on both arms were to receive adjuvant gemcitabine + cisplatin (GC). Primary endpoint: rate of freedom from DM at 3 years (DMF3). DMF3 was 78% and 84% for FCT and GD, respectively. Postinduction CR rates were 88% and 78%, respectively. In the FCT arm, 64% experienced treatment-related grade 3/4 acute toxicities, majority hematologic. In the GD arm, grade 3/4 acute toxicity was 55%, majority hematologic. **Conclusion: Both regimens exceeded the primary endpoint demonstrating a DMF3 greater than 75%. The trial was not powered to compare regimens. Fewer toxicities seen in the GD arm. Either arm would be acceptable to use as a base in future trials.**

Do target volumes need to include the entire bladder? Is there a benefit to ENI?

Given the difficulties with tumor localization as well as the propensity for multifocality of bladder cancer, standard RT techniques included the entire bladder in the target volume, even in localized disease. However, sparing the uninvolved bladder could potentially reduce toxicity, leading to interest in partial bladder-sparing techniques, which was assessed by the BC2001 trial. Most RTOG trials incorporate ENI using a "minipelvis" field, with the superior border at S2 to S3 to allow sparing of bowel in the potential future event of a urinary diversion. BC2001 did not intentionally target elective nodes, but did include the low pelvis/obturator nodes given the field design of whole bladder + 1.5 cm margin. Only 10 of 76 LRRs were in the pelvic nodes. A recent multi-RR of 599 MIBC patients including 369 who underwent whole pelvic radiation suggests a potential survival benefit to pelvic RT.[45]

Huddart, BC2001 (*IJROBP* 2013, PMID 23958147): A total of 219 patients (subset of BC2001) randomized to standard whole bladder RT (PTV included outer bladder wall + extravesical extent of tumor + 1.5 cm) vs. reduced high-dose volume RT (2 PTVs defined: PTV1 was the same as the control group and was treated to 80% of the prescribed dose, and PTV2 was defined as GTV + 1.5 cm). Patients were simulated with bladder empty. No difference in 2-year LRFS (61% vs. 64%), grades 3 to 4 acute toxicities (23% vs. 23%), 2-year grades 3 to 4 late toxicities (2% vs. 5%), or reduction in bladder capacity (76 mL difference favoring the reduced RT volume group; NS). **Conclusion: No differences in 2-year LRFS or late toxicity with reduced high-dose volume RT.**

Marcq, Canadian Multi-Institutional Cohort (*JCO* 2024, PMID 39361935): An inverse-probability treatment weighted analysis of 599 patients with cT2–4aN0–2M0 MIBC who underwent whole pelvic RT (WPRT) or bladder-only (BO) RT. Receipt of WPRT (369/599 patients, 62%) was associated with improved CSS (HR 0.66, *p* = .016) and OS (HR 0.68, *p* = .002), although patients who received WPRT were younger with better ECOG PS but also had more N+ disease and LVI. These patients were also more likely to receive neoadjuvant and concurrent CHT. **Conclusion: WPRT potentially confers improved CSS and OS, particularly in fit patients with N+ disease or with LVI, although randomized controlled trials are necessary for confirmation.**

Is there a benefit to hypofractionation?

The two most common fractionation schemes, 64 Gy/32 fx and 55 Gy/20 fx, have not been directly compared head-to-head in an RCT; however, a meta-analysis of the BC2001 and BCON trials supports the use of the hypofractionated schedule.[30]

Choudhury, BC2001/BCON Meta-Analysis (*Lancet Oncol* 2021, PMID 33539743): An individual patient data meta-analysis of 782 patients from the BC2001 trial (456 patients) and the BCON trial (326 patients) who had undergone SBP with either 64 Gy/32 fx or 55 Gy/20 fx (48% and 52% of the total cohort, respectively). With an MFU of 10 years, 55 Gy/20 fx was noninferior to 64 Gy/32 fx with respect to invasive LRR and bowel or bladder toxicity. The hypofractionated schedule was superior with regard to invasive LRR (HR 0.71, 95% CI 0.52–0.96). **Conclusion: SBP with hypofractionation, 55 Gy/20 fx, has superior invasive locoregional control and is iso-toxic compared with 64 Gy/32 fx.**

Is there a benefit to hyperfractionation?

Evidence for hyperfractionation is mixed, as two older PRTs showed improved outcomes with hyperfractionation over standard fractionation, while a more recent PRT demonstrated no benefit and increased toxicity.[46] None of these trials included concurrent CHT, and thus the role of hyperfractionation is unclear in this setting. However, hyperfractionated CRT was one of the arms in the completed RTOG 0712 phase II randomized trial and may be considered in select patients.

Is there a benefit to adjuvant RT after cystectomy?

Adjuvant RT after cystectomy is rarely utilized. However, certain patient populations are known to have high rates of LF (~30% for T3–4, ~70% for positive margins).[17] A randomized trial published in 1992 demonstrated an LC and DFS benefit in patients with T3–T4 disease; however, 80% of the patients on this study had SCC.[47] A patterns-of-failure analysis showed that in patients with negative margins and >pT3 disease, 76% of all LF sites would have been covered within a small CTV covering only the iliac/obturator nodes, which would limit dose to the bowel and neobladder. In patients with positive margins, failure in the cystectomy bed and presacral nodes increases substantially, necessitating larger CTV and the subsequent increase in potential toxicity, leading to consensus contouring guidelines.[30,48] An NCDB analysis found that PORT was associated with improved OS, although this must be confirmed in prospective trials.[33] Two randomized phase II trials have reported a potential LRFS benefit to adjuvant RT compared with observation[49] or adjuvant CHT as part of a sandwich approach with low rates of grade 3 toxicity.[50] The acute and late toxicities from the BART trial have shown ~10% risk of grades 3 to 4 late toxicities and cumulative 23% risk of grade 2+ toxicity, although oncologic outcomes have not yet been reported.[51] RT in this trial was delivered within 8 weeks of surgery or last adjuvant CHT.

Is there a role for RT in select cases of T1 non–muscle-invasive disease?

TURBT followed by intravesical therapy is the standard of care for most patients with high-grade NMIBC. However, many will still recur locally after this approach. For recurrent disease, standard therapy is cystectomy, although novel therapies are being explored (see Table 43.1). RT may offer a bladder-sparing option for some patients with high-grade T1 or recurrent T1 cancers after BCG.

Dahl, RTOG 0926 (*JCO* 2024, PMID 39226514): Single-arm phase II trial of 37 patients with recurrent high-grade non-MIBC (T1Nx/0M0) after TURBT followed by intravesicular BCG or CHT. All patients underwent TURBT followed by concurrent CRT (41.4 Gy/23 fx to pelvis and whole bladder boost to 61.2 Gy/34 fx + cisplatin or MMC/5-FU). MFU 5.1 years. The 3-year freedom from cystectomy rate was 88%, meeting the primary endpoint. OS at 3 and 5 years was 69% and 56%, respectively. Twelve patients (32%) had LR at 3 years. Eighteen patients (48%) had grade 3 AEs and one grade 4 AEs. **Conclusion: Trimodality therapy is a bladder preservation option for patients with recurrent high-grade, NMIBC, and will be the basis for the forthcoming NRG GU014 phase II study randomizing high grade T1 bladder cancers to pembrolizumab + RT vs. CRT.**

Is there a role for palliative radiation?

Duchesne, MRC BA09 (*IJROBP* 2000, PMID 10802363): PRT of 500 patients (272 evaluable) with symptomatic MIBC considered unsuitable for curative treatment due to staging (T4b, N1, or M1) or comorbidity. Randomized to 21 Gy/3 fx QOD vs. 35 Gy/10 fx QD. Primary endpoint was symptomatic improvement at 3 months. Results: At 3 months, there was no statistically significant difference in symptomatic improvement between the two arms (71% for 35 Gy vs. 64% for 21 Gy). **Conclusion: 21 Gy/3 fx delivered QOD is a reasonable option for palliation of MIBC.**

REFERENCES

1. National Comprehensive Cancer Network. *NCCN Clinical Practice Guidelines in Oncology: Bladder Cancer.* Version 6.2024. Published January 17, 2025. https://www.nccn.org/professionals/physician_gls/pdf/bladder.pdf

2. Steinberg GD, Shore ND, Redorta JP, et al. CREST: phase III study of sasanlimab and Bacillus Calmette-Guérin for patients with Bacillus Calmette-Guérin-naïve high-risk non-muscle-invasive bladder cancer. *Future Oncol.* 2024;20(14):891–901. doi:10.2217/fon-2023-0271

3. Siegel RL, Giaquinto AN, Jemal A. Cancer statistics, 2024. *CA Cancer J Clin.* 2024;74(1):12–49. doi:10.3322/caac.21820

4. Scosyrev E, Noyes K, Feng C, Messing E. Sex and racial differences in bladder cancer presentation and mortality in the US. *Cancer.* 2008;115(1):68–74. doi:10.1002/cncr.23986

5. Pelucchi C, Bosetti C, Negri E, Malvezzi M, La Vecchia C. Mechanisms of disease: the epidemiology of bladder cancer. *Nat Clin Pract Urol.* 2006;3(6):327–340. doi:10.1038/ncpuro0510

6. Edge SB, Byrd DR, Compton CC, Fritz AG, Greene FL, Trotti A, eds. *AJCC Cancer Staging Manual.* 7th ed. Springer; 2010. doi:10.1007/978-0-387-88441-7

7. Lotan Y, Roehrborn CG. Sensitivity and specificity of commonly available bladder tumor markers versus cytology: results of a comprehensive literature review and meta-analyses. *Urology.* 2003;61(1):109–118. doi:10.1016/s0090-4295(02)02136-2

8. Bryan RT, Liu W, Pirrie SJ, et al. Randomized comparison of magnetic resonance imaging versus transurethral resection for staging new bladder cancers: results from the prospective BladderPath trial. *J Clin Oncol.* 2025;43(1):JCO.23.02398. doi:10.1200/JCO.23.02398

9. Holzbeierlein J, Bixler BR, Buckley DI, et al. Treatment of non-metastatic muscle-invasive bladder cancer: AUA/ASCO/SUO guideline (2017; amended 2020, 2024). *J Urol.* 2024;212(1):3–10. doi:10.1097/ju.0000000000003981

10. Hall E, Hussain SA, Porta N, et al. Chemoradiotherapy in muscle-invasive bladder cancer: 10-yr follow-up of the phase 3 randomised controlled BC2001 trial. *Eur Urol.* 2022;82(3):273–279. doi:10.1016/j.eururo.2022.04.017

11. Moussa MJ, Tabet GC, Siefker-Radtke AO, et al. Histopathologic progression and metastatic relapse outcomes in small cell neuroendocrine carcinomas of the urinary tract. *Cancer Med.* 2025;14(2):e70594. doi:10.1002/cam4.70594

12. Sood A, Rudzinski JK, Labbate CV, et al. Long-term oncological outcomes in patients diagnosed with non-metastatic plasmacytoid variant of bladder cancer: a 20-year University of Texas MD Anderson Cancer Center experience. *J Urol.* 2024;211(2):241–255. doi:10.1097/JU.0000000000003778

13. Vlachou E, Johnson BA, Baraban E, Nadal R, Hoffman-Censits J. Current advances in the management of nonurothelial subtypes of bladder cancer. *Am Soc Clin Oncol Educ Book.* 2024;44(3):e438640. doi:10.1200/EDBK_438640

14. Kanaroglou A, Shayegan B. Management of the urethra in urothelial bladder cancer. *CUAJ.* 2013;3(6-S4):S211–S214. doi:10.5489/cuaj.1198

15. Portner R, Bajaj A, Elumalai T, et al. A practical approach to bladder preservation with hypofractionated radiotherapy for localised muscle-invasive bladder cancer. *Clin Transl Radiat Oncol.* 2021;31:1–7. doi:10.1016/j.ctro.2021.08.003

16. Feldman AS, Kulkarni GS, Bivalacqua TJ, et al. Surgical challenges and considerations in tri-modal therapy for muscle invasive bladder cancer. *Urol Oncol.* 2022;40(10):442–450. doi:10.1016/j.urolonc.2021.01.013

17. Herr HW, Faulkner JR, Grossman HB, et al. Surgical factors influence bladder cancer outcomes: a cooperative group report. *J Clin Oncol.* 2004;22(14):2781–2789. doi:10.1200/jco.2004.11.024

18. Lerner SP, Tangen C, Svatek RS, et al. Standard or extended lymphadenectomy for muscle-invasive bladder cancer. *N Engl J Med.* 2024;391(13):1206–1216. doi:10.1056/NEJMoa2401497

19. Sylvester RJ, van der Meijden APM, Witjes JA, Kurth K. Bacillus Calmette-Guérin versus chemotherapy for the intravesical treatment of patients with carcinoma in situ of the bladder: a meta-analysis of the published results of randomized clinical trials. *J Urol.* 2005;174(1):86–91. doi:10.1097/01.ju.0000162059.64886.1c

20. Shelley MD, Court JB, Kynaston H, Wilt TJ, Fish RG, Mason M. Intravesical Bacillus Calmette-Guérin in Ta and T1 bladder cancer. *Cochrane Database Syst Rev.* 2000;(4):CD001986. doi:10.1002/14651858.CD001986

21. Vale CL. Neoadjuvant chemotherapy in invasive bladder cancer: a systematic review and meta-analysis. *Lancet.* 2003;361(9373):1927–1934. doi:10.1016/s0140-6736(03)13580-5

22. Coen JJ, Zhang P, Saylor PJ, et al. Bladder preservation with twice-a-day radiation plus fluorouracil/cisplatin or once daily radiation plus gemcitabine for muscle-invasive bladder cancer: NRG/RTOG 0712—a randomized phase II trial. *J Clin Oncol.* 2019;37(1):44–51. doi:10.1200/JCO.18.00537

23. Choudhury A, Swindell R, Logue JP, et al. Phase II study of conformal hypofractionated radiotherapy with concurrent gemcitabine in muscle-invasive bladder cancer. *J Clin Oncol.* 2011;29(6):733–738. doi:10.1200/JCO.2010.31.5721

24. James ND, Hussain SA, Hall E, et al. Radiotherapy with or without chemotherapy in muscle-invasive bladder cancer. *N Engl J Med.* 2012;366(16):1477–1488. doi:10.1056/nejmoa1106106

25. Song YP, Mistry H, Irlam J, et al. Long-term outcomes of radical radiation therapy with hypoxia modification with biomarker discovery for stratification: 10-year update of the BCON (Bladder Carbogen Nicotinamide) phase 3 randomized trial (ISRCTN45938399). *Int J Radiat Oncol Biol Phys.* 2021;110(5):1407–1415. doi:10.1016/j.ijrobp.2021.03.001

26. Galsky MD, Witjes JA, Gschwend JE, et al. Adjuvant nivolumab in high-risk muscle-invasive urothelial carcinoma: expanded efficacy from CheckMate 274. *J Clin Oncol.* 2025;43(1):15–21. doi:10.1200/JCO.24.00340

27. Apolo AB, Ballman KV, Sonpavde G, et al. Adjuvant pembrolizumab versus observation in muscle-invasive urothelial carcinoma. *N Engl J Med.* 2025;392(1):45–55. doi:10.1056/NEJMoa2401726

28. Bellmunt J, Hussain M, Gschwend JE, et al. Adjuvant atezolizumab versus observation in muscle-invasive urothelial carcinoma (IMvigor010): a multicentre, open-label, randomised, phase 3 trial. *Lancet Oncol.* 2021;22(4):525–537. doi:10.1016/S1470-2045(21)00004-8

29. Powles T, Valderrama BP, Gupta S, et al. Enfortumab vedotin and pembrolizumab in untreated advanced urothelial cancer. *N Engl J Med.* 2024;390(10):875–888. doi:10.1056/NEJMoa2312117

30. Baumann BC, Bosch WR, Bahl A, et al. Development and validation of consensus contouring guidelines for adjuvant radiation therapy for bladder cancer after radical cystectomy. *Int J Radiat Oncol Biol Phys.* 2016;96(1):78–86. doi:10.1016/j.ijrobp.2016.04.032

31. Choudhury A, Porta N, Hall E, et al. Hypofractionated radiotherapy in locally advanced bladder cancer: an individual patient data meta-analysis of the BC2001 and BCON trials. *Lancet Oncol.* 2021;22(2):246–255. doi:10.1016/S1470-2045(20)30607-0

32. Videtic GMM, Woody NM, Vassil AD. *Handbook of Treatment Planning in Radiation Oncology.* 3rd ed. Springer Publishing Company; 2020.

33. Shipley WU. Treatment of invasive bladder cancer by cisplatin and radiation in patients unsuited for surgery. *JAMA.* 1987;258(7):931. doi:10.1001/jama.1987.03400070069037

34. Kaufman DS, Shipley WU, Griffin PP, Heney NM, Althausen AF, Efird JT. Selective bladder preservation by combination treatment of invasive bladder cancer. *N Engl J Med.* 1993;329(19):1377–1382. doi:10.1056/nejm199311043291903

35. Tester W, Porter A, Asbell S, et al. Combined modality program with possible organ preservation for invasive bladder carcinoma: results of RTOG protocol 85–12. *Int J Radiat Oncol Biol Phys.* 1993;25(5):783–790. doi:10.1016/0360-3016(93)90306-g

36. Tester W, Caplan R, Heaney J, et al. Neoadjuvant combined modality program with selective organ preservation for invasive bladder cancer: results of Radiation Therapy Oncology Group phase II trial 8802. *J Clin Oncol.* 1996;14(1):119–126. doi:10.1200/jco.1996.14.1.119

37. Kaufman DS, Winter KA, Shipley WU, et al. The initial results in muscle-invading bladder cancer of RTOG 95-06: phase I/II trial of transurethral surgery plus radiation therapy with concurrent cisplatin and 5-fluorouracil followed by selective bladder preservation or cystectomy depending on the initial response. *Oncologist.* 2000;5(6):471–476. doi:10.1634/theoncologist.5-6-471

38. Hagan MP, Winter KA, Kaufman DS, et al. RTOG 97-06: initial report of a phase I-II trial of selective bladder conservation using TURBT, twice-daily accelerated irradiation sensitized with cisplatin, and adjuvant MCV combination chemotherapy. *Int J Radiat Oncol Biol Phys.* 2003;57(3):665–672. doi:10.1016/s0360-3016(03)00718-1

39. Kaufman DS, Winter KA, Shipley WU, et al. Phase I-II RTOG study (99-06) of patients with muscle-invasive bladder cancer undergoing transurethral surgery, paclitaxel, cisplatin, and twice-daily radiotherapy followed by selective bladder preservation or radical cystectomy and adjuvant chemotherapy. *Urology.* 2009;73(4):833–837. doi:10.1016/j.urology.2008.09.036

40. Shipley WU, Kaufman DS, Zehr E, et al. Selective bladder preservation by combined modality protocol treatment: long-term outcomes of 190 patients with invasive bladder cancer. *Urology.* 2002;60(1):62–67. doi:10.1016/s0090-4295(02)01650-3

41. Efstathiou JA, Bae K, Shipley WU, et al. Late pelvic toxicity after bladder-sparing therapy in patients with invasive bladder cancer: RTOG 89-03, 95-06, 97-06, 99-06. *J Clin Oncol.* 2009;27(25):4055–4061. doi:10.1200/JCO.2008.19.5776

42. Huddart RA, Hall E, Lewis R, et al. Patient-reported quality of life outcomes in patients treated for muscle-invasive bladder cancer with radiotherapy ± chemotherapy in the BC2001 phase III randomised controlled trial. *Eur Urol.* 2020;77(2):260–268. doi:10.1016/j.eururo.2019.11.001

43. Kool R, Dragomir A, Kulkarni GS, et al. Benefit of neoadjuvant cisplatin-based chemotherapy for invasive bladder cancer patients treated with radiation-based therapy in a real-world setting: an inverse probability treatment weighted analysis. *Eur Urol Oncol.* 2024;7(6):1350–1357. doi:10.1016/j.euo.2024.01.014

44. Coppin CM, Gospodarowicz MK, James K, et al. Improved local control of invasive bladder cancer by concurrent cisplatin and preoperative or definitive radiation. The National Cancer Institute of Canada Clinical Trials Group. *J Clin Oncol.* 1996;14(11):2901–2907. doi:10.1200/jco.1996.14.11.2901

45. Marcq G, Kool R, Dragomir A, et al. Benefit of whole-pelvis radiation for patients with muscle-invasive bladder cancer: an inverse probability treatment weighted analysis. *J Clin Oncol.* 2025;43(3):308–317. doi:10.1200/JCO.23.02718

46. Horwich A, Dearnaley D, Huddart R, et al. A randomised trial of accelerated radiotherapy for localised invasive bladder cancer. *Radiother Oncol.* 2005;75(1):34–43. doi:10.1016/j.radonc.2004.11.003

47. Zaghloul MS, Awwad HK, Akoush HH, Omar S, Soliman O, Attar IE. Postoperative radiotherapy of carcinoma in bilharzial bladder: improved disease free survival through improving local control. *Int J Radiat Oncol Biol Phys.* 1992;23(3):511–517. doi:10.1016/0360-3016(92)90005-3

48. Baumann BC, Guzzo TJ, He J, et al. Bladder cancer patterns of pelvic failure: implications for adjuvant radiation therapy. *Int J Radiat Oncol Biol Phys.* 2013;85(2):363–369. doi:10.1016/j.ijrobp.2012.03.061

49. Zaghloul MS, Alnagmy AK, Kasem HA, et al. The value and safety of adjuvant radiation therapy after radical cystectomy in locally advanced urothelial bladder cancer: a controlled randomized study. *Int J Radiat Oncol Biol Phys.* 2024;120(3):658–666. doi:10.1016/j.ijrobp.2024.05.012

50. Zaghloul MS, Christodouleas JP, Smith A, et al. Adjuvant sandwich chemotherapy plus radiotherapy vs adjuvant chemotherapy alone for locally advanced bladder cancer after radical cystectomy: a randomized phase 2 trial. *JAMA Surg.* 2018;153(1):e174591. doi:10.1001/jamasurg.2017.4591

51. Murthy V, Maitre P, Bakshi G, et al. Bladder adjuvant radiation therapy (BART): acute and late toxicity from a phase III multicenter randomized controlled trial. *Int J Radiat Oncol Biol Phys.* 2024. doi:10.1016/j.ijrobp.2024.09.040c

44 TESTICULAR CANCER

Zachary S. Mayo, Omar Y. Mian, and Rahul D. Tendulkar

QUICK HIT Testicular cancer is a relatively uncommon GU malignancy with excellent prognosis. The majority of testicular malignancies are germ cell tumors (GCT) (95%), of which approximately 50% to 60% are seminomatous and 40% to 50% are nonseminomatous GCT (NSCGT). Eighty-five percent of seminomas present as clinical stage I disease. Initial management is inguinal orchiectomy with high ligation of the spermatic cord (not trans-scrotal biopsy). Treatment paradigm for seminomatous testicular cancer is summarized in Table 44.1. Depending on stage, adjuvant therapy for NSGCT after inguinal orchiectomy is surveillance, nerve-sparing retroperitoneal lymph node dissection (nsRPLND), or CHT.

Table 44.1 General Treatment Paradigm for Testicular Seminoma		
Seminoma	Initial Treatment	Adjuvant Treatment Options
Stage I	Radical inguinal orchiectomy with high ligation of the spermatic cord	Active surveillance preferred (NCCN)[1]: 15%–20% relapse Carboplatin (AUC 7 × 1–2C): <5% relapse (TE19 trial) RT (PA strip, 20 Gy/10 fx): <5% relapse (TE10/TE18 trials)
Stage II		Stage IIA: Modified dogleg RT, 20 Gy/10 fx with boost to 30 Gy EP × 4C or BEP × 3C nsRPLND Stage IIB: CHT preferred (NCCN)[1]: EP × 4C or BEP × 3C RT for select nonbulky disease (nodes ≤3 cm): Modified dogleg RT, 20 Gy/10 fx with boost to 36 Gy Stage IIC: EP × 4C or BEP × 3C RT/surgery for salvage
Stage III		EP × 4C or BEP × 3C RT/surgery for salvage

EPIDEMIOLOGY: Approximately 9,760 cases diagnosed annually, with 500 deaths.[2] Accounts for 1% of male cancers overall but is the most common solid tumor in men 15 to 34 years of age. NSGCTs typically present between 20 and 30 years of age, while seminomas present between 30 and 40 years of age. Up to 5% are bilateral (synchronous or metachronous). Excellent prognosis with 10-year survival >95%. Worldwide incidence has more than doubled in the past four decades. Lymphoma is the most common testicular tumor in men over 60.[3]

RISK FACTORS: Abdominal cryptorchid testes have 1/20 (5%) risk of cancer and must be resected. Inguinal cryptorchid testes have 1/80 (1.3%) risk of cancer and should undergo orchiopexy before puberty. Risk of cancer increases with age at which cryptorchidism is detected/reversed. Twenty percent of GCTs in patients with a history of cryptorchidism occur in the contralateral, normally descended testicle. Intratubular germ cell neoplasia of unclassified type (ITGCNU) has a 50% risk of progression to invasive malignancy at 5 years.[4] Other risk factors include hypospadias, androgen insensitivity syndrome, gonadal dysgenesis, previous contralateral testicular cancer, extragonadal GCT, family history, White race, HIV, marijuana use, and Peutz–Jeghers syndrome.[5]

ANATOMY: Layers (from external to internal): skin, dartos fascia, external spermatic fascia, cremasteric fascia, internal spermatic fascia, parietal layer of tunica vaginalis, visceral layer of tunica vaginalis, and tunica albuginea. Seminiferous tubules merge to form the rete testis. Testicular arteries arise directly from abdominal aorta. Right testicular vein joins the IVC inferior to the right renal vein; left testicular vein joins the left renal vein. Lymphatic drainage is from rete testes via the spermatic cord along testicular veins to retroperitoneal/PA LNs at vertebral levels T11 to L4, then via cisterna chyli and thoracic duct to posterior mediastinum, left SCV, and axilla. Inguinal nodes are not involved in testicular cancer unless the scrotum is surgically disrupted (usually by trans-scrotal biopsy, hernia repair, vasectomy, etc.).

PATHOLOGY[6]: Majority (95%) of testicular cancers are GCTs: seminomas (50%–60%) and NSGCTs (40%–50%). Minority (5%) are non-GCTs including Leydig cell, Sertoli cell, rhabdomyosarcoma, or lymphoma. Seminomas include classic (85%), anaplastic (10%), or spermatocytic (5%), which are all treated the same. Anaplastic has a high mitotic activity but does not have worse outcomes. Spermatocytic type occurs in older men (age >50) and has a favorable prognosis. Pure seminomas with syncytiotrophoblastic cells (still considered pure) may have elevated β-hCG in 10% to 15%. NSGCTs include embryonal, teratoma, choriocarcinoma, yolk sac (endodermal sinus tumors), and mixed tumors (see Table 44.2). CIS precedes invasive GCTs by 3 to 5 years and is found adjacent to invasive tumor in nearly 100% of cases (except spermatocytic seminoma and infant tumors). AFP is elevated in many NSGCT but is not elevated in pure seminoma. AFP can also be elevated in HCC and liver disease. β-hCG is very high with choriocarcinoma but can also be elevated with high LH, or GI, GU, lung and breast cancers. LDH is nonspecific and can be elevated in about half of GCT.

Table 44.2 Characteristics of Testicular Histologies				
GCT Histology	Age	Characteristics	% With AFP Elevation	% With β-hCG Elevation
Seminoma (50%–60%)	30–40	Radiosensitive; 80% local at presentation; lymphatic spread; relapse occurs later	0%	10%
NSGCTs (40%–50%)	20–30	Radioresistant; 70% distant at presentation; often hematogenous spread; relapse occurs earlier	50%	60%
• Embryonal	25–35	Most common pure NSGCT; more aggressive, >60% DM (lung, liver) at presentation	70%	60%
• Teratoma	25–35	Second most common NSGCT; multiple germ layers; mature vs. immature; >75% NSGCTs have teratoma component	40%	25%
• Choriocarcinoma	20–30	Rare; very high β-hCG (gynecomastia), AFP always normal; most aggressive; spreads hematogenously; may hemorrhage	0%	100%
• Yolk sac	<10	Most common pediatric GCT, 80% <2 yrs old; in adults, presents in mediastinum and is chemoresistant; Schiller–Duval bodies	75%	25%

CLINICAL PRESENTATION: Classically presents as a painless testicular mass or painless testicular swelling. Other presentations include a dull ache, heavy sensation in lower abdomen or perianal area, or fullness of the scrotum. A minority (10%) will present with acute pain. Symptoms associated with DM are seen in 10%. Infertility seen in 50%. Gynecomastia (5%) secondary to estrogenic effect of β-hCG. Tumor size and epididymal invasion are associated with higher risk of metastatic disease at the time of presentation.[7]

DIFFERENTIAL DIAGNOSIS: Testicular cancer, testicular torsion, epididymitis, hydrocele, varicocele, hernia, hematoma, or spermatocele.

WORKUP: H&P with bimanual exam of scrotal contents. A firm or fixed mass is cancer until proven otherwise. Palpate abdomen for nodal disease or visceral involvement. Examine chest for gynecomastia and palpate for SCV nodes.

Labs: CBC, CMP, serum tumor markers (AFP, β-hCG, LDH).

Imaging: Bilateral scrotal Doppler ultrasound demonstrates a hypoechoic mass. Seminomas are well-defined without cystic areas, while NSGCTs are inhomogeneous with calcifications, cystic areas, and indistinct margins. Surgery is required for staging as ultrasound is insufficient.[8] CXR and CT abdomen/pelvis (add CT chest if abnormal CXR or positive abdominal CT). PET is of limited utility for workup, may be more useful for seminoma than NSGCTs and alters staging in 10%.[9] Brain imaging if symptomatic, high burden of lung metastases, nonpulmonary visceral metastases (NPVM), or high β-hCG.

Other: Trans-scrotal biopsy or orchiectomy is absolutely contraindicated due to risk of tumor seeding into the scrotal sac, lymphatic disruption, or metastatic spread of tumor into the inguinal LN. Repeat post-orchiectomy serum tumor markers (AFP, β-hCG, and LDH) since S stage in the AJCC system is based on post-orchiectomy values. The half-life of β-hCG is 24 to 36 hours and AFP 5 to 7 days.[10]

PROGNOSTIC FACTORS

Seminoma: Stage, LVSI, elevated LDH and β-hCG, NPVM.[11]

NSGCT: LVI, NPVM, S3, mediastinal primary, embryonal predominant.[12,13]

NATURAL HISTORY: Risk for relapse after orchiectomy is approximately 12% for stage I seminoma with size <3 cm and 20% with size ≥3 cm. However, for patients who do not relapse in the first 2 years, risk of relapse in the next 5 years is 4% and 6%, respectively.[14] Ninety percent of nodal relapses on surveillance occur in the PA LN ("landing zone") and 10% also have positive pelvic LN.[15] Nodal crossover may occur from right to left (~15%), but rarely from left to right. Late distant relapses are possible.

STAGING: See Table 44.3.

Table 44.3 AJCC 8th Edition (2017): Staging for Testicular Cancer[16]							
pT		**cN**		**pN**		**M**	
Tis	• Germ cell neoplasia in situ	N1	• Regional LNs ≤2 cm (single or multiple)	N1	• Regional LN ≤2 cm • ≤5 LNs positive	M1a	• Nonretroperitoneal LNs • Pulmonary metastasis
T1	**a.** Limited to testis (including rete testis invasion), no LVSI, <3 cm **b.** Limited to testis (including rete testis invasion), no LVSI, ≥3 cm	N2	• Regional LN >2 cm and ≤5 cm	N2	• Regional LN >2 cm and ≤5 cm • >5 regional LNs, ≤5 cm • ECE	M1b	• Nonpulmonary visceral metastasis
T2	• Limited to testis (including rete testis) with LVSI or involves hilar soft tissue or involves epididymis or penetrating visceral mesothelial layer covering the external surface of tunica albuginea	N3	• Regional LNs >5 cm	N3	• Regional LN >5 cm		
T3	• Invasion of spermatic cord*			**S Staging (Serum Tumor Markers)**			

(continued)

Table 44.3 AJCC 8th ed. (2017): Staging for Testicular Cancer[16] (*continued*)					
pT		**cN**	**pN**		**M**
T4	• Invasion of scrotum			**AFP (ng/mL)**	**β-hCG (mIU/mL)**	**LDH**
			S0	WNL	WNL	WNL
			S1	<1,000	<5,000	<1.5 × normal
			S2	1,000–10,000	5,000–50,000	1.5–10 × normal
			S3	>10,000	>50,000	> 10 × normal

*Discontinuous involvement of the spermatic cord is considered M1.

Stage Grouping				
IA	T1	N0	M0	S0
IB	T2–4	N0	M0	S0
IS	Any T	N0	M0	S1–3
IIA	Any T	N1	M0	S0–1
IIB	Any T	N2	M0	S0–1
IIC	Any T	N3	M0	S0–1
IIIA	Any T	Any N	M1a	S0–1
IIIB	Any T	N1–3	M0	S2
	Any T	Any N	M1a	S2
IIIC	Any T	N1–3	M0	S3
	Any T	Any N	M1a	S3
	Any T	Any N	M1b	Any S

Source: Adapted from Amin MB, Edge SB, Greene FL, et al, eds. *AJCC Cancer Staging Manual.* 8th ed. Springer; 2017.

SEMINOMA TREATMENT PARADIGM: Mixed seminomas/NSGCTs are treated based on the NSGCT component. In NSGCT, RT is reserved for salvage/palliation. Seminomas may have an indication for RT and therefore this discussion will focus on the treatment of seminoma.

Surgery: The standard surgery is a radical inguinal orchiectomy with high ligation of the spermatic cord. This is both diagnostic and therapeutic. Per NCCN, nsRPLND is now an adjuvant treatment option for stage IIA seminoma.

Active Surveillance: Recommended option for stage I patients after orchiectomy. Must be compliant with follow-up. NCCN recommends H&P every 3 to 6 months for year 1, every 6 months for year 2, every 6 to 12 months for year 3, and then annually.[1] Serum tumor markers are optional and testicular ultrasound is recommended for an equivocal exam. CT abdomen/pelvis or MRI is recommended at 4 to 6 months and 12 months in year 1, every 6 months in year 2, every 6 to 12 months in year 3, then every 12 to 24 months in years 4 and 5. CXR as clinically indicated in years 1 to 5. Consider CT chest if symptomatic.[1]

Chemotherapy: Adjuvant CHT is based on stage. Single-agent carboplatin (AUC 7) × 1–2 cycles is an option for stage I patients. BEP (bleomycin, etoposide, cisplatin) × 3 cycles or EP (etoposide, cisplatin) × 4 cycles are options for stage II to III patients. CHT is preferred for stages IIB, IIC, and III.

Radiation Therapy: For stage I patients, a PA strip may be treated to 20 Gy/10 fx for those preferring adjuvant treatment. CHT may be preferred over RT in stage I patients due to less risk of impaired fertility. For stage IIA patients, a modified dogleg field to include the PA and ipsilateral internal iliac LNs can be delivered to 20 Gy/10 fx with a boost to 30 Gy for gross disease. For stage IIB patients, a modified dogleg field to 20 Gy/10 fx is followed by boost to 36 Gy to the gross disease.[6] Most recommend coverage of the left renal hilum (see TE10 in the following). Contraindications to RT include horseshoe kidney, inflammatory bowel disease, prior RT, and genetic syndromes with an increased risk of further malignancies. Side effects include fatigue, nausea, vomiting, skin changes, diarrhea, temporary oligospermia or azoospermia, infertility, and second malignancy. Offer sperm banking prior to treatment.

Procedure: See *Treatment Planning Handbook,* Chapter 8 for details.

EVIDENCE-BASED Q&A

STAGE I SEMINOMA

What data support active surveillance as an option for patients with stage I seminoma?

The risk of relapse and death from a stage I seminoma is low. A systematic literature review (14 studies with 2,060 men) showed that relapse occurred in 17% (9% relapsed >2 years) and mortality from seminoma was 0.3% due to effective salvage therapies.[17] Another study demonstrated that the risk of relapse can be as low as 6% if the tumor size is <4 cm and no rete testis invasion.[18] A Danish retrospective cohort study of 1,954 men showed that the median time to relapse was 14 months, with 73% of patients developing relapse during the first 2 years, 22% between years 3 and 5, and 4% after year 5. The 15-year DSS and OS rates were 99% and 92%, respectively.[19] The TRISST trial demonstrated a 12% relapse rate at 6 years, with stage ≥IIC relapse seen in only 1.5% of patients.[20]

Joffe, TRISST (*JCO* 2022, PMID 35298280): Phase III noninferiority trial of 669 patients with stage I seminoma s/p orchiectomy (no adjuvant treatment) randomized to one of four surveillance arms: (a) seven CTs (6, 12, 18, 24, 36, 48, 60 months after randomization), (b) seven MRIs (same schedule), (c) three CTs (6, 18, 36 months), and (d) three MRIs (same schedule). The primary outcome was 6-year incidence of stage ≥IIC relapse. Secondary outcomes included ≥3 cm relapse, DFS, and OS. MFU was 72 months. Overall relapse rate was 12%, but only 10 patients (1.5%) had stage ≥IIC relapse. Numerically higher stage ≥IIC relapses in three-scan group compared with seven-scan group (9 relapses vs. 1; 2.5% absolute increase from 0.3% to 2.8%), but noninferior based on study criteria (noninferiority threshold of 5.7%). Numerically fewer stage ≥IIC relapses in MRI group compared with CT group (2 relapses vs. 8; 1.9% absolute decrease from 0.6% vs. 2.6%). Only 5 of 82 relapses occurred beyond 3 years. No SS differences in incidence of ≥3 cm relapse, 5-year DFS (87% across groups), or 5-year OS (99% across groups). **Conclusion: In stage I seminoma s/p orchiectomy, relapse is uncommon and surveillance is a safe management approach regardless of imaging modality (CT or MRI). Reduced schedule of imaging had no adverse impact on long-term outcomes.**

Is a full dogleg field necessary for stage I patients treated with adjuvant RT or will a PA strip suffice?

For stage I patients, pelvic relapse is rare. MRC TE10 showed that PA strip is the appropriate RT field, and dogleg fields should be reserved for patients with prior inguinal or scrotal surgery due to altered lymphatic drainage.

Fossa, MRC TE10 (*JCO* 1999, PMID 10561173): Equivalence study of 478 patients with stage I (T1–T3) seminoma randomized to dogleg (DL: PA strip plus ipsilateral iliac LN) vs. PA strip (PAS; T11–L5) fields. All treated to 30 Gy/15 fx. MFU 4.5 years. No difference in 3-year RFS or OS (see Table 44.4). Each group had nine relapses, although the PAS group had four pelvic relapses compared with none in the DL group. PAS had less acute toxicity (nausea/vomiting, diarrhea, leukopenia) and higher sperm counts than DL fields. One patient in the PAS arm died of seminoma. **Conclusion: PA strip RT is considered standard treatment for stage I (T1–T3), with dogleg fields reserved for patients with prior inguinal or scrotal surgery.**

Table 44.4 Results of MRC TE10				
MRC TE10	**3-Yr RFS**	**3-Yr OS**	**Number of Pelvic Relapses**	**Azoospermia**
PAS	96%	99%	4 (2%)	11%
DL	97%	100%	0 (0%)	35%
p value	NS	NS	–	<.001

What is the optimal RT dose for patients with stage I seminoma?

Based on MRC TE18, the standard dose for stage I seminoma is 20 Gy in 10 fx.

Jones, MRC TE18 (*JCO*** 2005, PMID 15718317):** Noninferiority trial of 625 patients with stage I seminoma (pT1–3N0) randomized to 20 Gy/10 fx vs. 30 Gy/15 fx, all to PA strip (T11–L5). Designed to assess noninferiority and powered to exclude a 4% difference in 2-year relapse rates. MFU 61 months. No difference in OS or RFS; the 30 Gy arm had 10 relapses, compared with 11 relapses in the 20 Gy arm (*p* = NS); the 20 Gy arm had less acute side effects (moderate-severe fatigue and inability to conduct normal work) at 4 weeks, but differences returned to baseline by 12 weeks (see Table 44.5). Six new primary cancers diagnosed, all in the 30 Gy arm. **Conclusion: 20 Gy/10 fx is as effective as 30 Gy/15 fx with less acute side effects.**

Table 44.5 Results of MRC TE18			
MRC TE18	**2-Yr RFS**	**Moderate–Severe Lethargy**	**Inability to Work at 4 Weeks**
20 Gy	97%	5%	28%
30 Gy	97%	20%	46%
p value	NS	<.001	<.001

What is the role of CHT in patients with stage I seminoma?

Based on MRC TE19, carboplatin is noninferior to RT and has reduced side effects. Single-agent carboplatin is given for one to two cycles.[21]

Oliver, MRC TE19 (*Lancet*** 2005, PMID 16039331; Oliver, ***JCO*** 2011, PMID 21282539):** PRT of 1,477 patients with stage I seminoma s/p orchiectomy randomized to adjuvant carboplatin (1 cycle, AUC 7) vs. adjuvant RT (20 Gy/10 fx [36%] or 30 Gy/15 fx [54%]) or an intermediate dose (10%); 87% treated with PA strip and 13% with dogleg. Powered to exclude absolute differences in 2-year relapse rates of >3%. MFU 6.5 years. Carboplatin had more PA node-only relapses, but fewer pelvic, mediastinal, or SCV relapses compared with RT, with no difference in RFS (see Table 44.6). Carboplatin arm had fewer second GCTs (carboplatin *n* = 2, RT *n* = 15; HR 0.22, *p* = .03) and significantly less acute dyspepsia (8% vs. 17%), moderate-severe lethargy (7% vs. 24%), and inability to do normal work (19% vs. 38%), but more thrombocytopenia (12% vs. 2%). Only one seminoma death, which was in the RT arm. Those getting more of the prescribed CHT (>99% AUC 7) had improved RFS (96% vs. 93%) than those who received less CHT. **Conclusion: Adjuvant carboplatin is not inferior to RT for stage I seminoma, and it has fewer acute side effects.**

Table 44.6 Results of MRC TE19			
MRC TE19	**2-Yr RFS**	**5-Yr RFS**	**Contralateral GCT**
RT	97%	96%	15 (1.7%)
Carboplatin	98%	95%	2 (0.3%)

What are the outcomes in patients with stage I seminoma who experience a relapse?

Mead, UK TE Pooled Analysis (*JNCI*** 2011, PMID 21212385):** Pooled analysis of 3,049 patients on the TE10, TE18, and TE19 noninferiority trials. MFU 6.4 to 12 years; 99.8% CSS overall. There were 98 relapses, but only 4 (0.2%) relapsed after 3 years. Four died of metastatic failure. Among patients treated with dogleg who relapsed, 11 out of 16 (65%) failed in the mediastinum or neck. Of those treated with a PA strip who relapsed, 20 out of 54 (37%) failed in the pelvis and 14 out of 54 (26%) failed in the mediastinum or neck. In patients treated with carboplatin who relapsed, 18 out of 27 (67%) failed in the retroperitoneum. **Conclusion: Patterns of relapse depend on adjuvant treatment received.**

STAGE II SEMINOMA

What are the potential advantages of RT over CHT in patients with stage IIA/B seminoma?

Per the 2024 NCCN guidelines, either adjuvant RT to the PA and ipsilateral pelvic LN or CHT is recommended for stage II seminoma. RT is given to 30 Gy for stage IIA and 36 Gy for stage IIB. CHT is BEP × 3C or EP × 4C. Per NCCN, CHT is preferred for stage IIB or higher and is Category 1 for stage IIC or III.[1] RT is not considered a preferred option for bulky nodal disease due to higher failure rates. The GTCSG published a phase II trial of carboplatin in stage IIA/B patients and achieved a CR of 81% but with an overall failure rate of 18%. Single-agent carboplatin was not effective in eradicating retroperitoneal metastases in stage IIA/B seminoma.

Given excellent outcomes of single modality adjuvant treatment for stage IIA/B seminoma, can de-escalated, combination CHT and RT be utilized to reduce toxicity while maintaining efficacy?

Papachristofilou, SAKK 01/10 (*Lancet Oncol* 2022, PMID 36228644): Single-arm, multicenter, phase II study of de-escalated adjuvant treatment for stage IIA/B (either at diagnosis or first relapse after active surveillance) classic seminoma. Adjuvant regimen was one cycle of carboplatin AUC7 followed by involved-node RT, 30 Gy for IIA or 36 Gy for IIB. Primary endpoint was 3-year PFS target of 95%. 116 patients (40% IIA, 60% IIB) with MFU of 4.5 years. The 3-year PFS was 94%, which did not meet the prespecified PFS target. Grades 3 to 4 toxicities occurred in 8% and four patients developed a second primary tumor. **Conclusion: Combination de-escalated adjuvant treatment for stage IIA/B seminoma offers favorable LC and acute toxicity but did not meet the prespecified PFS target.**

Can primary surgical management with RPLND be used instead of CHT or RT to avoid long-term side effects associated with treatment?

The use of RPLND in stage IIA seminoma was recently added to NCCN guidelines. The single-arm SEMS (Surgery in Early Metastatic Seminoma) treated 55 patients with seminoma and isolated retroperitoneal lymphadenopathy (<3 cm) with RPLND and found a 2-year RFS of 81%. CHT and additional surgery were used as salvage therapy and the 2-year OS was 100%.[22] The PRIMETEST trial investigated RPLND in patients with unilateral retroperitoneal lymphadenopathy (<5 cm) and found a PFS of 70% at 32 months.[23]

TOXICITY AND SECONDARY MALIGNANCY RISK

What is the risk of developing secondary malignancy after adjuvant therapy for testicular cancer?

After adjuvant therapy (CHT or RT), patients with testicular cancer are at higher risk of developing secondary malignancy. Given the increased risk of mortality from secondary malignancies, it is important to appropriately select patients for adjuvant therapy.

Travis, NIH (*JNCI* 2005, PMID 16174857): Population-based registries of >40,000 testicular cancer survivors used to calculate relative and absolute risks of second solid cancers. Among 10-year survivors diagnosed at age 35, the relative risk of a second solid tumor was 1.9 and remained statistically significantly elevated for 35 years. Cancers of the lung (RR = 1.5), colon (RR = 2), bladder (RR = 2.7), pancreas (RR = 3.6), and stomach (RR = 4) accounted for ~60% of the excess malignancies. There was also an increased risk of pleural (malignant mesothelioma; RR = 3.4) and esophagus (RR = 1.7) cancers. Overall relative risk of second solid malignancy for patients treated with RT alone was 2, CHT alone 1.9, and both 2.9. For patients diagnosed with seminoma and NSGCT at 35 years of age, cumulative risk of solid cancer in the next 40 years was 36% and 31%, respectively (corresponding risk of solid cancer in the general population was 23%). Note that the authors estimate about 16% of the evaluated patients received chest RT. **Conclusion: Testicular cancer survivors treated with RT and/or CHT are at increased risk of solid tumors for at least 35 years.**

Kier, Danish Nationwide Cohort (*JAMA Oncology* 2016, PMID 27711914): Danish nationwide cohort of 5,190 patients (2,804 seminoma, 2,386 nonseminoma) treated with adjuvant therapy. Patients underwent surveillance, retroperitoneal RT, BEP CHT, or MTOL (more than one line) of CHT. MFU 14.4 years. The 20-year cumulative incidence of second malignancy (death used as a competing risk) was 8% for surveillance, 8% for BEP (HR 1.7), 14% for RT (HR 1.8), 9% for MTOL (HR 3.7), and 7% for controls. Excess mortality due to second malignancy was found with BEP (HR 1.6), RT (HR 2.1), and MTOL (HR 5.8). **Conclusion: Excess mortality due to second malignancy from adjuvant therapy suggests that approaches to define the best candidates for adjuvant therapy are needed.**

REFERENCES

1. National Comprehensive Cancer Network. *NCCN Clinical Practice Guidelines in Oncology: Testicular Cancer*. Version 1.2024. Accessed April 4, 2024. https://www.nccn.org/professionals/physician_gls/pdf/testicular.pdf

2. Siegel RL, Giaquinto AN, Jemal A. Cancer statistics, 2024. *CA Cancer J Clin*. 2024;74(1):12–49. doi:10.3322/caac.21820

3. Yacoub JH, Oto A, Allen BC, et al. ACR appropriateness criteria® staging of testicular malignancy. *J Am Coll Radiol*. 2016;13(10):1203–1209. doi:10.1016/j.jacr.2016.06.026

4. von der Maase H, Rørth M, Walbom-Jørgensen S, et al. Carcinoma in situ of contralateral testis in patients with testicular germ cell cancer: study of 27 cases in 500 patients. *BMJ*. 1986;293(6559):1398–1401. doi:10.1136/bmj.293.6559.1398

5. Fosså SD, Chen J, Schonfeld SJ, et al. Risk of contralateral testicular cancer: a population-based study of 29,515 U.S. men. *J Natl Cancer Inst*. 2005;97(14):1056–1066. doi:10.1093/jnci/dji185

6. Wilder RB, Buyyounouski MK, Efstathiou JA, Beard CJ. Radiotherapy treatment planning for testicular seminoma. *Int J Radiat Oncol Biol Phys*. 2012;83(4):e445–e452. doi:10.1016/j.ijrobp.2012.01.044

7. Scandura G, Wagner T, Beltran L, Alifrangis C, Shamash J, Berney DM. Pathological risk factors for metastatic disease at presentation in testicular seminomas with focus on the recent pT changes in AJCC TNM eighth edition. *Hum Pathol*. 2019;94:16–22. doi:10.1016/j.humpath.2019.10.004

8. Marth D, Scheidegger J, Studer UE. Ultrasonography of testicular tumors. *Urol Int*. 1990;45(4):237–240. doi:10.1159/000281715

9. Ng SP, Duchesne G, Tai KH, Toner G, Hicks R, Williams SG. Can Positron Emission Tomography (PET) complement conventional staging of early-stage testicular seminoma? *Int J Radiat Oncol Biol Phys*. 2016;96(2):E253. doi:10.1016/j.ijrobp.2016.06.1258

10. Amin MB, Edge SB, Greene FL, et al, eds. *AJCC Cancer Staging Manual*. 8th ed. Springer; 2017.

11. Wagner T, Toft BG, Lauritsen J, et al. Prognostic factors for relapse in patients with clinical stage I testicular seminoma: a nationwide, population-based cohort study. *J Clin Oncol*. 2024;42(1):81–89. doi:10.1200/JCO.23.00959

12. International Germ Cell Cancer Collaborative Group. International Germ Cell Consensus Classification: a prognostic factor-based staging system for metastatic germ cell cancers. *J Clin Oncol*. 1997;15(2):594–603. doi:10.1200/JCO.1997.15.2.594

13. Beyer J, Collette L, Sauve N, et al. Survival and new prognosticators in metastatic seminoma: results from the IGCCCG-update consortium. *J Clin Oncol*. 2021;39(14):1553–1562. doi:10.1200/JCO.20.03292

14. Nayan M, Jewett MAS, Hosni A, et al. Conditional risk of relapse in surveillance for clinical stage I testicular cancer. *Eur Urol*. 2016;70(6):1208–1214. doi:10.1016/j.eururo.2016.07.013

15. von der Maase H, Specht L, Jacobsen GK, et al. Surveillance following orchidectomy for stage I seminoma of the testis. *Eur J Cancer*. 1993;29A(14):1931–1934. doi:10.1016/0959-8049(93)90446-m

16. Amin MB, Edge SB, Greene FL, et al, eds. *AJCC Cancer Staging Manual*. 8th ed. Springer; 2017.

17. Groll RJ, Warde P, Jewett MAS. A comprehensive systematic review of testicular germ cell tumor surveillance. *Crit Rev Oncol Hematol*. 2007;64(3):182–197. doi:10.1016/j.critrevonc.2007.04.014

18. Albers P, Albrecht W, Algaba F, et al. Guidelines on testicular cancer: 2015 update. *Eur Urol*. 2015;68(6):1054–1068. doi:10.1016/j.eururo.2015.07.044

19. Mortensen MS, Lauritsen J, Gundgaard MG, et al. A nationwide cohort study of stage I seminoma patients followed on a surveillance program. *Eur Urol*. 2014;66(6):1172–1178. doi:10.1016/j.eururo.2014.07.001

20. Joffe JK, Cafferty FH, Murphy L, et al. Imaging modality and frequency in surveillance of stage I seminoma testicular cancer: results from a randomized, phase III, noninferiority trial (TRISST). *J Clin Oncol*. 2022;40(22):2468–2478. doi:10.1200/JCO.21.01199

21. Dieckmann KP, Dralle-Filiz I, Matthies C, et al. Testicular seminoma clinical stage 1: treatment outcome on a routine care level. *J Cancer Res Clin Oncol*. 2016;142(7):1599–1607. doi:10.1007/s00432-016-2162-z

22. Daneshmand S, Cary C, Masterson T, et al. Surgery in early metastatic seminoma: a phase II trial of retroperitoneal lymph node dissection for testicular seminoma with limited retroperitoneal lymphadenopathy. *J Clin Oncol*. 2023;41(16):3009–3018. doi:10.1200/JCO.22.00624

23. Hiester A, Che Y, Lusch A, et al. Phase 2 single-arm trial of primary retroperitoneal lymph node dissection in patients with seminomatous testicular germ cell tumors with clinical stage IIA/B (PRIMETEST). *Eur Urol*. 2023;84(1):25–31. doi:10.1016/j.eururo.2022.10.021

45 PENILE CANCER

Cole Billena, Rahul D. Tendulkar, and Omar Y. Mian

QUICK HIT Penile cancer is rare. Inguinal LNs are the primary nodal drainage site, and ~50% of clinically enlarged LNs are pathologically involved (the rest are reactive). Surgical management can include a partial or total penectomy, with inguinal and/or pelvic LND depending on stage and clinical risk factors (Table 45.1). Organ preservation can be performed for select early-stage patients with either EBRT or brachytherapy (ideally for T1–T2 tumors <4 cm with <1 cm of corpora invasion). Locally advanced patients should be evaluated for neoadjuvant CHT (TIP × 4 cycles) followed by surgery or definitive CRT.

Table 45.1 General Treatment Paradigms for Penile Cancer	
Stage	**Treatment Options**
Tis or Ta	Topical therapy, WLE, laser therapy, glansectomy, Mohs surgery
T1	Grades 1–2: WLE, glansectomy, Mohs, laser therapy, RT Grade 3: WLE, partial penectomy, total penectomy, RT, CRT
T2–T4	Partial penectomy, total penectomy, RT, CRT, neoadjuvant CHT (TIP), and surgery

EPIDEMIOLOGY: Rare cancer in the United States, accounting for ~0.1% of all solid tumors, with ~2,100 new cases and 500 deaths annually.[1] More common in the less developed world.[2] Mean age 60. A significant proportion of men have delayed treatment due to incorrect diagnosis or perceptions of social stigma.

RISK FACTORS[3]**:** Epidemiologic factors: single, never married, lack of circumcision. Medical factors: HPV exposure, genital warts, UTI, penile injury, urethral stricture, phimosis (circumferential fibrosis of the prepuce causing inability to retract the foreskin over the glans), HIV, tobacco exposure, psoralen, and UVA photochemotherapy. About 30% to 50% are HPV+ (most commonly 16 and 18).

ANATOMY: Generally divided into the root, shaft, and glans. Penis is anchored to the pubic ramus. Two corporal bodies share a perforated midline septum terminating at the glans. The urethra is surrounded by the corpus spongiosum. Two layers of fascia cover the corpora: the superficial fascia is continuous with the dartos fascia of the scrotum, and the deep fascia (Buck's) surrounds the erectile bodies (acts as barrier to corporal invasion). Blood supply is from the common penile artery from the internal pudendal artery, which is a branch of the internal iliac. LN drainage occurs bilaterally and sequentially, from the superficial inguinal to the deep femoral LNs, then into the pelvis. Regional LNs include superficial inguinal, deep inguinal, and iliac LNs. The sentinel LNs (Cloquet) are located anteromedial to the superficial epigastric and saphenous vessels.

PATHOLOGY: Ninety-five percent are squamous cell carcinoma (SCC). Other rarer subtypes include melanoma, TCC, BCC, Kaposi sarcoma, lymphoma, extramammary Paget disease, or metastasis from other sites. Penile SCCs can be subclassified by microscopic histologic features: usual type SCC (most common), papillary, warty, basaloid, verrucous, and sarcomatoid subgroups. Low-grade (1–2) carcinomas comprise 80% of cases. Poorly differentiated (grade 3), basaloid, and sarcomatoid subgroups have poorer prognosis. Verrucous and low-grade tumors are more commonly local diseases and rarely metastasize.

CLINICAL PRESENTATION: Often presents with a penile mass or skin abnormality, occurring typically on the glans, in the coronal sulcus, or prepuce (involvement of the shaft is rare, <10%). Presenting symptoms include rash, ulceration, bleeding, or secondary infection. May be mistaken for premalignant lesions such as bowenoid papulosis (papules on the penile shaft), Bowen disease (plaque on follicle-bearing epithelium of penile shaft), erythroplasia of Queyrat (red lesion on mucocutaneous epithelium of the glans or prepuce), lichen sclerosis, condylomas, Buschke–Lowenstein (giant condyloma), and Kaposi sarcoma. Bowenoid papulosis, Bowen disease, and erythroplasia of Queyrat are associated with HPV and are considered in situ lesions. Locoregionally advanced cases typically progress in an orderly fashion to the inguinal LNs, followed by spread to pelvic or retroperitoneal LNs. Only 50% of clinically apparent inguinal lymphadenopathies are due to metastatic nodal disease (other 50% are reactive adenopathy, often from infection); <10% have DM at presentation.

WORKUP: H&P with careful examination of penile lesion and inguinal LNs. If infection is suspected, consider 4 to 6 weeks of antibiotics.

Labs: CBC, CMP, alkaline phosphatase.

Imaging: CT abdomen/pelvis and CXR are standard. MRI and ultrasound may clarify depth of invasion. MRI should be performed if corporal involvement is suspected. Bone scan if advanced disease is suspected. PET/CT should be considered in high-risk patients, particularly those with LN+ by FNA or LND.

Procedures: Punch or incisional biopsy of the penile lesion can usually be performed, reserving excisional biopsy if the initial biopsy is not diagnostic. Assessment of HPV status is recommended. Cystourethroscopy should be performed to examine lower urinary tract.

PROGNOSTIC FACTORS: T stage,[4] grade,[5,6] LVSI,[5] PNI,[7] LN+, ENE. There is some suggestion that HPV may have better prognosis (but not reproducible across series).

STAGING: See Table 45.2.

Table 45.2 AJCC 8th Edition (2017): Staging for Penile Cancer[8]						
T/M	**N**	**N0**	**N1**	**N2**	**N3**	
Tis	Carcinoma in situ (penile intraepithelial neoplasia [PeIN])	0is				
Ta	Noninvasive localized SCC	0a				
T1[1]	a. No LVSI, PNI, or grade 3/sarcomatoid	I	IIIA	IIIB	IV	
	b. LVSI, PNI, or grade 3/sarcomatoid	IIA				
T2	• Invades corpus spongiosum with or without urethral invasion					
T3	• Invades corpus cavernosum with or without urethral invasion	IIB				
T4	• Invades adjacent structures (scrotum, prostate, pubic bone)	IV				
M1	• Distant metastasis					

Notes: T1[1] = glans: tumor invades lamina propria; foreskin: tumor invades dermis, lamina propria, or dartos fascia; shaft: tumor invades connective tissue between epidermis and corpora.
cN1: palpable, mobile unilateral inguinal LN; cN2: palpable, mobile, ≥2 unilateral inguinal or bilateral inguinal LN; cN3: palpable, fixed inguinal nodal mass, or pelvic lymphadenopathy.
pN1: ≤2 unilateral inguinal metastases, no ENE; pN2: ≥3 unilateral inguinal metastases or bilateral metastases; pN3: ENE of regional LN metastases or pelvic LN metastases, no ENE.

TREATMENT PARADIGM: The European Association of Urology/American Society of Clinical Oncology published updated guidelines in 2023, which are summarized along with recommendations from NCCN below.[9]

Surgery: In general, men with low-risk operable tumors (Tis, Ta, T1–2) are candidates for organ-preserving treatment (Table 45.3) with strict follow-up. A systematic review found that organ-sparing surgery for invasive disease confined to the glans has a 5-year recurrence-free rate (RFR) of 82% but carries slightly higher risk of recurrence compared with partial amputation.[10] LR risk is increased when deep surgical margins were <1 mm, and the overall LR rate was 4%.[11] Frozen section intraoperatively can assist in cases where sufficient margins may be difficult to obtain. NCCN recommends organ-sparing approaches only for Tis, Ta, and T1 penile lesions. High-risk patients with locally advanced T3–T4 tumors should undergo penile amputation with either a total penectomy or partial penectomy (removal of the glans ± underlying corpora cavernosa), depending on extent of disease and location of tumor. Distal T2–3 tumors can be treated with limited excision if a negative margin can be attained (need to leave >2 cm for standing void). In a large review, most patients are able to undergo partial penectomy (total penectomy accounted for 23%).[12] LR is <10% in most series. Those with unresectable primary tumors or bulky lymphadenopathy should receive neoadjuvant CHT ± RT prior to consideration of surgery. For patients who refuse surgery, interstitial brachytherapy can be considered. The most common side effect is meatal stenosis (4%–9%). Psychological trauma is also common, and some patients have attempted or committed suicide after penectomy. Men should be counseled about penile reconstruction options.

Table 45.3 Management Options for Early-Stage Penile Cancer		
Candidates	**Treatment**	**Notes**
Tis, Ta, or T1–2	Wide local excision	Goal is to preserve penile length and sexual function
Tis	Topical therapy	5-FU cream and imiquimod cream for 4–6 weeks
Tis, Ta, or T1	Laser ablation	CO_2, argon, Nd:YAG, or potassium titanyl phosphate laser ablation; high rate of preserving sexual activity and satisfaction
Tis, Ta, or T1–2	Total glans resurfacing	Removal of epithelial and subepithelial layers of glans down to corpus spongiosum, followed by skin graft
Tis or T1	Mohs surgery	Layer-by-layer excision to maximize organ preservation
T1–2	RT	Brachytherapy or EBRT

LN Assessment: In addition to assessment of the primary tumor, evaluation of LNs should be performed, noting high rates of false positives and negatives on clinical exam (Tables 45.4 and 45.5).[5] Factors such as T stage, grade, differentiation, and LVSI predict for LN involvement, and risk categories have been identified to guide management of the inguinal LNs. If no palpable or radiographic adenopathy, consider dynamic SLNB (high sensitivity, but requires expertise in technique).[6] A superficial inguinal LND or modified inguinal LND may be performed by clinicians without experience in dynamic SLNB, but they have higher complication rates than SLNB. For patients with palpable inguinal adenopathy or enlarged LNs on imaging, perform FNA first. If FNA is positive, perform a complete (superficial and deep) ipsilateral inguinal node dissection. All patients with pLN+ should also undergo a contralateral superficial inguinal LND and cross-sectional imaging for staging. After inguinal LND, if only 1–2 LNs are positive (pN1) without ENE, no pelvic LND is needed. If ≥3 LN+ (pN2–3) or ENE is present, then pelvic LND is indicated. For N2 disease, consider neoadjuvant CHT (TIP × 4 cycles) ± RT followed by surgery. For patients who are ineligible for neoadjuvant CHT, LND (pelvic and inguinal), RT, or CRT is recommended.

Table 45.4 Inguinal Node Evaluation in cN0 Patients		
Risk Category	**Primary Tumor Factors (All cN0)**	**Management of cN0 Inguinal LNs**
Low risk	pTis, Ta, or T1a	Surveillance (consider SLNB, or superficial or modified inguinal LND for noncompliant patients)
Intermediate/ high risk	pT1b or higher (T1 G3, >50% poorly differentiated, or LVSI)	SLNB or superficial or modified inguinal LND • If pN0 → surveillance • If 1–2 LN+, no ENE → complete inguinal LND • If ≥3 LN+ or ENE → complete inguinal and pelvic LND

Table 45.5 Inguinal Node Evaluation in cN+ Patients After Initial FNA of Suspicious LN(s)	
Clinical Scenario (All cN+)	**Management of cN+ inguinal LNs**
Nonbulky palpable inguinal LNs	If percutaneous LN biopsy negative → excisional biopsy of enlarged LN If percutaneous LN biopsy positive → complete inguinal LND • If 1–2 LN+, no ENE → surveillance • If ≥3 LN+ or ENE → pelvic LND

(continued)

Table 45.5 Inguinal Node Evaluation in cN+ Patients After Initial FNA of Suspicious LN(s) *(continued)*	
Clinical Scenario (All cN+)	Management of cN+ inguinal LNs
Bulky palpable inguinal LNs • >4 cm • Fixed • Bilateral	If percutaneous LN biopsy negative → excisional biopsy of enlarged LN If percutaneous LN biopsy positive → neoadjuvant TIP CHT followed by completion inguinal LND and PLND
Enlarged pelvic LNs	If percutaneous LN biopsy negative → management per status of inguinal LNs If percutaneous LN biopsy positive → neoadjuvant TIP followed by consolidation surgery or CRT

Chemotherapy: CHT options and indications are summarized in Table 45.6. Adjuvant CHT recommendations are largely extrapolated from the neoadjuvant and metastatic setting but may be applied to men with high-risk features.

Table 45.6 CHT Options for Penile Cancer		
Type	Indications	CHT Options
Neoadjuvant	Unresectable primary tumor (T4) Bulky inguinal LN+	• TIP (paclitaxel [175 mg/m^2 d1], ifosfamide [1,200 mg/m^2 d1–3], cisplatin [25 mg/m^2 d1–3]) q3–4 weeks × 4C
Adjuvant	Pelvic LN+ ENE Bilateral inguinal LN+ >4 cm tumor in LNs	• TIP • Cisplatin + 5-FU
Metastatic	Able to tolerate CHT	• TIP • Cisplatin (100 mg/m^2 d1) + 5-FU (1,000 mg/m^2/day d1–5) q3–4 weeks • Cisplatin (80 mg/m^2 on day 1) + irinotecan (60 mg/m^2 d1/8/15) on a 28-day cycle • Consider panitumumab, cetuximab alone, or in combination with CHT

Radiation: Used in the definitive setting for organ preservation (either RT alone or concurrent CRT, extrapolating from cervical and anal cancer), in the neoadjuvant setting for locally advanced unresectable disease, or for symptom palliation in those with metastatic disease (Table 45.7). First step in management is circumcision, which allows for full exposure and can prevent radiation balanitis and phimosis. Definitive RT for organ preservation of early-stage lesions can consist of either EBRT (LC 44%–65%, penile preservation 58%–86%) or brachytherapy (LC 70%–86%, penile preservation 74%–88%). Brachytherapy alone can be considered for lower risk (T1–T2) lesions <4 cm with corpora invasion <1 cm. For more advanced lesions, either EBRT alone or combined CRT or brachytherapy boost may be considered.

Table 45.7 General Principles of RT for Penile Cancer	
Group	RT Treatment Options
Early stage (T1–T2, N0) <4 cm	Definitive brachytherapy alone or EBRT alone or CRT to primary site ± LNs
Early stage (T1–T2, N0) >4 cm	Definitive CRT (primary site + LNs)
Locally advanced (T3–4 or N+)	Definitive CRT (primary site + LNs)
Resected with positive margins	Adjuvant EBRT to primary site and surgical scar ± LNs if inadequate LND
Resected LN+	Adjuvant CRT to primary site and regional LNs, including pelvic LNs (extrapolating from vulvar cancer trials)

EBRT: Setup may be prone or supine with immobilizing bolus to position the penis (wax mold, Perspex block, plastic cylinder, water bath, etc.). Setup frog-leg if planning inguinal node treatment via AP/PA technique (wide AP fields with electron supplementation). The entire length of the penis should be covered, with LNs included if clinically involved or at risk.

Dose: Historically, doses of 50 to 55 Gy were used,[13,14] but in the modern era 45 to 50 Gy is given to the entire penile shaft followed by a boost to 65 to 70 Gy to treat gross disease. A hypofractionated schedule of 52.5 Gy/16 fx may be considered.[15] When electively treating LNs, uninvolved nodes should receive 45 to 50 Gy and gross/unresected groin nodes should be boosted to 65 to 70 Gy.

Brachytherapy: ABS-GEC-ESTRO guidelines have been summarized by Crook et al.[16] Brachytherapy is ideally restricted to lesions <4 cm with <1 cm invasion of the corpora cavernosa (typically T1–T2 lesions and select T3 cases). Larger size associated with higher LR and increased risk of late effects. Superficial molds may be created to contain sources or interstitial implant. Patient placed under general anesthesia or penile block with systemic sedation. Foley catheter is placed to aid in urethral identification. Templates placed on either side of the penis for stabilization. Up to six needles inserted perpendicular to the penis, 1 cm apart and in planes. Target volume includes tumor + 1.5- to 2-cm margin for small lesions; include glans and shaft for larger lesions. Needles are loaded after edema has subsided.

Dose: LDR dose is 60 to 65 Gy, limiting urethra to 50 Gy over 6 to 7 days. Dose rates with PDR technique are typically ~50 to 60 cGy/hr. If using HDR brachytherapy, no consensus standard dosing exists. Common HDR doses are 54 Gy BID in 3 Gy/fx delivered over 9 days and 38.4 Gy BID in 3.2 Gy/fx over 6 days. Interfraction interval should be ≥6 hours. To reduce risk of penile necrosis, limit V125 <40% and V150 <20%. To decrease risk of urethral strictures, limit urethra V115 <10% and V90 <95%. Minimize confluent areas of 125%.

Toxicity: Dermatitis, dysuria, skin telangiectasia, urethral stricture (10%–40%), urethral fistula, impotence, penile fibrosis, penile necrosis (3%–15%, higher with interstitial technique), bowel obstruction.

Procedure: See *Handbook of Treatment Planning in Radiation Oncology*, Chapter 8.[17]

EVIDENCE-BASED Q&A

What are the general outcomes of penile cancer? Does surgery or RT provide better outcomes?

Surgery and RT are both appropriate modalities. Some retrospective series suggest better LC with surgical resection; however, psychosexual morbidity with penectomy is high.[18]

Sakalis (*Eur Urol Open Sci* 2022, PMID 35540709): Systematic review of 9,578 men from 88 studies, of which 72 were from case series and 16 from nonrandomized comparative studies, evaluating various treatment modalities. Using nonrandomized comparative studies only, the 5-year RFR was 77% for penile-sparing surgery and 93% for amputative surgery. From case series, the cumulative mean 5-year RFR for penile-sparing surgery was 82%, amputative surgery 84%, brachytherapy 79%, EBRT 55%, 70% lasers, and Moh's microsurgery 88%. Both penile-sparing and amputative surgery affect all aspects of psychosocial well-being. Amputative surgery and penile-sparing surgery, respectively, impact appearance and sexual function. **Conclusion: Organ-sparing techniques appear to have similar LC rates to amputation, with the caveat that most available data are of low quality.**

Ozsahin (*IJROBP* 2006, PMID 16949770): RR of 60 men with SCC s/p either surgery alone (*n* = 27), definitive RT (*n* = 29), or postoperative RT (*n* = 22); 70% cN0. Median EBRT dose 52 Gy (26–74.5 Gy) with brachytherapy boost given in seven patients (range 15–25 Gy). One patient treated with brachytherapy alone. Of 29 patients, 19 received nodal RT (36–66 Gy). LF was 13% in the surgery group and 56% in the organ-sparing. Seventy-three percent of LF salvaged with surgery; ultimate penis preservation rate of 52%. The 5-year OS was 43% and the 10-year OS was 25%. No survival difference between those treated with definitive RT vs. primary surgery (56% vs. 53%, *p* = .16). **Conclusion: LC is superior with surgery, but there is no difference in OS between surgery and definitive RT with an organ preservation rate of 52%.**

What are the expected outcomes with limited excision?

Limited excision has been used more recently for patients with early-stage disease with a low risk for LR (Tis, Ta, or T1a). Recent long-term data show low rates of LR. Importantly, the historical standard was for a 2-cm margin, but in the current era, negative margin excision with a goal of 5 mm is appropriate.

Philippou (*J Urol* 2012, PMID 22818137): UK study of 179 patients with invasive penile cancer treated from 2002 to 2010 with organ-preserving surgery: circumcision (involving skin shaft), WLE with primary closure, removal of the glans, or removal of the glans and distal corpora. Median distance to resection margin was 5 mm. After excision, LR in 9%, regional recurrence in 11%, and DM in 5%. The 5-year DSS rate after recurrence was 55%. For patients with isolated LR, the 5-year DSS was 92% vs. 38% for those with a regional recurrence. The 5-year local recurrence-free rate was 86%. On MVA, tumor grade, stage, and LVSI were independent predictors of LR. Distance to margin was not a significant predictor of recurrence. **Conclusion: Penile-conserving surgery is safe, and excision with 5-mm margin is still associated with low risk of LR. LR has no impact on OS.**

Is RT alone an adequate modality for early-stage lesions?

RT alone is an option for organ preservation. Nodal disease has poor prognosis. Close follow-up is required as relapses are frequent.

Zouhair (*Eur J Cancer* 2001, PMID 11166146): RR of 41 patients with nonmetastatic invasive penile carcinoma treated from 1962 to 1994. Stage distribution was as follows: T1 (29%), T2 (59%), T3 (10%), and Tx (2%); N0 (71%), N1 (20%), N2 (7%), and N3 (1%). Eighteen patients underwent surgical resection, 16 of whom received partial penectomy and 2 total penectomy. Postoperative RT was delivered in 37 out of 41 patients. Twenty-three patients received definitive RT alone. EBRT was used in 22 patients, followed by brachytherapy boost in 4, and brachytherapy alone was used in 1. With MFU of 70 months in the entire cohort, 5- and 10-year OS rates were 57% and 38%, respectively. The 5-year local and locoregional rates were 57% and 48%, respectively. Among patients who received RT alone, survival with penis preservation at 5 and 10 years was 36% and 18%, respectively. **Conclusion: Similar OS between patients treated with surgery and definitive RT +/– salvage surgery.**

What is the efficacy of brachytherapy for early-stage penile cancer?

Brachytherapy is effective with high rates of LC and penile preservation for early-stage tumors as shown in multiple RRs.[19,20]

Hasan, Meta-Analysis (*Brachytherapy* 2015, PMID 25944394): Meta-analysis of 19 retrospective studies published between 1984 and 2012 of 2,178 males treated for penile cancer. 1,505 patients treated with surgery and 673 with brachytherapy. The 5-year LC was improved with surgery (84% vs. 79%, $p = .009$). The 5-year OS with surgery was 76% vs. 73% with brachytherapy (OR 1.17, 95% CI 0.95–1.44). Organ preservation rate for brachytherapy was 74%. Among an early-stage subset stage I/II, 5-year OS and LC rates were 80% and 86% in the surgery arm vs. 79% and 84% in the brachytherapy arm. **Conclusion: In early-stage tumors, there is no LC or OS difference between surgery and brachytherapy.**

Are there data to support adjuvant RT in patients with LN+ penile cancer?

Given the rarity of penile cancer, data on the benefit of adjuvant RT in patients with LN+ disease are often extrapolated from vulvar cancer trials, which showed a benefit in LC and OS to pelvic RT. One series from the Netherlands[21] provides support, but also highlights shortcomings of RT in patients with ENE and pelvic LN+ disease.

Graafland, Netherlands (*J Urol* 2010, PMID 20723934): RR of 156 patients with LN+ penile cancer s/p therapeutic regional LND. PORT (50 Gy/25 fx) was given to inguinal ± pelvic nodes if >1 pLN+ and was performed in 45% of patients. The 5-year CSS was 61%. Patients with ENE had decreased 5-year CSS (42% vs. 80%). On MVA, ENE and pelvic LN+ disease were associated with decreased CSS. **Conclusion: Despite RT, ENE and pelvic LN+ disease are associated with inferior survival.**

Robinson, UK (*Eur Urol* 2018, PMID 29703686): Systematic review of seven retrospective studies including 1,605 patients with positive inguinal LNs. Due to wide variability in data, there was insufficient evidence to assess whether adjuvant inguinal nodal RT improved outcomes. Regional recurrence rates were high (10%–92%), and toxicity assessments were limited. **Conclusion: There is no good quality evidence to support the benefit of adjuvant RT in node-positive penile cancer following LND.**

REFERENCES

1. Siegel RL, Giaquinto AN, Jemal A. Cancer statistics, 2024. *CA Cancer J Clin.* 2024;74(1):12–49. doi:10.3322/caac.21820

2. Fu L, Tian T, Yao K, et al. Global pattern and trends in penile cancer incidence: population-based study. *JMIR Public Health Surveill.* 2022;8(7):e34874. doi:10.2196/34874

3. Douglawi A, Masterson TA. Penile cancer epidemiology and risk factors: a contemporary review. *Curr Opin Urol.* 2019;29(2):145–149. doi:10.1097/MOU.0000000000000581

4. Sun M, Djajadiningrat RS, Alnajjar HM, et al. Development and external validation of a prognostic tool for prediction of cancer-specific mortality after complete loco-regional pathological staging for squamous cell carcinoma of the penis. *BJU Int.* 2015;116(5):734–743. doi:10.1111/bju.12677

5. Ficarra V, Akduman B, Bouchot O, Palou J, Tobias-Machado M. Prognostic factors in penile cancer. *Urology.* 2010;76(2 suppl 1):S66–S73. doi:10.1016/j.urology.2010.04.008

6. Ornellas AA, Kinchin EW, Nobrega BL, Wisnescky A, Koifman N, Quirino R. Surgical treatment of invasive squamous cell carcinoma of the penis: Brazilian National Cancer Institute long-term experience. *J Surg Oncol.* 2008;97(6):487–495. doi:10.1002/jso.20980

7. Velazquez EF, Ayala G, Liu H, et al. Histologic grade and perineural invasion are more important than tumor thickness as predictor of nodal metastasis in penile squamous cell carcinoma invading 5 to 10 mm. *Am J Surg Pathol.* 2008;32(7):974–979. doi:10.1097/PAS.0b013e3181641365

8. Amin MB, Edge SB, Greene FL, et al, eds. *AJCC Cancer Staging Manual.* 8th ed. Springer; 2017.

9. Brouwer OR, Albersen M, Parnham A, et al. European Association of Urology-American Society of Clinical Oncology collaborative guideline on penile cancer: 2023 update. *Eur Urol.* 2023;83(6):548–560. doi:10.1016/j.eururo.2023.02.027

10. Sakalis VI, Campi R, Barreto L, et al. What is the most effective management of the primary tumor in men with invasive penile cancer: a systematic review of the available treatment options and their outcomes. *Eur Urol Open Sci.* 2022;40:58–94. doi:10.1016/j.euros.2022.04.002

11. Sri D, Sujenthiran A, Lam W, et al. A study into the association between local recurrence rates and surgical resection margins in organ-sparing surgery for penile squamous cell cancer. *BJU Int.* 2018;122(4):576–582. doi:10.1111/bju.14222

12. Solsona E, Bahl A, Brandes SB, et al. New developments in the treatment of localized penile cancer. *Urology.* 2010;76(2 suppl 1):S36–S42. doi:10.1016/j.urology.2010.04.009

13. Neave F, Neal AJ, Hoskin PJ, Hope-Stone HF. Carcinoma of the penis: a retrospective review of treatment with iridium mould and external beam irradiation. *Clin Oncol (R Coll Radiol).* 1993;5(4):207–210. doi:10.1016/S0936-6555(05)80230-4

14. Munro NP, Thomas PJ, Deutsch GP, Hodson NJ. Penile cancer: a case for guidelines. *Ann R Coll Surg Engl.* 2001;83(3):180–185. PMID: 11432137

15. Azrif M, Logue JP, Swindell R, Cowan RA, Wylie JP, Livsey JE. External-beam radiotherapy in T1-2 N0 penile carcinoma. *Clin Oncol (R Coll Radiol).* 2006;18(4):320–325. doi:10.1016/j.clon.2006.01.004

16. Crook JM, Haie-Meder C, Demanes DJ, Mazeron JJ, Martinez AA, Rivard MJ. American Brachytherapy Society-Groupe Européen de Curiethérapie-European Society of Therapeutic Radiation Oncology (ABS-GEC-ESTRO) consensus statement for penile brachytherapy. *Brachytherapy.* 2013;12(3):191–198. doi:10.1016/j.brachy.2013.01.167

17. Videtic GMM, Vassil AD, Woody NM. *Handbook of Treatment Planning in Radiation Oncology.* Springer Publishing Company; 2020.

18. Sarin R, Norman AR, Steel GG, Horwich A. Treatment results and prognostic factors in 101 men treated for squamous carcinoma of the penis. *Int J Radiat Oncol Biol Phys.* 1997;38(4):713–722. doi:10.1016/S0360-3016(97)00068-0

19. Crook J, Ma C, Grimard L. Radiation therapy in the management of the primary penile tumor: an update. *World J Urol.* 2009;27(2):189–196. doi:10.1007/s00345-008-0309-5

20. de Crevoisier R, Slimane K, Sanfilippo N, et al. Long-term results of brachytherapy for carcinoma of the penis confined to the glans (N- or NX). *Int J Radiat Oncol Biol Phys.* 2009;74(4):1150–1156. doi:10.1016/j.ijrobp.2008.09.054

21. Graafland NM, van Boven HH, van Werkhoven E, Moonen LM, Horenblas S. Prognostic significance of extranodal extension in patients with pathological node positive penile carcinoma. *J Urol.* 2010;184(4):1347–1353. doi:10.1016/j.juro.2010.06.016

Winston Vuong, Rahul D. Tendulkar, and Omar Y. Mian

QUICK HIT   Rare tumor that often presents with locally advanced disease, particularly proximal tumors, which have a worse prognosis. Urothelial carcinomas are the most common, followed by squamous cell carcinomas (SCC). Management involves surgery for early-stage disease (with organ preservation if possible) and combined modality therapy for advanced stage. Unfortunately, no prospective randomized trials guide management. Adjuvant RT (CRT preferred) is indicated for positive margins and pT3–4N+ disease. See Table 46.1 for general treatment paradigm of urethral cancer.

Table 46.1 General Treatment Paradigm for Urethral Cancer	
Ta, Tis, T1	Transurethral (endoscopic) resection followed by intraurethral CHT or BCG (in select cases)
T2 (male, pendulous urethra)	Distal urethrectomy (consider neoadjuvant CHT or CRT) or partial penectomy
T2 (male, bulbar urethra)	Urethrectomy (consider neoadjuvant CHT or CRT) ± cystoprostatectomy
T2 (female)	CRT or urethrectomy + cystectomy or distal urethrectomy depending on tumor location; for surgical approaches, consider neoadjuvant CHT or CRT
T3/T4 or LN+	Definitive CRT preferred (especially for SCC) or neoadjuvant CHT ± RT followed by surgery; inguinal LN dissection for patients with cN+ disease
Urothelial carcinoma of the prostate	Surgical management akin to bladder cancer, i.e., TUR + BCG for mucosal disease, cystoprostatectomy ± urethrectomy and neoadj CHT for more invasive/locally advanced disease

EPIDEMIOLOGY: Very rare tumor (<1% of GU malignancies). In a SEER registry from 2004 to 2016, there were 1,645 cases, with 4.3 cases per million men and 1.5 cases per million women, with a peak incidence in those 75 years and older. Women are more likely to present with higher stage disease and have worse cancer-specific mortality.[1] Up to 50% of patients die of their disease.[2]

RISK FACTORS: Chronic inflammation: prior history of STD, urethritis, urethral strictures (potentially secondary to trauma), urethral diverticuli, urinary stasis, recurrent infection. HPV, prior urothelial cancer, or prior RT.[3]

ANATOMY

Men: Male urethra extends from the bladder neck proximally to the urethral meatus distally (~20–21 cm in length), and is divided into the prostatic urethra (10% of cancer cases; composed of transitional epithelium), bulbomembranous (60%; transitional epithelium), and penile (30%; pseudostratified columnar epithelium) portions, with squamous epithelium at the meatus.

Women: Female urethra is shorter than males (3–4 cm) and is divided into the posterior segment (proximal one-third, transitional cells) and anterior segment (distal two-thirds, squamous epithelium).

PATHOLOGY: In general, the majority of urethral cancers are urothelial carcinomas, followed by SCC. Adenocarcinomas are rare and typically arise from periurethral glandular tissue (Skene's glands). Mixed tumors can also be seen. Unconventional histologies include mullerian type, melanocytic, neuroendocrine, lymphoma, sarcoma/mesenchymal, and spindle cell.[4]

CLINICAL PRESENTATION: May present with symptoms of a urethral stricture (urinary retention, difficulty voiding, dysuria), hematuria, urethral discharge, pain, swelling, priapism, irritative urinary symptoms, or dyspareunia. Often presents late because symptoms can be attributed to benign causes (e.g., UTI or strictures). Cancers can extend locally into the penis, and spread to the pelvic LNs (primary drainage for the proximal one-third urethra) or to inguinal LNs (primary drainage for the distal two-thirds urethra), which can present with palpable nodal metastasis. Clinically suspicious LNs are usually involved by urethral cancer metastases (in contrast to penile cancer where only ~50% of cN+ are pN+). DM present in only 10% at diagnosis (lung, liver, bone).

WORKUP: H&P with full GU exam (also GYN exam for women). EUA (palpation of the genitalia, urethra, rectum, perineum) and cystourethroscopy to evaluate extent of disease. Consider retrograde urethrogram.

Labs: CBC, CMP, urine cytology (more sensitive for urothelial carcinomas in pendulous urethra).

Imaging: CT or MRI of the primary site and pelvis. CT chest ± bone scan. PET/CT is not standard.

Biopsy: Transurethral biopsy.

PROGNOSTIC FACTORS: Poor prognosis associated with advanced age, tumor location (proximal worse than distal), tumor size (>2 cm vs. <2 cm), higher clinical nodal stage, higher histologic grade, presence of metastatic disease.[1,5-7]

STAGING: See Table 46.2 and Table 46.3 for AJCC staging summaries.

Table 46.2 AJCC 8th Edition (2017): Staging for Male Penile Urethra and Female Urethra		cN0	cN1	cN2
T/M	N			
T1	• Invades subepithelial connective tissue	I	III	
T2	• Invades corpus spongiosum or periurethral muscle	II		
T3	• Invades corpus cavernosum or anterior vagina			IV
T4	• Invades other adjacent organs (bladder)			
M1	• Distant metastasis			

Notes: Regional LNs include inguinal (superficial or deep), perivesical, obturator, internal iliac, external iliac, and presacral. cN1: single regional LN; cN2: multiple regional LNs.

Table 46.3 AJCC 8th Edition (2017): Staging for Prostatic Urethra	
Tis	Carcinoma in situ involving prostatic urethra or periurethral or prostatic ducts without stromal invasion
T1	Invades subepithelial connective tissue
T2	Invades prostatic stroma surrounding ducts by direct extension from urothelial surface or prostatic ducts
T3	Invades periprostatic fat
T4	Invades other adjacent organs (e.g., bladder wall, rectal wall)

Source: Adapted from AJCC Cancer Staging Manual. 8th ed. Springer International Publishing; 2017.

TREATMENT PARADIGM: Without prospective trials to guide management, only retrospective series are available. Treatment based on gender, location, extent of disease, and histology (Table 46.1).

General Principles

Localized Disease: Surgical management, with transurethral resection for small lesions or segmental resection for larger lesions (partial or total urethrectomy). Consider RT for organ preservation.

Locally Advanced Disease: Definitive CRT preferred (especially for SCC). Alternatively, neoadjuvant CHT or CRT can be used followed by consolidation surgery particularly for cT3–4N0 urothelial carcinoma.

Metastatic disease: CHT ± immunotherapy ± palliative local therapy.

Surgery: If attempting urethra-sparing/penile-preserving surgery or partial urethrectomy, a complete circumferential assessment is recommended. In both men and women, inguinal LND is generally recommended in patients with clinically or radiographically positive LNs. No definitive data on SLNB, although performed at some centers.

Men: For small Tis–T1 tumors, endoscopic resection is appropriate. Distal tumors can undergo distal urethrectomy. For larger tumors or if unable to obtain a negative margin resection endoscopically, perform a segmental resection with anastomosis. Subtotal urethrectomy and perineal urethrostomy for T2 cancers (spongiosum but not cavernosa involvement). T3–T4 tumors often require total penectomy, cystoprostatectomy, and anterior exenteration with perineal reconstruction.

Women: T1 tumors can be treated with endoscopic resection (must maintain urethral sphincter to preserve continence). More advanced tumors are treated by total urethrectomy with bladder neck closure and urinary diversion. Extensive locoregional disease may require pelvic exenteration and vaginectomy.

Chemotherapy: Neoadjuvant CHT indicated for locally advanced disease ± RT prior to surgery based on histology. SCC often treated with 5-FU + cisplatin or 5-FU + MMC. Urothelial carcinomas typically receive cisplatin-based regimens such as gemcitabine + cisplatin or ddMVAC (dose-dense methotrexate, vinblastine, doxorubicin, and cisplatin).

Radiation: Prior to RT, consider circumcision in men to prevent balanitis and phimosis.

Definitive: Consider organ preservation for distal tumors in men and proximal tumors in women. T1–T2 tumors can potentially be treated with RT alone, but for more advanced disease consider sequential or concurrent CRT.

Adjuvant: Consider postop RT (PORT) for patients with locally advanced (pT3–4/N+) disease.

Neoadjuvant: Consider preop RT or CRT to reduce tumor burden and/or extent of surgery required.

Palliative: Indicated for symptomatic locally advanced disease not amenable to curative therapy.

Dose: EBRT dose is 45 to 50.4 Gy to primary site and inguinal, external, and internal iliac LNs (strongly recommended even in cT2N0 disease). Positive margins or areas of ENE should be boosted to 54 to 60 Gy. Gross disease can be treated up to 66 to 70 Gy. Recurrent disease can be treated 66 to 74 Gy. Brachytherapy may be considered for lesions <2 to 3 cm with negative LNs or prior to EBRT for patients with larger tumors or LN+ disease. Brachytherapy dose is generally ~20 to 25 Gy after EBRT.

Toxicities: Acute: radiation dermatitis, local pain, fibrosis, radiation cystitis, urethritis. Late: chronic penile edema, fistula, hemorrhage, and urethral stricture (consider biopsy to rule out recurrent disease).

Procedure: See *Handbook of Treatment Planning in Radiation Oncology*, Chapter 8.[8]

EVIDENCE-BASED Q&A

Can an organ preservation approach be used for patients with early-stage urethral cancer?

Select series show promising outcomes with definitive RT (brachytherapy ± EBRT) as an alternative to surgery.

Garden, MDACC (*Cancer 1993*, PMID 8490839): RR of 97 women with primary carcinomas of the female urethra. Eighty-six patients received RT: 35 with combined EBRT + brachytherapy, 21 with EBRT alone, and 30 with brachytherapy alone. Cumulative doses ranged from 40 to 106 Gy, with a median of 65 Gy. The 5-year LC was 64%, 5-year OS 41%, and 5-year DSS 49%. Ninety-seven percent of recurrences occurred within the first 2 years. Among those with LC, 40% experienced moderate or severe complications. The type of treatment was not correlated with outcome. The only prognostic factor was the involved length of urethra ($p = .008$). **Conclusion: RT alone can be potentially curative for early-stage urethral cancer; however, treatment is associated with high rates of morbidity.**

Can an organ preservation approach be used for patients with locally advanced urethral cancer?

Select series show promising outcomes with definitive CRT for patients who refuse surgery or are not surgical candidates (as an alternative to surgery). However, those who do not respond to therapy have dismal outcomes (despite salvage surgery).

Kent, Lahey Clinic (*J Urol* 2015, PMID 25088950): RR of 26 male patients treated with two cycles of 5-FU 1,000 mg/m^2 + MMC 10 mg/m^2 with concurrent EBRT 45–55 Gy/25 fx to the genitals, perineum, and inguinal and external iliac LNs. All but one patient had SCC histology; 88% had at least T3 or LN+ disease; 79% had CR and 21% had no response to treatment (all of these patients died of their disease, regardless of salvage surgery). Of the CR patients, 42% had disease recurrence at a median of 12.5 months. The 5-year DSS was 68%, DFS 43%, and OS 52%. **Conclusion: CRT may allow for organ preservation in select patients.**

Are there any data supporting the use of neoadjuvant CHT or CRT in patients with locally advanced urethral cancer?

For significant locally advanced disease, neoadjuvant therapy can decrease the burden of disease and reduce the extent of surgery needed.

Gakis, Multi-Institutional (*Ann Oncol* 2015, PMID 25969370): Multicenter RR of 124 patients (86 men, 38 women) with urethral cancer treated at 10 centers from 1993 to 2012. Thirty-one percent received neoadjuvant CHT, 15% neoadjuvant CRT + adjuvant CHT, and 54% received adjuvant CHT. Neoadjuvant therapy was more likely to be used in patients with LN+ disease and reduced extent of surgery (avoiding cystectomy). Relative response to neoadjuvant CHT was 25% and to neoadjuvant CRT was 33%. The 3-year OS was 100% for those who received neoadjuvant CHT or neoadjuvant CRT, but only 50% after surgery and 20% after surgery + adjuvant CHT. Neoadjuvant treatment was associated with improved 3-year RFS and OS. **Conclusion: Neoadjuvant CHT or CRT for patients with T3 or LN+ disease was associated with improved outcomes compared with upfront surgery or surgery + CHT.**

What is the role of adjuvant RT in patients with locally advanced urethral cancer?

Son, Multi-Institutional (*IJROBP* 2018, PMID 29908944): RR of 2,614 patients, with 5-year OS of 54%. Among 501 patients with locally advanced urethral cancer, surgery + RT was associated with improved OS compared with surgery alone (especially for adenocarcinomas HR 0.20 and transitional cell carcinomas HR 0.45). For 1,705 patients with early-stage disease, no OS difference was noted with the addition of PORT.

Are there consensus guideline papers for urethral cancer?

Gakis, EAU Guidelines (*Eur Urol* 2020, PMID 32605889): An international multidisciplinary group of the European Association of Urology has compiled best-practice guidelines on the management of urethral cancer, published in 2020 but subsequently updated online at uroweb.org/guidelines/primary-urethral-carcinoma.

REFERENCES

1.   Wenzel M, Nocera L, Collà Ruvolo C, et al. Sex-related differences include stage, histology, and survival in urethral cancer patients. *Clin Genitourin Cancer*. 2021;19(2):135–143. doi:10.1016/j.clgc.2020.12.001

2.   Visser O, Adolfsson J, Rossi S, et al. Incidence and survival of rare urogenital cancers in Europe. *Eur J Cancer*. 2012;48(4):456–464. doi:10.1016/j.ejca.2011.10.031

3.   Neuzillet Y, Witjes JA, Bruins HM, Carrion A, Cathomas R. *EAU Guidelines on Primary Urethral Carcinoma*; 2024. European Association of Urology. Accessed June 7, 2025. https://uroweb.org/guidelines/primary-urethral-carcinoma/chapter/introduction

4.   Wenzel M, Collà Ruvolo C, Würnschimmel C, et al. Epidemiology of unconventional histological subtypes of urethral cancer. *Urol Int*. 2023;107(1):15–22. doi:10.1159/000525673

5.   Rabbani F. Prognostic factors in male urethral cancer. *Cancer*. 2011;117(11):2426–2434. doi:10.1002/cncr.25787

6.   Champ CE, Hegarty SE, Shen X, et al. Prognostic factors and outcomes after definitive treatment of female urethral cancer: a population-based analysis. *Urology*. 2012;80(2):374–381. doi:10.1016/j.urology.2012.02.058

7.   Gakis G, Morgan TM, Efstathiou JA, et al. Prognostic factors and outcomes in primary urethral cancer: results from the international collaboration on primary urethral carcinoma. *World J Urol*. 2016;34(1):97–103. doi:10.1007/s00345-015-1583-7

8.   Videtic GMM, Woody NM, Vassil AD. *Handbook of Treatment Planning in Radiation Oncology*. 3rd ed. Demos Medical; 2020.

47 RENAL CELL CARCINOMA

Salem Alfaifi, Omar Y. Mian, and Rahul D. Tendulkar

QUICK HIT   Renal cell carcinoma (RCC) is a relatively common primary tumor of the kidney. Surgical resection alone is recommended for localized disease. Adjuvant RT has had a minimal role due to the rarity of locoregional failure and the frequency of distant failure. Historically, radical nephrectomy was performed even in the setting of metastatic disease based on randomized data showing a survival benefit. With the advent of targeted therapy and immunotherapy, survival has been dramatically extended, and surgical resection in the setting of metastatic disease may not be necessary. For medically inoperable patients, definitive SBRT is an emerging option with growing evidence to support its efficacy and safety. Other options include RFA or cryotherapy for small tumors. In the metastatic setting, the role of SBRT to the primary tumor and/or to oligometastatic and oligoprogressive sites in combination with systemic therapy is evolving.

EPIDEMIOLOGY: Primary kidney and renal pelvis cancers have an annual incidence of ~81,000 cases and ~14,000 deaths in the United States.[1,2] Incidence has increased by 1.5% per year predominately for early localized disease likely related to incidental findings on imaging. Despite this increase, there is a 1% to 2% mortality decline likely related to advances in treatment.[1,3] Median age at diagnosis is 65 years, with a slight male preponderance.

RISK FACTORS: Cigarette smoking (risk increased 50% in males and 20% in females as compared with nonsmokers), obesity, phenacetin-containing analgesics (cancer usually follows prolonged and heavy use, with resultant renal papillary necrosis), and low fruit/vegetable diet.[4-7]

ANATOMY: The kidneys and renal pelvis are retroperitoneal structures surrounded by perinephric fat and encapsulated by Gerota's fascia. They are centered at L1 or L2 and lie between T12 and L3, with the right kidney slightly more inferior due to the liver. The minor and major calyces drain urine into the renal pelvis, which then conveys urine into the ureters. The right kidney drains to renal hilar, paracaval, and interaortocaval nodes, while the left kidney drains to renal hilar and para-aortic nodes.

PATHOLOGY: RCC arises within the renal cortex and represents 80% to 85% of primary renal neoplasms. Several RCC subtypes exist, including clear cell (75%–85%), papillary (10%–15%), chromophobe (5%–10%), oncocytic (3%–5%), and collecting duct (Bellini duct, <1%).[8] The distinct sarcomatoid subtype, representing <10% of renal tumors, is associated with worse OS than other subtypes, and 50% to 70% of patients with sarcomatoid tumors present with bone metastases.[9] While tumors <3 cm have historically been characterized as renal adenomas, data have shown small tumors can still represent malignancy and often require definitive management.[10]

GENETICS: Hereditary diseases: (a) von Hippel–Lindau (VHL): mutation/deletion in the *VHL* gene located on the short arm of chr 3 (3p25) that predisposes the development of characteristic red birthmarks, renal cancer, CNS hemangioblastoma, retinal angioma, pheochromocytoma, epididymal cystadenoma, and pancreatic tumors; 30%–45% of patients develop clear cell RCC. The VHL protein is responsible for ubiquitinating HIF-1α under normoxic conditions marking it for proteasomal degradation. The absence of functional VHL simulates hypoxia, causing upregulation of hypoxia-responsive genes such as *VEGF, PDGF, EGFR, GLUT-1, TGF-β*, and *EPO*. (b) Hereditary clear cell renal carcinoma (HCRC): rare, AD disease associated with mutation in the *VHL* gene. (c) Hereditary papillary cell renal carcinoma (HPRC): rare, AD disease associated with germline abnormality in the MET proto-oncogene.[11,12]

CLINICAL PRESENTATION: Common symptoms are painless gross or microscopic hematuria. Uncommon symptoms are pain, flank mass, and paraneoplastic syndromes. The classic triad of *gross hematuria, flank mass, and pain* occurs in only 10% of patients and usually indicates advanced disease. Up to 25% to 40% of patients with RCC are asymptomatic and discovered incidentally.

Paraneoplastic syndromes may cause anemia, polycythemia (EPO), pyrexia, amyloidosis, liver dysfunction, hypertension, or hypercalcemia (PTH-rp). The sudden onset of a left-sided varicocele should raise the possibility of a renal tumor obstructing the testicular vein at its entry point into the left renal vein (occurs in 2% of male patients).

WORKUP: H&P.

Labs: CBC, CMP.

Imaging: Ultrasound or abdominal CT based on presenting symptoms. MRI is useful when US and CT are inconclusive or if patient is unable to receive IV contrast. CT chest for staging. Bone scan indicated only in patients with symptoms or elevated alkaline phosphatase.

Biopsy: CT-guided biopsy may be performed for indeterminate tumor on radiographic workup. Surgery is often done without obtaining tissue biopsy if the diagnosis is obvious from radiographic workup. Selective renal arteriogram should be done if considering a partial nephrectomy.

PROGNOSTIC FACTORS: Stage is the most important factor. Other factors associated with poor survival include KPS <80, time from diagnosis to initiation of targeted therapy <1 year, low hemoglobin, high calcium, high neutrophil count, and high platelet count.[13]

STAGING: AJCC 8th edition (Table 47.1).

Table 47.1 AJCC 8th Edition: Staging for RCC			cN0	cN1
T/M		**N**		
T1	a. ≤4 cm, limited to kidney		I	III
	b. >4 and ≤7 cm, limited to kidney			III
T2	a. >7–10 cm, limited to kidney		II	
	b. >10 cm, limited to kidney			
T3	a. Tumor extends into the renal vein or its segmental branches, or invades the pelvicalyceal system, or invades perirenal and/or renal sinus fat but not beyond Gerota's fascia		III	
	b. Tumor extends into the vena cava below the diaphragm			
	c. Tumor grossly extends into the vena cava above the diaphragm or invades the wall of the vena cava			
T4	Tumor invades beyond Gerota's fascia (including contiguous extension to the ipsilateral adrenal gland)		IV	
M1	Distant metastasis			

TREATMENT PARADIGM

Active Surveillance: Active surveillance may be appropriate for small renal masses (<4 cm) as this approach has demonstrated slow linear growth rates, low rates of surgical intervention, and very low rates of metastatic progression in appropriately selected patients.[14]

Surgery: Mainstay of treatment for nonmetastatic disease. Surgical choice depends on tumor and patient factors.

Radical Nephrectomy (RN): En bloc removal of the kidney along with Gerota's fascia and its contents (including adrenal gland, kidney, perinephric fat, and often hilar lymph nodes). RN has not been compared with a simple nephrectomy in a randomized trial, but it allows a more reliable margin around the tumor. The surgical approach depends on the patient's body habitus, position of tumor, and comorbidities. Tumor within the IVC does NOT preclude a curative resection.

Partial Nephrectomy (PN): Indicated for early-stage (IA/IB) disease and in those with poor renal reserve, absence of a normally functioning contralateral kidney, or bilateral renal cancer with PN performed on the lesser involved kidney. PN may be considered electively for small tumors

(<4 cm) as well as for patients with VHL disease, renal artery stenosis, hydronephrosis, ureteral reflux, and nephrosclerosis. Compared with radical nephrectomy, PN is associated with similar oncologic outcomes, a lower risk of chronic renal dysfunction, but a greater risk of bleeding.[15] PN patients are candidates for salvage nephrectomy in the event of a local failure (<10% of cases).

Palliative Nephrectomy: Indicated for intractable bleeding and pain. Debulking nephrectomy prior to systemic therapy in patients with metastatic disease has improved survival compared with IFN-α alone in two randomized trials.[16,17] However, with more effective systemic therapy, there appears to be a more limited role for this approach in the modern era.[18,19] Debulking surgery induces spontaneous regression of metastases in <1% of cases. LN dissection remains controversial as it provides staging information but has no impact on survival.

Cryoablation/RFA: Minimally invasive option for localized disease especially in those with a single kidney or comorbidities. Contraindications include tumor >5 cm, DM, and hilar or central tumors.

Systemic Therapy: Multiple trials have investigated the role of adjuvant therapy in nonmetastatic disease. Sunitinib has been approved for adjuvant treatment in high-risk disease after resection based on an improvement in DFS, although it is associated with toxicity and no OS benefit.[20] Various immunotherapies are currently under investigation in the adjuvant setting, with pembrolizumab demonstrating promising preliminary results.[21] Several targeted therapy and immunotherapy options are available for the first-line treatment of metastatic disease, including nivolumab plus ipilimumab, pembrolizumab plus axitinib, or avelumab plus axitinib.[22]

Radiation

Adjuvant RT: After radical nephrectomy, the risk of LR is <5%, and thus adjuvant RT is not generally recommended. Two early randomized trials of postoperative RT (50–55 Gy) vs. observation showed no benefit in LC or OS with the addition of RT with a significant increase in toxicity and complications.[23,24] Although these studies were done in the 2D era, there have not been data to support adjuvant RT in more modern series. Some retrospective series suggest a potential LC benefit for adjuvant RT in patients with T3–T4 disease, positive margins, or positive LNs; however, given low rates of LR without RT, adjuvant treatment is generally not employed.

Definitive SBRT: Evidence for using SBRT in the definitive setting is growing, including prospective trials showing excellent rates of LC with favorable toxicity profiles in patients who are inoperable or have unresectable RCC. A recent ISRS practice guideline supported the practice of definitive SBRT for RCC as a safe and effective standard treatment option.[25]

Dose: 25–26 Gy/1 fx for tumors ≤4 cm and 42–48 Gy/3 fx for tumors >4 cm.[25,26]

Toxicity: Common acute side effects may include fatigue, nausea, vomiting, diarrhea, flank pain, hematuria, gastritis, peptic ulcer, and dermatitis. Late side effects may include reduced renal function.

EVIDENCE-BASED Q&A

What data are available to support the use of SBRT for the treatment of inoperable RCC?

The IROCK multi-institutional pooled analysis demonstrated excellent LC with SBRT for RCC with acceptable toxicity, even in large-sized tumors.[27–30] More recently, a large nonrandomized phase II study, FASTRACK-II/TROG15.03, confirmed the efficacy and safety of this approach.[26] A recent ISRS practice guideline supported using SBRT for inoperable RCC as a safe and effective standard treatment option.[25]

Siva, IROCK (*Lancet Oncology* 2022, PMID 36400098): Meta-analysis of 190 patients from 12 institutions treated with definitive SBRT. MFU 5 years. Eighty-one patients treated with single-fx SBRT (median 25 Gy/1 fx), and 109 patients treated with multi-fx regimens (42 Gy/2–10 fx). Median tumor diameter was 4 cm. The 5-year LF, CSS, and PFS rates were 6%, 92%, and 64%, respectively. Multi-fx SBRT (vs. single), larger tumor (>4 cm), and poor KPS were associated with worse outcomes. Grades 1 to 2 toxicities were reported in 37% of patients and no grade 3 toxicity. One patient had acute grade 4 duodenal ulcer and late grade 4 gastritis. Mean GFR decreased 14 mL/min at 5 years, and the incidence of ESRD after SBRT was only 7% despite >50% of patients having GFR <60 at baseline (for comparison, partial nephrectomy yields a 4%–36% incidence of ESRD in patients with GFR <60). **Conclusions: SBRT for inoperable RCC has excellent durable LC with acceptable toxicity and minimal effect on kidney function.**

Siva, FASTRACK-II/TROG15.03 (*Lancet Oncology* 2024, PMID 38423047): Single-arm, multi-institutional, phase II trial of definitive SBRT for biopsy-confirmed RCC of a single kidney lesion for patients with ECOG ≤2 and who were medically inoperable, high risk, or declined surgery. Tumors ≤4 cm received 26 Gy/1 fx and tumors >4 cm to 10 cm received 42 Gy/3 fx. Seventy patients enrolled with median age of 77 years and median tumor size of 4.6 cm (IQR: 3.7–5.5 cm). MFU was 43 months. LC and CSS were both 100% at 1 year. FFDM at 1 and 3 years was 97%; 1- and 3-year OS rates were 99% and 82%, respectively. Baseline mean eGFR was 61 mL/min and reduced by 10.8 and 14.6 at 1 and 2 years before plateauing. Ten percent of patients had grade 3 toxicity, and there was no grade 4 or 5 toxicity. **Conclusion: Definitive SBRT for solitary biopsy-confirmed RCC is well-tolerated, with 100% 1-year LC.**

Siva, ISRS (*Lancet Oncology* 2024, PMID 38181809): Systematic review of 36 studies (822 patients) with median tumor size of 4.4 cm. MFU was 31 months. Median LC was 94% (range 70–100), 5-year PFS was 80% (95% CI 72–92), and 5-year OS was 77% (95% CI 65–89). Four percent were reported to undergo post-SBRT dialysis, and 5%, 3%, and <1% had grades 2, 3, and 4 toxicities, respectively. **Conclusion: SBRT for primary RCC is a safe and effective standard treatment option.**

Is there a role for SBRT to the primary tumor in patients with metastatic RCC?

NRG-GU012 is an ongoing randomized trial evaluating SBRT as an alternative approach for treatment of the primary tumor in patients with metastatic RCC receiving immunotherapy who are not recommended for surgery or who decline surgery.[31]

Is there a role for SBRT to oligometastatic and oligoprogressive RCC?

A recent ESTRO/EAU project provided consensus guidelines on the management of oligometastatic and oligoprogressive RCC. They considered an upper threshold of three to five lesions to offer ablative SBRT in the oligoprogressive setting, and they agreed on the concomitant (within 30 days) administration of immunotherapy during SBRT.[32] *This consensus indicated SBRT as a treatment modality of choice for bone oligometastasis (24 Gy/2 fx spine, 30 Gy/3 fx nonspine) and adrenal oligometastasis (40 Gy/5 fx).*

REFERENCES

1. Siegel RL, Giaquinto AN, Jemal A. Cancer statistics, 2024. *CA Cancer J Clin.* 2024;74(1):12–49. doi:10.3322/caac.21820
2. Chen YW, Wang L, Panian J, et al. Treatment landscape of renal cell carcinoma. *Curr Treat Options Oncol.* 2023;24(12):1889–1916. doi:10.1007/s11864-023-01161-5
3. King SC, Pollack LA, Li J, King JB, Master VA. Continued increase in incidence of renal cell carcinoma, especially in young patients and high grade disease: United States 2001 to 2010. *J Urol.* 2014;191(6):1665–1670. doi:10.1016/j.juro.2013.12.046
4. Scelo G, Larose TL. Epidemiology and risk factors for kidney cancer. *J Clin Oncol.* 2018;36(36):3574–3581. doi:10.1200/JCO.2018.79.1905
5. Chow W-H, Dong LM, Devesa SS. Epidemiology and risk factors for kidney cancer. *Nat Rev Urol.* 2010;7(5):245–257. doi:10.1038/nrurol.2010.46
6. Zeegers MPA, Tan FES, Dorant E, Van Den Brandt PA. The impact of characteristics of cigarette smoking on urinary tract cancer risk. *Cancer.* 2000;89(3):630–639. doi:10.1002/1097-0142(20000801)89:3<630::AID-CNCR19>3.3.CO;2-H
7. Oh SW, Yoon YS, Shin S-A. Effects of excess weight on cancer incidences depending on cancer sites and histologic findings among men: Korea National Health Insurance Corporation Study. *J Clin Oncol.* 2005;23(21):4742–4754. doi:10.1200/JCO.2005.11.726
8. Athanazio DA, Amorim LS, Da Cunha IW, et al. Classification of renal cell tumors—current concepts and use of ancillary tests: recommendations of the Brazilian Society of Pathology. *Surg Exp Pathol.* 2021;4(1). doi:10.1186/s42047-020-00084-x
9. Shuch B, Bratslavsky G, Linehan WM, Srinivasan R. Sarcomatoid renal cell carcinoma: a comprehensive review of the biology and current treatment strategies. *Oncologist.* 2012;17(1):46–54. doi:10.1634/theoncologist.2011-0227
10. Bosniak MA, Birnbaum BA, Krinsky GA, Waisman J. Small renal parenchymal neoplasms: further observations on growth. *Radiology.* 1995;197(3):589–597. doi:10.1148/radiology.197.3.7480724
11. Haas NB, Nathanson KL. Hereditary kidney cancer syndromes. *Adv Chronic Kidney Dis.* 2014;21(1):81–90. doi:10.1053/j.ackd.2013.10.001

12. Maher ER. Hereditary renal cell carcinoma syndromes: diagnosis, surveillance and management. *World J Urol.* 2018;36(12):1891–1898. doi:10.1007/s00345-018-2288-5

13. Heng DY, Xie W, Regan MM, et al. External validation and comparison with other models of the International Metastatic Renal-Cell Carcinoma Database Consortium prognostic model: a population-based study. *Lancet Oncol.* 2013;14(2):141–148. doi:10.1016/S1470-2045(12)70559-4

14. McIntosh AG, Ristau BT, Ruth K, et al. Active surveillance for localized renal masses: tumor growth, delayed intervention rates, and >5-yr clinical outcomes. *Eur Urol.* 2018;74(2):157–164. doi:10.1016/j.eururo.2018.03.011

15. Maclennan S, Imamura M, Lapitan MC, et al. Systematic review of perioperative and quality-of-life outcomes following surgical management of localised renal cancer. *Eur Urol.* 2012;62(6):1097–1117. doi:10.1016/j.eururo.2012.07.028

16. Flanigan RC, Salmon SE, Blumenstein BA, et al. Nephrectomy followed by interferon alfa-2b compared with interferon alfa-2b alone for metastatic renal-cell cancer. *N Engl J Med.* 2001;345(23):1655–1659. doi:10.1056/NEJMoa003013

17. Mickisch GH, Garin A, van Poppel H, et al. Radical nephrectomy plus interferon-alfa-based immunotherapy compared with interferon alfa alone in metastatic renal-cell carcinoma: a randomised trial. *Lancet.* 2001;358(9286):966–970. doi:10.1016/S0140-6736(01)06103-7

18. Méjean A, Ravaud A, Thezenas S, et al. Sunitinib alone or after nephrectomy in metastatic renal-cell carcinoma. *N Engl J Med.* 2018;379(5):417–427. doi:10.1056/NEJMoa1803675

19. Studentova H, Spisarova M, Kopova A, Zemankova A, Melichar B, Student V. The evolving landscape of cytoreductive nephrectomy in metastatic renal cell carcinoma. *Cancers.* 2023;15(15):3855. doi:10.3390/cancers15153855

20. Ravaud A, Motzer RJ, Pandha HS, et al. Adjuvant sunitinib in high-risk renal-cell carcinoma after nephrectomy. *N Engl J Med.* 2016;375(23):2246–2254. doi:10.1056/NEJMoa1611406

21. Powles T, Tomczak P, Park SH, et al. Pembrolizumab versus placebo as post-nephrectomy adjuvant therapy for clear cell renal cell carcinoma (KEYNOTE-564): 30-month follow-up analysis of a multicentre, randomised, double-blind, placebo-controlled, phase 3 trial. *Lancet Oncol.* 2022;23(9):1133–1144. doi:10.1016/S1470-2045(22)00487-9

22. Bosma NA, Warkentin MT, Gan CL, et al. Efficacy and safety of first-line systemic therapy for metastatic renal cell carcinoma: a systematic review and network meta-analysis. *Eur Urol Open Sci.* 2022;37:14–26. doi:10.1016/j.euros.2021.12.007

23. Finney R. The value of radiotherapy in the treatment of hypernephroma—a clinical trial. *Br J Urol.* 1973;45(3):258–269. doi:10.1111/j.1464-410X.1973.tb12152.x

24. Micheletti E, Favardi U, Cozzoli A. Role of postoperative adjuvant radiotherapy in the treatment of class T2-3 N0 M0 adenocarcinoma of the kidney. *Radiol Med.* 1991;81(6):887–892. PMID: 1857798

25. Siva S, Louie AV, Kotecha R, et al. Stereotactic body radiotherapy for primary renal cell carcinoma: a systematic review and practice guideline from the International Society of Stereotactic Radiosurgery (ISRS). *Lancet Oncol.* 2024;25(1):e18–e28. doi:10.1016/S1470-2045(23)00513-2

26. Siva S, Bressel M, Sidhom M, et al. Stereotactic ablative body radiotherapy for primary kidney cancer (TROG 15.03 FASTRACK II): a non-randomised phase 2 trial. *Lancet Oncol.* 2024;25(3):308–316. doi:10.1016/S1470-2045(24)00020-2

27. Correa RJM, Louie AV, Staehler M, et al. Stereotactic radiotherapy as a treatment option for renal tumors in the solitary kidney: a multicenter analysis from the IROCK. *J Urol.* 2019;201(6):1097–1104. doi:10.1097/JU.0000000000000111

28. Siva S, Ali M, Correa RJM, et al. 5-year outcomes after stereotactic ablative body radiotherapy for primary renal cell carcinoma: an individual patient data meta-analysis from IROCK (the International Radiosurgery Consortium of the Kidney). *Lancet Oncol.* 2022;23(12):1508–1516. doi:10.1016/S1470-2045(22)00656-8

29. Siva S, Correa RJM, Warner A, et al. Stereotactic ablative radiotherapy for ≥T1b primary renal cell carcinoma: a report from the International Radiosurgery Oncology Consortium for Kidney (IROCK). *Int J Radiat Oncol Biol Phys.* 2020;108(4):941–949. doi:10.1016/j.ijrobp.2020.06.014

30. Siva S, Louie AV, Warner A, et al. Pooled analysis of stereotactic ablative radiotherapy for primary renal cell carcinoma: a report from the International Radiosurgery Oncology Consortium for Kidney (IROCK). *Cancer.* 2018;124(5):934–942. doi:10.1002/cncr.31156

31. McKay R. NRG-GU012: randomized phase II stereotactic ablative radiation therapy (SABR) for metastatic unresected Renal Cell Carcinoma (RCC) receiving immunotherapy (SAMURAI). *Oncologist.* 2023;28(suppl 1). doi:10.1093/oncolo/oyad216.020

32. Marvaso G, Jereczek-Fossa BA, Zaffaroni M, et al. Delphi consensus on stereotactic ablative radiotherapy for oligometastatic and oligoprogressive renal cell carcinoma—a European Society for Radiotherapy and Oncology study endorsed by the European Association of Urology. *Lancet Oncol.* 2024;25(5):e193–e204. doi:10.1016/S1470-2045(24)00023-8

PART VIII: Gynecologic

48 CERVICAL CANCER

Adannia N. Ufondu, Sheen Cherian, and Sudha R. Amarnath

QUICK HIT   The vast majority of cervical cancer cases are HPV-mediated. Incidence and mortality significantly declined with the introduction of screening with Pap smears. Three FDA-approved vaccines are available that prevent the development of cervical cancer. Treatment at early stages is often surgical, while RT ± CHT is employed in later stages. For locally advanced cervical cancer, induction CHT has been shown to have an OS and PFS benefit, and concurrent and adjuvant pembrolizumab has been shown to have a PFS benefit. When treating definitively, EBRT is followed by an intracavitary or interstitial brachytherapy boost. Postoperative RT ± CHT is occasionally indicated for adverse pathologic features. See Table 48.1 for details on general treatment paradigm.

Table 48.1 Cervical Cancer General Treatment Paradigm[1]	
Early Stage	
IA1 (non–fertility-sparing)	Simple hysterectomy or modified radical hysterectomy + SLN mapping/PLND OR Brachytherapy alone ± EBRT
IA1 (fertility-sparing)	*No LVSI:* CKC with at least 1-mm negative margins *LVSI:* CKC with 3-mm negative margins + SLN mapping/PLND OR Radical trachelectomy + PLND (± PA-LND)
IA2 (non–fertility-sparing)	Simple hysterectomy or modified radical hysterectomy + SLN mapping/PLND (± PA-LND) OR Pelvic EBRT + brachytherapy ± concurrent CHT (for high-risk features)
IA2 (fertility-sparing)	CKC with at least 1-mm negative margins + SLN mapping/PLND (± PA-LND) OR Radical trachelectomy + PLND (± PA-LND)
IB1 or IB2 or IIA1 (non–fertility-sparing)	Radical hysterectomy + SLN mapping/PLND (± PA-LND) (For IB1 consider simple hysterectomy) OR Pelvic EBRT + brachytherapy ± concurrent CHT
IB1 and select IB2 (fertility-sparing)	Radical trachelectomy + SLN mapping/PLND (± PA-LND)
Locally Advanced	
IB3, IIA2–IVA	Concurrent CHT/IO (cisplatin/pembrolizumab) + pelvic EBRT + brachytherapy → adjuvant pembrolizumab OR Induction CHT → pelvic EBRT + concurrent CHT + brachytherapy

Source: Adapted from AJCC Cancer Staging Manual. 8th ed. Springer International Publishing; 2017.

EPIDEMIOLOGY: In the United States, there were an estimated 13,820 new cases and 4,360 deaths due to invasive cervical cancer in 2024.[2] Disease burden in less developed countries is much higher as ~85% of all new cervical cancer cases occur in low- and middle-income countries.[3] With screening, precancerous lesions are diagnosed far more often than invasive lesions, and the incidence and death rates have decreased steadily over decades. The median age at diagnosis is 49.

RISK FACTORS: HPV infection is associated with >90% of cervical cancer cases. HPV 16/18 confer the highest risk of carcinogenesis and account for ~70% of cases (other cancer-causing strains are

31, 33, 45, 52, and 58).[4] Other risk factors include smoking, immunocompromised status (transplant, AIDS), history of STDs, young age at first intercourse, multiple sexual partners, multiparity, low SES, and diethylstilbestrol (DES) exposure in utero (associated with clear cell adenocarcinoma of cervix/vagina).

ANATOMY: Cervix: lower part of the uterus that is cylindrical in shape. The endocervical canal, lined by columnar epithelium, runs through it and connects the uterine cavity to the vagina. The distal part of the cervix projects into the vagina (called ectocervix) and is lined by squamous epithelium. The squamocolumnar junction is located at the external os and is the most common site for carcinogenesis. The broad and cardinal ligaments attach the uterus and cervix, respectively, to the pelvic sidewall. The uterosacral ligament attaches the lower uterus to the sacrum. Lymphatic drainage of the cervix is through these ligaments to the following lymphatic beds: presacral, obturator, internal iliac, external iliac, common iliac, and para-aortic LNs. The most common sites of distant spread are the lungs, supraclavicular LNs (via thoracic duct), bones, and liver.

PATHOLOGY: Squamous cell carcinoma (SCC; 70%–75%), adenocarcinoma (ACA; 20%–25%), adenosquamous (5%). There is a higher incidence of ACA in younger patients and often presents with larger tumors ("barrel cervix") with increased risk of LF. The incidence of ACA is increasing, and Pap screening is less sensitive for this histology. HPV testing may increase sensitivity. Less common histologies: clear cell ACA, small cell, neuroendocrine, sarcoma (rhabdomyosarcoma in adolescents), melanoma, and adenoid cystic carcinoma.

SCREENING: ACOG, SGO, and ASCCP have all adopted the USPSTF cervical screening recommendations as follows[5]:

Ages 21–29: Pap test alone q3 years, but high-risk HPV testing can be considered in high-risk patients 25 to 29 years old q5 years.

Ages 30–65: Pap test with high-risk HPV test (cotesting) q5 years, high-risk HPV testing alone q5 years, or Pap test alone q3 years.

≥65 years: No further screening after three consecutive negative cytology results, two consecutive negative cotesting results, or two consecutive negative high-risk HPV test results within 10 years before stopping screening.

Patients with hysterectomy and no history of high-grade cervical precancerous lesions or cervical cancer do not require screening.

CLINICAL PRESENTATION: Can be asymptomatic and detected on screening. However, abnormal vaginal discharge, postcoital bleeding, dyspareunia, and pelvic pain are also common symptoms. Differential diagnosis includes cervicitis, Paget disease, and vaginal and endometrial cancer.

WORKUP: H&P with focus on the GYN history and a careful abdominal/pelvic exam with attention to the inferior extension into the vagina, lateral extension into parametria, posterior extension into uterosacral ligament or rectum. Examine supraclavicular and inguinal LNs. Smoking cessation counseling.

Labs: CBC/CMP, pregnancy test; consider HIV testing.

Procedures: Colposcopy with cervical biopsy, cold-knife conization (CKC) if cervical biopsy is inadequate to determine depth of invasion (DOI) or if part of the lesion is not well-visualized on colposcopy. CKC can be the definitive procedure in select early cases desiring fertility preservation. EUA with cystoscopy/rectosigmoidoscopy (for advanced disease or if bladder or rectal extension is suspected); ureteral stent placement if necessary.

Imaging: PET/CT (nodal and metastatic staging),[6] pelvic MRI (to delineate local disease extent and guide decisions on fertility vs. non–fertility-sparing approaches).

PROGNOSTIC FACTORS: Stage, age, tumor size (≥4 cm worse), LN involvement, lymphovascular space invasion (LVSI), persistent uptake on posttreatment PET/CT,[7] prolonged treatment time (>56 days), low hemoglobin (<10 g/dL).

STAGING: See Table 48.2.

Table 48.2 AJCC 9th Edition (2021) and FIGO 2018: Staging for Cervical Cancer		
AJCC		**FIGO**
T1	Confined to cervix, microscopic lesion **1A1** ≤3 mm DOI **1A2** >3 and ≤5 mm DOI	I
	Confined to cervix, >5 mm DOI **1B1** ≤2 cm **1B2** >2 and ≤4 cm **1B3** >4 cm	
T2	Extension beyond uterus, but not to side wall or lower one-third vagina **2A1** ≤4 cm, no parametrial invasion **2A2** >4 cm, no parametrial invasion **2B** Parametrial invasion	II
T3	**3A** Involves the lower one-third vagina, no extension to pelvic side wall **3B** Extends to pelvic side wall and/or causes hydronephrosis or nonfunctioning kidney	III
T4	Invasion of bladder, rectum, and/or extends beyond true pelvis	IVA
N0	No regional LNs	
N0 (i +)	Isolated tumor cells ≤0.2 mm	
N1a	Pelvic LN metastases only	IIIC1
N2	Para-aortic LN metastases with or without positive pelvic LNs	IIIC2
M0	No distant metastasis	
M1	Distant metastasis	IVB

Notes: When in doubt, the lower staging should be assigned.
FIGO 2018 staging update: IA no longer includes horizontal spread; IB does not need to be visible; prior staging had only IB1 (<4 cm) and IB2 (>4cm), now there is IB1–IB3; IIIC added; advanced imaging can now be used with extra annotation ("r" for imaging and "p" for pathology). AJCC 9th edition was updated in 2021 to mirror FIGO 2018 staging changes.
Source: Adapted from AJCC 9th Edition (2021) and FIGO 2018.

TREATMENT PARADIGM

Observation: Refer to current ACOG guidelines on management for ASCUS, LSIL, HSIL, ASC-H, and AGC.

Prevention: ACS, CDC, and ACOG recommend routine vaccination of 11- to 12-year-old boys and girls with the nine-valent HPV vaccine (covers: 6, 11, 16, 18, 31, 33, 45, 52, 58). Vaccination can start at age 9, with "catch-up" vaccination through age 26.[8] HPV 6 and 11 cause ~90% cases of anogenital warts.

Surgery: Mainly reserved for IA1 to IB1 and IIA1. Bilateral salpingo-oophorectomy (BSO) is optional but spared when fertility preservation is desired. Goal of upfront surgery is to select patients at low risk for needing additional treatment due to increased morbidity with combined modality therapy. Minimally invasive radical hysterectomy is associated with lower rates of DFS and OS when compared with open abdominal radical hysterectomy.[9] Although radical hysterectomy has been the standard of care for cervical cancer surgery for many years, the recently published SHAPE trial found that simple hysterectomy with LN sampling was noninferior to radical hysterectomy in patients with low-risk cervical cancer (lesions ≤2 cm with limited stromal invasion) with respect to pelvic recurrence.[10]

CKC: Removal of cone-shaped piece of tissue containing the ectocervix and endocervical canal en bloc with scalpel to avoid electrosurgical artifact to facilitate margin status assessment.

Radical Trachelectomy: Fertility-sparing surgery that removes the cervix, upper vagina, and parametria, while leaving uterine body in place. Cerclage or "purse-string stitch" is made at the distal end of the uterine body.

Class I or "Simple" or "Extra-Fascial" Hysterectomy: Removal of the uterus and cervix, parametria left intact.

Class II or "Modified-Radical" Hysterectomy: Removes the uterus, cervix, 1 to 2 cm vagina, and wide local excision (WLE) of parametria.

Class III Hysterectomy or "Radical" Hysterectomy: Removal of the uterus, cervix, one-fourth to one-third of vagina, parametria divided at pelvic sidewall or sacral origin.

Adjuvant Hysterectomy: Not generally performed. No additional benefit seen in DFS and OS.[11] Caveat: If patient has persistent metabolic activity following upfront RT or CRT and is otherwise nonmetastatic, surgery is often performed as salvage in hopes of improving outcomes.

Chemotherapy

Induction: Historical studies on the role of neoadjuvant CHT are mixed, and outcomes vary based on dose intensity and time to definitive local therapy.[12,13] Two large phase III trials of neoadjuvant CHT before surgery and CRT alone demonstrated no OS benefit and a detriment to PFS,[14,15] likely due to the failure to control the interval between CHT completion and definitive treatment allowing for accelerated repopulation. Recent results of the INTERLACE trial showed PFS and OS benefit to the addition of compressed induction CHT with 6 weeks of carboplatin/paclitaxel 80 mg/m^2 followed by definitive CRT for locally advanced disease.[16]

Concurrent: Concurrent CHT with RT for locally advanced disease improves DFS and OS survival over RT alone (see below). Weekly cisplatin 40 mg/m^2 has become standard of care.[17] Common alternative is cisplatin/5-FU. Other concurrent regimens: weekly cisplatin + gemcitabine (increased pCR rate, PFS, and OS compared with cisplatin alone at the cost of very high acute toxicity)[18] and weekly cisplatin + bevacizumab (evaluated in RTOG 0417, proved to be tolerable with OS of 81%).[19] The recently published KEYNOTE-A18 showed a 2-year PFS benefit to the addition of concurrent and adjuvant pembrolizumab to definitive CRT for high-risk locally advanced disease.[20]

Adjuvant: Concurrent CHT with postoperative RT (PORT) improves OS in patients with positive margins, parametrial involvement, and positive LNs[21] (see below). Adjuvant CHT following definitive CRT was evaluated in the OUTBACK trial (definitive cisplatin with RT randomized to ± adjuvant carboplatin/paclitaxel × 4 cycles) with no OS or PFS benefit.

Metastatic: Doublet CHT shows better outcomes than single-agent therapy.[22] GOG 240 showed significant improvement in PFS (2 months) and OS (3.7 months) with the addition of bevacizumab to cisplatin/paclitaxel or topotecan/paclitaxel.[23] Pembrolizumab has shown an OS benefit over placebo for patients with metastatic, recurrent, or persistent cervical cancer (2-year OS 53% vs. 42%, $p < .001$), and is often added to first-line chemotherapy.[24]

Radiation

Definitive EBRT

Indicated in all cases stage ≥IA2 (and IA1 with LVSI) when treated nonoperatively. Ensure coverage of the uterus, cervix, parametria, uterosacral ligament, and LNs at risk determined by imaging and/or surgical nodal staging. Give sufficient vaginal margin (2–3 cm below the inferior most extent of gross disease). Cover external and internal iliacs, obturator, presacral LNs (superior border L4–5), and common iliac LNs. For high pelvic LN+ or high burden of nodal disease, elective PA coverage to renal vessels or higher should be considered. Include PA LNs for stage IIIC2, and add inguinal coverage for distal one-third vaginal extension.

Dose: 45 Gy/25 fx to the pelvis. Grossly involved unresected nodes can be boosted an additional 10 to 15 Gy. For bulky LNs theoretically requiring ≥65 to 66 Gy to control, consider excision followed by microscopic dose RT. The primary tumor is boosted to 85 to 95 Gy with brachytherapy[25] (see below). Use of IMRT for intact cervix is standard and requires special attention to contouring and must account for pelvic organ motion due to bowel/bladder filling with ITVs.[26]

Postoperative EBRT

Recommended following hysterectomy for those at higher risk for recurrence. PORT alone recommended for any two of three Sedlis risk factors: LVSI, middle or deep one-third stromal invasion, or tumor size ≥4 cm.[27] Rotman update showed RT improved outcomes in ACA or adenosquamous histology as well.[28] Consider vaginal brachytherapy boost for close or positive vaginal margin or deep one-third stromal invasion.

Dose: 45–50.4 Gy/25–28 fx. IMRT reduces small bowel and iliac crest (bone marrow) dose, especially when treating extended field to cover PA LNs and/or when boosting grossly involved nodes.[29] See RTOG 1203 and NRG Oncology/RTOG consensus on postop IMRT for further details on target volumes and constraints.

Brachytherapy

Can be used as monotherapy for select early-stage cases (IA1), but it is more commonly employed following pelvic EBRT to boost gross residual primary to a curative intent dose. Vaginal cuff brachytherapy is considered postoperatively following EBRT as a vaginal apex boost in cases of close or positive vaginal margin or other high-risk features. In cases of definitive CRT, EBRT + brachytherapy improves OS over EBRT alone even in the setting of concurrent CHT.[30] Proper applicator placement and dosing are critical to achieving optimal outcomes, and the goal is to complete the entire treatment course within 8 weeks.[31] Repeat clinical exam and imaging prior to first insertion allows selection of applicator; obtain MRI at week 5 of EBRT to evaluate response. Plan for one to two insertions per week (at least 72 hours between fxs) or interdigitate with EBRT by giving 4 fxs of EBRT per week with one HDR treatment per week. Generally, intracavitary therapy is employed (tandem and ring or tandem and ovoids), but interstitial technique may be necessary in certain circumstances (e.g., narrow anatomy not accommodating intracavity applicator, wide lateral extent of disease, distal vaginal involvement, inaccessible cervical os, etc.). Hybrid devices exist that combine intracavitary and interstitial components. Anesthesia is often needed for patient comfort and to achieve high-quality insertion, and anesthesia type varies widely among institutions.[32,33] Options include conscious sedation, epidural/spinal, general, and/or paracervical block. The 2012 ABS guidelines recommend 3D imaging with US, CT, and/or MR for planning and use of normal-tissue dosimetry for DVH evaluation.[34] However, MRI-based planning is preferred for better coverage of tumor, while potentially limiting dose to the bladder, sigmoid, and rectum as compared with conventional planning.[35] GEC-ESTRO guidelines define high-risk CTV (HR-CTV) and intermediate-risk CTV (IR-CTV) for 3D planning. HR-CTV includes the residual visible and palpable tumor on gynecologic exam plus any abnormal thickened or irregular vaginal mucosa/wall within the initial tumor extent on exam or imaging. IR-CTV includes all potentially significant microscopic disease adjacent to the HR-CTV. The IR-CTV should at least include the area of the initial extent of disease at the time of diagnosis plus at least a 5-mm margin on the HR-CTV, while taking into consideration previously unaffected anatomic barriers to microscopic spread, such as the pubic bone, pelvic wall, and so on.[36] Note, the vagina is both a target volume and an OAR.

Dose: HDR and LDR have comparable rates of cancer outcomes and toxicity. LDR utilizes manual afterloading Cs-137 at <2 Gy/hr. HDR utilizes Ir-192, >12 Gy/hr. Intended dose should cover ≥90% of HR-CTV (D90). Per EMBRACE II, the D90 for the HR-CTV is 90 to 95 Gy and D98 for GTV is >95 Gy. The vast majority of patients should have D90 for HR-CTV of at least 85 Gy and D98 for GTV ≥90 Gy. Localization with CT pelvis and dosimetry should be done for every fraction.

Brachytherapy Dose Constraints: Constraints per EMBRACE trials.[25] Bladder D2cc <80 Gy, rectum D2cc <65 Gy, sigmoid D2cc <70 Gy, bowel D2cc <70 Gy, and rectovaginal D2cc <65 Gy.

Toxicity: Acute: fatigue, diarrhea, rectal urgency, bloating/cramping, bladder/urethral irritation, skin erythema, and possible desquamation if inguinal LNs or distal vagina/vulva covered in fields. Late: rectal bleeding, bowel obstruction, hematuria, fistula (GI or urinary), vaginal ulceration/ necrosis, vaginal stenosis, infertility (~2 Gy), premature ovarian failure (5–10 Gy), and osteopenia leading to hip and sacral insufficiency fractures.

Procedure: See *Handbook of Treatment Planning in Radiation Oncology*, Chapter 9.[37]

EVIDENCE-BASED Q&A

SURGICAL MANAGEMENT

Can low-risk early-stage patients be managed with a simple hysterectomy?

Plante, SHAPE (*NEJM* 2024, PMID 38416430): Multicenter, randomized, noninferiority trial comprising 700 patients with early-stage disease (lesions ≤2 cm with limited stromal invasion). The majority had stage IB1 (92%), SCC (62%), and grade 1 or 2 (59%). Patients were randomized to radical hysterectomy or simple hysterectomy both with LN assessment. The primary outcome was pelvic recurrence at 3 years, which was found to be 2.2% vs. 2.5% (90% CI –1.62 to 2.32). Lower incidence of urinary retention (0.6% vs. 11%, $p < .001$) and urinary incontinence (2% vs. 6%, $p = .05$) within 4 weeks of surgery and after 4 weeks of surgery (urinary retention: 0.6% vs. 10%; urinary incontinence: 5% vs. 11%) with simple hysterectomy. **Conclusion: Simple hysterectomy is a safe and viable surgical option in patients with early-stage cervical cancer with lower risk of urinary incontinence or retention.**

What factors portend higher risk of pelvic LN involvement or unfavorable outcome?

Delgado, GOG 49 (*Gynecol Oncol* 1989, PMID 2599466; *Gynecol Oncol* 1990, PMID 2227547): Prospective registry of stage I cervical cancer patients with ≥3 mm invasion treated with radical hysterectomy with pelvic and PA nodal dissection. 645 SCC patients with negative PA LNs were included in this report. Factors associated with positive LNs included DOI, parametrial invasion, tumor grade, and gross vs. occult tumors. The 3-year disease-free interval (DFI) for positive nodes was 74% and for negative nodes was 86% ($p = .04$). Factors associated with worse 3-year DFI were DOI (deep one-third < middle one-third < superficial one-third invasion), tumor size (occult vs. <3 cm vs. ≥3 cm), parametrial invasion, and LVSI. Led to the development of GOG 92 (Sedlis) trial (see below).

What are the indications for adjuvant RT after hysterectomy?

The Sedlis trial defined these risk factors. Although inclusion criteria are challenging to remember, "any 2 of 3 risk factors" is a good way of simplifying it and will often be correct. Risk factors: LVSI, middle or deep one-third stromal invasion, and tumor size ≥4 cm. An ancillary analysis of GOG 49, 92, and 141 suggests that there may be histologic-specific risk factors defining risk of recurrence. DOI is most associated with recurrence (16% risk) in those with SCC; for ACA, tumor size ≥4 cm confers a 15% risk of recurrence with negative LVSI vs. 25% risk with LVSI.[38]

Sedlis, GOG 92 (*Gynecol Oncol* 1999, PMID 10329031; Update Rotman, *IJROBP* 2006, PMID 16427212): Phase III PRT of 277 patients with FIGO IB cervical cancer randomized to radical hysterectomy + pelvic LND ± adjuvant RT. Postoperatively, patients had negative nodes and (a) +LVSI and deep one-third stromal invasion; (b) +LVSI, middle one-third stromal invasion, and tumor ≥2 cm; (c) +LVSI, superficial one-third, and tumor ≥5 cm; or (d) no LVSI, deep or middle one-third, and tumor ≥4 cm. Whole pelvis RT given 4 to 6 weeks postoperatively to 46–50.4 Gy/23–28 fx. RT decreased LR (28% vs. 15%, $p = .019$) and improved RFS (79% vs. 88%, $p = .008$). At longer term follow-up, the LR benefit persisted and PORT also decreased the risk of recurrence for ACA/adenosquamous histologies (44% vs. 9%, $p = .019$). **Conclusion: Adjuvant pelvic RT reduces the risk of LR and prolongs PFS in women with stage IB cervical cancer who meet the "Sedlis" criteria.**

What factors postoperatively are indications for adjuvant CRT rather than RT alone?

The Peters criteria include any one of three factors ("3 P's")—positive margins, parametrial involvement, and positive nodes—and serve as indications for adjuvant CRT.

Peters, GOG 109 (*JCO* 2000, PMID 10764420; Update *Gynecol Oncol* 2005, PMID 15721417): Phase III PRT of 243 patients with FIGO IA2 to IIA cervical cancer with positive margins, positive pelvic nodes, or microscopic parametrial involvement randomized to adjuvant RT 49.3 Gy/29 fx ± concurrent cisplatin 70 mg/m^2 and 5-FU 1,000 mg/m^2/day over 96 hours × 4 cycles. Ninety-five percent were FIGO IB. CHT improved OS (81% vs. 71%, $p = .007$) and PFS (80% vs. 63%, $p = .003$). Subsequent retrospective analysis by Monk questioned CHT benefit for smaller (≤2 cm) tumors and for patients with only one LN+. **Conclusion: Addition of CHT to RT improves PFS and OS for early-stage cervical cancer patients s/p hysterectomy with positive margins, positive pelvic nodes, and microscopic parametrial involvement.**

Should FIGO IB to IIA patients be managed with surgery or RT?

Stage IA patients can easily be managed with extrafascial hysterectomy and stage IIB to IVA patients are typically better candidates for CRT given extent of disease. However, management of stage IB to IIA tumors is challenging and patient-specific. Main advantages of surgery over RT are preserved sexual and ovarian function and elimination of secondary malignancy risk.

Landoni, Italian Trial (*Lancet* 1997, PMID 9284774): Phase III PRT of 343 patients with FIGO stage IB or IIA cervical cancer randomized to radical hysterectomy or definitive RT. Sixty-nine percent of IBs were ≤4 cm. EBRT was 40 to 53 Gy followed by Cs-137 LDR implant to 70 to 90 Gy to point A. When lymphangiography showed common iliac or PA LNs+, 45 Gy was given to these beds; involved LNs boosted another 5 to 10 Gy. In surgical arm, adjuvant RT recommended for >pT2a disease, <3 mm of "safe" cervical stroma, tumor cut-through, or positive nodes. Adjuvant RT was 50.4 Gy to whole pelvis (± 45 Gy to PA LNs based on pathologic involvement). MFU 87 months. Identical 5-year OS and DFS in both groups, 83% and 74%, respectively. Recurrence rates were 25% in the surgery group and 26% in the RT group. Severe toxicity was seen in 28% of the surgery group and 12% of the RT group ($p = .0004$). ACA had inferior outcomes with RT as compared with surgery (DFS 47% vs. 66%, $p = .05$; OS 59% vs. 70%, $p = .02$). **Conclusion: Both surgery and definitive RT are options for stage IB to IIA cervical cancer. Although RT may be better tolerated, surgery may improve outcomes for ACA. Toxicity with combined treatment is worse than RT alone.** *Note: In the surgical arm, adjuvant RT was required in 64% (84% for those with tumors >4 cm). Those who received surgery + RT had significantly increased toxicity (29% G2–3 long term). However, surgical and RT techniques have since improved.*

Does adjuvant hysterectomy following RT improve overall survival?

Keys, GOG 71 (*Gynecol Oncol* 2003, PMID 12798694): Phase III PRT of 256 patients with FIGO IB "suboptimal or bulky" (current IB2) cervical cancer randomized to RT ± adjuvant simple extrafascial hysterectomy. Whole pelvis RT was 40 Gy for the RT arm and 45 Gy for the hysterectomy arm; both were followed by intracavitary boost to 40 Gy (RT only arm) or 30 Gy (hysterectomy arm) to point A. Extrafascial hysterectomy was performed 2 to 6 weeks later. No difference in OS (58% vs. 56%, $p = .26$) or PFS (62% vs. 53%, $p = .09$). Ten percent grades 3 to 4 toxicities in both arms. Interaction was demonstrated with tumor sizes of 4, 5, and 6 cm possibly benefitting from surgery. **Conclusion: Adjuvant hysterectomy did not improve survival.**

Is there benefit to IMRT in postoperative setting?

Phase III data confirm the benefit, safety, and efficacy of IMRT for gynecologic malignancies after hysterectomy[39,40] and is recommended as standard of care by ASTRO guidelines.[41]

DEFINITIVE MANAGEMENT

Is there benefit to concurrent CHT in addition to RT compared with RT (EFRT) alone? Which patients should receive concurrent CRT?

Yes. Based on mounting evidence, NCI issued clinical alert in 1999 recommending concurrent cisplatin be administered with RT for invasive cervical cancer. Several randomized trials (RTOG 9001, GOG 123) and meta-analyses have demonstrated DFS and OS benefit for concurrent CRT over RT alone in invasive cervical cancer.[42,43] NCCN recommends addition of concurrent platinum-based CHT for "bulky" tumors (stage IB2, IIA2, and higher). For stage IB1 and IIA1, CHT is optional. For IA1 with LVSI or IA2 tumors, surgery is a good option, but if treated nonoperatively, CHT can be omitted.[44]

Morris, RTOG 9001 (*NEJM* 1999, PMID 10202164; Update *JCO* 2004, PMID 14990643): Phase III PRT of 389 cervical cancer patients, stage IIB to IV or stage IB/IIA with tumor size ≥5 cm or biopsy-proven pelvic nodal metastasis randomized to extended field RT (EFRT) alone or whole pelvis RT with concurrent cisplatin 75 mg/m² and 5-FU 4,000 mg/m² over 96 hours for three cycles given every 3 weeks. Patients in CHT arm were treated from L4/5 interspace down to mid-pubis or 4 cm below the distal edge of the tumor. Patients in EFRT arm received RT to L1/2 interspace. Both arms received 45 Gy/25 fx. Updated results with MFU of 6.6 years showed 8-year OS improved from 41% to 67% with CHT ($p < .0001$). Late toxicity was similar. The 5-year LR and DM also improved with CHT. **Conclusions: Concurrent cisplatin/5-FU improved OS without significant increase in late effects.**

Keys, GOG 123 (*NEJM* 1999, PMID 10202166): Phase III PRT of 369 women with bulky IB cervical cancer (current IB2) without radiographic lymphadenopathy treated with RT (45 Gy + LDR boost) ± concurrent CHT (weekly cisplatin 40 mg/m² for up to six cycles) followed by extrafascial hysterectomy. PFS and OS were improved in CHT group (PFS HR 0.51, OS HR 0.54, both $p < .01$). **Conclusion: Concurrent cisplatin improves OS.**

Shrivastava, Tata Memorial (*JAMA Onc* 2018, PMID 29423520): Phase III PRT of 850 women with FIGO IIIB cervical cancer randomized to RT ± weekly cisplatin. Primary endpoint of 5-year DFS was significantly improved with RT + cisplatin vs. RT alone (52% vs. 44%, respectively, $p = .03$), as well as 5-year OS (54% vs. 46%, $p = .04$). **Conclusion: For women with stage IIIB cervical cancer, the addition of cisplatin to RT improves DFS and OS.**

What is standard concurrent CHT regimen?

Multiple single- and multiagent regimens have been studied, but currently single-agent cisplatin given weekly is the most common. Cisplatin/5-FU is common alternative. Concurrent and adjuvant gemcitabine/ cisplatin was shown to improve OS and PFS but with a significant increase in grades 3 to 4 toxicities.[45] Of note, KEYNOTE-A18 (discussed below) has shown a PFS benefit with the addition of concurrent and adjuvant pembrolizumab to definitive CRT.

Rose, GOG 120 (*NEJM* 1999, PMID 10202165; Update *JCO* 2007, PMID 17502627): Three-arm PRT of 526 women with stage IIB to IVA cervical carcinoma without para-aortic involvement randomized to either concurrent cisplatin (40 mg/m^2 weekly for 6 weeks), concurrent hydroxyurea, or combination cisplatin, 5-FU, and hydroxyurea. EBRT dose 40.8 Gy/24 fx (or 51 Gy/30 fx for stages IIB, IIIB–IVA) followed by brachytherapy boost. Superior border of pelvic field was L4/5 interspace. MFU 35 months. Hydroxyurea-alone arm demonstrated worse PFS and OS, but cisplatin and multiagent arms were similar. Acute toxicity was worse in three-drug arm. **Conclusion: Cisplatin-based CRT improves PFS and OS. No increased late toxicity seen at long-term follow-up.**

What is the role of immunotherapy in cervical cancer?

Data are mixed. The CALLA trial below showed no benefit to adding concurrent and adjuvant durvalumab to definitive CRT. A Chinese phase II trial showed patients with PD-L1 positivity had high response rates to induction CHT + camrelizumab followed by surgery.[46] KEYNOTE-A18 revealed significant PFS benefit with the addition of current and adjuvant pembrolizumab to CRT and is now considered a Category 1 recommendation in the NCCN 2025 guidelines.[1,20]

Monk, CALLA (*Lancet* 2023, PMID 38039991): Phase III RCT of 770 women with locally advanced cervical cancer (node-positive IB2–IIB or IIIA–IVA) undergoing CRT (platinum-based) randomized to concurrent and adjuvant durvalumab vs. placebo with a primary endpoint of PFS. MFU 18.5 months; 12-month PFS 76% with durvalumab vs. 73% with placebo ($p = .17$). **Conclusion: No PFS benefit to concurrent and adjuvant durvalumab with CRT.**

Lorusso, KEYNOTE-A18 (*Lancet*, 2024, PMID 38521086): Phase III double-blind RCT of 1,060 high-risk locally advanced cervical cancer patients (stage IB2–IIB N+ and stage III–IVA) receiving definitive CRT. Patients were randomly assigned to concurrent and adjuvant pembrolizumab vs. placebo. Median PFS at 24 months for the pembrolizumab group was 68% vs. 57% in the placebo group, with HR for disease progression or death of 0.70 (95% CI 0.55–0.89). OS at 24 months in pembrolizumab vs. placebo group was 87% vs. 81%, respectively (HR for death 0.73, 0.49–1.07). First safety report was published and showed grade 3+ adverse events rate of 63% vs. 58% in the pembrolizumab vs. placebo groups. **Conclusion: Addition of pembrolizumab to definitive CRT in high-risk locally advanced cervical cancer improves PFS without significant increase in toxicity.**

Is there a role for adjuvant CHT after definitive CRT?

No clear role based on the phase III OUTBACK trial.

Mileshkin, OUTBACK (*Lancet Oncol* 2023, PMID 37080223): Phase III RCT of 919 women with locally advanced cervical cancer (stage IB1 and N+, IB2, II, IIIB, or IVA) randomized to definitive CRT (cisplatin) ± adjuvant carboplatin/paclitaxel (four cycles) with a primary endpoint of 5-year OS. At MFU of 60 months, there was no significant difference in 5-year OS between those who received adjuvant CHT and those who did not (72% vs. 71%, $p = .81$) and no significant difference in 5-year PFS (63% vs. 61%), although there was an increase in G3+ AE from 62% to 81% with adjuvant CHT ($p < .0001$). **Conclusion: Adjuvant CHT adds toxicity without an OS or PFS benefit for locally advanced cervical cancer patients undergoing definitive CRT.**

Is there a role for induction CHT prior to definitive CRT?

Two large phase III trials of neoadjuvant CHT before surgery and CRT alone demonstrated no OS benefit and a detriment to PFS,[14,15] likely due to the failure to control the interval between CHT completion and definitive treatment allowing for accelerated repopulation. The INTERLACE trial, published in October 2024, showed PFS and OS benefit to the addition of compressed induction CHT with 6 weeks of carboplatin/paclitaxel 80 mg/m² followed by definitive CRT for locally advanced disease.[16] It has not yet been incorporated into the NCCN guidelines.

McCormack, GCIG INTERLACE Trial (*Lancet* 2024, PMID 39419054): A phase III trial of locally advanced cervical cancer patients randomized to weekly induction CHT (6 weeks of carboplatin/paclitaxel) followed by CRT vs. standard CRT alone. MFU 64 months; 5-year PFS and OS improved with induction CHT, 72% vs. 64% (p = .013) and 80% vs. 72% (p = .04), respectively. **Conclusion: Induction CHT followed by standard CRT improves PFS and OS in locally advanced cervical cancer.** Note: *The interval from completion of induction CHT to CRT start was ≤7 days in 78% of patients and ≤14 days in 93%.*

Is there a role for neoadjuvant CHT followed by surgical resection for locally advanced cervical cancer?

Randomized phase III data[14,15] suggest a DFS improvement with concurrent CRT over neoadjuvant CHT followed by surgical resection for locally advanced cervical cancer. No difference in OS.

What is the impact of overall treatment time (OTT) on outcomes of patients treated definitively?

OTT for EBRT + brachytherapy should be ≤56 days.[47] Other OTT limits have been identified: ≤49 days[48]; ≤63 days.[49] Brachytherapy should begin no more than 1 to 7 days post-EBRT if downsizing of bulky disease is required. Alternatively, for favorable anatomy or small primary tumor, practitioners can interdigitate brachytherapy during the last couple of weeks of EBRT. It is generally recommended to avoid CHT and EBRT administration on brachytherapy days.

What are the differences between high-dose rate (HDR) and low-dose rate (LDR) brachytherapy?

LDR is generally administered over 1 to 2 fx, each over 1 to 3 days, during which the patient stays on strict bed rest with the applicator and sources held in place. Despite best efforts, it is difficult to keep patients comfortable and immobilized for a prolonged period of time. Change in applicator position can lead to changes in dose distribution. RT exposure to healthcare personnel is also a major issue. The main theoretical advantage to LDR over HDR is much lower dose rate, which allows for enhanced sublethal damage repair. Concerns about HDR leading to increased toxicity have not consistently borne out in studies.[50] HDR, used by 85% of surveyed U.S. institutions in 2010,[51] requires more frequent insertions, but treatment time is short (~10 minutes). Remote afterloading by and large eliminates exposure risk to healthcare personnel. Several different dwell positions and times allow for shaping of dose to treat target and avoid OARs. On the recent clinical trial GY006,[52] HDR was used in 98% of cases. Pulsed dose rate used in some institutions combines the advantages of LDR and HDR. LDR: Dose rate 0.6 to 0.8 Gy/hr, generally with Cs-137 source, T½ = 30 years, β-decay, energy 662 keV. HDR: Dose rate >12 Gy/hr with Ir-192 source, T½ = 74 days, γ-decay with ~380 keV.

What is the difference between brachytherapy dose prescriptions to HR-CTV vs. point A?

Before CT/MRI were readily available, applicator placement was confirmed via AP and lateral films. Dose prescription was to 2D point A (2 cm superior and 2 cm lateral to os, in plane of tandem), roughly corresponding to the medial aspect of broad ligament (where uterine artery and ureter cross). Dose was estimated to point B (5 cm lateral to midline at level of point A), which represented pelvic sidewall/obturator LNs. Based on the ICRU 38 report, max doses to bladder and rectum were recorded at the following points: bladder: posterior surface of Foley balloon on lateral film; rectum: 0.5 cm posterior to the vaginal wall at intersection of tandem and ovoids/ring. CT/MRI studies have shown that adequate dose to point A does not always indicate good coverage of HR-CTV,[53] and ICRU bladder and rectal points do not always accurately estimate max doses to these OARs.[54,55] In the volumetric planning era, targets (HR-CTV, IR-CTV) and OARs (bladder, rectum, sigmoid, small bowel) can be accurately contoured in 3D and dose to these structures evaluated spatially and quantitatively using DVHs. Dose distribution during planning can be modified to adequately cover target while avoiding OARs. This is now the preferred method of planning/reporting.

REFERENCES

1. National Comprehensive Cancer Network. *NCCN Clinical Practice Guidelines in Oncology: Cervical Cancer.* Accessed November 2024. https://www.nccn.org/professionals/physician_gls/pdf/cervical.pdf
2. National Cancer Institute Surveillance, Epidemiology, and End Results Program. *Cancer Stat Facts: Cervix Uteri Cancer.* Accessed November 2024. https://seer.cancer.gov/statfacts/html/cervix.html
3. Hull R, Mbele M, Makhafola T, et al. Cervical cancer in low and middle-income countries. *Oncol Lett.* 2020;20(3):2058–2074. doi:10.3892/ol.2020.11754
4. National Cancer Institute. *HPV and Cancer.* Accessed November 2024. https://www.cancer.gov/about-cancer/causes-prevention/risk/infectious-agents/hpv-fact-sheet
5. American College of Obstetricians and Gynecologists. *Updated Cervical Cancer Screening Guidelines.* Published April 2021. Accessed November 2024. https://www.acog.org/clinical/clinical-guidance/practice-advisory/articles/2021/04/updated-cervical-cancer-screening-guidelines
6. Tsai CS, Lai CH, Chang TC, et al. A prospective randomized trial to study the impact of pretreatment FDG-PET for cervical cancer patients with MRI-detected positive pelvic but negative para-aortic lymphadenopathy. *Int J Radiat Oncol Biol Phys.* 2010;76(2):477–484. doi:10.1016/j.ijrobp.2009.02.020
7. Schwarz JK, Siegel BA, Dehdashti F, Grigsby PW. Metabolic response on post-therapy FDG-PET predicts patterns of failure after radiotherapy for cervical cancer. *Int J Radiat Oncol Biol Phys.* 2012;83(1):185–190. doi:10.1016/j.ijrobp.2011.05.053
8. Saslow D, Andrews KS, Manassaram-Baptiste D, Smith RA, Fontham ETH; American Cancer Society Guideline Development Group. Human papillomavirus vaccination 2020 guideline update: American Cancer Society guideline adaptation. *CA Cancer J Clin.* 2020;70(4):274–280. doi:10.3322/caac.21616
9. Nitecki R, Ramirez PT, Frumovitz M, et al. Survival after minimally invasive vs open radical hysterectomy for early-stage cervical cancer: a systematic review and meta-analysis. *JAMA Oncol.* 2020;6(7):1019–1027. doi:10.1001/jamaoncol.2020.1694
10. Plante M, Kwon JS, Ferguson S, et al. Simple versus radical hysterectomy in women with low-risk cervical cancer. *N Engl J Med.* 2024;390(9):819–829. doi:10.1056/NEJMoa2308900
11. Keys HM, Bundy BN, Stehman FB, et al. Radiation therapy with and without extrafascial hysterectomy for bulky stage IB cervical carcinoma: a randomized trial of the Gynecologic Oncology Group. *Gynecol Oncol.* 2003;89(3):343–353. doi:10.1016/s0090-8258(03)00173-2
12. Nguyen VT, Winterman S, Playe M, et al. Dose-intense cisplatin-based neoadjuvant chemotherapy increases survival in advanced cervical cancer: an up-to-date meta-analysis. *Cancers (Basel).* 2022;14(3):842. doi:10.3390/cancers14030842
13. Neoadjuvant Chemotherapy for Locally Advanced Cervical Cancer Meta-analysis Collaboration. Neoadjuvant chemotherapy for locally advanced cervical cancer: a systematic review and meta-analysis of individual patient data from 21 randomised trials. *Eur J Cancer.* 2003;39(17):2470–2486. doi:10.1016/s0959-8049(03)00425-8
14. Gupta S, Maheshwari A, Parab P, et al. Neoadjuvant chemotherapy followed by radical surgery versus concomitant chemotherapy and radiotherapy in patients with stage IB2, IIA, or IIB squamous cervical cancer: a randomized controlled trial. *J Clin Oncol.* 2018;36(16):1548–1555. doi:10.1200/JCO.2017.75.9985
15. Kenter GG, Greggi S, Vergote I, et al. Randomized phase III study comparing neoadjuvant chemotherapy followed by surgery versus chemoradiation in stage IB2-IIB cervical cancer: EORTC-55994. *J Clin Oncol.* 2023;41(32):5035–5043. doi:10.1200/JCO.22.02852
16. McCormack M, Eminowicz G, Gallardo D, et al. Induction chemotherapy followed by standard chemoradiotherapy versus standard chemoradiotherapy alone in patients with locally advanced cervical cancer (GCIG INTERLACE): an international, multicentre, randomised phase 3 trial. *Lancet.* 2024;403(10434):1341–1350. doi:10.1016/S0140-6736(24)01438-7
17. Mileshkin LR, Moore KN, Barnes EH, et al. Adjuvant chemotherapy following chemoradiotherapy as primary treatment for locally advanced cervical cancer versus chemoradiotherapy alone (OUTBACK): an international, open-label, randomised, phase 3 trial. *Lancet Oncol.* 2023;24(5):468–482. doi:10.1016/S1470-2045(23)00147-X
18. Dueñas-Gonzalez A, Cetina-Perez L, Lopez-Graniel C, et al. Pathologic response and toxicity assessment of chemoradiotherapy with cisplatin versus cisplatin plus gemcitabine in cervical cancer: a randomized phase II study. *Int J Radiat Oncol Biol Phys.* 2005;61(3):817–823. doi:10.1016/j.ijrobp.2004.07.676
19. Schefter T, Winter K, Kwon JS, et al. RTOG 0417: efficacy of bevacizumab in combination with definitive radiation therapy and cisplatin chemotherapy in untreated patients with locally advanced cervical carcinoma. *Int J Radiat Oncol Biol Phys.* 2014;88(1):101–105. doi:10.1016/j.ijrobp.2013.10.022
20. Lorusso D, Xiang Y, Hasegawa K, et al. Pembrolizumab or placebo with chemoradiotherapy followed by pembrolizumab or placebo for newly diagnosed, high-risk, locally advanced cervical cancer (ENGOT-cx11/GOG-3047/KEYNOTE-A18): a randomised, double-blind, phase 3 clinical trial. *Lancet.* 2024;403(10434):1341–1350. doi:10.1016/S0140-6736(24)00317-9

21. Peters WA 3rd, Liu PY, Barrett RJ 2nd, et al. Concurrent chemotherapy and pelvic radiation therapy compared with pelvic radiation therapy alone as adjuvant therapy after radical surgery in high-risk early-stage cancer of the cervix. *J Clin Oncol.* 2000;18(8):1606–1613. doi:10.1200/JCO.2000.18.8.1606

22. Long HJ 3rd, Bundy BN, Grendys EC Jr, et al. Randomized phase III trial of cisplatin with or without topotecan in carcinoma of the uterine cervix: a Gynecologic Oncology Group Study. *J Clin Oncol.* 2005;23(21):4626–4633. doi:10.1200/JCO.2005.10.021

23. Tewari KS, Sill MW, Long HJ 3rd, et al. Improved survival with bevacizumab in advanced cervical cancer. *N Engl J Med.* 2014;370(8):734–743. doi:10.1056/NEJMoa1309748

24. Colombo N, Dubot C, Lorusso D, et al. Pembrolizumab for persistent, recurrent, or metastatic cervical cancer. *N Engl J Med.* 2021;385(20):1856–1867. doi:10.1056/NEJMoa2112435

25. Potter R, Tanderup K, Schmid MP, et al. MRI-guided adaptive brachytherapy in locally advanced cervical cancer (EMBRACE-I): a multicentre prospective cohort study. *Lancet Oncol.* 2021;22(4):538–547. doi:10.1016/S1470-2045(20)30753-1

26. Lim K, Small W Jr, Portelance L, et al. Consensus guidelines for delineation of clinical target volume for intensity-modulated pelvic radiotherapy for the definitive treatment of cervix cancer. *Int J Radiat Oncol Biol Phys.* 2011;79(2):348–355. doi:10.1016/j.ijrobp.2009.10.075

27. Sedlis A, Bundy BN, Rotman MZ, Lentz SS, Muderspach LI, Zaino RJ. A randomized trial of pelvic radiation therapy versus no further therapy in selected patients with stage IB carcinoma of the cervix after radical hysterectomy and pelvic lymphadenectomy: a Gynecologic Oncology Group Study. *Gynecol Oncol.* 1999;73(2):177–183. doi:10.1006/gyno.1999.5387

28. Rotman M, Sedlis A, Piedmonte MR, et al. A phase III randomized trial of postoperative pelvic irradiation in stage IB cervical carcinoma with poor prognostic features: follow-up of a Gynecologic Oncology Group study. *Int J Radiat Oncol Biol Phys.* 2006;65(1):169–176. doi:10.1016/j.ijrobp.2005.10.019

29. Vargo JA, Kim H, Choi S, et al. Extended field intensity modulated radiation therapy with concomitant boost for lymph node-positive cervical cancer: analysis of regional control and recurrence patterns in the positron emission tomography/computed tomography era. *Int J Radiat Oncol Biol Phys.* 2014;90(5):1091–1098. doi:10.1016/j.ijrobp.2014.08.013

30. Gill BS, Lin JF, Krivak TC, et al. National Cancer Data Base analysis of radiation therapy consolidation modality for cervical cancer: the impact of new technological advancements. *Int J Radiat Oncol Biol Phys.* 2014;90(5):1083–1090. doi:10.1016/j.ijrobp.2014.07.017

31. Viswanathan AN, Moughan J, Small W Jr, et al. The quality of cervical cancer brachytherapy implantation and the impact on local recurrence and disease-free survival in radiation therapy oncology group prospective trials 0116 and 0128. *Int J Gynecol Cancer.* 2012;22(1):123–131. doi:10.1097/IGC.0b013e31823ae3c9

32. Rivera A, Barrios DM, Herbach E, et al. Analgesia and anesthesia practice patterns for gynecologic brachytherapy procedures and potential impact on women's procedural experience: a national survey. *Int J Radiat Oncol Biol Phys.* 2025;121(1):118–127. doi:10.1016/j.ijrobp.2024.07.2150

33. Petitt MS, Ackerman RS, Hanna MM, et al. Anesthetic and analgesic methods for gynecologic brachytherapy: a meta-analysis and systematic review. *Brachytherapy.* 2020;19(3):328–336. doi:10.1016/j.brachy.2020.01.006

34. Viswanathan AN, Thomadsen B; American Brachytherapy Society Cervical Cancer Recommendations Committee. American Brachytherapy Society consensus guidelines for locally advanced carcinoma of the cervix. Part I: general principles. *Brachytherapy.* 2012;11(1):33–46. doi:10.1016/j.brachy.2011.07.003

35. Zwahlen D, Jezioranski J, Chan P, et al. Magnetic resonance imaging-guided intracavitary brachytherapy for cancer of the cervix. *Int J Radiat Oncol Biol Phys.* 2009;74(4):1157–1164. doi:10.1016/j.ijrobp.2008.09.010

36. Kamrava M, Leung E, Bachand F, et al. GEC-ESTRO (ACROP)-ABS-CBG consensus brachytherapy target definition guidelines for recurrent endometrial and cervical tumors in the vagina. *Int J Radiat Oncol Biol Phys.* 2023;115(3):654–663. doi:10.1016/j.ijrobp.2022.09.072

37. Videtic GMM, Woody N, Vassil AD. *Handbook of Treatment Planning in Radiation Oncology.* 2nd ed. Demos Medical; 2015.

38. Levinson K, Beavis AL, Purdy C, et al. Beyond Sedlis—a novel histology-specific nomogram for predicting cervical cancer recurrence risk: an NRG/GOG ancillary analysis. *Gynecol Oncol.* 2021;162(3):532–538. doi:10.1016/j.ygyno.2021.06.017

39. Klopp AH, Yeung AR, Deshmukh S, et al. Patient-reported toxicity during pelvic intensity-modulated radiation therapy: NRG Oncology-RTOG 1203. *J Clin Oncol.* 2018;36(24):2538–2544. doi:10.1200/JCO.2017.77.4273

40. Shih KK, Hajj C, Kollmeier M, et al. Impact of postoperative intensity-modulated radiation therapy (IMRT) on the rate of bowel obstruction in gynecologic malignancy. *Gynecol Oncol.* 2016;143(1):18–21. doi:10.1016/j.ygyno.2016.07.116

41. Chino J, Annunziata CM, Beriwal S, et al. Radiation therapy for cervical cancer: executive summary of an ASTRO clinical practice guideline. *Pract Radiat Oncol.* 2020;10(4):220–234. doi:10.1016/j.prro.2020.04.002

42. Green JA, Kirwan JM, Tierney JF, et al. Survival and recurrence after concomitant chemotherapy and radiotherapy for cancer of the uterine cervix: a systematic review and meta-analysis. *Lancet.* 2001;358(9284):781–786. doi:10.1016/S0140-6736(01)05965-7

43. Chemoradiotherapy for Cervical Cancer Meta-Analysis Collaboration. Reducing uncertainties about the effects of chemoradiotherapy for cervical cancer: a systematic review and meta-analysis of individual patient data from 18 randomized trials. *J Clin Oncol.* 2008;26(35):5802–5812. doi:10.1200/JCO.2008.16.4368

44. National Comprehensive Cancer Network. *Cervical Cancer* (Version 1.2017). Accessed February 10, 2017. https://www.nccn.org/professionals/physician_gls/pdf/cervical.pdf

45. Dueñas-Gonzalez A, Zarba JJ, Patel F, et al. Phase III, open-label, randomized study comparing concurrent gemcitabine plus cisplatin and radiation followed by adjuvant gemcitabine and cisplatin versus concurrent cisplatin and radiation in patients with stage IIB to IVA carcinoma of the cervix. *J Clin Oncol.* 2011;29(13):1678–1685. doi:10.1200/JCO.2009.25.9663

46. Chen J, Han Y, Hu Y, et al. Neoadjuvant camrelizumab plus chemotherapy for locally advanced cervical cancer (NACI Study): a study protocol of a prospective, single-arm, phase II trial. *BMJ Open.* 2023; 13(5):e067767. doi:10.1136/bmjopen-2022-067767

47. Song S, Rudra S, Hasselle MD, et al. The effect of treatment time in locally advanced cervical cancer in the era of concurrent chemoradiotherapy. *Cancer.* 2013;119(2):325–331. doi:10.1002/cncr.27652

48. Perez CA, Grigsby PW, Castro-Vita H, Lockett MA. Carcinoma of the uterine cervix. I. Impact of prolongation of overall treatment time and timing of brachytherapy on outcome of radiation therapy. *Int J Radiat Oncol Biol Phys.* 1995;32(5):1275–1288. doi:10.1016/0360-3016(95)00220-S

49. Chen SW, Liang JA, Yang SN, Ko HL, Lin FJ. The adverse effect of treatment prolongation in cervical cancer by high-dose-rate intracavitary brachytherapy. *Radiother Oncol.* 2003;67(1):69–76. doi:10.1016/s0167-8140(02)00439-5

50. Liu R, Wang X, Tian JH, et al. High dose rate versus low dose rate intracavity brachytherapy for locally advanced uterine cervix cancer. *Cochrane Database Syst Rev.* 2014;(10):CD007563. doi:10.1002/14651858.CD007563.pub3

51. Viswanathan AN, Erickson BA. Three-dimensional imaging in gynecologic brachytherapy: a survey of the American Brachytherapy Society. *Int J Radiat Oncol Biol Phys.* 2010;76(1):104–109. doi:10.1016/j.ijrobp.2009.01.043

52. Leath CA, Deng W, Mell LK, et al. Incorporation of triapine (T) with cisplatin chemoradiation (CRT) for locally advanced cervical and vaginal cancer: results from NRG-GY006, a phase III randomized trial. *J Clin Oncol.* 2023;41(16_suppl):5502. doi:10.1200/JCO.2023.41.16_suppl.5502

53. Potter R, Kirisits C, Fidarova EF, et al. Present status and future of high-precision image guided adaptive brachytherapy for cervix carcinoma. *Acta Oncol.* 2008;47(7):1325–1336. doi:10.1080/02841860802282794

54. Pelloski CE, Palmer M, Chronowski GM, Jhingran A, Horton J, Eifel PJ. Comparison between CT-based volumetric calculations and ICRU reference-point estimates of radiation doses delivered to bladder and rectum during intracavitary radiotherapy for cervical cancer. *Int J Radiat Oncol Biol Phys.* 2005;62(1):131–137. doi:10.1016/j.ijrobp.2004.09.059

55. Hashim N, Jamalludin Z, Ung NM, Ho GF, Malik RA, Phua VC. CT based 3-dimensional treatment planning of intracavitary brachytherapy for cancer of the cervix: comparison between dose-volume histograms and ICRU point doses to the rectum and bladder. *Asian Pac J Cancer Prev.* 2014;15(13):5259–5264. doi:10.7314/apjcp.2014.15.13.5259

49 UTERINE CANCER: ENDOMETRIAL CANCER AND UTERINE SARCOMA

David S. Buchberger, Sarah M. C. Sittenfeld, Sheen Cherian, and Sudha R. Amarnath

QUICK HIT Endometrial cancer is the most common gynecologic malignancy in the United States. Medically operable patients should undergo TAH/BSO (or radical hysterectomy if cervical stromal involvement) with peritoneal cytology and sentinel lymph node mapping. Postoperative management is dictated by pathologic features. Early-stage patients are grouped into low-, intermediate-, or high-risk groups, which were defined by GOG 33, GOG 99, and PORTEC studies. The management paradigm for locally advanced endometrial cancer is evolving but generally consists of surgery followed by CHT ± IO or combination CRT followed by additional CHT ± IO (Table 49.1). Increasingly, molecular analysis and subtyping is being used for further risk stratification and treatment delineation, which is reflected in the updated FIGO 2023 staging system.

Table 49.1 General Treatment Paradigm for Endometrial Cancer (See ASCO/ASTRO Guidelines for Details)[1–3]

Stage	Adjuvant Treatment Options (After TAH/BSO)
Stage IA, grades I–II	Observation*
Stage IA, grade III or stage IB, grades I–II	Favor vaginal cuff brachytherapy (VBT)†
Stage IB, grade III	Favor pelvic RT
Stage II	Pelvic RT + VBT boost ± CHT
Stages III–IV	CRT, CHT ± IO vs. CHT/IO ± consolidative pelvic RT vs. CHT alone
Medically inoperable	EBRT to uterus, cervix, upper vagina, pelvic LN, other involved areas (45–50.4 Gy) + intracavitary boost ± CHT

*Can consider vaginal cuff brachytherapy if higher risk features (age >60, LVSI).
†Can consider pelvic RT if other high-risk factors are present (age >60, LVSI, p53abn) and surgical staging was inadequate.

EPIDEMIOLOGY: Malignancy of the uterine corpus is the most common gynecologic malignancy in the United States, with >67,000 new cases and >13,000 deaths projected in 2024 (now the most common cause of gynecologic cancer deaths).[4] Uterine cancer accounts for 3.4% of all new cancer cases in the United States.[5] Median age at diagnosis is 64, with ~7% of cases occurring in patients <45 years of age.[5]

RISK FACTORS: Main risk factor is excess endogenous/exogenous estrogen without opposing progestin: (a) *physiologic*: obesity, nulliparity, early menarche, and late menopause[6–9]; (b) *pathologic*: diabetes mellitus, polycystic ovarian syndrome[6,8]; (c) *exposure*: unopposed estrogen therapy, tamoxifen[10]; (d) *protective*: combined OCPs, progestin, exercise[6,11]; (e) *family history/genetics*: Lynch II, subset of HNPCC, has been associated with increased risk of endometrial cancer. HNPCC is an autosomal dominant mutation in DNA *MMR* genes and increases the lifetime risk of endometrial cancer to 27% to 71% as compared with the 3% lifetime risk in general population.[12,13] In patients diagnosed with endometrial cancer <50 years of age, consider screening for HNPCC.[14] Prophylactic TAH/BSO can be considered for HNPCC carriers.[15]

ANATOMY: Uterine corpus is defined as the upper two-thirds of the uterus above the internal cervical os (composed of fundus and body). Cervix and lower uterine segment comprise the lower one-third of the uterus. Oviducts (fallopian tubes) and round ligaments enter the uterus at the upper outer corners (cornu). The fundus and the body of uterus are separated by the line connecting the tubouterine orifices. Uterine wall is composed of endometrium, myometrium, and serosa from innermost to outermost layers. Cancer arising from the epithelial lining of the uterine cavity is referred to as endometrial cancer. The first site of local extension for endometrial cancer is into the myometrium. Cancers arising from the stromal and muscle tissues of the myometrium are referred to as uterine sarcomas.[16] There are three major ligaments that support the uterus: the broad ligament, uterosacral ligament, and transverse (Mackenrodt's or cardinal) ligament.

Lymphatics: Regional lymphatics include bilateral parametrial, obturator, internal iliac (hypogastric), external iliac, common iliac, para-aortic (PA), presacral, and sacral.[17] Fundal lesions can drain directly to PA LNs, but are uncommon, whereas cervical lesions drain laterally to parametrium, obturator, and pelvic nodes.[16]

PATHOLOGY: Two distinct pathologic types have been described:

- **Type I** (~80%): Favorable course, presents at early stage. Grades 1 to 2. Endometrioid histology. Estrogen responsive (and therefore main risk factors are related to excess of estrogen without opposing progestin as described previously). Diploid. Type I malignancies are thought to have multistep process leading to carcinogenesis: simple endometrial hyperplasia progresses to complex atypical hyperplasia, which becomes precursor lesion, and subsequently develops into endometrial intraepithelial neoplasia, which ultimately becomes endometrial carcinoma.[18]
- **Type II** (10%–20%): Aggressive course. Grade 3. Nonendometrioid histologies including serous and clear cell. Independent of estrogen or endometrial hyperplasia and develops from atrophic endometrium. Aneuploid. *TP53* is mutated early (81% of cases) and may account for the different rates of progression in these two subtypes.[6,16,19]

In addition to appropriate staging, grade of tumor must also be reported. Grading system reports the degree of glandular differentiation (which is described as the percentage of nonsquamous or nonmorular solid growth pattern) and corresponds to the aggressiveness of the tumor. Grades 1, 2, and 3 tumors have ≤5%, 6% to 50%, and >50% nonsquamous or nonmorular solid growth patterns, respectively. In addition, papillary serous and clear cell histologies are considered grade 3. Note: Nuclear atypia out of proportion to architectural grade raises grade by 1 for grade 1 and 2 tumors.[16] "MELF" pattern (microcystic, elongated, and fragmented) has been described as correlating with more advanced pathologic features and may necessitate nodal staging, although its impact on survival outcomes is unclear.[20,21]

GENETICS AND MOLECULAR SUBGROUPS: Many genetic mutations have been identified, most commonly in *PIK3CA* pathway and more specifically *PTEN* mutations, which are thought to be early events in carcinogenesis.[6,16,22,23] Four molecular subgroups have been identified (see Table 49.2) and are being increasingly used for prognostication and treatment decisions.[23–27] They include DNA polymerase-epsilon mutated tumors (POLE mutated), mismatch repair deficient tumors (MMRd), p53 mutated tumors (p53abn), and no specific molecular profile tumors (NSMP).

Table 49.2 Endometrial Cancer Molecular Subtypes[23–27]		
Molecular Subtype	**General Prognosis**	**Features**
POLE mutated	Good	~10% of endometrial cancers; younger patients, earlier stages, giant cells, and prominent lymphocytic infiltrates
MMRd	Intermediate	~25%–30% of endometrial cancers; Lynch syndrome association, although majority are sporadic
P53abn	Poor	More common in high-grade cancers
NSMP	Stage-dependent	Associations with the *PI3K/PTEN/AKT/mTOR* signaling pathway

SCREENING: Cancer Genetics Consortium recommends screening for patients with HNPCC with annual endometrial sampling and TVUS beginning at 30 to 35 years of age or 5 to 10 years prior to the earliest Lynch-associated cancer diagnosed in a family member.[28]

CLINICAL PRESENTATION: The most common presenting symptom is postmenopausal vaginal bleeding (~90%). Other symptoms including abdominal/pelvic pain, abdominal distension, urinary/rectal bleeding, and constipation may be symptoms of advanced disease.[6,14,17]

WORKUP

H&P: Careful inspection of external genitalia, vagina, and cervix; rectal exam; and bimanual pelvic exam. Attention for enlargement of uterus or tumor extension to cervix, vagina, or parametrium.

Labs: CBC; optional: LFTs and CA 125 for high-risk subtypes.[14]

Imaging: Goal is to guide surgical approach based on risk of recurrence as estimated per myometrial/cervical invasion and LN metastases. Endometrial stripe should be assessed with TVUS. If endometrial stripe is abnormally thickened, it should be further evaluated with a biopsy. Chest imaging with CXR. MRI pelvis is the preferred imaging modality for assessing preoperative local extent of disease; however, it is *not* particularly helpful in detecting LN or peritoneal involvement. It is performed only for suspicion of locally advanced disease or in the medically inoperable setting. PET/CT remains the best imaging modality for detecting LN metastases but is not routinely performed. May consider CT chest/abdomen/pelvis for high-grade tumors.[6,14]

Procedures: Gold standard is biopsy under hysteroscopy. Endometrial biopsy for histologic information as preoperative evaluation. If endometrial biopsy is nondiagnostic and a concern for malignancy persists, fractional D&C should be performed.[6,14]

PROGNOSTIC FACTORS: Poor prognostic factors include age, grade, tumor size, LVSI, depth of invasion, clear cell/papillary or serous histology, LN involvement, tumor involvement of lower uterine segment, and p53abn tumors.[29,30] Since the mid-1970s, survival has improved for all of the most common cancers except uterine corpus and cervix cancers, likely due to the lack of major treatment advances at the time of disease recurrence or development of metastatic disease.[4]

NATURAL HISTORY: May arise from background of hyperplasia. Simple hyperplasia is associated with ~1% risk of malignancy, complex hyperplasia ~3%, simple atypia ~10%, and complex atypia ~30% to 40%. In general, complexity refers to glandular structure, whereas atypia refers to cellular morphology. At diagnosis, disease is localized/organ confined in 67%, spread to regional LN and organs in 21%, and metastatic in 8%.[6] The most common metastatic sites are the vagina, ovaries, and lung.[16] Clear cell tumors have been associated with metastases to abdominal or pelvic peritoneal surfaces or to the omentum. The most common site of locoregional recurrence is the vagina.[31]

STAGING: AJCC staging system is both clinical and pathologic. The FIGO staging system was updated in 2023 to include surgical, pathologic, and molecular data (Tables 49.3 and 49.4).[32] Currently, there is significant institutional variation in the application of the 2023 FIGO staging system to routine practice, and treatment patterns continue to change as molecular subtyping becomes more widely available and studied. The clinical staging system is assigned before CHT or RT if those are the initial modalities of therapy.[33]

Table 49.3 AJCC 8th Edition (2017): Staging for Corpus Uteri Carcinoma and Carcinosarcoma[33]		
AJCC		**FIGO**
T1	**T1a** Tumor limited to endometrium or invades <50% of myometrium	**IA**
	T1b Tumor invades ≥50% of myometrium	**IB**
T2	Invades cervical stroma, but does not extend beyond uterus	**II**
T3	**T3a** Invades serosa and/or adnexa via direct extension or metastasis*	**IIIA**
	T3b Invades vagina via direct extension or metastasis; or parametrial involvement*	**IIIB**
N0 (i+)	Isolated tumor cells ≤0.2 mm	
N1mi	Positive pelvic LNs (0.2–2.0 mm)	**IIIC1**
N1a	Positive pelvic LNs (>2.0 mm)	
N2mi	Positive PA LNs (with or without pelvic LNs; 0.2–2.0 mm)	**IIIC2**
N2a	Positive PA LNs (with or without pelvic LNs; >2.0 mm)	
T4	Invasion of bladder and/or bowel mucosa (bullous edema not sufficient)	**IVA**
M1	Distant metastasis	**IVB**

*Positive cytology should be reported, but it does not change stage.
Source: Adapted from AJCC Cancer Staging Manual. 8th ed. Springer International Publishing; 2017.

Table 49.4 2023 FIGO Staging for Endometrial Cancer[32]	
Stage	**Description**
I	Confined to the uterine corpus and ovary
IA	Disease limited to the endometrium OR nonaggressive histologic type (i.e., low-grade endometroid) with invasion of <50% of myometrium with no or focal LVSI OR good prognosis disease **IA1:** Nonaggressive histologic type limited to an endometrial polyp OR confined to the endometrium **IA2:** Nonaggressive histologic types involving <50% of the myometrium with no or focal LVSI **IA3:** Low-grade endometrioid carcinomas limited to the uterus and ovary
IB	Nonaggressive histologic types with invasion of ≥50% of the myometrium, and with no or focal LVSI
IC	Aggressive histologic types limited to a polyp or confined to the endometrium
II	Invasion of cervical stroma without extrauterine extension OR with substantial LVSI OR aggressive histologic types with myometrial invasion
IIA	Invasion of the cervical stroma of nonaggressive histologic types
IIB	Substantial LVSI of nonaggressive histologic types
IIC	Aggressive histologic types with any myometrial involvement
III	Local and/or regional spread of the tumor of any histologic subtype
IIIA	Invasion of uterine serosa, adnexa, or both by direct extension or metastasis **IIIA1:** Spread to ovary or fallopian tube (except when meeting stage IA3 criteria) **IIIA2:** Involvement of uterine subserosa or spread through the uterine serosa
IIIB	Metastasis or direct spread to the vagina and/or to the parametria or pelvic peritoneum **IIIB1:** Metastasis or direct spread to the vagina and/or the parametria **IIIB2:** Metastasis to the pelvic peritoneum
IIIC	Metastasis to the pelvic or PA LNs or both **IIIC1:** Metastasis to the pelvic LNs **IIIC1i:** Micrometastasis **IIIC1ii:** Macrometastasis **IIIC2:** Metastasis to PA LNs up to the renal vessels, with or without metastasis to the pelvic LNs **IIIC2i:** Micrometastasis **IIIC2ii:** Macrometastasis
IV	Spread to the bladder mucosa and/or intestinal mucosa and/or DMs
IVA	Invasion of the bladder mucosa and/or the intestinal/bowel mucosa
IVB	Abdominal peritoneal metastasis beyond the pelvis
IVC	DM, including metastasis to any extra- or intra-abdominal LNs above the renal vessels, lungs, liver, brain, or bone

Source: Berek JS, Matias-Guiu X, Creutzberg C, et al. FIGO staging of endometrial cancer: 2023. *Int J Gynaecol Obstet.* 2023;162(2):383–394. doi:10.1002/ijgo.14923.

TREATMENT PARADIGM

Surgery: TAH/BSO (simple or type I hysterectomy) is standard of care for early stage disease. Minimally invasive (laparoscopic) approaches are preferred. Radical hysterectomy is done for cases of gross cervical invasion. Surgical staging requires evaluation of peritoneal surfaces. Omental and peritoneal biopsies are performed for high-risk disease.[6] SLN mapping is preferred for LN assessment in patients with uterine-confined disease even for high-risk histologies. Lymphadenectomy used in instances of failed SLN mapping and/or enlarged/suspicious nodes. PA evaluation commonly done for high-risk patients.[34,35]

Complications: Lymphedema (8%–50% risk depending on the number of LNs removed, adjuvant CHT/RT, preoperative NSAID use).[36]

Chemotherapy: Adjuvant CHT is standard in patients with stage III/IV disease, but generally is not indicated in patients with low- or intermediate-risk disease. High-risk patients should be encouraged to participate in ongoing clinical trials. Carboplatin/paclitaxel is the most common adjuvant regimen. Cisplatin is the most common therapy given concurrently with RT (see the following trials).[14]

Immunotherapy: Recent prospective randomized trials established a PFS and OS benefit to the addition of PD-1 inhibitors (pembrolizumab, dostarlimab) to CHT in patients with "advanced stage" endometrial cancer, which included stages III/IVA/IVB and recurrent disease of all histologies (most patients had not received prior RT on these trials, and most patients had gross residual disease).[37,38] IO in addition to CHT has been incorporated into the latest NCCN guidelines for the treatment of this patient population.[14]

Radiation

Indications: RT is used as adjuvant therapy after TAH/BSO or as primary therapy for patients who are not surgical candidates. Indications for VBT include high intermediate risk (HIR) disease, generally defined as grades 1 to 2 tumors with ≥50% myometrial invasion (MI) or grade 3 tumors with <50% invasion (see the following trials and ABS guidelines),[1,2,39] or as boost following pelvic EBRT (not generally warranted except with risk factors such as cervical stromal invasion or positive margin). Pelvic EBRT is given to early-stage patients at high risk (grade 3 tumors with ≥50% invasion) and can additionally be considered in stage III disease.

Dose: To treat the whole pelvis adjuvantly, 45 to 50.4 Gy is given via EBRT with IMRT.[14] For adjuvant VBT alone, PORTEC-2 (see the following) used 21 Gy/3 fx prescribed to 0.5 cm depth given weekly, but there are multiple acceptable regimens (see ABS guidelines). For a VBT boost following EBRT, 18 Gy/3 fx prescribed to the vaginal surface is acceptable among other regimens. For medically inoperable patients, see ABS consensus statement for guidelines.[40]

Toxicity: Acute: fatigue, diarrhea, nausea, myelosuppression, dysuria, urinary frequency. Late: vaginal stenosis, vaginal dryness, rarely RT cystitis, proctitis, sacral insufficiency fractures, bowel obstruction, fistula.

Procedure: See *Handbook of Treatment Planning in Radiation Oncology*, Chapter 9.[41]

EVIDENCE-BASED Q&A

EARLY-STAGE ENDOMETRIAL CANCER

How are women with endometrial cancer categorized?

Endometrial cancers are historically classified into low-, intermediate-, and high-risk groups. The Aalders trial was one of the first to demonstrate differences by risk group.[42] GOG 33 was a surgical study that demonstrated noninvasive (old stage IA) tumors were "low" risk, invasive cancers (old stage IB, IC, and occult stage IIA–B) were "intermediate" risk, and any stage III or IV or invasive clear cell/papillary were "high" risk. GOG 33 further subdivided "intermediate" risk into low- and high-intermediate risk (see GOG 99). The HIR group benefitted from adjuvant therapy as demonstrated in GOG 99 and PORTEC-1/2. Increasingly, molecular status is becoming a routine part of endometrial cancer categorization, reflected in the recently published "Molecular PORTEC" analysis of studies PORTEC-1 and PORTEC-2, as well as the molecular analysis of PORTEC-3.

What pathologic findings correlate with risk of nodal involvement?

Early studies from GOG suggest that depth of invasion (DOI) and grade highly correlate with nodal involvement.

Creasman, GOG 33 Staging (*Cancer* **1987, PMID 3652025):** Prospective observational study of 681 women treated with TAH/BSO, pelvic, and PA dissection with peritoneal cytology from 1977 to 1983. See Table 49.5. **Conclusion: On MVA, grade, DOI, and intraperitoneal disease were predictive of LN metastasis.**

Table 49.5 Results of GOG 33 for Endometrial Cancer						
Depth of Invasion	% PA and Pelvic LN Involvement					
	Grade 1		Grade 2		Grade 3	
	PA	Pelvic	PA	Pelvic	PA	Pelvic
Endometrium only	0%	0%	3%	3%	0%	0%
Superficial myometrial invasion	1%	3%	4%	5%	4%	9%
Middle myometrial invasion	5%	0%	0%	9%	0%	4%
Deep myometrial invasion	6%	11%	14%	19%	23%	34%

Note: Risk of PA LN involvement is two-thirds the risk of pelvic LN involvement; 30%–55% of +pelvic LNs have +PA LNs.

Morrow, GOG 33 (*Gynecol Oncol* 1991, PMID 1989916): Same study as the preceding but correlated surgical pathology findings and recurrence patterns prospectively; 895 patients with FIGO stage I and II (occult), endometrioid type. Isolated positive PA LNs in the setting of negative pelvic LNs are uncommon (2.2%). Only 5.4% (*n* = 48) had positive PA LNs. Of these, 47 had >1 grossly positive pelvic LNs, grossly positive adnexal metastases, or deep myometrial penetration (accounted for 98% of cases with positive PA LNs and could be used to select patients for nodal staging). Among M0 patients, LVSI, DOI, and grade correlate with recurrence-free interval. LRF rate (32% vs. 48%) appears to favor adjuvant RT for patients with greater than one-third MI and grades 2 to 3 tumors. **Conclusion: The greatest determinant of recurrence was grade 3 histology.**

Katsoulakis, SEER (*Int J Gynaecol Obstet* 2014, PMID 25194213): SEER analysis from 1998 to 2003 ("contemporary era") including 4,052 patients using FIGO 1988 stage classification. Pelvic nodal metastases identified as per Table 49.6.

Table 49.6 SEER Patterns of Nodal Spread						
	Grade 1		Grade 2		Grade 3	
	Pelvic	PA	Pelvic	PA	Pelvic	PA
IA	1%	0%	2%	0%	1%	1%
IB	2%	0%	3%	1%	3%	2%
IC	3%	3%	8%	5%	12%	8%
IIA	7%	3%	10%	4%	10%	5%
IIB	8%	4%	13%	8%	19%	12%

Is pelvic nodal dissection necessary in early-stage disease? What is the role of SLN mapping?

Without suspicious intraoperative LNs, elective pelvic and PA nodal dissection likely does not change oncologic outcomes. Two trials failed to show a difference in RFS/DFS or OS with the addition of lymphadenectomy to TAH/BSO for early-stage disease.[43,44] More recently, SLN mapping has become the preferred LN assessment technique for patients with uterine-confined disease (including high-risk histologies) based on numerous prospective and retrospective studies suggesting that SLN mapping with ultrastaging may even increase the detection rate of LN metastasis with low false-negative rates relative to lymphadenectomy. The increasing use of SLN mapping in early-stage patients has resulted in an increasing detection of isolated tumor cells (ITCs) with no consensus guidelines about treatment approaches for these patients.[45]

Which patients benefit from adjuvant RT after TAH/BSO?

Early-stage patients with adverse path features are at risk of extrauterine disease and recurrence. High-risk features vary but overall include deep myometrial invasion (MI), tumor grade, cervical involvement, older age, LVSI, and tumor size (from GOG 33).

Keys, GOG 99 (*Gynecol Oncol* 2004, PMID 14984936): PRT of 392 patients with "intermediate-risk" endometrial cancer s/p TAH/BSO with pelvic/PA nodal sampling and cytology randomized to no adjuvant therapy vs. whole pelvic RT (WPRT). Eligibility: 1988 FIGO IB to occult stage II (2009 FIGO stages IA, IB, and occult II) disease. Inclusion criteria were revised during the trial to include only HIR subgroup (based on GOG 33): (a) age >70 years with one risk factor (grade 2 or 3, LVSI, outer one-third MI); (b) age >50 years with two risk factors; and (c) any age with three risk factors. All others were LIR. RT 50.4 Gy/28 fx. Primary endpoint was cumulative incidence of recurrence (CIR), and the study was not powered for OS. MFU 69 months. Fifty-nine percent of patients had stage IA disease, and 82% had grade 1 or 2 disease. Greatest benefit in LR was in HIR patients from 26% vs. 6% vs. LIR patients from 6% vs. 2% (Table 49.7). Of three pelvic and vaginal recurrences in the RT arm, two had refused RT. RT had worse hematologic, GI, GU, and cutaneous toxicities. **Conclusion: Adjuvant RT in early-stage intermediate-risk endometrial cancer decreases the risk of recurrence in HIR patients.** *Comment: Grade 2 was grouped with grade 3 even though grade 2 tends to behave more similarly to grade 1.*

Table 49.7 Results of GOG 99

GOG 99	2-Yr Any Recurrence (All Patients)	2-Yr Any Recurrence for HIR Patients	4-Yr OS
Surgery	12%	26%	86%
Surgery + RT	3%	6%	92%
p value	.007	.007	.557

Scholten, PORTEC-1 (*IJROBP* 2005, PMID 15927414; Update Creutzberg, *IJROBP* 2011, PMID 21640520; QOL Update Nout, *JCO* 2011, PMID 21444867): PRT of 714 patients with stage I disease evaluating TAH/BSO + cytology ± pelvic RT (no PLND). Eligibility: <50% MI and G2–3 OR ≥50% MI and G1–2 (stage IB/IC at time); 99 patients with stage IC, G3 disease not randomized, but received adjuvant WPRT. RT 46 Gy/23 fx in two to four fields within 8 weeks postop. MFU 97 months. On MVA, RT and age <60 were favorable prognostic factors for LRR. Patients with two or more of the three risk factors (age ≥60, >50% MI, and grade 3) had the highest benefit from RT. In patients with isolated vaginal relapse, CR was obtained in 31 out of 35 patients (89%), and 24 patients (77%) still had CR after further follow-up; 3-year OS after vaginal relapse was 73%. On MVA of 15-year data (MFU 13.3 years), grade 3, age >60, and >50% MI were prognostic for both LRR and endometrial cancer death (Table 49.8). **Conclusion: Adjuvant WPRT in stage IB, G1–2 or stage IA, G2–3 endometrial cancer reduces LRR with no impact on OS.** *Note: ~75% of LRs were in the vaginal vault. On central pathology review, there was a significant shift from G2 to G1. WPRT is not indicated in patients with stage IA, G2 disease, or for patients <60 years of age with stage IB, G1–2 or stage IA, G2–3 disease. OS after relapse is significantly better in the group without prior RT. Treatment for vaginal relapse is effective. Patients with stage IB, G3 disease have high risk of early DM and endometrial cancer-related death. Adjuvant WPRT should be avoided in patients at low or intermediate risk of recurrence.*

Table 49.8 Results of PORTEC-1

15-Yr Data	LRR	OS	DM	Physical Functioning	Urinary/Bowel Symptoms	Second Malignancy
No RT	16%	60%	7%	62%	24%/14%	13%
WPRT	6%	52%	9%	51%	28%/20%	19%
p value	<.0001	.14	.26	.004	<.001	.12

Is there benefit to adding pelvic RT to vaginal brachytherapy?

Aalders, Norway (*Obstet Gynecol* 1980, PMID 6999399): PRT of 540 patients with stage I disease evaluating TAH/BSO (without LND or peritoneal cytology) followed by VBT, then randomized to no further treatment or pelvic EBRT (4,000 rads *[sic]* to pelvic LNs with midline block at 2,000 rads *[sic]*). See Table 49.9 for results. Overall, pelvic RT decreased 9-year LR (7% vs. 2%, *p* < .01) but more DM (5% vs. 10%). There was no difference in 5-year OS. On subset analysis, pelvic RT improved 9-year OS for patients with G3 and >50% MI or LVSI (72% vs. 82%). **Conclusion: Only patients with grade 3 tumors and >50% MI or LVSI may benefit from pelvic RT. All other stage I patients should receive VBT alone.**

Table 49.9 Results of Aalders (Norway) Trial of Pelvic RT for Endometrial Cancer					
	5-Yr OS	9-Yr OS	LRR	DM	Deaths From DM
No pelvic RT	91%	90%	7%	5%	5%
Pelvic RT	89%	87%	2%	10%	10%
p value	NS	NS	<.01	NS	.10 > p > .05

Blake, MRC ASTEC-NCIC EN.5 Pooled Results (*Lancet* 2009, PMID 19070891): PRT of 905 patients with intermediate-risk or *high-risk* early-stage endometrial cancer treated with TAH/BSO ± adjuvant EBRT. Lymphadenectomy was optional (29% of patients underwent LND, of which 4% had positive LN) and intracavitary was optional but had to be stated upfront whether the institution would deliver it, and it had to be offered to both arms if given (used in 51% vs. 52%). High-risk disease: grade 3, stage IB, endocervical glandular involvement, serous papillary, or clear cell type; +PA nodes excluded. RT was 40–46 Gy/20–25 fx. Median age 65. EBRT had higher any acute (57% vs. 26%) and any late (61% vs. 45%) toxicity; 5-year OS 84%, DSS 89%, RFS 78%. No difference between arms. Isolated vaginal/pelvic relapse (3% vs. 6% favoring EBRT, *p* = .038). **Conclusion: EBRT should not be routinely recommended for intermediate- or high-risk patients, and although EBRT reduces LR it is not without toxicity.** *Note: LR rate in the observation group with brachytherapy was 6%.*

Kong (*J Natl Cancer Inst* 2012, PMID 22962693): Meta-analysis of seven RCTs comparing EBRT vs. no EBRT (included VBT) and one trial comparing VBT with no additional treatment. EBRT significantly reduced LRR (HR 0.36, 95% CI 0.25–0.52) but did not improve OS (HR 0.99, 0.82–1.20), CSS, or DM. EBRT associated with increased severe acute and late toxicity. **Conclusion: EBRT, compared with observation or VBT alone, reduces LRR but has no impact on survival and is associated with significant morbidity and reduction in QOL.**

Sorbe, Swedish Intermediate Risk (*IJROBP* 2012, PMID 21676554): PRT of 527 medium-risk patients (stage I endometrioid histology with one risk factor: G3, ≥50% MI, or DNA aneuploidy) randomized to TAH/BSO + VBT ± WPRT. Treated with 46 Gy + VBT or VBT alone (3 Gy × 6, 5.9 Gy × 3, or 20 Gy × 1 to 5 mm). Fifteen pelvic recurrences in VBT-alone arm, one in WPRT + VBT (LR 5% vs. 2% at 5 years); 5-year OS was 89% and 90% (*p* = .548). Deep MI was prognostic but not grade or DNA ploidy. WPRT had low toxicity (<2%) but difference favored VBT alone. **Conclusion: Even with LR benefit for WPRT + VBT, combined RT should be reserved for high-risk cases with ≥2 high-risk factors given toxicity and no OS benefit. VBT alone should be the adjuvant treatment option for purely medium-risk cases.**

Does vaginal brachytherapy reduce recurrences in low-risk women?

Sorbe, Swedish Low Risk (*Int J Gyn Cancer* 2009, PMID 19574776). PRT of 645 patients randomized to TAH/BSO ± VBT (HDR or LDR). Eligibility: FIGO 1988 stage IA/B and G1–2. RT with Perspex applicators or ovoids, Rx 3 to 8 Gy × 3 to 6 fx prescribed to 5 mm depth. Vaginal recurrence 1% with VBT and 3% without (*p* = .114). Few side effects with G1–2 toxicity of 2.8% with VBT and 0.6% without. **Conclusion: VBT is associated with a nonsignificant reduction in recurrence. Observation is appropriate for this subgroup.** *Comment: Possible that certain other subgroups of low- or medium-risk patients (only stage IB, grade 2 or tumors with LVSI, or patients with higher age) may benefit from VBT.*

How should one select between adjuvant VBT and adjuvant EBRT?

Appropriate patient selection is key. Most recurrences in GOG 99 and PORTEC were in the vaginal vault, although 28% were noncentral (sidewall). GOG 99 patients were surgically staged, whereas LND was not standard on PORTEC.

Nout, PORTEC-2 (*Lancet* 2010, PMID 20206777; 10-Year Update *Br J Cancer* 2018, PMID 30356126): PRT of 427 HIR patients s/p TAH/BSO (no PLND) randomized to EBRT (46 Gy/23 fx) vs. VBT (21 Gy/3 fx HDR or 30 Gy LDR). Eligibility: age ≥60 and IB G1–2; or IA G3; or endocervical glandular involvement grades 1 to 3, any age; >50% MI with G3 excluded. MFU 45 months. Central path review: G2 tumors showed poor reproducibility and on re-review, many patients considered grade 1 (see Table 49.10). QOL better in VBT (sexual function, diarrhea, fecal incontinence, and restriction of ADLs). Acute grades 1 to 2 GI toxicities were lower in the VBT group (13% vs. 54%).

On MVA, high-risk profile and LVSI were the only risk factors for OS and RFS. At 10-year update, no significant difference in vaginal recurrence (VR), isolated pelvic recurrence, or OS. Pelvic recurrence more common in the VBT group (6% vs. 1%, p = .004) and was usually combined with DM. L1CAM expression, p53abn, and substantial LVSI were risk factors for pelvic recurrence and DM. **Conclusion: No difference in vaginal recurrence, OS, and DFS for VBT vs. EBRT. In view of QOL benefit, VBT should be the treatment of choice for HIR endometrial cancer.**

Table 49.10 Results of PORTEC-2 for Endometrial Cancer

5-Yr Results	VR	LRR	Pelvic-Only Recurrence	DFS	OS	Gr 1–2 GI Toxicity	Path Distribution	G1	G2	G3
EBRT	1.6%	2%	1.5%	83%	85%	54%	Original	48%	45%	7%
VBT	1.8%	5%	0.5%	78%	80%	13%	Review	79%	9%	12%
p value	.74	.17	.30	.74	.57	NS after 24 months				

Randall, GOG 249 (*JCO* 2019, PMID 30995174): Phase III PRT of 601 patients with FIGO stage I endometrioid meeting HIR criteria as per GOG 99, all stage II, or stage I/II serous/clear cell carcinoma randomized after surgery to whole-pelvis EBRT (45–50.4 Gy/25–28 fx) vs. VBT followed by carboplatin/paclitaxel for three cycles given q3 weeks (VBT/C). Optional cuff boost allowed on the EBRT arm for stage II patients or papillary serous/clear cell histology; 74% of patients stage I, 71% endometrioid, and 20% serous/clear cell. Eighty-nine percent underwent LND. MFU 53 months; 60-month RFS 76% for both arms. The 5-year OS was not statistically different between EBRT and VBT/C (87% and 85%, respectively). No differences were seen for vaginal or distant failures. However, there was a significant differential in the cumulative incidence of pelvic or PA nodal recurrences within 5 years of entry, with more failures seen in the VBT/C arm (9% vs. 4%). Acute grade ≥3 toxicity significantly increased in the VBT/C group. Grade ≥3 late toxicity was similar in both groups. No clear subset benefitted from either regimen. **Conclusion: VBT/C is not superior to pelvic RT in terms of RFS or OS and is associated with more acute toxicity (but similar late toxicity). VBT/C has higher rate of pelvic and PA nodal recurrences compared with EBRT, while both modalities have similar rates of vaginal and distant recurrence. Pelvic RT remains an effective adjuvant treatment modality for patients with high-risk, early-stage endometrial cancer of all histologies.**

How much does age, LVSI, and molecular status impact outcomes?

LVSI has consistently been shown to be a strong risk factor for local and distant recurrence, as evidenced in the first pooled analysis of PORTEC-1 and PORTEC-2 patients described below. A second pooled analysis of these two trials published in 2023 provides insight into the outcomes through the lens of molecular classification, adding to similar data previously published on the PORTEC-3 cohort (see below). Regardless of histopathologic or molecular risk factors, further pooled analyses of these trials suggest that older patients have worse outcomes and treatment should be tailored accordingly.

Bosse, LVSI PORTEC-1 and PORTEC-2 (*Eur J Cancer* 2015, PMID 26049688): Pooled analysis from PORTEC-1 and PORTEC-2 showed that substantial LVSI (diffuse or multifocal LVSI as opposed to focal or no LVSI) was the strongest independent prognostic factor for pelvic regional recurrence (HR 6.2), DM (HR 3.6), and OS (HR 2.0); the 5-year risk of pelvic failure was 1.7%, 2.5%, and 15% for no, focal, and substantial LVSI, respectively. In patients with substantial LVSI, the 5-year pelvic recurrence was 4% after EBRT vs. 27% with VBT alone and 31% after no additional treatment. **Conclusion: Substantial LVSI is a strong risk factor for pelvic recurrence and more comprehensive treatment seems to be of benefit.** *Comment: LND was not required on the PORTEC studies.*

Horeweg, Molecular PORTEC-1 and PORTEC-2 (*J Clin Oncol* 2023, PMID 37487144): Pooled analysis from PORTEC-1 and PORTEC-2 assessing locoregional RFS by molecular classification and receipt of RT. With an MFU of 11.3 years, no LRR was observed in POLEmut patients. For MMRd patients, LRR was similar regardless of adjuvant treatment (EBRT 94%, VBT 94%, observation 90%, p = .74). For p53abn patients, LRR was significantly improved with EBRT vs. VBT vs. observation (97% vs. 64% vs. 72%, p = .048). In patients with NSMP, both EBRT and VBT resulted in improved LRR rates compared with observation (98%, 96%, 88%, p < .0001). **Conclusion: Outcomes differ by subgroup, and molecular classification can be used to potentially guide treatment decisions.**

Wakkerman, Age PORTEC-1, PORTEC-2, and PORTEC-3 (*Lancet Oncol* 2024, PMID 38701815): Pooled analysis of PORTEC-1, PORTEC-2, and PORTEC-3 patients assessing age as an independent risk factor in endometrial cancer vs. the accumulation of risk factors in older endometrial cancer patients. Data analyzed from over 1,800 women. Recurrence and death from endometrial cancer were significantly associated with age. There was an increased frequency of deep MI, serous histology, and p53abn tumors in older women. Despite this, age remained an independent risk factor for recurrence (HR 1.02 per year, 95% CI 1.01–1.04, $p = .0012$) and endometrial cancer-specific death (HR 1.03 per year, 95% CI 1.02–1.05, $p = .0012$). **Conclusion: Age is an independent risk factor for poor outcomes in endometrial cancer, and it is also associated with more aggressive histology.**

Does postoperative IMRT reduce treatment-related toxicity while maintaining control rates?

RTOG 0418 and RTOG 0921 suggest that IMRT is safe and effective for pelvic RT in combination with systemic therapy with an acceptable toxicity profile.[46,47] RTOG 1203 (below) has since shown that IMRT decreases GI and GU toxicity with no decrease in efficacy compared with conventional four-field RT and is now standard of care.

Klopp, RTOG 1203/TIME-C (*JCO* 2018, PMID 29989857; Toxicity Update Yeung, *JCO* 2022, PMID 35960897): Phase III PRT of patient-reported toxicity and QOL during PORT in 278 patients with cervical or endometrial cancer randomized to IMRT vs. conventional four-field RT. Between baseline and end of RT, mean EPIC bowel score declined 23.6 points with standard RT vs. 18.6 points with IMRT ($p = .048$); mean EPIC urinary score declined 10.4 points with standard RT vs. 5.6 points with IMRT ($p = .03$). At the end of RT, 52% in standard RT vs. 34% in IMRT arm reported frequent or almost constant diarrhea ($p = .01$). Update showed no difference in treatment efficacy (DFS, LRF, OS) at 3 years between IMRT and 3D conformal techniques. Initial differences in GI symptoms resolved, with worsening GU symptoms in the 3D conformal arm relative to the IMRT arm at 3 years. **Conclusion: IMRT improves acute toxicity and QOL and reduces late GI and urinary toxicity with no difference in treatment efficacy at 3 years.**

Is there a role for hypofractionated pelvic EBRT?

Leung, SPARTACUS (*JAMA Oncol* 2022, PMID 35420695): The Stereotactic Pelvic Adjuvant Radiation Therapy in Cancers of the Uterus (SPARTACUS) trial was a phase I/II nonrandomized controlled trial of 61 patients with endometrial cancer, stages I to III, treated posthysterectomy with hypofractionated pelvic RT, 30 Gy/5 fx, delivered QOD or once weekly. Toxicity and QOL were the primary endpoints. Only one grade 3 GI side effect (diarrhea), which resolved at subsequent follow-up. Patient reported diarrhea scores were the only toxicity domain worse at fraction 5 than baseline, all of which resolved at follow-up. **Conclusion: Hypofractionated postoperative pelvic RT for the treatment of endometrial cancer appears to be well-tolerated with acceptable toxicity and further study is warranted.**

ADVANCED ENDOMETRIAL CANCER

What is the definition of advanced endometrial cancer?

The clearest definition of advanced endometrial cancer is any stage III to IVA, although multiple trials also included high-risk early-stage patients typically defined by GOG 99 and PORTEC-1 as stage IB grade 3, stage II, or those with aggressive histologies (papillary serous or clear cell).

Is adjuvant CHT alone superior to adjuvant RT alone for locally advanced disease?

Numerous studies have compared the use of CHT with RT in the locally advanced setting. GOG 122 randomized patients with stage III/IV endometrial cancer postsurgery to whole-abdomen irradiation (WAI) or doxorubicin-cisplatin, finding that patients treated with CHT had improved OS and PFS but increased toxicity.[48] A subset analysis of high-risk patients from JGOG233 also showed improved OS and PFS with CHT compared with RT,[49] while a similar study from Italy showed no difference in outcomes between modalities.[50] Multiple meta-analyses[51,52] combining the above trials have also suggested oncologic benefit to the use of CHT in this population, with one analysis finding an increased survival of ~25% with CHT vs. RT at the expense of increased toxicity.[52] Direct comparisons (see below) of CHT to CRT show improved LC with CRT, a trend to better distant control with CHT, and no difference in OS. After the recent publication of multiple landmark trials showing a benefit to the addition of IO in stage III (with measurable disease) and IV patients, IO is being increasingly utilized in this setting (see below).[37,38]

Is it safe and effective to give RT along with CHT?

Multiple studies have demonstrated the safety of various forms of systemic therapy along with RT, and compared with previous results these regimens may be more effective. In addition to RTOG 0418[46] *and RTOG 0921,*[47] *RTOG 9708 showed that pelvic RT with concurrent cisplatin was safe with excellent LRC.*[53,54] *GOG 184 randomized patients to pelvic/extended-field RT (50.4 Gy to pelvis, 43.5 Gy to PAs when +PA or inadequate LND) with cisplatin and doxorubicin ± paclitaxel and found that the addition of paclitaxel to cisplatin was not associated with improved RFS but was associated with increased toxicity (note: difficult to compare to GOG 122, as stage IV patients became ineligible early in GOG 184).*[55]

Is combined CRT superior to either modality alone?

The preceding trials seemed to support that RT reduces LRF, whereas CHT reduces DM. Therefore, combined CRT may be the superior regimen, although this has not been demonstrated clearly, and details on optimal sequencing are in flux.

De Boer, PORTEC-3 (*Lancet Oncol* 2018, PMID 29449189; Update *Lancet Oncol* 2019, PMID 31345626): Phase III trial of 660 women with high-risk endometrial cancer (FIGO stage I grade 3 endometrioid with deep MI and/or LVSI, stage II/III endometrioid, or stage I–III serous or clear cell histology) randomized to RT (48.6 Gy/27fx) vs. CRT-CHT (RT/cisplatin → carbo/taxol × 4 cycles). MFU 72.6 months. Co-primary endpoints were OS and FFS. The 5-year OS was significantly higher for CRT-CHT vs. RT (81% vs. 76%, *p* = .034). Similarly, the 5-year FFS was 75% for CRT-CHT vs. 68% for RT (*p* = .01). Stage III patients had lower 5-year FFS and OS compared with stage I to II (FFS 64% vs. 79%, OS 74% vs. 83%, *p* < .0001). Stage III had the greatest benefit to CRT-CHT with 5-year FFS of 69% vs. 58% for RT (*p* = .031) and 5-year OS of 79% vs. 70% (Cox-adjusted *p* = .074). Serous histology had similar improvements with CRT-CHT with 5-year FFS and OS of 60% and 71% vs. 53% and 48% with RT alone (*p* = .037 and .008). Interestingly, patients ≥70 years old had significantly better OS and FFS with CRT-CHT. **Conclusion: CHT given during and after pelvic RT significantly improved 5-year OS and FFS compared with RT alone in high-risk endometrial cancer patients. Subgroup analysis showed the most benefit in stage III patients and serous histology, with stage I to II patients not benefitting, although this may be attributed to low numbers.**

De Boer, PORTEC-3 QOL (*Lancet Oncol* 2016, PMID 27397040): Phase III PRT detailed above. Secondary endpoints of health-related QOL as assessed by EORTC QLC-C30 and symptom scales from CX 24 and OV28. During treatment, grade ≥2 and grade ≥3 toxicities occurred in 94% and 61% of patients in the CRT arm vs. 44% and 13% in the RT-alone arm, respectively (SS). At 12 and 24 months, there were no significant differences in grade ≥3 toxicity; only grade ≥2 neuropathy persisted in 10% of the CRT group vs. 1% of the RT-alone group (SS). **Conclusion: At completion of RT and at 6 months, QOL was worse for the CRT group. But at 12 and 24 months, QOL was similar and only physical functioning scores remained slightly lower in the CRT arm.**

Matei, GOG 258 (*NEJM* 2019, PMID 31189035; 10-Year Update *JCO* 2024, PMID 39700442): Phase III trial of stage III and IVA with <2 cm residual OR those with positive cytology and serous/clear cell histology randomized to CHT alone (carbo/taxol × 6C) vs. CRT (EBRT + cisplatin, then carbo/taxol × 4C); 707 patients, MFU 47 months, with 75% completing CRT and 85% completing CHT; 5-year RFS 59% in CRT vs. 58% in CHT (NS). CRT significantly reduced 5-year vaginal recurrence (2% vs. 7% in CHT arm) and significantly reduced pelvic/PA nodal recurrence at 5 years to 11% vs. 20% in the CHT arm. Distant recurrences more common with CRT vs. CHT (27% vs. 21%; HR 1.36, 95% CI 1.00–1.86); 5-year OS 70% in the CRT arm vs. 73% in the CHT arm. Long-term results (MFU 112 months) show no difference in OS between the two arms, with more LR recurrences in the CHT group and more distant recurrences with CRT. **Conclusions: Although CRT reduced the rate of vaginal and nodal recurrence compared with CHT, the combined-modality regimen did not increase RFS in optimally debulked, stage III/IVA endometrial cancer patients.**

Hogberg, Pooled Results of MaNGO ILIADE-III and EORTC 55991 (*Eur J Cancer* 2010, PMID 20619634): Data from two PRTs of sequential adjuvant CHT and RT. Arm 1—adjuvant RT; Arm

2—adjuvant CHT and RT. Patients with serous, clear cell, or anaplastic carcinomas were eligible regardless of risk factors; however, serous/clear cell carcinoma was excluded in ILIADE-III. RT was 45 Gy/25 fx. VBT was allowed if cervical stromal involvement. CHT was doxorubicin 60 mg/m^2 and cisplatin 50 mg/m^2 q3 weeks × 3 cycles; 5-year PFS was 69% vs. 78% and 5-year OS was 75% vs. 82% (p = .07) for Arms 1 and 2, respectively. CSS was SS for CRT. Subset analysis showed no benefit to CHT for serous/clear cell carcinoma. **Conclusion: Addition of adjuvant CHT improves PFS with trend to OS improvement.** *Comment: Subset analysis was not planned and not powered to address question of endometrioid vs. serous/clear cell histology.*

What is the ideal sequencing of CHT with RT?

Optimal sequencing of CHT is unclear and varies widely depending on institutional preferences, but Geller and Secord demonstrated the benefit of "sandwich" regimen (CHT → RT → CHT); however, these were small and retrospective evaluations, with imbalances in histologic subtypes between treatment groups requiring complex modeling. In addition to the study outlined below, Secord published another RR in 2009 finding significantly better 3-year PFS and OS with a sandwich approach compared with CHT followed by RT or vice versa.[56]

Geller (*Gynecol Oncol* 2011, PMID 21239048): Phase II trial of carboplatin and docetaxel followed by RT and then consolidation CHT given in "sandwich" method; 42 patients with surgically staged III to IV (excluding IIIA from cytology alone) or biopsy-proven recurrent disease were eligible; three cycles of docetaxel and carboplatin followed by IFRT (45 Gy) ± VBT and three additional cycles of docetaxel and carboplatin; seven patients expired with MFU of 28 months. Kaplan–Meier estimates of OS at 1, 3, and 5 years were 95%, 90%, and 71%, respectively. KM estimates of PFS at 1, 3, and 5 years were 87%, 71%, and 64%, respectively. **Conclusion: "Sandwiching" RT between CHT for advanced or recurrent endometrial cancer should be further investigated in PRTs.**

Secord (*Gynecol Oncol* 2007, PMID 17688923): RR of 356 patients from 1975 to 2006 at Duke/UNC with surgical stage III/IV with TAH/BSO ± pelvic/PA LND followed with CHT ± RT. The subset of 51 patients treated with "sandwich regimen" CHT → RT → CHT had the highest 3-year OS (91%) and PFS (69%) compared with 9 patients treated with CHT → RT (47% and 19%) or 15 patients treated with RT → CHT (65% and 60%), respectively. **Conclusion: Promising results warrant further investigation on sequencing of therapy.** *Comment: Retrospective study, small number of patients, histology imbalance, and complex modeling of study are significant limitations.*

Can genetic or molecular features guide CHT treatment planning?

In conjunction with other recent publications (see the molecular analysis of PORTEC-1 and PORTEC-2 above), the data below offer further support to the prognostic and predictive value of molecular classification in endometrial cancer. The results of ongoing prospective clinical trials (PORTEC-4a, NCT03469674) investigating optimal treatment regimens based on molecular subtype are eagerly awaited.

Leon-Castillo, PORTEC-3 Molecular Classification (*JCO* 2020, PMID 32749941): Molecular analysis of 410 evaluable tissue samples from PORTEC-3 analyzed for association of RFS after adjuvant CRT vs. adjuvant RT alone with molecular features as defined by TCGA prognostic molecular classification. Tumors were classified as p53 abnormal (p53abn, 23%), POLE-ultramutated (POLEmut, 12%), MMR-deficient (MMRd, 33%), or no specific molecular profile (NSMP, 32%). Primary endpoint: RFS. For p53abn patients, 5-year RFS 59% for CRT vs. 36% RT alone (p = .019). No significant difference in RFS after CRT vs. RT for the other molecular classes. Furthermore, regardless of treatment modality, molecular class was prognostic for RFS at 5 years, RFS 48% for p53abn, 98% for POLEmut, 72% for MMRd, 74% for NSMP. **Conclusion: In high-risk endometrial cancer, molecular classification is strongly prognostic for RFS. In patients with p53abn disease, adjuvant CRT improves RFS over adjuvant RT alone.**

What is the role of immunotherapy in advanced endometrial cancer?

The recent publications of RUBY and GY-018 established the role of IO (in addition to CHT) in the treatment of advanced endometrial cancer. Notably, patients eligible for these trials represented a particularly advanced group with the majority having measurable disease at the time of enrollment as well as being deemed not amendable to curative therapy. Despite this, the addition of IO significantly improved outcomes, particularly in MMRd patients. Presently, the role of RT remains unclear in this population, and additional studies that elucidate its application are awaited.

Mirza, RUBY (*NEJM* 2023, PMID 36972026): International phase III PRT of patients with stage III/IV (stage IIIA–IIIC1, measurable disease required) or recurrent endometrial cancer (all histologies) randomized to carboplatin/paclitaxel × 6 C ± dostarlimab (given concurrently and adjuvantly q6 weeks for up to 3 years). 494 patients randomized, 24% of which were MMRd, the vast majority of which had no prior pelvic RT. For the entire cohort, 24-month PFS was 36% in the dostarlimab arm vs. 18% in the placebo arm (*p* < .001), while OS was 71% in the dostarlimab group and 56% in the placebo group (*p* = .0021). For the MMRd population, 24-month PFS was 61% vs. 16% in the placebo group (*p* < .001). Serious adverse event rate was 38% in the dostarlimab group and 28% in the placebo group. Of note, there was no difference in PFS on subgroup analysis for stage III patients. **Conclusion: CHT-IO (with dostarlimab) improves PFS in primary advanced or recurrent endometrial cancer, particularly in MMRd patients.**

Eskander, GY-018 (*NEJM* 2023, PMID 36972022): Phase III PRT of 816 patients (28% MMRd, 40% with prior pelvic RT) with stage III/IV (stage III–IVA, with measurable disease) or recurrent endometrial cancer (excluding carcinosarcoma) were randomized to carboplatin/paclitaxel × 6 C ± pembrolizumab (given concurrently and adjuvantly every 6 weeks for up to 14 maintenance cycles). Stratified for analysis by MMR status. At 12-month analysis, PFS in the MMRd group receiving pembrolizumab was 74% vs. 38% for placebo (*p* < .001). For the MMRp group, median PFS was 13.1 months in pembrolizumab arm vs. 8.7 months for placebo (*p* < .001). **Conclusion: CHT-IO improves PFS in stage III/IV (with residual disease) and recurrent endometrial cancer regardless of MMR status, although the effect seems more pronounced in MMRd patients.** *Note: Outcomes not separately reported for patients by stage.*

What about medically inoperable endometrial cancer?

The primary treatment for endometrial cancer is upfront surgery, which also serves as a means of staging. However, it is estimated that ~10% of patients are medically inoperable at presentation.[57,58] While prospective data are limited, several retrospective series demonstrate promising outcomes with a risk-stratified approach involving various combinations of HDR brachytherapy, EBRT, and CHT.[57,58] A systematic review including 25 studies with over 2,500 patients treated with RT alone for inoperable endometrial cancer (47% treated with EBRT + brachytherapy, 51% treated with brachytherapy alone, 1% treated with EBRT alone) reported a 5-year DSS rate of 79% with a G3+ toxicity rate of 3.7% in patients treated with EBRT + brachytherapy, 2.8% for brachytherapy alone, and 1.2% for EBRT alone.[59] Guidelines exist to guide treatment planning, especially brachytherapy.[40]

CARCINOSARCOMA

What is carcinosarcoma, and how does its management differ from that of other endometrial carcinomas?

Carcinosarcoma is a high-grade carcinoma mixed with mesenchymal elements. Historically named "malignant mixed Müllerian tumor," it was considered one of the uterine sarcomas (see uterine sarcoma studies below) but now is often treated like a high-grade carcinoma and staged as an endometrial cancer. General management is similar to that of other high-grade endometrial cancers: thorough workup followed by surgery, including omentectomy, peritoneal washings, and pelvic and PA nodal dissection.

These are rare tumors, and often present at advanced stages, so evidence for adjuvant treatment is primarily retrospective. Carcinosarcomas were included in the EORTC 55874 study,[60] which demonstrated an LC benefit to adjuvant pelvic RT (47% vs. 24%) compared with observation. Similarly, the French SARCGYN[61] also included carcinosarcoma and demonstrated a DFS improvement to CRT over pelvic RT alone. Others prefer multiagent CHT alone based on GOG 150 in the following. However, multiple retrospective series, including NCDB and SEER, have demonstrated a benefit to either pelvic RT or VBT in addition to CHT, so the optimal adjuvant treatment remains unclear.[62–68]

Wolfson, GOG 150 (*Gynecol Oncol* 2007, PMID 17822748): PRT of stages I to IV uterine carcinosarcoma with <1 cm residual disease randomized to either WAI or cisplatin/ifosfamide/mesna (CIM) × 3 cycles. WAI delivered AP/PA, 30 Gy/30 fx BID, then due to slow accrual, changed to 30 Gy/20 fx QD. After WAI, whole-pelvis boost to 20 Gy/20 fx BID but then changed to 19.8 Gy/11 fx

QD boost (total 49.8 Gy); 232 patients, 44% stage I/II, 57% stage III/IV. MFU 5 years. After adjustment for age and stage, recurrence rate was 21% lower for CIM than WAI and the death rate was 29% lower for CIM than for WAI (relative hazard 0.712, p = .085). **Conclusion: The results favor multiagent CHT for carcinosarcoma.** *Comment: Trial used older obsolete RT techniques and does not answer the question in the modern era about combined CHT and pelvic RT.*

UTERINE SARCOMA

Uterine sarcomas are rare tumors, comprising ~3% of all uterine malignancies. They are stromal neoplasms arising from the myometrium and connective tissue elements (in contrast to endometrial carcinomas, which are epithelial), and generally behave more aggressively. They are broadly divided into nonepithelial tumors, including endometrial stromal sarcomas (ESS, low grade), leiomyosarcomas (LMS, high grade), and undifferentiated endometrial sarcoma (UDES), and mixed epithelial–nonepithelial tumors, which include adenosarcomas. A separate staging system is used (Table 49.11). In general, patients with resectable disease should undergo total hysterectomy and BSO followed by adjuvant therapy depending on risk factors (Table 49.12).

Table 49.11 AJCC 8th Edition (2017) and FIGO Staging for Uterine Sarcoma[33]			
AJCC	LMS and ESS	Adenosarcoma	FIGO
T1	a. ≤5 cm in greatest dimension	Limited to endometrium/endocervix	IA
	b. >5 cm in greatest dimension	Invades ≤½ myometrium	IB
	c. Not applicable	Invades >½ myometrium	IC
T2	a. Involves adnexa	Involves adnexa	IIA
	b. Involves other pelvic tissue	Involves other pelvic tissue	IIB
T3	a. Tumor infiltrates abdominal tissues (1 site)	Tumor infiltrates abdominal tissues (1 site)	IIIA
	b. Tumor infiltrates abdominal tissues (>1 site)	Tumor infiltrates abdominal tissues (>1 site)	IIIB
N1	• Regional LNs	• Regional LNs	IIIC
T4	• Invades bladder or rectum	• Invades bladder or rectum	IVA
M1	• Distant metastasis	• Distant metastasis	IVB

Source: Adapted from AJCC Cancer Staging Manual. 8th ed. Springer International Publishing; 2017.

Table 49.12 General Adjuvant Treatment Guidelines for Uterine Sarcoma Following Hysterectomy		
	LMS/UDES	ESS/Adenosarcoma
Stage I	Observation (CHT under investigation)	Observation vs. endocrine therapy
Stage II	Observation (CHT under investigation)	Endocrine therapy ± RT
Stages III–IVA	CHT ± RT	Endocrine therapy ± RT
Stage IVB	CHT ± palliative RT	Endocrine therapy ± palliative RT

Should RT be offered as adjuvant treatment for patients with uterine sarcoma?

Evidence supporting the use of RT in uterine sarcomas is sparse and generally limited to RRs. These generally show small benefits in LC and no difference in survival, although much of the benefit was derived from patients with carcinosarcoma who were included on these trials.

Sampath, UC Davis (*IJROBP* 2010, PMID 19700247): RR of 3,650 patients with uterine sarcoma identified from the NODB (proprietary data set). Patients with sarcoma, myomatous neoplasm, and complex/mixed neoplasm identified. Of those included, 51% were carcinosarcomas, 25% LMS, 15% ESS, 4% adenosarcoma, and 5% other; 30% were stage I, 37% unknown stage; 7%, 12%, and 13% were stages II to IV, respectively. Adjuvant RT improved LC in the entire cohort as well as in all subgroups (see Table 49.13). No difference in OS (5-year OS 37%). On MVA, age, stage, grade, histology, and nodal status significantly influenced OS. **Conclusion: RT may improve LRFS for patients with uterine sarcoma.**

Table 49.13 Results of Sampath Study: RT for Uterine Sarcoma			
Group	5-Yr LRFS		Log-Rank p value
	No RT	RT	
Carcinosarcoma	80%	90%	<.001
LMS	84%	98%	<.01
ESS	93%	97%	<.05
Overall	85%	93%	<.01

Reed, EORTC 55874 (*Eur J Cancer* 2008, PMID 18378136): Phase III PRT of 224 patients with stage I to II uterine sarcoma (99 LMS, 92 CS, 30 ESS, 3 other) s/p TAH BSO randomized to adjuvant pelvic RT (50.4 Gy/28 fx) vs. observation. Required 13 years to accrue. In all patients, the addition of RT decreased the rate of LR (40% vs. 24%) with no impact on DFS or OS. On subgroup analysis, the improvement in LF was driven by CS (47% vs. 24%), and there was no benefit in LR in patients with LMS (24% vs. 20%). **Conclusion: The addition of adjuvant RT improves LC in patients with stage I to II carcinosarcoma, but not LMS. RT does not impact survival.**

Is CRT more effective than RT alone?

Pautier, SARCGYN French Study (*Ann Oncol* 2013, PMID 23139262): Phase III PRT of 81 patients. Stage I to III CS (19), LMS (53), and UDES (9) randomized to adjuvant CHT (four cycles of doxorubicin, ifosfamide, cisplatin) followed by pelvic RT (45 Gy/25 fx) vs. RT alone. Primary endpoint DFS. Fifty patients also received VBT. Stopped early due to poor accrual (planned 256 patients). The addition of CHT improved 3-year DFS (55% vs. 41%, p = .048). OS improved but not statistically (81% vs. 69%, p = .41). Two toxic deaths; 76% grades 3 to 4 thrombocytopenia in the CHT arm. **Conclusion: Adjuvant CRT improves DFS for uterine sarcoma**. *Comment: Approximately 25% were carcinosarcoma.*

REFERENCES

1. Klopp A, Smith BD, Alektiar K, et al. The role of postoperative radiation therapy for endometrial cancer: executive summary of an American Society for radiation oncology evidence-based guideline. *Pract Radiat Oncol.* 2014;4(3):137–144. doi:10.1016/j.prro.2014.01.003
2. Harkenrider MM, Abu-Rustum N, Albuquerque K, et al. Radiation therapy for endometrial cancer: an American Society for radiation oncology clinical practice guideline. *Pract Radiat Oncol.* 2023;13(1):41–65. doi:10.1016/j.prro.2022.09.002
3. Meyer LA, Bohlke K, Powell MA, et al. Postoperative radiation therapy for endometrial cancer: American Society of clinical oncology clinical practice guideline endorsement of the American Society for radiation oncology evidence-based guideline. *J Clin Oncol.* 2015;33(26):2908–2913. doi:10.1200/JCO.2015.62.5459
4. Siegel RL, Giaquinto AN, Jemal A. Cancer statistics, 2024. *CA Cancer J Clin.* 2024;74(1):12–49. doi:10.3322/caac.21820
5. National Cancer Institute. *Cancer Stat Facts: Endometrial Cancer.* https://seer.cancer.gov/statfacts/html/corp.html
6. Morice P, Leary A, Creutzberg C, Abu-Rustum N, Darai E. Endometrial cancer. *Lancet.* 2016;387(10023):1094–1108. doi:10.1016/S0140-6736(15)00130-0
7. Renehan AG, Tyson M, Egger M, Heller RF, Zwahlen M. Body-mass index and incidence of cancer: a systematic review and meta-analysis of prospective observational studies. *Lancet.* 2008;371(9612):569–578. doi:10.1016/S0140-6736(08)60269-X
8. Hernandez AV, Pasupuleti V, Benites-Zapata VA, Thota P, Deshpande A, Perez-Lopez FR. Insulin resistance and endometrial cancer risk: a systematic review and meta-analysis. *Eur J Cancer.* 2015;51(18):2747–2758. doi:10.1016/j.ejca.2015.08.031
9. Katagiri R, Iwasaki M, Abe SK, et al. Reproductive factors and endometrial cancer risk among women. *JAMA Netw Open.* 2023;6(9):e2332296. doi:10.1001/jamanetworkopen.2023.32296
10. Shapiro S, Kelly JP, Rosenberg L, et al. Risk of localized and widespread endometrial cancer in relation to recent and discontinued use of conjugated estrogens. *N Engl J Med.* 1985;313(16):969–972. doi:10.1056/NEJM198510173131601

11. Beavis AL, Smith AJ, Fader AN. Lifestyle changes and the risk of developing endometrial and ovarian cancers: opportunities for prevention and management. *Int J Womens Health*. 2016;8:151–167. doi:10.2147/IJWH.S88367

12. Barrow E, Robinson L, Alduaij W, et al. Cumulative lifetime incidence of extracolonic cancers in Lynch syndrome: a report of 121 families with proven mutations. *Clin Genet*. 2009;75(2):141–149. doi:10.1111/j.1399-0004.2008.01125.x

13. Koornstra JJ, Mourits MJ, Sijmons RH, Leliveld AM, Hollema H, Kleibeuker JH. Management of extra-colonic tumours in patients with Lynch syndrome. *Lancet Oncol*. 2009;10(4):400–408. doi:10.1016/S1470-2045(09)70041-5

14. National Comprehensive Cancer Network. *NCCN Clinical Practice Guidelines in Oncology: Uterine Neoplasms*. 2024. Accessed January 5, 2025. https://www.nccn.org

15. Schmeler KM, Lynch HT, Chen LM, et al. Prophylactic surgery to reduce the risk of gynecologic cancers in the Lynch syndrome. *N Engl J Med*. 2006;354(3):261–269. doi:10.1056/NEJMoa052627

16. Amant F, Mirza MR, Koskas M, Creutzberg CL. Cancer of the corpus uteri. *Int J Gynaecol Obstet*. 2018;143(suppl 2):37–50. doi:10.1002/ijgo.12612

17. Halperin EC, Wazer DE, Perez CA, Brady LW. *Perez and Brady's Principles and Practice of Radiation Oncology*. 6th ed. Lipincott Williams; 2013.

18. Owings RA, Quick CM. Endometrial intraepithelial neoplasia. *Arch Pathol Lab Med*. 2014;138(4):484–491. doi:10.5858/arpa.2012-0709-RA

19. Kuhn E, Wu RC, Guan B, et al. Identification of molecular pathway aberrations in uterine serous carcinoma by genome-wide analyses. *J Natl Cancer Inst*. 2012;104(19):1503–1513. doi:10.1093/jnci/djs345

20. Kihara A, Yoshida H, Watanabe R, et al. Clinicopathologic association and prognostic value of microcystic, elongated, and fragmented (MELF) pattern in endometrial endometrioid carcinoma. *Am J Surg Pathol*. 2017;41(7):896–905. doi:10.1097/PAS.0000000000000856

21. Sanci M, Gungorduk K, Gulseren V, et al. MELF pattern for predicting lymph node involvement and survival in grade I-II endometrioid-type endometrial cancer. *Int J Gynecol Pathol*. 2018;37(1):17–21. doi:10.1097/PGP.0000000000000370

22. Mutter GL, Lin MC, Fitzgerald JT, et al. Altered PTEN expression as a diagnostic marker for the earliest endometrial precancers. *J Natl Cancer Inst*. 2000;92(11):924–930. doi:10.1093/jnci/92.11.924

23. Cancer Genome Atlas Research Network, Kandoth C, Schultz N, et al. Integrated genomic characterization of endometrial carcinoma. *Nature*. 2013;497(7447):67–73. doi:10.1038/nature12113

24. Huvila J, McAlpine JN. Endometrial cancer: pathology and classification. In: Chakrabarti A, ed. UpToDate. 2024.

25. Crosbie EJ, Kitson SJ, McAlpine JN, Mukhopadhyay A, Powell ME, Singh N. Endometrial cancer. *Lancet*. 2022;399(10333):1412–1428. doi:10.1016/S0140-6736(22)00323-3

26. Talhouk A, McConechy MK, Leung S, et al. A clinically applicable molecular-based classification for endometrial cancers. *Br J Cancer*. 2015;113(2):299–310. doi:10.1038/bjc.2015.190

27. Talhouk A, McConechy MK, Leung S, et al. Confirmation of ProMisE: A simple, genomics-based clinical classifier for endometrial cancer. *Cancer*. 2017;123(5):802–813. doi:10.1002/cncr.30496

28. Lindor NM, Petersen GM, Hadley DW, et al. Recommendations for the care of individuals with an inherited predisposition to Lynch syndrome: a systematic review. *JAMA*. 2006;296(12):1507–1517. doi:10.1001/jama.296.12.1507

29. Benedetti Panici P, Basile S, Salerno MG, et al. Secondary analyses from a randomized clinical trial: age as the key prognostic factor in endometrial carcinoma. *Am J Obstet Gynecol*. 2014;210(4):363.e1–363.e10. doi:10.1016/j.ajog.2013.12.025

30. Doll KM, Tseng J, Denslow SA, Fader AN, Gehrig PA. High-grade endometrial cancer: revisiting the impact of tumor size and location on outcomes. *Gynecol Oncol*. 2014;132(1):44–49. doi:10.1016/j.ygyno.2013.10.023

31. Creutzberg CL, van Putten WL, Koper PC, et al. Surgery and postoperative radiotherapy versus surgery alone for patients with stage-1 endometrial carcinoma: multicentre randomised trial. PORTEC Study Group. *Lancet*. 2000;355(9213):1404–1411. doi:10.1016/s0140-6736(00)02139-5

32. Berek JS, Matias-Guiu X, Creutzberg C, et al. FIGO staging of endometrial cancer: 2023. *Int J Gynaecol Obstet*. 2023;162(2):383–394. doi:10.1002/ijgo.14923

33. Amin MB, Edge SB, Greene FL, et al, eds. *AJCC Cancer Staging Manual*. 8th ed. Springer International Publishing; 2017.

34. Milam MR, Java J, Walker JL, et al. Nodal metastasis risk in endometrioid endometrial cancer. *Obstet Gynecol*. 2012;119(2 Pt 1):286–292. doi:10.1097/AOG.0b013e318240de51

35. Neubauer NL, Lurain JR. The role of lymphadenectomy in surgical staging of endometrial cancer. *Int J Surg Oncol*. 2011;2011:814649. doi:10.1155/2011/814649

36. Beesley VL, Rowlands IJ, Hayes SC, et al. Incidence, risk factors and estimates of a woman's risk of developing secondary lower limb lymphedema and lymphedema-specific supportive care needs in women treated for endometrial cancer. *Gynecol Oncol*. 2015;136(1):87–93. doi:10.1016/j.ygyno.2014.11.006

37. Mirza MR, Chase DM, Slomovitz BM, et al. Dostarlimab for primary advanced or recurrent endometrial cancer. *N Engl J Med*. 2023;388(23):2145–2158. doi:10.1056/NEJMoa2216334
38. Eskander RN, Sill MW, Beffa L, et al. Pembrolizumab plus chemotherapy in advanced endometrial cancer. *N Engl J Med*. 2023;388(23):2159–2170. doi:10.1056/NEJMoa2302312
39. Small W Jr, Beriwal S, Demanes DJ, et al. American Brachytherapy Society consensus guidelines for adjuvant vaginal cuff brachytherapy after hysterectomy. *Brachytherapy*. 2012;11(1):58–67. doi:10.1016/j.brachy.2011.08.005
40. Schwarz JK, Beriwal S, Esthappan J, et al. Consensus statement for brachytherapy for the treatment of medically inoperable endometrial cancer. *Brachytherapy*. 2015;14(5):587–599. doi:10.1016/j.brachy.2015.06.002
41. Videtic GMM, Woody NM, Vassil AD. *Handbook of Treatment Planning in Radiation Oncology*. 3rd ed. Demos Medical; 2020.
42. Aalders J, Abeler V, Kolstad P, Onsrud M. Postoperative external irradiation and prognostic parameters in stage I endometrial carcinoma: clinical and histopathologic study of 540 patients. *Obstet Gynecol*. 1980; 56(4):419–427. PMID: 6999399
43. Kitchener H, Swart AM, Qian Q, Amos C, Parmar MK; ASTEC Study Group. Efficacy of systematic pelvic lymphadenectomy in endometrial cancer (MRC ASTEC trial): a randomised study. *Lancet*. 2009; 373(9658):125–136. doi:10.1016/S0140-6736(08)61766-3
44. Benedetti Panici P, Basile S, Maneschi F, et al. Systematic pelvic lymphadenectomy vs. no lymphadenectomy in early-stage endometrial carcinoma: randomized clinical trial. *J Natl Cancer Inst*. 2008;100(23): 1707–1716. doi:10.1093/jnci/djn397
45. Musunuru HB, Keller A, Olawaiye A, Sukumvanich P, Beriwal S. Indications for adjuvant radiation therapy in patients with pN0(i +) adenocarcinoma of the endometrium. *Pract Radiat Oncol*. 2022;12(4):348–353. doi:10.1016/j.prro.2022.01.014
46. Klopp AH, Moughan J, Portelance L, et al. Hematologic toxicity in RTOG 0418: a phase 2 study of postoperative IMRT for gynecologic cancer. *Int J Radiat Oncol Biol Phys*. 2013;86(1):83–90. doi:10.1016/j.ijrobp.2013.01.017
47. Viswanathan AN, Moughan J, Miller BE, et al. NRG Oncology/RTOG 0921: a phase 2 study of postoperative intensity-modulated radiotherapy with concurrent cisplatin and bevacizumab followed by carboplatin and paclitaxel for patients with endometrial cancer. *Cancer*. 2015;121(13):2156–2163. doi:10.1002/cncr.29337
48. Randall ME, Filiaci VL, Muss H, et al. Randomized phase III trial of whole-abdominal irradiation versus doxorubicin and cisplatin chemotherapy in advanced endometrial carcinoma: a Gynecologic Oncology Group Study. *J Clin Oncol*. 2006;24(1):36–44. doi:10.1200/JCO.2004.00.7617
49. Susumu N, Sagae S, Udagawa Y, et al. Randomized phase III trial of pelvic radiotherapy versus cisplatin-based combined chemotherapy in patients with intermediate- and high-risk endometrial cancer: a Japanese Gynecologic Oncology Group study. *Gynecol Oncol*. 2008;108(1):226–233. doi:10.1016/j.ygyno.2007.09.029
50. Maggi R, Lissoni A, Spina F, et al. Adjuvant chemotherapy vs radiotherapy in high-risk endometrial carcinoma: results of a randomised trial. *Br J Cancer*. 2006;95(3):266–271. doi:10.1038/sj.bjc.6603279
51. Johnson N, Bryant A, Miles T, Hogberg T, Cornes P. Adjuvant chemotherapy for endometrial cancer after hysterectomy. *Cochrane Database Syst Rev*. 2011;2011(10):CD003175. doi:10.1002/14651858.CD003175.pub2
52. Galaal K, Al Moundhri M, Bryant A, Lopes AD, Lawrie TA. Adjuvant chemotherapy for advanced endometrial cancer. *Cochrane Database Syst Rev*. 2014;2014(5):CD010681. doi:10.1002/14651858.CD010681.pub2
53. Greven K, Winter K, Underhill K, et al. Preliminary analysis of RTOG 9708: adjuvant postoperative radiotherapy combined with cisplatin/paclitaxel chemotherapy after surgery for patients with high-risk endometrial cancer. *Int J Radiat Oncol Biol Phys*. 2004;59(1):168–173. doi:10.1016/j.ijrobp.2003.10.019
54. Greven K, Winter K, Underhill K, Fontenesci J, Cooper J, Burke T. Final analysis of RTOG 9708: adjuvant postoperative irradiation combined with cisplatin/paclitaxel chemotherapy following surgery for patients with high-risk endometrial cancer. *Gynecol Oncol*. 2006;103(1):155–159. doi:10.1016/j.ygyno.2006.02.007
55. Homesley HD, Filiaci V, Gibbons SK, et al. A randomized phase III trial in advanced endometrial carcinoma of surgery and volume directed radiation followed by cisplatin and doxorubicin with or without paclitaxel: a Gynecologic Oncology Group study. *Gynecol Oncol*. 2009;112(3):543–552. doi:10.1016/j.ygyno.2008.11.014
56. Secord AA, Havrilesky LJ, O'Malley DM, et al. A multicenter evaluation of sequential multimodality therapy and clinical outcome for the treatment of advanced endometrial cancer. *Gynecol Oncol*. 2009;114(3): 442–447. doi:10.1016/j.ygyno.2009.06.005
57. Wegner RE, Beriwal S, Heron DE, et al. Definitive radiation therapy for endometrial cancer in medically inoperable elderly patients. *Brachytherapy*. 2010;9(3):260–265. doi:10.1016/j.brachy.2009.08.013
58. Shen JL, O'Connor KW, Moni J, Zweizig S, Fitzgerald TJ, Ko EC. Definitive radiation therapy for medically inoperable endometrial carcinoma. *Adv Radiat Oncol*. 2023;8(1):101003. doi:10.1016/j.adro.2022.101003

59. van der Steen-Banasik E, Christiaens M, Shash E, et al. Systemic review: radiation therapy alone in medical non-operable endometrial carcinoma. *Eur J Cancer*. 2016;65:172–181. doi:10.1016/j.ejca.2016.07.005

60. Reed NS, Mangioni C, Malmstrom H, et al. Phase III randomised study to evaluate the role of adjuvant pelvic radiotherapy in the treatment of uterine sarcomas stages I and II: an European Organisation for research and treatment of cancer gynaecological cancer group study (protocol 55874). *Eur J Cancer*. 2008;44(6):808–818. doi:10.1016/j.ejca.2008.01.019

61. Pautier P, Floquet A, Gladieff L, et al. A randomized clinical trial of adjuvant chemotherapy with doxorubicin, ifosfamide, and cisplatin followed by radiotherapy versus radiotherapy alone in patients with localized uterine sarcomas (SARCGYN study). A study of the French Sarcoma Group. *Ann Oncol*. 2013;24(4):1099–1104. doi:10.1093/annonc/mds545

62. Seagle BL, Kanis M, Kocherginsky M, Strauss JB, Shahabi S. Stage I uterine carcinosarcoma: Matched cohort analyses for lymphadenectomy, chemotherapy, and brachytherapy. *Gynecol Oncol*. 2017;145(1):71–77. doi:10.1016/j.ygyno.2017.01.010

63. Odei B, Boothe D, Suneja G, Werner TL, Gaffney DK. Chemoradiation versus chemotherapy in uterine carcinosarcoma: patterns of care and impact on overall survival. *Am J Clin Oncol*. 2018;41(8):784–791. doi:10.1097/COC.0000000000000360

64. Cha J, Kim YS, Park W, et al. Clinical significance of radiotherapy in patients with primary uterine carcinosarcoma: a multicenter retrospective study (KROG 13-08). *J Gynecol Oncol*. 2016;27(6):e58. doi:10.3802/jgo.2016.27.e58

65. Zwahlen DR, Schick U, Bolukbasi Y, et al. Outcome and predictive factors in uterine carcinosarcoma using postoperative radiotherapy: a rare cancer network study. *Rare Tumors*. 2016;8(2):6052. doi:10.4081/rt.2016.6052

66. Manzerova J, Sison CP, Gupta D, et al. Adjuvant radiation therapy in uterine carcinosarcoma: a population-based analysis of patient demographic and clinical characteristics, patterns of care and outcomes. *Gynecol Oncol*. 2016;141(2):225–230. doi:10.1016/j.ygyno.2016.02.013

67. Sozen H, Ciftci R, Vatansever D, et al. Combination of adjuvant chemotherapy and radiotherapy is associated with improved survival at early stage type II endometrial cancer and carcinosarcoma. *Aust N Z J Obstet Gynaecol*. 2016;56(2):199–206. doi:10.1111/ajo.12449

68. Guttmann DM, Li H, Sevak P, et al. The impact of adjuvant therapy on survival and recurrence patterns in women with early-stage uterine carcinosarcoma: a multi-institutional study. *Int J Gynecol Cancer*. 2016;26(1):141–148. doi:10.1097/IGC.0000000000000561

Jana M. Kobeissi, Sheen Cherian, and Sudha R. Amarnath

QUICK HIT Vulvar cancers are rare, most commonly squamous cell carcinoma (SCC), and occur in older women with a history of either HPV or lichen sclerosis. Primary therapy is surgical with risk-adapted adjuvant RT as indicated. Neoadjuvant concurrent CRT is recommended for unresectable disease or locally advanced disease where surgery has high morbidity (Table 50.1). IMRT use is becoming more routine, but it is technically challenging. Prospective data guiding the use of concurrent CHT are lacking except in the neoadjuvant setting.

Table 50.1 General Treatment Paradigm for Vulvar Cancer[1]		
Stage	**Initial Treatment**	**Subsequent Therapy**
VIN	Local excision, skinning vulvectomy, imiquimod, topical 5-FU, laser ablation	N/A
Stage IA	Wide local excision (WLE)	Excision alone appropriate if final pathology demonstrates ≤1 mm of invasion, negative margins, and no additional risk factors
Stage IB–II	Radical local resection or modified radical vulvectomy with inguinal SLNB (can be unilateral SLNB for well-lateralized primary >2 cm from midline)	*RT to vulva if* margins <8 mm (also consider for LVSI, depth of invasion >5 mm, tumor size, diffuse or spray histology) *RT to inguinal and pelvic nodes* if ≥2 positive nodes or ECE; consider treatment for 1 positive node, particularly if <12 nodes were dissected without SLNB; consider concurrent CHT based on risk factors (no clear indications described)
Stage III/IVA	Surgical resection preferred if feasible If unresectable disease or locally advanced with high surgical morbidity, neoadjuvant CRT with concurrent weekly cisplatin	Risk-adapted adjuvant RT to primary and/or LNs as in the preceding case Biopsy for pathologic confirmation of CR and consider groin dissection; if PR, organ-sparing surgery if possible vs. definitive CRT alone

Source: Data from Network NCCN. *Vulvar Cancer* (Version 4.2024). Accessed August 2024. https://www.nccn.org/professionals/physician_gls/pdf/vulvar.pdf.

EPIDEMIOLOGY: Rare cancer, ~6,900 new cases and 1,630 deaths in 2024.[1] White women are at slightly higher risk than Black or Hispanic women.[2] Peak incidence is in the seventh decade of life.

RISK FACTORS: The two major etiologies are HPV infection and vulvar dystrophy.[2] Risk factors relating to HPV: younger age at first intercourse, number of sexual partners, genital warts. Vulvar intraepithelial neoplasm (VIN) is related to HPV. The most common high-risk HPV subtypes are HPV 16, 18, and 33. Vaginal dystrophies, such as lichen sclerosis, are chronic inflammatory lesions and are associated with vulvar cancer in older patients. Risk of malignant transformation of lichen sclerosis is ~5%.[2] Risk of malignant transformation of VIN III is 80%.[3]

ANATOMY: The vulva consists of the mons pubis, clitoris, labia majora, and labia minora. The fourchette is the merging of the labia minora posteriorly. The vulva is bounded posteriorly by the perineal body. Innervation is provided by the pudendal nerve (S2–S4). Bartholin glands are in the posterior labia majora; Skene's glands are periurethral. Lymphatic drainage is to the superficial inguinal nodes but can travel directly to the deep inguinal nodes. In addition to inguinal nodes, clitoral lesions can drain directly to pelvic nodes (obturator, internal, or external).[2] Cloquet's/Rosenmüller's node is the superior-most deep inguinal node classically associated with additional pelvic metastases.[4] As per AJCC, pelvic nodes are distant (FIGO stage IVB), a finding supported by poor outcomes on GOG 37 but is questioned in the modern era.[5]

PATHOLOGY: Approximately 90% are SCC and 5% to 10% are melanoma. The remaining are rare types, such as adenocarcinomas arising from the Bartholin gland. Basaloid carcinoma is associated with HPV; keratinizing is associated with vulvar dystrophy. Verrucous carcinoma is a squamous variant that is warty in appearance and rarely metastasizes.[6,7] Among SCCs, two patterns of invasion have been identified by NCCN as risk factors requiring adjuvant treatment after surgery: spray and diffuse.[8] Spray pattern is associated with "fingers" of the tumor extending deeper than the main tumor and into the dermis. Diffuse pattern is connected tumor of >1 mm in dimension and is often deeply invasive with stromal desmoplasia.[2] Extramammary Paget disease of the vulva may be associated with invasive carcinoma in ~80%.[9] Risk of inguinal LN metastasis is related to tumor thickness (as measured in GOG 36, similar but not identical to depth of stromal invasion). The risk of inguinal LN metastasis with tumor thickness <1, 2, 3, 4, 5, and >5 mm is 3%, 9%, 19%, 31%, 33%, and 48%, respectively.[10] For unilateral lesions, the risk of contralateral inguinal involvement was 8% on GOG 36. Ipsilateral inguinal LN positive-to-sampled ratio >20% is associated with a 53% risk of contralateral nodal metastases.[11]

CLINICAL PRESENTATION: Erythematous ulcerated lesion that may be associated with bleeding, pruritus, or pain. Inguinal/groin nodes may be palpable and/or ulcerated. Dark discoloration should raise concern for melanoma. Lung is the most common site of DM. Differential includes epidermal inclusion cyst, lentigo, benign Bartholin gland disorders, acrochordons, seborrheic keratoses, hidradenomas, lichen scleroses, and condyloma acuminata.

WORKUP: H&P with pelvic and rectal exam.

Labs: CBC, LFTs. Pregnancy test as indicated.

Pathology: Biopsy with HPV testing. Consider EUA with proctoscopy or cystoscopy if concerning.

Imaging: CXR is sufficient if early-stage/local disease unless symptoms suggest metastatic disease. MRI pelvis with and without contrast for surgical or RT planning. Contrast MRI yields ~85% accuracy in tumor staging and in detecting LN metastases.[12] Consider PET/CT or CT CAP for clinically advanced disease (stage II+); PET/CT for positive SLNB to assess undissected LNs.[8]

PROGNOSTIC FACTORS: The most important factor for nonmetastatic patients is LN involvement. Other factors: margin status, depth of invasion (DOI), extracapsular extension (ECE), tumor grade, LVSI, tumor size, perineural invasion, and p16 status.[13]

STAGING: See Table 50.2.

Table 50.2 AJCC 9th Edition (2023)[14] and FIGO 2021[15] Staging for Vulvar Cancer			
AJCC			**FIGO**
T1	**a**	Confined to vulva/perineum, ≤2 cm in size, stromal invasion* ≤1 mm	**IA**
	b	Confined to vulva/perineum, >2 cm in size, stromal invasion* >1 mm	**IB**
T2		Adjacent spread to distal one-third urethra and/or distal one-third vagina or anus	**II**
T3		Extension to proximal two-thirds urethra and/or proximal two-thirds vagina, bladder/rectal mucosa	**IIIA**
T4		Fixation to pelvic bones	**IVA**
N0 (i+)		Isolated tumor cells ≤0.2 mm in LNs[†], or single cells or cluster ≤200 tumor cells in a single cross-section of an LN	
N1		Nonfixed, nonulcerated, involved LNs[†]	**III**
	mi	>0.2 mm but ≤2 mm in diameter	**IIIA**
	a	>2 mm but ≤5 mm	
	b	>5 mm	**IIIB**
	c	Any LN with ECE	**IIIC**
N2		Fixed or ulcerated involved LNs[†]	**IVA**
M1		Distant metastasis	**IVB**

Note: Vulvar melanoma is staged separately.
*Depth of stromal invasion is the distance from the basement membrane of the deepest tumor-free rete ridge to the deepest point of invasion.
[†]Regional nodes include the inguinal and femoral LNs.

TREATMENT PARADIGM

Surgery: Surgical excision prior to RT is standard and is determined by size and location of the lesion. For small T1 lesions, WLE is appropriate. For T2 or higher lesions, consider modified radical vulvectomy (also called "radical local excision"; spares the uninvolved parts of the vulva, whereas radical vulvectomy removes the entire vulva). For select well-localized lesions, hemivulvectomy is appropriate. For large T3 lesions in which the degree of necessary resection would not be tolerated, definitive nonoperative management is appropriate. For primary resection, the gross tumor should be excised to the deep fascia and periosteum with at least 1-cm clinical margin and 8-mm pathologic margin (see Heaps below).[16] For close or positive margins, re-excision should be considered. For cN0 patients with DOI ≤1 mm (FIGO stage IA), nodal dissection is likely unnecessary. For cN0 stage IB to II patients, SLNB is usually appropriate. If both Tc-99m and blue dye are used, SLNB sensitivity is 91%, with NPV of 96%.[17] Unilateral nodal staging with SLNB can be performed for well-lateralized lesions (≥2 cm from midline). If SLN+, NCCN recommends RT, CRT, or completion dissection followed by risk-adapted RT (see the following for indications).[8] For cN+ patients, at least SLNB is recommended as even MRI is inaccurate in predicting inguinal LN involvement in ~15% (in pre-MRI era, false-negative rate of clinical exam was 24% on GOG 36).[10,12] If a positive SLN ≤2 mm is identified, adjuvant EBRT is appropriate per GROINS-V-II. If the positive SLN is >2 mm, a complete inguinofemoral lymphadenectomy is indicated with risk-adapted adjuvant EBRT.[18] If there are fixed nodal metastases, definitive RT is recommended, and surgical management is variable based on surgeon preference. Historically, radical vulvectomy with bilateral groin dissection was common but associated with high wound complication rates (~50%). Today, for those requiring full groin dissection, the primary tumor is often managed independently from groin dissection with two to three separate incisions, thus improving recovery. Tumor recurrence between primary and groin incision is possible but rare.

Chemotherapy: No prospective randomized data exist to confirm the benefit of concurrent CHT with RT for vulvar cancer in the adjuvant setting, but NCDB data suggest a survival benefit for N+ patients.[19] Although patterns of practice vary, the most common regimen is concurrent weekly cisplatin (typically 40 mg/m²).[20] For locally advanced tumors, neoadjuvant CRT is an option and has been prospectively evaluated with various regimens, including cisplatin/5-FU, 5-FU/MMC, and gemcitabine/cisplatin.[21,22] NCCN suggests adjuvant CRT for stage Ib to II tumors with microscopic positive nodes on SLNB and recommends neoadjuvant CRT for tumors >4 cm or patients requiring resection of visceral organs.[8]

Radiation

Indications: RT to the primary tumor is indicated for close (<8 mm) or positive margins,[23] LVSI, tumor size, DOI (cutoff unclear, some use >5 mm), and/or diffuse or spray histology.[8] Adjuvant RT to groin and pelvic nodes is indicated for ≥2 positive groin nodes (GOG 37 in the following),[23] ECE, or clinically node-positive groin. Data are less clear for those with a single positive node, but RT may be beneficial when ≤12 nodes are removed on groin dissection (may not apply in sentinel era).[24]

Dose (Per NCCN and Consensus Guideline[8,25]): For postoperative RT (PORT) in patients with negative margins, the recommended vulvar dose is 45 to 50.4 Gy, but higher doses may be necessary for LVSI. For positive margins, consider 54 to 60 Gy.[26] For gross disease, 60 to >70 Gy is recommended (consider site, size, response, CHT, and toxicity when deciding dose). For clinically and/or radiographically uninvolved LNs, 45 to 50 Gy is recommended. For gross unresectable nodal disease, 60 to 70 Gy is recommended based on size and safety.[8] For neoadjuvant CRT, dose is classically 45 Gy to regional nodes with cone-down boost to a total of 57.6 Gy/32 fx to primary disease (as per GOG 205 in the following),[27] although the recently published GOG 279 boosts gross tumor to 64 Gy/34 fx (60 Gy to high-risk groin and 45 Gy to low-risk nodes).[22] For ECE, consider 54 to 64 Gy.

Toxicity: Acute: wound breakdown, skin moist desquamation, cystitis, and proctitis. Late: pelvic insufficiency fracture, vaginal and skin fibrosis, lymphedema, RT proctitis, cystitis, and bowel obstruction.

Procedure: See *Handbook of Treatment Planning in Radiation Oncology*, Chapter 9.[28]

Other Modalities: Laser ablation, topical 5-FU, and imiquimod (immune response modulator) are options for VIN.

EVIDENCE-BASED Q&A

ADJUVANT THERAPY

Which resected patients benefit from adjuvant RT to the vulva?

Classically, adjuvant RT to the vulva is indicated for patients with close (<8 mm) or positive margins given multiple RR showing a reduction in LR.[23,29,30] LVSI, tumor size, DOI, and diffuse or spray histology are also factors to consider per NCCN.[8] Note that node-negative patients with risk factors are often treated to the vulva alone rather than comprehensively.

Heaps, UCLA (*Gynecol Oncol* 1990, PMID 2227541): RR of 135 patients with vulvar SCC treated surgically between 1957 and 1985. Ninety-one patients had margin ≥8 mm, and none had LR. Forty-four patients had margin <8 mm, and 21 recurred locally. Other factors associated with higher LR included LVSI, DOI (>9.1 mm), tumor thickness (>9.97 mm), and spray histologic pattern. **Conclusion: Final surgical margin of <8 mm is associated with 50% chance of recurrence.**

Bedell, Minnesota (*Gynecol Oncol* 2019, PMID 31171409): RR of 150 patients with FIGO stage I vulvar SCC treated with resection between 1995 and 2017. Forty-seven patients had close (<8 mm) or positive margins. Of these, 21 (45%) underwent re-excision or vulvar RT, while the rest were observed. The 2-year recurrence rates were not statistically different between the no further therapy group vs. the re-excision/RT groups (12% vs. 5%, *p* = .62), with no difference in RFS or OS. **Conclusion: For resected stage I vulvar cancer with close/positive margins, adjuvant RT or re-excision is associated with numerically lower rates of LR, although not statistically significant when compared with observation.**

Which patients benefit from adjuvant RT to inguinal and pelvic nodes after inguinal dissection?

GOG 37 provides the strongest data supporting comprehensive nodal RT to groin and pelvic nodes for those with ≥2 positive nodes after inguinal dissection.[33] Adjuvant RT may also be considered in patients with a single positive node, specifically when ≤12 nodes are dissected as supported by SEER data.

Homesley, GOG 37 (*Obstet Gynecol* 1986, PMID 3785783; Update *Obstet Gynecol* 2009, PMID 19701032): Phase III PRT from 1977 to 1984 that recruited patients with vulvar SCC and ≥1 pathologically positive inguinal node after radical vulvectomy and bilateral groin dissection. (Of note, 51% were cN+; GOG 36 was overarching study looking at inguinal metastases[9]; if positive, patient was eligible for GOG 37.) Patients were intraoperatively randomized to either ipsilateral pelvic LN dissection or adjuvant RT to groins and pelvis with 45 to 50 Gy. Groin dose prescribed to 2 to 3 cm depth. Fields were from L5/S1 interspace to the top of the obturator foramen. Primary vulvar site was omitted. In the surgery arm, 28% were found to have positive pelvic LNs (14% of those with N0–1 and 1 positive groin node; 45% of those with N2–3 and 2+ positive groin nodes). Trial closed early due to significant survival difference; 2-year OS from 54% to 68% (*p* = .03) with RT. See Table 50.3 for results. Benefit from RT was particularly significant for those with ≥2 positive groin LNs. In the updated report with MFU of 74 months, 6-year OS difference was not evident for all patients, but it remained significant for those with ≥2 positive inguinal LNs or with fixed/ulcerated groin LNs. Isolated vulvar recurrence noted in 9% in the RT arm (vulva not targeted) vs. 7% in the surgery arm. The 2-year OS for those with positive pelvic nodes was 23%, and hence pelvic nodes are staged as FIGO IVB (this has been questioned in the modern era[7]). Rates of acute and late side effects were similar. **Conclusion: Adjuvant pelvic RT improves OS for patients with ≥2 positive groin LNs, and pelvic nodal dissection is not routinely indicated.**

Table 50.3 Results of GOG 37 for Vulvar Cancer				
	2-Yr OS	6-Yr OS	MS (N2/3)	2-Yr Groin Relapse
RT	68%	51%	40 months	5%
Pelvic LND	54%	41%	12 months	24%
p value	.03	.18	.01	.02

Parthasarathy, SEER Analysis (*Gynecol Oncol* 2006, PMID 16889821): SEER data from 1988 to 2001 identified 208 patients with vulvar SCC with one positive inguinal node, 92% of whom were treated with radical vulvectomy with either unilateral or bilateral inguinal dissection. Median of 13 nodes removed; 102 (49%) underwent adjuvant RT. The 5-year DSS was 77% vs. 61% (p = .02) in favor of RT. RT was particularly beneficial in those with ≤12 nodes removed (DSS 77% vs. 55%, p = .035), but in those with >12 nodes removed the difference did not reach significance (77% RT vs. 67% no RT, p = .23). **Conclusion: Adjuvant RT may improve DSS for patients with a single positive node, particularly when ≤12 nodes are resected.**

Is RT alone sufficient to treat inguinals or is an inguinal dissection necessary?

Given the morbidity associated with an inguinal dissection, GOG 88 investigated the omission of inguinal dissection in those with clinically negative/nonsuspicious nodes and found that inguinal dissection is superior to RT alone.[31] However, review of 50 cases demonstrated subpar delivery of RT.[34] Single-arm phase II prospective data from GROINS-V-II suggest that inguinofemoral RT may be sufficient for patients with micrometastases on SLNB.[18]

Stehman, GOG 88 (*IJROBP* 1992, PMID 1526880): Phase III PRT of 52 patients with vulvar SCC and clinically negative/nonsuspicious nodes treated with radical vulvectomy and randomized to either inguinal dissection or RT. T1–3 tumors were included, but T1 tumors required LVSI or >5 mm DOI to be eligible. RT dose was 50 Gy/25 fx to 3-cm depth with photons allowed but electrons recommended; only inguinal nodes were treated (omitted pelvic nodes and primary). Patients in the surgery arm with positive groin nodes received PORT to ipsilateral groin and hemipelvis (based on GOG 37). Trial stopped early due to excessive recurrences in the RT arm. Of the 25 patients in the inguinal dissection arm, 5 had positive LNs. PFS and OS were both inferior in the RT arm. Lymphedema (28% vs. 0%) and acute episodes of grades 3 to 4 toxicities (22 vs. 10) were both worse in the inguinal dissection arm. See Table 50.4 for results. **Conclusion: RT, as delivered in this study, is inferior to inguinal dissection.** *Comment: Review of 50 cases by Koh et al.[34] demonstrated median femoral vessel depth of 6.1 cm (range 2.0–18.5 cm); thus, RT may have undertreated patients as dose was prescribed to only 3 cm.*

Table 50.4 Results of GOG 88		
	2-Yr OS	**2-Yr PFS**
Radical vulvectomy + groin RT	60%	65%
Radical vulvectomy + LND (with PORT if LN+)	85%	90%
p value	.035	.033

Oonk, GROINSS-V-II (*JCO* 2021, PMID 34432481): Phase II single-arm PRT of 1,535 patients with early-stage vulvar SCC with tumors <4 cm and no suspicious nodes >15 mm on preoperative imaging. Patients underwent local excision and SLNB. If positive sentinel nodes (SLN+), 50 Gy inguinofemoral RT was given. Primary endpoint was isolated groin recurrence at 2 years. Twenty-one percent of patients had SLN+. Of note, protocol was amended after 91 SLN+ patients to mandate inguinofemoral lymphadenectomy (IFL) for patients with macrometastases (>2 mm) due to excessive LRs among patients with macrometastases receiving RT only. Of the 160 patients with micrometastases (≤2 mm), 126 received RT, with a 2-year ipsilateral isolated groin recurrence rate of 2%. Of the 162 patients with macrometastases, isolated groin recurrence rate with RT alone (n = 51) was 22% vs. 7% for IFL (n = 105; 56% also received adjuvant RT). The 2-year disease-specific death risk was 2% for N0 patients, 7% for micrometastases, and 26% for macrometastases. Treatment-related lymphedema at 12 months was less common with RT vs. IFL, 11% vs. 23%, respectively. **Conclusion: Inguinofemoral RT may be a safe alternative to inguinofemoral lymphadenectomy for patients with micrometastases (≤2 mm) on SLNB but not for those with macrometastases.**

For whom is SLNB sufficient compared with groin dissection?

Groin dissection is associated with high rates of postoperative morbidity including wound complications and lymphedema. Per NCCN guidelines, SLNB is an alternative standard of care to groin dissection for patients with a clinically node negative physical exam, negative imaging, unifocal vulvar tumor <4 cm in diameter, and no previous vulvar surgery that may have altered lymphatic drainage. If only unilateral SLNB is performed and is positive, the contralateral side should be considered for RT.[8] The GROINNS-V-II study (see above) suggests adjuvant RT may be beneficial for a single positive node (≤2 mm and no ENE) if inguinal dissection is omitted. Inguinal dissection is still recommended for macrometastasis (>2mm or ENE).[18]

Levenback, GOG 173 (*JCO* 2012, PMID 22753905): Single-arm trial of 452 women with vulvar SCC with ≥1 mm of invasion, tumor size of 2 to 6 cm, and clinically negative groin. Patients underwent SLNB followed by inguinal dissection; sentinel nodes were identified in 418 of 452 patients (92%). Incidence of nodal metastasis was 32%, with a false-negative rate of 8% and sensitivity of 92%. False-negative predictive value (1-negative predictive value) was 4% in all-comers and 2% in tumors <4 cm. **Conclusion: SLNB is a potential alternative to inguinal dissection.**

Van der Zee, GROINSS-V (*JCO* 2008, PMID 18281661): Single-arm trial of 403 patients with T2 unifocal vulvar SCC with tumor size of <4 cm and DOI >1 mm, all cN0, treated from 2000 to 2006. Patients underwent radical excision with SLNB. If SLNB was negative, groin dissection was omitted. PORT to 50 Gy was recommended if ≥2 nodes were positive or if ECE present. After a negative SLNB, the rate of groin recurrence was 2%, with a 3-year OS of 97%. **Conclusion: Negative SLNB is associated with a low rate of groin recurrence, and groin dissection may be omitted.**

Which patients benefit from adjuvant CRT after surgical resection?

Adjuvant CRT may be considered in N+ patients. Benefits to the addition of CHT are unclear given the absence of prospective data. If done, weekly cisplatin is recommended as the concurrent CHT regimen.[25]

Gill, NCDB Analysis (*Gynecol Oncol* 2015, PMID 25868965): NCDB analysis from 1998 to 2011 of ~1,800 patients with vulvar SCC who underwent surgery with confirmed inguinal nodes and were treated with adjuvant RT. Overall, 26% received adjuvant CHT (use of CHT increased with time, 41% of patients received CHT in 2006), particularly those with a greater number of positive nodes, stage IVA disease, and positive margins. CHT was associated with improved OS on propensity-adjusted modeling. **Conclusion: Adjuvant CRT may benefit N+ patients.**

NEOADJUVANT/DEFINITIVE THERAPY FOR ADVANCED DISEASE

Is neoadjuvant therapy a feasible option for patients whose disease would require radical surgery?

Multiple prospective trials and retrospective data[32] *have demonstrated the safety and feasibility of this approach for both unresectable vulvar primary tumors and unresectable adenopathy.*

Moore, GOG 101 Unresectable Primary Cohort (*IJROBP* 1998, PMID 9747823): Multipart phase II study of 73 patients with stage III to IV vulvar SCC (T3–4 regardless of nodal status) requiring more than just radical vulvectomy. This cohort included unresectable primary tumors, while the Montana cohort (the following study) included unresectable inguinal nodes. Both cohorts received CRT with a split-course RT via AP/PA fields to 47.6 Gy to primary tumor, with inguinal/pelvic nodes included for N2–N3 disease. RT was delivered BID (1.7 Gy/fx) for the first 4 days during CHT (cisplatin 50 mg/m² on day 1 + infusion of 5-FU 1,000 mg/m²/day on days 1–4) and QD thereafter for a total of 12 treatment days and 23.8 Gy per course. Courses were separated by 1.5 to 2.5 weeks. Surgery was performed 4 to 8 weeks later. RT boost was given for residual unresectable disease (20 Gy) or for microscopically positive margins (10–15 Gy). Complete clinical response was observed in 47%, while 54% had gross residual disease. Only two patients (3%) had residual unresectable disease, and only three required surgery sacrificing their bowel/bladder continence. **Conclusion: Preoperative CRT is feasible for unresectable primary tumors and may reduce rates of pelvic exenteration.**

Montana, GOG 101 Unresectable Lymph Node Cohort (*IJROBP* 2000, PMID 11072157): Second part of the phase II study included 46 patients who underwent the same treatment regimen per Moore (described above) except with fields including inguinal and pelvic nodes. After CRT, disease was resectable in 38 of 40 patients, and LN pCR rate was 41%. Control of lymphatic disease was ultimately achieved in 36 of 37 patients (97%). **Conclusion: Preoperative CRT is feasible for unresectable LNs, and high rates of control may be achieved.**

Moore, GOG 205 (*Gynecol Oncol* 2012, PMID 22079361): Single-arm phase II trial of locally advanced (T3/T4) vulvar SCC treated with CRT using 57.6 Gy/32 fx with weekly cisplatin 40 mg/m² followed by resection of residual disease. Fifty-eight evaluable patients and 69% completed treatment. Thirty-seven (64%) had complete clinical response, and 29 (78% of those 37) had complete pathologic response. Of note, overall pathologic response rate was 50% in GOG 205 and 31% in GOG 101. **Conclusion: Induction with concurrent cisplatin and RT yields high response rates with acceptable toxicity.**

Horowitz, GOG 279 (*JCO* 2024, PMID 38574312): Single-arm phase II trial evaluating concurrent CRT for patients with locally advanced, unresectable vulvar SCC with a primary endpoint of complete pathologic response. RT was delivered with IMRT, 64 Gy to the vulva and 50 to 64 Gy to the groins/low pelvis, concurrent with weekly 40 mg/m^2 cisplatin and 50 mg/m^2 gemcitabine. Out of 57 enrolled patients, 52 were evaluable, and 77% had stage II/III disease. Most RT plans (85%) were centrally reviewed, and all complied with protocol. Out of 52 patients, 38 (73%) had a complete pathologic response. With MFU of 51 months, 1-year PFS was 74% and 2-year OS was 70%. G3/4 toxicity was most commonly hematologic or RT dermatitis; only one reported G5 toxicity, which was unlikely treatment-induced. **Conclusion: Dual-agent radiosensitization with weekly cisplatin/gemcitabine given concurrently with RT is associated with a high complete pathologic response rate.**

Is there a role for re-irradiation in locally recurrent vulvar cancer?

Bockel, Systematic Review (*Cancers* 2021, PMID 33799617): Systematic review of 15 studies investigating the feasibility of re-RT using image-guided brachytherapy for locally recurrent GYN cancers. Most were retrospective, and only four included patients with vulvar cancer. In those studies, patients underwent either CT-planned HDR or LDR interstitial brachytherapy, with a median dose of 20 to 30 Gy for HDR and 30 to 50 Gy for LDR. At 1 to 2 years after re-RT, LC rates ranged from 50% to 73% and OS rates from 52% to 82%. Grade 3 toxicity ranged from 8% to 29%, with no reported grade 5 toxicity. **Conclusion: For locally recurrent GYN cancers, including vulvar cancer, re-RT with brachytherapy is feasible, particularly in inoperable patients or those who refuse surgery.**

What is the significance of *p16* and *p53* expression in vulvar SCC?

A meta-analysis found p16 overexpression to be associated with improved 5-year OS, possibly an independent prognostic factor. Women with p53-positive vulvar SCC were found to have lower OS than those with p53-negative tumors, but p53 significance remains inconclusive.[13]

Sand, Meta-Analysis (*Gynecol Oncol* 2018, PMID 30415992): A systematic review and meta-analysis of 18 studies analyzing the significance of p16 and p53 expression. For the p16 analysis, 475 cases were included, and 38% of patients were p16-positive. p16 expression was associated with improved 5-year OS (HR 0.40, 95% CI 0.29–0.55) and remained significant on adjusted analysis. The analysis for p53 included 310 cases, and 54% were p53-positive. p53 expression was associated with worse 5-year OS (HR 1.81, 1.22–2.68). Unlike p16, p53 was not significant on adjusted analysis, so the value remains inconclusive. **Conclusion: p16 and possibly p53 are of prognostic importance in women diagnosed with vulvar SCC.**

REFERENCES

1. Siegel RL, Giaquinto AN, Jemal A. Cancer statistics, 2024. *CA Cancer J Clin.* 2024;74(1):12–49. doi:10.3322/caac.21820
2. Chino JP, Hsu L, Montana GS. Carcinoma of the vulva. In: *Perez and Brady's Principles and Practice of Radiation Oncology.* 6th ed. Lippincott Williams & Wilkins; 2013.
3. Alkatout I, Schubert M, Garbrecht N, et al. Vulvar cancer: epidemiology, clinical presentation, and management options. *Int J Womens Health.* 2015;7:305–313. doi:10.2147/IJWH.S68979
4. Chu CK, Zager JS, Marzban SS, et al. Routine biopsy of Cloquet's node is of limited value in sentinel node-positive melanoma patients. *J Surg Oncol.* 2010;102(4):315–320. doi:10.1002/jso.21635
5. Thaker NG, Klopp AH, Jhingran A, Frumovitz M, Iyer RB, Eifel PJ. Survival outcomes for patients with stage IVB vulvar cancer with grossly positive pelvic lymph nodes: time to reconsider the FIGO staging system? *Gynecol Oncol.* 2015;136(2):269–273. doi:10.1016/j.ygyno.2014.12.013
6. Kurman RJ, Toki T, Schiffman MH. Basaloid and warty carcinomas of the vulva: distinctive types of squamous cell carcinoma frequently associated with human papillomaviruses. *Am J Surg Pathol.* 1993;17(2):133–145. doi:10.1097/00000478-199302000-00005
7. Alkatout I, Schubert M, Garbrecht N, et al. Vulvar cancer: epidemiology, clinical presentation, and management options. *Int J Womens Health.* 2015;7:305–313. doi:10.2147/IJWH.S68979
8. National Comprehensive Cancer Network. *NCCN Clinical Practice Guidelines in Oncology: Vulvar Cancer.* Version 4.2024. Accessed August 2024. https://www.nccn.org/professionals/physician_gls/pdf/vulvar.pdf
9. van der Linden M, Meeuwis KA, Bulten J, Bosse T, van Poelgeest MI, de Hullu JA. Paget disease of the vulva. *Crit Rev Oncol Hematol.* 2016;101:60–74. doi:10.1016/j.critrevonc.2016.03.008

10. Homesley HD, Bundy BN, Sedlis A, et al. Prognostic factors for groin node metastasis in squamous cell carcinoma of the vulva (a Gynecologic Oncology Group study). *Gynecol Oncol.* 1993;49(3):279–283. doi:10.1006/gyno.1993.1127

11. Kunos C, Simpkins F, Gibbons H, Tian C, Homesley H. Radiation therapy compared with pelvic node resection for node-positive vulvar cancer: a randomized controlled trial. *Obstet Gynecol.* 2009;114(3):537–546. doi:10.1097/AOG.0b013e3181b12f99

12. Kataoka MY, Sala E, Baldwin P, et al. The accuracy of magnetic resonance imaging in staging of vulvar cancer: a retrospective multi-centre study. *Gynecol Oncol.* 2010;117(1):82–87. doi:10.1016/j.ygyno.2009.12.017

13. Sand FL, Nielsen DMB, Frederiksen MH, Rasmussen CL, Kjaer SK. The prognostic value of p16 and p53 expression for survival after vulvar cancer: a systematic review and meta-analysis. *Gynecol Oncol.* 2019; 152(1):208–217. doi:10.1016/j.ygyno.2018.10.015

14. Olawaiye AB, Hagemann I, Bhoshale P, et al. Vulva. In: *AJCC Cancer Staging Manual.* 9th ed. American College of Surgeons; 2023.

15. Olawaiye AB, Cotler J, Cuello MA, et al. FIGO staging for carcinoma of the vulva: 2021 revision. *Int J Gynaecol Obstet.* 2021;155(1):43–47. doi:10.1002/ijgo.13880

16. Heaps JM, Fu YS, Montz FJ, Hacker NF, Berek JS. Surgical-pathologic variables predictive of local recurrence in squamous cell carcinoma of the vulva. *Gynecol Oncol.* 1990;38(3):309–314. doi:10.1016/0090-8258(90)90064-r

17. Meads C, Sutton AJ, Rosenthal AN, et al. Sentinel lymph node biopsy in vulval cancer: systematic review and meta-analysis. *Br J Cancer.* 2014;110(12):2837–2846. doi:10.1038/bjc.2014.205

18. Oonk MHM, Slomovitz B, Baldwin PJW, et al. Radiotherapy versus inguinofemoral lymphadenectomy as treatment for vulvar cancer patients with micrometastases in the sentinel node: results of GROINSS-V II. *J Clin Oncol.* 2021;39(32):3623–3632. doi:10.1200/JCO.21.00006

19. Gill BS, Bernard ME, Lin JF, et al. Impact of adjuvant chemotherapy with radiation for node-positive vulvar cancer: a National Cancer Data Base (NCDB) analysis. *Gynecol Oncol.* 2015;137(3):365–372. doi:10.1016/j.ygyno.2015.03.056

20. Gaffney DK, Du Bois A, Narayan K, et al. Patterns of care for radiotherapy in vulvar cancer: a Gynecologic Cancer Intergroup study. *Int J Gynecol Cancer.* 2009;19(1):163–167. doi:10.1111/IGC.0b013e3181996ac3

21. Reade CJ, Eiriksson LR, Mackay H. Systemic therapy in squamous cell carcinoma of the vulva: current status and future directions. *Gynecol Oncol.* 2014;132(3):780–789. doi:10.1016/j.ygyno.2013.11.025

22. Horowitz NS, Deng W, Peterson I, et al. Phase II trial of cisplatin, gemcitabine, and intensity-modulated radiation therapy for locally advanced vulvar squamous cell carcinoma: NRG Oncology/GOG Study 279. *J Clin Oncol.* 2024;42(16):1914–1921. doi:10.1200/JCO.23.02235

23. Faul CM, Mirmow D, Huang Q, Gerszten K, Day R, Jones MW. Adjuvant radiation for vulvar carcinoma: improved local control. *Int J Radiat Oncol Biol Phys.* 1997;38(2):381–389. doi:10.1016/S0360-3016(97)82500-X

24. Parthasarathy A, Cheung MK, Osann K, et al. The benefit of adjuvant radiation therapy in single-node-positive squamous cell vulvar carcinoma. *Gynecol Oncol.* 2006;103(3):1095–1099. doi:10.1016/j.ygyno.2006.06.030

25. Gaffney DK, King B, Viswanathan AN, et al. Consensus recommendations for radiation therapy contouring and treatment of vulvar carcinoma. *Int J Radiat Oncol Biol Phys.* 2016;95(4):1191–1200. doi:10.1016/j.ijrobp.2016.02.043

26. Chapman BV, Gill BS, Viswanathan AN, Balasubramani GK, Sukumvanich P, Beriwal S. Adjuvant radiation therapy for margin-positive vulvar squamous cell carcinoma: defining the ideal dose-response using the National Cancer Data Base. *Int J Radiat Oncol Biol Phys.* 2017;97(1):107–117. doi:10.1016/j.ijrobp.2016.09.023

27. Moore DH, Ali S, Koh WJ, et al. A phase II trial of radiation therapy and weekly cisplatin chemotherapy for the treatment of locally advanced squamous cell carcinoma of the vulva: a Gynecologic Oncology Group study. *Gynecol Oncol.* 2012;124(3):529–533. doi:10.1016/j.ygyno.2011.11.003

28. Videtic GMM, Woody N, Vassil AD. *Handbook of Treatment Planning in Radiation Oncology.* 3rd ed. Demos Medical; 2020.

29. Ignatov T, Eggemann H, Burger E, Costa SD, Ignatov A. Adjuvant radiotherapy for vulvar cancer with close or positive surgical margins. *J Cancer Res Clin Oncol.* 2016;142(2):489–495. doi:10.1007/s00432-015-2060-9

30. Bedell SM, Hedberg C, Griffin A, et al. Role of adjuvant radiation or re-excision for early stage vulvar squamous cell carcinoma with positive or close surgical margins. *Gynecol Oncol.* 2019;154(2):276–279. doi:10.1016/j.ygyno.2019.05.028

31. Stehman FB, Bundy BN, Thomas G, et al. Groin dissection versus groin radiation in carcinoma of the vulva: a Gynecologic Oncology Group study. *Int J Radiat Oncol Biol Phys.* 1992;24(2):389–396. doi:10.1016/0360-3016(92)90699-I

32. Beriwal S, Coon D, Heron DE, et al. Preoperative intensity-modulated radiotherapy and chemotherapy for locally advanced vulvar carcinoma. *Gynecol Oncol.* 2008;109(2):291–295. doi:10.1016/j.ygyno.2007.10.026

33. Homesley HD, Bundy BN, Sedlis A, Adcock L. Radiation therapy versus pelvic node resection for carcinoma of the vulva with positive groin nodes. *Obstet Gynecol.* 1986;68(6):733–740. PMID: 3785783

34. Koh WJ, Chiu M, Stelzer KJ, et al. Femoral vessel depth and the implications for groin node radiation. *Int J Radiat Oncol Biol Phys.* 1993;27(4):969–974. doi:10.1016/0360-3016(93)90476-c

51 VAGINAL CANCER

Erik M. Davies, Sheen Cherian, and Sudha R. Amarnath

QUICK HIT Vaginal cancer is a rare malignancy that arises as a primary in the vagina without involvement of the cervix or vulva. The majority (>80%) are squamous cell carcinomas, arise in the posterior aspect of the upper third of the vagina (60%–80%),[1,2] and are not amenable to organ-sparing surgical resection due to proximity of the urethra, bladder, and rectum. Thus, treatment typically consists of definitive RT with or without CHT (Table 51.1). Brachytherapy boost is often recommended, and choice of intracavitary cylinder vs. interstitial is based on depth of invasion (≤0.5 cm for cylinder vs. >0.5 cm for interstitial).

Table 51.1 General Treatment Paradigm for Vaginal Cancer[1,2]	
Stage	**Treatment**
VAIN 1–2	Close surveillance as ~80% of lesions will spontaneously regress.[3]
CIS (VAIN 3)	Surgery (local excision, partial or complete vaginectomy), topical 5-FU, or RT. RT usually delivered via intracavitary brachytherapy, 60 Gy to the entire vagina + 70 Gy boost to the involved vaginal mucosa.[4-6]
Stage I	RT preferred over surgery per 2024 NCCN guidelines. For lesions measuring <2 cm and <5 mm thickness, treat with HDR intracavitary brachytherapy to an EQD2 of 50–60 Gy (commonly 8 Gy × 5 fx twice weekly). Otherwise treat using EBRT to 45–50.4 Gy with brachytherapy boost of 25–35 Gy (interstitial if residual tumor thickness >5 mm) ± concurrent platinum-based CHT. If ineligible for RT, consider partial or total vaginectomy ± inguinal nodal dissection.
Stage II (subvaginal infiltration only, ≤0.5 cm depth)	Treat whole pelvis to 45–50.4 Gy and boost with intracavitary implant 25–35 Gy.
Stage II–IVA (paravaginal/parametrial invasion)	Treat whole pelvis to 45–50.4 Gy and boost with interstitial implant 25–35 Gy to achieve total dose of 75–80 Gy. For tumors involving the lower one-third of the vagina, inguinal nodes should be treated 45–50.4 Gy. Boost clinically positive nodes an additional 20–25 Gy. Evaluate candidacy for concurrent platinum-based CHT. Surgical option is total exenteration with bilateral inguinal lymphadenectomy (although a highly morbid surgery).

EPIDEMIOLOGY: Vaginal cancer is rare and accounts for <3% of all gynecologic cancers, with ~8,600 cases in the United States annually.[7] The most common histology is SCC (≥80%), followed by ACA (~10%), with several other uncommon histologies including melanoma, small cell, lymphoid, and carcinoid.[8] Median age of diagnosis of vaginal SCC is 65 years.

ANATOMY: The vagina is a fibromuscular tube lined with mucous membrane and extends from the uterus to the vestibule. The urethra and bladder are located directly anterior to the vagina. Posteriorly, the superoposterior vaginal wall is separated from the rectum by a fold of peritoneum called the "rectouterine pouch" (pouch of Douglas). Extending caudally, the vagina runs adjacent to the rectum with the perineal body separating the two at their inferior most location. The pelvic fascia, ureters, and levator ani run lateral to the vagina. The posterior wall (~9 cm) is longer than the anterior wall (~7 cm) because the vagina joins the uterus at an angle of ~90 degrees. The cervix projects into the vaginal lumen, thus creating the anterior, posterior, and lateral fornices. Layers of the vagina are as follows: *inner mucosa* (nonkeratinizing, stratified squamous epithelium, no glands) → *lamina propria* (connective tissue) → *muscularis* (inner circular and outer longitudinal layers) → *adventitia* (thin, outer connective tissue). The vagina has two embryologic origins: the upper one-third derives from the uterine canal and the lower two-thirds from the urogenital sinus (implications for lymphatic drainage). The upper one-third drains similar to cervix (parametrial, obturator, and pelvic nodes). The lower one-third drains to inguinal nodes and then to external iliacs. Lesions in the middle one-third can go either direction. Common sites of metastasis are the para-aortic LNs, lungs, liver, and bone.

PATHOLOGY[9]: See Table 51.2 for details.

Table 51.2 Summary of Pathologic Types of Vaginal Cancer		
Vaginal Cancer Subtype	Prevalence	Notes
CIS a.k.a. VAIN3	Rare	Most are multifocal and can involve all vaginal surfaces.
SCC	75%–95%	Most are nonkeratinizing and moderately differentiated.
ACA (non-clear cell)	5%–10%	May be associated with another primary (ovarian, endometrial, renal, etc.). Otherwise, non-clear cell ACA of vagina has a very poor prognosis.[10]
ACA (clear cell)		Related to in utero DES exposure; 1/1,000 risk if exposed. Younger age. Preceded by vaginal adenosis in up to 95% of cases.
Melanoma	<5%	Projects into the lumen, tends to involve the vaginal surface rather than invade into the wall. Melanin differentiates this from sarcoma. More common in White individuals than Black individuals. OS <20%.
Sarcoma botryoides (embryonal rhabdomyosarcoma)	Rare	Most common vaginal neoplasm in infants and children. Characteristic "grape-like" exophytic mass. Aggressive. Treat with surgery, multiagent CHT, and RT. OS 90%.
Verrucous carcinoma (variant of SCC), serous papillary ACA, small cell, spindle cell epithelioma, other sarcoma, *and* lymphoma	Rare	Verrucous carcinoma presents as a large, warty, fungating mass. Locally aggressive but rarely metastasizes and thus has favorable prognosis.

RISK FACTORS: Risk factors are similar to cervical cancer: current smoker, multiple lifetime sexual partners, and early age at first intercourse.[11,12] The latter two correlate with exposure to HPV, and multiple studies have shown that HPV DNA can be found in at least 75% of VAIN/invasive vaginal cancers, specifically the HPV 16 and 18 subtypes.[13,14] Additionally, previous gynecologic malignancy, DES exposure in utero (clear cell ACA), and alcohol consumption have all been associated with vaginal cancer, with some controversy regarding exposure to prior pelvic RT.[11,15,16]

CLINICAL PRESENTATION: Vaginal bleeding, often postcoital, is the most common presenting symptom (~50%–60% of patients), although as many as 20% of patients may be asymptomatic.[17] Additional symptoms include vaginal discharge, dysuria, or GI symptoms (tenesmus, constipation, melena). Frank vaginal and/or pelvic pain are often late presenting symptoms, suggestive of invasion to surrounding tissues.[17,18] If vaginal cancer is diagnosed <5 years after previous gynecologic malignancy, the new diagnosis should be categorized as a recurrence. Differential diagnosis includes cervical cancer, vulvar cancer, and metastasis from ovarian, renal cell, or other primaries.

WORKUP: H&P including thorough abdominopelvic exam. Speculum exam can miss anterior and posterior lesions; to avoid this, rotate the speculum upon exiting the vault. Pelvic exam should include bimanual exam, rectovaginal exam, EUA with vaginal and cervical biopsies, and colposcopy. Perform cystoscopy and proctosigmoidoscopy for more advanced lesions.

Labs: CBC, CMP (with particular attention to creatinine and LFTs).

Imaging: MRI with and without gadolinium to assess local extent. MRI has excellent sensitivity (95%) and specificity (90%).[19] Lesions are best seen on the T2 phase. Insertion of gel into the vagina can improve measurement of tumor thickness. For more advanced presentations, CT chest/abdomen/pelvis or PET to evaluate for metastatic disease.

PROGNOSTIC FACTORS: See Table 51.3 for details.

Table 51.3 Prognostic Factors for Vaginal Cancer	
Better	HPV+, SCC, involving <⅓ length of vagina (5-yr DFS 61% vs. 25%),[20] location in the upper one-third of the vagina, >75 Gy total dose (2-yr PFS 76% vs. 40%).[21] Smaller size (<4–5 cm),[10,22,23] DES exposure.[21] Prior hysterectomy also appears to be protective perhaps due to patterns of tumor spread.[10,19,24]
Worse	Advanced clinical stage, larger size (≥4–5 cm), presence of symptoms, LN involvement, ACA, nonepithelial tumors, posterior wall location, overexpression of *HER-2/neu* in SCC, mutated p53, prolonged treatment time, HIV.[25]

STAGING: AJCC 8th edition and FIGO staging system are outlined in Table 51.4.

Table 51.4 AJCC 8th Edition (2017) and FIGO Staging for Vaginal Cancer[8,22,26–28]			
AJCC		**FIGO**	**Risk of LNs**
T1	a. Confined to vagina, ≤2 cm	I	6%–14%
	b. Confined to vagina, >2 cm		
T2	a. Invades paravaginal tissues but not pelvic wall, ≤2 cm*	II	23%–32%
	b. Invades paravaginal tissues but not pelvic wall, >2 cm*		
T3	• Extends to pelvic side wall* • Involves the lower one-third of the vagina • Hydronephrosis or nonfunctioning kidney	III	78%
N1	• Pelvic or inguinal LNs		
T4	• Invasion into bladder, rectum, and/or extends beyond true pelvis†	IVA	83%
M1	• Distant metastasis	IVB	

AJCC Group Staging	
IA	T1aN0M0
IB	T1bN0M0
IIA	T2aN0M0
IIB	T2bN0M0
III	T3N0M0, T1–3N1M0
IVA	T4N0–1M0
IVB	M1

*Pelvic wall is muscle, fascia, neurovascular structures, or skeletal portions of bony pelvis.
†Bullous edema is not sufficient to classify tumor as T4.

TREATMENT PARADIGM[1,2,9]

Surgery: Wide local excision may be possible for VAIN 3/CIS. For lesions in the superior one-third of the vagina, radical hysterectomy with pelvic lymphadenectomy and partial vaginectomy may be feasible. For distal one-third lesions, total vaginectomy or vulvovaginectomy with reconstruction (e.g., split thickness skin graft) may be possible, but often exenteration (either total or anterior, including the vagina and bladder only but sparing the rectum) will be necessary. Multiple surgical series have demonstrated pathologic nodal involvement of ~10% for stage I lesions and ~30% for stage II lesions.[26,27] Thus, pelvic LN dissection is often performed, and inguinofemoral nodes are also dissected if lesion is in the distal vagina. Because of the extent of surgery often required in these cases, RT is the preferred definitive treatment modality.

Chemotherapy: Indication for CHT is an extrapolation from cervical cancer data. Concurrent weekly cisplatin 40 mg/m^2 can be considered with other retrospective series using various multi-agent combinations such as cisplatin/5-FU.

Radiation

Indications: RT delivered definitively typically for stage I to IVA lesions.

Dose: EBRT to whole pelvis, 45 Gy/25 fx (50.4 Gy/28 fx also common). In the postoperative setting or when treating inguinal LN, IMRT improves toxicity compared with traditional four-field box.[29] HDR brachytherapy is given as a boost, which may be intracavitary (≤0.5 cm depth of invasion) or interstitial (>0.5 cm). Following 45 Gy EBRT to the vagina and elective nodes, a variety of interstitial brachytherapy dose fractionation schemes are plausible; 25 Gy/5 fx BID is commonly prescribed. Refer to ABS guidelines for details.[1] If brachytherapy boost is not feasible, boost with EBRT to a cumulative dose of 64 to 70 Gy to primary and 55 to 66 Gy to involved lymphadenopathy.

Toxicity: Acute: vaginitis, pain, dysuria, proctitis. Late: vaginal stenosis, proctitis, fistulae, bleeding, bowel obstruction, incontinence, hemorrhagic cystitis, urethral stricture, sexual dysfunction. Risk factors include location, stage, and smoking.[21] Late RT toxicity is ~5% for bowel and bladder (each) with "vaginal morbidity" of 64%.[30]

Procedure: See *Handbook of Treatment Planning in Radiation Oncology*, Chapter 9.[31]

EVIDENCE-BASED Q&A

What evidence supports current treatment approaches and outcomes for vaginal cancer?

Most data for vaginal cancer treatment are retrospective. The most commonly cited series are listed below.

Frank, MDACC (*IJROBP* 2005, PMID 15850914). RR of 193 patients with SCC of the vagina and no prior gynecologic cancers. FIGO I (26%), II (50%), III (20%), and IVA (4%), treated from 1970 to 2000. 119 (62%) patients had EBRT + brachytherapy (median 85 Gy to surface, 81 Gy to depth), 63 (32%) had EBRT alone (median 66 Gy), and 11 (6%) had brachytherapy alone (median 65 Gy); 18 patients had gross excision. EBRT alone more likely for advanced lesions, bulky, or comorbid disease; 22% of advanced stage received CHT. In more recent years, EBRT was used in addition to brachytherapy even for stage I disease (see Table 51.5). Three of nine patients with stage I treated with brachytherapy alone failed in regional LN. Four patients were treated with neoadjuvant CHT; all died of progressive disease. To the contrary, four of nine treated with concurrent CHT were NED. **Conclusion: Size was significantly associated with DSS (82% vs. 60% for <4 or >4 cm lesions, *p* = .027). Stage predictive of survival and toxicity. Predominant pattern of relapse was locoregional (I–II: 68%; III–IVA: 83%). Concurrent CRT reasonable for advanced disease.**

Table 51.5 Summary of MDACC Series on Vaginal Cancer				
FIGO Stage	5-Yr DSS	5-Yr Vaginal Control	5-Yr Pelvic Control	Severe Toxicity
I	85%	91%	86%	4%
II	78%		84%	9%
III	58%*	83%*	71%*	21%*
IVA				

*Statistically significant.

Tran, Stanford (*Gynecol Oncol* 2007, PMID 17363046): RR of 78 patients with SCC of the vagina treated with RT between 1959 and 2005. Median age 65 years. FIGO I (42%), II (29%), III (17%), and IVA/B (11%); 62% treated with EBRT + brachytherapy, 22% EBRT alone, and 13% with brachytherapy alone. Intracavitary RT (46%) delivered to a mean dose of 41 Gy; interstitial RT (31%) delivered to a mean dose of 33 Gy. Sixty-two percent treated with EBRT + brachytherapy to the whole vagina. On MVA, stage, Hgb (<12.5 mg/dL), and prior hysterectomy were prognostic for DSS (*p* < .02). These three factors and tumor size (<4 cm) were all prognostic for LRC (*p* = .01). Twenty-six patients failed:

13 of 26 local, 9 of 26 regional, 10 of 26 distant; 16 of 26 failed in the pelvis only. MS after LF was 14 months. Clinical outcomes by FIGO stage shown in Table 51.6. Of 35 patients with lower one-third vaginal involvement, 22 (63%) received elective inguinofemoral RT with no treatment failures. Of 13 patients with lower one-third vaginal involvement who did *not* receive elective inguinofemoral RT, one patient failed. Toxicity: 14% grade 3/4 complications. Tumor size (≥4 cm) and tumor dose (70 Gy) were independently predictive ($p < .05$). **Conclusion: RT is an effective treatment for stage I/II disease. Advanced disease necessitates a combined modality given poor outcomes. Most failures are local, and most cancer-related deaths are due to LF, not DM. Hgb level at the time of treatment appears to be prognostic.** *Comment: The authors suggested that studies evaluating correction of anemia may be warranted; however, extrapolating from cervical cancer literature, transfusion may not be associated with improved prognosis for anemic patients.*[32]

Table 51.6 Stanford Vaginal Cancer Series			
FIGO Stage	5-Yr LRC	5-Yr DMFS	5-Yr DSS
I	83%	100%	92%
II	76%	95%	68%
III	62%	65%	44%
IVA	30%	18%	13%

Should concurrent CHT be utilized?

No prospective trials are available to answer this question. Nevertheless, given the similarities in epidemiology, risk factors, histology, and anatomy between vaginal cancer and cervical cancer, many argue for extrapolation from multiple cervical cancer randomized trials to support the addition of concurrent CHT to improve PFS and OS. In the absence of randomized data, the following RRs provide support for concurrent CHT.

Rajagopalan, UPMC (*Gynecol Oncol* 2014, PMID 25281493): NCDB analysis of ~14,000 patients treated for vaginal cancer between 1998 and 2011. Sixty percent received RT. Of these, 48% received concurrent CHT, with increasing use from 1998 to 2011. Median survival was longer with use of concurrent CHT, improved from 41 to 56 months ($p < .0005$). On MVA, the following factors were independently prognostic for improved OS: younger age, higher facility volume, squamous histology, concurrent CHT, use of brachytherapy, and lower stage. **Conclusion: Concurrent CHT may improve OS.**

Miyamoto, Harvard (*PLoS One* 2013, PMID 23762284): Single-institution RR of 71 primary vaginal cancer patients treated with definitive RT ($n = 51$) or CRT ($n = 20$). MFU 3 years; 3-year OS improved from 56% with RT alone to 79% with CRT ($p = .037$). The 3-year DFS also improved with CHT, from 43% with RT alone to 73% with CRT ($p = .011$). On MVA, use of concurrent CHT remained a significant predictor of DFS (HR 0.31, 95% CI 0.10–0.97). **Conclusion: Concurrent CHT leads to improved outcomes in vaginal cancer patients.**

REFERENCES

1. Beriwal S, Demanes DJ, Erickson B, et al. American Brachytherapy Society consensus guidelines for interstitial brachytherapy for vaginal cancer. *Brachytherapy*. 2012;11(1):68–75. doi:10.1016/j.brachy.2011.06.008
2. Lee LJ, Jhingran A, Kidd E, et al. ACR Appropriateness criteria management of vaginal cancer. *Oncology (Williston Park)*. 2013;27(11):1166–1173. PMID: 24575547
3. Aho M, Vesterinen E, Meyer B, Purola E, Paavonen J. Natural history of vaginal intraepithelial neoplasia. *Cancer*. 1991;68(1):195–197. doi:10.1002/1097-0142(19910701)68:1<195::AID-CNCR2820680135>3.0.CO;2-L
4. National Comprehensive Cancer Network. *NCCN Clinical Practice Guidelines in Oncology: Vaginal Cancer*. Updated August 8, 2024. Accessed September 11, 2024. https://www.nccn.org/professionals/physician_gls/pdf/vaginal.pdf
5. Blanchard P, Monnier L, Dumas I, et al. Low-dose-rate definitive brachytherapy for high-grade vaginal intraepithelial neoplasia. *Oncologist*. 2011;16(2):182–188. doi:10.1634/theoncologist.2010-0326
6. Zolciak-Siwinska A, Gruszczynska E, Jonska-Gmyrek J, Kulik A, Michalski W. Brachytherapy for vaginal intraepithelial neoplasia. *Eur J Obstet Gynecol Reprod Biol*. 2015;194:73–77. doi:10.1016/j.ejogrb.2015.08.018

7. American Cancer Society. *Cancer Facts and Figures 2024*. American Cancer Society; 2024.

8. Creasman WT, Phillips JL, Menck HR. The National Cancer Data Base report on cancer of the vagina. *Cancer*. 1998;83(5):1033–1040. PMID: 9731908

9. Halperin EC, Perez CA, Wazer DE, Brady LW, eds. *Principles and Practice of Radiation Oncology*. 6th ed. Wolters Kluwer/Lippincott Williams & Wilkins; 2013.

10. Chyle V, Zagars GK, Wheeler JA, Wharton JT, Delclos L. Definitive radiotherapy for carcinoma of the vagina: outcome and prognostic factors. *Int J Radiat Oncol Biol Phys*. 1996;35(5):891–905. doi:10.1016/0360-3016(95)02394-1

11. Madsen BS, Jensen HL, van den Brule AJ, Wohlfahrt J, Frisch M. Risk factors for invasive squamous cell carcinoma of the vulva and vagina—population-based case-control study in Denmark. *Int J Cancer*. 2008;122(12):2827–2834. doi:10.1002/ijc.23446

12. Daling JR, Madeleine MM, Schwartz SM, et al. A population-based study of squamous cell vaginal cancer: HPV and cofactors. *Gynecol Oncol*. 2002;84(2):263–270. doi:10.1006/gyno.2001.6502

13. Alemany L, Saunier M, Tinoco L, et al. Large contribution of human papillomavirus in vaginal neoplastic lesions: a worldwide study in 597 samples. *Eur J Cancer*. 2014;50(16):2846–2854. doi:10.1016/j.ejca.2014.07.018

14. Sinno AK, Saraiya M, Thompson TD, et al. Human papillomavirus genotype prevalence in invasive vaginal cancer from a registry-based population. *Obstet Gynecol*. 2014;123(4):817–821. doi:10.1097/AOG.0000000000000171

15. Lee JY, Perez CA, Ettinger N, Fineberg BB. The risk of second primaries subsequent to irradiation for cervix cancer. *Int J Radiat Oncol Biol Phys*. 1982;8(2):207–211. doi:10.1016/0360-3016(82)90515-6

16. Boice JD Jr, Engholm G, Kleinerman RA, et al. Radiation dose and second cancer risk in patients treated for cancer of the cervix. *Radiat Res*. 1988;116(1):3–55. PMID: 3186929

17. Gallup DG, Talledo OE, Shah KJ, Hayes C. Invasive squamous cell carcinoma of the vagina: a 14-year study. *Obstet Gynecol*. 1987;69(5):782–785. PMID: 3574807

18. Rubin SC, Young J, Mikuta JJ. Squamous carcinoma of the vagina: treatment, complications, and long-term follow-up. *Gynecol Oncol*. 1985;20(3):346–353. doi:10.1016/0090-8258(85)90216-1

19. Chang YC, Hricak H, Thurnher S, Lacey CG. Vagina: evaluation with MR imaging. Part II. Neoplasms. *Radiology*. 1988;169(1):175–179. doi:10.1148/radiology.169.1.3420257

20. Stock RG, Chen AS, Seski J. A 30-year experience in the management of primary carcinoma of the vagina: analysis of prognostic factors and treatment modalities. *Gynecol Oncol*. 1995;56(1):45–52. doi:10.1006/gyno.1995.1008

21. Frank SJ, Jhingran A, Levenback C, Eifel PJ. Definitive radiation therapy for squamous cell carcinoma of the vagina. *Int J Radiat Oncol Biol Phys*. 2005;62(1):138–147. doi:10.1016/j.ijrobp.2004.09.032

22. Shah CA, Goff BA, Lowe K, Peters WA III, Li CI. Factors affecting risk of mortality in women with vaginal cancer. *Obstet Gynecol*. 2009;113(5):1038–1045. doi:10.1097/AOG.0b013e31819fe844

23. Rajagopalan MS, Xu KM, Lin JF, Sukumvanich P, Krivak TC, Beriwal S. Adoption and impact of concurrent chemoradiation therapy for vaginal cancer: a National Cancer Data Base (NCDB) study. *Gynecol Oncol*. 2014;135(3):495–502. doi:10.1016/j.ygyno.2014.09.018

24. Tran PT, Su Z, Lee P, et al. Prognostic factors for outcomes and complications for primary squamous cell carcinoma of the vagina treated with radiation. *Gynecol Oncol*. 2007;105(3):641–649. doi:10.1016/j.ygyno.2007.01.033

25. Merino MJ. Vaginal cancer: the role of infectious and environmental factors. *Am J Obstet Gynecol*. 1991;165(4 Pt 2):1255–1262. doi:10.1016/S0002-9378(12)90738-3

26. Al-Kurdi M, Monaghan JM. Thirty-two years experience in management of primary tumours of the vagina. *Br J Obstet Gynaecol*. 1981;88(11):1145–1150. doi:10.1111/j.1471-0528.1981.tb01770.x

27. Davis KP, Stanhope CR, Garton GR, Atkinson EJ, O'Brien PC. Invasive vaginal carcinoma: analysis of early-stage disease. *Gynecol Oncol*. 1991;42(2):131–136. doi:10.1016/0090-8258(91)90332-Y

28. Amin MB, Edge SB, Greene FL, et al, eds. *AJCC Cancer Staging Manual*. 8th ed. Springer; 2017.

29. Wortman BG, Post CCB, Powell ME, et al. Radiation therapy techniques and treatment-related toxicity in the PORTEC-3 trial: comparison of 3-dimensional conformal radiation therapy versus intensity-modulated radiation therapy. *Int J Radiat Oncol Biol Phys*. 2022;112(2):390–399. doi:10.1016/j.ijrobp.2021.09.042

30. Lian J, Dundas G, Carlone M, Ghosh S, Pearcey R. Twenty-year review of radiotherapy for vaginal cancer: an institutional experience. *Gynecol Oncol*. 2008;111(2):298–306. doi:10.1016/j.ygyno.2008.07.007

31. Videtic G, Woody N, Vassil AD. *Handbook of Treatment Planning in Radiation Oncology*. 3rd ed. Demos Medical; 2020.

32. Bishop AJ, Allen PK, Klopp AH, Meyer LA, Eifel PJ. Relationship between low hemoglobin levels and outcomes after treatment with radiation or chemoradiation in patients with cervical cancer: has the impact of anemia been overstated? *Int J Radiat Oncol Biol Phys*. 2015;91(1):196–205. doi:10.1016/j.ijrobp.2014.09.023

PART IX: Hematologic

Sean M. Parker, Matthew C. Ward, and Sheen Cherian

QUICK HIT Hodgkin lymphoma (HL) accounts for 10% of lymphomas in the United States and is broadly grouped into classic and nodular lymphocyte predominant types. Risk stratification of classic Hodgkin determines treatment and includes early-stage favorable, early-stage unfavorable, and advanced (stages III–IV) disease. Each major study group (EORTC, German HSG, UK RAPID, Stanford) defines risk stratification differently. Most recent trials use PET response as judged by Deauville criteria to guide treatment. For early-stage favorable disease, multiple large trials confirm CHT alone is inferior to combined CRT (in terms of PFS). Despite this, many still favor CHT alone due to favorable salvage rates with autologous SCT and equivalent OS. Late effects with RT are of particular concern due to the disease's excellent prognosis. Although most trials delivered IFRT, ISRT is well-accepted internationally and may reduce toxicity. Early nodular lymphocyte predominant patients are treated with definitive RT. Treatment paradigms are different in children and adolescents (see Chapter 66 for details). See Table 52.1 for general treatment paradigm of adult Hodgkin Lymphoma.

Table 52.1 General Treatment Paradigm for Adult Hodgkin Lymphoma			
	Stage/Status	**Example Treatment Options (See Trials for Specifics)**[1]	**Recent Trials Defining Paradigm**
Classic HL	**Stage IA/IIA favorable**	Combined CRT: ABVD × 2–4C and ISRT to 20–30 Gy or CHT alone: ABVD × 3–4C (if PET– after 2–3C) or Stanford V × 8 weeks + ISRT to 30 Gy	HD10, HD16, UK RAPID, EORTC H10F, Stanford G4
	Stage I/II unfavorable	ABVD × 2C then If PET–: ABVD × 2C and ISRT 30 Gy or AVD alone × 4C If PET+: BEACOPP × 2C and ISRT 30 Gy or BEACOPP alone × 4C	HD11, HD14, HD17, EORTC H10U, RATHL, CALGB 50801
	Stage III–IV*	BV-AVD or BEACOPP × 6C or BV-AVD or ABVD × 2C then If PET–: AVD × 4C If PET+: BEACOPP × 4C or BEACOPP × 4–6C based on PET response	RATHL, HD12, HD15, HD18, ECHALON-1, AHL2011
NLP-HL	**Stage IA/IIA**	ISRT alone to 30 Gy (consider + 6 Gy boost for bulky disease)	
	Stage IA/IIA bulky or IB/IIB	CHT + rituximab + ISRT	
	Stage III–IV	CHT + rituximab ± ISRT OR local RT for palliation only	

*Consider ISRT to initially bulky or select PET+ sites.

EPIDEMIOLOGY: Relatively uncommon; 0.4% of new cancer diagnoses, ~8,570 cases and ~910 deaths in 2024.[2] Accounts for 10% of all lymphomas diagnosed in the United States. Slight male predominance, rare under age 10. Bimodal age distribution with peaks around 25 and 60 to 70 years of age.

RISK FACTORS: HL is associated with EBV. EBV DNA has been isolated within Reed–Sternberg (RS) cells, and patients with history of infectious mononucleosis are at higher risk of developing HL. EBV tied most closely with mixed cellularity subtype and pediatric HL in developing countries. Other risk factors include HIV and immunosuppression.

ANATOMY: Primarily nodal disease with predictable spread. Extranodal spread is rare. Eighty percent of patients present with cervical nodes and >50% with mediastinal nodes. The most common site of extranodal disease is the spleen; 13 individual lymphatic regions identified in 1965 now define Ann Arbor staging and include Waldeyer's ring, cervical/SCV/occipital/preauricular, infraclavicular, axillary/pectoral, mediastinal, hilar, para-aortic, spleen, mesenteric, iliac, inguinal/femoral, popliteal, and epitrochlear/brachial. Right and left hilar and cervical regions are counted as separate regions. Waldeyer's ring and spleen are considered lymphatic but extranodal regions for staging purposes. EORTC and German groups count differently than the classic Ann Arbor system: EORTC includes the axilla and infraclavicular as one site. German HSG includes cervical and infraclavicular regions as one site. Both EORTC and German HSG consider mediastinum and hilar areas as one site. These definitions have implications in risk stratification.

PATHOLOGY: Classic diagnostic cells are RS cells, although these account for only 1% to 2% of tumor volume, with the rest being infiltration of lymphocytes, eosinophils, and plasma cells. An RS cell is classically binucleate with two prominent nucleoli, well-demarcated nuclear membrane, and eosinophilic cytoplasm with perinuclear halo. Likely origin is precursor B-cell. Monoclonal EBV DNA has been identified in RS cells in classic HL. Several subtypes of HL have slightly different pathologic markers (Table 52.2).

Table 52.2 Histologic Characteristics of Hodgkin Lymphoma

	Histology	Frequency	Clinicopathologic Features	Markers
CLASSIC HL	Nodular sclerosis (NS-HL)	≥70%	Broad bands of birefringent collagen surrounding nodules of lymphocytes, eosinophils, plasma cells, and tissue histiocytes, intermixed w/ atypical mononuclear cells and RS cells. No gender predilection. Median age ~26. Mediastinum often involved. One-third have B symptoms.	CD15+, CD30+, CD20−, CD45−
	Mixed cellularity (MC-HL)	~20%	Less favorable than NS. Diffuse effacement of LNs by lymphocytes, eosinophils, plasma cells, and relatively abundant atypical mononuclear and RS cells. Males and older patients more common. Often have abdominal involvement or advanced disease. One-third with B symptoms.	
	Lymphocyte-rich (LR-HL)	5%	Best prognosis. Occasional RS cell but mostly diffusely effaced with normal-appearing lymphocytes. Males more common. Median age 30. Frequently stages I–II, <10% have B symptoms. Uncommon mediastinal/abdominal involvement.	
	lymphocyte-depleted (LD-HL)	<5%	Worst prognosis. Paucity of normal-appearing cells and abundance of abnormal mononuclear cells, RS cells, and variants. Difficult to differentiate from anaplastic large cell lymphoma. Males and older patients more common. Usually advanced disease. Two-thirds with B symptoms.	
Nodular lymphocyte predominant (NLP-HL)		5%	Likely distinct entity from other HLs with natural history similar to low-grade NHL. Lacks RS cells. Significant rate of transformation to DLBCL and frequent late relapse. Some response to rituximab. EBV-negative.	CD19+, CD20+, CD45+, CD15−, CD30−

CLINICAL PRESENTATION: Painless adenopathy most common. B symptoms: drenching night sweats, fever >38.0°C, weight loss >10% in 6 months (B symptoms present at diagnosis in one-third of patients; combination of weight loss and fever carries poor prognosis). Generalized pruritus/alcohol-induced pain in infiltrated tissues. Disease foci contiguous in 90% of patients (including connection of SCV nodes to upper celiac/splenic nodes via thoracic duct). Visceral involvement is most frequently splenic, and there is a correlation between burden of splenic disease and likelihood of hematogenous spread. Marrow and liver involvement occurs almost exclusively in the setting of splenic disease. HL in HIV+ patients often behaves more aggressively.

WORKUP: H&P with attention to LN regions and B symptoms, chest and abdominal (spleen/liver) exam.

Labs: Pregnancy test, HIV, CBC, ESR, albumin, BMP, LFT, LDH, PFTs including DLCO, fertility preservation.

Imaging: CXR, PET/CT (≥90% sensitivity, changes treatment in 14%–25%), echocardiogram/MUGA (if doxorubicin CHT considered).

Biopsy: Excisional biopsy recommended vs. core needle biopsy (may be adequate if diagnostic of HL). FNA is inadequate. Bone marrow biopsy only recommended for PET-positive marrow or PET-negative with unexplained cytopenia (overall frequency of bone marrow involvement 5% or less).[1,3]

PROGNOSTIC FACTORS: Several prognostic factors including stage, age, ESR, number of nodal sites involved, extranodal involvement, and LN bulk have been identified. In addition to Ann Arbor stage, these factors have defined risk stratification into early-stage favorable and early-stage unfavorable, which define treatment. GHSG, EORTC, and NCCN have defined unfavorable risk factors for early-stage (stage I-II) classical Hodgkin's lymphoma with some discrepancies among groups. All groups take into consideration ESR, bulky disease, and number of nodal sites. GHSG considers patients unfavorable for elevated ESR (>30 if B symptoms present, >50 otherwise), mediastinal mass/intrathoracic diameter >0.33, >2 nodal regions involved, and presence of ENE. EORTC designates patients unfavorable if age is ≥50, ESR (>30 if B symptoms present, >50 otherwise), mass width/intrathoracic diameter >0.35 at level of T5-6, and >3 nodal regions involved. NCCN specifies unfavorable patients as ESR ≥50, presence of B symptoms, mediastinal mass/intrathoracic diameter >0.33, >3 nodal sites involved, and mass ≥10 cm.

International Prognostic Score (IPS): Prognostic scoring system for advanced HL is composed of seven factors: albumin <4 g/dL, Hgb <10.5 g/dL, male gender, age ≥45, Ann Arbor stage IV, leukocytes ≥15,000, and lymphocytes <600/mm³ or <8% of white count. Initial publication stratified PFS from 84% to 42% going from 0 to 7 points.[4] Scoring system was reanalyzed in 2012 and remained valid with PFS ranging between 69% and 88%.[5]

STAGING: See Table 52.3.

Table 52.3 Ann Arbor (Lugano Update) Staging System for Lymphoma[†6]		
I	One node or group of adjacent nodes *OR* single extranodal lesions without nodal involvement (IE)	**A:** No systemic symptoms **B:** Unexplained weight loss >10% in 6 months before diagnosis; unexplained fever with temperatures above 38°C; drenching night sweats **E*:** Extralymphatic involvement **X*:** Bulky disease (≥10 cm or >1/3 of thoracic diameter)
II	≥2 nodal groups on same side of diaphragm OR stage I or II by nodal extent with limited contiguous extranodal involvement	
III	Nodes on both sides of diaphragm; nodes above diaphragm with spleen involvement	
IV	Additional noncontiguous extralymphatic involvement	

*Note that the 2014 Lugano update suggests "X" and "A/B" modifiers are necessary only for HL and "E" unnecessary for stage III–IV disease.[6]
†Number of involved regions may be designated with subscript (i.e., II3).
Source: Cheson BD, Fisher RI, Barrington SF, et al. Recommendations for initial evaluation, staging, and response assessment of Hodgkin and non-Hodgkin lymphoma: the Lugano classification. *J Clin Oncol.* 2014;32(27):3059–3067. doi:10.1200/JCO.2013.54.8800.

TREATMENT PARADIGM

Surgery: There is typically no role for surgery in the treatment of adult HL. In children with NLP-HL, resection followed by observation with CHT at progression has been investigated.[7]

Systemic Therapy: Several CHT regimens have been used in HL. Historical regimen MOPP (mustard, vincristine, procarbazine, prednisone) resulted in sterility (80% of men, age-linked in women) and secondary acute nonlymphocytic leukemia. Modern regimens are associated with less sterility and secondary malignancy risk.

ABVD: Adriamycin, bleomycin, vinblastine, dacarbazine. Toxicities include nausea, vomiting, hair loss, and marrow suppression. Long-term toxicities include cardiac and pulmonary toxicity. Each cycle is generally 1 month with two infusions per cycle. German HD13 study examined if bleomycin, dacarbazine, or both could be omitted (ABV, AVD, and AV arms) in early-stage HL. All alternative regimens were associated with inferior outcomes relative to ABVD.[8]

BEACOPP: Bleomycin, etoposide, doxorubicin, cyclophosphamide, vincristine, procarbazine, prednisone. Intensified treatment studied in the setting of poor response or for unfavorable patients. Associated with higher response rates but also higher incidence of marrow suppression and alopecia.[9]

Stanford V: Nitrogen mustard, doxorubicin, vinblastine, vincristine, bleomycin, etoposide, prednisone. Quicker treatment (8–12 weeks vs. 16–24 weeks for 4–6C of ABVD) and includes lower cumulative doses of doxorubicin and bleomycin.[10] Designed as combined modality therapy with RT, and therefore RT should not be omitted. Other studies suggest similar outcomes as ABVD assuming RT is delivered.[11–13] Stanford V regimen was not superior to ABVD on ECOG E2496 for advanced HL.[14] Despite demonstrated efficacy, the regimen is not included in the NCCN guidelines.

Number of Cycles: Number of cycles delivered on trials varies by study group and risk group. Treatment should proceed per trials evaluating response and outcomes in that risk group (Table 52.1).

Targeted Therapy/Immunotherapy: Brentuximab vedotin (BV) is an antibody–drug conjugate against CD30. For patients with advanced disease, substitution of BV for bleomycin (BV-AVD) on the ECHELON-1 trial improved PFS and OS. PD-1 inhibitors have demonstrated response in relapsed/refractory disease[15,16] Furthermore, the SWOG-S1826 trial demonstrated improved PFS with 6C of nivolumab-AVD compared with BV-AVD for advanced HL. Phase III studies evaluating the integration of BV and immune checkpoint inhibition into treatment of early-stage HL are underway.

Response Evaluation: Favorable (rapid/early) response to CHT, determined by PET, has become an important predictor of outcome and is increasingly being used to determine treatment paradigm. Deauville score (named after conference in Deauville, France) is the standardized method of evaluating PET response (Table 52.4). Typically, trials consider early response of Deauville 1 to 2 to be a CR with favorable outcomes, Deauville 3 to 4 to be a PR with need to initiate adaptive treatment, and Deauville 5 to define refractory disease. However, Deauville 3 is considered a favorable response in some trials.

Table 52.4 Deauville (5-Point) Score[1,17,18]

Score		Definition
Negative	1	No uptake (background)
	2	Uptake ≤ mediastinum
	3	Uptake > mediastinum but ≤ liver
Positive	4	Uptake moderately > liver
	5	Uptake markedly > liver and/or new lesions
	X	Not attributable to lymphoma

Radiation: RT, once the only curative treatment for HL, continues to play an important role in the combined treatment of HL together with CHT. For early-stage favorable disease, multiple large trials have confirmed CHT alone is not noninferior to combined CHT and RT in terms of PFS. An NCDB study of utilization of RT in stage I/II HL between 1998 and 2011 revealed that RT use had declined from 55% to 44% and receipt of RT was associated with significant improvement in 5-year OS (95% vs. 89%).[19]

Indications: RT is used in combined modality treatment of early-stage patients and consolidation for select advanced-stage patients. The rationale for combined modality is to lower the intensity of CHT required for cure. For early-stage patients, RT use is defined by CHT paradigms set by accompanying clinical trials. RT is delivered after CHT to pre-CHT sites. Historically, large RT fields such as mantle, inverted-Y, or total nodal RT (mantle + inverted Y) were used alone to doses >40 Gy. Most recent trials used IFRT, but now ISRT is well-accepted. ILROG guidelines define ISRT and involved node RT (INRT, less common in the United States).[20] Studies have shown that appropriate use of these techniques results in equivalent outcomes.[20,21] For advanced (stages III–IV) disease, although controversial, RT can be considered for initially bulky or select sites that remain PET-positive after CHT.[1] If given, initiate RT within 3 to 6 weeks of completion of CHT.

Dose: RT dose should follow the paradigm of the clinical trial that applies based on PET response and number of CHT cycles given. Typically, for early-stage favorable disease following CHT, 20–30 Gy/10–15 fx is sufficient after PET CR. For early-stage unfavorable disease, 30 Gy is recommended, and for bulky disease 30–36 Gy/15–20 fx. For advanced HL patients with residual disease on PET/CT or for consolidation of initially bulky disease, consider 30–36 Gy/15–20 fx.

Toxicity: Acute: fatigue, RT dermatitis, esophagitis, odynophagia, cough, xerostomia, nausea, mucositis. Late: site/age-dependent but may include hypothyroidism, pneumonitis, cardiac disease, xerostomia, infertility. Second malignancy is of significant concern and may include leukemia (CHT-related), breast cancer, and lung cancer. Historical data show that cause of death in HL at 25 years is most commonly Hodgkin (24% cumulative incidence), followed by second malignancy (13.5%) and cardiovascular disease (6.9%).[22] Note that late effects data are generally based on obsolete RT techniques and doses; late effects data in combined modality/ISRT era are evolving.

Procedure: See *Handbook of Treatment Planning in Radiation Oncology*, Chapter 10.[23]

EVIDENCE-BASED Q&A

EARLY-STAGE FAVORABLE HODGKIN LYMPHOMA

What trials define current standard of care in early-stage favorable HL?

Through much effort over many years, Hodgkin has transitioned treatment from the 1950s' standard of large-field RT alone to modern PET-adapted combined modality therapy.[13,24–30] The most recent trials define the current "standard" of care and have focused mainly on the role of PET and omission of IFRT from CHT. Most physicians prefer to pick an approach as defined by the following trials to guide treatment. Omission of RT from ABVD remains controversial, but because of excellent OS results due to salvage autologous SCT, many argue that RT for all is overtreatment and may increase late effects, although this has not been validated with modern RT techniques, volumes, and doses.

Engert, German HD10 (*NEJM* 2010, PMID 20818855; Update Sasse, *JCO* 2017, PMID 28418763): A total of 1,370 patients with early-stage favorable (by German criteria); 2 × 2 design randomized to ABVD × 4C vs. ABVD × 2C + IFRT 20 Gy vs. 30 Gy. Primary endpoint FFTF. PET was not used to assess response. MFU at update 98 months. No significant differences in initial report or follow-up between either randomization. Noninferiority was confirmed for both (10-year PFS of ABVD × 4C + 30 Gy vs. ABVD × 2C + 20 Gy was 87.4% vs. 87.2%). **Conclusion: ABVD for 2C and IFRT to 20 Gy are standard as per German paradigm.**

Fuchs, German HD16 (*JCO* 2019, PMID 31498753; Update *Leukemia* 2023, PMID 37845285): Randomized phase III trial for early-stage favorable HL. Patients assigned to combined modality therapy (CMT) with ABVD × 2C and 20 Gy consolidation RT or single modality therapy (SMT) omitting RT with PET guidance (Deauville score <3); MFU at update 64 months; 5-year PFS 94% CMT vs. 87% SMT (HR 2.05, 95% CI 1.20–3.51). **Conclusion: In early-stage favorable HL, omitting RT results in reduced tumor control.**

Raemaekers, EORTC H10F (*JCO* 2014, PMID 24637998; Update André, *JCO* 2023, PMID 37967311): PRT of PET-adapted therapy including both favorable (H10F stratum) and unfavorable (H10U stratum) early-stage HL patients as defined by EORTC criteria. Trial evaluated both the ability to omit INRT in those with rapid PET response and utility of escalating to BEACOPP in early nonresponders on PET. In H10F, patients were randomized to PET-adapted treatment vs. standard treatment and received ABVD × 2C followed by PET. In the standard arm, patients received one additional cycle of ABVD with INRT to 30 Gy (6 Gy boost allowed for residual disease). In the experimental PET-adapted arm, patients received two additional cycles of ABVD (total of four) if PET-negative (Deauville 1–2). If PET-positive, patients received escalated BEACOPP × 2C and INRT to 30 Gy (6 Gy boost allowed for residual). Primary endpoint PFS, designed as noninferiority, powered to detect 5-year PFS decrease from 95% (H10F) to 85%. Randomization to PET-adapted therapy was stopped early as noninferiority was unlikely. 1,950 patients were recruited; 18.5% of PET scans were positive. Noninferiority of ABVD alone could not be established (H10F

10-year PFS 99% vs. 85%; HR 13.2, 95% CI 3.1–55.8; noninferiority margin was 3.2). Although significant on initial analysis, escalation to BEACOPP no longer improved PFS on 10-year update (HR 0.67, 95% CI 0.37–1.20; p = .18). **Conclusion: Even in patients with excellent PET response, omission of INRT is associated with increased risk of progression (but no difference in OS).**

Radford, UK RAPID (*NEJM* 2015, PMID 25901426): Noninferiority trial of patients with classic HL stages IA or IIA (baseline PET not performed) without bulk (≥33% thoracic diameter at T5–6). Patients received 3C of ABVD, then underwent PET and if negative (Deauville 1–2) randomized to 30 Gy IFRT vs. no further treatment. If positive, received a total of 4C of ABVD and 30 Gy IFRT. Noninferiority trial designed to exclude a difference in 3-year PFS with a 7% decrease from the assumed 95% PFS. Overall, 32% were unfavorable per German criteria and 31% had ≥3 nodal sites. MFU 60 months; 3-year PFS 95% in the RT group and 91% in the no additional therapy group (difference −3.8%, 95% CI −8.8% to 1.3%). **Conclusion: ABVD alone is not noninferior to ABVD + IFRT, although prognosis is excellent regardless.**

EARLY-STAGE UNFAVORABLE HODGKIN LYMPHOMA

The following trials are the most recent to define "standard" of care in early-stage unfavorable HL. Note that many trials define subsets of early-stage patients with high-risk features such as bulk, B symptoms, or extranodal disease as advanced rather than early-stage unfavorable, so it is important to identify the inclusion criteria for each paradigm when deciding treatment.

What trials define current standard of care in early-stage unfavorable HL?

Eich, German HD11 (*JCO* 2010, PMID 20713848; Update Sasse, *JCO* 2017, PMID 28418763): Precursor trial to the following HD14. PRT of patients with early-stage unfavorable (by German criteria) HL randomized in 2 × 2 fashion to either ABVD × 4C or BEACOPP × 4C as well as 20 Gy IFRT or 30 Gy IFRT; 1,395 patients included, FFTF primary endpoint, updated MFU 106 months. BEACOPP + 20 Gy was initially more effective than ABVD + 20 Gy, but not confirmed on long-term follow-up. No difference in FFTF between BEACOPP + 30 Gy and ABVD + 30 Gy. Similarly, after BEACOPP, 20 Gy was noninferior to 30 Gy, but after ABVD, 20 Gy was not noninferior to 30 Gy (10-year PFS difference −8.3%, 95% CI −15.2 to −1.3%). **Conclusion: ABVD × 4C + 30 Gy is standard for early-stage unfavorable HL.**

von Tresckow, German HD14 (*JCO* 2012, PMID 22271480; Update *Lancet Haematol* 2021, PMID 33770483): Follow-up to HD11. Prospective superiority trial of patients <60 years of age with early-stage unfavorable (by German criteria) randomized to either ABVD × 4C or BEACOPP × 2C followed by ABVD × 2C ("2 + 2" regimen). No PET. Both arms received 30 Ga IFRT following CHT. Primary endpoint FFTF; 1,528 patients, MFU 74 months. FFTF improved with "2 + 2" regimen (FFTF HR 0.44, p < .001) at 5 years; 10-year difference in PFS 5.6% (91.2%–85.6%, p < .001). No difference in OS. **Conclusion: In patients <60 years of age, escalated "2 + 2" + 30 Gy is standard German HSG treatment for early-stage unfavorable patients.**

Borchmann, German HD17 (*Lancet Oncol* 2021, PMID 33539742): 1,100 patients with early unfavorable disease randomized to BEACOPP × 2C + ABVD × 2C with 30 Gy (standard arm) vs. the same CHT without RT if cycle 4 PET showed Deauville of 1 to 2; 5-year PFS primary endpoint, designed as noninferiority with 8% margin. Results: 68% in the PET arm were negative at C4 and omitted RT. The 5-year PFS was 97.3% (standard) vs. 95.1% (PET4 arm; 95% CI −0.9% to 5.3%), meeting the criteria for noninferiority. **Conclusions: PET4 negativity allowed for omission of RT, essentially exchanging BEACOPP escalation for RT in about two-thirds of patients.**

Raemaekers, EORTC H10U (*JCO* 2014, PMID 24637998; Update *JCO* 2023, PMID 37967311): Patients with unfavorable early-stage disease randomized to standard arm of 4C of ABVD + INRT vs. either ABVD × 6C for PET-negative patients (Deauville 1–2) or ABVD × 2C, BEACOPP × 2C, and INRT if PET-positive. PET completed after first 2C of ABVD. H10U stratum powered to detect PFS decrease from 90% to 80%. Similar to favorable group, if PET was negative, 10-year PFS was not noninferior in ABVD-alone group (ABVD + INRT 91.4% vs. ABVD alone 86.5%; HR 1.52, 95% CI 0.8–2.75; noninferiority margin was 2.1). As noted previously, although significant on initial analysis, escalation to BEACOPP no longer improved PFS (HR 0.67, 95% CI 0.37–1.20; p = .1777). **Conclusion: In unfavorable HL, omission of INRT is associated with increased risk of recurrence even after excellent PET response (but no difference in OS).**

LaCasce, CALGB 50801/Alliance (*JCO* 2023, PMID 36269899): Phase II PRT of 98 stage I to II HL patients with bulky disease (>10 cm or >0.33 max intrathoracic diameter on CXR) randomized to ABVD × 2C followed by interim PET. PET-negative (Deauville 1–3) patients received additional ABVD × 4C, and PET-positive (Deauville 4–5) patients BEACOPP × 4C + 30 Gy ISRT. The 3-year PFS (primary endpoint) and OS rates were 93.1% and 98.6% for PET-negative patients and 89.7% and 94.4% for PET-positive patients. **Conclusion: In this phase II study, excellent PFS outcomes were observed in all patients using a PET-adapted approach that allowed omission of RT in 78% of patients.**

ADVANCED-STAGE HODGKIN LYMPHOMA

What trials define current standard of care in advanced HL?

Advanced HL is primarily treated with systemic therapy, and four trials are commonly cited to define treatment (HD15, UK RATHL, AHL2011, and ECHELON-1). Note that some unfavorable stage I to II patients were included in these trials. German HD15 found that BEACOPP × 6C followed by PET-guided RT should be standard compared with BEACOPP × 8C or BEACOPP-14.[31] AHL2011 demonstrated the benefit of PET adaptive therapy and found that those with PET response after 2C of BEACOPP could be de-escalated to 4C ABVD with no detriment in PFS when compared with BEACOPP × 6C.[32,33] UK RATHL reported that omission of bleomycin (AVD) is possible in patients who have an interim PET response (Deauville 1–3) after cycle 2 of ABVD.[34] ECHELON-1 demonstrated that brentuximab-AVD improves PFS and OS when compared with ABVD, with a decreased risk of pulmonary toxicity but an increased risk of neuropathy.[35,36] Alternative nivolumab-AVD and BrECADD regimens have demonstrated early promise in phase III PRTs.

What is the role of consolidative RT for advanced disease in the modern era?

Multiple trials have investigated this question directly. Older meta-analysis and trials in MOPP era suggested no benefit.[37–39] More recent trials in the ABVD/BEACOPP era have suggested improvement.[40,41] The German HD12 study completed in the pre-PET era with BEACOPP found that omitting consolidation RT in those with initial bulk or residual disease led to inferior FFTF and PFS. The HD0607 study (below) shows that consolidative RT in those with a negative PET at cycles 2 and 6 may not be beneficial. Overall, it seems that consolidative RT to sites not responding on PET/CT or RT to initially bulky sites may be of value, although this is controversial and institution-dependent.

Gallamini, Italian HD0607 Analysis (*JCO* 2020, PMID 32946355): PRT with substudy randomizing 296 advanced (IIB–IVB) Hodgkin patients with nodal mass ≥5 cm and negative PET (at cycles 2 and 6) to either consolidation RT or no treatment after 6C of ABVD. Median dose 30.6 Gy. Results: No change in PFS regardless of nodal size. **Conclusion: Consolidation RT may not be necessary in patients with negative cycles 2 and 6 PETs.**

RELAPSED/REFRACTORY HODGKIN LYMPHOMA

What treatment options are considered for refractory/relapsed patients?

There is no consensus regarding optimal management of relapsed/refractory patients. Treatment typically involves salvage systemic therapy and autologous SCT ± consolidation RT and adjuvant systemic therapy. Brentuximab vedotin and immune checkpoint inhibition have demonstrated promise on phase III trials.[42,43] Anti-CD30 CAR-T cell therapy has also shown benefit in patients failing many lines of salvage systemic therapy.[44]

Is there a role for adjuvant RT in refractory patients undergoing autologous SCT?

This is controversial and is without significant modern data. Some authors recommend consolidation RT prior to SCT to induce response if CR is not obtained on PET or consolidation RT after SCT for bulky disease, but this is informed by small retrospective series.[45,46] See ILROG guidelines for details.[47]

REFERENCES

1. National Comprehensive Cancer Network. *NCCN Clinical Practice Guidelines in Oncology: Hodgkin Lymphoma.* Version 4.2024. Accessed September 2024. https://www.nccn.org
2. Siegel RL, Giaquinto AN, Jemal A. Cancer statistics, 2024. *CA Cancer J Clin.* 2024;74(1):12–49. doi:10.3322/caac.21820

3. El-Galaly TC, d'Amore F, Mylam KJ, et al. Routine bone marrow biopsy has little or no therapeutic conse-quence for positron emission tomography/computed tomography–staged treatment-naive patients with Hodgkin lymphoma. *J Clin Oncol.* 2012;30(36):4508–4514. doi:10.1200/JCO.2012.42.4036

4. Hasenclever D, Diehl V, Armitage JO, et al. A prognostic score for advanced Hodgkin's disease. *N Engl J Med.* 1998;339(21):1506–1514. doi:10.1056/NEJM199811193392104

5. Moccia AA, Donaldson J, Chhanabhai M, et al. International Prognostic Score in advanced-stage Hodgkin's lymphoma: altered utility in the modern era. *J Clin Oncol.* 2012;30(27):3383–3388. doi:10.1200/JCO.2011.41.0910

6. Cheson BD, Fisher RI, Barrington SF, et al. Recommendations for initial evaluation, staging, and response assessment of Hodgkin and non-Hodgkin lymphoma: the Lugano classification. *J Clin Oncol.* 2014;32(27):3059–3067. doi:10.1200/JCO.2013.54.8800

7. Mauz-Körholz C, Gorde-Grosjean S, Hasenclever D, et al. Resection alone in 58 children with limited stage, lymphocyte-predominant Hodgkin lymphoma–experience from the European Network Group on pediat-ric Hodgkin lymphoma. *Cancer.* 2007;110(1):179–185. doi:10.1002/cncr.22762

8. Behringer K, Goergen H, Hitz F, et al. Omission of dacarbazine or bleomycin, or both, from the ABVD regimen in treatment of early-stage favourable Hodgkin's lymphoma (GHSG HD13): an open-label, ran-domised, non-inferiority trial. *Lancet.* 2015;385(9976):1418–1427. doi:10.1016/S0140-6736(14)61469-0

9. Federico M, Luminari S, Iannitto E, et al. ABVD compared with BEACOPP compared with CEC for the ini-tial treatment of patients with advanced Hodgkin's lymphoma: results from the HD2000 Gruppo Italiano per lo Studio dei Linfomi trial. *J Clin Oncol.* 2009;27(5):805–811. doi:10.1200/JCO.2008.17.0910

10. Advani RH, Hoppe RT, Baer D, et al. Efficacy of abbreviated stanford V chemotherapy and involved-field radiotherapy in early-stage Hodgkin lymphoma: mature results of the G4 trial. *Ann Oncol.* 2013;24(4):1044–1048. doi:10.1093/annonc/mds542

11. Chisesi T, Bellei M, Luminari S, et al. Long-term follow-up analysis of HD9601 trial comparing ABVD versus Stanford V versus MOPP/EBV/CAD in patients with newly diagnosed advanced-stage Hodgkin's lymphoma: a study from the Intergruppo Italiano Linfomi. *J Clin Oncol.* 2011;29(32):4227–4233. doi:10.1200/JCO.2010.30.9799

12. Gobbi PG, Levis A, Chisesi T, et al. ABVD versus modified Stanford V versus MOPPEBVCAD with optional and limited radiotherapy in intermediate- and advanced-stage Hodgkin's lymphoma: final results of a multicenter randomized trial by the Intergruppo Italiano Linfomi. *J Clin Oncol.* 2005;23(36):9198–9207. doi:10.1200/JCO.2005.02.907

13. Hoskin PJ, Smith P, Maughan TS, et al. Long-term results of a randomised trial of involved field radio-therapy vs extended field radiotherapy in stage I and II Hodgkin lymphoma. *Clin Oncol (R Coll Radiol).* 2005;17(1):47–53. doi:10.1016/j.clon.2004.07.004

14. Gordon LI, Hong F, Fisher RI, et al. Randomized phase III trial of ABVD versus Stanford V with or without radiation therapy in locally extensive and advanced stage Hodgkin lymphoma: an intergroup study coor-dinated by the Eastern Cooperative Oncology Group (E2496). *J Clin Oncol.* 2012;31(6):684–691. doi:10.1200/JCO.2012.43.4803

15. Armand P, Engert A, Younes A, et al. Nivolumab for relapsed/refractory classic Hodgkin lymphoma after failure of autologous hematopoietic cell transplantation: extended follow-up of the multicohort single-arm phase II CheckMate 205 trial. *J Clin Oncol.* 2018;36(14):1428–1439. doi:10.1200/JCO.2017.76.0793

16. Ansell SM, Lesokhin AM, Borrello I, et al. PD-1 blockade with nivolumab in relapsed or refractory Hodgkin's lymphoma. *N Engl J Med.* 2015;372(4):311–319. doi:10.1056/NEJMoa1411087

17. Gallamini A, Fiore F, Sorasio R, Meignan M. Interim positron emission tomography scan in Hodgkin lym-phoma: definitions, interpretation rules, and clinical validation. *Leuk Lymphoma.* 2009;50(11):1761–1764. doi:10.3109/10428190903308072

18. Meignan M, Gallamini A, Haioun C. Report on the First International Workshop on interim-PET scan in lymphoma. *Leuk Lymphoma.* 2009;50(8):1257–1260. doi:10.1080/10428190903040048

19. Parikh RR, Grossbard ML, Harrison LB, Yahalom J. Early-stage classic Hodgkin lymphoma: the utilization of radiation therapy and its impact on overall survival. *Int J Radiat Oncol Biol Phys.* 2015;93(3):684–693. doi:10.1016/j.ijrobp.2015.06.039

20. Specht L, Yahalom J, Illidge T, et al. Modern radiation therapy for Hodgkin lymphoma: field and dose guidelines from the International Lymphoma Radiation Oncology Group (ILROG). *Int J Radiat Oncol Biol Phys.* 2014;89(4):854–862. doi:10.1016/j.ijrobp.2013.05.005

21. Campbell BA, Voss N, Pickles T, et al. Involved-nodal radiation therapy as a component of combina-tion therapy for limited-stage Hodgkin's lymphoma: a question of field size. *J Clin Oncol.* 2008;26(32):5170–5174. doi:10.1200/JCO.2007.15.1001

22. Aleman BM, van den Belt-Dusebout AW, Klokman WJ, van't Veer MB, Bartelink H, van Leeuwen FE. Long-term cause-specific mortality of patients treated for Hodgkin's disease. *J Clin Oncol.* 2003;21(18):3431–3439. doi:10.1200/JCO.2003.07.131

23. Videtic GM, Woody NW, Vassil AD. Lymphoma and myeloma radiotherapy. In: *Handbook of Treatment Planning in Radiation Oncology.* 3rd ed. Demos Medical; 2020.

24. Arakelyan N, Jais JP, Delwail V, et al. Reduced versus full doses of irradiation after 3 cycles of combined doxorubicin, bleomycin, vinblastine, and dacarbazine in early stage Hodgkin lymphomas. *Cancer.* 2010;116(17):4054–4062. doi:10.1002/cncr.25295

25. Dühmke E, Franklin J, Pfreundschuh M, et al. Low-dose radiation is sufficient for the noninvolved extended-field treatment in favorable early-stage Hodgkin's disease: long-term results of a randomized trial of radiotherapy alone. *J Clin Oncol.* 2001;19(11):2905–2914. doi:10.1200/JCO.2001.19.11.2905

26. Engert A, Schiller P, Josting A, et al. Involved-field radiotherapy is equally effective and less toxic compared with extended-field radiotherapy after four cycles of chemotherapy in patients with early-stage unfavorable Hodgkin's lymphoma: results of the HD8 trial of the German Hodgkin's Lymphoma Study Group. *J Clin Oncol.* 2003;21(19):3601–3608. doi:10.1200/JCO.2003.03.023

27. Fermé C, Eghbali H, Meerwaldt JH, et al. Chemotherapy plus involved-field radiation in early-stage Hodgkin's disease. *N Engl J Med.* 2007;357(19):1916–1927. doi:10.1056/NEJMoa064601

28. Noordijk EM, Carde P, Dupouy N, et al. Combined-modality therapy for clinical stage I or II Hodgkin's lymphoma: long-term results of the European Organisation for Research and Treatment of Cancer H7 randomized controlled trials. *J Clin Oncol.* 2006;24(19):3128–3135. doi:10.1200/JCO.2005.05.2746

29. Sasse S, Bröckelmann PJ, Goergen H, et al. Long-term follow-up of contemporary treatment in early-stage Hodgkin lymphoma: updated analyses of the German Hodgkin Study Group HD7, HD8, HD10, and HD11 trials. *J Clin Oncol.* 2017;35(18):1999–2007. doi:10.1200/JCO.2016.70.9410

30. Zittoun R, Audebert A, Hoerni B, et al. Extended versus involved fields irradiation combined with MOPP chemotherapy in early clinical stages of Hodgkin's disease. *J Clin Oncol.* 1985;3(2):207–214. doi:10.1200/JCO.1985.3.2.207

31. Engert A, Haverkamp H, Kobe C, et al. Reduced-intensity chemotherapy and PET-guided radiotherapy in patients with advanced stage Hodgkin's lymphoma (HD15 trial): a randomised, open-label, phase 3 non-inferiority trial. *Lancet.* 2012;379(9828):1791–1799. doi:10.1016/S0140-6736(11)61940-5

32. Casasnovas RO, Bouabdallah R, Brice P, et al. PET-adapted treatment for newly diagnosed Advanced Hodgkin Lymphoma (AHL2011): a randomised, multicentre, non-inferiority, phase 3 study. *Lancet Oncol.* 2019;20(2):202–215. doi:10.1016/S1470-2045(18)30784-8

33. Casasnovas RO, Bouabdallah R, Brice P, et al. Positron emission tomography-driven strategy in advanced Hodgkin lymphoma: prolonged follow-up of the AHL2011 phase III Lymphoma Study Association study. *J Clin Oncol.* 2022;40(10):1091–1101. doi:10.1200/JCO.21.01777

34. Johnson P, Federico M, Kirkwood A, et al. Adapted treatment guided by interim PET-CT scan in advanced Hodgkin's lymphoma. *N Engl J Med.* 2016;374(25):2419–2429. doi:10.1056/NEJMoa1510093

35. Connors JM, Jurczak W, Straus DJ, et al. Brentuximab vedotin with chemotherapy for stage III or IV Hodgkin's lymphoma. *N Engl J Med.* 2018;378(4):331–344. doi:10.1056/NEJMoa1708984

36. Ansell SM, Radford J, Connors JM, et al. Overall survival with brentuximab vedotin in stage III or IV Hodgkin's lymphoma. *N Engl J Med.* 2022;387(4):310–320. doi:10.1056/NEJMoa2206125

37. Aleman BM, Raemaekers JM, Tirelli U, et al. Involved-field radiotherapy for advanced Hodgkin's lymphoma. *N Engl J Med.* 2003;348(24):2396–2406. doi:10.1056/NEJMoa022628

38. Aleman BM, Raemaekers JM, Tomišić R, et al. Involved-field radiotherapy for patients in partial remission after chemotherapy for advanced Hodgkin's lymphoma. *Int J Radiat Oncol Biol Phys.* 2007;67(1):19–30. doi:10.1016/j.ijrobp.2006.08.041

39. Loeffler M, Brosteanu O, Hasenclever D, et al. Meta-analysis of chemotherapy versus combined modality treatment trials in Hodgkin's disease. International Database on Hodgkin's Disease Overview Study Group. *J Clin Oncol.* 1998;16(3):818–829. doi:10.1200/JCO.1998.16.3.818

40. Borchmann P, Haverkamp H, Diehl V, et al. Eight cycles of escalated-dose BEACOPP compared with four cycles of escalated-dose BEACOPP followed by four cycles of baseline-dose BEACOPP with or without radiotherapy in patients with advanced-stage Hodgkin's lymphoma: final analysis of the HD12 trial of the German Hodgkin Study Group. *J Clin Oncol.* 2011;29(32):4234–4242. doi:10.1200/JCO.2010.33.9549

41. Laskar S, Gupta T, Vimal S, et al. Consolidation radiation after complete remission in Hodgkin's disease following six cycles of doxorubicin, bleomycin, vinblastine, and dacarbazine chemotherapy: is there a need? *J Clin Oncol.* 2004;22(1):62–68. doi:10.1200/JCO.2004.01.021

42. Kuruvilla J, Ramchandren R, Santoro A, et al. Pembrolizumab versus brentuximab vedotin in relapsed or refractory classical Hodgkin lymphoma (KEYNOTE-204): an interim analysis of a multicentre, randomised, open-label, phase 3 study. *Lancet Oncol.* 2021;22(4):512–524. doi:10.1016/S1470-2045(21)00005-X

43. Moskowitz CH, Walewski J, Nademanee A, et al. Five-year PFS from the AETHERA trial of brentuximab vedotin for Hodgkin lymphoma at high risk of progression or relapse. *Blood.* 2018;132(25):2639–2642. doi:10.1182/blood-2018-07-861641

44. Ramos CA, Grover NS, Beaven AW, et al. Anti-CD30 CAR-T cell therapy in relapsed and refractory Hodgkin lymphoma. *J Clin Oncol.* 2020;38(32):3794–3804. doi:10.1200/JCO.20.01342

45. Mundt AJ, Sibley G, Williams S, Hallahan D, Nautiyal J, Weichselbaum RR. Patterns of failure following high-dose chemotherapy and autologous bone marrow transplantation with involved field radiotherapy for relapsed/refractory Hodgkin's disease. *Int J Radiat Oncol Biol Phys.* 1995;33(2):261–270. doi:10.1016/0360-3016(95)00180-7

46. Poen JC, Hoppe RT, Horning SJ. High-dose therapy and autologous bone marrow transplantation for relapsed/refractory Hodgkin's disease: the impact of involved field radiotherapy on patterns of failure and survival. *Int J Radiat Oncol Biol Phys.* 1996;36(1):3–12. doi:10.1016/S0360-3016(96)00277-5

47. Constine LS, Yahalom J, Ng AK, et al. The role of radiation therapy in patients with relapsed or refractory Hodgkin lymphoma: guidelines from the International Lymphoma Radiation Oncology Group. *Int J Radiat Oncol Biol Phys.* 2018;100(5):1100–1118. doi:10.1016/j.ijrobp.2018.01.011

53 AGGRESSIVE NON-HODGKIN LYMPHOMA

Anirudh Bommireddy, Chirag Shah, and Sheen Cherian

QUICK HIT Non-Hodgkin lymphoma (NHL) is a heterogeneous disease. Aggressive NHL is a loosely defined group of B- and T-cell histologies with survival measured in months if untreated. T-cell histologies are aggressive but uncommon. Multiagent CHT is indicated in almost all cases of aggressive NHL. Diffuse large B-cell lymphoma (DLBCL) is the most common aggressive NHL and the subject of the majority of clinical data. Limited-stage DLBCL is typically treated with R-CHOP for either three cycles followed by ISRT to 30 to 36 Gy or R-CHOP for four to six cycles (Table 53.1). After six to eight cycles, the role of consolidative RT is controversial in the setting of a CR. Advanced-stage DLBCL can be treated with R-CHOP for six to eight cycles with consideration of consolidation RT. When selecting for consolidative RT, risk factors such as bulk (≥7.5 cm), skeletal involvement, inability to tolerate full CHT, residual disease after CHT on PET/CT, and perhaps mutational burden can be considered, although no clear standard exists. Relapsed or refractory DLBCL is typically managed with salvage chemoimmunotherapy followed by autologous stem cell transplant (SCT). Further relapse may be managed with CAR T-cell therapy or allogeneic SCT. RT can be considered in patients with oligopersistent disease considering SCT before or after transplant.

Table 53.1 General Overview of Treatment Paradigm for DLBCL	
Limited (stage I–II)	R-CHOP × 3C followed by 30–36 Gy for CR 40–50 Gy for PR or R-CHOP × 6–8C or CHOP × 4C and R × 6C
Advanced (stage III–IV)	R-CHOP × 6–8C ± ISRT 30–36 Gy
Relapsed/refractory	High-dose CHT + autologous SCT ± RT pre- or posttransplant

EPIDEMIOLOGY: There were ~80,620 cases of NHL expected in the United States in 2024 and ~20,140 deaths.[1] NHL is the seventh most common noncutaneous cancer and ninth most common cause of death. It is slightly more common in males (lifetime risk 1.26:1). Approximately 50% to 60% of NHLs are classified as aggressive. The most common forms of NHL are DLBCL (29%), follicular (26%), SLL/CLL (7%), MZL/MALT (9%), mantle cell (8%), MZL/nodal (3%), and primary mediastinal DLBCL (2%), among others.[2,3] Aggressive NHL is more common in low- and middle-income countries.

RISK FACTORS: NHL is a heterogeneous disease with a multitude of risk factors, including older age, race, family history,[4] geographic region,[3] viral infection (*EBV* [NK-T-cell, Burkitt], *HTLV-1, HHV8* [Kaposi sarcoma and various lymphomas in HIV+], *hepatitis C* [DLBCL and splenic MZL]), bacterial infection (*Helicobacter pylori* [gastric MALT], *Chlamydia psittaci* [orbital MALT], *Borrelia burgdorferi* [tick bite, mantle cell],[5] *Campylobacter jejuni* [intestinal MALT]), autoimmune disease (rheumatoid arthritis, Sjögren syndrome, lupus), immune suppression (HIV, organ transplant), medication (immunosuppressants, alkylating agents), chemicals (hair dye, pesticides), and previous CLL/hairy cell leukemia (Richter transformation into DLBCL in 5%–10%).[6]

ANATOMY: Thirteen individual nodal groups identified in 1965 now define staging and include Waldeyer's ring, cervical/supraclavicular/occipital/preauricular, infraclavicular, axillary/pectoral, mediastinal, hilar, para-aortic, spleen, mesenteric, iliac, inguinal/femoral, popliteal, and epitrochlear/brachial. Waldeyer's ring and the spleen are considered lymphatic but extranodal regions for staging purposes.

PATHOLOGY: NHL includes cancers originating from cells that normally differentiate into T or B lymphocytes, whether originating from the bone marrow or peripheral nodal tissues. Approximately 85% to 90% of NHLs derive from B-cell origins.[6] In contrast, leukemias derive from cells that differentiate into erythrocytes, monocytes, or granulocytes. Originally, it was thought that leukemia arose from the bone marrow and lymphoma from a mass lesion. Today, cell lineage, morphology, genetics, and immunotyping classify leukemia and lymphomas. Over 60 types of NHL are identified in the WHO 2016 classification, which does not attempt to differentiate into aggressive/indolent due to variable clinical behavior.[7] Additionally, many treat grade 3B follicular lymphoma similar to DLBCL.[8]

GENETICS: See Table 53.2.

Table 53.2 Common Translocations, Immunotype, and Clinical Pearls for Select "Aggressive" Non-Hodgkin Lymphomas				
Histology		**Classic Genetics and Implications**	**Classic Immunotype**	**Pearls**
B-cell	**DLBCL**	t(14:18), BCL2, BCL6, ALK, many others	CD19+, CD20+, CD45+	Most common NHL. WHO 2016 subtypes: EBV+, germinal center, activated, primary cutaneous, ALK+, HHV8+, "double-hit" (rearrangements of MYC and BCL2 or BCL6). Rare "triple-hit" subtype (MYC, BCL2, and BCL6) associated with dismal prognosis. Gray zone lymphoma is intermediate between DLBCL and HL.
	Primary mediastinal (thymic) DLBCL	No classic translocations	CD19+, CD20+, CD5–	Anterior mediastinal (thymic) mass most common in young women. Treatment different from DLBCL.
	Mantle cell	t(11:14), cyclin D1	CD19+, CD20+, CD5+	Older age and advanced stage more common. Radiosensitive.
	Burkitt	t(8:14) → C-MYC (transcription factor)	CD19+, CD20+, CD5–, CD10+	Classic "starry sky" appearance. Most common NHL in children, endemic type in Africa (jaw, EBV+). Also, nonendemic (abdomen, visceral organs) and immune-deficient types.
	Follicular (FL), grade 3B	Grade 3B genetically distinct from grades 1–3A	CD19+, CD20+	High-grade FL (especially grade 3B) is often treated per DLBCL paradigm (grades 1–3A managed as per low-grade NHL paradigm).
T-cell	**Peripheral T-cell, NOS (PTCL)**	t(7:14), t(11:14), or t(14:14)	Variable T-cell (±CD 2, 3, 4, 5, 7)	Most common peripheral T-cell, older adults.
	Anaplastic large cell	t(2:5) → ALK	CD30+, EMA+	More common in kids, good prognosis with ALK+. T-cell neoplasm.
	Angioimmunoblastic	No classic translocations	CD4+	Older adults.
	Extranodal NK-T-cell, nasal type	LOH 6q	CD2+, CD56+	More common in Asian males. EBV+ (EBER by FISH).
Either	**Lymphoblastic lymphoma/leukemia**	t(1:19), t(9:22)	TdT+	Nodal presentation of ALL and treated similarly. Can be T- or B-cell presentation.

CLINICAL PRESENTATION: Most commonly presents with a painless enlarging LN. B symptoms (fever >38°C, drenching night sweats, weight loss >10% in 6 months) or numerous other symptoms may be present (fatigue, anemia, pain, cord compression, SVC syndrome, etc.) depending on location and degree of involvement.

WORKUP: H&P with attention to constitutional symptoms (B symptoms), enlarged LNs, or hepatosplenomegaly.

Labs: CBC, CMP, β2 microglobulin, LDH, uric acid, hepatitis B testing (reactivation with rituximab), pregnancy test. LP with flow cytometry if symptomatic, testicular involvement, double-hit, HIV-associated, or epidural lymphoma (see CNS prognostic model for risk factors).[9]

Imaging: PET/CT is standard in almost all lymphoma histologies except certain low-grade histologies (extranodal MZL and SLL).[8,10,11] Uptake (SUV >10) in indolent lymphoma suggests transformation.[12,13] CT with contrast should also be obtained. Echocardiogram or MUGA if CHT dictates. EBV viral load for extranodal NK/T-cell, nasal type.

Biopsy: At least a core needle biopsy but preferably excisional biopsy should be performed for adequate pathologic evaluation, including morphology, nodal architecture, genomic profiling, and immunoprofiling. FNA is insufficient. A negative PET is usually sufficient at ruling out bone marrow involvement of DLBCL.[14,15] Bone marrow biopsy remains standard for most other NHLs (~20% risk of BM involvement for aggressive NHL vs. 50%–80% of indolent NHLs).

PROGNOSTIC FACTORS: Age, bulk (classically defined as ≥10 cm or >⅓ thoracic diameter, but more recently defined as ≥7.5 cm), and stage (see Table 53.5). DLBCL with *MYC* plus *BCL2* and/or *BCL6* rearrangements are classified as "double-hit" or "triple-hit" lymphomas and are associated with poor prognosis.[7] Germinal center subtype is more favorable than nongerminal center as defined by tissue microarray (combination of CD10, BCL6, and MUM1).[16] Multiple prognostic models exist for patients with aggressive NHL treated with CHT (Tables 53.3 and 53.4). The IPI[17] is classic (mnemonic "LEAPS": **L**DH, **e**xtranodal sites, **a**ge, **p**erformance status, and **s**tage). While the original IPI remains standard, modified indices such as the age-adjusted IPI, stage-adjusted IPI, and NCCN-IPI may have improved prognostic utility. For DLBCL, a prognostic index using baseline metabolic tumor volume, age, and stage performed better than IPI and was also better at defining a high-risk group (3-year PFS 46% vs. 58% and 3-year OS 52% vs. 66% for the new model and IPI, respectively).[18] Mantle cell may be best classified using the MIPI.[19] The Deauville (5-point) score is used to interpret PET scans and is prognostic, particularly at the end of treatment. This consists of five levels. Level 1 includes no uptake above background; level 2 is uptake less than or equal to mediastinal blood pool; level 3 is uptake above mediastinal blood pool but less than or equal to liver uptake; level 4 is uptake moderately above liver; and level 5 is uptake markedly greater than liver or new lesions.[20]

NATURAL HISTORY: Aggressive lymphoma, loosely defined, includes cancers with survival measured in months if untreated, as compared with indolent lymphoma, with survival measured in years. Compared with Hodgkin lymphoma (HL), the pattern of spread is less predictable and can skip nodal levels/sites.

Table 53.3 Classic IPI Prognostic System (1993[17]) and NCCN-IPI (2014[21]) for Aggressive NHL					
	IPI		**Age-Adjusted IPI**		**NCCN-IPI**	
	Factor	**Score**	**Factor**	**Score**	**Factor**	**Score**
Age	>60	1	*N/A*	1	>40 to ≤60 >60 to <75 ≥75	1 2 3
LDH	High	1	High	1	>1× ULN but ≤3× ULN >3× ULN	1 2
Extranodal sites	≥2	1	*N/A*	1	Bone marrow, CNS, liver/GI tract, lung	1
Performance status (ECOG)	≥2	1	≥2	1	≥2	1
Stage (Ann Arbor)	III–IV	1	III–IV	1	I–II vs. III–IV	1

Source: International Non-Hodgkin's Lymphoma Prognostic Factors P. A predictive model for aggressive non-Hodgkin's lymphoma. *N Engl J Med.* 1993;329(14):987–994. doi:10.1056/NEJM199309303291402; Zhou Z, Sehn LH, Rademaker AW, et al. An enhanced International Prognostic Index (NCCN-IPI) for patients with diffuse large B-cell lymphoma treated in the rituximab era. *Blood.* 2014;123(6):837–842. doi:10.1182/blood-2013-09-524108.

Table 53.4 Aggressive NHL Outcome by IPI Score (See Table 53.3 for Risk Factors)

Risk Group	Original IPI (Pre-Rituximab)[17]			Age-Adjusted IPI[17]				IPI in Rituximab Era[22]			NCCN-IPI[21]		
	Score	5-Yr OS	5-Yr RFS	Score	5-Yr OS (≤60 Yrs Old)	5-Yr OS (>60 Yrs Old)	5-Yr RFS	Score	3-Yr OS	3-Yr PFS	Score	5-Yr OS	5-Yr PFS
Low	0–1	73%	70%	0	83%	56%	86%	0–1	91%	87%	0–1	96%	91%
Low–intermediate	2	51%	50%	1	69%	44%	66%	2	81%	75%	2–3	82%	74%
High–intermediate	3	43%	49%	2	46%	37%	53%	3	65%	59%	4–5	64%	51%
High	4–5	26%	40%	3	32%	21%	58%	4–5	59%	56%	6	33%	30%

STAGING: See Table 53.5.

Table 53.5 Ann Arbor (Lugano) Staging System for Lymphoma[†]

I	One node or a group of adjacent nodes OR single extranodal lesions without nodal involvement (IE)	**A*:** No systemic symptoms **B*:** Unexplained weight loss >10% in 6 months before diagnosis; unexplained fever with temperatures above 38°C; drenching night sweats **E*:** Extranodal involvement **X*:** Bulky disease (*Hodgkin: >10 cm or mediastinal mass more than one-third the maximum thoracic diameter at T5–6 on PA CXR*)
II	≥2 nodal groups on the same side of the diaphragm OR stage I or II by nodal extent with limited contiguous extranodal involvement	
III	Nodes on both sides of the diaphragm; nodes above the diaphragm with spleen involvement	
IV	Additional noncontiguous extralymphatic involvement	

*Note that 2014 Lugano update suggests "X" and "A/B" modifiers are no longer necessary for NHL, and "E" is unnecessary for stages III–IV disease.[23]
†Number of involved regions may be designated with a subscript (i.e., II_3).
Source: Adapted from Cheson BD, Fisher RI, Barrington SF, et al. Recommendations for initial evaluation, staging, and response assessment of Hodgkin and non-Hodgkin lymphoma: the Lugano classification. *J Clin Oncol.* 2014;32(27): 3059–3068. doi:10.1200/JCO.2013.54.8800.

TREATMENT PARADIGM

Observation: Unlike indolent lymphomas, there is generally no role for observation of aggressive lymphomas. Notable exceptions may include mantle cell with a low tumor burden.[24]

Surgery: Generally, the role of surgery is limited to excisional biopsy.

Chemotherapy: CHT is the backbone of treatment for NHL. See Table 53.6 for regimens. Rituximab is an anti-CD20 antibody that consistently demonstrated in the early 2000s improvement in 5-year OS for DLBCL by approximately 10%, with minimal increase in toxicity.[25–27] R-CHOP: rituximab, cyclophosphamide, doxorubicin, vincristine, and prednisone, often given q21 days for 6C. Per FLYER trial, CHOP × 4C and R × 6C is equivalent to R-CHOP × 6C, reducing toxicity from CHOP.[28] R-EPOCH consists of the same agents as R-CHOP but with etoposide and overall, across subtypes of DLBCL, did not demonstrate a benefit compared with R-CHOP in the CALGB/Alliance 50303 trial (although it is still an option in other subtypes; e.g., primary mediastinal DLBCL or double-hit DLBCL). Pola-R-CHP was shown to have an improved PFS compared with standard R-CHOP (77% vs. 70%) in previously untreated DLBCL with no difference in OS (88.7% vs. 88.6%).[29] Consolidation with autologous SCT is not routinely recommended for DLBCL but can be considered for "double-hit" type.[30] CNS prophylaxis can be delivered to high-risk patients via systemic MTX, intrathecal MTX, or cytarabine.[8–10]

Table 53.6 Example Regimens for Aggressive Non-Hodgkin Lymphoma

Diagnosis	Common/Example CHT Regimens	Notes
DLBCL, germinal center type	R-CHOP × 6C ± RT	Good outcomes with standard R-CHOP; Pola-R-CHP improved PFS compared with R-CHOP without difference in OS
	R-CHOP × 3C + RT	
	Pola-R-CHP × 6C + R × 2C ± RT	

(continued)

Table 53.6 Example Regimens for Aggressive Non-Hodgkin Lymphoma (*continued*)

Diagnosis	Common/Example CHT Regimens	Notes
DLBCL, activated B-cell type	R-CHOP × 6–8C ± RT	Studies suggest inferior outcomes with standard R-CHOP, some intensify CHT
	R-ACVBP + MTX/Leucovorin[31]	
	R-CHOP + lenalidomide[32]	
	Pola-R-CHP × 6C + R × 2C ± RT	
DLBCL, "double-hit" (MYC and BCL2 or BCL6) or "triple-hit" (MYC, BCL2, and BCL6)	R-EPOCH	Outcomes with standard R-CHOP are inferior, consider CNS prophylaxis or autologous SCT
	R-Hyper-CVAD	
	Pola-R-CHP × 6C + R × 2C ± RT	
DLBCL, transformed follicular	R-CHOP × 6C ± RT	Diagnosis: Biopsy regions of PET SUV >10[13]
Follicular, grade 3B	R-CHOP ± RT	Per DLBCL paradigm
Primary mediastinal DLBCL	R-EPOCH × 6C ± RT[33]	
	R-CHOP × 6C + RT	
Mantle cell	R-CHOP + autologous SCT[34]	
	R-Hyper-CVAD/cytarabine/MTX[35]	
	R-CHOP + RT	Select stages I–II patients
	R-CHOP	Not curative
	Bendamustine + rituximab	
	Many others	
Burkitt	CODOX-M[36]	
	CALGB regimen[37]	
	R-EPOCH[38]	
	Hyper-CVAD[39]	
Extranodal NK-T-cell, nasal type	SMILE + RT[40]	
	DeVIC + concurrent RT[41]	
	GELOX + sandwich RT[42]	

Radiation

Definitions: Involved-field RT (IFRT) preceded the standard use of CT simulation and was based on fluoroscopy and bony landmarks. Involved-nodal RT (INRT) was introduced in Europe for HL and markedly reduced the irradiated volume. INRT design requires accurate pre-CHT or pre-biopsy information obtained in the treatment position. Involved-site RT (ISRT) evolved because detailed pre-CHT information and imaging is not always optimal in standard clinical practice. Compared with INRT, ISRT volumes are slightly larger to ensure coverage of all initially involved tissue. In most situations, ISRT will include significantly smaller volumes than IFRT.

Indications: The role of RT in aggressive NHL is either for consolidation or for palliation. For select patients unable to receive CHT or in early-stage mantle cell lymphoma, definitive RT may be appropriate. RT decisions should incorporate the CHT regimen chosen and response to induction therapy. Historical technique was IFRT; the modern technique is now ISRT (when treated after CHT). ILROG guidelines delineate the technique for ISRT.[43] See Table 53.7 for RT dosing.

Dose

Table 53.7 NCCN RT Dose Guidelines for Aggressive Non-Hodgkin Lymphoma[8,10]

Mantle cell, stage I–II	RT alone	30–36 Gy
DLBCL*	Consolidation after CR	30–36 Gy
	Consolidation after PR	40–50 Gy

(*continued*)

Table 53.7 NCCN RT Dose Guidelines for Aggressive Non-Hodgkin Lymphoma[8,10] (*continued*)		
	Primary treatment (non-CHT candidate)	40–55 Gy
	Combined with SCT	20–36 Gy
	Scrotal RT after CHT	25–30 Gy
Peripheral T-cell lymphoma	Consolidation	30–40 Gy
Extranodal NK-T-cell, nasal type	Concurrent with DeVIC	50 Gy
	Sequential after SMILE	45–50.4 Gy
	After GELOX	56 Gy
	RT alone	≥50 Gy

*Note that grade 3B follicular lymphoma is often managed according to DLBCL paradigm.
Source: NCCN Clinical Practice Guidelines: B-Cell Lymphoma. Version 2.2025; NCCN Clinical Practice Guidelines: T-Cell Lymphomas. Version 1.2025.

Toxicity: Acute: fatigue, skin erythema, other sequelae are site-dependent. Late: site-dependent but includes second malignancy, xerostomia, fibrosis, cardiotoxicity, and so on.

Procedure: See *Handbook of Treatment Planning in Radiation Oncology*, Chapter 10.[44]

EVIDENCE-BASED Q&A

Historically, what data exist regarding the role of RT in DLBCL?

Three cooperative groups (SWOG, ECOG, French GELA) investigated the role of consolidative IFRT after CHT with variable results in the pre-rituximab era.[45–49] RT was effective at reducing in-field relapses but only improved OS in the initial results of one trial (SWOG), although these studies used higher doses and older RT techniques. Overall, it appears that less intense CHT with RT is comparable to intensive CHT alone. Toxicity is significant with intense CHT; therefore, combined modality treatment may be ideal for some patients.

What was the impact of rituximab on outcomes with CHT alone?

The preceding historical trials evaluating the role of RT were performed in the pre-rituximab era. The introduction of rituximab in the early 2000s markedly improved outcomes above CHOP alone, with ~10% improvement in OS at 5 years.[25–27,50] Therefore, many argue consolidation with RT is unnecessary, although there is no level I evidence to support this conclusion at this time.

How many cycles of R-CHOP are necessary for DLBCL?

Trials performed either six or eight cycles for DLBCL given every 21 days. The RICOVER-60 trial directly addressed this question.

Pfreundschuh, RICOVER-60 (*Lancet Oncol* 2008, PMID 18226581): PRT of 1,222 patients, 61 to 80 years, with aggressive B-cell lymphoma; 2 × 2 randomization: CHOP vs. R-CHOP and 6C vs. 8C (both q14 days, rather than conventional q21 days). IFRT to 36 Gy was recommended to sites initially ≥7.5 cm (bulky) or extranodal sites regardless of response. R-CHOP improved DFS and OS with no difference between 6C vs. 8C. **Conclusion: 6C of R-CHOP is the preferred regimen for older adult patients.**

Can R-CHOP be de-escalated to reduce toxicity in early-stage aggressive B-cell NHL?

In the FLYER trial, CHOP × 4C and R × 6C maintained efficacy compared with R-CHOP × 6C while reducing toxicity rates. No RT was planned except for treatment of testicular lymphoma.[28]

Poeschel, FLYER (*Lancet* 2019, PMID 31868632): Phase III noninferiority trial of patients aged 18 to 60 years with stage I to II disease, normal serum LDH concentration, ECOG performance status 0 to 1, and without bulky disease randomized to receive either 6C of R-CHOP or 4C of R-CHOP plus two additional cycles of rituximab. No RT was planned except for treatment of testicular lymphoma. *N* = 592; MFU = 66 months. The 3-year PFS was 96% for 4C of R-CHOP plus two doses of rituximab vs. 93% for 6C of R-CHOP. Adverse events were lower in the 4C group

(294 hematologic and 1,036 nonhematologic for 4C vs. 426 hematologic and 1,280 nonhematologic for 6C). **Conclusion: 4C of CHOP and 6C of rituximab are noninferior in terms of PFS to 6C of R-CHOP, with reduced toxicity.**

Is consolidative RT necessary for early-stage DLBCL in the rituximab era?

This is a controversial question and use of RT is limited to selected patients.[51] No high-quality data exist to guide decisions. Multiple retrospective studies, including data from NCDB, SEER, and NCCN, support the role of RT.[51–58] The UNFOLDER trial found that consolidative RT to extralymphatic and bulky disease confers an EFS benefit in patients with intermediate prognosis aggressive B-cell lymphoma, but response was assessed without PET/CT and therefore results are difficult to apply in the modern era.[59] Consolidative RT should be considered in patients with bulky disease (most commonly defined as >7.5 cm), limited skeletal involvement, inability to tolerate full CHT, residual disease after CHT on PET/CT, and perhaps genetic factors.[60]

Held, RICOVER-60 NoRTh (*JCO* 2014, PMID 24493716): After the completion of the RICOVER-60 trial (see above), the protocol was amended, and another 166 patients were accrued to the best arm of the RICOVER-60 trial (R-CHOP × 6C q14 days) but omitting RT. The arm from the original trial (RT arm) was compared with the no-RT cohort. MFU 39 months. MVA in the per-protocol population demonstrated worse EFS, PFS, and OS in those with bulky disease not treated with RT. **Conclusion: RT should be used in all patients with bulky disease.**

Held, German Pooled Analysis (*JCO* 2013, PMID 24062391): Pooled analysis of data from nine randomized trials including 3,840 patients with aggressive B-cell lymphoma; 8% had skeletal involvement. Skeletal involvement was associated with worse EFS after R-CHOP (EFS HR 1.5, p = .05). Rituximab was not found to improve the outcome for patients with skeletal involvement. RT did improve EFS for patients with skeletal involvement (EFS HR 0.3, p = .001; OS HR 0.5, p = .111). **Conclusion: RT may benefit those with skeletal involvement.**

Lamy, 02–03 Lysa/Goelams Group (*Blood* 2018, PMID 29061568): Patients with nonbulky (<7 cm) stage I to II DLBCL treated with R-CHOP for 4C (IPI of 0) or 6C (IPI >0) and then randomized to 40 Gy IFRT or observation. Patients with PR (PET-assessed) after 4C received 6C total and RT. At an MFU of 64 months, intention-to-treat analysis showed no difference in primary endpoint 5-year EFS (89% no RT vs. 92% with RT; p = .18). **Conclusion: Among patients with nonbulky stage I to II DLBCL who achieve CR after R-CHOP × 4–6C, observation is noninferior to consolidative RT.**

Intergroup National Clinical Trials Network Study S1001 (*JCO* 2020, PMID PMC7479758): Phase II trial including 132 eligible patients with nonbulky (<10 cm) stage I to II DLBCL who underwent R-CHOP × 3C followed by interim PET/CT. Those with negative PET/CT (Deauville 1–3) received R-CHOP × 1C without consolidative RT, while those with positive PET/CT (Deauville 4–5) received IFRT (36–45 Gy) followed by ibritumomab tiuxetan. PET negativity rate was 86% after R-CHOP × 3C. The 5-year PFS was 89% among patients who were PET-negative and received R-CHOP × 4C and 86% among patients who were PET/CT-positive and received consolidative RT followed by ibritumomab tiuxetan. **Conclusion: Consolidative RT can be considered for patients with low-risk DLBCL with residual PET-positive disease after R-CHOP × 3C, achieving similar PFS to patients who PET-negativize.**

Is there a role for consolidative RT for advanced-stage DLBCL?

This is also a controversial question with less data available. NCCN suggests R-CHOP for 6C and, if CR is confirmed on PET, to consider RT to initially bulky sites or areas of skeletal involvement. RICOVER-60 provides the best data for this, as it included all stages (60% in the no-RT cohort were stage III–IV). Retrospective data from MD Anderson,[61] Duke,[54] and observational data from the NCCN database also suggest a benefit.[58]

What is the optimal RT dose?

Classic trials often used doses >40 Gy, but modern doses are lower. NCCN guidelines recommend 40 to 55 Gy for primary treatment without chemoimmunotherapy or for refractory disease. Consolidation after chemoimmunotherapy include doses of 30 to 36 Gy for CR or 36 to 50 Gy for PR. Current studies are investigating dose de-escalation with doses as low as 20 Gy.[62]

Lowry, UK (*Radiother Oncol* 2011, PMID 21664710): PRT with any histologic subtype of NHL requiring RT for LC; 640 sites were randomized to either high-dose RT to 40–45 Gy/20–23 fx vs. low-dose RT (30 Gy/15 fx for aggressive histologies and 24 Gy/12 fx for indolent histologies). MFU 5.6 years. No difference in response rates, in-field progression, PFS, or OS. Toxicity was reduced (but not SS) in the low-dose arm. **Conclusion: 24 Gy and 30 Gy are sufficient for indolent and aggressive NHL, respectively.**

How should response to treatment be evaluated for patients with NHL? Is interim PET predictive of outcome?

The updated Lugano classification[23] defines both staging and response assessment. See the manuscript for details, but in brief a CR should be defined as Deauville 1 to 3, without new lesions, no abnormal bone marrow uptake, regression of the nodal size to ≤1.5 cm in longest diameter, and no organomegaly. A Deauville 3 is usually sufficient but may be considered abnormal if reduced-intensity CHT is used. Of note, a midtreatment PET is not clearly predictive of outcome (as opposed to HL), and it is not recommended that therapy be altered due to the midtreatment PET.[60]

How is primary mediastinal DLBCL managed?

Primary mediastinal DLBCL is a different entity from other forms of DLBCL and has a natural history between NHL and HL. It should be managed with either R-EPOCH CHT for 6 to 8C or R-CHOP for 6C + RT.[8,33] There are minimal data investigating the omission of RT in these patients. Like HL, midtreatment PET/CT is prognostic.[63]

Martelli, IELSG37 (*JCO* 2024, PMID 39159403): PRT of 545 patients with primary mediastinal DLBCL who received standard immunochemotherapy, and those with complete metabolic response randomized to observation vs. 30 Gy consolidative RT. Those without complete metabolic response received RT. PFS at 30 months for complete responders (*n* = 268, 49%) was 98.5% with RT and 96% with observation. The 5-year OS was 99% in both arms of complete responders. **Conclusion: About half of the patients with primary mediastinal DLBCL had a CR to chemoimmunotherapy, and those patients had excellent early outcomes with omission of consolidative RT.**

How is primary cutaneous B-cell lymphoma leg type managed?

PCLBCL leg type is a rare and highly aggressive form of cutaneous lymphoma and typically presents with nodules on one or both legs, although 10% to 15% may present outside of the lower extremities. Typical management for limited-stage disease includes R-CHOP × 3–6C followed by 30 to 36 Gy for CR or 40 to 45 Gy for PR.

How is testicular DLBCL managed?

Primary testicular DLBCL is an uncommon disease comprising just 1% to 2% of NHL cases. Although most patients present with early-stage disease, outcomes are generally poor. Relapse in extranodal sites including the CNS and contralateral testis remains a clinical challenge. The current treatment paradigm defined by the phase II IELSG-10 trial consists of orchiectomy, R-CHOP, CNS prophylaxis, and prophylactic RT to the contralateral testis.[64] No testicular relapses were observed on trial. RT typically consists of 30 Gy to the entire scrotum.

How is primary bone DLBCL managed?

Primary lymphoma of the bone accounts for <2% of adult lymphomas and the vast majority are DLBCL of the germinal center subtype. Treatment historically consisted of multiagent CHT followed by RT, although the role of RT in the rituximab era is less clear. Typical management for limited-stage disease includes R-CHOP × 3–6C followed by 30 to 36 Gy for CR or 40 to 45 Gy for PR.

How is CAR T-cell therapy delivered and what role does it play in relapsed refractory DLBCL? What role does RT play as bridging therapy?

CAR T-cell therapy is a form of adoptive cellular transfer immunotherapy, whereby autologous T-cells are harvested from a patient and genetically engineered to express chimeric antigen receptor molecules targeting a specific antigen of interest on malignant cells, in particular CD19 for DLBCL. The workflow begins with leukapheresis (collection of T-cells); CAR T-cell production, which can take a minimum of 2 weeks; and lympho-depleting CHT for several days prior to CAR T-cell infusion. CD19-directed CAR T-cell therapies are FDA-approved for relapsed refractory DLBCL. Phase II trials (JULIET [NCT02445248], ZUMA-1 [NCT02348216], and TRANSCEND-NHL-001 [NCT02631044]) show ORR of 52% to 82% and CR rates of 40% to 54%.

During the period of time between leukapheresis and infusion, bridging therapies, such as steroids, CHT, targeted therapy, immunotherapy, and RT, may be used for palliation and prevent disease progression. Several single institutional series show that RT is feasible and does not compromise CAR T-cell outcomes. Indications for bridging RT include palliation of symptomatic disease, cytoreduction of bulky disease, and treatment of localized refractory disease.[65,66]

REFERENCES

1. Siegel RL, Giaquinto AN, Jemal A. Cancer statistics, 2024. *CA Cancer J Clin.* 2024;74(1):12–49. doi:10.3322/caac.21820
2. Armitage JO, Weisenburger DD. New approach to classifying non-Hodgkin's lymphomas: clinical features of the major histologic subtypes. Non-Hodgkin's lymphoma classification project. *J Clin Oncol.* 1998;16(8):2780–2795. doi:10.1200/JCO.1998.16.8.2780
3. Perry AM, Diebold J, Nathwani BN, et al. Non-Hodgkin lymphoma in the developing world: review of 4539 cases from the International non-Hodgkin lymphoma classification project. *Haematologica.* 2016; 101(10):1244–1250. doi:10.3324/haematol.2016.148809
4. Cerhan JR, Slager SL. Familial predisposition and genetic risk factors for lymphoma. *Blood.* 12 2015; 126(20):2265–2273. doi:10.1182/blood-2015-04-537498
5. Schollkopf C, Melbye M, Munksgaard L, et al. Borrelia infection and risk of non-Hodgkin lymphoma. *Blood.* 2008;111(12):5524–5529. doi:10.1182/blood-2007-08-109611
6. Armitage JO, Gascoyne RD, Lunning MA, Cavalli F. Non-Hodgkin lymphoma. *Lancet.* 2017;390(10091): 298–310. doi:10.1016/S0140-6736(16)32407-2
7. Swerdlow SH, Campo E, Pileri SA, et al. The 2016 revision of the World Health Organization classification of lymphoid neoplasms. *Blood.* 2016;127(20):2375–2390. doi:10.1182/blood-2016-01-643569
8. NCCN Clinical Practice Guidelines: B-Cell Lymphoma . Version 2.2025. Accessed January 2025. https://www.nccn.org/professionals/physician_gls/pdf/b-cell.pdf
9. Savage KJZS, Kansara RR, et al. Validation of a prognostic model to assess the risk of CNS disease in patients with aggressive B-Cell lymphoma. *Blood.* 2014;124(21):394. doi:10.1182/blood.v124.21.394.394
10. NCCN Clinical Practice Guidelines: T-Cell Lymphomas. Version 1.2025. Accessed January 2025. https://www.nccn.org/professionals/physician_gls/pdf/t-cell.pdf
11. Weiler-Sagie M, Bushelev O, Epelbaum R, et al. (18)F-FDG avidity in lymphoma readdressed: a study of 766 patients. *J Nucl Med.* 2010;51(1):25–30. doi:10.2967/jnumed.109.067892
12. Noy A, Schoder H, Gonen M, et al. The majority of transformed lymphomas have high Standardized Uptake Values (SUVs) on Positron Emission Tomography (PET) scanning similar to Diffuse Large B-Cell Lymphoma (DLBCL). *Ann Oncol.* 2009;20(3):508–512. doi:10.1093/annonc/mdn657
13. Schoder H, Noy A, Gonen M, et al. Intensity of 18fluorodeoxyglucose uptake in positron emission tomography distinguishes between indolent and aggressive non-Hodgkin's lymphoma. *J Clin Oncol.* 2005; 23(21):4643–4651. doi:10.1200/JCO.2005.12.072
14. Khan AB, Barrington SF, Mikhaeel NG, et al. PET-CT staging of DLBCL accurately identifies and provides new insight into the clinical significance of bone marrow involvement. *Blood.* 2013;122(1):61–67. doi:10.1182/blood-2012-12-473389
15. Alzahrani M, El-Galaly TC, Hutchings M, et al. The value of routine bone marrow biopsy in patients with diffuse large B-cell lymphoma staged with PET/CT: a Danish-Canadian study. *Ann Oncol.* 2016;27(6):1095–1099. doi:10.1093/annonc/mdw137
16. Hans CP, Weisenburger DD, Greiner TC, et al. Confirmation of the molecular classification of diffuse large B-cell lymphoma by immunohistochemistry using a tissue microarray. *Blood.* 2004;103(1):275–282. doi:10.1182/blood-2003-05-1545
17. International Non-Hodgkin's Lymphoma Prognostic Factors P. A predictive model for aggressive non-Hodgkin's lymphoma. *N Engl J Med.* 1993;329(14):987–994. doi:10.1056/NEJM199309303291402
18. Mikhaeel NG, Heymans MW, Eertink JJ, et al. Proposed new dynamic prognostic index for diffuse large B-cell lymphoma: international metabolic prognostic index. *J Clin Oncol.* 2022;40(21):2352–2360. doi:10.1200/JCO.21.02063
19. Hoster E, Dreyling M, Klapper W, et al. A new prognostic index (MIPI) for patients with advanced-stage mantle cell lymphoma. *Blood.* 2008;111(2):558–565. doi:10.1182/blood-2007-06-095331
20. Meignan M, Gallamini A, Meignan M, Gallamini A, Haioun C. Report on the First International Workshop on Interim-PET-scan in lymphoma. *Leuk Lymphoma.* 2009;50(8):1257–1260. doi:10.1080/10428190903040048

21. Zhou Z, Sehn LH, Rademaker AW, et al. An enhanced International Prognostic Index (NCCN-IPI) for patients with diffuse large B-cell lymphoma treated in the rituximab era. *Blood*. 2014;123(6):837–842. doi:10.1182/blood-2013-09-524108

22. Ziepert M, Hasenclever D, Kuhnt E, et al. Standard International prognostic index remains a valid predictor of outcome for patients with aggressive CD20+ B-cell lymphoma in the rituximab era. *J Clin Oncol*. 2010;28(14):2373–2380. doi:10.1200/JCO.2009.26.2493

23. Cheson BD, Fisher RI, Barrington SF, et al. Recommendations for initial evaluation, staging, and response assessment of Hodgkin and non-Hodgkin lymphoma: the Lugano classification. *J Clin Oncol*. 2014;32(27):3059–3068. doi:10.1200/JCO.2013.54.8800

24. Martin P, Chadburn A, Christos P, et al. Outcome of deferred initial therapy in mantle-cell lymphoma. *J Clin Oncol*. 2009;27(8):1209–1213. doi:10.1200/JCO.2008.19.6121

25. Habermann TM, Weller EA, Morrison VA, et al. Rituximab-CHOP versus CHOP alone or with maintenance rituximab in older patients with diffuse large B-cell lymphoma. *J Clin Oncol*. 2006;24(19):3121–3127. doi:10.1200/JCO.2005.05.1003

26. Feugier P, Van Hoof A, Sebban C, et al. Long-term results of the R-CHOP study in the treatment of elderly patients with diffuse large B-cell lymphoma: a study by the Groupe d'Etude des Lymphomes de l'Adulte. *J Clin Oncol*.2005;23(18):4117–4126. doi:10.1200/JCO.2005.09.131

27. Coiffier B, Lepage E, Briere J, et al. CHOP chemotherapy plus rituximab compared with CHOP alone in elderly patients with diffuse large-B-cell lymphoma. *N Engl J Med*. 2002;346(4):235–242. doi:10.1056/NEJMoa011795

28. Poeschel V, Held G, Ziepert M, et al. Four versus six cycles of CHOP chemotherapy in combination with six applications of rituximab in patients with aggressive B-cell lymphoma with favourable prognosis (FLYER): a randomised, phase 3, non-inferiority trial. *Lancet*. 2019;394(10216):2271–2281. doi:10.1016/S0140-6736(19)33008-9

29. Tilly H, Morschhauser F, Sehn LH, et al. Polatuzumab vedotin in previously untreated diffuse large B-cell lymphoma. *N Engl J Med*. 2022;386(4):351–363. doi:10.1056/NEJMoa2115304

30. Greb A, Bohlius J, Schiefer D, Schwarzer G, Schulz H, Engert A. High-dose chemotherapy with autologous stem cell transplantation in the first line treatment of aggressive Non-Hodgkin Lymphoma (NHL) in adults. *Cochrane Database Syst Rev*. 2008;2008(1):CD004024. doi:10.1002/14651858.CD004024.pub2

31. Recher C, Coiffier B, Haioun C, et al. Intensified chemotherapy with ACVBP plus rituximab versus standard CHOP plus rituximab for the treatment of diffuse large B-cell lymphoma (LNH03-2B): an open-label randomised phase 3 trial. *Lancet*. 2011;378(9806):1858–1867. doi:10.1016/S0140-6736(11)61040-4

32. Vitolo U, Chiappella A, Franceschetti S, et al. Lenalidomide plus R-CHOP21 in elderly patients with untreated diffuse large B-cell lymphoma: results of the REAL07 open-label, multicentre, phase 2 trial. *Lancet Oncol*. 2014;15(7):730–737. doi:10.1016/S1470-2045(14)70191-3

33. Dunleavy K, Pittaluga S, Maeda LS, et al. Dose-adjusted EPOCH rituximab therapy in primary mediastinal B-cell lymphoma. *N Engl J Med*. 2013;368(15):1408–1416. doi:10.1056/NEJMoa1214561

34. Fenske TS, Zhang MJ, Carreras J, et al. Autologous or reduced-intensity conditioning allogeneic hematopoietic cell transplantation for chemotherapy-sensitive mantle-cell lymphoma: analysis of transplantation timing and modality. *J Clin Oncol*. 2014;32(4):273–281. doi:10.1200/JCO.2013.49.2454

35. Khouri IF, Romaguera J, Kantarjian H, et al. Hyper-CVAD and high-dose methotrexate/cytarabine followed by stem-cell transplantation: an active regimen for aggressive mantle-cell lymphoma. *J Clin Oncol*. 1998;16(12):3803–3809. doi:10.1200/JCO.1998.16.12.3803

36. Evens AM, Carson KR, Kolesar J, et al. A multicenter phase II study incorporating high-dose rituximab and liposomal doxorubicin into the CODOX-M/IVAC regimen for untreated Burkitt's lymphoma. *Ann Oncol*. 2013;24(12):3076–3081. doi:10.1093/annonc/mdt414

37. Rizzieri DA, Johnson JL, Byrd JC, et al. Improved efficacy using rituximab and brief duration, high intensity chemotherapy with filgrastim support for Burkitt or aggressive lymphomas: cancer and Leukemia Group B study 10 002. *Br J Haematol*. 2014;165(1):102–111. doi:10.1111/bjh.12736

38. Dunleavy K, Pittaluga S, Shovlin M, et al. Low-intensity therapy in adults with Burkitt's lymphoma. *N Engl J Med*. 2013;369(20):1915–1925. doi:10.1056/NEJMoa1308392

39. Thomas DA, Faderl S, O'Brien S, et al. Chemoimmunotherapy with hyper-CVAD plus rituximab for the treatment of adult Burkitt and Burkitt-type lymphoma or acute lymphoblastic leukemia. *Cancer*. 2006;106(7):1569–1580. doi:10.1002/cncr.21776

40. Yamaguchi M, Kwong YL, Kim WS, et al. Phase II study of SMILE chemotherapy for newly diagnosed stage IV, relapsed, or refractory extranodal Natural Killer (NK)/T-cell lymphoma, nasal type: the NK-cell tumor study group study. *J Clin Oncol*. 2011;29(33):4410–4416. doi:10.1200/JCO.2011.35.6287

41. Yamaguchi M, Tobinai K, Oguchi M, et al. Concurrent chemoradiotherapy for localized nasal natural killer/T-cell lymphoma: an updated analysis of the Japan Clinical Oncology group study JCOG0211. *J Clin Oncol*. 2012;30(32):4044–4046. doi:10.1200/JCO.2012.45.6541

42. Bi XW, Xia Y, Zhang WW, et al. Radiotherapy and PGEMOX/GELOX regimen improved prognosis in elderly patients with early-stage extranodal NK/T-cell lymphoma. *Ann Hematol*. 2015;94(9):1525–1533. doi:10.1007/s00277-015-2395-y

43. Wirth A, Mikhaeel NG, Aleman BMP, et al. Involved site radiation therapy in adult lymphomas: an overview of International Lymphoma Radiation Oncology group guidelines. *Int J Radiat Oncol Biol Phys*. 2020;107(5):909–933. doi:10.1016/j.ijrobp.2020.03.019

44. Videtic GNM WN, Vassil AD. *Handbook of Treatment Planning in Radiation Oncology*. 3rd ed. Demos Medical; 2020.

45. Stephens DM, Li H, LeBlanc ML, et al. Continued risk of relapse independent of treatment modality in limited-stage diffuse large B-cell lymphoma: final and long-term analysis of southwest oncology group study S8736. *J Clin Oncol*. 2016;34(25):2997–3004. doi:10.1200/JCO.2015.65.4582

46. Horning SJ, Weller E, Kim K, et al. Chemotherapy with or without radiotherapy in limited-stage diffuse aggressive non-Hodgkin's lymphoma: eastern cooperative oncology group study 1484. *J Clin Oncol*. 2004;22(15):3032–3038. doi:10.1200/JCO.2004.06.088

47. Miller TP, Dahlberg S, Cassady JR, et al. Chemotherapy alone compared with chemotherapy plus radiotherapy for localized intermediate- and high-grade non-Hodgkin's lymphoma. *N Engl J Med*. 1998;339(1): 21–26. doi:10.1056/NEJM199807023390104

48. Reyes F, Lepage E, Ganem G, et al. ACVBP versus CHOP plus radiotherapy for localized aggressive lymphoma. *N Engl J Med*. 2005;352(12):1197–1205. doi:10.1056/NEJMoa042040

49. Bonnet C, Fillet G, Mounier N, et al. CHOP alone compared with CHOP plus radiotherapy for localized aggressive lymphoma in elderly patients: a study by the Groupe d'Etude des Lymphomes de l'Adulte. *J Clin Oncol*. 2007;25(7):787–792. doi:10.1200/JCO.2006.07.0722

50. Pfreundschuh M, Kuhnt E, Trumper L, et al. CHOP-like chemotherapy with or without rituximab in young patients with good-prognosis diffuse large-B-cell lymphoma: 6-year results of an open-label randomised study of the MabThera International Trial (MInT) group. *Lancet Oncol*. 2011;12(11):1013–1022. doi:10.1016/S1470-2045(11)70235-2

51. Vargo JA, Gill BS, Balasubramani GK, Beriwal S. Treatment selection and survival outcomes in early-stage diffuse large B-cell lymphoma: do we still need consolidative radiotherapy? *J Clin Oncol*. 2015;33(32):3710–3717. doi:10.1200/JCO.2015.61.7654

52. Gill BS, Vargo JA, Pai SS, Balasubramani GK, Beriwal S. Management trends and outcomes for stage I to II mantle cell lymphoma using the National Cancer Data Base: ascertaining the ideal treatment paradigm. *Int J Radiat Oncol Biol Phys*. 2015;93(3):668–676. doi:10.1016/j.ijrobp.2015.07.2265

53. Marcheselli L, Marcheselli R, Bari A, et al. Radiation therapy improves treatment outcome in patients with diffuse large B-cell lymphoma. *Leuk Lymphoma*. 2011;52(10):1867–1872. doi:10.3109/10428194.2011.585526

54. Dorth JA, Prosnitz LR, Broadwater G, et al. Impact of consolidation radiation therapy in stage III-IV diffuse large B-cell lymphoma with negative post-chemotherapy radiologic imaging. *Int J Radiat Oncol Biol Phys*. 2012;84(3):762–767. doi:10.1016/j.ijrobp.2011.12.067

55. Shi Z, Das S, Okwan-Duodu D, et al. Patterns of failure in advanced stage diffuse large B-cell lymphoma patients after complete response to R-CHOP immunochemotherapy and the emerging role of consolidative radiation therapy. *Int J Radiat Oncol Biol Phys*. 2013;86(3):569–577. doi:10.1016/j.ijrobp.2013.02.007

56. Kwon J, Kim IH, Kim BH, Kim TM, Heo DS. Additional survival benefit of involved-lesion radiation therapy after R-CHOP chemotherapy in limited stage diffuse large B-cell lymphoma. *Int J Radiat Oncol Biol Phys*. 2015;92(1):91–98. doi:10.1016/j.ijrobp.2014.12.042

57. Haque W, Dabaja B, Tann A, et al. Changes in treatment patterns and impact of radiotherapy for early stage diffuse large B cell lymphoma after rituximab: a population-based analysis. *Radiother Oncol*. Jul 2016;120(1):150–155. doi:10.1016/j.radonc.2016.05.027

58. Dabaja BS, Vanderplas AM, Crosby-Thompson AL, et al. Radiation for diffuse large B-cell lymphoma in the rituximab era: analysis of the national comprehensive cancer network lymphoma outcomes project. *Cancer*. 2015;121(7):1032–1039. doi:10.1002/cncr.29113

59. Thurner L, Ziepert M, Berdel C, et al. Radiation and dose-densification of R-CHOP in aggressive B-cell lymphoma with intermediate prognosis: the UNFOLDER study. *Hemasphere*. 2023;7(7):e904. doi:10.1097/HS9.0000000000000904

60. Moskowitz CH, Schoder H, Teruya-Feldstein J, et al. Risk-adapted dose-dense immunochemotherapy determined by interim FDG-PET in advanced-stage diffuse large B-Cell lymphoma. *J Clin Oncol*. 2010;28(11):1896–1903. doi:10.1200/JCO.2009.26.5942

61. Phan J, Mazloom A, Medeiros LJ, et al. Benefit of consolidative radiation therapy in patients with diffuse large B-cell lymphoma treated with R-CHOP chemotherapy. *J Clin Oncol*. 2010;28(27):4170–4176. doi:10.1200/JCO.2009.27.3441

62. Kelsey CR, Broadwater G, James O, et al. Phase 2 study of dose-reduced consolidation radiation therapy in diffuse large B-cell lymphoma. *Int J Radiat Oncol Biol Phys*. 2019;105(1):96–101. doi:10.1016/j.ijrobp.2019.02.055

63. Martelli M, Ceriani L, Zucca E, et al. [18F]fluorodeoxyglucose positron emission tomography predicts survival after chemoimmunotherapy for primary mediastinal large B-cell lymphoma: results of the international extranodal lymphoma study group IELSG-26 study. *J Clin Oncol*. 2014;32(17):1769–1775. doi:10.1200/JCO.2013.51.7524

64. Vitolo U, Chiappella A, Ferreri AJ, et al. First-line treatment for primary testicular diffuse large B-cell lymphoma with rituximab-CHOP, CNS prophylaxis, and contralateral testis irradiation: final results of an international phase II trial. *J Clin Oncol*. 2011;29(20):2766–2772. doi:10.1200/JCO.2010.31.4187

65. Saifi O, Breen WG, Lester SC, et al. Don't put the CART before the horse: the role of radiation therapy in peri-CAR T-cell therapy for aggressive B-cell non-Hodgkin Lymphoma. *Int J Radiat Oncol Biol Phys*. 2023;116(5):999–1007. doi:10.1016/j.ijrobp.2022.12.017

66. Saifi O, Breen WG, Rule WG, et al. Comprehensive bridging radiotherapy for limited pre-CART Non-hodgkin lymphoma. *JAMA Oncol*. 2024;10(7):979–981. doi:10.1001/jamaoncol.2024.1113

Jenna E. Kocsis, Aryavarta M. S. Kumar, and Christopher W. Fleming

QUICK HIT   Indolent NHLs are a diverse group of diseases with survival measured in years to decades. Most common histologies are grades 1 to 2 follicular lymphoma and extranodal mucosa-associated lymphoid tissue (MALT) lymphoma. Limited-stage disease (stages I–II) is typically treated with definitive RT alone. Advanced disease (stages III–IV) is not curable and is typically treated with initial observation, with initiation of CHT for symptomatic disease and RT for palliation. ILROG guidelines are useful for treatment selection and field design (Table 54.1).

Table 54.1 General Treatment Paradigm for Indolent NHLs[1]		
	Treatment Options	**Common RT Regimens**
Stage I–II	Definitive RT	Follicular and MZL: 24–30 Gy/12–15 fx Gastric MALT: 30 Gy/20 fx
		Orbital and Salivary gland MZL: 24 Gy/12 fx 4 Gy/2 fx if providing regular follow-up
Stage III–IV	Observation, CHT, and/or palliative RT	24–30 Gy/12–15 fx
		4 Gy/2 fx (i.e., "boom boom")

Source: Data from National Comprehensive Cancer Network. *B-Cell Lymphomas* (Version 2.2024). Accessed June 3, 2024. https://www.nccn.org/professionals/physician_gls/pdf/b-cell.pdf.

EPIDEMIOLOGY: Estimated 80,620 of new NHL cases annually in the United States, with ~20,140 deaths. It is the eighth leading cause of death.[2] Indolent NHLs usually occur in older adults, with a median age of 64 and peak incidence at >65.[3] It is more common in North America, Europe, and Australia.[4] Follicular type represents ~21% of all NHLs (second most common NHL after DLBCL), MALT/MZL represents approximately ~9% and CLL/SLL ~7%.[5] Other subtypes are less common.

RISK FACTORS: There are four broad risk factors: immunosuppression, autoimmune diseases, infections, and environmental exposures. See Chapter 53 for details.

ANATOMY: Indolent NHLs can present as nodal or extranodal. Nodal anatomy is detailed further in Chapter 53. Common extranodal lymphoid sites include the thymus, spleen and tonsils, and adenoids (Waldeyer's ring). Extralymphatic sites include the bone marrow, skin, CNS, ovary, testicle, salivary glands, ocular adnexae, liver, stomach, bowel, breast, and lung.

PATHOLOGY/GENETICS: B-cell indolent NHLs are more common than T-cell. The WHO 2016 classification defines subtypes of lymphoid neoplasms.[6] *Follicular NHL is* graded by the number of centroblasts per high-powered field (HPF): grade 1: 0 to 5/HPF; grade 2: 6 to 15/HPF; grade 3: >15/HPF. It can be subdivided into 3A (centrocytes present) and 3B (solid aggregates of centroblasts with no centrocytes). 3B is often treated as DLBCL.[7] t(14:18) is a classic translocation and results in overexpression of BCL-2, which inhibits apoptosis. *Marginal zone NHL* can occur in LNs (nodal MZL), spleen (splenic MZL), or extranodal (ENMZL, i.e., MALT). See Table 54.2 for details.

Table 54.2 Pathology, Immunophenotype, and Genetics of Common Indolent Non-Hodgkin Lymphomas				
Disease	**Common Immunotype**		**Common Genetics**	**Notes**
Follicular NHL[7]	CD19+, CD20+	CD10+, CD21+, CD22+, CD79a+, PAX5, CD5−, CD43−	t(14:18) in up to 90% of cases	BCL2 expression result of t(14:18), marrow involvement common, risk of transformation 28% at 10 yrs[8]

(continued)

Table 54.2 Pathology, Immunophenotype, and Genetics of Common Indolent Non-Hodgkin Lymphomas (*continued*)

Disease	Common Immunotype	Common Genetics	Notes
Nodal marginal zone (MZL)[9]	CD22+, CD79a+, CD3–, 5–, 10–, 23–	Trisomy 3, t(14;18), t(11:18)	Less common than extranodal
Extranodal MZL (MALT)			Frequently localized, t(11:18) associated with triple-antibiotic therapy failure for gastric MALT[10]
SLL/CLL[11,12]	CD5+, 23+, CD22–, low levels of immunoglobulins	Common chromosomal abnormalities seen on FISH: 17p deletion, 11q deletion, 13q deletion, trisomy 12	Initial leukemic phase represents CLL, progression to the lymphoma phase represents SLL

CLINICAL PRESENTATION: Indolent NHLs often present only with slow-growing lymphade-nopathy, hepatosplenomegaly, cytopenias, or nonspecific constitutional symptoms such as fatigue, malaise, or low-grade fever. Lymphadenopathy most commonly presents in the neck, groin, axilla, and abdomen. Less commonly, NHL may involve the skin, manifesting as rash or pruritus. Bone marrow involvement is common. Follicular NHLs commonly present as stage III to IV with involve-ment of the spleen (in 40% of cases), liver (50%), and bone marrow (60%–70%), whereas marginal zone NHL more commonly presents as localized disease.[13] B symptoms are usually associated with aggressive histologies or extensive disease.

WORKUP: Workup includes an H&P with attention to lymphatic, liver, spleen, and skin exam. An excisional/incisional or core biopsy of an LN is preferred for adequate histologic, immuno-logic, and molecular biological assessment. FNA is insufficient for final diagnosis, but it may dis-tinguish benign lymphadenopathy from clonal B-cell proliferation via flow cytometry. Endoscopic ultrasound, biopsy, and testing for *H. pylori* is recommended for gastric MALT. Per NCCN, despite advances in PET-CT, bone marrow biopsy is still recommended for indolent NHL (except for extran-odal MZL).[1] LP should be performed in those with testicular, paravertebral, parameningeal, or bone marrow involvement and in those with neurologic symptoms or HIV.

Labs: CBC, peripheral smear, ESR, CMP, LDH, HIV, albumin, SPEP (CLL/SLL), hepatitis B, hepati-tis C, $\beta 2$ microglobulin (see the following FLIPI2 prognostic model), urea breath test for *Helicobacter pylori* (gastric MALT), pregnancy test.

Imaging: Contrast-enhanced CT chest, abdomen, and pelvis or PET/CT (preferred) is indicated for peripheral lymphadenopathy. PET/CT is used for staging in all nodal lymphomas, but it is less sensitive and not indicated in CLL/SLL and extranodal MZL. PET SUV >10 in patients with indo-lent NHL may suggest transformation to high-grade histology and can be used to target biopsy (i.e., Richter transformation from CLL/hairy cell leukemia to DLBCL).[14] Obtain MRI brain/spine for symptoms. Obtain echocardiogram or MUGA scan if anthracycline CHT planned.

PROGNOSTIC FACTORS: FLIPI and updated FLIPI2 are useful prognostic assessment tools for follicular patients. FLIPI was designed pre-rituximab but remains prognostic in the rituximab era.[15] See Table 54.3. Grade is prognostic for follicular with grade 3B often treated as a DLBCL.[7] Other prognostic factors for MALT lymphoma include age, stage, and performance status.[16]

Table 54.3 FLIPI and FLIPI2 Risk Factors

Original FLIPI Risk Factors[15,17]	FLIPI2 Risk Factors[18]
Hemoglobin <12 ng/dL	Hemoglobin <12 ng/dL
Age >60	Age >60
Stage III–IV	Serum $\beta 2$ microglobulin elevated
Nodal sites >4	Bone marrow involvement
LDH elevated	Maximal diameter of lymph node >6 cm

(*continued*)

Table 54.3 FLIPI and FLIPI2 Risk Factors (*continued*)						
		FLIPI Pre-Rituximab[17]			FLIPI2[18]	
Score	Risk Group	5-Yr OS	10-Yr OS	Score	Risk Group	5-Yr PFS
0–1	Low	91%	71%	0	Low	80%
2	Intermediate	78%	51%	1–2	Intermediate	51%
≥3	High	52%	36%	3–5	High	19%

STAGING: See Chapter 53 for Lugano modification of Ann Arbor staging.

TREATMENT PARADIGM

Observation: Considered for elderly or asymptomatic patients with stage III/IV indolent NHLs; see CHT paradigm in the following for discussion on observation vs. treatment.

Surgery: Minimal role for NHL and is used mostly for biopsy. Rarely, for small intestinal MZL it can be therapeutic.

Medical: Triple therapy is the first-line treatment for *H. pylori*-positive, t(11;18)-negative gastric MALT, and it includes proton pump inhibitor, clarithromycin, and either amoxicillin or metronidazole. Give triple therapy as first line with endoscopic biopsy at 3 months to confirm resolution. If *H. pylori*-negative and lymphoma-negative, observe. If *H. pylori*-positive and lymphoma-negative, give second-line antibiotics. If *H. pylori*-negative and lymphoma-positive, can either continue observation with repeat biopsy or treat with RT for symptoms. If both remain positive, treat with second-line antibiotics with immediate or delayed RT. Response to doxycycline has been noted (65%) for ocular and cutaneous MZL.[19]

Chemotherapy: Systemic therapy usually reserved for noncontiguous stage II or advanced stage III/IV. Note that grade 3B follicular NHL is often treated as per DLBCL regimens (see Chapter 53). GELF criteria are used in stage III or IV follicular lymphoma patients to determine when to initiate treatment. Factors include nodal or extranodal tumor mass with a diameter ≥7 cm, involvement of ≥3 nodal sites with a diameter ≥3 cm, B symptoms, splenomegaly, pleural effusions or peritoneal ascites, risk of local compression (epidural, ureteral, etc.), cytopenias, or leukemia.[20] If none, then NCCN suggests observation.[1] If indications are present, treatment can be initiated and may consist of regimens such as bendamustine + rituximab, R-CHOP, R-CVP (rituximab, cyclophosphamide, vincristine, prednisone), lenalidomide + rituximab, or rituximab alone. Rituximab is a chimeric monoclonal antibody against CD20. The most serious toxicities include infusion reactions, hepatitis B reactivation, and progressive multifocal leukoencephalopathy.[21] Obinutuzumab is an alternative anti-CD20 monoclonal antibody with similar effects as rituximab, but it binds a slightly different epitope of CD20.[22]

Radiation

Indications: In limited-stage indolent NHLs (stage I–II), RT is treatment of choice for cure and is usually delivered to the whole organ, particularly for gastric, thyroid, orbit (but not conjunctiva), breast, and salivary gland extranodal indolent NHL. Per ILROG 2015 guidelines, when disease is limited to the conjunctiva, the CTV should include the entire conjunctival sac and local extensions to the eyelid.[23] In advanced disease, RT is typically used for focal palliation. ILROG guidelines exist for both nodal and extranodal NHLs, and these guidelines support the use of ISRT, limiting the volume to either the entire organ involved or to the involved lesion, plus an expansion to encompass potential adjacent microscopic disease sites.[23–25]

Dose: See Table 54.4 for NCCN dosing guidelines. Doses are usually delivered at 1.8 to 2 Gy/fx, but 1.5 Gy/fx may be given for gastric MALT to minimize acute GI toxicity.[1] Effective palliation can be provided via "boom boom" regimen of 4 Gy/2 fx (see the following data).

Table 54.4 NCCN Dosing Guidelines for Indolent Non-Hodgkin Lymphomas	
Follicular	24–30 Gy
Gastric MALT	24–30 Gy (can use 1.5 Gy/fx to minimize GI toxicity)
Other extranodal sites (orbit, salivary, skin, etc.)	24–30 Gy or 4 Gy/2 fx
Nodal MZL	24–30 Gy
Palliation of indolent lymphoma	4 Gy (i.e., "boom boom")

Toxicity: Generally, toxicity mild, given in low total doses. Fatigue is common; others are related to location of delivery.

Procedure: See *Handbook of Treatment Planning in Radiation Oncology*, Chapter 10.[26]

Unsealed Sources: Y-90 ibritumomab tiuxetan (Zevalin®) and I-131 tositumomab (Bexxar®) are radiolabeled antibodies against CD20 that were recently discontinued by the FDA and no longer indicated per NCCN guidelines.

EVIDENCE-BASED Q&A

What data suggest that follicular NHL (grades 1–2) can be cured with RT alone?

Multiple RRs are available, but one example is as follows.

Campbell, British Columbia (*Cancer* 2010, PMID 20564082): RR of 237 patients with stage I to II grades 1 to 3A follicular NHL treated with RT alone. Doses ranged from 20 to 40 Gy. Involved regional RT included LN group with ≥1 adjacent uninvolved LN group (60%) or INRT (40%). MFU 7.3 years; 10-year PFS 49%, OS 66%. Distant recurrence alone was the most common pattern of failure, occurring in 38% of involved regional RT and 32% of INRT. **Conclusion: Cure is possible with RT, and reducing field size does not compromise outcome.**

For limited-stage follicular NHL, is there detriment to initial observation as compared with initial RT?

Indolent lymphoma is slowly progressive, and no treatment may be a reasonable first approach. However, for early-stage disease, this is not supported by observational data, and definitive treatment with RT should remain standard of care.

Pugh, SEER (*Cancer* 2010, PMID 20564102): SEER analysis of 6,568 patients with stage I to II, grades 1 to 2 follicular NHL diagnosed from 1973 to 2004; 34% received initial RT. Those observed were younger, stage I, and without extranodal disease. RT was associated with improved 20-year DSS (63% vs. 51%; HR 0.61, $p < .0001$) and OS (35% vs. 23%; HR 0.68, $p < .0001$). **Conclusion: Initial RT is standard for early-stage follicular NHL, and deferring treatment until time of salvage is associated with worse outcomes.**

Vargo, NCDB (*Cancer* 2015, PMID 26042364): NCDB analysis of 35,961 patients with stage I to II, grades 1 to 2 follicular NHL. RT use decreased from 37% to 24% between 1999 and 2012. The 10-year OS was 68% for RT patients compared with 54% for no-RT patients ($p < .0001$). **Conclusion: RT is significantly underutilized and is associated with improved survival in early-stage follicular lymphoma. RT should remain standard.**

What RT dose is optimal for indolent NHL?

For definitive RT of early-stage indolent lymphoma, 24 to 30 Gy is usually sufficient, with some advocating for 36 Gy in rare case of bulky disease. For palliation, 4 Gy/2 fx and 24 Gy/12 fx are both reasonable. Note that the "boom boom" regimen of 4 Gy/2 fx was inferior for definitive treatment of limited-stage patients in the FoRT trial and should not be extrapolated to aggressive NHL.

Lowry, British National Lymphoma Investigation (*Radiother Oncol* 2011, PMID 21664710): PRT including any subtype and stage of NHL requiring RT for LC. 361 sites of indolent NHL randomized to either 40–45 Gy/20–23 fx (standard) vs. 24 Gy/12 fx (low-dose). For indolent patients, 59% were grades 1 to 2 follicular NHL, 19% MZL/MALT, and 69% were stage I to II. MFU 5.6 years. ORR no different: 93% vs. 92% in standard vs. low-dose groups, respectively. PFS and OS were also not significantly different. **Conclusion: 24 Gy is sufficient for indolent lymphomas.**

Hoskin, FoRT Trial (*Lancet Oncol* 2014, PMID 24572077; Update *Lancet Oncol* 2021, PMID 33539729): Noninferiority trial of patients with either follicular NHL or MZL requiring RT for either definitive or palliative treatment. Randomized between 4 Gy/2 fx (i.e., "boom boom") and 24 Gy/12 fx. Primary endpoint LC. Trial closed early with 548 patients at 614 sites. MFU 74 months; 60% stage I to II; 5-year local progression-free rate was 90% for 24 Gy and 70% for 4 Gy (HR 3.46, $p < .0001$). No difference in OS. **Conclusion: 24 Gy is more effective when durable LC is the goal. However, "boom boom" is useful in palliation and often induces a response.**

Is there benefit to adjuvant CHT after definitive RT for early-stage indolent NHL?

Adjuvant CHT does not appear to improve OS based on the results of at least five randomized trials from the pre-rituximab era (Denmark, Milan, British, EORTC, MSKCC)[27–31] as well as the more recent TROG study outlined below. Given around 25% of patients will develop DM,[32] some have advocated for the addition of rituximab to RT in indolent lymphoma patients. NCCN still recommends ISRT alone as the preferred initial treatment option.

MacManus, TROG 99.03 (*JCO* 2018, PMID 29975623): Multicenter PRT enrolling 150 patients with stage I to II low-grade follicular NHL after CT and bone marrow biopsies. PET was not mandatory. Patients randomized to 30 Gy IFRT alone vs. IFRT plus 6C CVP. After 2006, rituximab was added to CVP (41% of CVP arm); 75% stage I. MFU 9.6 years; 10-year PFS superior with CVP (59% vs. 41%; HR 0.57, *p* = .033) and markedly improved with R-CVP (HR 0.26, *p* = .045). However, 10-year OS was not significantly different (87% vs. 95%, *p* = .40). **Conclusion: Systemic therapy with R-CVP after IFRT significantly improved PFS without a benefit in OS.**

What data inform treatment of gastric MALT?

Multiple small institutional retrospective studies have shown excellent LC with 25 to 30 Gy.[33–36] The study by Wündisch informs treatment of H. pylori-positive gastric MALT and supports observation when H. pylori is eradicated. NCCN recommends ISRT for H. pylori-positive patients who are resistant to medical therapy and those with H. pylori-negative or t(11;18)-positive disease. Given excellent outcomes with 24 to 30 Gy, some are investigating dose de-escalation.

Wündisch, Germany (*JCO* 2005, PMID 16204012): Prospective trial tracking the outcomes of *H. pylori*-positive gastric MALT; 120 patients, all with stage IE disease treated with antibiotics and observed after *H. pylori* eradication. MFU 75 months. Eighty percent achieved complete histologic remission (CR), with 80% of those experiencing long-term complete histologic remission. Three percent of CR patients relapsed and were referred for alternative treatment, 17% of CR patients had histologic residual disease on follow-up and were observed, and all ultimately entered into a second CR. Fifteen percent of patients were t(11;18)-positive, and t(11;18) and ongoing monoclonality were associated with no response or relapse. **Conclusion: Eradication of *H. pylori* results in continuous CR in most patients. Observation is appropriate for most when close follow-up is possible.**

Gunther, MDACC (*Lancet Haematology* 2024, PMID 38843856): Single-center, single-arm, prospective trial investigating response-adapted ultra-low dose RT in newly diagnosed or relapsed *H. pylori*-negative gastric MALT lymphoma stage I to IV patients. Twenty-four patients received 4 Gy/2 fx and those with CR were observed, those with PR were re-evaluated in 6 to 9 months, and those with residual disease at 9 to 13 months or progressive disease received an additional 20 Gy. MFU 36 months. Twenty patients had CR, two patients received the additional 20 Gy for symptomatic stable disease, and two received 20 Gy for residual disease at 9 to 13 months. The 3-year LC was 96%. **Conclusion: Most patients had CR to 4 Gy. Response-adapted approach could be used to select patients who would benefit from additional dose and spare others potential toxicity.**

What data inform treatment of other MALT NHL?

Common RT regimens include 24 to 30 Gy. NCCN now recommends 4 Gy/2 fx as an alternative for orbital and salivary gland MZL, with careful regular follow-up and definitive doses for incomplete responses or relapsed disease.

Teckie, MSKCC (*IJROBP* 2015, PMID 25863760): A total of 244 patients with stage IE or IIE MZL treated with RT alone; 92% were stage IE. MFU 5.2 years. Stomach (50%), orbit (18%), nonthyroid head and neck (8%), skin (8%), and breast (5%). Median RT dose 30 Gy; 5-year OS 92%, RFS 74%. Most common relapse site was distant. Disease-specific death 1% at 5 years. All sites except H&N demonstrated worse RFS compared with gastric. Transformation to aggressive histology was rare (1.6%). **Conclusion: OS and DSS are high in early-stage extranodal MZL. Gastric MALT has improved prognosis compared with other sites.**

MacManus, TROG 05.22 (*Eur J Cancer* 2021, PMID 34098462): Phase II prospective trial of 68 stage I to II nongastric MZL patients treated with IFRT or ISRT 24 to 30.6 Gy. Orbital (26%), conjunctiva (19%), lacrimal (12%), skin (12%), salivary (10%), and muscle (6%). MFU 5 years; PFS 79% and OS 95%. Apart from cataracts (26%), three treatment-related late grade ≥3 adverse events (dry mouth, dyspnea, and skin atrophy). **Conclusion: RT provides a potentially curative treatment with low toxicity for localized nongastric MZL.**

Pinnix, MDACC (*JAMA Oncol* 2024, PMID 38990564): Single-institution phase II trial of 50 patients with stage I to IV indolent B-cell lymphoma of the ocular adnexa. Patients were treated with ultra-low dose RT 4 Gy/2 fx and assessed for response at 3-month intervals. Those with persistent disease were offered an additional 20 Gy/10 fx to complete response-adapted treatment. Primary endpoint 2-year local orbital control after response-adapted therapy. MFU 37.4 months; 2-year local control rate of 89% and 2-year OS rate of 98%. Forty-five patients had a CR to response-adapted RT, including 44 patients with a CR to ultra-low dose RT. No local recurrences in those with CR. No grade 3 or higher toxicity noted. **Conclusion: Response-adapted ultra-low dose RT for indolent B-cell lymphoma of the ocular adnexa results in high response rates with minimal toxicity.**

REFERENCES

1. National Comprehensive Cancer Network. *B-Cell Lymphomas* (Version 2.2024). Accessed June 3, 2024. https://www.nccn.org/professionals/physician_gls/pdf/b-cell.pdf
2. Siegel RL, Miller KD, Wagle NS, Jemal A. Cancer statistics, 2023. *CA Cancer J Clin*. 2023;73(1):17–48. doi:10.3322/caac.21763
3. National Cancer Institute. *Cancer Stat Facts: NHL - Follicular Lymphoma*. Accessed June 13, 2024. https://seer.cancer.gov/statfacts/html/follicular.html
4. Sun H, Xue L, Guo Y, et al. Global, regional and national burden of non-Hodgkin lymphoma from 1990 to 2017: estimates from Global Burden of disease study in 2017. *Ann Med*. 2022;54(1):633–645. doi:10.1080/07853890.2022.2039957
5. Cerhan JR, Maurer MJ, Link BK, et al. The lymphoma epidemiology of outcomes cohort study: design, baseline characteristics, and early outcomes. *Am J Hematol*. 2024;99(3):408–421. doi:10.1002/ajh.27202
6. Swerdlow SH, Campo E, Pileri SA, et al. The 2016 revision of the World Health Organization classification of lymphoid neoplasms. *Blood*. 2016;127(20):2375–2390. doi:10.1182/blood-2016-01-643569
7. Khanlari M, Chapman JR. Follicular lymphoma: updates for pathologists. *J Pathol Transl Med*. 2022;56(1):1–15. doi:10.4132/jptm.2021.09.29
8. Montoto S, Davies AJ, Matthews J, et al. Risk and clinical implications of transformation of follicular lymphoma to diffuse large B-cell lymphoma. *J Clin Oncol*. 2007;25(17):2426–2433. doi:10.1200/JCO.2006.09.3260
9. Angelopoulou MK, Kalpadakis C, Pangalis GA, Kyrtsonis MC, Vassilakopoulos TP. Nodal marginal zone lymphoma. *Leuk Lymphoma*. 2014;55(6):1240–1250. doi:10.3109/10428194.2013.840888
10. Yepes S, Torres MM, Saavedra C, Andrade R. Gastric mucosa-associated lymphoid tissue lymphomas and *Helicobacter pylori* infection: a Colombian perspective. *World J Gastroenterol*. 2012;18(7):685–691. doi:10.3748/wjg.v18.i7.685
11. Scarfo L, Ferreri AJ, Ghia P. Chronic lymphocytic leukaemia. *Crit Rev Oncol Hematol*. 2016;104:169–182. doi:10.1016/j.critrevonc.2016.06.003
12. Mukkamalla SKR, Taneja A, Malipeddi D, Master SR. Chronic lymphocytic leukemia. In: *StatPearls*. StatPearls Publishing; 2024.
13. Shankland KR, Armitage JO, Hancock BW. Non-Hodgkin lymphoma. *Lancet*. 2012;380(9844):848–857. doi:10.1016/S0140-6736(12)60605-9
14. Noy A, Schoder H, Gonen M, et al. The majority of transformed lymphomas have high Standardized Uptake Values (SUVs) on Positron Emission Tomography (PET) scanning similar to Diffuse Large B-Cell Lymphoma (DLBCL). *Ann Oncol*. 2009;20(3):508–512. doi:10.1093/annonc/mdn657
15. Nooka AK, Nabhan C, Zhou X, et al. Examination of the Follicular Lymphoma International Prognostic Index (FLIPI) in the National LymphoCare study (NLCS): a prospective US patient cohort treated predominantly in community practices. *Ann Oncol*. 2013;24(2):441–448. doi:10.1093/annonc/mds429
16. Qi S, Liu X, Noy A, et al. Predictors of survival in patients with MALT lymphoma: a retrospective, case-control study. *Blood Adv*. 2023;7(8):1496–1506. doi:10.1182/bloodadvances.2022007772
17. Solal-Celigny P, Roy P, Colombat P, et al. Follicular lymphoma international prognostic index. *Blood*. 2004;104(5):1258–1265. doi:10.1182/blood-2003-12-4434
18. Federico M, Bellei M, Marcheselli L, et al. Follicular lymphoma international prognostic index 2: a new prognostic index for follicular lymphoma developed by the international follicular lymphoma prognostic factor project. *J Clin Oncol*. 2009;27(27):4555–4562. doi:10.1200/JCO.2008.21.3991
19. Ferreri AJ, Govi S, Pasini E, et al. *Chlamydophila psittaci* eradication with doxycycline as first-line targeted therapy for ocular adnexae lymphoma: final results of an international phase II trial. *J Clin Oncol*. 2012;30(24):2988–2994. doi:10.1200/JCO.2011.41.4466
20. Brice P, Bastion Y, Lepage E, et al. Comparison in low-tumor-burden follicular lymphomas between an initial no-treatment policy, prednimustine, or interferon alfa: a randomized study from the Groupe d'Etude des Lymphomes Folliculaires. *J Clin Oncol*. 1997;15(3):1110–1117. doi:10.1200/JCO.1997.15.3.1110

21. Hanif N, Anwer F. Rituximab. *StatPearls*. 2024. https://pubmed.ncbi.nlm.nih.gov/33232044/

22. Marcus R, Davies A, Ando K, et al. Obinutuzumab for the first-line treatment of follicular lymphoma. *N Engl J Med*. 2017;377(14):1331–1344. doi:10.1056/NEJMoa1614598

23. Yahalom J, Illidge T, Specht L, et al. Modern radiation therapy for extranodal lymphomas: field and dose guidelines from the International Lymphoma Radiation Oncology Group. *Int J Radiat Oncol Biol Phys*. 2015;92(1):11–31. doi:10.1016/j.ijrobp.2015.01.009

24. Illidge T, Specht L, Yahalom J, et al. Modern radiation therapy for nodal non-Hodgkin lymphoma-target definition and dose guidelines from the International Lymphoma Radiation Oncology Group. *Int J Radiat Oncol Biol Phys*. 2014;89(1):49–58. doi:10.1016/j.ijrobp.2014.01.006

25. Wirth A, Mikhaeel NG, Aleman BMP, et al. involved site radiation therapy in adult lymphomas: an overview of International Lymphoma Radiation Oncology Group guidelines. *Int J Radiat Oncol Biol Phys*. 2020; 107(5):909–933. doi:10.1016/j.ijrobp.2020.03.019

26. Videtic GMM, WN, Vassil AD. *Handbook of Treatment Planning in Radiation Oncology*. 3rd ed. Demos Medical; 2020.

27. Monfardini S, Banfi A, Bonadonna G, et al. Improved five year survival after combined radiotherapy-chemotherapy for stage I–II non-Hodgkin's lymphoma. *Int J Radiat Oncol Biol Phys*. 1980;6(2):125–134. doi:10.1016/0360-3016(80)90027-9

28. Nissen NI, Ersboll J, Hansen HS, et al. A randomized study of radiotherapy versus radiotherapy plus chemotherapy in stage I–II non-Hodgkin's lymphomas. *Cancer*. 1983;52(1):1–7. doi:10.1002/1097-0142(19830701) 52:1<1::aid-cncr2820520102>3.0.co;2-m

29. Carde P, Burgers JM, van Glabbeke M, et al. Combined radiotherapy-chemotherapy for early stages non-Hodgkin's lymphoma: the 1975-1980 EORTC controlled lymphoma trial. *Radiother Oncol*. 1984;2(4):301–312. doi:10.1016/s0167-8140(84)80072-9

30. Kelsey SM, Newland AC, Hudson GV, Jelliffe AM. A British national lymphoma investigation randomised trial of single agent chlorambucil plus radiotherapy versus radiotherapy alone in low grade, localised non-Hodgkins lymphoma. *Med Oncol*. 1994;11(1):19–25. doi:10.1007/BF02990087

31. Yahalom J, Varsos G, Fuks Z, Myers J, Clarkson BD, Straus DJ. Adjuvant cyclophosphamide, doxorubicin, vincristine, and prednisone chemotherapy after radiation therapy in stage I low-grade and intermediate-grade non-Hodgkin lymphoma. Results of a prospective randomized study. *Cancer*. 1993;71(7):2342–2350. doi:10.1002/1097-0142(19930401)71:7<2342::aid-cncr2820710728>3.0.co;2-i

32. Brady JL, Binkley MS, Hajj C, et al. Definitive radiotherapy for localized follicular lymphoma staged by (18)F-FDG PET-CT: a collaborative study by ILROG. *Blood*. 2019;133(3):237–245. doi:10.1182/blood-2018 -04-843540

33. Tsai HK, Li S, Ng AK, Silver B, Stevenson MA, Mauch PM. Role of radiation therapy in the treatment of stage I/II mucosa-associated lymphoid tissue lymphoma. *Ann Oncol*. 2007;18(4):672–678. doi:10.1093/ annonc/mdl468

34. Goda JS, Gospodarowicz M, Pintilie M, et al. Long-term outcome in localized extranodal mucosa-associated lymphoid tissue lymphomas treated with radiotherapy. *Cancer*. 2010;116(16):3815–3824. doi:10.1002/ cncr.25226

35. Ono S, Kato M, Takagi K, et al. Long-term treatment of localized gastric marginal zone B-cell mucosa associated lymphoid tissue lymphoma including incidence of metachronous gastric cancer. *J Gastroenterol Hepatol*. 2010;25(4):804–809. doi:10.1111/j.1440-1746.2009.06204.x

36. Schechter NR, Portlock CS, Yahalom J. Treatment of mucosa-associated lymphoid tissue lymphoma of the stomach with radiation alone. *J Clin Oncol*. 1998;16(5):1916–1921. doi:10.1200/JCO.1998.16.5.1916

55 MULTIPLE MYELOMA AND PLASMACYTOMA

Anirudh Bommireddy, Kailin Yang, and Sheen Cherian

QUICK HIT Multiple myeloma (MM) is not considered curable with conventional treatment modalities. It is sensitive to a variety of cytotoxic and biological drugs, and treatment has evolved due to therapeutics such as thalidomide, lenalidomide, bortezomib, and daratumumab. The primary management of MM is CHT ± autologous SCT. RT is reserved for symptomatic bone metastases, prevention of pathologic fractures, and spinal cord compression. Solitary plasmacytoma is a rare plasma cell dyscrasia that can occur locally in the bone (SBP) or soft tissue (SEP). Thorough workup to exclude systemic disease is necessary. Definitive RT to a total dose of 35 to 50 Gy with 1.8 to 2 Gy daily fractions is the primary treatment for SBP and SEP (Table 55.1).

Table 55.1 Overview of MM, SBP, and SEP			
Feature	MM	SBP	SEP
Common location	Axial skeleton	Vertebral body and pelvic bone	Head and neck region
Progression to MM	NA	>75%	10%–30%
Local control	Not curable	80%–100%	90%–100%
Radiation	Palliative RT (25–30 Gy/10 fx, 20 Gy/5 fx, 8 Gy/1 fx)	35–40 Gy (<5 cm) 40–50 Gy (≥5 cm)	40–50 Gy
Primary treatment	CHT ± autologous SCT	RT	RT

EPIDEMIOLOGY: MM accounts for 1% of all cancer cases. In the United States, there are ~36,000 new diagnoses of MM and 13,000 myeloma-related deaths per year.[1] Incidence in Black people is two to three times the incidence seen in Caucasians. Incidence in men to women is 1.4:1. Median age at diagnosis is 66 years.

RISK FACTORS: A small number of cases are believed to be familial.[2] Risk of developing MM is approximately 3.7-fold higher in those with a first-degree relative diagnosed with the disease. Other risk factors include older age, immunosuppression, and exposure to radiation, benzene, or herbicide.[3]

PATHOLOGY: MM is caused by clonal proliferation of plasma cells, a type of terminally differentiated B lymphocytes. Plasma cells appear in an ovoid shape with abundant blue cytoplasm and eccentric nucleus with coarse chromatin. They can produce a large amount of monoclonal immunoglobulin (M protein), which can be detected in urine or serum studies: urine protein electrophoresis (UPEP) or serum protein electrophoresis (SPEP). For most patients, the increased immunoglobulin is either IgG (52%) or IgA (21%). Some patients (16%) have kappa or lambda light chain only disease (Bence Jones protein). A small fraction (7%) of patients present with nonsecretory myeloma.[4]

Pathogenesis of normal B lymphocytes → MGUS (monoclonal gammopathy of undetermined significance): MGUS is the precursor to MM and results from cumulative damage leading to primary cytogenetic abnormalities in a single B-cell lineage.

Pathogenesis of MGUS → MM: Progressive genetic alterations (Ras mutation, secondary translocations, Cdk1 methylation, and Myc abnormalities) and alteration in bone marrow microenvironment (increased angiogenesis, apocrine IL-6 activity, which is a growth factor for MM) lead to transformation of MGUS into MM at a rate of 1% per year.

GENETICS: Chromosomal abnormality is common in MM.[5] Abnormalities associated with a poor prognosis include 17p deletion, translocation 14:16, translocation 14:20, 1p deletion, translocation 4:14, and 1q gain.[6]

CLINICAL PRESENTATION: Symptoms include anemia, bone pain, elevated serum creatinine, fatigue, hypercalcemia, and weight loss. These presenting symptoms are typically associated with infiltration of myeloma cells into the bone or other organs or are the effect of excess light chains (such as kidney injury).

WORKUP: H&P.

Labs: CBC with differential, peripheral blood smear (increased rouleaux formation in 50% of patients), serum BUN/creatinine, albumin, calcium, LDH, and β2 microglobulin. Serum quantitative immunoglobulin, SPEP, and free light chain ratio. 24-hour urine for total protein and UPEP. Bone marrow biopsy with cytogenetic and FISH studies.

Imaging: Skeletal survey. PET/CT, MRI, and/or CT if bone pain or neurologic symptoms are concerning for spinal cord compression. For patients with suspected smoldering myeloma (presence of M protein but without myeloma-defining events) or solitary plasmacytoma, PET/CT and MRI should be performed to confirm the absence of more than one focal lytic lesion.

PROGNOSTIC FACTORS: Age, performance status, comorbidity, albumin concentration, and high-risk cytogenetic abnormalities (del[17p], t[4;14], t[14;16], t[14;20], 1q+) have been associated with prognosis.[4,7]

STAGING: Diagnosis of MM requires clonal bone marrow plasma cells (≥10%) with biopsy-proven bony or extramedullary plasmacytoma and at least one of the myeloma-defining events, which include evidence of end-organ damage that can be attributed to the underlying plasma cell proliferative disorder (hypercalcemia, renal insufficiency, anemia, or bone lesion) or a biomarker of malignancy (clonal bone marrow plasma cells ≥60%, involved:uninvolved serum free light chain ratio ≥100, or >1 focal lesions on MRI studies). Absence of a myeloma-defining event is referred to as smoldering myeloma. The Revised International Staging System (R-ISS) is the preferred staging system for MM, and it stratifies patients into three risk groups using β2 microglobulin (B2M), serum albumin, LDH, and bone marrow FISH (see Table 55.2).[7,8] OS for R-ISS stages I, II, and III is 82%, 62%, and 40% at 5 years, respectively.

Table 55.2 Staging for Multiple Myeloma (R-ISS)

Stage I	Stage II	Stage III
All of the following: • B2M <3.5 mg/L • Serum albumin ≥3.5 g/dL • Normal LDH • del(17p), t(4;14), or t(14;16) by FISH	Neither stage I nor stage III	Both of the following: • B2M ≥3.5 mg/L • Elevated LDH **and/or** del(17p), t(4;14), or t(14;16) by FISH

Source: Data from Palumbo A, Avet-Loiseau H, Oliva S, et al. Revised international staging system for multiple myeloma: a report from International Myeloma Working Group. *J Clin Oncol.* 2015;33(26):2863–2869. doi:10.1200/JCO.2015.61.2267; Greipp PR, San Miguel J, Durie BG, et al. International staging system for multiple myeloma. *J Clin Oncol.* 2005;23(15):3412–3420. doi:10.1200/JCO.2005.04.242.

TREATMENT PARADIGM

Surgery: Prophylactic internal fixation should be used for weight-bearing long bone lesions that are at risk for impending fracture. Vertebroplasty and kyphoplasty can also reduce pain and improve function for patients with compression fracture from a lytic lesion in the vertebral body. See Chapter 69 for details.

Chemotherapy: High-dose CHT followed by autologous HCT is considered standard of care for eligible patients with newly diagnosed active MM. Autologous HCT is associated with improved OS and therefore assessment for eligibility is critical for pretreatment evaluation.[9] Patients eligible for autologous HCT are typically treated with three to six cycles of induction CHT followed by autologous stem cell collection. For standard-risk patients, the decision is then made to either proceed with autologous HCT (early HCT strategy) or continue the same CHT regimen and reserve HCT for the first relapse (delayed HCT strategy). Early single or tandem HCT is preferred in high-risk patients after induction CHT. Patients who are ineligible for HCT typically receive 8 to 12 cycles of triplet induction therapy followed by maintenance therapy. Primary induction CHT agents with high response rates include **bortezomib** (proteasome inhibitor; side effects: herpes zoster, neuropathy, and GI disturbance), **thalidomide** (immunomodulator that increases natural killer cells, IL-2, and INF-γ), and **lenalidomide** (analogue of thalidomide). Anti-CD38 monoclonal antibody **daratumumab** has also been added to the initial regimen in some circumstances (side effects: GI disturbance, cytopenias, fatigue, musculoskeletal pain, cough, and infusion reaction). VRd (bortezomib, lenalidomide, and dexamethasone) is a commonly used regimen for induction, although Rd is an acceptable alternative for frail patients.[10] Active treatment is not routinely indicated for patients with MGUS or smoldering MM. However, in a high-risk subgroup of patients with smoldering MM who are at increased risk of progression to symptomatic disease, treatment with lenalidomide plus dexamethasone followed by maintenance lenalidomide delays progression to active disease and increases OS.[11]

Radiation: For patients with MM, RT is indicated for palliative management of pain, prevention of pathologic fracture particularly for weight-bearing bones, or relief of spinal cord compression. Typical palliative doses such as 20–30 Gy/10 fx, 20 Gy/5 fx, or 8 Gy/1 fx are commonly used for bony metastasis and spinal cord compression. For large volume or retreatment, 20 to 30 Gy in 10 to 15 daily fractions may be preferred to reduce side effects on bone marrow and other critical structures.[12]

RT is the primary definitive management for SBP and SEP. For SBP, RT is commonly directed to the involved bone and areas of soft tissue involvement with a margin to 40 to 50 Gy in 1.8–2 Gy/fx. The ILROG consensus recommends 35 to 40 Gy for SBP <5 cm and 40 to 50 Gy for SBP ≥5 cm.[12] RT dose is similar for SEP (40–50 Gy per ILROG consensus), although the treatment volume depends on the site of involvement.[12] For SEP of the head and neck area, treatment of regional LNs can be considered despite limited data. RT planning typically involves a GTV to CTV expansion based on tumor location: 0.5 to 1 cm for microscopic disease in soft tissue and 2 to 3 cm for long bones at proximal and distal expansions. When there is uncertainty regarding the extent of involvement and minimal additional toxicity, whole bone RT can be considered. SBP has a high risk of progression to MM: 65% to 85% at 10 years and 100% at 15 years. The risk of progression to MM for SEP is 10% to 30% at 10 years, although LF can occur in ~20% of patients.[13]

EVIDENCE-BASED Q&A

What is the role of RT in the era of CAR T-cell therapy?

CAR T-cell therapy is increasingly being considered in the treatment of relapsed or refractory MM. A study involving 128 patients showed a 73% objective response rate, with 33% obtaining a CR with idecabtagene vicleucel CAR T-cell therapy.[14] Combining RT with CAR T-cells can induce immunostimulatory genes and enhance signals for CAR T-cell activation and proliferation. RT is being used as bridging treatment to CAR T-cell therapy and has been shown to increase LC rates when compared with salvage RT.[15]

What is the role of combined CHT in addition to RT for solitary plasmacytoma?

The role of CHT for solitary plasmacytoma is controversial, but it can be considered for SBP given high risk of progression to MM. One historical prospective study of 53 patients demonstrated improved DFS and OS when adding combined melphalan and prednisone to RT.[16] Multiple retrospective studies using newer agents showed mixed results.[17–19] Ongoing phase III randomized clinical trials are investigating the efficacy of systemic therapy after RT for SBP.

REFERENCES

1. Siegel RL, Giaquinto AN, Jemal A. Cancer statistics, 2024. *CA Cancer J Clin.* 2024;74(1):12–49. doi:10.3322/caac.21820
2. Lynch HT, Sanger WG, Pirruccello S, Quinn-Laquer B, Weisenburger DD. Familial multiple myeloma: a family study and review of the literature. *J Natl Cancer Inst.* 2001;93(19):1479–1483. doi:10.1093/jnci/93.19.1479
3. Dores GM, Landgren O, McGlynn KA, Curtis RE, Linet MS, Devesa SS. Plasmacytoma of bone, extramedullary plasmacytoma, and multiple myeloma: incidence and survival in the United States, 1992–2004. *Br J Haematol.* 2009;144(1):86–94. doi:10.1111/j.1365-2141.2008.07421.x
4. Kyle RA, Gertz MA, Witzig TE, et al. Review of 1027 patients with newly diagnosed multiple myeloma. *Mayo Clin Proc.* 2003;78(1):21–33. doi:10.4065/78.1.21
5. Palumbo A, Anderson K. Multiple myeloma. *N Engl J Med.* 2011;364(11):1046–1060. doi:10.1056/NEJMra1011442

6. Rajan AM, Rajkumar SV. Interpretation of cytogenetic results in multiple myeloma for clinical practice. *Blood Cancer J.* 2015;5(10):e365. doi:10.1038/bcj.2015.92

7. Palumbo A, Avet-Loiseau H, Oliva S, et al. Revised international staging system for multiple myeloma: a report from International Myeloma Working Group. *J Clin Oncol.* 2015;33(26):2863–2869. doi:10.1200/JCO.2015.61.2267

8. Greipp PR, San Miguel J, Durie BG, et al. International staging system for multiple myeloma. *J Clin Oncol.* 2005;23(15):3412–3420. doi:10.1200/JCO.2005.04.242

9. Goldschmidt H, Lokhorst HM, Mai EK, et al. Bortezomib before and after high-dose therapy in myeloma: long-term results from the phase III HOVON-65/GMMG-HD4 trial. *Leukemia.* 2018;32(2):383–390. doi:10.1038/leu.2017.211

10. Palumbo A, Bringhen S, Mateos MV, et al. Geriatric assessment predicts survival and toxicities in elderly myeloma patients: an International Myeloma Working Group report. *Blood.* 2015;125(13):2068–2074. doi:10.1182/blood-2014-12-615187

11. Mateos MV, Hernandez MT, Giraldo P, et al. Lenalidomide plus dexamethasone for high-risk smoldering multiple myeloma. *N Engl J Med.* 2013;369(5):438–447. doi:10.1056/NEJMoa1300439

12. Tsang RW, Campbell BA, Goda JS, et al. Radiation therapy for solitary plasmacytoma and multiple myeloma: guidelines from the International Lymphoma Radiation Oncology Group. *Int J Radiat Oncol Biol Phys.* 2018;101(4):794–808. doi:10.1016/j.ijrobp.2018.05.009

13. Ozsahin M, Tsang RW, Poortmans P, et al. Outcomes and patterns of failure in solitary plasmacytoma: a multicenter rare cancer network study of 258 patients. *Int J Radiat Oncol Biol Phys.* 2006;64(1):210–217. doi:10.1016/j.ijrobp.2005.06.039

14. Munshi NC, Anderson LD Jr, Shah N, et al. Idecabtagene Vicleucel in Relapsed and Refractory Multiple Myeloma. *N Engl J Med.* 2021;384(8):705–716. doi:10.1056/NEJMoa2024850

15. Saifi O, Breen WG, Lester SC, et al. Don't put the CART before the horse: the role of radiation therapy in peri-CAR T-cell therapy for aggressive B-cell non-Hodgkin lymphoma. *Int J Radiat Oncol Biol Phys.* 2023;116(5):999–1007. doi:10.1016/j.ijrobp.2022.12.017

16. Aviles A, Huerta-Guzman J, Delgado S, Fernandez A, Diaz-Maqueo JC. Improved outcome in solitary bone plasmacytomata with combined therapy. *Hematol Oncol.* 1996;14(3):111–117. doi:10.1002/(SICI)1099-1069(199609)14:3<111::AID-HON575>3.0.CO;2-G

17. Mignot F, Schernberg A, Arsene-Henry A, Vignon M, Bouscary D, Kirova Y. Solitary plasmacytoma treated by lenalidomide-dexamethasone in combination with radiation therapy: clinical outcomes. *Int J Radiat Oncol Biol Phys.* 2020;106(3):589–596. doi:10.1016/j.ijrobp.2019.10.043

18. Le Ray E, Belin L, Plancher C, et al. Our experience of solitary plasmacytoma of the bone: improved PFS with a short-course treatment by IMiDs or proteasome inhibitors combined with intensity-modulated radiotherapy. *Leuk Lymphoma.* 2018;59(7):1756–1758. doi:10.1080/10428194.2017.1393667

19. Katodritou E, Terpos E, Symeonidis AS, et al. Clinical features, outcome, and prognostic factors for survival and evolution to multiple myeloma of solitary plasmacytomas: a report of the Greek myeloma study group in 97 patients. *Am J Hematol.* 2014;89(8):803–808. doi:10.1002/ajh.23745

56 LEUKEMIA

Erik M. Davies, Erin S. Murphy, and Sheen Cherian

QUICK HIT Leukemias are hematologic malignancies defined by clonal proliferation of immature cells of myeloid or lymphoid origin. The hallmark of acute leukemias is more than 20% blasts in the peripheral blood, while chronic leukemias have less than 20%. Workup includes peripheral blood smear, bone marrow biopsy, and in some (such as ALL) an LP for CNS involvement. Systemic therapy is the cornerstone of therapy and guided by molecular subtypes. Treatment paradigm includes an induction phase to achieve remission, a consolidation phase, and a maintenance phase. Total body irradiation (TBI) is often part of the conditioning regimens prior to hematopoietic stem cell transplant (HSCT). Involvement of the CNS at diagnosis or relapse is highly morbid, and prophylactic cranial irradiation (PCI) or craniospinal irradiation (CSI) can be delivered to patients at high risk of CNS involvement or in whom the CNS is involved at relapse. The testicles are a sanctuary site for relapse of B-ALL and may receive RT (24 Gy) if there is incomplete response to systemic agents.

EPIDEMIOLOGY: Leukemias are a heterogeneous group of hematologic malignancies with an incidence in the United States of ~67,000 in 2017. They are the 10th most common cancer diagnosis.[1] Leukemias represent ~3% of new cancer diagnoses in the United States and have a slight male predominance.[2] While leukemias represent ~4% of all cancer deaths, the survival has markedly improved from ~33% at 5 years in 1975 to 66% in 2012, attributable to earlier detection and new therapies.[3] Incidence is slightly higher among Caucasians and Native Americans relative to Asian and Black Americans.[2] Acute lymphoblastic leukemia (ALL) and acute myeloid leukemia (AML) are usually diagnosed in children and adults, with bimodal age distributions, while chronic myeloid leukemia (CML) and chronic lymphocytic leukemia (CLL) tend to affect older adults.[4]

RISK FACTORS: Many risk factors potentiate the development of leukemia. Broadly, they can be separated into genetic predispositions and environmental factors:

Genetic: Fanconi anemia, Bloom syndrome, trisomy 21, Li–Fraumeni, dyskeratosis congenita, severe congenital neutropenia.[5,6]

Environmental: Exposure to ionizing radiation, prior CHT (particularly alkylating agents and topoisomerase II inhibitors), prior cancer diagnosis, exposure to benzene, virus exposure (HTLV, Epstein–Barr).[4,7–9]

ANATOMY: The bone marrow is a complex tissue that serves as the primary site of hematopoiesis, the process through which hematopoietic stem cells (HSCs) differentiate into blood cell lineages. Key sites of adult hematopoiesis are the pelvis (~34% of the blood constituents), vertebrae (28%), sternum (10%), femur (4%), and tibia (2%).[10,11] The bone marrow microenvironment consists of cellular and molecular components that regulate self-renewal, differentiation, and proliferation of HSCs. Leukemias arise from the clonal proliferation of HSC or progenitor cells within the bone marrow. Genetic mutations or cytogenetic abnormalities disrupt normal hematopoiesis, leading to growth of aberrant lymphoid cells.[12] Leukemias are classified according to the cell line lineage and the extent to which the cells are differentiated in the peripheral blood. The myeloid cell line gives rise to erythrocytes (red blood cells), megakaryocytes (platelets), granulocytes (neutrophils, eosinophils, and basophils), monocytes, and macrophages. The lymphoid cell line consists of B-cells, T-cells, and natural killer (NK) cells.[13,14]

PATHOLOGY: The leukemia diagnosis is further classified by the maturity of the respective cell lines present in the blood. Blasts are dysfunctional, immature cells that typically constitute 1% to 5% of the normal marrow. In acute leukemias, blasts constitute more than 20% of the peripheral blood smear or the bone marrow biopsy, corresponding to more pronounced symptoms. Chronic leukemias consist of less than 20% blasts, and more indolent symptoms. Table 56.1 further characterizes the epidemiology and pathologic features of various leukemias.

Table 56.1 Epidemiologic and Pathologic Characteristics of Leukemia[15-21]		
Leukemic Subtype	Epidemiology	Pathologic Features
Acute lymphoblastic leukemia (ALL)	Most common leukemia in children (70%). B-ALL most common in children (2–5 years), however with bimodal age distribution, with second peak after age 45. T-ALL with median age of onset 9 years in children and 30 in adults. Male predominance. Incidence 1.8 per 100,000 in the United States.	Proliferation of immature lymphoid cells of B- or T-cell lineages; B-ALL with t(12;21) and the ETV6-RUNX1 fusion. 50% of T-ALL with NOTCH1 mutations. T-ALL often presents as an anterior mediastinal mass. Early thymocyte precursor (ETP) phenotype in 15% of T-ALL with worse clinical outcomes. Therapy is guided by the presence or absence of the Philadelphia (Ph) chromosome, t(9;22).
Acute myeloid leukemia (AML)	Incidence increases with age. Higher incidence in males. Most common acute leukemia in the adult population.	Myeloid blasts in bone marrow. Auer rods, eosinophilic needle-shaped cytoplasmic bodies, may be present.
Chloroma (myeloid sarcoma)	Rare on presentation, occurs in ~10% of patients with AML. More common after multiple relapses and progression; often palliated with RT.	Extramedullary tumor of myeloid cells that precedes or accompanies AML.
Acute promyelocytic leukemia (APL)	Subtype of AML. No difference in incidence between men and women. Most commonly age 20–50. Slight predilection for Hispanic individuals. APL patients are more likely to be obese than individuals with AML.	Characteristic mutation is t(15;17) resulting in abnormal fusion product PML/RARα; high risk of coagulopathy. Treatment with all-trans-retinoic acid (ATRA) induces differentiation of APL cells and decreases incidence of disseminated intravascular coagulation (DIC).
Chronic lymphocytic leukemia (CLL)	Most common leukemia in adults; median age of diagnosis 65–70 years, increasing incidence with age.	Clonal proliferation of mature B cells. IGVH mutation status, TP53 mutation, and deletion of 17p dictate treatment. Indolent clinical course, although ~5% of cases can undergo Richter transformation to an aggressive lymphoma (associated with NOTCH1 gene mutation).
Chronic myeloid leukemia (CML)	Incidence rate 1–2 per 100,000; median age of diagnosis is 65 years.	Increased granulocytes on CBC. Ph chromosome t(9;22) with BCR-ABL1 fusion product. Three phases: chronic phase, accelerated phase, blast crisis.
Hairy cell leukemia	Rare; incidence ~0.3 per 100,000.	Pathognomonic feature is "hairy" cytoplasmic projections extending from B-cells; over 95% have BRAF V600E mutation.

SCREENING: There is no utility for routine screening for leukemia; however, some high-risk populations, such as individuals with genetic predispositions, may receive routine CBC with differential and possibly bone marrow evaluations.[22]

CLINICAL PRESENTATION

Acute Leukemias: Clinical presentation is dictated by the rapid accumulation of blasts in bone marrow, leading to bone marrow failure. Nonspecific symptoms follow, including fever, fatigue, weight loss, bone pain, petechiae, bleeding mucous membranes, recurrent infections, and pallor. DIC can occur in up to 77% of patients with APL due to the release of procoagulant and fibrinolytic moieties from leukemic promyelocytes that can precipitate life-threatening hemorrhagic complications.[23,24]

Chronic Leukemias: This class of disease is typically more indolent given relatively slower accumulation of blasts and fewer immature cells in circulation. CLL may present with fatigue, reduced exercise tolerance, lymphadenopathy, and splenomegaly. More advanced presentations may include frequent infections, unintentional weight loss, and fever. Enlarged LNs can be seen radiographically. CML is often asymptomatic and diagnosed with routine bloodwork showing increased granulocytes. When CML progresses from the chronic phase to the accelerated phase or blast crisis, symptoms can mirror acute leukemias with increasing numbers of blasts.[24,25] The diagnostic criteria of a blast crisis are >20% blasts in the blood or bone marrow or the presence of an extramedullary blast collection. Blast crises represent oncologic emergencies.

WORKUP

Labs: Obtain CBC with differential, peripheral smear, CMP, LFTs, uric acid, PT/PTT/INR, B_{12}/folate. While some chronic leukemias can be diagnosed solely on smear, often a bone marrow core biopsy is required with advanced analysis of the aspirate (FISH, cytogenetics, IHC, or whole genome analysis). If ALL is diagnosed or neurologic symptoms are noted, obtain LP with cell count (including blasts) and flow cytometry. In ALL, obtain Ph chromosome status to guide treatment. Assess for hepatitis B/C and HIV.[26–29]

Imaging: Imaging is guided by symptoms. If there is suspicion for extramedullary involvement/chloroma (such as a solid soft tissue mass), obtain CT imaging of the involved sites. In those with neurologic signs or symptoms, obtain MRI brain. Perform scrotal ultrasound in all male patients diagnosed with ALL. Echocardiogram if initiation of an anthracycline is planned or prior thoracic RT.[26–29]

Other: Referral to fertility preservation services according to patient preference prior to initiation of treatment.

PROGNOSTIC FACTORS: Leukemias have variable natural histories; thus, the prognostic features vary widely. Major risk factors are provided in Table 56.2. Refer to the NCCN guidelines for elaboration of molecular and genetic characteristics that influence prognosis.

Table 56.2 Overview of Prognostic Factors by Leukemic Subtype[4,26,28–30]	
Leukemic Type	**Prognostic Factors**
B-ALL	High-risk: age >35 in adults, age <1 or >10 in pediatrics; WBC >30 × 10^9/L in adults or >50 × 10^9/L in pediatrics Molecular/genetic markers subdivide into standard and poor risk: • Standard-risk: t(9;22) BCR::ABL1 without IKZF1^{plus} and no antecedent CML; hyperdiploidy; and trisomy 4, 10, and 17 (most favorable) • High-risk: hypodiploidy (<44 chromosomes); TP53 mutation; BCR::ABL1-like; and t(9;22) BCR::ABL1 with IKZF1^{plus} and/or antecedent CML
T-ALL	High-risk features: age >35, WBC >100 × 10^9/L, ETP-ALL phenotype, RAS/PTEN mutation, NOTCH/FBXW7 wild-type
AML	Molecular/genetic markers guide prognosis and include: • Favorable: IDH1/2 mut; NPM1 mut; myelodysplasia-related gene mutations including FLT3-ITD negative, NRAS wt, KRAS wt, TP53 wt (mOS 23–39 months) • Intermediate: myelodysplasia-related gene mutations including FLT3-ITD positive, NRAS mut, KRAS mut (mOS 12–13 months) • Adverse: TP53 mut (mOS 5–8 months)
APL	Low-risk: WBC ≤10 × 10^9/L High-risk: WBC >10 × 10^9/L
CLL	Poor prognostic mutations: ATM, BIRC3, NOTCH1, SF3B1, TP53 Genes implicated in resistance to systemic therapy: BTK, CARD11, PLCG2, BCL2
CML	Poor prognostic features: increasing age, spleen size (as measured by distance below costal margin), platelets >1,500 × 10^9/L, basophils >3%, increasing blast count

STAGING: A variety of staging systems are used to guide treatment decisions and to obtain prognostic information about each of the leukemias. WHO classifications were updated in 2016 to integrate immunophenotypic and genetic data into diagnoses. AML is most commonly staged by the WHO paradigm.[31] T-ALL is usually staged by the Murphy/St. Jude staging system, which resembles the Ann Arbor staging system for lymphoma. B-ALL is classified according to the Children's Oncology Group (COG) and NCCN risk groups as described above. CLL patients are stratified by the Rai system, which takes into account lymphadenopathy, splenomegaly, hepatomegaly, anemia, and thrombocytopenia; or the Binet system, which incorporates the number of involved lymphoid subsites and the presence of anemia and thrombocytopenia.[32] CML is staged according to the phase of the disease: chronic phase (<10% blasts in the peripheral blood and bone marrow), accelerated phase (10%–19% blasts), and blast phase (≥20% blasts). Several other scoring systems can be applied to the chronic phase to predict prognosis and guide therapy decisions.[33]

ALL has the greatest predilection for CNS involvement among the leukemia subtypes, and thus most indications for RT involve this disease. CNS risk classification for acute leukemias is based on the presence of WBCs in the CSF and flow cytometry findings as follows:[26]

- CNS1: no blasts in the CSF, negative flow cytometry
- CNS2: WBC <5/μL in CSF with presence of lymphoblasts
- CNS3: WBC ≥5/μL in CSF with presence of lymphoblasts or the presence of neurologic symptoms

CNS3 disease is an indication for CSI (see Evidence-Based Q&A).

TREATMENT PARADIGM

Prevention: Multidisciplinary oncologic teams limit exposure to ionizing radiation and chemo-therapies, especially in childhood, given the increased risk of developing leukemias.[34] Individuals should limit exposure to benzene.

Surgery: No role for surgery. Bone marrow biopsy and LP are performed as discussed above.

Systemic Therapy: CHT and targeted therapy are the mainstay of treatment for leukemia and are heavily dictated by the molecular and genetic markers of the malignant cells, as well as patient factors including age and performance status. Systemic therapy usually begins with an induction phase in which remission is obtained. Treatment is then intensified in a consolidative phase. The patient then continues on a maintenance regimen while on surveillance for residual or recurrent disease.

The cornerstone of treatment for AML is 7+3 CHT, which consists of 7 days of cytarabine and 3 days of an anthracycline. Favorable-risk patients then receive gemtuzumab ozogamicin, an anti-CD33 antibody–drug conjugate. HSCT is reserved for relapse. Intermediate-risk patients instead receive a tyrosine kinase inhibitor (TKI) depending on the molecular profile of their tumor, with 7+3. HSCT is considered following maintenance in this risk group.[4,27]

APL is a subtype of AML and often presents with hemorrhagic manifestations as well as a hypercoag-ulable milieu. The cornerstone of treatment is all-trans-retinoic acid (ATRA), which should be initiated when APL is clinically suspected prior to confirmatory testing.[4] The major complication of ATRA initiation is differentiation syndrome, a constellation of fever, respiratory distress with pulmonary infiltrates on imaging, hypotension, and renal failure that can mimic sepsis and results from the release of proinflammatory cytokines from differentiating leukemic cells. This causes a systemic inflammatory response and capillary leakage. The incidence of differentiation syndrome is as high as 37% with some treatment regimens. Appropriate management of differentiation syndrome is initiation of dexamethasone. In severe cases, ATRA may need to be suspended until the patient stabilizes.[35–37]

Treatment of ALL is determined by the presence or absence of the Ph chromosome. Second-generation oral TKIs such as imatinib or dasatinib are combined with CHT in the Ph-positive population. Younger patients (15–40 years) may be considered for intensified pediatric regimens such as peg-asparaginase. Patients over 40 years may be treated with hyper-CVAD (cyclophosphamide, vincristine, doxorubicin, and dexamethasone) alternated with high-dose methotrexate and cytarabine. Dose reductions may be used in patients older than 65 or with marginal performance status. There is no role for TKIs in the Ph-negative ALL patient population. All ALL regimens include CNS prophylaxis via systemic or intrathecal MTX or cytarabine.[18,26]

Chimeric Antigen Receptor (CAR) T-Cell Therapy: CAR T-cells are genetically modified autologous T-cells directed at leukemic cell-surface antigens, commonly CD19. Autologous T-cells are harvested from the patient, modified with chimeric tumor-specific transmembrane antibodies, replicated ex vivo, and reinfused into the patient. Use of CAR-T is indicated in relapsed/refractory disease among patients who show incomplete response to induction CHT. CAR T-cells can achieve complete remission through direct cell kill and serve as a bridge to HSCT.[26]

Radiation

Indications: The acute subtypes have a greater predilection for CNS penetration; thus ALL and, to a much lesser extent, AML are the most common indications for RT. Consider CSI for adult patients with known CNS3 disease without planned HSCT. Deliver CSI in adult patients with relapsed ALL or with CNS disease refractory to systemic or intrathecal therapies. Pediatric trials have usually administered PCI rather than CSI for CNS3 disease upfront or CNS relapse to mitigate the risk of growth restriction; however, the CSF is dynamic and thus WBRT may offer inadequate coverage of the presumed volume of disease spanning the neuroaxis. Many conditioning regimens require TBI prior to HSCT. For B-ALL relapsed to the testicles with incomplete response to systemic agents, intensify treatment with testicular RT. Chloromas are extramedullary, localized manifestation of systemic disease and can be treated with photons or electrons up to 24 Gy.[21]

Dose: A variety of doses are possible for TBI, but myeloablative regimens are often delivered in 12 Gy/6–8 fx BID. More truncated "mini" regimens are 2–4 Gy/1–2 fx. For high-risk ALL patients undergoing TBI as part of conditioning regimen, can consider cranial boost of 6 Gy/3 fx.[38] Administer testicular electron boost of 4 Gy/1 fx to men with ALL.[39] CSI for CNS3 disease is typically given 18–23.4 Gy/10–13 fx. If relapsed B-ALL in the testicles, treat to 24 Gy/12 fx. If delivering CSI for relapsed disease in a transplanted patient, incorporate prior TBI dose into treatment planning.

Toxicity: WBRT: neurocognitive decline (particularly for cranial doses to 24 Gy in children <8 years), dermatitis, alopecia, fatigue, nausea, cataract formation. Including spine as part of CSI can cause growth restriction (pediatrics) and acute nausea. Elevated risk of secondary malignancies. TBI: fatigue, nausea, parotitis, and secondary malignancies. Counsel all prepubescent patients and patients of childbearing age about the risk of permanent sterility (12 Gy in prepubescent girls and 2 Gy in premenopausal women; 2.5–3 Gy with fractionated RT or 6 Gy in a single dose for men).

Procedure: See *Handbook of Treatment Planning in Radiation Oncology*, Chapters 10 and 12.[40]

Follow-Up: Physical exam, CBC with differential q1–2 months for the first year following treatment, q3–6 months at year 2, and q6–12 months thereafter. LFTs until normalized. If ALL, bone marrow biopsy with molecular classification q3–6 months for at least 5 years.

EVIDENCE-BASED Q&A

When is CNS-directed RT indicated in the management of acute leukemia? Is there any utility to RT prior to HSCT?

CNS RT prophylaxis is reserved for only the highest risk populations (per ASTRO guidelines), typically when TBI is not planned.[41] The preponderance of evidence for the use of RT arises from the pediatric literature. RT is particularly toxic in pediatric patients, especially those <3 years, due to the risk of neurocognitive decline, radionecrosis, secondary malignancies, growth disturbances, and endocrinopathies. CNS-penetrant CHT such as MTX, cytarabine, and hyper-CVAD demonstrate excellent CNS control rates with a favorable toxicity profile. The meta-analysis by Vora et al. below comprising children with ALL suggests that systemic or intrathecal CHT affords excellent CNS control and that cranial RT benefits only a subset of CNS3 patients, which account for 2% to 3% of patients at diagnosis. Of note, PCI did not significantly improve 5-year OS.

ASTRO guidelines from 2018 recommend RT prior to HSCT among patients with CNS disease at diagnosis or relapse, regardless of degree of response to systemic or intrathecal agents.[41] The Mayadev RR below supports the addition of CNS-directed RT prior to transplant. PCI in patients with CNS1 or CNS2 disease planned for HSCT is not routine as relapse rates following transplant are <5%. Some institutions consider all T-cell leukemias high risk and administer CSI to these patients; however, the publication of AALL0434 indicates that CNS relapse rates are 1% to 2% in newly diagnosed T-ALL patients with CNS1 and CNS2 disease with CHT alone (CNS3 patients were excluded from this trial).[42] CNS-directed RT is typically delivered for CNS3 disease prior to planned HSCT.

Vora (*JCO* 2016, PMID 26755523): Meta-analysis of over 16,000 pediatric patients aged 1 to 18 treated from 1996 to 2007 on 10 cooperative study group trials for new diagnoses of ALL. Purpose was to determine which high-risk subgroups benefit from prophylactic WBRT. The primary endpoints were EFS and cumulative incidence of CNS relapse between patients who received WBRT and those who did not. Those with "overt" CNS disease at diagnosis (indications varied but typically CNS3) had significantly lower risk of isolated CNS relapse (4% vs. 17%, $p = .02$) with WBRT. However, EFS was not statistically different between groups (32% vs. 34%, NS). No survival benefit to WBRT. **Conclusion: WBRT reduces the rate of CNS relapse in pediatric patients with CNS3 ALL at diagnosis but does not lower EFS. Unclear whether CSI prophylaxis would further limit CNS relapse to justify the substantial late effects associated with therapy.**

Mayadev, University of Washington (*IJROBP* 2011, PMID 20584584): RR of 648 adult AML patients, of which 71 had CNS involvement (CNS1–3 classification not reported), who received a myeloablative HCT. Of those with CNS involvement, 52 had intrathecal CHT alone (ITC) and 19 had CNS RT boost in addition to intrathecal CHT (RT + ITC). Of the RT + ITC patients, 15 had WBRT and 4 had CSI at physician discretion. Sixty-one (86%) patients with CNS involvement received TBI as part of their conditioning regimen. RFS at 1 and 5 years was 15% and 6% in the ITC group vs. 37% and 32% in the RT + ITC group (SS). OS at 1 and 5 years was 21% and 6% in the ITC group vs. 53% and 42% in the RT + ITC group (SS). Survival at 1 and 5 years in the RT + ITC group was comparable to patients with no CNS disease. **Conclusion: Among adult AML patients with leukemia involving the CNS and planned HSCT, CNS-directed RT prior to transplant was associated with improved 1- and 5-year RFS and OS over intrathecal CHT alone.**

Can TBI prior to HSCT be omitted?

Data from the FORUM trial indicate that in pediatric patients in whom CR was achieved following induction, there is a survival advantage and lower incidence of recurrence among those treated with TBI vs. intensified CHT prior to transplant.

FORUM (*JCO* 2021, PMID 33332189): Multi-institutional noninferiority study of 417 patients with ALL age ≤18 at diagnosis who achieved CR prior to planned HSCT randomized to myeloablative TBI 12 Gy vs. intensified CHT conditioning. Primary endpoint 2-year OS, and secondary endpoints 2-year incidence of relapse and treatment-related mortality. The 2-year OS was significantly higher following TBI (91% vs. 75%, SS). The 2-year incidence of relapse and treatment-related mortality was 12% and 2% with TBI and 33% and 9% (both SS) with CHT conditioning, respectively. **Conclusion: In pediatric patients with ALL and CR to induction therapy, TBI prior to HSCT demonstrates improved 2-year OS, lower incidence of relapse, and lower treatment-related mortality than intensified CHT conditioning.**

What data support the use of CAR T-cells for relapsed/refractory ALL?

ELIANA (*NEJM* 2018, PMID 29385370; Update *JCO* 2023, PMID 36399695): Phase II multi-institutional study of tisagenlecleucel (anti-CD19 CAR T-cell therapy) with CD19+ relapsed or refractory B-ALL. Overall remission rate was 82% with MFU of 39 months. Median EFS is 24 months, and mOS was not reached. The 3-year EFS was 44% and the 3-year OS was 63%, with most events occurring within the first 2 years. Grade 3/4 adverse events reported in 29%. QOL improved up to 36 months following infusion. **Conclusion: CAR T-cells are a safe and effective therapy for induction of remission in young adults with relapsed/refractory B-ALL.**

What is the management approach for B-ALL relapsed in the testicles?

Barredo (*Pediatr Blood Cancer* 2018, PMID 29286562): Multicenter analysis of 40 patients with first isolated testicular relapse of B-ALL enrolled on AALL02P2 with at least 18 months prior to first relapse. Induction CHT preceded by one dose of HD-MTX. Following induction, 25 of 26 patients with persistent testicular enlargement underwent testicular biopsy. Twelve patients had biopsy-proven disease, and 11 then received bilateral testicular RT to 24 Gy. The remaining patients in the study did not receive testicular RT. The 5-year EFS was 62% vs. 73%, favoring testicular RT ($p = .64$). The 5-year OS and proportion of second relapses were similar among patients who did not receive testicular RT vs. those who did (72% in each). **Conclusion: For patients with B-ALL relapsed to the testicles with persistent disease following induction CHT, testicular RT to 24 Gy leads to acceptable EFS and OS.**

How should extramedullary leukemias/chloromas be managed?

Chloromas are extramedullary tumors that most commonly arise in the setting of AML, occurring in ~10% of cases. They are sometimes detectable on exam, and CT imaging should be obtained to delineate the extent of the lesion. Leukemia cutis is another extramedullary manifestation of AML and presents as painful or pruritic dermal or epidermal lesions. The appearance of leukemia cutis is often a manifestation of systemic disease, although it infrequently precedes systemic onset. The most common involved site are the lower extremities. These extramedullary lesions can be treated for palliation with 24 Gy in 2 Gy per fraction; however, responses are noted with as low as 6 Gy given the radiosensitivity of these tumors. For extensive skin involvement, consider TSET (see Chapter 23). Dermal toxicity following EBRT is most associated with anthracyclines; however, dermatitis can occur following other CHT, including cytarabine.[21]

REFERENCES

1. Siegel RL, Miller KD, Jemal A. Cancer statistics, 2017. *CA Cancer J Clin.* 2017;67(1):7–30. doi:10.3322/caac.21387
2. Bakhati B, Chamarti K, Sibi V, Dang T, Bajaj K. Trends of leukemia mortality in the United States, 1999–2018. *J Clin Oncol.* 2022;40(16_suppl):e19034. doi:10.1200/JCO.2022.40.16_suppl.e19034
3. Yang X, Chen H, Man J, et al. Secular trends in the incidence and survival of all leukemia types in the United States from 1975 to 2017. *J Cancer.* 2021;12(8):2326–2335. doi:10.7150/jca.52186
4. Chennamadhavuni A, Lyengar V, Mukkamalla SKR, Shimanovsky A. Leukemia. *StatPearls.* StatPearls Publishing; 2024.
5. Stieglitz E, Loh ML. Genetic predispositions to childhood leukemia. *Ther Adv Hematol.* 2013;4(4):270–290. doi:10.1177/2040620713498161
6. Savage SA, Dufour C. Classical inherited bone marrow failure syndromes with high risk for myelodysplastic syndrome and acute myelogenous leukemia. *Semin Hematol.* 2017;54(2):105–114. doi:10.1053/j.seminhematol.2017.04.004
7. Bispo JAB, Pinheiro PS, Kobetz EK. Epidemiology and etiology of leukemia and lymphoma. *Cold Spring Harb Perspect Med.* 2020;10(6):a034819. doi:10.1101/cshperspect.a034819
8. Snyder R. Leukemia and benzene. *Int J Environ Res Public Health.* 2012;9(8):2875–2893. doi:10.3390/ijerph9082875
9. Greim H, Kaden DA, Larson RA, et al. The bone marrow niche, stem cells, and leukemia: impact of drugs, chemicals, and the environment. *Ann N Y Acad Sci.* 2014;1310(1):7–31. doi:10.1111/nyas.12362
10. Le PM, Andreeff M, Battula VL. Osteogenic niche in the regulation of normal hematopoiesis and leukemogenesis. *Haematologica.* 2018;103(12):1945–1955. doi:10.3324/haematol.2018.197004
11. Ershler W, Longo D. Hematology in older persons. In: *Williams Hematology.* 8th ed. McGraw-Hill; 2010.
12. Pimenta DB, Varela VA, Datoguia TS, Caraciolo VB, Lopes GH, Pereira WO. The bone marrow microenvironment mechanisms in acute myeloid leukemia. *Front Cell Dev Biol.* 2021;9:764698. doi:10.3389/fcell.2021.764698
13. Weiskopf K, Schnorr PJ, Pang WW, et al. Myeloid cell origins, differentiation, and clinical implications. *Microbiol Spectr.* 2016;4(5). doi:10.1128/microbiolspec.MCHD-0031-2016
14. Kondo M. Lymphoid and myeloid lineage commitment in multipotent hematopoietic progenitors. *Immunol Rev.* 2010;238(1):37–46. doi:10.1111/j.1600-065X.2010.00963.x
15. Choi JK, Xiao W, Chen X, et al. Fifth edition of the World Health Organization classification of tumors of the hematopoietic and lymphoid tissues: acute lymphoblastic leukemias, mixed-phenotype acute leukemias, myeloid/lymphoid neoplasms with eosinophilia, dendritic/histiocytic neoplasms, and genetic tumor syndromes. *Mod Pathol.* 2024;37(5):100466. doi:10.1016/j.modpat.2024.100466
16. Dores GM, Devesa SS, Curtis RE, Linet MS, Morton LM. Acute leukemia incidence and patient survival among children and adults in the United States, 2001–2007. *Blood.* 2012;119(1):34–43. doi:10.1182/blood-2011-04-347872
17. Runjic E, Jelicic Kadic A, Bastian L, et al. Clinical and cytogenetic characteristics of children with leukemia: 20-year retrospective study. *J Pediatr Hematol Oncol.* 2023;45(2):e161–e166. doi:10.1097/MPH.0000000000002529
18. Brown PA, Shah B, Advani A, et al. Acute lymphoblastic leukemia, version 2.2021, NCCN Clinical Practice Guidelines in Oncology. *J Natl Compr Canc Netw.* 2021;19(9):1079–1109. doi:10.6004/jnccn.2021.0042
19. Kamath GR, Tremblay D, Coltoff A, et al. Comparing the epidemiology, clinical characteristics and prognostic factors of acute myeloid leukemia with and without acute promyelocytic leukemia. *Carcinogenesis.* 2019;40(5):651–660. doi:10.1093/carcin/bgz014
20. Arshad F, Ali A, Rehman G, et al. Comparative expression analysis of breakpoint cluster region-Abelson oncogene in leukemia patients. *ACS Omega.* 2023;8(6):5975–5982. doi:10.1021/acsomega.2c07885
21. Bakst RL, Dabaja BS, Specht LK, Yahalom J. Use of radiation in extramedullary leukemia/chloroma: guidelines from the International Lymphoma Radiation Oncology Group. *Int J Radiat Oncol Biol Phys.* 2018;102(2):314–319. doi:10.1016/j.ijrobp.2018.05.045

22. de Haas V, Ismaila N, Advani A, et al. Initial diagnostic work-up of acute leukemia: ASCO clinical practice guideline endorsement of the college of American pathologists and American Society of Hematology guideline. *J Clin Oncol.* 2019;37(3):239–253. doi:10.1200/JCO.18.01468

23. Chang H, Kuo MC, Shih LY, et al. Clinical bleeding events and laboratory coagulation profiles in acute promyelocytic leukemia. *Eur J Haematol.* 2012;88(4):321–328. doi:10.1111/j.1600-0609.2011.01747.x

24. Shephard EA, Neal RD, Rose PW, Walter FM, Hamilton W. Symptoms of adult chronic and acute leukaemia before diagnosis: large primary care case-control studies using electronic records. *Br J Gen Pract.* 2016;66(644):e182–e188. doi:10.3399/bjgp16X683989

25. Gbenjo JTC, McCrary GLM, Wilson SE. Leukemia: what primary care physicians need to know. *Am Fam Physician.* 2023;107(4):397–405. PMID: 37054416

26. National Comprehensive Cancer Network. *NCCN Clinical Practice Guidelines in Oncology: Acute Lymphoblastic Leukemia.* Version 3.2024. Accessed December 31, 2024. https://www.nccn.org/professionals/physician_gls/pdf/all.pdf

27. National Comprehensive Cancer Network. *NCCN Clinical Practice Guidelines in Oncology: Acute Myeloid Leukemia.* Version 1.2025. Accessed January 3, 2025. https://www.nccn.org/professionals/physician_gls/pdf/aml.pdf

28. National Comprehensive Cancer Network. *NCCN Clinical Practice Guidelines in Oncology: Chronic Lymphocytic Leukemia/Small Lymphocytic Lymphoma.* Version 1.2025. Accessed January 3, 2025. https://www.nccn.org/professionals/physician_gls/pdf/cll.pdf

29. National Comprehensive Cancer Network. *NCCN Clinical Practice Guidelines in Oncology: Chronic Myeloid Leukemia.* Version 3.2025. Accessed January 3, 2025. https://www.nccn.org/professionals/physician_gls/pdf/cml.pdf

30. Döhner H, DiNardo CD, Appelbaum FR, et al. Genetic risk classification for adults with AML receiving less-intensive therapies: the 2024 ELN recommendations. *Blood.* 2024;144(21):2169–2173. doi:10.1182/blood.2024025409

31. Arber DA, Orazi A, Hasserjian R, et al. The 2016 revision to the World Health Organization classification of myeloid neoplasms and acute leukemia. *Blood.* 2016;127(20):2391–2405. doi:10.1182/blood-2016-03-643544

32. Wierda WG, Brown J, Abramson JS, et al. Chronic lymphocytic leukemia/small lymphocytic lymphoma, version 2.2024, NCCN Clinical Practice Guidelines in Oncology. *J Natl Compr Canc Netw.* 2024;22(3): 175–204. doi:10.6004/jnccn.2024.0018

33. Shah NP, Bhatia R, Altman JK, et al. Chronic myeloid leukemia, version 2.2024, NCCN Clinical Practice Guidelines in Oncology. *J Natl Compr Canc Netw.* 2024;22(1):43–69. doi:10.6004/jnccn.2024.0007

34. Miranda-Filho A, Piñeros M, Ferlay J, Soerjomataram I, Monnereau A, Bray F. Epidemiological patterns of leukaemia in 184 countries: a population-based study. *Lancet Haematol.* 2018;5(1):e14–e24. doi:10.1016/S2352-3026(17)30232-6

35. Stahl M, Tallman MS. Differentiation syndrome in acute promyelocytic leukaemia. *Br J Haematol.* 2019; 187(2):157–162. doi:10.1111/bjh.16151

36. Woods AC, Norsworthy KJ. Differentiation syndrome in acute leukemia: APL and beyond. *Cancers (Basel).* 2023;15(19):4767. doi:10.3390/cancers15194767

37. Luesink M, Pennings JL, Wissink WM, et al. Chemokine induction by all-trans retinoic acid and arsenic trioxide in acute promyelocytic leukemia: triggering the differentiation syndrome. *Blood.* 2009;114(27):5512–5521. doi:10.1182/blood-2009-02-204834

38. Su W, Thompson M, Sheu RD, et al. Low-dose cranial boost in high-risk adult acute lymphoblastic leukemia patients undergoing bone marrow transplant. *Pract Radiat Oncol.* 2017;7(2):103–108. doi:10.1016/j.prro.2016.06.008

39. Wong JYC, Filippi AR, Dabaja BS, Yahalom J, Specht L. Total body irradiation: guidelines from the International Lymphoma Radiation Oncology Group (ILROG). *Int J Radiat Oncol Biol Phys.* 2018;101(3): 521–529. doi:10.1016/j.ijrobp.2018.04.071

40. Videtic GMM, Vassil AD. *Handbook of Treatment Planning in Radiation Oncology.* 3rd ed. Demos Medical; 2020.

41. Pinnix CC, Yahalom J, Specht L, Dabaja BS. Radiation in central nervous system leukemia: guidelines from the International Lymphoma Radiation Oncology Group. *Int J Radiat Oncol Biol Phys.* 2018;102(1):53–58. doi:10.1016/j.ijrobp.2018.05.067

42. Hayashi RJ, Winter SS, Dunsmore KP, et al. Successful outcomes of newly diagnosed T lymphoblastic lymphoma: results from Children's Oncology Group AALL0434. *J Clin Oncol.* 2020;38(26):3062–3070. doi:10.1200/JCO.20.00531

PART X: Sarcomas

57 SOFT TISSUE SARCOMA

Anirudh Bommireddy, Jacob G. Scott, and Shauna R. Campbell

QUICK HIT Soft tissue sarcomas (STS) are a heterogeneous group of tumors that include more than 100 histologic subtypes, with the majority originating in the extremities. Core needle biopsy should be performed by the treating surgeon, preferably a surgical/orthopedic oncologist. Surgical resection is required for cure and the role of systemic therapy is evolving in the targeted era. Positive margins confer a higher risk of LR, and high grade confers a higher risk of developing DM. The role of RT is to improve outcomes for localized disease when combined with surgery. General treatment paradigms are included in Table 57.1. For extremity STS, surgery alone may be considered for low-grade, stage I tumors resected with negative margins. For stage II to III STS of the extremity that are resectable with reasonable functional outcomes (limb-sparing), RT is recommended and can be delivered either preop or postop (PORT). RT improves LC and may improve OS. Retroperitoneal sarcoma (RPS) comprises 10% to 15% of STS and are most commonly liposarcoma (LS). Surgical resection is standard, and LR following gross total resection (GTR) is common. RT can be delivered preoperatively to improve LC.

Table 57.1 General Treatment Paradigm for Soft Tissue and Retroperitoneal Sarcoma[1]		
	Extremities/Superficial Trunk	**Retroperitoneal**
Stage I	Total en bloc excision alone. Add PORT if positive margins and consider for close (<5 mm) margin or high grade. PORT dose is 60 Gy/30 fx plus boost (66 Gy for microscopic positive margins and 70–76 Gy for gross residual). Preop RT (50 Gy/25 fx) can be considered if close or positive margins are anticipated.	Surgery alone OR Preop RT to 45–50.4 Gy/25–28 fx is considered *PORT is not recommended for RPS. Consider limited-field PORT when recurrence would be morbid and/or unresectable.*
Stage II–III	Preop RT (50 Gy/25 fx*). Postop EBRT boost for positive/close margins of 16 Gy is controversial. OR PORT (60 Gy/30 fx plus boost as above) OR Adjuvant brachytherapy alone (30–40 Gy given BID for 10 fx)	
Unresectable	Consider neoadjuvant RT, CHT, or CRT to facilitate surgery. Dose >70 Gy necessary for LC with RT alone.	Consider CHT or RT to facilitate surgery. If truly unresectable, treatment is palliative.
	Spatially fractionated RT (SFRT) combined with palliative RT or stereotactic body RT (SBRT) can be considered to improve LC for select cases.	
Desmoid	Observation may be reasonable. Primary management is surgical or medical. RT to 56–58 Gy if nonoperative. PORT for positive margins is controversial; many reserve RT for recurrence or unresectable disease. Consider nirogacestat, sorafenib, tamoxifen, sulindac, and imatinib for unresectable patients or those with familial adenomatous polyposis (FAP).	

*36 Gy/18 fx can be considered for myxoid LS.[2]
Source: Data from National Comprehensive Cancer Network . *NCCN Clinical Practice Guidelines in Oncology: Soft Tissue Sarcoma.* Version 1.2024. https://www.nccn.org.

EPIDEMIOLOGY: Sarcomas are rare, representing ~1% of malignancies, with 80% of these being STS and 20% originating in bone. Benign soft tissue masses are much more common than STS. In 2024, there were ~13,590 cases of STS diagnosed in the United States and ~5,200 deaths.[3] Median age of diagnosis is 45 to 55 years; ~20% are diagnosed before age 40, 30% between age 40 and 60, and 50% age >60.

RISK FACTORS: Male gender, genetic predisposition, prior exposure to RT or CHT, chemical carcinogens, chronic irritation or lymphedema, and HIV/HHV8 involvement in Kaposi's. In reported series from MSKCC, distribution of RT-induced sarcomas was 21% osteosarcoma, 16%

undifferentiated pleomorphic sarcoma (UPS), and 15% angiosarcoma. These were seen most commonly following treatment of breast cancer (26%), lymphoma (25%), and cervical cancer (14%), with median latency of 10.3 years.[4] FAP, or more specifically Gardner syndrome, is a risk factor for desmoid tumors.

ANATOMY: STS arise from a mesenchymal cell of origin and can occur in all body sites; however, approximately two-thirds occur in the extremities, most commonly in the proximal lower extremity. The remaining one-third are found in the retroperitoneum and trunk or H&N region, with slightly more retroperitoneal cases. At diagnosis, 90% of extremity STS are localized. Most common STS by site: extremities (LS, UPS, synovial, and fibrosarcoma [FS]) and retroperitoneum/intra-abdominal (well-differentiated and dedifferentiated LS, leiomyosarcoma [LMS], visceral gastrointestinal stromal tumor [GIST]). The tumor is usually surrounded by a pseudocapsule (region of compressed reactive tissue) and reactive zone (high MRI T2 signal) that can harbor microscopic disease, which is important for resection assessment. In one series, infiltrating tumor cells were found up to 4 cm from the pseudocapsule in 67% of patients, and all but one of which were found in the "edema" region.[5]

PATHOLOGY: Greater than 100 histologic subtypes have been reported. The most common subtypes in decreasing order are LS, LMS, high-grade UPS, GIST, synovial sarcoma, myxofibrosarcoma, and malignant peripheral nerve sheath tumor (MPNST). Certain subtypes have a propensity for metastasis, such as LMS. Histologic grade is determined by differentiation, mitotic count, and necrosis.[6] Of note, myogenic differentiation in pleomorphic sarcomas increases the risk of DM and is prognostic of many subtypes. Grade is less prognostic of MPNST, angiosarcoma, extraskeletal myxoid chondrosarcoma, and clear cell sarcoma.

GENETICS: Simple karyotypes and reciprocal translocations include alveolar rhabdomyosarcoma (t[2;13]), clear cell sarcoma (t[12;22]), myxoid LS (t[12;16]), synovial sarcoma (t[X;18]), dermatofibrosarcoma protuberans (ring [17;22]), and solitary fibrous tumor (fusion NAB2-STAT6). Characteristic amplifications: well-differentiated and undifferentiated LS (MDM2). Specific driver mutations: desmoid fibromatosis (CTNNB1), GIST (c-kit or PDGFRA), rhabdoid tumors (loss of INI1). Complex karyotypes may be found in some high-grade tumors. Classic genetic syndromes with their specific mutations that increase the risk of STS are characterized in Table 57.2.

Table 57.2 Genetic Syndromes Commonly Associated With Soft Tissue Sarcoma

Syndrome	Clinical Findings	Gene	Chromosome
Neurofibromatosis type 1 (NF1)	MPNST (5%), optic glioma, astrocytoma, neurofibromas, café au lait spots, Lisch nodules, axillary freckling	NF-1	17q11
Familial retinoblastoma (Rb)	STS, osteosarcoma, retinoblastoma	Rb-1	13q14
Li–Fraumeni	STS, osteosarcoma, leukemia, breast cancer, CNS tumors, adrenal tumors	TP53	17p13
Werner's (adult progeria)	STS, osteosarcoma, meningioma	WRN	8p12
Gardner's (subset of FAP)	FS, intraabdominal desmoid, colon cancer	APC	5q21
Gorlin's (nevoid BCC)	FS, rhabdomyosarcoma, BCC, CNS tumors	PTC	9q22
Carney's triad	GIST, extra-adrenal paraganglioma, pulmonary chondroma	c-KIT	Unknown

CLINICAL PRESENTATION: Symptoms are generally site-dependent. Typical presentation is an enlarging, painless mass. Symptoms of compression may be reported, including new-onset edema and/or paresthesia. Constitutional symptoms including fever and weight loss are rare. Metastatic disease is present at initial diagnosis in 6% to 10%, with increased risk in deep and high-grade tumors.[4]

WORKUP: As benign soft tissue disease is much more common, workup of a painless enlarging mass should include a thorough H&P with examination of the mass and draining LN regions to assess for adenopathy and rule out benign causes.

Labs: CBC and CMP.

Imaging: MRI with contrast of the affected area. On MRI, the tumor is typically hypointense on T1 and hyperintense on T2. CT chest to evaluate for metastatic disease once STS is confirmed. The role of FDG PET/CT is evolving, and according to NCCN it may be useful in prognostication, grading, and determining response to neoadjuvant CHT.[1] It may also be helpful to distinguish MPNST from neurofibroma as well as to evaluate areas of dedifferentiation in retroperitoneal LS. Whole-body MRI or at minimum MRI of the spine should be performed at diagnosis and annually for myxoid LS and round cell sarcomas.

Procedures: Core needle biopsy is preferred to determine grade and histology. If necessary, open biopsy incisions should be placed longitudinally along the extremity so the scar can be resected at the time of surgery. Ideally, the surgeon performing the biopsy should be the surgeon performing the resection, especially in complex anatomic locations, and they should be a trained surgical/orthopedic oncologist. For RPS, the use of CT-guided biopsy via retroperitoneal approach can avoid seeding of the peritoneum. FNA may be performed to detect recurrence or metastatic disease.

PROGNOSTIC FACTORS: Grade, size, and metastatic disease. Factors increasing risk of LF include age >50, recurrent disease, margins <1 cm, and high-grade histology. Factors increasing risk of DM include higher grade (G1: 5%–10%; G2: 25%–30%; G3: 50%–60%), size (>5 cm), deep-seated tumor, recurrence, and histology.

NATURAL HISTORY: The most common route of DM is hematogenous, with lungs the most common site in 75% of patients, especially for STS of extremity/trunk region. Other less common sites in decreasing order include bone, other soft tissues (including bone marrow; e.g., for myxoid/round cell LS), liver (e.g., from adjacent visceral sarcoma, RPS), and rarely brain metastasis (LMS, angiosarcoma, and alveolar soft part sarcoma). If there are ≤4 lung metastases and long disease-free interval without endobronchial invasion, ~25% can be cured with resection (3-year OS was 30%–50%).[7] This appears to be true regardless of ablative modality for metastasis.[8] LN involvement is rare (<5%), but more common in "CARE" histologies: clear cell (28%), angiosarcoma (24%), rhabdomyosarcoma (32%), and epithelioid (32%).[5,9] Some histologies have unique natural histories; for example, dermal spread for superficial malignant fibrous histiocytoma (MFH), lack of pseudocapsule and poorly defined margins for desmoid tumor, and dermal nodules or skip metastases for epithelioid sarcoma. Specific subtypes primarily recurring locally include desmoid, MPNST, atypical lipomatous or well differentiation LS, and dermatofibrosarcoma protuberans (DMFSP). Those with local and intermediate risk for DM include myxoid LS, myxofibrosarcoma, extraskeletal myxoid chondrosarcoma, and hemangiopericytoma. STS increases in size with direct local extension along tissue planes, which are not always superior/inferior, and may grow centrifugally. Myxoid LS are known to be the most radiosensitive. RPS of well-differentiated LS histology have a long natural history and may not require aggressive treatment.[10]

STAGING: AJCC 8th edition emphasizes the primary site of STS; thus, multiple separate staging systems exist (trunk/extremities, H&N, abdomen/thoracic visceral organs, GIST, and RPS).[6] Table 57.3 includes the staging for STS of trunk and extremities.

Table 57.3 AJCC 8th Edition (2017): Staging for Soft Tissue Sarcoma of Trunk and Extremities (H&N, Abdomen and Thoracic, Retroperitoneal, and GIST Not Included Here)							
Tumor		**Node**		**Distant Metastasis**		**Grade**	
T1	≤5 cm	N0	No regional LNs	M0	No distant metastasis	G1	Total differentiation, mitotic count, and necrosis score of 2–3
T2	5.1–10 cm	N1	Regional LNs	M1	Distant metastasis	G2	Total differentiation, mitotic count, and necrosis score of 4–5
T3	10.1–15 cm					G3	Total differentiation, mitotic count, and necrosis score of 6–8
T4	>15 cm						

(continued)

Table 57.3 AJCC 8th Edition (2017): Staging for Soft Tissue Sarcoma of Trunk and Extremities (H&N, Abdomen and Thoracic, Retroperitoneal, and GIST Not Included Here) (*continued*)		
TNM	**Grade**	**Group Stage**
T1N0M0	G1	IA
T2–4N0M0	G1	IB
T1N0M0	G2, G3	II
T2N0M0	G2, G3	IIIA
T3–4N0M0	G2, G3	IIIB
Any T, N1, M0 Any T, any N, M1	Any	IV

Source: Adapted from AJCC Cancer Staging Manual. 8th ed. Springer International Publishing; 2017.

TREATMENT PARADIGM

Surgery: Negative-margin resection with preservation of function is the goal of treatment for localized disease. En bloc excision encompasses the biopsy site, scar, and tumor achieving >1 cm margins ideally. Extent of surgical resection (originally described by Enneking): (a) *intralesional*; (b) *marginal*: plane of resection through reactive tissue surrounding sarcoma; (c) *simple*: narrow margin (LR 60%–90%); (d) *wide*: plane of resection through normal tissue (~2–3 cm margin) and within the compartment of STS origin (LR 30%–60%); (e) *radical/compartmental*: en bloc resection of anatomic compartment, includes amputation (LR 10%–20%).[11] Margin status is the most important variable for LC. Violation of tumor is associated with higher LR rates. It is usually unnecessary to resect adjacent bone in the absence of radiographic invasion. About 75% of patients with LR after limb-sparing surgery and RT can be salvaged by subsequent amputation. Consider free or rotational flap closures for large wounds requiring PORT. Indication for amputation (~5% of cases): (a) involvement of major neurovascular structures or multiple compartments such that a functional limb is not achievable; (b) RT dose and volume constraints; (c) recurrence not amenable to further surgery or RT; (d) severely compromised normal tissue (due to age, peripheral vascular disease, or other comorbidities). For RPS, en bloc resection of nearby organs (kidney, bowel, spleen) may be required.

Chemotherapy: There are conflicting data regarding the routine use of CHT in the definitive management of STS, for which it has primarily been evaluated in extremity STS and less commonly in sites such as RPS. For localized primary extremity STS, studies are conflicting regarding an OS benefit to neoadjuvant CHT, but there appears to be the greatest benefit when doxorubicin is combined with ifosfamide, and there is a trend to improved OS with single-agent doxorubicin based on an updated meta-analysis from the Sarcoma Meta-Analysis Collaboration (SMAC). Analysis of the U.S. Sarcoma Collaborative database found that patients with extremity and trunk STS tumors >10 cm derive a benefit from neoadjuvant CHT, and just over half of patients in that analysis received RT.[12] Sarculator is a validated nomogram that predicts OS of patients with resected, primary extremity STS. This tool may be used to prognostically stratify patients into high- vs. low-risk groups to predict which patients may benefit from CHT.[13,14]

Immunotherapy: The role of immunotherapy is emerging in STS. SARC028 evaluated the use of pembrolizumab in unresectable or metastatic soft tissue or bone sarcoma, and while the overall response endpoint was not met for the entire cohort those with UPS or dedifferentiated LS had a favorable response.[15] SARC032 evaluated the use of neoadjuvant and adjuvant pembrolizumab with preop RT and surgery for patients with stage III UPS or dedifferentiated LS of the extremity, and demonstrated an improved disease-free survival (DFS) with pembrolizumab.[16]

Radiation

EBRT for STS of Extremity: RT may be delivered preop or in the adjuvant setting. *Preop RT:* For extremity sarcoma, dose is 50 Gy/25 fx. The single-arm phase II DOREMY study demonstrates excellent LC of myxoid LS of the trunk and extremity treated with preop RT 36 Gy/18 fx.[2] Postop EBRT boost 10 to 16 Gy (total 60–66 Gy) was performed on historical trials for patients with close/positive margins after preop RT, but is rarely used currently; a small retrospective study showed that postop boost with EBRT did not improve LRFS.[17] Other options for close margins include IORT (10–16 Gy) or brachytherapy (12–20 Gy). Preop hypofractionated RT is becoming more commonly utilized, and the HYPORT-STS phase II trial demonstrated that 42.75 Gy/15 fx was safe with 2-year MFU.[18] Ultra-hypofractionation with 30–35 Gy/5 fx followed by resection can be considered for select patients.[19] *PORT:* If RT is given in the adjuvant setting, typical dosing and fractionation is 50 Gy/25 fx followed by a cone down to 60 Gy for negative margins, 66 Gy for microscopically positive margins, and 70 to 76 Gy for gross residual disease.

EBRT for RPS: Doses of 45–50.4 Gy/25–28 fx are recommended when treating preop, although indications for preop RT are controversial. PORT is most beneficial in decreasing LF for well-differentiated LS and recurrent tumors. Consensus statements exist for treatment selection and contouring for RPS.[10]

Brachytherapy: Advantages include conformal tumor bed irradiation, short overall treatment time, and less dose to surrounding normal tissue (may yield better functional outcome). Brachytherapy alone may be used as adjuvant treatment for intermediate- to high-grade sarcomas of the extremity or superficial trunk with negative margins and has been shown to improve LC.[20] ABS guidelines are available to guide dose and technique.[21] Brachytherapy implemented following primary wound closure should be delayed to postop day 5 to decrease the risk of wound complications; however, when using negative pressure wound therapy as a temporary closure, brachytherapy can be initiated immediately. Most commonly, HDR brachytherapy with Ir-192 is used as a boost, 12 to 20 Gy BID over 2 to 3 days in conjunction with EBRT. Brachytherapy may also be utilized as adjuvant therapy alone (30–40 Gy BID over 5 days) and is preferred after resection of LR in previously irradiated patients.[21,22]

Procedure: See *Handbook of Treatment Planning in Radiation Oncology*, Chapter 11.[23]

EVIDENCE-BASED Q&A

PRIMARY EXTREMITY STS

Can the addition of PORT to limb salvage surgery (LSS) avoid amputation?

Historically, high recurrence rates after local excision alone led to the use of radical compartment excisions or amputations. This generated the idea behind the Rosenberg NCI trial.

Rosenberg, NCI (*Ann Surg* 1982, PMID 7114936): PRT of 43 patients with extremity, high-grade STS treated from 1975 to 1981 randomized to amputation (*n* = 16) vs. LSS + PORT (*n* = 27) consisting of 50 Gy with 10 to 20 Gy boost to the tumor bed. All patients received postop CHT with doxorubicin, cyclophosphamide, and methotrexate. LR was 15% in the LSS arm vs. 0% in the amputation arm (*p* = .06); 5-year DFS 71% vs. 78% (NS) and OS 82% vs. 88% (NS) for LSS vs. amputation, respectively. QOL similar in both cohorts. On MVA, only positive margins were correlated with LR, even in the setting of PORT. **Conclusion: LSS + PORT is safe and effective, and it has become standard of care.**

With limited randomized data showing PORT + LSS is as effective as amputation, is PORT necessary in those who undergo LSS alone? Does grade matter?

Although LSS + PORT became standard after the NCI study, morbidity with PORT is not trivial, and there were only historical comparisons to suggest it improved LR rates over LSS alone. This led to the NCI trial, which confirmed an LC benefit with no OS benefit to the addition of PORT in both low- and high-grade STS. A large SEER study suggests an OS benefit that is limited to high-grade STS.

Yang, NCI (*JCO* 1998, PMID 9440743): Phase III PRT including 91 patients with high-grade extremity STS s/p LSS with negative or minimal microscopic margins randomized to postop CHT alone (*n* = 44) vs. CHT + PORT (*n* = 47) to 63 Gy (45 Gy + 18 Gy boost at 1.8 Gy/fx) assessing LC, OS, and QOL. Additional 50 patients with low-grade sarcomas were enrolled to receive PORT (*n* = 26) vs. LSS alone (*n* = 24). MFU 9.6 years. See Table 57.4. LC was significantly improved with the addition of RT for both low- and high-grade patients with no OS benefit. PORT resulted in significantly worse limb strength, edema, and range of motion, but these deficits were often transient and had little effect on ADLs or QOL. **Conclusion: PORT confers a significant LC benefit with no OS benefit.**

Table 57.4 Results of NCI Trial

High-Grade (*n* = 91)	10-Yr LC	10-Yr OS	Low-Grade (*n* = 50)	10-Yr LC
Postop CHT	78%	74%	No adjuvant treatment	67%
Postop CRT	100%	75%	Postop RT	96%
p value	.0028	.71	*p* value	.016

Koshy, SEER (*IJROBP* 2010, PMID 19679403): SEER retrospective analysis from 1988 to 2005 including 6,960 patients with both low-/high-grade extremity STS assessing OS benefit of RT after LSS; 47% of patients received RT, primarily postop (86%). For high-grade STS, addition of RT was associated with 3-year OS benefit (73% vs. 63%, *p* < .001). There was no OS benefit for low-grade STS. **Conclusion: This large retrospective analysis showed improved OS with the addition of RT after LSS for high-grade STS.**

Can the addition of adjuvant brachytherapy improve LC?

Compared with surgery alone, there appears to be a significant LC benefit to brachytherapy, which is confined to high-grade histology, but there is no improvement in disease-specific survival (DSS) or DM.

Pisters, MSKCC (*JCO* 1996, PMID 8622034): PRT of 164 patients with STS of the extremity or superficial trunk randomized intraop to adjuvant brachytherapy vs. no further treatment after R0 resection. Brachytherapy via Ir-192 implant delivering 42 to 45 Gy over 4 to 6 days. MFU 76 months. Equivalent DSS and no difference in DM. The 5-year actuarial LC was 82% vs. 69% (*p* = .04) in favor of brachytherapy. However, on further analysis, this improvement in LC was found only for high-grade lesions (see Table 57.5). There was no difference in wound complication rates among patients who were loaded after postop day 5 (modified timing midtrial from loading <5 days to ≥6 days). **Conclusion: Brachytherapy improves LC for high-grade STS with no difference in DSS or DM.**

Table 57.5 Results of MSKCC Trial of Adjuvant Brachytherapy for Soft Tissue Sarcoma

	5-Yr LC	5-Yr DSS	LC	
			Low-Grade	High-Grade
Observation	69%	81%	72%	66%
Brachytherapy	82%	84%	73%	89%
p value	.04	.65	.49	.0025

What is the optimal sequencing of RT when indicated for the management of STS?

Both pre- and postop EBRT are reasonable, with trade-offs. Preop RT allows for smaller field sizes and lower doses, which are associated with better long-term functional outcomes. This comes at the expense of higher rates of acute wound complications.

O'Sullivan, NCIC SR2 (*Lancet* 2002, PMID 12103287; *Radiother Oncol* 2005, PMID 15948265): PRT of 190 patients with STS stratified by tumor size (≤10 cm vs. >10 cm) and randomized to preop RT (50 Gy/25 fx) vs. PORT (66–70 Gy; 50 Gy/25 fx to initial field + 16–20 Gy boost). Preop arm was treated with additional 16 to 20 Gy for positive margins. Primary endpoint: acute wound complications and erythema, with later analyses assessing 2-year late effects of grades 2 to 4 fibrosis, edema, and joint stiffness. Study terminated early at interim analysis. Updated MFU 6.9 years. Median RT field size was smaller in the preop arm. Complete results in Table 57.6. LC was identical between the two arms. Initial trend toward improved OS in the preop arm was lost at later follow-up. Tumor size and grade predicted for OS; grade predicted for RFS; margin status predicted for LC. Preop RT was associated with lower rates of acute skin erythema, late fibrosis, joint stiffness, and edema, albeit none were statistically significant. Preop RT had higher rates of acute wound complications (35% vs. 17%, highest in proximal lower extremity). **Conclusion: No difference in LC, RFS, or OS between preop and PORT. Preop RT for extremity STS may be preferred due to lower rates of irreversible late fibrosis, at the cost of higher, but generally reversible, acute wound complications.**

Table 57.6 Results of NCIC SR2 Trial of Preoperative vs. Postoperative RT for STS

	Acute Wound Complications	2-Yr Grade 2–4 Fibrosis	2-Yr Grade 2–4 Edema	2-Yr Joint Stiffness	5-Yr LC	5-Yr RFS	5-Yr Mets RFS	5-Yr OS	5-Yr CSS
Preop RT	35%	32%	15%	18%	93%	58%	67%	73%	78%
PORT	17%	48%	23%	23%	92%	59%	69%	67%	73%
p value	.01	.07	.26	.51	NS	NS	NS	.47	.64

Al-Absi, Ontario (*Ann Surg Oncol* 2010, PMID 20217260): Systematic review and meta-analysis of five eligible studies of preop vs. PORT for localized, resectable STS including 1,098 patients. Significant improvement in LC with preop RT despite larger average tumor size in the preop group (OR 0.61, 95% CI 0.42–0.89 by means of fixed-effects method; OR 0.67, 0.39–1.15 by means of random-effects method). Time-dependent survival averaged across all studies was 76% (range 62%–88%) preop vs. 67% (range 41%–83%) postop, NS. **Conclusion: Findings must be interpreted with caution due to heterogeneity but suggest that delay in surgery due to preop RT does not confer increased DM rate vs. PORT and may provide superior LC.**

Can preop hypofractionated EBRT be given with comparable outcomes?

Data are limited to single-institution series, although it appears that neoadjuvant hypofractionated RT with or without CHT can be given prior to surgical resection; however, further investigation is needed.

Pennington, UCLA (*Am J Clin Oncol* 2018, PMID 29664796): RR of 116 patients from single institution treated between 1990 and 2013 with neoadjuvant hypofractionated RT (28 Gy/8 fx daily) with ifosfamide-based CHT. RT given concurrently with ifosfamide or sequentially with combined doxorubicin and ifosfamide. Resection 2 to 3 weeks after RT. MFU 5.9 years; actuarial LRR 11% and 17% at 3 and 6 years, respectively. On MVA, positive margin was associated with increased risk of LR. Fifteen percent of patients experienced acute and long-term toxicity, including 10% with acute wound complications. **Conclusion: Ifosfamide-based neoadjuvant CHT with hypofractionated RT provides acceptable tumor control with LF 17% at 6 years.**

Kalbasi, UCLA (*Clin Cancer Res* 2020, PMID 32054730): Phase II single-institution study of 52 patients evaluating safety of 5-day preop RT (30 Gy/5 fx) with standard margins. Primary endpoint was grade ≥2 late RT toxicity. MFU 29 months; 7 of 44 (16%) evaluable patients developed grade ≥2 late RT toxicity. Major wound complications in 16 patients (32%), associated with lower extremity tumor location and a signature germline biomarker. **Conclusion: 5 fx neoadjuvant RT demonstrates favorable rates of wound complications and late toxicity, which may be predictive with a germline biomarker if further validated.**

Bedi, MCW (*Adv Radiat Oncol* 2022, PMID 35647402): Single-arm, prospective phase II trial of 32 patients receiving preoperative 35 Gy/5 fx followed by resection 4 to 6 weeks later. CHT was optional. At MFU 36 months, there were no LRs; 3-year OS 82% and 3-year MFS 69%. Major wound complications seen in 25% of patients, while late grade 2 and 3 fibrosis was seen in 22% and 13%, respectively. **Conclusion: 5 fx preoperative RT leads to excellent LC and OS with acceptable toxicity.**

Mayo, CCF (*Radiother Oncol* 2022, PMID 36481382): RR of 22 patients treated with preoperative 30 Gy/5 fractions followed by immediate resection (within 7 days) for STS of the extremity or trunk. MFU 24 months. The median time from RT completion to surgery was 1 day, and the median time from biopsy to surgery 34 days; 2-year LC 100%, MFS 71%, and OS 77%. Major wound complications in 41% of patients, with reoperation (eight of nine) being the most common. Late grade ≥2 toxicity seen in four patients (18%) and included grade 3 fracture and grade 2 fibrosis, stiffness, and lymphedema. **Conclusion: Ultra-hypofractionated preoperative RT followed by immediate resection permits expedited completion of oncologic therapy, with early results demonstrating excellent LC and acceptable toxicity.**

Guadagnolo, HYPORT-STS (*Lancet Oncol* 2022, PMID 36343656): Single-arm phase II trial of 120 patients receiving moderately hypofractionated 42.75 Gy/15 fx followed by resection at a median of 5.7 weeks. MFU 24 months. At a median of 16 months, LR was 5% in evaluable patients. Major wound complications were seen in 31% at a median time of 37 days from surgery. No patients had acute grade ≥3 toxicity. Grade 2 fibrosis occurred in three patients (3%). Four patients (3%) had grade ≥3 late toxicity, including two femur fractures, one lymphedema, and one skin ulceration. **Conclusion: Moderately hypofractionated neoadjuvant RT for STS is safe, and late toxicity and wound complication risk are comparable to historical conventional rates.**

Can dose-reduced preoperative EBRT be given for myxoid LS?

A phase II nonrandomized trial demonstrated that preop 36 Gy/18 fx had excellent LC with low risk of wound healing complications.

Lansu, DOREMY (*JAMA Oncol* 2020, PMID 33180100): International single-arm phase II trial of 79 patients with resectable extremity or trunk myxoid LS. Patients received 36 Gy/18 fx preop IMRT. Primary outcome was extensive pathologic treatment response in definitive resection specimen, defined as <50% vital tumor cells, with trial being positive if ≥70% of patients achieved this. Of 77 patients resected, 91% had extensive pathologic response. Wound complications of any severity were observed in 22%, of which 17% needed any intervention. With MFU 25 months, LC was 100% regardless of extent of pathologic response. **Conclusion: Dose-reduced preop EBRT can be considered for myxoid LS, which may lead to decreased wound complications without a detriment in LC.**

What is the role of postoperative boost with EBRT in patients who receive preoperative RT and undergo surgical resection with positive surgical margins?

Data are limited to small RRs with no PRT to answer this question. There is suggestion that EBRT boost may not be effective in preventing LR in patients with positive margins after preop RT.

Al Yami (*IJROBP* 2010, PMID 20056340): RR of 216 extremity STS patients treated from 1986 to 2003 who had positive surgical margins. Ninety-three patients had been treated with preop RT (50 Gy), while 41 additionally received a postop boost (80% received boost dose of 16 Gy with EBRT to a total dose of 66 Gy). The 5-year LRFS estimates were 90% for no boost vs. 74% for boost (*p* = .13). **Conclusion: Postop boost with EBRT did not improve LRFS in this small retrospective analysis.**

Can modern image-guided RT improve morbidity?

Part of the rationale for preop RT is to decrease late effects by reducing the irradiated volume. Image-guided RT (IGRT) may be able to reduce the volume even further without compromising tumor control.

Wang, RTOG 0630 (*JCO* 2015, PMID 25667281): Multi-institutional phase II trial assessing the utility of preop IGRT (3DCRT or IMRT) in reducing CTV margins and toxicity compared with the O'Sullivan NCIC trial. Primary endpoint: 2-year grade ≥2 late RT morbidity. Ninety-eight patients were accrued to two cohorts: Cohort A (12 patients; intermediate- to high-grade STS ≥8 cm who received CHT; results not reported) and Cohort B (79 evaluable patients; all treated without CHT). RT: 50 Gy/25 fx with postop boost suggested for positive margins (16 Gy/8 fx EBRT, 16 Gy LDR, 13.6 Gy/4 fx HDR, or 10–12.5 Gy IORT); 2 or 3 cm longitudinal CTV expansion and 1 or 1.5 cm radial (<8 or ≥8 cm, respectively), including suspicious edema with IGRT. MFU 3.6 years. Most patients had UPS (23%), LS (22%), or myxofibrosarcoma (22%). The most common primary site was the thigh (42%), and 75% were treated with IMRT. Five patients did not undergo surgery due to progression; 56 (76%) had R0 resection and 11 (15%) received postop boost. Five patients had in-field LF (three with positive margins and two treated with postop boost). Overall rate of grade ≥2 late toxicity was significantly improved compared with O'Sullivan preop arm (11% vs. 37%, *p* < .001). Individual toxicities compared favorably: fibrosis (5% vs. 32%), joint stiffness (4% vs. 18%), edema (5% vs. 15%). Thirty-seven percent of patients experienced at least one wound complication, all in lower extremity tumors, and most commonly in proximal lower extremity. **Conclusion: Significant reduction of late toxicities and absence of marginal-field recurrences suggest that smaller target volumes are appropriate for preop RT with IGRT.**

O'Sullivan, Canada (*Cancer* 2013, PMID 23423841): Single-arm phase II trial using IMRT with image guidance to deliver preop RT with primary endpoint of acute wound complications compared with NCIC trial: 59 evaluable patients. RT: 50 Gy/25 fx without boost; 4-cm longitudinal and 1.5-cm radial expansions, including edema with IGRT; dose restricted to "future surgical skin flaps" and bone. MFU 49 months. Most patients had UPS (36%), myxoid LS (32%), or pleomorphic LS (10%). R1 resection in four patients. Buttock was the most common site of wound complications

(45%), followed by adductor (44%) and hamstring (44%). Overall rate of complications was not different from NCIC trial, but primary closure was more frequent (93% vs. 71%, $p = .002$). Number of secondary operations was numerically less but not SS. Flap/PTV overlap was improved on MVA (<1% overlap, 14% vs. 40%). Four patients had LF (7%), none near surgical flaps, and two had positive margins. No grade >2 late toxicities in patients surviving longer than 2 years with no fractures. **Conclusion: Preop IMRT with IGRT significantly diminished the need for tissue transfer, with NS reduction in acute wound complications, chronic morbidities, and need for subsequent secondary operations, while maintaining good limb function.**

With respect to IMRT and brachytherapy, does one have a better therapeutic ratio compared with the other?

Data are limited to RRs and comparisons of modern control rates of each separately, but there is suggestion of superior LC with IMRT.

Alektiar, MSKCC (*Cancer* 2011, PMID 21264834): RR of 134 patients with high-grade extremity STS who were treated with LSS + either brachytherapy (1995–2003) or IMRT (2002–2006). LDR brachytherapy ($n = 71$) was administered postop with a median dose of 45 Gy. IMRT ($n = 63$) was delivered preop ($n = 10$) with a median dose of 50 Gy, and postop ($n = 53$) to a median dose of 63 Gy. MFU 46 months for IMRT and 47 months for brachytherapy. There were statistically higher risk tumors in the IMRT cohort, such as positive/close margins (<1 mm), large tumors (>10 cm), and requiring bone or nerve stripping/resection. The 5-year LC favored IMRT (92% vs. 81%, $p = .04$). On MVA, IMRT was the only significant predictor of improved LC ($p = .04$). **Conclusion: LC with IMRT was significantly better than brachytherapy despite higher rates of adverse features for IMRT in this nonrandomized comparison.**

Does the addition of adjuvant CHT improve outcomes for resected STS?

This has been an area of controversy based on risk vs. benefit of such therapy, but due to the risk of local and distant failures adjuvant CHT was often administered historically, typically with doxorubicin-based therapy. SMAC updated their meta-analysis in 2008 of RCTs including adjuvant CHT following surgical resection confirming the efficacy of doxorubicin-based CHT with greater benefit when given with ifosfamide.

Pervaiz, Sarcoma Meta-Analysis Collaboration (*Cancer* 2008, PMID 18521899): Comprehensive meta-analysis of 18 RCTs including 1,953 patients assessing failures and survival outcomes with doxorubicin-based adjuvant CHT in resectable STS. LR rates were improved with the addition of CHT (OR 0.73, 95% CI 0.56–0.94). DM and overall recurrence were also improved with CHT (OR 0.67, 0.56–0.82). On survival analysis, doxorubicin alone was not statistically significant (OR 0.84, 0.68–1.03), but doxorubicin + ifosfamide was associated with improved survival (OR 0.56, 0.36–0.85) **Conclusion: CHT is associated with reduced rates of LR and DM. The addition of ifosfamide to doxorubicin demonstrated a significant survival benefit.**

In the preoperative setting, what is the role of the addition of CHT?

DM continues to be the driving factor limiting OS in STS. Previous small pilot studies of neoadjuvant CHT or CRT appeared promising, leading to RTOG 9514, which assessed the feasibility of neoadjuvant CHT interdigitated with RT prior to surgery followed by additional adjuvant CHT alone or following additional RT for positive margin. Neoadjuvant CHT is not a standard of care approach at this time but can be considered for large, high-grade tumors.

Kraybill, RTOG 9514 (*JCO* 2006, PMID 16446334): Phase II trial of 66 patients evaluating neoadjuvant CHT with preop RT followed by CHT postop in multi-institutional setting. Patients with high-grade extremity/body wall STS ≥8 cm were eligible. CHT consisted of MAID regimen (modified mesna, doxorubicin, ifosfamide, and dacarbazine), which was given for three cycles, with interdigitated RT 44 Gy/22 fx split course (MAID → RT → MAID → RT → MAID) followed by resection 3 weeks later. Postop therapy was based on margin status. If positive margins, additional 16 Gy/8 fx given to postop bed + 1 cm margin, followed by MAID for three cycles. If negative margins, MAID × 3 cycles alone. Sixty-four patients were evaluable; 79% completed preop CHT, with only 59% receiving full CHT course due to toxicity, 5% experiencing grade 5 fatal toxicity, and 83% experiencing grade 4. Sixty-one patients underwent surgery, with 58 R0 resections (five amputations). At 3 years, the estimated DFS was 57%, DMFS 65%, and OS 75%. There were five amputations leading to 92% limb preservation rate. Estimated 3-year LRF of 18% if amputation considered failure and 10% if not. **Conclusion: Just over 50% of patients received planned treatment course due to substantial toxicity, but regimen does appear to show activity.**

Zaidi, U.S. Sarcoma Collaborative (*Ann Surg Oncol* 2019, PMID 31342400): RR of 770 patients from the U.S. Sarcoma Collaborative database treated from 2000 to 2016 with curative-intent resection of high-grade, primary truncal, and extremity STS ≥5 cm. Primary endpoints were RFS and OS. The most common histology was UPS (42%). A total of 216 patients (28%) received neoadjuvant CHT (NACT) and were more likely to have deeper and larger tumors ($p < .001$). For patients with tumors ≥10 cm, NACT improved 5-year RFS (51% vs. 40%, $p = .053$) and 5-year OS (58% vs. 47%, $p = .043$). When evaluating location, tumors ≥10 cm in the extremity had improved 5-year RFS (54% vs. 42%, $p = .042$) and 5-year OS (61% vs. 47%, $p = .015$) with NACT, but the truncal cohort did not; however, it was likely underpowered. **Conclusion: NACT improves RFS and OS for extremity tumors ≥10 cm, and further investigation is required to determine role in large truncal tumors.**

Is there a role for immunotherapy in localized STS?

SARC028 evaluated the use of pembrolizumab in unresectable or metastatic soft tissue or bone sarcoma and demonstrated a favorable response for those with UPS or dedifferentiated LS.[15] SARC032 evaluated the use of neoadjuvant and adjuvant pembrolizumab with preop RT and surgery for patients with stage III UPS or dedifferentiated LS of the extremity and demonstrated improved DFS with pembrolizumab.

Mowery, SARC032 (*Lancet* 2024, PMID 39547252): Phase II randomized trial of 143 patients with stage III UPS (including deep myxofibrosarcoma) or dedifferentiated LS of the extremity randomized to preop RT then surgery vs. preop pembrolizumab + RT then surgery with postop pembrolizumab. Primary endpoint was DFS. RT 50 Gy/25 fx. The 2-year DFS was 67% with pembrolizumab vs. 52% in the control group ($p = .035$). Grade 3+ toxicity was 56% with pembrolizumab vs. 31% in the control group. In subgroup analysis, benefit was greatest in patient with grade 3 tumors. **Conclusion: Pre- and postoperative pembrolizumab for stage III extremity UPS and dedifferentiated LS improves DFS.**

RETROPERITONEAL SARCOMA (RPS)

What is the general approach to managing RPS?

Primary management is based on achieving an R0 surgical resection. As with primary extremity STS, RPS data are limited mainly to small RRs. The EORTC STRASS trial failed to demonstrate a benefit to preop RT; however, the LS subgroup may benefit. If RT is given, it is delivered in the preoperative setting as toxicity can be significant postoperatively.

What current data suggest benefit, including OS, to the addition of RT for RPS?

Based on SEER/NCDB datasets, there appears to be a survival benefit with the addition of RT (given either preop or postop), with usual limitations of such nonrandomized registry studies; however, the results of the randomized EORTC STRASS trial did not demonstrate an RFS benefit in all patients.

Zhou, SEER (*Arch Surg* 2010, PMID 20479339): SEER analysis evaluating the effect of surgical resection and RT for 1,901 patients with localized RPS and nonvisceral abdominal sarcoma from 1988 to 2005. Eighty-two percent underwent surgical resection and 24% received RT. Combined therapy was associated with improved OS vs. single modality therapy, and surgery or RT was better than no therapy ($p < .001$). Cox analysis demonstrated surgical resection (HR 0.24, 95% CI 0.21–0.29) and RT (HR 0.78, 0.63–0.95) independently predicted improved OS in locoregional disease only. In adjusted analyses stratified for stage, for stage I disease ($n = 694$), RT provided additional benefit (HR 0.49, 0.25–0.96) independent of that from resection (HR 0.35, 0.21–0.58). For stage II/III ($n = 552$), resection remained significant (HR 0.24, 0.18–0.32); however, RT was not associated with significant benefit (HR 0.78, 0.58–1.06). **Conclusion: In this retrospective cohort, surgical resection was associated with significant survival benefits for AJCC stage I to III RPS, and RT provided additional benefit in stage I disease.**

Nussbaum, NCDB Analysis (*Lancet Oncol* 2016, PMID 27210906): Case–control, propensity score-matched analyses of 9,068 NCDB patients who were diagnosed with RPS from 2003 to 2011.

Included patients with local RPS undergoing resection and either preop RT or PORT, but not both, and no additional therapy or IORT. Primary objective was OS for patients who received preop RT or PORT compared with those who received no RT within propensity score-matched datasets. 563 patients received preop RT (MFU 42 months), 2,215 received PORT (MFU 54 months), and 6,290 received no RT (MFU 43 months when compared with preop and 47 months when compared with postop). Negligible differences in all demographics, clinic-pathologic, and treatment-level variables. MS was 110 months for preop cohort vs. 66 months for matched no-RT cohort. MS was 89 months for postop cohort vs. 64 months for matched no-RT cohort. Both preop (HR 0.70, 95% CI 0.59–0.82) and PORT (HR 0.78, 0.71–0.85) were significantly associated with higher OS compared with surgery alone. **Conclusion: RT is associated with higher OS compared with surgery alone when delivered either preop or postop.**

Bonvalot, EORTC STRASS (*Lancet* 2020, PMID 32941794): International phase III trial of 266 patients with RPS (75% had LS) randomized to preop RT (50.4 Gy) vs. surgery alone. Primary endpoint: abdominal RFS defined as local relapse after complete resection, peritoneal carcinomatosis, progression during RT, or unresectable disease. Designed to demonstrate 20% increase in abdominal RFS at 5 years from 50% to 70%. There was no significant increase in rate of inoperable tumors or reoperations in the RT + surgery group. Twice as many LR observed in surgery-alone group, specifically in the LS group. The 3-year abdominal RFS was 60% in RT + surgery vs. 59% surgery alone (NS). **Conclusion: There is no abdominal RFS benefit with preop RT in RPS; however, a subset of patients with LS may benefit and further follow-up is needed.**

Callegro, STRASS vs. STREXIT (*Ann Surg* 2023, PMID 35833413): Pooled analysis of patients enrolled on STRASS as well as patients treated off-trial with curative-intent surgery for primary RPS ± preoperative RT (STREXIT cohort). Primary endpoint was abdominal RFS defined as macroscopically incomplete resection, abdominal recurrence, or death of any cause. After 1:1 propensity score matching, there were 266 patients in the STRASS cohort and 202 in the STREXIT cohort. Patients with well-differentiated LS and G1–2 dedifferentiated LS treated with preop RT had better abdominal RFS (HR 0.63, 95% CI 0.40–0.97). There was no association between RT and OS or DMFS. **Conclusion: Preop RT may be of value for patients with retroperitoneal well-differentiated LS or grades 1 to 2 dedifferentiated LS. It did not benefit patients with LMS or grade 3 dedifferentiated LS.**

Does the addition of IORT to PORT improve outcomes following surgically resected RPS?

Retrospective data exist; however, only one small PRT has addressed this question. In the NCI trial, addition of IORT reduced LRR, but this did not translate into an OS benefit. Bowel toxicity was also reduced.[24]

Is IORT combined with preoperative IMRT safe and effective?

Roeder (*BMC Cancer* 2014, PMID 25163595): Unplanned interim analysis of phase I/II single-arm trial assessing the feasibility of preop IMRT with IORT in 27 patients with primary/recurrent RPS (>5 cm, M0, at least marginally resectable) from 2007 to 2013. Preop IMRT delivered using SIB with doses of 45 to 50 Gy to PTV and 50 to 56 Gy to GTV in 25 fx, followed by surgery and IORT (10–12 Gy). Primary endpoint 5-year LC. Majority of patients had high-grade lesions (82% grades 2–3), predominantly LS (70%), with median tumor size of 15 cm (6–31 cm). MFU 33 months. Preop IMRT performed as planned in 93%. GTR with contiguous-organ resection was feasible in 96%, with 22% achieving R0 and 74% R1 resections. IORT was performed in 23 patients (85%) with a median dose of 12 Gy (10–20 Gy). There were seven recurrences; 3- and 5-year LC rates of 72%. Grade 3 acute toxicity in four patients (15%) and severe postop complications in nine patients (33%). Grade 3 late toxicity in 6% of surviving patients after 1 year and none after 2 years. **Conclusion: Combination preop IMRT, surgery, and IORT is feasible with acceptable toxicity and yields favorable results in terms of LC and OS in patients with high-risk RPS. Long-term follow-up is needed.**

Does preoperative RT improve outcomes compared with postoperative RT?

In theory, preop RT may reduce toxicity due to lower dose, smaller volumes of normal tissue in the irradiated volume due to better target delineation, normal tissue displacement, and subsequent smaller treatment fields. Additionally, it may be more effective from a radiobiological standpoint due to improved vascularity and oxygenation. Most do not recommend PORT for RPS.

Ballo, MDACC (*IJROBP* 2007, PMID 17084545): RR of 83 patients with localized RPS treated with complete surgical resection and RT; 60 patients presented with primary disease, and 23 having LR following previous surgery. MFU 47 months. Actuarial overall DSS, LC, and DMFS were 44%, 40%, and 67%, respectively. Of 38 deaths, local progression was the only site of recurrence for 16 patients and was a component of progression for another 11 patients. MVA indicated histologic grade was associated with 5-year rates of DSS (low grade, 92%; intermediate grade, 51%; high grade, 41%; $p = .006$) and indicated an inferior 5-year LC for patients presenting with recurrent disease, positive margins or uncertain margin status, and age >65. Higher doses of RT or IORT were not associated with improved LC. RT-related complications (10% at 5 years) in five patients, with all complications limited to those who received PORT (23%) vs. preop RT (0%). **Conclusion: Preoperative RT may be preferred over PORT.**

What are the current recommendations for unresectable RPS?

According to NCCN, treatment may include CHT or RT alone or in combination to facilitate resection, if possible.[1] For large tumors, spatially fractionated RT (SFRT) combined with palliative RT or SBRT can be considered to optimize symptom control and LC.

Kepka, Poland (*IJROBP* 2005, PMID 16199316): RR of 112 patients treated with definitive RT for unresectable STS; 43% extremities, 26% retroperitoneal, 24% H&N, and 7% trunk; 89% grades 2 to 3. Median RT dose 64 Gy (range, 25–87.5 Gy). CHT was given in 20%. MFU 139 months; 5-year LC, DFS, and OS 45%, 24%, 35%, respectively; 5-year LC affected by tumor size (51%, 45%, and 9% for tumors <5, 5–10, and >10 cm, respectively) and RT dose (<63 Gy: 22%; >63 Gy: 60%). Dose >68 Gy vs. <68 Gy was associated with higher risk of complications (27% vs. 8%). **Conclusion: Definitive RT should be considered for inoperable STS including RPS. Higher RT doses improve LC but at the risk of increasing toxicity with doses >68 Gy.**

Duriseti, LITE SABR M1 (*Radiother Oncol* 2022, PMID 34875286): Single-arm phase I trial of 22 patients with tumors >4.5 cm treated with SFRT via Lattice to 20 Gy/5x with SIB to 66.7 Gy in a defined geometric arrangement delivered every other day. Primary outcome was 90-day grade ≥3 toxicity. There was no likely treatment-associated grade ≥3 toxicity in the 90-day period, but one case of possibly treatment-associated grade 4 toxicity. **Conclusion: Lattice SFRT appears to be a safe treatment option for patients with large tumors.**

Ahmed, Mayo Clinic (*Adv Radiat Oncol* 2023, PMID 38495033): RR of 53 patients (61 SFRT treatments) with soft tissue (75%) and bone (25%) sarcomas. SFRT dose was 16–20 Gy/1 fx. Consolidative EBRT was delivered in 90% of treatment courses with a median time interval of 5 days (range 0–14). Median EBRT dose was 40 Gy (range 9–73.5 Gy) delivered in a median of 10 fx (range 3–33 fx). Symptom relief was observed in 60% of treatment courses, and stable or partial response was observed in 90%. The 1-year LC and OS rates were 82% and 53%, respectively. There were four (8%) grades 3 to 4 acute and subacute toxicities related to SFRT. **Conclusion: Combined SFRT with EBRT yields high rates of symptomatic and radiographic response, with acceptable toxicity.**

REFERENCES

1. National Comprehensive Cancer Network . *NCCN Clinical Practice Guidelines in Oncology: Soft Tissue Sarcoma.* Accessed October 16, 2024. Version 1.2024. https://www.nccn.org
2. Lansu J, Bovee J, Braam P, et al. Dose reduction of preoperative radiotherapy in myxoid liposarcoma: a nonrandomized controlled trial. *JAMA Oncol.* 2021;7(1):e205865. doi:10.1001/jamaoncol.2020.5865
3. Siegel RL, Giaquinto AN, Jemal A. Cancer statistics, 2024. *CA Cancer J Clin.* 2024;74(1):12–49. doi:10.3322/caac.21820
4. Brady MS, Gaynor JJ, Brennan MF. Radiation-associated sarcoma of bone and soft tissue. *Arch Surg.* 1992;127(12):1379–1385. doi:10.1001/archsurg.1992.01420120013002
5. White LM, Wunder JS, Bell RS, et al. Histologic assessment of peritumoral edema in soft tissue sarcoma. *Int J Radiat Oncol Biol Phys.* 2005;61(5):1439–1445. doi:10.1016/j.ijrobp.2004.08.036
6. Amin MB, Edge SB, Greene FL, et al, eds. *AJCC Cancer Staging Manual.* 8th ed. Springer; 2017.
7. van Geel AN, Pastorino U, Jauch KW, et al. Surgical treatment of lung metastases: the European Organization for research and treatment of cancer-soft tissue and bone sarcoma group study of 255 patients. *Cancer.* 1996;77(4):675–682. doi:10.1002/(SICI)1097-0142(19960215)77:4<675::AID-CNCR13>3.0.CO;2-H

8. Falk AT, Moureau-Zabotto L, Ouali M, et al. Effect on survival of local ablative treatment of metastases from Sarcomas: a study of the French Sarcoma Group. *Clin Oncol (R Coll Radiol).* 2015;27(1):48–55. doi:10.1016/j.clon.2014.09.010

9. Baratti D, Pennacchioli E, Casali PG, et al. Epithelioid sarcoma: prognostic factors and survival in a series of patients treated at a single institution. *Ann Surg Oncol.* 2007;14(12):3542–3551. doi:10.1245/s10434-007-9628-9

10. Baldini EH, Wang D, Haas RL, et al. Treatment guidelines for preoperative radiation therapy for retroperitoneal sarcoma: preliminary consensus of an international expert panel. *Int J Radiat Oncol Biol Phys.* 2015;92(3):602–612. doi:10.1016/j.ijrobp.2015.02.013

11. Enneking WF, Spanier SS, Goodman MA. A system for the surgical staging of musculoskeletal sarcoma. *Clin Orthop Relat Res.* 1980;(153):106–120. PMID: 7449206

12. Zaidi MY, Ethun CG, Tran TB, et al. Assessing the role of neoadjuvant chemotherapy in primary high-risk truncal/extremity soft tissue sarcomas: an analysis of the multi-institutional U.S. Sarcoma collaborative. *Ann Surg Oncol.* 2019;26(11):3542–3549. doi:10.1245/s10434-019-07639-7

13. Pasquali S, Palmerini E, Quagliuolo V, et al. Neoadjuvant chemotherapy in high-risk soft tissue sarcomas: a Sarculator-based risk stratification analysis of the ISG-STS 1001 randomized trial. *Cancer.* 2022;128(1):85–93. doi:10.1002/cncr.33895

14. Voss RK, Callegaro D, Chiang YJ, et al. Sarculator is a good model to predict survival in resected extremity and trunk sarcomas in US patients. *Ann Surg Oncol.* 2022. doi:10.1245/s10434-022-11442-2

15. Tawbi HA, Burgess M, Bolejack V, et al. Pembrolizumab in advanced soft-tissue sarcoma and bone sarcoma (SARC028): a multicentre, two-cohort, single-arm, open-label, phase 2 trial. *Lancet Oncol.* 2017;18(11):1493–1501. doi:10.1016/S1470-2045(17)30624-1

16. Mowery YM, Ballman KV, Hong AM, et al. Safety and efficacy of pembrolizumab, radiation therapy, and surgery versus radiation therapy and surgery for stage III soft tissue sarcoma of the extremity (SU2C-SARC032): an open-label, randomised clinical trial. *Lancet.* 2024;404(10467):2053–2064. doi:10.1016/S0140-6736(24)01812-9

17. Al Yami A, Griffin AM, Ferguson PC, et al. Positive surgical margins in soft tissue sarcoma treated with preoperative radiation: is a postoperative boost necessary? *Int J Radiat Oncol Biol Phys.* 2010;77(4):1191–1197. doi:10.1016/j.ijrobp.2009.06.074

18. Guadagnolo BA, Bassett RL, Mitra D, et al. Hypofractionated, 3-week, preoperative radiotherapy for patients with soft tissue sarcomas (HYPORT-STS): a single-centre, open-label, single-arm, phase 2 trial. *Lancet Oncol.* 2022;23(12):1547–1557. doi:10.1016/S1470-2045(22)00638-6

19. Mayo ZS, Fan C, Jia X, et al. Meta-analysis of 5-fraction preoperative radiotherapy for soft tissue sarcoma. *Am J Clin Oncol.* 2024;47(9):412–418. doi:10.1097/COC.0000000000001110

20. Pisters PW, Harrison LB, Leung DH, Woodruff JM, Casper ES, Brennan MF. Long-term results of a prospective randomized trial of adjuvant brachytherapy in soft tissue sarcoma. *J Clin Oncol.* 1996;14(3):859–868. doi:10.1200/JCO.1996.14.3.859

21. Campbell SR, Shah C, Scott JG, et al. American Brachytherapy Society (ABS) consensus statement for soft-tissue sarcoma brachytherapy. *Brachytherapy.* 2021;20(6):1200–1218. doi:10.1016/j.brachy.2021.05.011

22. Pearlstone DB, Janjan NA, Feig BW, et al. Re-resection with brachytherapy for locally recurrent soft tissue sarcoma arising in a previously radiated field. *Cancer J Sci Am.* 1999;5(1):26–33. PMID: 10188058

23. Videtic GMM, Woody N, Vassil AD. *Handbook of Treatment Planning in Radiation Oncology.* 2nd ed. Demos Medical; 2015. doi:10.1891/9781617051975

24. Sindelar WF, Kinsella TJ, Chen PW, et al. Intraoperative radiotherapy in retroperitoneal sarcomas. Final results of a prospective, randomized, clinical trial. *Arch Surg.* 1993;128(4):402–410. doi:10.1001/archsurg.1993.01420160040005

PART XI: Pediatric

Adannia N. Ufondu and Erin S. Murphy

QUICK HIT Medulloblastoma (MB) is the most common malignant pediatric CNS tumor, accounting for 20% of all childhood brain cancers.[1] MB typically arises in the cerebellum, most commonly in the cerebellar vermis, leading to obstruction of CSF flow and hydrocephalus. Presenting symptoms are related to elevated ICP. Surgery alone leads to poor outcomes, with multiple studies showing an improvement with the use of RT and CHT.[2,3] Attempts to reduce CSI dose and its associated growth, endocrine, and neurocognitive toxicities have been facilitated by optimized CHT regimens.[4] The recommended treatment paradigm is determined by patients' risk status (average vs. high; see Table 58.1). In the average-risk setting, clinicians have transitioned to CSI + involved field (IF) boost vs. historical standard of complete posterior fossa (PF) boost based on promising results from ACNS0331.[5] The role of molecular pathways and associated subgrouping is evolving with prognosis falling on a spectrum: Wnt group conferring best prognosis, SHH-TP53wt and group 4 conferring intermediate prognosis, and a worse prognosis is seen for group 3/SHH-TP53mt.

Table 58.1 General Treatment Paradigm for MB Following Maximal Safe Resection

Classic Risk Group	CSI	Boost	Post-RT CHT	5-Yr OS
Average-risk (two-thirds of pts at presentation) • ≥3 years of age AND • M0 AND • ≤1.5 cm² of residual disease postop • Favorable histology (classic, desmoplastic/nodular, extensive nodularity)	23.4 Gy in 13 fx (1.8 Gy/fx) +/− concurrent vincristine (VCR)	IF boost: 30.6 Gy in 17 fx (54 Gy total)	COG: • Cycle A: cisplatin, lomustine (CCNU), VCR • Cycle B: cyclophosphamide (CYC), VCR • Cadence: AABAABAAB St. Jude protocol: • Cisplatin, CYC, VCR	80%
High-risk (one-third of pts at presentation) • <3 years of age* OR • M+ OR • >1.5 cm² residual disease postop • Poor histology (large cell, anaplastic)	36 Gy in 20 fx (1.8 Gy/fx) with concurrent VCR For high-risk group 3 patients, consider adding daily carboplatin per ACNS 0332	PF boost: 18–19.8 Gy in 10 fx (54–55.8 Gy total)†	COG/St. Jude protocol: • Six cycles of cisplatin, CYC, VCR	60%

*Infants <3 years old warrant a risk-adapted approach combining maximal safe resection, CHT, second-look surgery with delayed CSI, or focal RT given poor neurocognitive outcomes with standard CSI. See below for details.
†For lesions of the spinal cord, boost to 45 Gy. For lesions below the spinal cord, boost to 50.4 Gy.

EPIDEMIOLOGY: MB accounts for 40% of all PF tumors and 20% of all pediatric CNS tumors, with ~500 cases per year in the United States.[6] Most commonly presents between 5 and 7 years of age with distribution as follows: 10% before age 1, 60% to 70% before age 9, and 30% above age 10. When present in adults, the histology is typically desmoplastic. It is about three times more common in males than females.

RISK FACTORS: The majority arise sporadically, but ~5% are thought to be secondary to familial syndromes.

- *Gorlin syndrome* (also known as "nevoid basal cell carcinoma syndrome"): AD condition associated with basal cell carcinoma, skeletal anomalies, and macrocephaly. MB develops in ~5% of patients. Associated with a 9q22.3 germline mutation, which confers inactivation of PTCH1, a protein that functions as the receptor for sonic hedgehog (SHH) whose pathway is important for the development of the cerebellum.[7]

- *Turcot syndrome:* AD; characterized by polyposis, colorectal cancers, gliomas, and MBs. 92-fold higher relative risk of developing MB than the unaffected population.[8] Associated with APC mutation on chr 5q. The APC complex is in part responsible for degrading cytoplasmic β-catenin and is regulated by the Wingless pathway (Wnt). These molecular pathways help underpin the evolving biomolecular paradigm of MB.
- *Li–Fraumeni and NF-1:* Associated with TP53 mutation, and both occasionally associated with MB.

ANATOMY: Most commonly presents in the PF, with ~75% occurring in the midline vermis. Hemispheric location is associated with older age and desmoplastic histology. The boundaries of the PF are as follows: anterior: clivus and posterior clinoid; posterior: inion (bony prominence at confluence of straight and sagittal sinuses); inferior: occipital bone; lateral: temporal, occipital, and parietal bones; superior: tentorium cerebellum. CSF flow: lateral ventricles to third ventricle via foramen of Monro, then to the fourth ventricle via aqueduct of Sylvius, then into the subarachnoid space via the medial foramen of Magendie and the lateral foramina of Luschka. The tendency for MB to obstruct CSF efflux leads to symptoms associated with elevated ICP.[6]

PATHOLOGY: MBs are classified according to both histopathologic and molecular features (MB, genetically defined and MB, histologically defined). In the 2021 WHO classification update, the SHH molecular group is now further subdivided into four methylome-based subgroups SHH-1, SHH-2, SHH-3, and SHH-4. The non-Wnt/non-SHH groups have also been subdivided into eight methylome-based subgroups.[9] IHC demonstrates neuronal markers (neurofilament, neuron-specific enolase, synaptophysin) in most cases and occasionally stains positive for GFAP (glial fibrillary acidic protein). Rare subtypes: melanotic (<1%) and medullomyoblastoma (<1%; contains striated muscle differentiation). See Table 58.2 for a summary of the morphologic classification.

Table 58.2 Morphologic Classification of Medulloblastoma			
Histopathologic Subtype	**Prognosis**	**Relative Frequency**	**Features**
Desmoplastic/ nodular	Good	15%–20%, more common in older patients	Biphasic with dense cellular areas surrounded by stromal component. Desmoplastic variant is associated with Gorlin syndrome and resultant inactivation of PTCH1.
Extensive nodularity	Good		Nodules dominate and are typically large and irregularly shaped.
Classic	Intermediate	80%–90%	Densely cellular, undifferentiated small round blue cells. Classically associated with Homer-Wright rosettes (rings of neuroblasts surrounding eosinophilic neuropil), but these are observed in the minority of cases.
Large cell/ anaplastic	Poor	~5%–10%, rare	Large cells with large nuclei, prominent nucleoli, many mitoses, and nuclear polymorphism. More cytoplasm than classic; associated with amplification of MYC, bulky spinal metastases.

GENETICS: Historically, risk stratification has relied primarily on clinicopathologic variables. A molecularly driven risk stratification system was initially established at a 2015 consensus that supports the development of biomarker-driven clinical trials.[10,11] C-MYC amplification and alterations in chr 17 confer poor prognosis.[12] Note that different molecular subgroups may have different CNS origins; for example, Wnt appears to originate mostly from the dorsal brainstem/lower rhombic lip, SHH is mostly found in cerebellar hemispheres, and groups 3/4 are found in the subventricular zone.[13,14] Please refer to Tables 58.3 and 58.4 for a summary of the WHO 2021 molecular classification and the molecular-based risk stratification, respectively.

Table 58.3 WHO 2021 Molecular Classification of Medulloblastoma[9,10,15]					
Molecular Subgroup	**Incidence**	**Age**	**5-Yr OS**	**Associated Histology**	**Pathogenesis**
Wingless (Wnt)	10%	Older children and adults	~100% in children	Classic	Mutation in *CTNNB1* gene upregulates Wnt pathway, which increases accumulation of nuclear β-catenin and promotes cell division and proliferation.

(continued)

Table 58.3 WHO 2021 Molecular classification of Medulloblastoma[9,10,15] (continued)

Molecular Subgroup	Incidence	Age	5-Yr OS	Associated Histology	Pathogenesis
Sonic hedgehog, TP53-wild-type (SHH-wt)	30%	Bimodal: <5 years and adolescent/ young adults	~80% in the absence of high-risk features[†]	Desmoplastic/ nodular	Mutation in *PTCH1* gene, which upregulates SHH pathway and promotes DNA transcription, decreases cell–cell adhesion, and increases angiogenesis.
Sonic hedgehog, TP53-mutant (SHH-mt)	10%–15% of SHH MBs	Older children	~40%	Large cell/ anaplastic	Similar to SHH-wt, but with associated TP53 mutation.
Group 3*	25%	Infants and young children	20%–30%	Classic/large cell/anaplastic	Not well-defined. Upregulation of OTX2 transcription factor upregulates *C-Myc* oncogene and associated overexpression. High genomic instability and isodicentric 17q.
Group 4*	35%	Median age 9 years	75%–90%	Classic	Overexpression of histone methylases/acetylases. Oncogene *MYCN* and **CDK6** amplifications. Isodicentric 17q. Chr X loss in 80% of females with group 4 MB.

*New evidence suggests that growth factor independent-1 (Gfi1 and Gfi1B) proto-oncogene activation is implicated in group 3 and group 4 MB.[16]
[†]MYCN amplification is independently associated with a poor prognosis.

Table 58.4 Molecular-Based Risk Stratification: 2016 International Consensus[11]

	Survival Rates	Criteria	Clinical Significance
Low risk	>90%	• WNT subgroup • Nonmetastatic group 4 with whole chr 11 loss or whole chr 17 gain	May qualify for reduced-intensity therapy
Average risk	75%–90%	• Others	May warrant intensification of therapy
High risk	50%–75%	• MYCN amplified SHH tumors • Metastatic SHH tumors • Metastatic group 4 tumors	May warrant intensification of therapy
Very high risk	<50%	• Metastatic group 3 • SHH with TP53 mutation	

Source: Data from Ramaswamy V, Remke M, Bouffet E, et al. Risk stratification of childhood medulloblastoma in the molecular era: the current consensus. *Acta Neuropathol.* 2016;131(6):821–831. doi:10.1007/s00401-016-1569-6.

CLINICAL PRESENTATION: Tumors usually grow into/fill the fourth ventricle with signs and symptoms related to increased ICP: headaches, morning emesis, papilledema, diplopia due to CN VI palsy. Infants may manifest bulging anterior fontanelle and splitting of cranial sutures. Destruction of the vermis can cause truncal ataxia. Other cerebellar symptoms include dysmetria, dysdiadochokinesia, and spasticity. Although most commonly seen in pineal gland tumors, Parinaud syndrome (upward gaze palsy, pseudo-Argyll Robertson pupils, convergence-retraction nystagmus, eyelid retraction) can be observed, as can the "setting sun sign" (conjugate down gaze). Extraneural metastases are uncommon (<5%) but most commonly involve bone.[6] Differential diagnosis of a pediatric PF mass: BEAM (brainstem glioma, ependymoma, astrocytoma, medulloblastoma), hemangioblastoma, lymphoma, and dysplastic cerebellar ganglioma.

WORKUP: H&P with detailed neurologic exam. Preoperatively, obtain MRI brain with contrast (MB appears as an isointense/hypointense mass with patchy contrast enhancement on T1; isointense on FLAIR and hyperintense on DWI) and establish baseline neuropsychiatric testing, neuroendocrine testing, growth curves, CBC, and audiologic evaluation. If imaging suggests MB or other brain tumor, upfront resection (not biopsy) is indicated. Obtain postoperative MRI brain with contrast *within* 72 hours (inflammation of the meninges and residual blood products in the CSF can become pronounced beyond 72 hours and falsely suggest M+ disease). Obtain MRI spinal axis 10 to 14 days postop to avoid confounding due to artifactual changes that can be seen in the immediate postop period. LP with cytology should be performed after MRI spinal axis is obtained to avoid confounding inflammation from the procedure. Usually, LP cannot be safely performed preoperatively due to increased ICP. False-positive LPs can occur within 10 days and can be repeated if positive. Systemic staging not routinely performed.

PROGNOSTIC FACTORS: Factors associated with worse prognosis: age <3 years, M+, STR (>1.5 cm² residual), group 3 or SHH-mt molecular profile, anaplastic/large cell morphology.

STAGING: MB follows the Modified Chang system (Table 58.5), which is based on preoperative MRI, postoperative MRI, operative findings, and CSF analysis. Note: T stage is no longer thought to be prognostic, but it is included here for reference.

Table 58.5 Modified Chang System for Medulloblastoma Staging[17]	
Extent of Tumor	
T1	≤3 cm diameter
T2	>3 cm diameter
T3a	>3 cm with extension into the aqueduct of Sylvius and/or foramen of Luschka
T3b	>3 cm with unequivocal extension into the brainstem
T4	>3 cm with extension past the aqueduct of Sylvius and/or down past the foramen magnum (beyond posterior fossa)
Degree of Metastasis	
M0	No CSF, cerebral, or spinal involvement
M1	Positive CSF Cytology
M2	Gross nodular seeding along cerebellar/cerebral subarachnoid space or in the third or lateral ventricles
M3	Gross nodular seeding in the spinal subarachnoid space
M4	Metastasis outside the cerebrospinal axis

Source: Data from Chang CH, Housepian EM, Herbert C Jr. An operative staging system and a megavoltage radiotherapeutic technic for cerebellar medulloblastomas. *Radiology.* 1969;93(6):1351–1359. doi:10.1148/93.6.1351.

TREATMENT PARADIGM

Multimodality therapy is currently the standard of care as surgery alone confers dismal prognosis with only 1 out of 61 patients surviving this single modality approach in Cushing's original paper.[18] Adjuvant RT was introduced in the 1950s, with some improvement in survival, although still dismal compared with current standards. Improvements in outcome were finally observed with modern RT techniques including craniospinal target volumes and the addition of CHT.[19,20] Several cooperative trials have helped delineate the current treatment paradigm, which generally includes maximal safe resection followed by CSI + PF/IF boost with concurrent weekly VCR followed by approximately eight cycles of CHT.

Surgery: Suboccipital craniotomy with maximal safe resection. The goal is to achieve GTR/NTR with <1.5 cm² residual disease on postop MRI. Previous studies have indicated essentially equivalent outcomes between GTR and NTR[21] but worse PFS when compared with STR (~70% vs. 50%),[22] although this is evolving in the molecular era.[23] Stereotactic or open biopsy is rarely indicated. Preoperatively, vasogenic tumor edema may be managed with steroids. Obstructive hydrocephalus is typically relieved by removal of the tumor, but intraoperative ventriculostomy may be indicated to relieve pressure. *Complications:* PF syndrome in up to 25% (also known as cerebellar mutism: manifested by mutism, truncal ataxia, dysphagia, emotional lability; usually self-resolves over weeks to months and should not delay adjuvant treatment). Operative mortality is <2%.

Chemotherapy: MB is one of the most chemosensitive brain tumors. The incorporation of platinum agents is standard given their efficacy. Usually initiated ~4 weeks following CSI with eight to nine cycles delivered. Per the German HIT91 RCT, immediate postoperative CSI/VCR followed by adjuvant CHT became standard (as opposed to postop CHT followed by CSI).[24] In young children, CHT is used to delay or avoid the use of RT in order to decrease associated neurocognitive risks (treatment paradigm: induction CHT followed by surgery and then additional consolidation CHT, with RT offered only for salvage).[25] *Complications:* ototoxicity, infertility (related to CYC; affects males > females), myelosuppression, second malignancy.

Radiation: CSI indicated for all patients (aside from the very young, as noted above) and should start within ~30 days of surgery. *Average risk*: After maximal safe resection: CSI to 23.4 Gy/13 fx with IF boost to 54 Gy (tumor bed + margin) based on ACNS 0331.[5] Concurrent single-agent VCR is used at some institutions but considered too toxic at others. *High risk*: After maximal resection: CSI to 36–39.6 Gy/20–22 fx with PF boost to 55.8 Gy with concurrent VCR during CSI followed by adjuvant CHT. If M+, boost metastatic disease as follows (per ACNS 0332): 50.4 Gy: intracranial metastasis; 50.4 Gy: focal spinal metastasis below cord; 45 Gy: focal spine metastasis above cord terminus; 39.6 Gy: diffuse spinal disease. Both IMRT[26] and proton therapy[27] have been shown to reduce ototoxicity as compared with 3D-CRT regimens.

St. Jude is actively investigating treating select low-risk patients to a lower dose CSI of 15 Gy (M0, GTR, NTR [≤1.5 cm^2], WNT subgroup, classic histology, presence of monosomy 6 by FISH, presence of B catenin by IHC, no MYC or MYCN amplification).

Note that historical RR data suggest a boost dose <50 Gy is associated with 33% LC as opposed to 79% LC with at least 50 Gy, albeit using whole PF.[28]

Complications of CSI

Acute: myelosuppression, nausea/vomiting, diarrhea, fatigue.

Chronic: neurocognitive (mnemonic "I am able" / I M ABL – **I**Q, **m**emory, **a**ttention, **b**ehavior, **l**earning), neuroendocrine deficits (particularly GH deficiency, hypothyroidism, gonadal dysfunction), impaired soft tissue/bone growth, ototoxicity (RT and/or cisplatin), second neoplasms, Lhermitte syndrome, cataracts, CNS necrosis (2%–5%).[29,30]

Impact on Neurocognition

4.2 point IQ decrease per year (conventional photon CSI)[31,32] prior to modern dose reduction and boost volumes; we are now seeing IQ point decrease of about 2.4 per year.[33]

1.5 point IQ decrease per year (conventional proton CSI).[34]

Odds of worsening associative memory (23%–26% per 1 Gy mean hippocampal dose).[35]

Odds of worsening processing speed (10%–15% per 1 Gy mean to frontal white matter or corpus callosum).[35]

There is evidence that proton plans facilitate decreased dose to the cochlea and temporal lobes compared with IMRT (~2% for protons, ~20% for IMRT) with essentially zero exit dose through the abdomen, chest, heart, and pelvis.[26,34] Additional data show that when administered to adults needing CSI, proton-based treatment was associated with essentially one-third the rates of nausea, vomiting, and weight loss, and 10-fold less esophagitis.[36] The risk for brainstem injury in patients treated with protons to PF tumors has been shown to be ~2% at 5 years, which is roughly in line with the incidence reported for patients treated with photons; this evidence helps dispel prior concerns that the dose uncertainty associated with protons leads to higher rates of brainstem injury than seen with photons.[30] In a report of long-term survivors (adults who were treated as children) with an MFU of 10 years, 12 of 17 patients were able to live without assistance. The most common long-term side effects included executive dysfunction ($n = 15$), weakness/ataxia ($n = 14$), and depression/anxiety ($n = 9$).

Procedure: See *Handbook of Treatment Planning in Radiation Oncology,* Chapter 12[37]

EVIDENCE-BASED Q&A

AVERAGE RISK MB

What historical data led to the current treatment paradigm of maximal safe resection followed by combined concurrent CHT-CSI with boost and adjuvant CHT?

In the premolecular era, CCG 942[38] and SIOP 1[39] did not find benefit to the addition of CHT after 36 Gy CSI in an unselected population but did find an OS and EFS benefit in those with T3–T4 and M1–3 disease. Attempts were then made to modify the extent of RT fields to minimize toxicity. However, omission of supratentorial RT led to a 6-year EFS of <20% with 64% of failures occurring supratentorially, therefore establishing the need for whole brain coverage.[40] The POG8631/CCG 923 trial tested 23.4 Gy vs. 36 Gy CSI (both with 54 Gy PF boost) without CHT in patients with <1.5 cc residual disease with no difference in 5-year PFS, albeit there were more early neuroaxis failures in the 23.4 Gy arm and higher toxicity with 36 Gy CSI, suggesting that 23.4 Gy with CHT may be warranted.[41] The use of CHT with RT was re-established with the PNET-3 trial (see below) showing an EFS benefit to pre-RT CHT, and CCG 9892 (see below) demonstrated that reduced-dose CSI with concurrent and adjuvant CHT has favorable outcomes for average-risk disease.

Taylor, PNET-3 (*JCO* 2003, PMID 12697884): PRT of pre-RT CHT (VCR, etoposide, carboplatin, CYC × 4 cycles) vs. RT alone for nonmetastatic MB. RT: 35 Gy CSI followed by PF boost to 55 Gy. Results: 179 evaluable patients. The 3-year EFS improved in the CHT arm (79% vs. 65% with RT alone, SS), as did 5-year EFS (74% vs. 60%, SS). There was no significant difference in 3- or 5-year OS. **Conclusion: First PRT to show improved EFS with the addition of CHT. The authors added that this non–cisplatin-containing regimen could also reduce ototoxicity and nephrotoxicity.**

Packer, CCG 9892 (*JCO* 1999, PMID 10561268): Phase II trial of 65 patients 3 to 10 years old with M0 MB enrolled following maximal surgical resection. Patients received RT within 28 days postop with concurrent weekly VCR. RT was delivered as CSI to 23.4 Gy with PF boost to 55.8 Gy. Six weeks following RT, patients received CCNU, VCR, and cisplatin for eight cycles (q6 weeks). Results: MFU 56 months. No prognostic factors identified; ~33% RT protocol violation rate. The 3-year PFS was 88% and the 3-year OS was 85%. **Conclusions: These results suggest that reduced-dose CSI and adjuvant cisplatin-based CHT during and after RT are feasible for M0 MB.**

Can patients with average-risk MB receive a lower CSI dose? Can any average-risk patient receive IF boost rather than whole PF boost?

Michalski, COG ACNS0331 (*JCO* 2021, PMID 34110925): Enrolled patients ages 3 to 21 years with average-risk MB. Primary endpoint EFS. Patients from ages 3 to 7 years underwent two randomizations (CSI dose of 18 Gy vs. 23.4 Gy; IF vs. PF boost). Patients from 8 to 21 years were eligible only for the IF vs. PF question; all received CSI dose of 23.4 Gy. Note that this is the first multi-institution RCT that was sufficiently powered to address the question of IF vs. full PF boost. Protocol: max safe resection followed by initiation of RT within 31 days delivered with weekly VCR followed by cisplatin/VCR and either CCNU or CYC (alternating AABAABAAB pattern). Results: 464 patients. MFU 6.6 years. IF was not inferior to PF RT and low dose (18 Gy) was inferior to standard dose. The 5-year EFS was 83% (95% CI 77–88) and 81% (95% CI 75–86) for the IF and PF regimens, respectively, and 71% (95% CI 63–80) and 83% (95% CI 76–90) for the 18 Gy and 23.4 Gy regimens, respectively. Children receiving 23.4 Gy CSI exhibited greater late declines in IQ (estimate = 5.87; $p = .02$). See Table 58.6. **Conclusion: IF boost is noninferior to full PF boost for average-risk patients ages 3 to 21 years. However, reduced-dose CSI (18 Gy) is associated with worse 5-year EFS and OS, and thus average-risk MB patients should continue to receive 23.4 Gy as the standard CSI dose unless enrolled on a clinical trial.**

Table 58.6 Results of COG ACNS 0331 Medulloblastoma			
	5-Yr LF	5-Yr EFS	5-Yr OS
All patients ages 3–21:			
IF boost	2%	83%	85%
PF boost	4%	81%	85%
	$p = .18$	$p = .44$; IF-RT was deemed noninferior to PF-RT.	

(continued)

Table 58.6 Results of COG ACNS 0331 Medulloblastoma (*continued*)			
	5-Yr LF	5-Yr EFS	5-Yr OS
Patients ages 3–7:			
Low dose (18 Gy)		71%	78%
Standard dose (23.4 Gy)		83%	86%
		Noninferiority of low-dose CSI was not established.	

Can cyclophosphamide (CYC) replace CCNU in the adjuvant CHT portion of treatment?

COG A9961 was a large PRT randomizing average-risk MB patients (all of whom were postop and received 23.4 Gy CSI) to two different adjuvant CHT regimens, one with CYC and another with CCNU. The rationale was that data supporting the use of CCNU in pediatric tumors were scant, whereas xenograft and early clinical data for the use of CYC were more promising.[42] Ultimately, there was no significant difference between the two regimens, with 5-year OS ~85% in both arms. Authors concluded that, although neither CHT regimen was superior, the favorable outcomes seen with both regimens offer additional support to the use of reduced dose CSI.

When treating average-risk MB, does hyperfractionation of CSI affect outcomes or reduce toxicity?

MSFOP 98 was a phase I/II average-risk trial using hyperfractionated RT, 36 Gy CSI with tumor bed boost to 68 Gy at 1 Gy/fx BID.[43] It showed excellent long-term EFS in the absence of CHT and full-scale IQ drop was less pronounced compared with other standard RT reports. This led to a large European PRT (HIT-SIOP PNET-4), which enrolled average-risk MB patients and randomized them to standard fractionation (23.4 Gy CSI with PF boost to 54 Gy at 1.8 Gy/fx) vs. hyperfractionation (36 Gy CSI with PF boost to 60 Gy and tumor bed boost to 68 Gy at 1 Gy/fx BID with 8-hr interfx interval).[44] Results published in the JCO in 2012 showed equivalent outcomes for EFS and OS with no difference in ototoxicity; IQ measurements were not reported in their final publication. Based on these results, hyperfractionation is typically not employed in average-risk MB.

HIGH-RISK MB

What data initially supported the use of CHT in high-risk disease?

CCG 942 (discussed above in the average-risk section) and SIOP I were both PRTs evaluating postoperative patients who received CSI who were then randomized to CHT or no CHT.[38,39] For both studies, there was no difference in outcome between the two groups, but when limited to those with more advanced disease (T3–T4, M+, or STR), an improvement in EFS was observed.

Can outcomes be improved by intensifying the CHT regimen with additional agents?

CCG 921 included patients with a variety of high-risk pediatric brain tumors to see if "8 in 1" CHT (8 types of CHT in 1 day: cisplatin, procarbazine, CCNU, VCR, CYC, methylprednisolone, hydroxyurea, cytarabine) was better than a combination of VCR/CCNU/prednisone (VCP). 421 children enrolled, of which 203 had MB. Subset analysis of this group showed better outcomes with VCP than 8 in 1 CHT (5-year PFS 63% vs. 45%, p = .006).[22]

Is there a benefit to altering the sequence of CHT (e.g., delivering CHT immediately postop followed by RT)?

Four PRTs have evaluated this question: SIOP II, SIOP III, POG 9031, and HIT 91 from Germany. All of them except for SIOP III showed no benefit to immediate postop CHT; both POG 9031 and SIOP II showed 5-year EFS to be about 60% to 70% and 5-year OS ~75% in both groups (NS), and HIT 91 actually showed an improvement in 3-year EFS with immediate RT (78% vs. 65%, p = .03).[4,24,45] SIOP III is the only exception and showed improved 3- and 5-year EFS with upfront CHT.[3] Therefore, with three of these four studies showing no benefit to upfront CHT, standard of care is to perform maximal safe resection followed by RT (with concurrent VCR) followed by adjuvant CHT.

Does the use of carboplatin as a radiosensitizer during CSI lead to better outcomes?

This was addressed in COG 99701, a phase I/II trial that evaluated the role of adding radiosensitizing carbo-platin to VCR during CSI and the 5-year OS was ~75%.[46] This carboplatin-containing regimen was tested in the phase III PRT, ACNS 0332, which is summarized below.

Leary, ACNS 0332 (*JAMA Oncology* 2021, PMID 34292305): Phase III PRT evaluated 261 children (3–21 years) with high-risk MB. High-risk features included M+ (72% of patients), diffuse anaplasia histology (22%), or incomplete surgical resection defined as >1.5 cm^3 residual tumor (5%). Patients were randomized to receive 36 Gy CSI and weekly VCR ± daily carboplatin followed by 6 cycles of maintenance CHT with cisplatin, CYC, and VCR ± 12 cycles of isotretinoin during and following maintenance. Primary endpoint was EFS. The 5-year EFS was 66% with carboplatin vs. 59% without ($p = .11$), with the benefit exclusively observed in group 3 subgroup patients: 73% with carboplatin vs. 54% without ($p = .047$). **Conclusion: Addition of concurrent daily carboplatin to standard 36 Gy CSI and weekly VCR should be considered in high-risk group 3 MB as it improves 5-year EFS.**

Is there any detriment to interrupting RT?

SIOP III (Table 58.7) showed better 3-year OS when RT was delivered within 50 days, suggesting that avoid-ing RT interruption can lead to better outcomes.[3] These results confirm earlier findings from the University of Florida that duration of RT is associated with outcomes (used a cut point of 45 days).[47]

Table 58.7 SIOP III RT Duration Results	
RT Duration	**3-Yr OS**
<50 days	84%
>50 days	71%
p value	.036

Is there a role for re-irradiation?

Recurrent MB is rarely cured and has a dismal prognosis with 2-year OS historically <25%. However, several salvage treatments have been considered, including surgical resection, brachytherapy, radiosurgery, high-dose CHT with autologous stem cell transplant, and re-RT. Re-RT may be a reasonable option to con-sider in both average-risk and high-risk patients.

Wetmore, St. Jude (*Cancer* 2014, PMID 25080363): RR of 38 patients with recurrent MB. Of these patients, 14 received re-RT (8 repeat CSI, 3 spinal only re-RT, and 3 primary only). Median re-RT dose was 36 Gy (range, 18–54 Gy), and median max cumulative dose was 91.9 Gy (range, 73.8–109.8 Gy). For patients who initially had average-risk MB, the 5-year OS with RT was 55% vs. 33% without RT; 10-year OS 46% with RT vs. 0% without ($p = .003$). Similarly, high-risk individuals also benefit-ted ($p = .003$). Re-RT did result in an increased rate of necrosis ($p = .047$).

Is there a neurocognitive toxicity benefit to using proton RT (PBT)?

PBT offers several dosimetric advantages over photon therapy. Because protons deposit near the terminus of the Bragg peak, a modulated posterior beam can limit anterior dose. This greatly limits integral dose, the sum of ionizing RT deposited in the body. Models of treatment planning with protons in children with MB have estimated a reduction in lifetime incidence of secondary malignancies by a factor ranging from 8 to 15; however, prospective data on the true incidence of secondary malignancies are limited. In one retrospective study of pediatric patients receiving either proton or photon CSI, protons reduced grade 2 vomiting and nau-sea.[48] Vertebral-sparing approaches to mitigate growth impairment have been retrospectively reported with a dramatic reduction of grade 4 lymphopenia from 77% to 33% with the use of protons and significantly fewer red blood cell transfusions.[49] ASTRO 2018 guidelines caution that high-RBE protons tend to occur at the distal edge of the Bragg peak, thus they recommend placing the distal edge of the Bragg peak within the center of the vertebral bodies.[50] Retrospective data suggest an intellectual sparing advantage with PBT compared with photon RT.

Kahalley, Multi-Institutional (*JCO* 2020, PMID 31774710): RR of 79 children with MB treated with either PBT or photon RT for MB at eight different cancer centers. Primary endpoints were various longitudinal intelligence composite scores. Demographic/clinical variables were similar between patients except for boost dose ($p < .01$) and boost margin ($p = .01$). The PBT group exhibited superior long-term outcomes in global IQ, perceptual reasoning, and working memory compared with photons (all $p < .05$). **Conclusion: Authors concluded that PBT may significantly improve long-term neurocognitive toxicity from CSI.** *Comment: This study performed unplanned comparison between nonrandomized patients treated in different countries, had variable PF boost volume, and used whole brain fields that should have delivered equivalent biological doses regardless of treatment modality.*

MB IN INFANTS

What is the recommended treatment for infants (<3 years)?

CSI can lead to significant neurocognitive toxicity, which is dose- and age-dependent (younger is worse).[32,51] Therefore, CHT has been evaluated as a stop-gap to delay RT. "Baby POG #1" showed this was possible with a 5-year OS of 40%.[52] An unintended consequence of this study was complete parent refusal of RT, which showed that in a select group of MB infants there may not be a need for RT at all. As described earlier, the CCG group tried eight CHT drugs ("8-in-1") with worse outcomes but confirmed the approach of CHT before RT was feasible. Follow-up trials including the Head Start I and II for infant MB used intensive CHT and used RT only in a salvage setting.[53] This approach eliminated CSI in 52% of patients and may preserve quality of life and intellectual function. However, the intense CHT is not without cost and 4 out of 21 infants died of treatment-related death. The findings of "Baby POG#1" have been further bolstered by Rutkowski et al. using surgery and subsequent CHT, with 5-year OS for those with GTR of 93%, 56% if STR, and 38% for those with macroscopic metastases.[25]

REFERENCES

1. Louis DN, Ohgaki H, Wiestler OD, et al. The 2007 WHO classification of tumours of the central nervous system. *Acta Neuropathol.* 2007;114(2):97–109. doi:10.1007/s00401-007-0243-4
2. Thomas CC. *Brain Tumors of Childhood. Medulloblastoma.* 1952 .
3. Taylor RE, Bailey CC, Robinson KJ, et al. Impact of radiotherapy parameters on outcome in the International Society Of Paediatric Oncology/United Kingdom children's cancer study group PNET-3 study of preradiotherapy chemotherapy for M0-M1 medulloblastoma. *Int J Radiat Oncol Biol Phys.* 2004;58(4):1184–1193. doi:10.1016/j.ijrobp.2003.08.010
4. Bailey CC, Gnekow A, Wellek S, et al. Prospective randomised trial of chemotherapy given before radiotherapy in childhood medulloblastoma. International Society of Paediatric Oncology (SIOP) and the (German) Society of Paediatric Oncology (GPO): SIOP II. *Med Pediatr Oncol.* 1995;25(3):166–178. doi:10.1002/mpo.2950250303
5. Michalski J. Results of COG ACNS0331: a phase III trial of Involved-Field Radiotherapy (IFRT) and Low Dose Craniospinal Irradiation (LD-CSI) with chemotherapy in average-risk medulloblastoma: a report from the Children's Oncology Group. *Int J Radiat Oncol Biol Phys.* 2016;96(5):937. doi:10.1016/j.ijrobp.2016.09.046
6. Dhall G. Medulloblastoma. *J Child Neurol.* 2009;24(11):1418–1430. doi:10.1177/0883073809341668
7. Stone DM, Hynes M, Armanini M, et al. The tumour-suppressor gene patched encodes a candidate receptor for Sonic hedgehog. *Nature.* 1996;384(6605):129–134. doi:10.1038/384129a0
8. Hamilton SR, Liu B, Parsons RE, et al. The molecular basis of Turcot's syndrome. *N Engl J Med.* 1995;332(13):839–847. doi:10.1056/NEJM199503303321302
9. Louis DN, Perry A, Wesseling P, et al. The 2021 WHO classification of tumors of the central nervous system: a summary. *Neuro Oncol.* 2021;23(8):1231–1251. doi:10.1093/neuonc/noab106
10. Khatua S. Evolving molecular era of childhood medulloblastoma: time to revisit therapy. *Future Oncol.* 2016;12(1):107–117. doi:10.2217/fon.15.284
11. Ramaswamy V, Remke M, Bouffet E, et al. Risk stratification of childhood medulloblastoma in the molecular era: the current consensus. *Acta Neuropathol.* 2016;131(6):821–831. doi:10.1007/s00401-016-1569-6
12. Pan E, Pellarin M, Holmes E, et al. Isochromosome 17q is a negative prognostic factor in poor-risk childhood medulloblastoma patients. *Clin Cancer Res.* 2005;11(13):4733–4740. doi:10.1158/1078-0432.CCR-04-0465
13. Smith KS, Bihannic L, Gudenas BL, et al. Unified rhombic lip origins of group 3 and group 4 medulloblastoma. *Nature.* 2022;609(7929):1012–1020. doi:10.1038/s41586-022-05208-9
14. Gibson P, Tong Y, Robinson G, et al. Subtypes of medulloblastoma have distinct developmental origins. *Nature.* 2010;468(7327):1095–1099. doi:10.1038/nature09587
15. National Comprehensive Cancer Network. *Pediatric Central Nervous System Cancers* (Version 1.2024). https://www.nccn.org/professionals/physician_gls/pdf/ped_cns.pdf

16. Northcott PA, Lee C, Zichner T, et al. Enhancer hijacking activates GFI1 family oncogenes in medulloblastoma. *Nature*. 2014;511(7510):428–434. doi:10.1038/nature13379

17. Chang CH, Housepian EM, Herbert C Jr. An operative staging system and a megavoltage radiotherapeutic technic for cerebellar medulloblastomas. *Radiology*. 1969;93(6):1351–1359. doi:10.1148/93.6.1351

18. Cushing H. Experiences with the cerebellar medulloblastomas: a critical review. *Acta Pathologica et Microbiologica Scandinavica*. 1930;7:1–86. doi:10.1111/j.1600-0463.1930.tb06503.x

19. Lampe I, Mac IR. Medulloblastoma of the cerebellum. *Arch Neurol Psychiatry*. 1949;62(3):322-329. doi:10.1001/archneurpsyc.1949.02310150069008

20. Tomlinson FH, Scheithauer BW, Meyer FB, et al. Medulloblastoma: I. Clinical, diagnostic, and therapeutic overview. *J Child Neurol*. 1992;7(2):142–155. doi:10.1177/088307389200700203

21. Gajjar A, Sanford RA, Bhargava R, et al. Medulloblastoma with brain stem involvement: the impact of gross total resection on outcome. *Pediatr Neurosurg*. 1996;25(4):182–187. doi:10.1159/000121121

22. Zeltzer PM, Boyett JM, Finlay JL, et al. Metastasis stage, adjuvant treatment, and residual tumor are prognostic factors for medulloblastoma in children: conclusions from the Children's Cancer Group 921 randomized phase III study. *J Clin Oncol*. 1999;17(3):832–845. doi:10.1200/jco.1999.17.3.832

23. Thompson EM, Hielscher T, Bouffet E, et al. Prognostic value of medulloblastoma extent of resection after accounting for molecular subgroup: a retrospective integrated clinical and molecular analysis. *Lancet Oncol*. 2016;17(4):484–495. doi:10.1016/S1470-2045(15)00581-1

24. Kortmann RD, Kuhl J, Timmermann B, et al. Postoperative neoadjuvant chemotherapy before radiotherapy as compared to immediate radiotherapy followed by maintenance chemotherapy in the treatment of medulloblastoma in childhood: results of the German prospective randomized trial HIT '91. *Int J Radiat Oncol Biol Phys*. 2000;46(2):269–279. doi:10.1016/s0360-3016(99)00369-7

25. Rutkowski S, Bode U, Deinlein F, et al. Treatment of early childhood medulloblastoma by postoperative chemotherapy alone. *N Engl J Med*. 2005;352(10):978–986. doi:10.1056/NEJMoa042176

26. Huang E, Teh BS, Strother DR, et al. Intensity-modulated radiation therapy for pediatric medulloblastoma: early report on the reduction of ototoxicity. *Int J Radiat Oncol Biol Phys*. 2002;52(3):599–605. doi:10.1016/s0360-3016(01)02641-4

27. Moeller BJ, Chintagumpala M, Philip JJ, et al. Low early ototoxicity rates for pediatric medulloblastoma patients treated with proton radiotherapy. *Radiat Oncol*. 2011;6:58. doi:10.1186/1748-717X-6-58

28. Hughes EN, Shillito J, Sallan SE, Loeffler JS, Cassady JR, Tarbell NJ. Medulloblastoma at the joint center for radiation therapy between 1968 and 1984. The influence of radiation dose on the patterns of failure and survival. *Cancer*. 1988;61(10):1992–1998. doi:10.1002/1097-0142(19880515)61:10<1992::aid-cncr2820611011>3.0.co;2-j

29. Murphy ES, Merchant TE, Wu S, et al. Necrosis after craniospinal irradiation: results from a prospective series of children with central nervous system embryonal tumors. *Int J Radiat Oncol Biol Phys*. 2012; 83(5):e655–e660. doi:10.1016/j.ijrobp.2012.01.061

30. Gentile MS, Yeap BY, Paganetti H, et al. Brainstem injury in pediatric patients with posterior fossa tumors treated with proton beam therapy and associated dosimetric factors. *Int J Radiat Oncol Biol Phys*. 2018;100(3):719–729. doi:10.1016/j.ijrobp.2017.11.026

31. Merchant TE, Schreiber JE, Wu S, Lukose R, Xiong X, Gajjar A. Critical combinations of radiation dose and volume predict intelligence quotient and academic achievement scores after craniospinal irradiation in children with medulloblastoma. *Int J Radiat Oncol Biol Phys*. 2014;90(3):554–561. doi:10.1016/j.ijrobp.2014.06.058

32. Ris MD, Packer R, Goldwein J, Jones-Wallace D, Boyett JM. Intellectual outcome after reduced-dose radiation therapy plus adjuvant chemotherapy for medulloblastoma: a children's cancer group study. *J Clin Oncol*. 2001;19(15):3470–3476. doi:10.1200/jco.2001.19.15.3470

33. Merchant TE, Kun LE, Krasin MJ, et al. Multi-institution prospective trial of reduced-dose craniospinal irradiation (23.4 Gy) followed by conformal posterior fossa (36 Gy) and primary site irradiation (55.8 Gy) and dose-intensive chemotherapy for average-risk medulloblastoma. *Int J Radiat Oncol Biol Phys*. 2008; 70(3):782–787. doi:10.1016/j.ijrobp.2007.07.2342

34. Yock TI, Yeap BY, Ebb DH, et al. Long-term toxic effects of proton radiotherapy for paediatric medulloblastoma: a phase 2 single-arm study. *Lancet Oncol*. 2016;17(3):287–298. doi:10.1016/S1470-2045(15)00167-9

35. Acharya S, Guo Y, Patni T, et al. Association between brain substructure dose and cognitive outcomes in children with medulloblastoma treated on SJMB03: a step toward substructure-informed planning. *J Clin Oncol*. 2022;40(1):83–95. doi:10.1200/jco.21.01480

36. Fossati P, Ricardi U, Orecchia R. Pediatric medulloblastoma: toxicity of current treatment and potential role of protontherapy. *Cancer Treat Rev*. 2009;35(1):79–96. doi:10.1016/j.ctrv.2008.09.002

37. Videtic GMM, Woody NM, Vassil AD. *Handbook of Treatment Planning in Radiation Oncology*. 3rd ed. Demos Medical; 2020.

38. Evans AE, Jenkin RD, Sposto R, et al. The treatment of medulloblastoma. Results of a prospective randomized trial of radiation therapy with and without CCNU, vincristine, and prednisone. *J Neurosurg*. 1990; 72(4):572–582. doi:10.3171/jns.1990.72.4.0572

39. Tait DM, Thornton-Jones H, Bloom HJ, Lemerle J, Morris-Jones P. Adjuvant chemotherapy for medullo-blastoma: the first multi-centre control trial of the International Society of Paediatric Oncology (SIOP I). *Eur J Cancer*. 1990;26(4):464–469. PMID: 2141512

40. Bouffet E, Bernard JL, Frappaz D, et al. M4 protocol for cerebellar medulloblastoma: supratentorial radio-therapy may not be avoided. *Int J Radiat Oncol Biol Phys*. 1992;24(1):79–85. doi:10.1016/0360-3016(92)91025-i

41. Thomas PR, Deutsch M, Kepner JL, et al. Low-stage medulloblastoma: final analysis of trial comparing standard-dose with reduced-dose neuraxis irradiation. *J Clin Oncol*. 2000;18(16):3004–3011. doi:10.1200/jco.2000.18.16.3004

42. Packer RJ, Gajjar A, Vezina G, et al. Phase III study of craniospinal radiation therapy followed by adjuvant chemotherapy for newly diagnosed average-risk medulloblastoma. *J Clin Oncol*. 2006;24(25):4202–4208. doi:10.1200/JCO.2006.06.4980

43. Carrie C, Grill J, Figarella-Branger D, et al. Online quality control, hyperfractionated radiotherapy alone and reduced boost volume for standard risk medulloblastoma: long-term results of MSFOP 98. *J Clin Oncol*. 2009;27(11):1879–1883. doi:10.1200/JCO.2008.18.6437

44. Lannering B, Rutkowski S, Doz F, et al. Hyperfractionated versus conventional radiotherapy followed by chemotherapy in standard-risk medulloblastoma: results from the randomized multicenter HIT-SIOP PNET 4 trial. *J Clin Oncol*. 2012;30(26):3187–3193. doi:10.1200/JCO.2011.39.8719

45. Tarbell NJ, Friedman H, Polkinghorn WR, et al. High-risk medulloblastoma: a pediatric oncology group randomized trial of chemotherapy before or after radiation therapy (POG 9031). *J Clin Oncol*. 2013;31(23): 2936–2941. doi:10.1200/JCO.2012.43.9984

46. Jakacki RI, Burger PC, Zhou T, et al. Outcome of children with metastatic medulloblastoma treated with carboplatin during craniospinal radiotherapy: a Children's Oncology Group Phase I/II study. *J Clin Oncol*. 2012;30(21):2648–2653. doi:10.1200/JCO.2011.40.2792

47. del Charco JO, Bolek TW, McCollough WM, et al. Medulloblastoma: time-dose relationship based on a 30-year review. *Int J Radiat Oncol Biol Phys*. 1998;42(1):147–154. doi:10.1016/s0360-3016(98)00197-7

48. Uemura S, Demizu Y, Hasegawa D, et al. The comparison of acute toxicities associated with craniospinal irradiation between photon beam therapy and proton beam therapy in children with brain tumors. *Cancer Med*. 2022;11(6):1502–1510. doi:10.1002/cam4.4553

49. Chou B, Hopper A, Elster J, et al. Volumetric de-escalation and improved acute toxicity with proton craniospinal irradiation using a vertebral body-sparing technique. *Pediatr Blood Cancer*. 2022;69(5):e29489. doi:10.1002/pbc.29489

50. Pinnix CC, Yahalom J, Specht L, Dabaja BS. Radiation in Central Nervous System Leukemia: Guidelines From the International Lymphoma Radiation Oncology Group. *Int J Radiat Oncol Biol Phys*. 2018;102(1): 53–58. doi:10.1016/j.ijrobp.2018.05.067

51. Fouladi M, Gilger E, Kocak M, et al. Intellectual and functional outcome of children 3 years old or younger who have CNS malignancies. *J Clin Oncol*. 2005;23(28):7152–7160. doi:10.1200/JCO.2005.01.214

52. Duffner PK, Horowitz ME, Krischer JP, et al. The treatment of malignant brain tumors in infants and very young children: an update of the Pediatric Oncology Group experience. *Neuro Oncol*. 1999;1(2):152–161. doi:10.1093/neuonc/1.2.152

53. Dhall G, Grodman H, Ji L, et al. Outcome of children less than three years old at diagnosis with non-meta-static medulloblastoma treated with chemotherapy on the "" "Head Start" I and II protocols. *Pediatr Blood Cancer*. 2008;50(6):1169–1175. doi:10.1002/pbc.21525

59 EPENDYMOMA

Adannia N. Ufondu, John H. Suh, and Erin S. Murphy

QUICK HIT Ependymomas are an uncommon CNS tumor originating from glial stem cells most commonly in the fourth ventricle (children) or filum terminale (myxopapillary type in adults). The 10-year OS in adults and children is approximately 79% and 66%, respectively. The treatment paradigm is maximal safe resection with attempted GTR; the degree of resection classically represents the most important prognostic factor. In the molecular era with a new classification system, genetic markers such as 1q gain and 6q loss are also associated with worse outcomes. RT should be given postoperatively, 50.4 to 59.4 Gy, to the resection bed and any residual disease, depending on location. There is no clearly established role for CHT, but it may be used in select cases to delay RT or attempt second-look surgery.

EPIDEMIOLOGY: Ependymomas are an uncommon tumor originating from glial stem cells that can occur in all age groups but are more common in children.[1] They represent ~6% of CNS tumors in children (235 cases per year) and 2% of CNS tumors in adults.[1-3] Intracranial ependymomas are more common in children, whereas spinal ependymomas are more common in adults, with a median age at diagnosis of 30 to 40 years.

RISK FACTORS: No risk factors have been clearly identified. NF2 patients may be at an increased risk for spinal ependymomas.[4]

ANATOMY: Ependymomas can originate from anywhere in the CNS and classification is broadly divided by location: supratentorial (ST), posterior fossa (PF), and spinal cord. ST includes the cerebrum, ventricles, choroid plexus, hypothalamus, pineal gland, pituitary gland, and optic nerve. PF contains the cerebellum, tectum, fourth ventricle, and brainstem. CSF enters the fourth ventricle from the cerebral aqueduct and exits via the foramen of Luschka laterally and foramen of Magendie medially. The obex is the most caudal aspect of the fourth ventricle. The spinal cord ends at approximately L3 in children and L1–2 in adults. The thecal sac (filum terminale) ends at approximately S2 in both children and adults.[5-7]

PATHOLOGY: The WHO 2021 update on ependymomas attempted to refine and enhance the classification of ependymomas using molecular characteristics and localization rather than histologic features alone (Table 59.1). Histopathologic variants such as papillary, tanycytic, and clear cell morphology are no longer listed as subtypes, and grade plays less of a role in classification. The new WHO classification recognizes eight specific types of ependymoma and two additional types that cannot be assigned to any of the molecular subtypes but have specific locations.[8] ST ependymomas, which do not have the ZFTA or YAP1 molecular classifications, are regarded as ST-NEC (not elsewhere classified). Similarly, PF ependymomas without the expected molecular classifications are regarded as PF-NEC. Spinal (SP)-MYCN shows pseudorosettes and has a papillary or pseudopapillary architecture on histology with microvascular proliferation, necrosis, and high mitotic cell count typically.[8] Myxopapillary ependymomas (MPE) stain positive for GFAP and are characterized by the presence of papillary structures.

Table 59.1 WHO 2021 Update[8]						
	Median Age	5-Yr PFS	5-Yr OS	Molecular Features	Criteria†	Characteristics
ST NEC					Supratentorial localization	
ST-ZFTA	8 years	Poor	Poor	ZFTA fusions; CDKN2A and/or CDKN2B loss	Supratentorial; ZFTA fusion	Methylation class ST-ZFTA; immunoreactivity for p65 (RELA) or LICAM

(continued)

Table 59.1 WHO 2021 Update[8] (*continued*)

	Median Age	5-Yr PFS	5-Yr OS	Molecular Features	Criteria[†]	Characteristics
ST-YAP1	1.4 years	Intermediate	Good	YAP1 fusions	Supratentorial; YAP1 fusion	Methylation class ST-YAP1; no p65 or LICAM reactivity
PF NEC					Posterior fossa localization	
PF-A	3 years	Poor	Poor	EZHIP mutations; chr 1q gain or 6q loss	PF location; global reduction of K27me3 in nuclei OR methylation class PFA	Stable genome on CNP
PF-B	30 years	Intermediate	Intermediate	Chromosomal instability	PF location; methylation class PFB	Chromosomal instability and aneuploidy on CNP
SP-EPN	41 years	Intermediate	Good	NF2 mutations; chr 22q loss	Spinal location; absence of MPE or SE	Methylation class SP-EPN; loss of chromosome 22q; NO MYCN amp
SP-MYCN	32 years	Poor	Poor	MYCN amp	Spinal location; MYCN amp	Methylation class SP-MYCN; high-grade histologic features
MPE	39 years	Intermediate	Good	Chromosomal instability	Papillary structures and perivascular myxoid change; GFAP immunoreactive; methylation class MP	Papillary arrangements of tumor cells around vascularized fibromyxoid cores; location in filum terminale/conus
SE	~50 years	Good*	Good	TERT mutations; loss of chr 6	Circumscribed glioma; clustering of tumor cell nuclei; no conspicuous nuclear atypia; absent/minimal mitotic activity; DNA methylation class SE	

MPE, myxopapillary ependymoma; NEC, not elsewhere classified; PF, posterior fossa; SE, subependymoma; SP-EPN, spinal ependymoma; ST, supratentorium.
*SE of the supratentorium has low progression rate; however, those of the PF have a tendency to progress.[9]
[†]The WHO update lists obligatory criteria for classification of each tumor type, as well as desirable criteria that can support the diagnosis of each tumor type.
Source: Data from Kresbach C, Neyazi S, Schuller U. Updates in the classification of ependymal neoplasms: the 2021 WHO Classification and beyond. *Brain Pathol.* 2022;32(4):e13068. doi:10.1111/bpa.13068.

GENETICS: ST ependymomas are divided into two main groups, comprising of ZFTA (formerly C11orf95) or YAP1 molecular markers. ZFTA fusion-positive type has replaced the former ST-RELA tumor type in the new classification.[8] ZFTA fusions result from chromothripsis of chr 11, which leads to activation of the NF-κB signaling pathway.[9] YAP1 is a transcriptional coactivator controlled by the Hippo signaling pathway, which is important in homeostasis and regeneration.[10] Other important molecular markers include K27me3 reduction, gain of 1q or loss of 6q, and hypermethylation of CpG islands, which diagnose PF-A ependymoma. On the contrary, PF-B tumors show retained H3K27me3 and display a host of chromosomal abnormalities including monosomy 6, 10, and 17, and trisomy 18, 5, and 8. Most SP-EPN have chr 22q losses, predisposing to neurofibromatosis type 2 (NF2).[11] As the name suggests, SP-MYCN tumors exhibit MCYN amplifications and may exhibit loss of chr 10 and focal losses on chr 11q. Subependymomas may have TERT promoter mutations of loss of chr 6.

CLINICAL PRESENTATION: Most common presenting symptoms are those of increased ICP (headache, nausea, ataxia, vertigo, papilledema) in children or back pain in adults, depending on location.

WORKUP: H&P, MRI brain and spine with and without contrast, consider ventriculostomy over shunt if symptomatic. Postoperative MRI to evaluate the extent of resection within 48 hours. CSF cytology at least 10 to 12 days postop. Heterogeneous enhancement (more pronounced with high grade) is usually appreciated on MRI, and there is often involvement of the foramen of Luschka in PF ependymomas. Risk of CSF seeding is ~10% for infratentorial tumors and 8% to 20% for high-grade tumors.

PROGNOSTIC FACTORS: Extent of surgical resection is the most important prognostic factor.[12,13] Others may include younger age, high grade, male gender, and intracranial location.[13] Gain of 1q and loss of 6q are markers of poor outcome within PF-A.[14] SP-MYCN appears to be more aggressive when compared with other spinal ependymomas. ZFTA fusion also has poor prognosis when compared with ST-YAP1 tumors.[8] Subependymoma subgroups located in the PF and those harboring TERT promoter mutations/loss of chr 6 have been identified to be more aggressive.

NATURAL HISTORY: Grade I tumors have excellent outcomes and failure is uncommon. For grades II to III tumors, LF is usually more common than distant failure (12% vs. 8% in original Merchant phase II).[15] Failure usually occurs within 2 years.[3] EFS and OS for children at 5 years were 63% and 84% in ACNS0121, respectively[16]

TREATMENT PARADIGM

Surgery: Maximal safe resection with attempt at GTR is standard of care. NTR defined as <5 mm max diameter of residual disease.[15]

Chemotherapy: There is no clear, standardized role for the routine use of CHT. Various multidrug regimens have been used to delay RT for infants or to attempt a second-look surgery for those with an initial STR.

Radiation

Indications: RT is indicated postoperatively in essentially all cases. A spinal myxopapillary ependymoma after GTR is controversial, with some recommending treatment to 54 Gy and others recommending observation. Proton therapy (PBT) has been shown to be effective and safe in the management of grades II/III pediatric ependymoma.[17]

Dose: For PF tumors, treat to 54 Gy (often if proton therapy is used), up to 59.4 Gy. For gross residual disease, there is no clear role for dose escalation. Spinal ependymomas typically treated to 50.4 to 54 Gy. For ependymoblastomas or those with craniospinal dissemination, treat 36Gy CSI with conformal RT boost to 54 to 59.4Gy.

Toxicity: Acute: alopecia, fatigue, headache, nausea, erythema. Late: cognitive decline, hearing loss, endocrinopathies (most commonly, GH, TSH, ACTH), microcephaly.

Procedure: See *Handbook of Treatment Planning in Radiation Oncology*, Chapter 12.[18]

EVIDENCE-BASED Q&A

Is there a role for craniospinal irradiation (CSI) for patients with limited disease at presentation?

Historically, pediatric trials through the early 1990s routinely delivered CSI to doses of 23.4 to 36 Gy with a boost to 54 to 55 Gy.[19,20] However, local relapse was found to be the most common site of failure, with distant CNS failure occurring in only 5% to 7% of patients. Subsequent protocols (see the following) demonstrated similar outcomes and patterns of failure treating only a CTV = GTV/postoperative bed + 1 cm. Therefore, limited-field RT is now standard of care except in the uncommon situation of leptomeningeal spread at the time of diagnosis.

Merchant, St. Jude (*IJROBP* 2002, PMID 11872277; Update Merchant, *JCO* 2004, PMID 15284268; Update Merchant, *Lancet Oncol* 2009, PMID 19274783): Phase II trial of 153 children

(2009 update) with ependymoma, 85 of which were grade III, evaluating the patterns of failure after conformal RT. The initial report included low-grade astrocytoma as well. CTV = GTV + 1 cm. GTV encompassed the postoperative bed and any residual tumor. PTV = CTV + 0.5 cm. Dose was 59.4 Gy except for those younger than 18 months with a GTR who received 54 Gy. Spinal cord limited to approximately 57.8 Gy (54 Gy limit for first 30 fx, then 70% of prescription for the final 3 fx). *Results*: The 7-year rates of LC, EFS, and OS were 87%, 69%, and 81%. Of the patients, 14 failed locally, 7 locally and distantly, and 15 failed distantly. Negative prognostic factors included anaplastic histology, non-White race, STR, and pre-RT CHT. **Conclusion: Limited-volume RT allowed for high rates of disease control and stable neurocognitive outcomes.**

How does the extent of resection affect outcome?

The extent of resection is a strong prognostic factor in nearly every study performed. On the more recent St. Jude studies, EFS/PFS ranged from 78% to 82% with GTR compared with 41% to 43% with STR.[3,15] One earlier retrospective study from the University of Pittsburgh demonstrated an even more marked difference, with 5-year PFS ranging from 9% without GTR to 68% with GTR.[21]

Is there a role for adjuvant CHT?

No trial has clearly demonstrated a benefit to the routine use of CHT. CCG942 and CCG921 found no benefit to adjuvant CHT after maximal safe resection and CSI.[19,20] COG 9942 studied CHT in those with an STR and showed a 40% CR rate.[22] This gave consideration to the idea of CHT prior to second-look surgery for responders, which was studied in the modern ACNS0121 trial.

Garvin, COG 9942 (*Pediatr Blood Cancer* 2012, PMID 22949057): Phase II study of 41 patients with residual tumor after surgery and treated with pre-RT CHT consisting of vincristine (VCR), etoposide, cisplatin, and cyclophosphamide (CYC). Results: 40% experienced CR, 17% PR, 29% stable disease, and 14% progression. The 5-year EFS and OS rates were 57% and 71%. **Conclusion: Patients with STR have inferior outcomes despite radiographic response to CHT and should be considered for second-look surgery.**

How should children who are too young for RT be managed?

Patients <3 years of age experience worse neurocognitive outcomes with RT (particularly CSI) and may benefit from alternate therapy. Patients on Dr. Merchant's study who were <18 months of age and had a GTR were treated with focal RT to 54 Gy rather than 59.4 Gy.[15] Other strategies include using CHT to delay RT. Multiple studies (Baby POG, CCG 9921, HIT-SKK 87 and 92, UKCCSG/SIOP, and POG 9233) delayed or omitted RT with the use of CHT, with mixed results.[23–26] CCG9921, UKCCSG/SIOP, and POG9233 found no detriment in EFS or OS when using CHT to avoid or delay RT in patients <3 years with ependymoma.[23,25,26] HIT-SKK 87 and 92 found that delaying RT until age 3 may jeopardize survival.[24] The SJYC07 trial below reports on the clinical characteristics, molecular grouping, and outcomes of children <3 years of age, which may help guide the intensity of treatment.[27]

Duffner, "Baby POG" (*NEJM* 1993, PMID 8388548; Update *Pediatr Neurosurg* 1998, PMID 9732252): Phase II trial of children <3 years old with malignant brain tumors (medulloblastoma, ependymoma, PNET, brainstem glioma, other gliomas). All patients were treated with CYC, VCR, cisplatin, and etoposide. This was continued until progression or for 2 years for patients <24 months old and for 1 year if 24 to 36 months old, at which time RT was delivered. RT was localized for ependymomas to 54 Gy, but for anaplastic ependymomas treatment was CSI to 35.2 Gy with a localized boost to 54 Gy. Results: 48 patients had ependymoma. The 5-year survival was 25% for those <23 months and 63% for those 24 to 36 months. **Conclusion: Delaying RT beyond 1 year for ependymomas may lead to inferior outcomes.**

Upadhyaya, SJYC07 (*Neuro Oncol* 2019, PMID 30976811): Phase II prospective trial of 54 children with ependymoma (≤3 years old) with maximal safe surgical resection, four cycles of systemic CHT, consolidation therapy using focal conformal RT (5 mm CTV), and 6 months of oral maintenance CHT. Most patients had anaplastic tumors (76%) and a PF primary site (78%). The 4-year PFS was 75% and OS was 93%. There was no difference in outcomes for children <1 year vs. ≥1 year. STR (vs. GTR/NTR) and PF-EPN-A tumors with 1q gain had inferior PFS. No difference in outcomes was seen between classic vs. anaplastic histopathology. **Conclusion: ST-EPN-RELA tumors had a more favorable outcome than previously reported. PF-EPN-A with 1q gain and STR were associated with inferior outcomes.**

In the modern era, can a stratified approach lead to comparable outcomes when utilizing CHT and RT selectively?

Merchant, COG ACNS0121 (*JCO*** 2019, PMID 30811284):** Prospective phase II trial of 356 children with ependymoma (aged 1–21) between 2003 and 2007 from 115 institutions. Enrolled into four strata based on degree of resection, histology, and location, and treated with either observation, immediate RT, or CHT with response adaptive therapy (+/− surgery with RT). Tumors were classified and graded according to the 2007 WHO criteria. In 2019, the authors further reported patient outcomes, updated and stratified by treatment and stratum, RELA fusion and chromosome 1q status, and molecular subgroup. The 5-year EFS rates for observation, STR, and NTR/GTR with immediate RT were 61%, 37%, and 69%, respectively. The 5-year EFS rates differed significantly by tumor grade but not by age, location, RELA fusion status, or PF-A/PF-B grouping. EFS was higher for patients with infratentorial tumors without 1q gain than with 1q gain (83% vs. 47%, $p = .0013$). **Conclusion: Children with GTR have the highest EFS and OS rates. Immediate conformal RT appeared beneficial in all strata (even children ages 1–3) and should remain standard of care.**

Massimino, AIEOP Italian Study (*Neuro Oncol*** 2016, PMID 27194148):** Prospective study stratifying patients by WHO grade and degree of resection. WHO grade II patients with a GTR/NTR received 59.4 Gy. Grade III patients with a GTR/NTR received 59.4 Gy followed by VCR, etoposide, and CYC. Patients with residual disease (either grade) received the same CHT for one to four4 cycles followed by second-look surgery, then 59.4 Gy with an 8 Gy boost if there was residual disease. Results: 160 children with an MFU of 67 months. PFS and OS were 58% and 69% in the 40 patients with incomplete resection. **Conclusion: These results were comparable to the best single-institution results, and the boost appeared effective. Repeat second-look surgery to achieve GTR/NTR can improve outcomes.**

Can proton therapy be safely and effectively used in the management of pediatric ependymomas?

Patteson, Mass Gen Hospital (*Neuro Oncol*** 2021, PMID 32514542):** Prospective study reviewing 145 ependymoma patients treated with adjuvant PBT from 2001 to 2019. Eighty-one percent of patients underwent GTR or NTR. Patients received a median dose of 54 Gy (50.4–59.4 Gy) using PBT. COG ACNS 0121 and ACNS 0831 guidelines were observed, but underdosing was favored when critical structures reached tolerance. At 7 years, one patient developed grade II+ brainstem injury/necrosis. Two patients developed progressive disease and later died. The 7-year incidence of secondary tumors was 2%. The 7-year EFS for the intracranial cohort with GTR/NTR vs. STR was 70% and 35%, respectively. There was no adverse effect on disease control if RT was initiated within 9 weeks of GTR/NRT. **Conclusion: Proton therapy is safe and effective in pediatric ependymoma. There was no LC benefit to escalating dose to >54Gy.**

Can dose-escalated hyperfractionation improve outcomes?

Three prospective trials (POG 9132, AIEOP, and SPO) have been performed in children, none of which clearly demonstrated a benefit to dose-escalated hyperfractionated RT.[28–30] The regimens included 69.6 Gy/58 fx at 1.2 Gy/fx (POG 9132), 70.4 Gy/64 fx at 1.1 Gy/fx BID (AIEOP), or 60–66 Gy/60–66 fx at 1 Gy/fx (SPO).

ADULT SPINAL EPENDYMOMA

Can RT be omitted for select myxopapillary ependymomas?

The standard recommendation after GTR for myxopapillary ependymomas is adjuvant RT to at least 50.4 Gy as omission of RT seems to confer increased risk of LF. An RR from Switzerland of 85 patients with spinal myxopapillary ependymomas showed worse PFS (50% vs. 75%) in those treated with surgery alone compared with surgery + RT. On MVA, a dose of 50.4 Gy or higher was an independent predictor of improved PFS. However, an RR from Cleveland Clinic in 2020 showed that RT did not improve RFS after surgery and the extent of resection was the most important factor.

Kotecha, Cleveland Clinic (*J Neurosurg Spine*** 2020, PMID 32357340):** RR of 59 patients with spinal myxopapillary ependymoma. Median age 34 years and MFU 6.2 years; 83% underwent initial surgery and 17% received postoperative RT to a median of 49 Gy (range 45–58 Gy). RFS was improved in the GTR group compared with STR (median 11.2 vs. 5.5 years, $p < .001$). RT did not improve RFS after GTR or STR. At the time of salvage surgery, RT did improve RFS (9.5 vs. 1.6 years, $p = .006$). **Conclusion: Initial GTR is recommended when possible; the role for adjuvant RT is undetermined. Postsalvage RT appears to improve RFS.**

REFERENCES

1. Wu J, Armstrong TS, Gilbert MR. Biology and management of ependymomas. *Neuro Oncol.* 2016;18(3). doi:10.1093/neuonc/now016
2. Imbach P, Kühne T, Arceci R. *Pediatric Oncology: A Comprehensive Guide.* 2nd ed. Springer; 2011.
3. Merchant TE, Mulhern RK, Krasin MJ, et al. Preliminary results from a phase II trial of conformal radiation therapy and evaluation of radiation-related CNS effects for pediatric patients with localized ependymoma. *J Clin Oncol.* 2004;22(15):3156–3162. doi:10.1200/JCO.2004.11.142
4. Rubio MP, Correa KM, Ramesh V, et al. Analysis of the neurofibromatosis 2 gene in human ependymomas and astrocytomas. *Cancer Res.* 1994;54(1):45–47. PMID: 8261460
5. Binokay F, Akgul E, Bicakci K, Soyupak S, Aksungur E, Sertdemir Y. Determining the level of the dural sac tip: magnetic resonance imaging in an adult population. *Acta Radiol.* 2006;47(4):397–400. doi:10.1080/02841850600557158
6. Scharf CB, Paulino AC, Goldberg KN. Determination of the inferior border of the thecal sac using magnetic resonance imaging: implications for radiation therapy treatment planning. *Int J Radiat Oncol Biol Phys.* 1998;41(3):621–624. doi:10.1016/s0360-3016(97)00562-2
7. Dunbar SF, Barnes PD, Tarbell NJ. Radiologic determination of the caudal border of the spinal field in cranial spinal irradiation. *Int J Radiat Oncol Biol Phys.* 1993;26(4):669–673. doi:10.1016/0360-3016(93)90286-5
8. Kresbach C, Neyazi S, Schuller U. Updates in the classification of ependymal neoplasms: the 2021 WHO Classification and beyond. *Brain Pathol.* 2022;32(4):e13068. doi:10.1111/bpa.13068
9. Gubbiotti MA, Madsen PJ, Tucker AM, et al. ZFTA-fused supratentorial ependymoma with a novel fusion partner, DUX4. *J Neuropathol Exp Neurol.* 2023;82(7):668–671. doi:10.1093/jnen/nlad038.
10. Szulzewsky F, Holland EC, Vasioukhin V. YAP1 and its fusion proteins in cancer initiation, progression and therapeutic resistance. *Dev Biol.* 2021;475:205–221. doi:10.1016/j.ydbio.2020.12.018
11. Patronas NJ, Courcoutsakis N, Bromley CM, Katzman GL, MacCollin M, Parry DM. Intramedullary and spinal canal tumors in patients with neurofibromatosis 2: MR imaging findings and correlation with genotype. *Radiology.* 2001;218(2):434–442. doi:10.1148/radiology.218.2.r01fe40434
12. Freeman CR, Farmer JP, Roger E. Central nervous system tumors in children. *Principles & Practice of Radiation Oncology.* 6th ed. Lippincott & Williams.
13. Rodríguez D, Cheung MC, Housri N, Quinones-Hinojosa A, Camphausen K, Koniaris LG. Outcomes of malignant CNS ependymomas: an examination of 2408 cases through the Surveillance, Epidemiology, and End Results (SEER) database (1973–2005). *J Surg Res.* 2009;156(2):340–351. doi:10.1016/j.jss.2009.04.024
14. Baroni LV, Sundaresan L, Heled A, et al. Ultra high-risk PFA ependymoma is characterized by loss of chromosome 6q. *Neuro Oncol.* 2021;23(8):1360–1370. doi:10.1093/neuonc/noab034.
15. Merchant TE, Li C, Xiong X, Kun LE, Boop FA, Sanford RA. Conformal radiotherapy after surgery for paediatric ependymoma: a prospective study. *Lancet Oncol.* 2009;10(3):258–266. doi:10.1016/s1470-2045(08)70342-5
16. Merchant TE, Bendel AE, Sabin ND, et al. Conformal radiation therapy for pediatric ependymoma, chemotherapy for incompletely resected ependymoma, and observation for completely resected, supratentorial ependymoma. *J Clin Oncol.* 2019;37(12):974–983. doi:10.1200/JCO.18.01765
17. Patteson BE, Baliga S, Bajaj BVM, et al. Clinical outcomes in a large pediatric cohort of patients with ependymoma treated with proton radiotherapy. *Neuro Oncol.* 2021;23(1):156–166. doi:10.1093/neuonc/noaa139
18. Videtic GMM, Vassil AD. *Handbook of Treatment Planning in Radiation Oncology.* 3rd ed. Demos Medical; 2020.
19. Robertson PL, Zeltzer PM, Boyett JM, et al. Survival and prognostic factors following radiation therapy and chemotherapy for ependymomas in children: a report of the Children's Cancer Group. *J Neurosurg.* 1998;88(4):695–703. doi:10.3171/jns.1998.88.4.0695
20. Evans AE, Anderson JR, Lefkowitz-Boudreaux IB, Finlay JL. Adjuvant chemotherapy of childhood posterior fossa ependymoma: cranio-spinal irradiation with or without adjuvant CCNU, vincristine, and prednisone: a Children's Cancer Group study. *Med Pediatr Oncol.* 1996;27(1):8–14. doi:10.1002/(SICI)1096-911X(199607)27:1<8::AID-MPO3>3.0.CO;2-K
21. Pollack IF, Gerszten PC, Martinez AJ, et al. Intracranial ependymomas of childhood: long-term outcome and prognostic factors. *Neurosurgery.* 1995;37(4):655–666. doi:10.1227/00006123-199510000-00008
22. Garvin JH Jr, Selch MT, Holmes E, et al. Phase II study of pre-irradiation chemotherapy for childhood intracranial ependymoma. Children's Cancer Group protocol 9942: a report from the Children's Oncology Group. *Pediatr Blood Cancer.* 2012;59(7):1183–1189. doi:10.1002/pbc.24274
23. Geyer JR, Sposto R, Jennings M, et al. Multiagent chemotherapy and deferred radiotherapy in infants with malignant brain tumors: a report from the Children's Cancer Group. *J Clin Oncol.* 2005;23(30):7621–7631. doi:10.1200/JCO.2005.09.095

24. Timmermann B, Kortmann RD, Kuhl J, et al. Role of radiotherapy in anaplastic ependymoma in children under age of 3 years: results of the prospective German brain tumor trials HIT-SKK 87 and 92. *Radiother Oncol.* 2005;77(3):278–285. doi:10.1016/j.radonc.2005.10.016

25. Grundy RG, Wilne SA, Weston CL, et al. Primary postoperative chemotherapy without radiotherapy for intracranial ependymoma in children: the UKCCSG/SIOP prospective study. *Lancet Oncol.* 2007;8(8): 696–705. doi:10.1016/S1470-2045(07)70208-5

26. Strother DR, Lafay-Cousin L, Boyett JM, et al. Benefit from prolonged dose-intensive chemotherapy for infants with malignant brain tumors is restricted to patients with ependymoma: a report of the Pediatric Oncology Group randomized controlled trial 9233/34. *Neuro Oncol.* 2014;16(3):457–465. doi:10.1093/neuonc/not163

27. Upadhyaya SA, Robinson GW, Onar-Thomas A, et al. Molecular grouping and outcomes of young children with newly diagnosed ependymoma treated on the multi-institutional SJYC07 trial. *Neuro Oncol.* 2019;21(10):1319–1330. doi:10.1093/neuonc/noz069

28. Kovnar E, Curran W, Tomato T, et al. Hyperfractionated irradiation for childhood ependymoma: improved local control in subtotally resected tumors. *Childs Nerv Syst.* 1998;14(9):489–490 .

29. Massimino M, Gandola L, Giangaspero F, et al. Hyperfractionated radiotherapy and chemotherapy for childhood ependymoma: final results of the first prospective AIEOP study. *Int J Radiat Oncol Biol Phys.* 2004;58(5):1336–1345. doi:10.1016/j.ijrobp.2003.08.030

30. Conter C, Carrie C, Bernier V, et al. Intracranial ependymomas in children: Society of Pediatric Oncology experience with postoperative hyperfractionated local radiotherapy. *Int J Radiat Oncol Biol Phys.* 2009; 74(5):1536–1542. doi:10.1016/j.ijrobp.2008.09.051

60 BRAINSTEM GLIOMA

Jenna E. Kocsis, Jason W. D. Hearn, and John H. Suh

QUICK HIT Brainstem gliomas (BSGs) are uncommon tumors arising predominantly in children. Prognosis varies between diffuse intrinsic tumors and more favorable types (focal, dorsally exophytic, or cervicomedullary). Diffuse midline glioma (DMG), previously known as diffuse intrinsic pontine glioma (DIPG), is the most common and carries a poor prognosis, with MS of <1 year. By definition, a DMG must be diffuse (infiltrating), midline, and have the H3 K27 mutation. Surgery is typically not feasible; therefore, standard treatment of these unresectable tumors is often RT alone (Table 60.1). Hyperfractionation, hypofractionation, dose escalation, and CHT have generally not proven beneficial. For other subtypes of BSGs, surgery may be feasible and prognosis is more favorable.

Table 60.1 General Treatment Paradigm for Brainstem Glioma	
BSG Location/Subtype	**Management**
DMG	RT alone, 54 Gy/30 fx; MS <1 yr
Focal, dorsally exophytic, cervicomedullary tumors	Surgery; RT for unresectable or recurrent disease
Focal tectal tumors	Indolent; CSF diversion and observation[1]; 5-yr OS >90%

EPIDEMIOLOGY: BSGs account for 10% to 15% of pediatric CNS tumors, with annual incidence of 1.8 per 100,000 population, but constitute <2% of adult CNS tumors.[2-5] DMG comprises 75% to 80% of pediatric BSGs and is most commonly diagnosed between 5 and 10 years of age.[6,7] Overall, BSGs are grouped into four categories based on imaging characteristics: diffusely infiltrating (typically pontine, a.k.a. DIPG/DMG), focal, dorsally exophytic, or cervicomedullary.[8]

RISK FACTORS: NF1 confers an increased risk of BSGs (second most common after optic pathway glioma). Despite the increased incidence of BSGs in NF1 patients, these tumors tend to be relatively favorable compared with those in patients without NF1.[9] Other risk factors include Li–Fraumeni syndrome, Turcot syndrome, Lynch syndrome, and exposure to ionizing radiation.[3,10]

ANATOMY: The brainstem comprises the midbrain, pons, and medulla oblongata. CN III to IV originate from the midbrain, CN V to VIII from the pons, and CN IX to XII from the medulla. The tectum (Latin for "roof"; also referred to as the "quadrigeminal plate") represents the dorsal midbrain and includes the paired superior and inferior colliculi. The tegmentum forms the floor of the midbrain (region ventral to the ventricular system) and continues inferiorly through the pons and into the medulla. The tegmentum includes the nuclei of CN III and IV, the red nucleus, and the substantia nigra. Approximately 80% of BSGs arise within the pons, and the remaining 20% arise in the medulla, midbrain, or cervicomedullary junction.[11]

PATHOLOGY: BSGs are classified based on WHO criteria integrating histologic and genetic parameters.[12] Approximately 50% of BSGs are low grade (WHO 1–2) and ~50% are high grade (WHO 3–4); nearly all are astrocytic. For pediatric BSGs, there is generally no difference in outcomes between tumors that are low grade vs. high grade at biopsy, perhaps due to a high tendency for malignant transformation as well as heterogeneity within the tumor.[13] In the 2021 WHO classification, there is a distinct subset of pediatric diffuse high-grade gliomas called diffuse midline glioma H3 K27-altered.[12] If pediatric high-grade gliomas do not have the H3 K27 alteration, then they are classified as diffuse pediatric-type high-grade glioma, H3-wild-type and IDH-wild-type. BSGs may be intrinsic or exophytic, and if intrinsic they may be diffuse or focal. Focal tumors are generally defined as well-circumscribed lesions <2 cm without edema or infiltration.[1] Cervicomedullary junction, focal, and dorsally exophytic tumors all tend to be low grade.[14] Focal tumors occur more frequently in the midbrain or medulla. Dorsally exophytic gliomas arise from subependymal glial tissue in the floor of the fourth ventricle, growing along the path of least resistance rather than infiltrating tissue, whereas cervicomedullary tumors can be more infiltrative and expand the medulla and upper cervical spinal cord.

GENETICS: Adult and pediatric gliomas are now recognized by distinct underlying genetic events. Although the etiology is unknown, genomic studies have identified alterations in *PDGFRA, MDM4, MYCN, EGFR, MET, KRAS, CDK4, H3F3A*, the Sonic Hedgehog (SHH) pathway, and others.[15-24] IDH1/2 mutations are rare in pediatric BSGs but may be present in adult BSGs and are associated with improved prognosis.[25] DMGs harbor a H3 K27 mutation or alteration and represent a distinct subset of midline gliomas now recognized in the WHO classification.[12] They are high-grade gliomas, WHO grade 4 by definition, and there is ongoing investigation of whether they may be amenable to targeted therapies.[17,26,27]

CLINICAL PRESENTATION: CN palsies (e.g., diplopia, facial weakness, and difficulty with speech or swallowing), ataxia, long tract signs (motor weakness), or symptoms of elevated ICP such as headache, nausea, and vomiting. Pontine CNs are most affected, followed by medullary CNs, and then midbrain CNs. DMGs typically have rapid symptom onset (median 1 month before diagnosis), generally including bilateral cranial neuropathies, ataxia, and long tract signs. Focal tumors are usually more indolent and typically present with limited cranial neuropathies. Dorsally exophytic lesions present insidiously with failure to thrive and symptoms of elevated ICP; long tract signs are uncommon. Depending on the epicenter of the tumor, cervicomedullary lesions may present with predominantly medullary dysfunction (failure to thrive due to nausea, vomiting, dysphagia, chronic aspiration, sleep apnea, and head tilt) or cervical spinal cord dysfunction (facial or neck pain, progressive weakness, spasticity, hand preference, motor regression, and sensory deficits).[14] Tectal tumors often present with elevated ICP secondary to hydrocephalus from stenosis of the cerebral aqueduct.

WORKUP: H&P with careful neurologic exam.

Imaging: MRI with gadolinium. DMG is often hypointense on T1 with little enhancement (although variable), but hyperintense on T2. Diffusion tensor imaging can also be useful to evaluate the relationship of the tumor to white matter tracts, which can influence surgical candidacy and planning.[14] Up to 10% to 15% of BSGs have leptomeningeal involvement. Dorsally exophytic lesions often fill the fourth ventricle, causing obstruction and hydrocephalus. Such lesions are typically juvenile pilocytic astrocytomas (JPAs), which intensely enhance despite being low grade. Cervicomedullary tumors cause expansion of the medulla toward the fourth ventricle and/or expansion of the cervical cord.

Procedures: Biopsy is generally not indicated for lesions radiologically consistent with DMG, since grade does not affect management. However, biopsy can be helpful in determining H3 K27 status. Since stereotactic biopsy techniques have reduced risks, biopsies may be done for research purposes and can be informative for cases with atypical radiologic or clinical features.[16,28,29] Notably, a biopsy may be more useful in adults, in whom histology and genetics (IDH1/2 mutation) have more prognostic importance. Differential diagnosis includes primitive neuroectodermal tumor (PNET), atypical teratoid/rhabdoid tumor (ATRT), vascular malformation, demyelinating disorders (e.g., multiple sclerosis), ganglioglioma, hamartoma (especially in patients with neurofibromatosis), metastasis, abscess, encephalitis, and parasitic cysts, among others.

PROGNOSTIC FACTORS: Tumor location and type are the most important prognostic factors, with DMG demonstrating worse outcomes than more favorable types (focal, dorsally exophytic, or cervicomedullary). Other favorable prognostic factors include long interval between onset of symptoms and diagnosis, lack of pontine CN palsies, and lack of enhancement.[30-34]

TREATMENT PARADIGM

DMG: There is no therapeutic role for surgery given morbidity, and there is no proven benefit to systemic therapy. Studies investigating cytotoxic CHT, concurrent etanidazole (hypoxic cell radiosensitizer), high-dose tamoxifen, high-dose CHT with bone marrow transplant, blood–brain barrier disruption, p-glycoprotein inhibition (for multidrug resistance), and other strategies have generally not demonstrated significant benefit.[4] Temozolomide (TMZ) has not shown any benefit in DMGs with concurrent RT; however, it should be considered for adult patients with IDH mutations.[35,36] RT alone remains the standard for DMG, as it is the only modality proven to extend survival. Recommended dose is 54 Gy/30 fx over 6 weeks with a cone-down to 59.4 Gy if able to meet constraints. LFs occur within the high-dose volume, and there has been no proven benefit to extending the CTV margin beyond 1 cm.[37] Other RT approaches such as hyperfractionation, hypofractionation, I-125 interstitial implants, and SRS have been attempted with no clear benefit over standard RT, although hypofractionation can diminish the time spent receiving treatment. Most patients improve clinically after RT; typical time to progression is 5 to 6 months, and MS in most studies is <10 to 12 months.[31,38] ONC201 is an investigational oral compound used in H3 K27-altered DMGs that is currently being investigated in a placebo-controlled randomized phase III trial.[39]

Focal: Surgical resection is indicated when feasible (e.g., for tumors that extend toward the surface of the brainstem laterally or at the floor of the fourth ventricle). Preservation of neurologic function is important for these often indolent tumors and may require judicious use of STR. RT is useful for progression after surgery and for unresectable lesions.[1] As in the case of DMG, RT dose is typically 54 Gy/30 fx, although smaller CTV margins are often appropriate.

Dorsally Exophytic or Cervicomedullary: Maximal safe resection is indicated when possible.[14,40,41] RT is a useful alternative for unresectable tumors and can be considered postoperatively for high-grade tumors or those with early progression after surgery. Those who have late progression may benefit from reoperation when feasible. CHT is occasionally a useful adjunct, and in some cases can yield tumor shrinkage followed by a more complete resection. CHT may produce disease stabilization or objective responses, although eventual progression is inevitable.[42] CHT is particularly helpful in very young children to delay RT and thereby enable more physical and neurocognitive development. The 5- and 10-year treatment-free survival estimates are 65% and 45%, respectively, with 5- and 10-year OS ~87%.[14]

Tectal: Focal tectal tumors of the midbrain tend to be very indolent and may require only CSF diversion with a third ventriculostomy or shunt.[43] Biopsy is not needed unless atypical features are present, and most can be observed after shunting. Most patients with these tumors remain free from progression for extended periods without surgical resection (which is associated with substantial risk in this location) or RT.[44] Thus, definitive intervention is reserved for patients with evidence of progression. The 10-year PFS and OS rates were 49% and 84%, respectively.[45]

Treatment-Related Complications: Complications of surgery may include impaired respiratory function (especially if medullary involvement), diplopia, facial palsy, dysphagia, vocal cord paralysis, loss of gag/cough reflexes, additional cranial neuropathies, long tract deficits, and death, among others. Complications of RT may include dermatitis (especially at the external auditory canal and retroauricular region), hearing loss, growth impairment, endocrine dysfunction, cognitive dysfunction, radiation necrosis, and radiation-induced tumors, among others.

EVIDENCE-BASED Q&A

Does RT dose escalation and/or altered fractionation improve outcomes?

No improvement with dose escalation or altered fractionation has been demonstrated (Table 60.2).

Table 60.2 Studies Evaluating Dose Escalation and/or Altered Fractionation in Brainstem Gliomas				
Author, Institution/ Group	**Study Design**	**Radiation Scheme**	**MS**	**Conclusion**
Freeman, POG 8495[46]	Phase I/II, dose escalation with hyperfractionation	66 Gy/60 fx BID 70.2 Gy/60 fx BID 75.6 Gy/60 fx BID	10 months	No differences in PFS or OS across dose levels
Packer, CCG 9882[47]	Phase I/II, hyperfractionation	72 Gy/72 fx BID	1-yr OS 38%	No benefit with hyperfractionation
Lewis, UKCCSG[48]	Pilot study, hyperfractionation	48.6–50.4 Gy/27–28 fx BID	8.5 months	No improvement with hyperfractionation
Mandell, POG 9239[49]	PRT, conventional vs. hyperfractionation with concurrent cisplatin	50.4 Gy/30 fx vs. 70.2 Gy/60 fx BID	8.5 months vs. 8 months	No significant improvement with hyperfractionation Similar toxicity in both arms

(continued)

Table 60.2 Studies Evaluating Dose Escalation and/or Altered Fractionation in Brainstem Gliomas (continued)				
Author, Institution/ Group	Study Design	Radiation Scheme	MS	Conclusion
Janssens, Netherlands[50]	Prospective, hypofractionation	39 Gy/13 fx or 33 Gy/6 fx, 4 days per week	8.6 months	Shorter RT course feasible, with similar toxicity; note: only nine patients enrolled
Zaghloul, Egypt[51]	PRT, hypofractionation vs. conventional fractionation	39 Gy/13 fx, 45 Gy/15 fx, and 54 Gy/30 fx	9.6 vs. 8.2 vs. 8.7 months (NS)	Hypofractionated RT noninferior to conventional RT
Chuba, Wayne State[52]	RR, conventional fraction → stereotactic radiosurgery boost → brachytherapy boost	50 Gy/25 fx → 12 Gy/4 fx stereotactic boost → LDR I-125 implant, 82.9 Gy	8.4 months	Tumor control not improved with stereotactic and/or brachytherapy boost

Does stereotactic radiosurgery (SRS) improve outcomes?

Data are very limited and do not imply any improvement relative to conventionally fractionated RT.

Fuchs, Austria (*Acta Neurochir Suppl* 2002, PMID 12379009): RR of 21 patients (8–56 years of age) treated with GKRS for BSG. Twelve lesions were located primarily in the pons, two in the medulla, and seven in the midbrain. Median SRS dose 12 Gy (9–20 Gy) to the tumor margin by the median isodose of 45%. Prior to SRS, four patients had received conventional RT, one had RT and CHT, one underwent CHT, and one was shunted due to hydrocephalus. Of the 19 patients with follow-up imaging, tumor progression was seen in two, stable disease in ten, and regression in three patients. MFU 29 months. Neurologic status improved in five patients. Microsurgical cyst fenestration was performed in one patient after SRS, and shunting was necessary for two. Nine patients died unrelated to SRS at a median of 20.7 months. **Conclusion: SRS may be feasible in select patients, but the very limited sample size and heterogeneity in treatment limit interpretation.**

Is there a role for re-irradiation?

Limited data show feasibility and suggest symptomatic benefit in select patients.[53–55]

Amsbaugh, MDACC (*IJROBP* 2019, PMID 30610915): Phase I/II trial of 12 patients with DIPG undergoing re-RT at three dose levels: 24 Gy/12 fx, 26.4 Gy/12 fx, and 30.8 Gy/14 fx, with co-primary endpoints of toxicity and efficacy. Five of six patients receiving 24 Gy showed improvement in two of three efficacy domains, one patient with improvement in all domains. Of the four patients who received 26.4 Gy, one patient without any improvement, while the others had varying improvement. Of the two patients who received 30.8 Gy, one demonstrated improvement in three efficacy domains and the other did not complete the survey. Median OS for all patients was 19.5 months from initial diagnosis, and mPFS was 4.5 months from the start of re-RT. **Conclusion: Re-RT can be safely delivered.**

Is there a benefit from systemic therapy in diffuse intrinsic tumors?

Given efficacy of TMZ in adults with high-grade gliomas, multiple studies have investigated the use of concurrent and adjuvant TMZ, but no improvement in outcomes has been noted (although it still is considered in cases with IDH mutations).[56–58] The preponderance of evidence has shown no benefit to systemic therapy (see Table 60.3). An exception was the French BSG 98 study, which suggested possible improvement in survival relative to historical controls; however, this regimen required protracted CHT, was quite toxic, and involved prolonged hospitalizations. More recently, an investigational oral compound ONC201 (dordaviprone) was tested in 50 patients with recurrent H3 K27-altered DMGs and yielded an overall response rate of 20%, with a median response duration of 11.2 months.[59] Additional trials investigating ONC201 are underway in children and adults.

Table 60.3 Studies Evaluating Systemic Therapy in Diffuse Intrinsic Tumors

Author, Institution/ Group	Study Design	Systemic Therapy	MS	Conclusion
Jenkin, CCSG[60]	PRT of 50–60 Gy RT ± adjuvant CHT	CCNU, vincristine, and prednisone	9 months	No benefit with CHT
Freeman, Cross Trial Comparison of POG 9239/8495[61]	POG 9239: 70.2 Gy + CHT POG 8495: 70.2 Gy alone	Concurrent cisplatin No CHT	1-yr OS 28% 1-yr OS 40% ($p = .723$)	Cisplatin does not improve OS and may be detrimental
Marcus, Harvard[62]	63–66 Gy/42–44 fx + radiosensitizer	Etanidazole	8.5 months	No benefit to etanidazole despite toxicity
Broniscer, St. Jude SJHG-98[63]	RT (median 55.8 Gy) + adjuvant CHT	TMZ	12 months	No benefit to adjuvant TMZ
Frappaz, French BSG 98[64]	CHT given at 30-day intervals to delay RT (given at progression)	Tamoxifen, BCNU, cisplatin, followed by two cycles of HD-MTX	17 months	Improved MS vs. historical controls but with significant toxicity and prolonged hospitalizations
Jalali, Tata Memorial[57]	54 Gy/30 fx + concurrent and adjuvant CHT	TMZ	9.2 months	No benefit to concurrent and adjuvant TMZ

Does histology have prognostic significance in adult diffuse intrinsic BSGs?

Adult BSGs appear to behave somewhat differently from those in children, particularly diffuse intrinsic low-grade gliomas, which carry a substantially better prognosis than those in children.

Guillamo, France (*Brain* 2001, PMID 11701605): French RR of 48 adult patients with BSG. Mean age 34 years (range 16–70). MRI demonstrated nonenhancing, diffusely infiltrative tumors (50%), contrast-enhancing localized masses (31%), isolated tectal tumors (8%), and other patterns (11%). Treatments included STR (8%), RT (94%), and CHT (56%). MS 5.4 years. Significant prognostic factors on MVA included histologic grade, duration of symptoms, and the appearance of "necrosis" on MRI. Eighty-five percent could be classified into one of the following three groups on the basis of clinical, histologic, and radiologic characteristics:

- Diffuse intrinsic low-grade gliomas (46%): In young adults with a long clinical history before diagnosis and a diffusely enlarged nonenhancing brainstem on MRI. Neurologic status improved with RT in 62% and MS was 7.3 years.
- Focal tectal gliomas (8%): In young adults, often presenting with isolated hydrocephalus. Indolent course with estimated MS >10 years (similar to children for this type of tumor).
- Malignant gliomas (31%): In older patients with short clinical history, as well as contrast enhancement and "necrosis" on MRI. Poor prognosis despite treatment: MS 11.2 months.

REFERENCES

1. Klimo P Jr, Pai Panandiker AS, Thompson CJ, et al. Management and outcome of focal low-grade brainstem tumors in pediatric patients: the St. Jude experience. *J Neurosurg Pediatr.* 2013;11(3):274–281. doi:10.3171/2012.11.PEDS12317
2. Hu J, Western S, Kesari S. Brainstem glioma in adults. *Front Oncol.* 2016;6:180. doi:10.3389/fonc.2016.00180
3. National Comprehensive Cancer Network (NCCN). *NCCN Clinical Practice Guidelines in Oncology: Pediatric Central Nervous System Cancers.* Accessed October 21, 2024. https://www.nccn.org/professionals/physician_gls/pdf/ped_cns.pdf
4. Pfister SM, Reyes-Mugica M, Chan JKC, et al. A summary of the inaugural WHO classification of pediatric tumors: transitioning from the optical into the molecular era. *Cancer Discov.* 2022;12(2):331–355. doi:10.1158/2159-8290.CD-21-1094
5. Ostrom QT, Patil N, Cioffi G, Waite K, Kruchko C, Barnholtz-Sloan JS. CBTRUS statistical report: primary brain and other central nervous system tumors diagnosed in the United States in 2013–2017. *Neuro Oncol.* 2020;22(12 suppl 2):iv1–iv96. doi:10.1093/neuonc/noaa200

6. Warren KE. Diffuse intrinsic pontine glioma: poised for progress. *Front Oncol.* 2012;2:205. doi:10.3389/fonc.2012.00205

7. Liu H, Qin X, Zhao L, Zhao G, Wang Y. Epidemiology and survival of patients with brainstem gliomas: a population-based study using the SEER database. *Front Oncol.* 2021;11:692097. doi:10.3389/fonc.2021.692097

8. Choux M, Lena G, Do L. *Pediatric Neurosurgery.* Churchill Livingstone; 2000.

9. Mahdi J, Shah AC, Sato A, et al. A multi-institutional study of brainstem gliomas in children with neurofibromatosis type 1. *Neurology.* 2017;88(16):1584–1589. doi:10.1212/WNL.0000000000003881

10. Ostrom QT, Adel Fahmideh M, Cote DJ, et al. Risk factors for childhood and adult primary brain tumors. *Neuro Oncol.* 2019;21(11):1357–1375. doi:10.1093/neuonc/noz123

11. Patil N, Kelly ME, Yeboa DN, et al. Epidemiology of brainstem high-grade gliomas in children and adolescents in the United States, 2000–2017. *Neuro Oncol.* 2021;23(6):990–998. doi:10.1093/neuonc/noaa295

12. Louis DN, Perry A, Wesseling P, et al. The 2021 WHO Classification of tumors of the central nervous system: a summary. *Neuro Oncol.* 2021;23(8):1231–1251. doi:10.1093/neuonc/noab106

13. Hoffman LM, DeWire M, Ryall S, et al. Spatial genomic heterogeneity in diffuse intrinsic pontine and midline high-grade glioma: implications for diagnostic biopsy and targeted therapeutics. *Acta Neuropathol Commun.* 2016;4:1. doi:10.1186/s40478-015-0269-0

14. McAbee JH, Modica J, Thompson CJ, et al. Cervicomedullary tumors in children. *J Neurosurg Pediatr.* 2015;16(4):357–366. doi:10.3171/2015.5.PEDS14638

15. Barrow J, Adamowicz-Brice M, Cartmill M, et al. Homozygous loss of ADAM3A revealed by genome-wide analysis of pediatric high-grade glioma and diffuse intrinsic pontine gliomas. *Neuro Oncol.* 2011;13(2):212–222. doi:10.1093/neuonc/noq158

16. Grill J, Puget S, Andreiuolo F, Philippe C, MacConaill L, Kieran MW. Critical oncogenic mutations in newly diagnosed pediatric diffuse intrinsic pontine glioma. *Pediatr Blood Cancer.* 2012;58(4):489–491. doi:10.1002/pbc.24060

17. Khuong-Quang DA, Buczkowicz P, Rakopoulos P, et al. K27M mutation in histone H3.3 defines clinically and biologically distinct subgroups of pediatric diffuse intrinsic pontine gliomas. *Acta Neuropathol.* 2012;124(3):439–447. doi:10.1007/s00401-012-0998-0

18. Li G, Mitra SS, Monje M, et al. Expression of epidermal growth factor variant III (EGFRvIII) in pediatric diffuse intrinsic pontine gliomas. *J Neurooncol.* 2012;108(3):395–402. doi:10.1007/s11060-012-0842-3

19. Paugh BS, Broniscer A, Qu C, et al. Genome-wide analyses identify recurrent amplifications of receptor tyrosine kinases and cell-cycle regulatory genes in diffuse intrinsic pontine glioma. *J Clin Oncol.* 2011;29(30):3999–4006. doi:10.1200/JCO.2011.35.5677

20. Paugh BS, Qu C, Jones C, et al. Integrated molecular genetic profiling of pediatric high-grade gliomas reveals key differences with the adult disease. *J Clin Oncol.* 2010;28(18):3061–3068. doi:10.1200/JCO.2009.26.7252

21. Warren KE, Killian K, Suuriniemi M, Wang Y, Quezado M, Meltzer PS. Genomic aberrations in pediatric diffuse intrinsic pontine gliomas. *Neuro Oncol.* 2012;14(3):326–332. doi:10.1093/neuonc/nor190

22. Wu G, Broniscer A, McEachron TA, et al. Somatic histone H3 alterations in pediatric diffuse intrinsic pontine gliomas and non-brainstem glioblastomas. *Nat Genet.* 2012;44(3):251–253. doi:10.1038/ng.1102

23. Zarghooni M, Bartels U, Lee E, et al. Whole-genome profiling of pediatric diffuse intrinsic pontine gliomas highlights platelet-derived growth factor receptor alpha and poly (ADP-ribose) polymerase as potential therapeutic targets. *J Clin Oncol.* 2010;28(8):1337–1344. doi:10.1200/JCO.2009.25.5463

24. Puget S, Philippe C, Bax DA, et al. Mesenchymal transition and PDGFRA amplification/mutation are key distinct oncogenic events in pediatric diffuse intrinsic pontine gliomas. *PLoS One.* 2012;7(2):e30313. doi:10.1371/journal.pone.0030313

25. Banan R, Stichel D, Bleck A, et al. Infratentorial IDH-mutant astrocytoma is a distinct subtype. *Acta Neuropathol.* 2020;140(4):569–581. doi:10.1007/s00401-020-02194-y

26. Himes BT, Zhang L, Daniels DJ. Treatment strategies in diffuse midline gliomas with the H3K27M mutation: the role of convection-enhanced delivery in overcoming anatomic challenges. *Front Oncol.* 2019;9:31. doi:10.3389/fonc.2019.00031

27. Cohen KJ, Jabado N, Grill J. Diffuse intrinsic pontine gliomas—current management and new biologic insights. Is there a glimmer of hope? *Neuro Oncol.* 2017;19(8):1025–1034. doi:10.1093/neuonc/nox021

28. Cage TA, Samagh SP, Mueller S, et al. Feasibility, safety, and indications for surgical biopsy of intrinsic brainstem tumors in children. *Childs Nerv Syst.* 2013;29(8):1313–1319. doi:10.1007/s00381-013-2101-0

29. Puget S, Beccaria K, Blauwblomme T, et al. Biopsy in a series of 130 pediatric diffuse intrinsic pontine gliomas. *Childs Nerv Syst.* 2015;31(10):1773–1780. doi:10.1007/s00381-015-2832-1

30. Veldhuijzen van Zanten SEM, Lane A, Heymans MW, et al. External validation of the diffuse intrinsic pontine glioma survival prediction model: a collaborative report from the International DIPG Registry and the SIOPE DIPG Registry. *J Neurooncol.* 2017;134(1):231–240. doi:10.1007/s11060-017-2514-9

31. Hoffman LM, Veldhuijzen van Zanten SEM, Colditz N, et al. Clinical, radiologic, pathologic, and molecular characteristics of long-term survivors of Diffuse Intrinsic Pontine Glioma (DIPG): a collaborative report from the International and European Society for Pediatric Oncology DIPG Registries. *J Clin Oncol.* 2018;36(19):1963–1972. doi:10.1200/JCO.2017.75.9308

32. Sanford RA, Freeman CR, Burger P, Cohen ME. Prognostic criteria for experimental protocols in pediatric brainstem gliomas. *Surg Neurol.* 1988;30(4):276–280. doi:10.1016/0090-3019(88)90299-6

33. Freeman CR, Bourgouin PM, Sanford RA, Cohen ME, Friedman HS, Kun LE. Long-term survivors of childhood brain stem gliomas treated with hyperfractionated radiotherapy: clinical characteristics and treatment-related toxicities. *Cancer.* 1996;77(3):555–562. doi:10.1002/(SICI)1097-0142(19960201)77:3<555::AID-CNCR19>3.0.CO;2-3

34. Jackson S, Patay Z, Howarth R, et al. Clinico-radiologic characteristics of long-term survivors of diffuse intrinsic pontine glioma. *J Neurooncol.* 2013;114(3):339–344. doi:10.1007/s11060-013-1189-0

35. Cohen KJ, Heideman RL, Zhou T, et al. Temozolomide in the treatment of children with newly diagnosed diffuse intrinsic pontine gliomas: a report from the Children's Oncology Group. *Neuro Oncol.* 2011;13(4):410–416. doi:10.1093/neuonc/noq205

36. Bailey S, Howman A, Wheatley K, et al. Diffuse intrinsic pontine glioma treated with prolonged temozolomide and radiotherapy—results of a United Kingdom phase II trial (CNS 2007 04). *Eur J Cancer.* 2013;49(18):3856-3862. doi:10.1016/j.ejca.2013.08.006

37. Tinkle CL, Simone B, Chiang J, et al. Defining optimal target volumes of conformal radiation therapy for diffuse intrinsic pontine glioma. *Int J Radiat Oncol Biol Phys.* 2020;106(4):838–847. doi:10.1016/j.ijrobp.2019.11.020

38. Hassan H, Pinches A, Picton SV, Phillips RS. Survival rates and prognostic predictors of high-grade brain stem gliomas in childhood: a systematic review and meta-analysis. *J Neurooncol.* 2017;135(1):13–20. doi:10.1007/s11060-017-2546-1

39. Arrillaga-Romany I, Lassman A, McGovern SL, et al. ACTION: a randomized phase 3 study of ONC201 (dordaviprone) in patients with newly diagnosed H3 K27M-mutant diffuse glioma. *Neuro Oncol.* 2024;26(suppl 2):S173–S181. doi:10.1093/neuonc/noae031

40. Robertson PL, Allen JC, Abbott IR, Miller DC, Fidel J, Epstein FJ. Cervicomedullary tumors in children: a distinct subset of brainstem gliomas. *Neurology.* 1994;44(10):1798–1803. doi:10.1212/wnl.44.10.1798

41. Di Maio S, Gul SM, Cochrane DD, Hendson G, Sargent MA, Steinbok P. Clinical, radiologic and pathologic features and outcome following surgery for cervicomedullary gliomas in children. *Childs Nerv Syst.* 2009;25(11):1401–1410. doi:10.1007/s00381-009-0956-x

42. Raabe E, Kieran MW, Cohen KJ. New strategies in pediatric gliomas: molecular advances in pediatric low-grade gliomas as a model. *Clin Cancer Res.* 2013;19(17):4553–4558. doi:10.1158/1078-0432.CCR-13-0662

43. Daglioglu E, Cataltepe O, Akalan N. Tectal gliomas in children: the implications for natural history and management strategy. *Pediatr Neurosurg.* 2003;38(5):223–231. doi:10.1159/000069823

44. Griessenauer CJ, Rizk E, Miller JH, et al. Pediatric tectal plate gliomas: clinical and radiological progression, MR imaging characteristics, and management of hydrocephalus. *J Neurosurg Pediatr.* 2014;13(1):13–20. doi:10.3171/2013.9.PEDS13347

45. Liu APY, Harreld JH, Jacola LM, et al. Tectal glioma as a distinct diagnostic entity: a comprehensive clinical, imaging, histologic and molecular analysis. *Acta Neuropathol Commun.* 2018;6(1):101. doi:10.1186/s40478-018-0602-5

46. Freeman CR, Krischer J, Sanford RA, et al. Hyperfractionated radiation therapy in brain stem tumors: results of treatment at the 7020 cGy dose level of Pediatric Oncology Group study #8495. *Cancer.* 1991;68(3):474–481. doi:10.1002/1097-0142(19910801)68:3<474::aid-cncr2820680305>3.0.co;2-7

47. Packer RJ, Boyett JM, Zimmerman RA, et al. Hyperfractionated radiation therapy (72 Gy) for children with brain stem gliomas: a Children's Cancer Group Phase I/II Trial. *Cancer.* 1993;72(4):1414–1421. doi:10.1002/1097-0142(19930815)72:4<1414::aid-cncr2820720442>3.0.co;2-c

48. Lewis J, Lucraft H, Gholkar A. UKCCSG study of accelerated radiotherapy for pediatric brain stem gliomas. *Int J Radiat Oncol Biol Phys.* 1997;38(5):925–929. doi:10.1016/s0360-3016(97)00134-x

49. Mandell LR, Kadota R, Freeman C, et al. There is no role for hyperfractionated radiotherapy in the management of children with newly diagnosed diffuse intrinsic brainstem tumors: results of a Pediatric Oncology Group phase III trial comparing conventional vs. hyperfractionated radiotherapy. *Int J Radiat Oncol Biol Phys.* 1999;43(5):959–964. doi:10.1016/s0360-3016(98)00501-x

50. Janssens GO, Gidding CE, Van Lindert EJ, et al. The role of hypofractionation radiotherapy for diffuse intrinsic brainstem glioma in children: a pilot study. *Int J Radiat Oncol Biol Phys.* 2009;73(3):722–726. doi:10.1016/j.ijrobp.2008.05.030

51. Zaghloul MS, Nasr A, Tolba M, et al. Hypofractionated radiation therapy for diffuse intrinsic pontine glioma: a noninferiority randomized study including 253 children. *Int J Radiat Oncol Biol Phys.* 2022;113(2):360–368. doi:10.1016/j.ijrobp.2022.01.054

52. Chuba PJ, Zamarano L, Hamre M, et al. Permanent I-125 brain stem implants in children. *Childs Nerv Syst.* 1998;14(10):570-577. doi:10.1007/s003810050274

53. Fontanilla HP, Pinnix CC, Ketonen LM, et al. Palliative reirradiation for progressive diffuse intrinsic pontine glioma. *Am J Clin Oncol.* 2012;35(1):51–57. doi:10.1097/COC.0b013e318201a2b7

54. Cacciotti C, Liu KX, Haas-Kogan DA, Warren KE. Reirradiation practices for children with diffuse intrinsic pontine glioma. *Neurooncol Pract.* 2021;8(1):68–74. doi:10.1093/nop/npaa063

55.   Amsbaugh MJ, Mahajan A, Thall PF, et al. A phase 1/2 trial of reirradiation for diffuse intrinsic pontine glioma. *Int J Radiat Oncol Biol Phys*. 2019;104(1):144–148. doi:10.1016/j.ijrobp.2018.12.043

56.   Cohen KJ, Pollack IF, Zhou T, et al. Temozolomide in the treatment of high-grade gliomas in children: a report from the Children's Oncology Group. *Neuro Oncol*. 2011;13(3):317–323. doi:10.1093/neuonc/noq191

57.   Jalali R, Raut N, Arora B, et al. Prospective evaluation of radiotherapy with concurrent and adjuvant temozolomide in children with newly diagnosed diffuse intrinsic pontine glioma. *Int J Radiat Oncol Biol Phys*. 2010;77(1):113–118. doi:10.1016/j.ijrobp.2009.04.031

58.   Chassot A, Canale S, Varlet P, et al. Radiotherapy with concurrent and adjuvant temozolomide in children with newly diagnosed diffuse intrinsic pontine glioma. *J Neurooncol*. 2012;106(2):399–407. doi:10.1007/s11060-011-0681-7

59.   Arrillaga-Romany I, Gardner SL, Odia Y, et al. ONC201 (Dordaviprone) in recurrent H3 K27M-mutant diffuse midline glioma. *J Clin Oncol*. 2024;42(13):1542–1552. doi:10.1200/JCO.23.01134

60.   Jenkin RD, Boesel C, Ertel I, et al. Brain-stem tumors in childhood: a prospective randomized trial of irradiation with and without adjuvant CCNU, VCR, and prednisone. *J Neurosurg*. 1987;66(2):227–233. doi:10.3171/jns.1987.66.2.0227

61.   Freeman CR, Kepner J, Kun LE, et al. A detrimental effect of a combined chemotherapy-radiotherapy approach in children with diffuse intrinsic brain stem gliomas? *Int J Radiat Oncol Biol Phys*. 2000;47(3):561–564. doi:10.1016/s0360-3016(00)00471-5

62.   Marcus KJ, Dutton SC, Barnes P, et al. A phase I trial of etanidazole and hyperfractionated radiotherapy in children with diffuse brainstem glioma. *Int J Radiat Oncol Biol Phys*. 2003;55(5):1182–1185. doi:10.1016/s0360-3016(02)04391-2

63.   Broniscer A, Iacono L, Chintagumpala M, et al. Role of temozolomide after radiotherapy for newly diagnosed diffuse brainstem glioma in children: results of a multiinstitutional study (SJHG-98). *Cancer*. 2005;103(1):133–139. doi:10.1002/cncr.20741

64.   Frappaz D, Schell M, Thiesse P, et al. Preradiation chemotherapy may improve survival in pediatric diffuse intrinsic brainstem gliomas: final results of BSG 98 prospective trial. *Neuro Oncol*. 2008;10(4):599–607. doi:10.1215/15228517-2008-029

61 CRANIOPHARYNGIOMA

Zachary S. Mayo, Timothy D. Smile, and Martin C. Tom

QUICK HIT Craniopharyngioma (CP) is a rare benign neoplasm arising from the hypophyseal duct (Rathke's pouch), most commonly arising from the suprasellar region in children and older adults. Presentation includes headache, visual disturbances, nausea/vomiting, and/or endocrine abnormalities, with imaging revealing a suprasellar solid and/or cystic (filled with classic "crankcase oil") enhancing mass. Treatment typically consists of either gross total resection (GTR) alone (can be morbid) or subtotal resection (STR) followed by adjuvant RT, which appear to have comparable long-term outcomes (PFS >65%, OS >90%). RT strategies include IMRT or proton beam RT to 54 Gy in 30 fractions with recommended on-treatment MRI to account for cyst volume fluctuation, or SRS. For patients with BRAF-V600E-mutant CP (majority of papillary CP), BRAF-MEK inhibition with vemurafenib–cobimetinib has high response rates, and it can be used prior to surgery or RT to allow for modification of surgical and radiotherapeutic approaches with the goal of mitigating toxicity. Multidisciplinary discussion is encouraged to individualize management.

EPIDEMIOLOGY: The incidence of CP in the United States is an estimated 617 per year and is similar between sexes, with a slightly higher rate in Black people.[1] CP represents 0.7% of all CNS tumors, 1% of all nonmalignant CNS tumors, and 4% of CNS tumors in children/adolescents ages 0 to 19 (153 per year).[1] There is a bimodal age distribution between 5 to 14 and 50 to 75 years of age.[2] The 5- and 10-year relative OS rates for tumors arising from the craniopharyngeal duct are 85% and 78%, respectively.[1]

RISK FACTORS: No proven risk factors.

ANATOMY: CPs arise from the hypophyseal duct (Rathke's pouch) or from its remnant in adults. They are typically suprasellar and can involve the optic chiasm, basal vasculature, hypothalamus, third ventricle, or pituitary stalk. They can appear grossly well-encapsulated but formation of multiple cysts is characteristic.[3]

PATHOLOGY: CPs are histologically benign epithelial tumors. The two major subtypes are adamantinomatous (85%–90%) and papillary (i.e., squamous papillary; 11%–14%). The adamantinomatous subtype is associated with children and appears solid and/or cystic with calcifications and dark brown/black fluid ("crankcase oil" appearance). They tend to be more adherent to surrounding structures, and on histology they demonstrate wet keratin nodules, Rosenthal fibers, and a palisading basal layer of cells with intense gliosis.[4] The papillary subtype appears more similar to Rathke's cleft cysts with squamous differentiation and pseudopapillae and is less likely to have calcification on imaging.[3,5]

GENETICS: The adamantinomatous subtype is related to Wnt pathway activation and almost always contains a CTNNB1 gene mutation, which codes for β-catenin.[6,7] The papillary subtype typically harbors the BRAF (V600E) mutation, which is susceptible to BRAF-MEK inhibition with vemurafenib–cobimetinib.[8,9]

CLINICAL PRESENTATION: Patients can present with headaches, visual deficits, nausea/vomiting, or hormonal abnormalities such as GH insufficiency or hypothyroidism (growth failure), ADH insufficiency (central diabetes insipidus), impotence, amenorrhea, or galactorrhea. Other symptoms can include depression, lethargy/somnolence, coma, seizures, hyperphagia, diencephalic syndrome, and changes in cognitive function or personality.[10,11]

WORKUP: H&P with attention to endocrine symptoms and a detailed neurologic exam that includes visual field testing, memory, personality, psychological, and cognitive function testing.

Labs: Endocrine workup to establish baseline function, electrolyte studies, and urinalysis.

Imaging: MRI and/or CT reveal a cystic, calcified (more common in adamantinomatous), enhancing, parasellar lesion with hydrocephalus.[8] MRI typically demonstrates a hyperintense abnormality on T1-weighted images, which differentiates CP from Rathke's cleft and tumor cysts. Upon contrast administration, both the solid and cystic components typically enhance. Diagnosis can be made based on radiographic appearance, cyst fluid analysis ("crankcase oil"), or histopathology.

PROGNOSTIC FACTORS: Negative prognostic factors include >53 years of age in adults, two or more prior surgeries, tumor size >5 cm, STR alone (vs. with RT), hydrocephalus, and RT dose <54 to 55 Gy.[10,12–15] Close observation with on-treatment MRI to monitor for cyst expansion is associated with improved control.[14]

TREATMENT PARADIGM

Surgery: Surgical resection with safe debulking is indicated in almost all patients. While some favor initial aggressive total resection, GTR can be morbid due to proximity to the hypothalamus, pituitary, optic pathways, circle of Willis, and other surrounding structures. Therefore, others advocate for limited resection followed by RT (adjuvant or salvage). STR alone has poor LC rates. Intrasellar tumors can be removed transsphenoidally, while suprasellar tumors can be removed via an extended transsphenoidal approach using an endoscope.[15] Many utilize a pterional craniotomy. Tumors with large cysts may be aspirated prior to surgery. For large BRAF-V600E mutant tumors, BRAF-MEK inhibitors may be used for tumor reduction prior to surgery. Ommaya reservoirs may be placed within cystic components and the cysts can be accessed for draining if expansion occurs.

Chemotherapy: Intracystic CHT with either bleomycin or IFN-α has been used, albeit with limited experience, for temporary tumor control with response rates of 62% to 100% and control rates of 59% to 71%. There is some suggestion that IFN-α has fewer side effects compared with bleomycin.[16] Patients with BRAF-V600E mutant papillary CP can be treated with the BRAF-MEK inhibitor combination vemurafenib-cobimetinib. In a small cohort of patients, BRAF-MEK inhibitor combination resulted in at least a partial response in 15 of 16 subjects, with a median 91% tumor volume reduction. However, grades 3 and 4 toxicities were seen in 75% and 17% of patients, respectively.[17] The results of this study are compelling and demonstrate the efficacy of BRAF-MEK inhibition, which can be used to modify the extent of surgery and/or RT in order to reduce toxicity.

Radiation

Indications: RT is indicated following STR (adjuvant), following targeted therapy with residual disease and no surgical intervention, or at tumor recurrence (salvage). Proton beam therapy (PBT) and photon therapy have demonstrated efficacy in small retrospective series with limited follow-up.[18–20] A prospective phase II study utilizing PBT reported similar rates of 5-year PFS and OS compared with a historical photon study with no difference in severe toxicity. However, PBT was associated with decreased RT dose to surrounding structures and improved cognitive outcomes.[21] With fractionated conformal techniques, interfraction imaging with noncontrast MRI every 1 to 2 weeks may be necessary to account for fluctuations in cyst volume.[15,22] For predominantly cystic lesions, intracavitary RT with rhenium-186, yttrium-90, or phosporus-32 has demonstrated response rates of 50% to 100% and control rates of 67%, although data are limited.[16,23–26]

Dose: Conventional EBRT dose is typically 54 Gy/30 fx. Doses of 54 of 55.8 Gy or greater have demonstrated improved LC compared with lower doses.[13–15] Several series of Gamma Knife® SRS used doses of 10 to 14.5 Gy with long-term control rates of 66% to 80%.[27–30]

Procedure: See *Handbook of Treatment Planning in Radiation Oncology, Chapter 12.*[31]

EVIDENCE-BASED Q&A

Does aggressive GTR improve outcomes compared with limited STR followed by RT?

This is controversial. Retrospective data and systematic reviews of the literature suggest GTR vs. STR + adjuvant RT have similar OS and LC, but GTR may cause more endocrine dysfunction (Tables 61.1 and 61.2).[11,32–36]

Table 61.1 Yang et al. (2010): All CP[34]

	2-Yr PFS	5-Yr PFS	5-Yr OS	10-Yr OS
GTR (n = 256)	88%	67%	98%	98%
STR + RT (n = 85)	91%	69%	99%	95%
	All NS			

Source: Data from Yang I, Sughrue ME, Rutkowski MJ, et al. Craniopharyngioma: a comparison of tumor control with various treatment strategies. *Neurosurg Focus.* 2010;28(4):E5. doi:10.3171/2010.1.focus09307.

Table 61.2 Clark et al. (2013): Pediatric CP[33]

n = 377	1-Yr PFS	5-Yr PFS
GTR	89%	77%
STR + RT	84%	73%
	All NS	

Source: Data from Clark AJ, Cage TA, Aranda D, et al. A systematic review of the results of surgery and radiotherapy on tumor control for pediatric craniopharyngioma. *Childs Nerv Syst.* 2013;29(2):231–238. doi:10.1007/s00381-012-1926-2.

Does proton RT lead to improved outcomes compared with photon RT?

Studies comparing the outcomes of pediatric patients with brain tumors treated with proton vs. photon RT have shown that PBT results in more favorable intellectual outcomes.[37,38] The RT2CR single-arm phase II study outlined below demonstrated that PBT results in less decline in IQ and adaptive behavior compared with a historical cohort of patients treated with photon RT with no differences in oncologic outcomes.[21]

Merchant, RT2CR (*Lancet Oncol* 2023, PMID 37084748): Single-arm, phase II study of 94 patients ages 0 to 21 with CP treated with passively scattered protons to 54 Gy with a 0.5-cm CTV and 0.3-cm PTV. Surgical treatment prior to RT was individualized. The co-primary endpoints were PFS and OS, and they were compared with a historical cohort of 101 patients treated with photon RT (over time the photon cohort CTV decreased from 1 to 0.5 cm or less, and the PTV from 0.5 to 0.3 cm). Median age was 9.4 years in the proton cohort. At MFU of 7.6 years, 10% of patients treated with protons had tumor progression. The 5-year PFS was 94% and the 5-year OS was 100%, which was not statistically different from photons. There was no difference in severe complications (necrosis, clinically important vasculopathy, permanent neurologic deficits). There were significantly worse outcomes in IQ (–1.09 points per year, $p = .007$) and adaptive behavior (–1.48 points per year, $p = .030$) in patients treated with photon therapy compared with PBT. **Conclusion: Passively scattered PBT leads to similar PFS, OS, and severe toxicity compared with photon RT. PBT leads to less decline in IQ and adaptive behavior compared with photon RT.**

Can RT be reserved for salvage treatment?

Most likely. Retrospective data from the University of Pennsylvania found that LC was worse with surgery alone vs. surgery + adjuvant RT, but after accounting for the surgery alone patients who ultimately received salvage RT, LC and OS were comparable.[39] Furthermore, retrospective data from the UK demonstrated similar outcomes among 87 patients treated with adjuvant RT vs. salvage RT.[40]

What are the late effects after treatment?

CP originates in a highly sensitive area of the brain, particularly in children, and late effects from treatment are common given the long natural history of the disease. Endocrine abnormalities due to altered pituitary function are common and can manifest as panhypopituitarism or as a single endocrine abnormality. Diabetes insipidus is common after aggressive surgical resection. Neuropsychological changes including disinhibition, perseveration, attention, and memory deficits are common. Additional effects of treatment near the hypothalamus include hypothalamic obesity, sleep disturbance, and defective thirst sensation. Visual impairment can occur from treatment or tumor progression. RT increases the risk of cerebrovascular changes, and stroke can occur due to proximity of the carotid artery. Radiation necrosis and secondary malignancy can also occur. Moyamoya syndrome (microvascular ischemia of the basal ganglia) is less common. Cognitive decline can occur after RT and can be mitigated by decreasing the RT dose to uninvolved brain with PBT.[21]

REFERENCES

1. Ostrom QT, Price M, Neff C, et al. CBTRUS statistical report: primary brain and other central nervous system tumors diagnosed in the United States in 2016–2020. *Neuro Oncol.* 2023;25(12)(suppl 2):iv1–iv99. doi:10.1093/neuonc/noad149

2. Bunin GR, Surawicz TS, Witman PA, Preston-Martin S, Davis F, Bruner JM. The descriptive epidemiology of craniopharyngioma. *J Neurosurg.* 1998;89(4):547–551. doi:10.3171/jns.1998.89.4.0547

3. Gunderson LL, Tepper JE, eds. *Clinical Radiation Oncology.* 4th ed. Elsevier; 2016.

4. Adamson TE, Wiestler OD, Kleihues P, Yasargil MG. Correlation of clinical and pathological features in surgically treated craniopharyngiomas. *J Neurosurg.* 1990;73(1):12–17. doi:10.3171/jns.1990.73.1.0012

5. Crotty TB, Scheithauer BW, Young WF Jr, et al. Papillary craniopharyngioma: a clinicopathological study of 48 cases. *J Neurosurg.* 1995;83(2):206–214. doi:10.3171/jns.1995.83.2.0206

6. Gaston-Massuet C, Andoniadou CL, Signore M, et al. Increased Wingless (Wnt) signaling in pituitary progenitor/stem cells gives rise to pituitary tumors in mice and humans. *Proc Natl Acad Sci U S A.* 2011; 108(28):11482–11487. doi:10.1073/pnas.1101553108

7. Hussain I, Eloy JA, Carmel PW, Liu JK. Molecular oncogenesis of craniopharyngioma: current and future strategies for the development of targeted therapies. *J Neurosurg.* 2013;119(1):106–112. doi:10.3171/2013 .3.jns122214

8. Brastianos PK, Taylor-Weiner A, Manley PE, et al. Exome sequencing identifies BRAF mutations in papillary craniopharyngiomas. *Nat Genet.* 2014;46(2):161–165. doi:10.1038/ng.2868

9. Larkin S, Karavitaki N. Recent advances in molecular pathology of craniopharyngioma. *F1000Res.* 2017;6:1202. doi:10.12688/f1000research.11549.1

10. Hetelekidis S, Barnes PD, Tao ML, et al. 20-year experience in childhood craniopharyngioma. *Int J Radiat Oncol Biol Phys.* 1993;27(2):189–195. doi:10.1016/0360-3016(93)90227-m

11. Merchant TE, Kiehna EN, Sanford RA, et al. Craniopharyngioma: the St. Jude Children's Research Hospital experience 1984–2001. *Int J Radiat Oncol Biol Phys.* 2002;53(3):533–542. doi:10.1016/s0360-3016(02)02799-2

12. Masson-Cote L, Masucci GL, Atenafu EG, et al. Long-term outcomes for adult craniopharyngioma following radiation therapy. *Acta Oncol.* 2013;52(1):153–158. doi:10.3109/0284186x.2012.685525

13. Regine WF, Kramer S. Pediatric craniopharyngiomas: long term results of combined treatment with surgery and radiation. *Int J Radiat Oncol Biol Phys.* 1992;24(4):611–617. doi:10.1016/0360-3016(92)90704-j

14. Habrand JL, Ganry O, Couanet D, et al. The role of radiation therapy in the management of craniopharyngioma: a 25-year experience and review of the literature. *Int J Radiat Oncol Biol Phys.* 1999;44(2):255–263. doi:10.1016/s0360-3016(99)00030-9

15. Varlotto JM, Flickinger JC, Kondziolka D, Lunsford LD, Deutsch M. External beam irradiation of craniopharyngiomas: long-term analysis of tumor control and morbidity. *Int J Radiat Oncol Biol Phys.* 2002;54(2):492–499. doi:10.1016/s0360-3016(02)02936-7

16. Steinbok P, Hukin J. Intracystic treatments for craniopharyngioma. *Neurosurg Focus.* 2010;28(4):E13. doi:10.3171/2010.1.focus09315

17. Brastianos PK, Twohy E, Geyer S, et al. BRAF-MEK inhibition in newly diagnosed papillary craniopharyngiomas. *N Engl J Med.* 2023;389(2):118–126. doi:10.1056/NEJMoa2213329

18. Luu QT, Loredo LN, Archambeau JO, Yonemoto LT, Slater JM, Slater JD. Fractionated proton radiation treatment for pediatric craniopharyngioma: preliminary report. *Cancer J.* 2006;12(2):155–159. doi:10.1097/00130404-200603000-00011

19. Fitzek MM, Linggood RM, Adams J, Munzenrider JE. Combined proton and photon irradiation for craniopharyngioma: long-term results of the early cohort of patients treated at Harvard Cyclotron Laboratory and Massachusetts General Hospital. *Int J Radiat Oncol Biol Phys.* 2006;64(5):1348–1354. doi:10.1016/j .ijrobp.2005.09.034

20. Rutenberg MS, Rotondo RL, Rao D, et al. Clinical outcomes following proton therapy for adult craniopharyngioma: a single-institution cohort study. *J Neurooncol.* 2020;147(2):387–395. doi:10.1007/s11060 -020-03432-9

21. Merchant TE, Hoehn ME, Khan RB, et al. Proton therapy and limited surgery for paediatric and adolescent patients with craniopharyngioma (RT2CR): a single-arm, phase 2 study. *Lancet Oncol.* 2023;24(5):523–534. doi:10.1016/S1470-2045(23)00146-8

22. Winkfield KM, Linsenmeier C, Yock TI, et al. Surveillance of craniopharyngioma cyst growth in children treated with proton radiotherapy. *Int J Radiat Oncol Biol Phys.* 2009;73(3):716–721. doi:10.1016/j .ijrobp.2008.05.010

23. Voges J, Sturm V, Lehrke R, Treuer H, Gauss C, Berthold F. Cystic craniopharyngioma: long-term results after intracavitary irradiation with stereotactically applied colloidal beta-emitting radioactive sources. *Neurosurgery.* 1997;40(2):263–269. doi:10.1097/00006123-199702000-00007

24. Pollock BE, Lunsford LD, Kondziolka D, Levine G, Flickinger JC. Phosphorus-32 intracavitary irradiation of cystic craniopharyngiomas: current technique and long-term results. *Int J Radiat Oncol Biol Phys.* 1995;33(2):437–446. doi:10.1016/0360-3016(95)00175-x

25. Hasegawa T, Kondziolka D, Hadjipanayis CG, Lunsford LD. Management of cystic craniopharyngio-mas with phosphorus-32 intracavitary irradiation. *Neurosurgery.* 2004;54(4):813–820. doi:10.1227/01.neu.0000114263.01949.26

26. Van den Berge JH, Blaauw G, Breeman WA, Rahmy A, Wijngaarde R. Intracavitary brachytherapy of cystic craniopharyngiomas. *J Neurosurg.* 1992;77(4):545–550. doi:10.3171/jns.1992.77.4.0545

27. Niranjan A, Kano H, Mathieu D, Kondziolka D, Flickinger JC, Lunsford LD. Radiosurgery for craniophar-yngioma. *Int J Radiat Oncol Biol Phys.* 2010;78(1):64–71. doi:10.1016/j.ijrobp.2009.07.1693

28. Lee CC, Yang HC, Chen CJ, et al. Gamma Knife surgery for craniopharyngioma: report on a 20-year experience. *J Neurosurg.* 2014;121(suppl):167–178. doi:10.3171/2014.8.gks141411

29. Kobayashi T. Long-term results of gamma knife radiosurgery for 100 consecutive cases of craniopharyngi-oma and a treatment strategy. *Prog Neurol Surg.* 2009;22:63–76. doi:10.1159/000163383

30. Xu Z, Yen CP, Schlesinger D, Sheehan J. Outcomes of gamma knife surgery for craniopharyngiomas. *J Neurooncol.* 2011;104(1):305–313. doi:10.1007/s11060-010-0494-0

31. Videtic GMM, Vassil AD. *Handbook of Treatment Planning in Radiation Oncology.* 3rd ed. Springer Publishing Company, LLC; 2020.

32. Clark AJ, Cage TA, Aranda D, Parsa AT, Auguste KI, Gupta N. Treatment-related morbidity and the man-agement of pediatric craniopharyngioma: a systematic review. *J Neurosurg Pediatr.* 2012;10(4):293–301. doi:10.3171/2012.7.peds11436

33. Clark AJ, Cage TA, Aranda D, et al. A systematic review of the results of surgery and radiotherapy on tumor control for pediatric craniopharyngioma. *Childs Nerv Syst.* 2013;29(2):231–238. doi:10.1007/s00381-012-1926-2

34. Yang I, Sughrue ME, Rutkowski MJ, et al. Craniopharyngioma: a comparison of tumor control with various treatment strategies. *Neurosurg Focus.* 2010;28(4):E5. doi:10.3171/2010.1.focus09307

35. Schoenfeld A, Pekmezci M, Barnes MJ, et al. The superiority of conservative resection and adjuvant radia-tion for craniopharyngiomas. *J Neurooncol.* 2012;108(1):133–139. doi:10.1007/s11060-012-0806-7

36. Sughrue ME, Yang I, Kane AJ, et al. Endocrinologic, neurologic, and visual morbidity after treatment for craniopharyngioma. *J Neurooncol.* 2011;101(3):463–476. doi:10.1007/s11060-010-0265-y

37. Kahalley LS, Peterson R, Ris MD, et al. Superior intellectual outcomes after proton radiotherapy compared with photon radiotherapy for pediatric medulloblastoma. *J Clin Oncol.* 2020;38(5):454–461. doi:10.1200/JCO.19.01706

38. Lassaletta A, Morales JS, Valenzuela PL, et al. Neurocognitive outcomes in pediatric brain tumors after treatment with proton versus photon radiation: a systematic review and meta-analysis. *World J Pediatr.* 2023;19(8):727–740. doi:10.1007/s12519-023-00726-6

39. Stripp DC, Maity A, Janss AJ, et al. Surgery with or without radiation therapy in the management of crani-opharyngiomas in children and young adults. *Int J Radiat Oncol Biol Phys.* 2004;58(3):714–720. doi:10.1016/s0360-3016(03)01570-0

40. Pemberton LS, Dougal M, Magee B, Gattamaneni HR. Experience of external beam radiotherapy given adjuvantly or at relapse following surgery for craniopharyngioma. *Radiother Oncol.* 2005;77(1):99–104. doi:10.1016/j.radonc.2005.04.015

62 RHABDOMYOSARCOMA

Cole Billena, Shauna R. Campbell, and Erin S. Murphy

QUICK HIT Rhabdomyosarcoma (RMS) is the most common malignant soft tissue sarcoma in children. Risk stratification is performed via preoperative staging, postoperative grouping, histology, and fusion status to determine treatment. Presence of metastatic disease and PAX/FOX01 gene fusion are the two most important negative prognostic factors. All patients require multiagent CHT (usually VAC-based: vincristine, actinomycin D, and cyclophosphamide). General treatment paradigm is biopsy or nonmorbid resection, followed by CHT, local therapy (surgery, RT, or a combination), and more CHT for up to ~1 year. RT is indicated for all patients except those with embryonal histology after GTR without nodal involvement. The timing of RT varies by protocol and presentation. Patients with intracranial extension, vision loss, or cord compression should be considered for urgent RT, especially if not responding to CHT; those with cranial nerve palsies and base of skull erosion can receive delayed RT without a compromise in outcomes. RT dose recommendations are listed in Table 62.1.

Table 62.1 Summary of RT Dosing Guidelines for RMS by Extent of Resection and Histology		
Disease Status	**Embryonal Histology**	**Alveolar Histology**
Margin negative	No RT	36 Gy
Margin positive	36 Gy	36 Gy
Node positive	41.4 Gy	41.4 Gy
Gross disease*	50.4 Gy	50.4 Gy

*Gross disease in the orbit: 45 Gy with VAC (if lower CYC dose given and response <CR, 50.4 Gy should be considered) or 50.4 Gy with VA CHT.[1,2] Dose escalation to 59.4 Gy can be considered for patients with diffuse anaplasia or bulky disease (>5 cm) with <CR after CHT per ARST1431.

EPIDEMIOLOGY: RMS is the most common pediatric soft tissue sarcoma, with ~4.5 cases per million per year and 350 cases total annually in the United States.[3,4] There is a slight male predominance, 1.4:1, and the peak incidence occurs at 3 to 5 years of age, with 70% of cases occurring before 10 years of age.[5,6]

RISK FACTORS: The majority of cases are sporadic, with no predisposing risk factor.[7] RMS has been associated with Li–Fraumeni,[7–9] NF-1,[10,11] Beckwith–Wiedemann syndrome,[12] Noonan syndrome,[13] and Costello syndrome.[14]

ANATOMY: RMS can arise anywhere in the body, with the most common locations in GU and H&N sites (Table 62.2).[6] It is a locally invasive tumor with the potential to spread along fascial planes. The overall risk of regional lymphatic spread varies with site of primary lesion; GU, abdominal/pelvic, extremity, and H&N tumors more commonly involve regional LNs, whereas trunk and female genital organs rarely involve LNs.[5] DM is present in 15% of cases at the time of diagnosis, with the lungs, bone, and bone marrow being most common.[15]

Table 62.2 Distribution of RMS by Anatomic Site		
Site[16]	**Distribution**	**Subdivisions**
H&N (nonparameningeal)	7%	Cheek, hypopharynx, larynx, oral cavity, oropharynx, parotid, scalp, face, pinna, neck, masseter muscle
Parameningeal (PM)	25%	Infratemporal fossa, mastoid, middle ear, nasal cavity, nasopharynx, paranasal sinus, parapharyngeal, pterygopalatine fossa

(continued)

Table 62.2 Distribution of RMS by Anatomic Site (*continued*)		
Site[16]	Distribution	Subdivisions
Orbit	9%	
GU	31%	Bladder, paratesticular, prostate, urethra, uterus/cervix, vagina, vulva
Extremity	13%	
Trunk	5%	Chest wall, paraspinal, abdominal wall
Retroperitoneum	7%	
Other	3%	Hepatobiliary tree, perineal, perianal

Note: Combined H&N (including PM and orbit) is the most common site.
Source: Data from Crist WM, Anderson JR, Meza JL, et al. Intergroup rhabdomyosarcoma study-IV: results for patients with nonmetastatic disease. *J Clin Oncol.* 2001;19(12):3091–3102. doi:10.1200/JCO.2001.19.12.3091.

PATHOLOGY: There are four distinct histologic subtypes recognized by the WHO: embryonal, alveolar, spindle cell/sclerosing, and pleomorphic/undifferentiated (Table 62.3).[17] Fusion status now overrides the prognosis of histologic subtypes.

Table 62.3 Pathologic Subtypes of RMS[5,6,17]						
Subtype	Frequency	Common Site	Histologic Appearance	Age	Prognosis	5-Yr OS
Botryoid (grape-like appearance, embryonal variant)	6%	Mucosa-lined organs: bladder, vagina, nasopharynx, nasal cavity, middle ear, biliary tree	Loose myxoid stroma with "cambium" tumor cell layer	Infants	Excellent	95%
Spindle cell/sclerosing (embryonal variant)	3%	Paratesticular	Predominant spindle cells pattern	Childhood		88%
Embryonal	70%–80%	Most commonly in H&N (~50%) and GU tract (~50%)	Small round mesenchymal cells on myxoid stroma; subset can demonstrate diffuse anaplasia	Childhood	Intermediate	66%
Alveolar	20%	Extremities, trunk, perianal, perineal region	Monomorphic round cells arranged in sheets or cords with pseudolining clefts, looks like lung alveoli	Adolescents and young adults	Poor	54%
Pleomorphic	2%	Extremity, trunk	Diffuse mesenchymal/primitive cell population; diagnosis of exclusion	Adults		40%
Other	9%					

GENETICS[5]

Embryonal: Eighty percent are associated with LOH 11p15.5. Absence of N-myc amplification in most, and 95% are PAX/FOX01 fusion-negative. TP53 portends worse prognosis.[17] *MYOD1* mutations confer poor prognosis and are associated with sclerosing/spindle cell RMS.[18]

Alveolar: Eighty percent are associated with PAX/FOXO1 gene fusion. N-myc amplification, found in 50% of cases, and 12q13–14 amplification resulting in CDK4 overexpression have both been associated with worse survival.[19,20] Two chromosomal translocations are commonly identified: **t(2;13) (PAX3/FOX01 fusion)** in 60% of cases and **t(1;13) (PAX7/FOX01 fusion)** in 20% of cases. Genes are FKHR (on chr 13), PAX3 (chr 2), and PAX7 (chr 1). Alveolar tumors that do not have PAX/FOX01 gene fusion have prognosis similar to embryonal.

CLINICAL PRESENTATION: Often presents as an asymptomatic mass but can have site-specific signs and symptoms (e.g., orbital tumors may cause proptosis and ophthalmoplegia, and GU tumors may cause hematuria or urinary obstruction).

WORKUP: H&P with exam of affected area (H&N, pelvic exam under anesthesia as indicated).

Labs: CBC, BMP, LFTs, urinalysis.

Imaging: For all sites: CT or MRI of primary tumor area, PET/CT (can replace CT chest/abdomen/pelvis and bone scan studies). Scrotal ultrasound is often the first step for a paratesticular tumor. MRI spine is optional if CSF is positive or if patient is symptomatic.

Procedures: Bone marrow biopsy and aspirate is considered for patients with high-risk presentation. For H&N primary tumor with intracranial extension, an LP with cytologic exam of CSF is indicated.

PROGNOSTIC FACTORS: For high-risk patients, Oberlin risk factors are predictive of outcome and include >10 years or <1 year of age, bone or bone marrow involvement, ≥3 metastatic sites, or unfavorable primary site. Patients with ≤1 Oberlin factor have a better outcome.[21] Table 62.4 compares favorable and unfavorable prognostic factors.

Table 62.4 Comparison of Favorable vs. Unfavorable Prognostic Factors in RMS		
Variable	Favorable	Unfavorable
Metastases	None	Present
Primary site	Orbit, non-PM H&N, GU (non-bladder/prostate)	Extremity, trunk, PM, bladder, prostate
Histology	Botryoid, spindle cell, embryonal	Alveolar, undifferentiated
Lymph node metastasis	No	Yes
Resectability	Complete	Microscopic < gross residual
Age	2–10 years old	<1 years, >10 years old
DNA proliferation	Low S-phase	High S-phase
DNA ploidy	Hyperdiploid	Diploid
PAX/FOX01	Fusion negative	Fusion positive

STAGING: The Intergroup Rhabdomyosarcoma Study Group (IRSG) pretreatment staging system (Table 62.5). Preop based on "SSN" (site, size, nodes). If favorable site and nonmetastatic, all are stage I. If unfavorable site, must be BOTH <5 cm AND node-negative to be stage II.

Table 62.5 IRSG Staging System					
Stage	Sites	Size	N	M	3-Yr Failure-Free Survival[15]
1: Favorable site	Orbit H&N (non-PM) GU (non-bladder/prostate)	Any size	Any N	M0	86%
2: Unfavorable site, N0, and ≤5 cm	Bladder/prostate Extremity Parameningeal Other (including retroperitoneum, perineal, perianal, intrathoracic, GI) Biliary tract/liver	≤5 cm	N0 or Nx	M0	80%

(continued)

Table 62.5 IRSG Staging System (*continued*)					
Stage	**Sites**	**Size**	**N**	**M**	**3-Yr Failure-Free Survival**[15]
3: Unfavorable site and either >5 cm or node positive	Same as stage II	≤5 cm	N1	M0	68%
		>5 cm	Any N	M0	
4: Metastatic	All	Any size	Any N	M1	25%

N0: not clinically involved; N1: clinically involved; Nx: clinical status unknown; M0: no distant metastases; M1: distant metastases.

IRSG Clinical Grouping Classification[4,6]

Group (Table 62.6) is assessed at the time of diagnosis based on resectability (i.e., patient unresectable at diagnosis, treated with CHT, then undergoes GTR remains group III). See Table 62.7 for COG Risk Stratification.

Table 62.6 IRSG Grouping Classification[4]	
Group I	Localized disease, completely resected A: Confined to muscle or organ of origin B: Infiltration outside the muscle or organ of origin
Group II	Gross total resection with: A: Microscopic residual disease B: Regional LN spread, completely resected C: Regional LN resected with microscopic residual disease
Group III	Incomplete resection with gross residual disease A: After biopsy only B: After major resection (>50%)
Group IV	Distant metastasis at diagnosis

Source: Adapted from Haduong JH, Heske CM, Allen-Rhoades W, et al. An update on rhabdomyosarcoma risk stratification and the rationale for current and future Children's Oncology Group clinical trials. *Pediatr Blood Cancer.* 2022;69(4):e29511. doi:10.1002/pbc.29511.

Table 62.7 COG Risk Stratification Based on Preop Staging + Postop Grouping[4]	
Risk Group	**Involved Groups**
Low (~35%)	• PAX/FOX01 fusion negative, stage 1–2, groups I–II • PAX/FOX01 fusion negative, stage 1, group III (orbit only)
Intermediate (~50%)	• PAX/FOX01 fusion negative, stage 1–2, group III (excluding orbit) • PAX/FOX01 fusion negative, stage 3, groups I–III • PAX/FOX01 fusion negative, stage 4, group IV, age >2 and <10 years • PAX/FOX01 fusion positive, stage 1–3, groups I–III
High (~15%)	• PAX/FOX01 fusion negative, stage 4, group IV, age >10 years • PAX/FOX01 fusion positive, stage 4, group IV

Source: Adapted from Haduong JH, Heske CM, Allen-Rhoades W, et al. An update on rhabdomyosarcoma risk stratification and the rationale for current and future Children's Oncology Group clinical trials. *Pediatr Blood Cancer.* 2022;69(4):e29511. doi:10.1002/pbc.29511.

TREATMENT PARADIGM

Surgery: Complete excision with 5-mm margin is preferable if functional and cosmetic outcomes are acceptable.[15] If not feasible (or if disease involves the orbit, vagina, bladder, or biliary tract), diagnostic incisional biopsy can be performed, followed by induction CHT and definitive local therapy. LC with organ preservation is the goal.[5] Delayed primary excision of group III patients after induction CHT permits reduced-dose RT and has equivalent or improved outcomes.[22] Current COG studies require LN evaluation for all extremity tumors (SLNB acceptable if clinically negative), and all boys ≥10 years of age with a paratesticular RMS should undergo routine ipsilateral nerve-sparing retroperitoneal LND. Consider ilioinguinal lymphadenectomy for perianal or anal tumors. In H&N primaries, neck dissection is not indicated, but suspicious nodes should be surgically evaluated.[5]

Chemotherapy: All patients require multiagent CHT, regardless of stage and group.[15] VAC (vincristine [VCR], actinomycin-D, cyclophosphamide [CYC]) is standard regimen. In sequential IRS trials, the addition of many individually active agents (e.g., doxorubicin, cisplatin, etoposide, ifosfamide, topotecan, and melphalan) did not improve outcomes compared with VAC, in any subgroup. In IRS-IV, VA was equivalent to VAC in low-risk/excellent prognosis group. ARST0331 added modest-dose CYC to VA while condensing therapy from 45 to 22 weeks with RT for low-risk patients, and there was no compromise in outcomes.[23] ARST0531 compared VAC with VAC/VI alternating for intermediate-risk patients and found no improvement in EFS or OS, but there was less hematologic toxicity and cumulative CYC dose, making VAC/VI an alternative.[24] VCR ± irinotecan can be continued concurrently during RT per ARST0431.

Radiation: Per COG ARST trials, RT is indicated in all cases except group I embryonal. RT dosing is outlined in Table 62.1. Patients with pulmonary metastases and/or pleural effusion can be treated with whole lung irradiation (15 Gy/10 fx). Clinical trials, such as ARST1431, include consolidation RT to metastases in patients with intermediate-risk stage IV disease using standard dose fractionation for sites >5 cm and SBRT dose fractionation for sites ≤5 cm.

Procedures: See *Handbook of Treatment Planning in Radiation Oncology*, Chapter 12.[25]

EVIDENCE-BASED Q&A

What did the IRS studies show?

The IRSG was formed in 1972 to investigate the biology and treatment of RMS; it was merged into the COG in 2000. They led a series of protocols (IRS I–V) that have dictated RMS management with a rise in OS seen for all patients from ~50% to >70%. Pertinent conclusions from the studies are summarized in Table 62.8.

Table 62.8 Summary of IRSG Trials	
	Key Takeaways
IRS-I (1988)[26]	• 5-yr OS for all groups I–IV was 55% • Best prognosis: orbit, GU tract • Worst prognosis: retroperitoneum • FH group 1: RT not needed if given 2 yrs of VAC • UH group 1: RT improves FFS and OS[27] • Limited RT volumes (GTV + 2 cm) had similar outcomes to big fields such as whole muscle bundle RT
IRS-II (1993)[28]	• 5-yr OS for all groups I–IV was 63%, improvement from IRS-I ($p < .001$) • 5-yr OS for all nonmetastatic patients was improved from 63% (IRS-I) to 71% • LC (93%) was improved with >40 Gy for orofacial and laryngopharyngeal sites[29] • CYC not needed in FH group I/II
IRS-III (1995)[30]	• 5-yr OS for all groups I–IV was 71%, improved from IRS-II ($p < .001$) • UH group 1 benefitted with addition of RT • For PM H&N sites with CN palsy or BOS erosion, limited RT volumes equivalent to WBRT (WBRT was still used for intracranial extension)
IRS-IV (2003)[15,16]	• Group IV patients with ≤2 metastatic sites had improved 3-yr OS and FFS on MVA ($p = .007$ and .006, respectively) • For group III disease, no benefit to hyperfractionated regimen (59.4 Gy with 1.1 Gy BID) over conventional regimen of 50.4 Gy in 1.8 Gy/fx • No benefit to VAI or VIE over VAC for nonmetastatic disease
IRS-V (2011)[31]	• Reduced RT dose (36 Gy for microscopic disease [stage 1/group IIa] and 45 Gy for group III orbit primaries if CYC is included in systemic therapy) does not compromise LC • An alkylating CHT agent (CYC or ifosfamide) may be important for FFS

What is the significance of the PAX/FOX01 gene fusion?

Using clinical trial data from six COG trials, investigators evaluated the prognostic value of the PAX/FOX01 gene fusion as a stratification factor. The first factor important for stratification was localized vs. metastatic disease (EFS 73% vs. 30%; OS 84% vs. 42%), and the second factor was PAX/FOX01 status (positive vs. negative), which was found to be the most important factor for patients with RMS, improving risk stratification for patients with localized RMS (Table 62.9).[32]

Table 62.9 Prognostic Value of PAX/FOX01 Fusion From Pooled COG Trials

	PAX/FOX01 Fusion Positive	PAX/FOX01 Fusion Negative
Localized disease EFS	52%	78%
OS	65%	88%
Metastatic disease EFS	6%	46%
OS	19%	58%

What is the benefit of RT and in whom is RT required?

There are no good prospective randomized data. RT is currently indicated for all patients except embryonal tumors after GTR without LN involvement. Wolden et al. reviewed patients treated on IRS I–III and showed that patients with alveolar/undifferentiated histology after GTR (group I) have improved EFS and OS with the addition of RT.[29] Further, when comparing outcomes between IRS-IV and MMT-89 (contemporary European International Society of Pediatric Oncology Malignant Mesenchymal Tumor study that attempted to avoid RT and radical surgery as much as possible by giving more CHT as necessary), RT appears to have significant benefits in LC, EFS, and OS.[29]

When should RT be initiated?

RT timing has varied by protocol and risk group through the years. On the most recent COG protocols, low-risk patients start RT at week 13, intermediate-risk at week 4, and high-risk at week 20. Metastatic sites may be treated at the end of CHT. Patients with cord compression, visual loss, or intracranial extension should be considered for urgent RT, on day 0, per high-risk COG ARST0431. ARST0531 moved RT earlier to week 4 for intermediate-risk patients with the hopes of improving LC, but results showed no advantage with this approach. Analysis from IRS II–IV[33] showed reduced LF if RT started within 2 weeks vs. >2 weeks for patients with meningeal impingement (18% vs. 33%, p = .03) and intracranial extension (16% vs. 37%, p = .07). An analysis from Spaulding et al. demonstrated similar clinical outcomes for patients with cranial nerve palsy or skull base erosion treated with immediate vs. delayed RT[27]; thus, it is acceptable to treat patients with these high-risk features at a later date (week 20 per COG ARST0431) but consider treating patients with intracranial extension or lack of CHT response earlier.

Does whole lung irradiation (WLI) improve outcomes in patients with lung metastases?

Luo (*JCO* 2024, PMID 39255438): Retrospective pooled analysis of four COG trials (D9802, D9803, ARST08P1, ARST0431) evaluating the benefit of WLI in patients with lung metastases. 143 patients were included, 65 of whom received WLI and 78 did not despite protocol requirements. The 5-year EFS and OS rates for those who received WLI vs. those who did not were 38% vs. 25% (*p* = .0496) and 46% vs. 32% (*p* = .08), respectively. In subgroup analysis, receipt of WLI significantly improved EFS (HR 1.9, 95% CI 1.14–3.16) and OS (HR 2.06, 1.21–3.52) in patients ≥10 years old. **Conclusion: WLI is associated with higher EFS and OS in retrospective pooled analysis.**

Is 45 Gy a sufficient dose for all orbital embryonal RMS?

Historically, patients with orbital embryonal RMS received VAC, followed by RT to 45 Gy. However, in a subset analysis of group III orbital embryonal RMS patients on ARST033, a higher risk of LR (16%) was seen in patients with less than a CR as compared with patients who achieved a CR (0%) after CHT. It is important to note that this trial used a lower dose of CYC. For patients with a PR after VAC (with low-dose CYC), 50.4 Gy should be considered.

Is there a benefit to proton therapy in RMS?

The rationale is to reduce late effects and protons are permitted on ongoing RMS trials. Small series demonstrating dosimetric advantages have been published for orbit, parameningeal, and pelvic sites.[34]

REFERENCES

1   Ermoian RP, Breneman J, Walterhouse DO, et al. 45 Gy is not sufficient radiotherapy dose for Group III orbital embryonal rhabdomyosarcoma after less than complete response to 12 weeks of ARST0331 chemotherapy: a report from the Soft Tissue Sarcoma Committee of the Children's Oncology Group. *Pediatr Blood Cancer.* 2017;64(5):e26540. doi:10.1002/pbc.26540

2   Walterhouse DO, Pappo AS, Meza JL, et al. Reduction of cyclophosphamide dose for patients with subset 2 low-risk rhabdomyosarcoma is associated with an increased risk of recurrence: a report from the Soft Tissue Sarcoma Committee of the Children's Oncology Group. *Cancer.* 2017;123(12):2368–2375. doi:10.1002/cncr.30613

3   Rajagopalan A, Christenberry SC, Ramachandran V. Rhabdomyosarcoma. *Pediatr Rev.* 2022;43(10):599–600. doi:10.1542/pir.2021-004977

4   Haduong JH, Heske CM, Allen-Rhoades W, et al. An update on rhabdomyosarcoma risk stratification and the rationale for current and future Children's Oncology Group clinical trials. *Pediatr Blood Cancer.* 2022;69(4):e29511. doi:10.1002/pbc.29511

5   Terezakis SA. Pediatric rhabdomyosarcoma. In: Merchant TE, Kieran MW, eds. *Pediatric Radiation Oncology.* Springer; 2018:127–142.

6   Halperin EC, Constine LS, Tarbell NJ, Kun LE. *Pediatric Radiation Oncology.* 5th ed. Lippincott Williams & Wilkins; 2011.

7   Diller L, Sexsmith E, Gottlieb A, Li FP, Malkin D. Germline p53 mutations are frequently detected in young children with rhabdomyosarcoma. *J Clin Invest.* 1995;95(4):1606–1611. doi:10.1172/JCI117834

8   Li FP, Fraumeni JF Jr. Rhabdomyosarcoma in children: epidemiologic study and identification of a familial cancer syndrome. *J Natl Cancer Inst.* 1969;43(6):1365–1373. PMID: 5396222

9   Trahair T, Andrews L, Cohn RJ. Recognition of Li Fraumeni syndrome at diagnosis of a locally advanced extremity rhabdomyosarcoma. *Pediatr Blood Cancer.* 2007;48(3):345–348. doi:10.1002/pbc.20795

10 Crucis A, Richer W, Brugieres L, et al. Rhabdomyosarcomas in children with neurofibromatosis type I: a national historical cohort. *Pediatr Blood Cancer.* 2015;62(10):1733–1738. doi:10.1002/pbc.25556

11 Ferrari A, Bisogno G, Macaluso A, et al. Soft-tissue sarcomas in children and adolescents with neurofibromatosis type 1. *Cancer.* 2007;109(7):1406–1412. doi:10.1002/cncr.22533

12 DeBaun MR, Tucker MA. Risk of cancer during the first four years of life in children from The Beckwith-Wiedemann Syndrome Registry. *J Pediatr.* 1998;132(3 pt 1):398–400. doi:10.1016/s0022-3476(98)70008-3

13 Kratz CP, Rapisuwon S, Reed H, Hasle H, Rosenberg PS. Cancer in Noonan, Costello, cardiofaciocutaneous and LEOPARD syndromes. *Am J Med Genet C Semin Med Genet.* 2011;157C(2):83–89. doi:10.1002/ajmg.c.30300

14 Gripp KW. Tumor predisposition in Costello syndrome. *Am J Med Genet C Semin Med Genet.* 2005;137C(1):72–77. doi:10.1002/ajmg.c.30065

15 Breneman JC, Lyden E, Pappo AS, et al. Prognostic factors and clinical outcomes in children and adolescents with metastatic rhabdomyosarcoma: a report from the Intergroup Rhabdomyosarcoma Study IV. *J Clin Oncol.* 2003;21(1):78–84. doi:10.1200/JCO.2003.06.129

16 Crist WM, Anderson JR, Meza JL, et al. Intergroup rhabdomyosarcoma study-IV: results for patients with nonmetastatic disease. *J Clin Oncol.* 2001;19(12):3091–3102. doi:10.1200/JCO.2001.19.12.3091

17 Dehner CA, Rudzinski ER, Davis JL. Rhabdomyosarcoma: updates on classification and the necessity of molecular testing beyond immunohistochemistry. *Hum Pathol.* 2024;147:72–81. doi:10.1016/j.humpath.2023.12.004

18 Kohsaka S, Shukla N, Ameur N, et al. A recurrent neomorphic mutation in MYOD1 defines a clinically aggressive subset of embryonal rhabdomyosarcoma associated with PI3K-AKT pathway mutations. *Nat Genet.* 2014;46(6):595–600. doi:10.1038/ng.2969

19 Williamson D, Lu YJ, Gordon T, et al. Relationship between MYCN copy number and expression in rhabdomyosarcomas and correlation with adverse prognosis in the alveolar subtype. *J Clin Oncol.* 2005;23(4):880–888. doi:10.1200/JCO.2005.11.078

20 Barr FG, Duan F, Smith LM, et al. Genomic and clinical analyses of 2p24 and 12q13-q14 amplification in alveolar rhabdomyosarcoma: a report from the Children's Oncology Group. *Genes Chromosomes Cancer.* 2009;48(8):661–672. doi:10.1002/gcc.20673

21 Weigel BJ, Lyden E, Anderson JR, et al. Intensive multiagent therapy, including dose-compressed cycles of ifosfamide/etoposide and vincristine/doxorubicin/cyclophosphamide, irinotecan, and radiation, in

patients with high-risk rhabdomyosarcoma: a report from the Children's Oncology Group. *J Clin Oncol.* 2016;34(2):117–122. doi:10.1200/JCO.2015.63.4048

22   Lautz TB, Chi YY, Li M, et al. Benefit of delayed primary excision in rhabdomyosarcoma: a report from the Children's Oncology Group. *Cancer.* 2021;127(2):275–283. doi:10.1002/cncr.33275

23   Walterhouse DO, Pappo AS, Meza JL, et al. Shorter-duration therapy using vincristine, dactinomycin, and lower-dose cyclophosphamide with or without radiotherapy for patients with newly diagnosed low-risk rhabdomyosarcoma: a report from the Soft Tissue Sarcoma Committee of the Children's Oncology Group. *J Clin Oncol.* 2014;32(31):3547–3552. doi:10.1200/JCO.2014.55.6787

24   Hawkins DS, Chi YY, Anderson JR, et al. Addition of vincristine and irinotecan to vincristine, dactinomy-cin, and cyclophosphamide does not improve outcome for intermediate-risk rhabdomyosarcoma: a report from the Children's Oncology Group. *J Clin Oncol.* 2018;36(27):2770-2777. doi:10.1200/JCO.2018.77.9694

25   Vassil AD, Videtic GMM. *Handbook of Treatment Planning in Radiation Oncology.* Springer Publishing Company; 2010.

26   Maurer HM, Beltangady M, Gehan EA, et al. The Intergroup Rhabdomyosarcoma Study-I. A final report. *Cancer.* 1988;61(2):209–220. doi:10.1002/1097-0142(19880115)61:2<209::AID-CNCR2820610202>3.0.CO;2-L

27   Spalding AC, Hawkins DS, Donaldson SS, et al. The effect of radiation timing on patients with high-risk features of parameningeal rhabdomyosarcoma: an analysis of IRS-IV and D9803. *Int J Radiat Oncol Biol Phys.* 2013;87(3):512–516. doi:10.1016/j.ijrobp.2013.07.003

28   Maurer HM, Gehan EA, Beltangady M, et al. The Intergroup Rhabdomyosarcoma Study-II. *Cancer.* 1993;71(5):1904–1922. doi:10.1002/1097-0142(19930301)71:5<1904::AID-CNCR2820710530>3.0.CO;2-X

29   Wolden SL, Anderson JR, Crist WM, et al. Indications for radiotherapy and chemotherapy after complete resection in rhabdomyosarcoma: a report from the Intergroup Rhabdomyosarcoma Studies I to III. *J Clin Oncol.* 1999;17(11):3468–3475. doi:10.1200/JCO.1999.17.11.3468

30   Crist W, Gehan EA, Ragab AH, et al. The Third Intergroup Rhabdomyosarcoma Study. *J Clin Oncol.* 1995;13(3):610–630. doi:10.1200/JCO.1995.13.3.610

31   Raney RB, Walterhouse DO, Meza JL, et al. Results of the Intergroup Rhabdomyosarcoma Study Group D9602 protocol, using vincristine and dactinomycin with or without cyclophosphamide and radiation ther-apy, for newly diagnosed patients with low-risk embryonal rhabdomyosarcoma: a report from the soft tis-sue sarcoma committee of the children's oncology group. *J Clin Oncol.* 2011;29(10):1312–1318. doi:10.1200/JCO.2010.30.4469

32   Hibbitts E, Chi YY, Hawkins DS, et al. Refinement of risk stratification for childhood rhabdomyosar-coma using FOXO1 fusion status in addition to established clinical outcome predictors: a report from the Children's Oncology Group. *Cancer Med.* 2019;8(14):6437–6448. doi:10.1002/cam4.2504

33   Michalski JM, Meza J, Breneman JC, et al. Influence of radiation therapy parameters on outcome in children treated with radiation therapy for localized parameningeal rhabdomyosarcoma in Intergroup Rhabdomyosarcoma Study Group trials II through IV. *Int J Radiat Oncol Biol Phys.* 2004;59(4):1027–1038. doi:10.1016/j.ijrobp.2004.02.064

34   Vennarini S, Colombo F, Mirandola A, et al. Clinical insight on proton therapy for paediatric rhabdomyo-sarcoma. *Cancer Manag Res.* 2023;15:1125–1139. doi:10.2147/CMAR.S362664

Salem Alfaifi, Praveen Pendyala, and Erin S. Murphy

QUICK HIT   Neuroblastoma (NB) is a small round blue cell tumor arising from the neural crest cells of the sympathetic nervous system. NB is the most common malignancy in infants and the most common pediatric extracranial solid tumor. Workup includes H&P, labs, urinary catecholamines (VMA/HVA), CT/MRI of primary site, CT chest/abdomen/pelvis, MIBG scan, and bilateral bone marrow biopsy. Patients are stratified into risk groups based on stage, age, N-myc status, DNA ploidy, and Shimada classification. Risk group determines treatment (Table 63.1).

Table 63.1 General Treatment Paradigm for Neuroblastoma		
INRG/Risk Group	**5-Yr OS**	**General Treatment Paradigm**
INRG L1 or low risk	>95%	Surgery alone. CHT for residual disease (if >18 months or unfavorable factors), recurrent, or symptomatic disease **OR** Observation for those with stage MS or infants <6 months with isolated adrenal masses <5 cm in diameter
INRG L2 or intermediate risk	90%–95%	Upfront resection if possible, depending on IDRFs and biological risk factors, followed by CHT **OR** CHT (2, 4, or 8 cycles depending on histology and M stage) with response assessment driving surveillance vs. surgery vs. additional CHT RT if persistent or worsening symptoms despite other therapy (per ANBL0531)
High risk	30%–50%	Induction CHT, then surgery, then myeloablative CHT and tandem autologous SCT, then consolidative RT, then oral isotretinoin + anti-GD2 antibody (per ANBL0532) RT: Treat primary post-CHT and presurgical volume to 21.6 Gy/12 fx if GTR (no boost for residual disease); treat metastatic sites active on post-CHT and pretransplant MIBG scan

Note: Regarding spinal cord compression: occurs in 5%–15% of patients. RT is reserved for those who fail initial CHT and/or surgery as RT is associated with late toxicity (e.g., scoliosis).

EPIDEMIOLOGY: Most common pediatric extracranial solid tumor, most common infant malignancy, and the third most common pediatric cancer overall (after leukemia, brain, lymphoma). It represents 6% to 10% of all childhood malignancies and 15% of deaths (most lethal pediatric solid tumor); 650 to 700 new cases per year, median age 17 months at diagnosis (90% are <5 years, 40% <1 year). Incidence is higher in males than females and higher in Caucasians than Blacks. Approximately 50% present with high-risk disease.[1]

RISK FACTORS: Poorly established. Increased incidence with maternal use of alcohol, diuretics, opioids/codeine, and paternal exposure to hydrocarbons/wood dust/solders.[2,3] There is suggestion of protective effect of vitamin/folic acid use and history of asthma/allergies. Majority of tumors are sporadic; hereditary in only 1% to 2% of cases. Associated with Hirschsprung disease and NF-1.[4]

ANATOMY: Can originate from anywhere along the sympathetic nervous system, most commonly along the paraspinal sympathetic ganglia (mediastinal or abdominal) or the adrenal glands.

PATHOLOGY: Spectrum ranges from benign ganglioneuroma (well-differentiated, favorable prognosis) to ganglioneuroblastoma (moderately differentiated, unfavorable prognosis), to neuroblastoma (poorly differentiated, favorable to poor prognosis), but 97% of neuroblastic tumors are NB.[5,6] Originates from neural crest cells of the sympathetic nervous system that migrate to form the adrenal medulla and spinal sympathetic ganglia. NB is a small round blue cell tumor with pathognomonic neuritic processes (neuropil) in almost all tumors except undifferentiated. Homer Wright pseudorosettes are neuroblasts surrounding areas of eosinophilic neuropil (15%–50% of cases). IHC positive for neuron-specific enolase, chromogranin A, neurofilament protein, S100, and synaptophysin can aid in distinction from other similar tumors (non-Hodgkin lymphoma, Ewing's, sarcomas).[7,8] Negative for leukocyte common antigen, vimentin, myosin, desmin, and actin.

Shimada Histopathologic System: Classifies tumors into favorable or unfavorable categories based on **S**tromal pattern, **A**ge, degree of neuroblastic **D**ifferentiation, **M**itosis-karyorrhexis index (MKI relating to fragmentation of the nucleus), a**n**d **N**odularity (mnemonic: **SADMaN**). Favorable Shimada: young age, low MKI, mature neuroblast differentiation, rich stroma with nonnodular pattern.[6]

GENETICS: N-myc protein amplification encoded by *MYCN* gene, proto-oncogene found on the short arm of chr 2 and identified by FISH. N-myc amplification found in 20% to 25% overall: 0% to 10% early stage, 40% to 50% advanced stage.[9] Other poor prognostic factors include deletion/loss of 1p or 11q, unbalanced gain of 17q, TERT rearrangements, ATRX deletion, or ALK mutation (accounts for up to 15% of hereditary NB).[5,7,8] Favorable factors are tumor cell hyperdiploidy or TRK-A amplification.[6,10–13]

SCREENING: Currently no role. Data from Japan, Canada, and Europe showed that screening urine for HVA/VMA at 3 weeks of age, 6 months of age, or 1 year increases detection overall; however, no change in detection of advanced-stage disease with unfavorable characteristics in older children. It also failed to reduce deaths from NB in infants.[10–12] Earlier detection can identify a higher incidence of NBs in infants, but these tend to be more favorable, spontaneously regress in early infancy, and may not have been detected otherwise.[13]

CLINICAL PRESENTATION: Abdominal mass, abdominal pain, fever, malaise, weight loss, micturition, dyspnea, and dysphagia. Approximately one-third experience fatigue, anorexia, irritability, and pallor. Bone pain frequent in patients with skeletal mets (most often skull/posterior orbit). Excess catecholamines can produce flushing, sweating, and hypertension (although rare). Can be confused with Wilms tumor (see Chapter 64, Table 64.3 comparing NB and Wilms presentation). IV pyelogram classically shows renal displacement ("drooping lily sign") without pelvocaliceal disruption seen in Wilms tumor. See Table 63.2 for associated classic signs and symptoms.

Table 63.2 Clinical Eponyms for Neuroblastoma Presentation	
Dumbbell tumor	Paraspinal sympathetic ganglia tumors with invasion through neural foramina
Raccoon eyes	Proptosis and periorbital ecchymosis from retrobulbar/orbital bone metastases
Blueberry muffin	Cutaneous metastasis causing a blue skin discoloration (usually infants)
Pepper syndrome	Liver metastases with hepatomegaly leading to respiratory distress
Horner syndrome	Ipsilateral ptosis, miosis, and anhidrosis due to cervical ganglion tumor
Hutchinson sign	Limping and irritability due to bone or bone marrow metastases
Opsoclonus–myoclonus	Paraneoplastic syndrome (antineural antibodies) of myoclonic jerking, random eye movement, and truncal ataxia; can persist even after cure
Kerner–Morrison sign	Intractable secretory diarrhea, hypokalemia, dehydration due to VIP secretion

WORKUP: H&P with attention to child development and signs/symptoms as in the preceding table.

Labs: CBC, CMP, LDH, serum ferritin, urinary catecholamines. Elevated urinary catecholamines (including HVA or VMA) can be detected in 90% to 95% of patients.

Imaging: CT and/or MRI of the primary site; CT chest, abdomen, pelvis. PET/CT is not standard. MIBG scintigraphy labeled with I-123 is recommended for assessment of the primary and metastatic sites (sensitivity 90%, specificity ~100%).[14,15] MIBG is a norepinephrine analogue that is concentrated in cells of neural crest origin. MIBG may distinguish residual active tumor from necrotic tumor or scar tissue and is more sensitive than Tc-99 bone scans for assessing the response of cortical bone mets to treatment.[16] The Curie score (CS) is an MIBG scoring method quantifying the extent of MIBG uptake in nine subdivided areas of the skeleton.[17,18] It has been adapted for use in COG trials, and postinduction CS ≥2 was associated with inferior EFS on COG A3973 in patients with stage 4 NB.[19] Bone scan is not required unless primary tumor is not MIBG-avid.

Pathology: Biopsy indicated when resection at diagnosis is not possible. FNA is not adequate. Bilateral bone marrow biopsy. Increased urinary HVA/VMA in conjunction with compatible tumor cells in the bone marrow can be sufficient for establishing diagnosis without biopsy.[20]

PROGNOSTIC FACTORS: See Table 63.3.

Table 63.3 Neuroblastoma Prognostic Factors[6,19,21-28]	
Favorable	**Unfavorable**
Younger age (<1 year)	Older age (>5 years)
Low MKI	High MKI
Differentiated neuroblasts	Undifferentiated neuroblasts
Stromal pattern: rich and nonnodular	Stromal pattern: poor and nodular
1p intact	1p deleted
MYCN nonamplified (MYCN-NA)	MYCN amplified (MYCN-A)
Hypo/hyperdiploid (DNA index <1 or >1)	Diploid (DNA index 1)
TRK amplification	17q gain; 11q LOH
Stage 1, 2, 4S	Stage 3, 4
Thorax primary, multifocal	H&N primary
Skin, liver, bone marrow mets	Bone, CNS, orbit, pleura, lung mets
Low NSE and ferritin	High NSE (>100) or ferritin (>143)

NATURAL HISTORY: Seventy percent of patients present with metastatic disease, with bone marrow mets seen in 80% to 90%. Positive LNs in 35%. The abdomen is the most common primary site (50%–80%). Other common sites include adrenal gland (35%), low-thoracic or abdominal paraspinal ganglia (30%–35%), posterior mediastinum (20%), pelvis (2%), cervical spine (1%), and other sites (12%).[29] Spontaneous regression may occur, especially in infants with 4S disease.[30] The 5-year OS is 71% in the modern era, but attributable mainly to increased cure rates in patients with less aggressive disease.[31] Relapsed patients can often be managed with chronic disease for years, but long-term DFS after relapse is rare.

STAGING: The International NB Risk Group Staging Systemic (INRGSS) is a simplified staging system based on preoperative evaluation and extent of disease determined by image-defined risk factors (IDRFs).[32] This is the staging system used in active protocols. The International NB Staging System (INSS) can be used for staging but is included mostly for historical perspective (Tables 63.4 and 63.5). The INSS staging system was further classified into low, intermediate, and high-risk groups by the COG, and treatment is determined by risk stratification (see protocols for details). Factors incorporated into the most recent COG risk grouping include **S**tage, **A**ge, **N**-myc, **D**NA ploidy, and **S**himada histology (mnemonic "**SANDS**": from trials ANBL00B1, ANBL0531, and ANBL0532). Patients with amplified N-myc are always high risk.

INRGSS Image-Defined Risk Factors (IDRFS)[28]

- Ipsilateral tumor extension within two body compartments: neck and chest, chest and abdomen, abdomen and pelvis
- Infiltration of adjacent organs/structures: pericardium, diaphragm, kidney, liver, duodenopancreatic block, mesentery
- Encasement of major vessels by tumor: vertebral artery, internal jugular vein, subclavian vessels, carotid artery, aorta, vena cava, major thoracic vessels, iliac vessels, branches of the superior mesenteric artery at its root and the celiac axis
- Compression of trachea or central bronchi
- Encasement of brachial plexus

- Infiltration of porta hepatis or hepatoduodenal ligament
- Infiltration of the costovertebral junction between T9 and T12
- Tumor crossing the sciatic notch
- Tumor invading renal pedicle
- Extension of tumor to base of skull
- Intraspinal tumor extension with more than one-third spinal canal invasion, leptomeningeal space obliteration, or abnormal spinal cord MRI signal

Table 63.4 Comparison of INSS[33] and More Recent INRGSS[32]

INSS (1993; Postoperative)		INRGSS (2009; Preoperative)	
1	Tumor on one side of the body. Complete resection (microscopic disease allowed). Ipsilateral LNs histologically negative (nodes adherent to and removed with the primary tumor may be positive).	L1	Localized tumor without vital structure involvement as defined by IDRF and limited to one body compartment (neck, chest, abdomen, pelvis).
2A	Same as stage I except residual disease after resection.	L2	Locoregional tumor with one or more IDRFs.
2B	Ipsilateral nonadherent LNs contain tumor. Contralateral LNs must be negative microscopically. Residual disease after resection allowed.		
3	Unresectable unilateral tumor extending across midline (beyond opposite side of the vertebral body) with or without involved regional LNs, OR unilateral tumor with contralateral regional LN involvement, OR midline tumor with bilateral extension by infiltration (unresectable) or by LN involvement.		
4	Dissemination to distant LNs, bone, bone marrow, liver, skin, and/or other organs (except as defined for 4S).	M	Distant metastatic disease (except stage MS).
4S	Localized primary tumor as in stage 1, 2A, or 2B, with dissemination limited to skin, liver, and/or bone marrow (<10% of total nucleated cells on bone biopsy/aspirate). **Limited to infants <1 years old.**	MS	Children <18 months with metastatic disease limited to skin, liver, and/or bone marrow (≤10% marrow cells positive).

Source: Monclair T, Brodeur GM, Ambros PF, et al. The international neuroblastoma risk group (INRG) staging system: an INRG Task Force report. *J Clin Oncol.* 2009;27(2):298–303. doi:10.1200/JCO.2008.16.6876.

Table 63.5 Previous Staging Systems for Neuroblastoma

Evans/Children's Cancer Study Group (CCSG) Clinical Staging		St. Jude/POG Surgical-Pathologic Staging	
I	Tumor confined to organ or structure of origin	A	GTR of primary, with or without microscopic residual; LNs not adherent to primary tumor are negative and liver is negative
II	Tumor extending beyond the organ or structure of origin but not crossing midline and/or involved ipsilateral LNs	B	Grossly unresected primary tumor; LNs not adherent to primary tumor are negative and liver is negative
III	Tumor extending in continuity beyond the midline; regional LN may be involved bilaterally	C	Complete or incomplete resection of primary, nonadherent LN+, liver is negative
IV	Remote disease involving bone, bone marrow, soft tissue, or distant LNs	D	Distant LN, bone, bone marrow, liver, or skin
IV–S	Stage I or II except for presence of mets confined to liver, skin, and/or marrow (does not include non-marrow bone mets)	D(S)	Infants <1 year with stage IV-S disease (as defined in CCSG system)

TREATMENT PARADIGM: See Table 63.6 for treatment overview by risk group.

Observation: Recommended initially for stage 4S, which may spontaneously resolve.

Surgery: Useful for diagnosis, staging, and treatment for LC. Goal is GTR of visible tumor, and regional LNs with maintenance of function as organ preservation is key. Uninvolved contralateral LNs should be sampled, and a liver biopsy should be obtained. Large tumors that encase regional organs or large vessels and "dumbbell" tumors that compress the spinal cord are considered unresectable. Intermediate- and high-risk patients with clinically unresectable disease should undergo initial biopsy/diagnostic surgery, induction CHT, and then delayed/second-look surgery. CR in 66% to 79% of patients after induction CHT. Piecemeal resection may be necessary and is acceptable. STR can still be attempted after CHT. Titanium clips are recommended at sites of residual disease. Note that resection of the primary is no longer required for stage 4S, but a biopsy should be obtained.

Chemotherapy: CHT is used in intermediate- and high-risk patients to shrink primary tumors to facilitate delayed surgery (vs. observation in intermediate risk). Generally, no role for CHT in low-risk patients except for persistent/recurrent disease. Consider CHT for 4S with hepatomegaly. CHT regimen is dependent on protocol (no universal standard). The most common agents are cyclophosphamide (CYC), cisplatin, doxorubicin, and etoposide; others include (but are not limited to) carboplatin, vincristine (VCR), vindesine, ifosfamide, dacarbazine, topotecan, and melphalan. Intensive doses of combination CHT with short intervals between courses should be delivered in high-risk patients. The preferred European regimen is rapid COJEC (cisplatin, VCR, carboplatin, etoposide, CYC) based on improved toxicity profile vs. the MSKCC-N5 regimen (48% vs. 68% grades 3–4 nonhematologic adverse events) with equivalent outcomes.[34] For intermediate-risk patients, disease response (RECIST criteria) is assessed following induction CHT, and the decision is made per protocol regarding additional systemic therapy, surgery, or surveillance. In high-risk patients, myeloablative CHT with autologous SCT improved survival over CHT alone, and tandem transplant improves EFS over single transplantation.[35,36] Single transplant consists of induction CHT with carboplatin/etoposide/melphalan followed by autologous SCT. Tandem transplantation consists of induction CHT with thiotepa/CYC followed by autologous SCT and then dose-reduced carboplatin/etoposide/melphalan followed by autologous SCT.

Differentiation Therapy: NB cell lines can be induced to terminally differentiate on exposure to retinoids. Risk of relapse is reduced in patients who receive isotretinoin, which is now part of standard therapy in high-risk patients.[37]

Immunotherapy: NB cells uniformly express disialoganglioside GD2 on their surface, which creates a target for immunotherapy (IO). Dinutuximab, a chimeric anti-GD2 antibody (ch14.18), is FDA-approved for adjuvant first-line therapy but is associated with significant acute toxicity in the form of capillary leak syndrome and pain. Human (rather than chimeric) forms are under evaluation and may improve tolerance.[38]

Radiation

Indications: RT is indicated for all cases of high-risk NB. The primary site is always irradiated. Persistently active metastatic sites (either MIBG uptake or soft tissue mass >1cm^3) prior to transplant are also irradiated. If there are more than five persistently active sites pretransplant, a repeat scan is recommended posttransplant. The primary and selected metastatic sites that meet criteria for treatment should be irradiated concurrently. In intermediate-risk patients, RT is delivered to recurrent or gross residual disease. Adjuvant RT is not indicated for low- or intermediate-risk disease unless urgent symptomatic (life/organ-threatening) concerns exist, and the patient is unable to receive CHT or has an insignificant response to CHT (i.e., liver mets with respiratory compromise or cord compression).

Dose: A dose of 21.6 Gy/12 fx daily (COG). High-risk protocol ANBL0532 allowed a boost to 36 Gy for gross residual disease after surgery >1 cc (21.6 Gy to preop GTV, then 14.4 Gy boost); however, this did not improve the 5-year cumulative incidence of local progression.[39] A recent study treated high-risk patients to 18 Gy at 1.5 Gy/fx BID, and this did not result in compromised LC or OS[40]; however, only 25 patients were enrolled and larger prospective studies for validation are warranted. As a result, the ongoing COG 2131 study allows for a dose reduction to 18 Gy for patients who undergo a GTR. Treatment volume is the *post-CHT GTV prior to attempted surgical resection.* If primary was grossly resected at diagnosis, GTV is the preop volume. Volume can be shaved out of normal tissues occupying space previously occupied by tumor (if the normal tissue was not infiltrated). CTV is the GTV + 1 cm margin (PTV is 0.3–0.8 cm). COG protocols recommend treating the vertebral body overlapping with the 10 Gy isodose line to at least 18 Gy. For hepatic metastases causing respiratory compromise or orbit/optic pathway disease leading to vision loss requiring emergent RT: 4.5 Gy/3 fx. For cord compression, CHT is preferred followed by surgical decompression.

Toxicity: Acute: diarrhea, nausea, vomiting, erythema, fatigue, myelosuppression. Late: bony/ soft tissue hypoplasia, scoliosis/kyphosis, slipped capital femoral epiphysis, short stature, second malignancy, renal impairment, renal insufficiency; others are location-dependent.

Targeted Radionuclides: I-131 MIBG therapy has shown response rates of 30% to 40% in otherwise refractory patients and is being investigated before resection or in combination with SCT for consolidation.[41]

Table 63.6 Neuroblastoma Treatment Overview by Risk Group

Low risk (5-yr OS >95%): Patients with stage 4S/MS disease may undergo spontaneous disease regression and can be observed (or given short-course CHT for hepatomegaly). No benefit from resection of primary (may biopsy skin nodule) for stage 4S. For other low-risk patients, *surgery alone* is usually recommended.[25,42] Adjuvant RT has not improved outcomes after GTR and is not indicated for STR or positive margins. CHT indicated for symptomatic patients or disease progression. RT reserved for CHT-resistant tumor.

Intermediate risk (3-yr OS 95%): Surgery first if possible and CHT (without RT) is standard. If primary is unresectable, biopsy → CHT → delayed surgery or observation. CHT is typically given for approximately four cycles for favorable histology tumors and eight cycles for unfavorable histology. RT if persistent or worsening symptoms despite other therapy (per ANBL0531).

High risk (3-yr OS 30%–50%): Paradigm includes combined modality therapy with intensive platinum-based multiagent induction CHT, delayed surgery, myeloablative CHT and autologous SCT (often twice, "tandem"), RT to primary site and residual mets, then isotretinoin and IO. CHT has a response rate of 70%–80%. Exact timing of RT is not well-established, but usually delivered after autologous SCT when disease burden is minimal. RT should be delivered to the primary site even if the patient has undergone GTR. RT should also be delivered to metastatic sites with persistent active disease (+ MIBG) after induction CHT. Adjuvant 13-cis-retinoic acid (isotretinoin) and anti-GD-2 monoclonal antibody improve EFS and OS, respectively, in those without progression.[35,36,43–45] Patients can have recurrent disease after completion of aggressive treatment.

EVIDENCE-BASED Q&A

HIGH RISK

What is the role of autologous SCT and adjuvant isotretinoin in high-risk disease?

Matthay, CCG 3891 (*NEJM* 1999, PMID 10519894; Update *JCO* 2009, PMID 19171716): Prospective study of 539 patients with high-risk NB. Induction CHT consisted of cisplatin, doxorubicin, etoposide, and CYC × 5 cycles, then patients without progression underwent delayed primary surgery with nodal assessment, followed by RT to gross residual disease. RT dose was 20 Gy/10 fx to extra-abdominal disease and 10 Gy/5 fx to mediastinal and intra-abdominal tumors. Patients were subsequently randomized to consolidation CHT or myeloablative CHT + TBI with SCT. Consolidation CHT consisted of three cycles of cisplatin, etoposide, doxorubicin, and ifosfamide. Myeloablative CHT was carboplatin and etoposide. TBI 10 Gy/3 fx daily. Following SCT or consolidation CHT, patients without disease progression were randomized to six cycles of 13-cis-retinoic acid (isotretinoin) or no further therapy. The 5-year EFS and OS rates for all patients were 26% and 36%, respectively. The 5-year LRR was 51% for patients treated with CHT vs. 33% for patients treated with SCT ($p = .0044$). The 3-year EFS improved with both SCT and the addition of 13-cis-retinoic acid (see Table 63.7). The 2009 update demonstrated improvement in 5-year EFS with SCT (30% vs. 19%, $p = .04$) and trended toward an EFS benefit with isotretinoin (42% vs. 31%, $p = .12$), **Conclusions: This study set the standard treatment regimen for high-risk NB, which includes both autologous SCT and isotretinoin.**

Table 63.7 Results of Matthay CCG 3891

CCG 3891	3-Yr EFS	5-Yr LRR	5-Yr OS	Second Randomization	3-Yr EFS	5-Yr OS
CHT	22%	51%	30%	13-cis-RA	46%	50%
HDC + ABMT	34%	33%	39%	No therapy	29%	39%
p value	.034	.004	.39	*p* value	.027	.19

Why are doses above 20 Gy recommended to control gross disease?

Historically, there appeared to be a benefit to the addition of 10 Gy TBI when only 10 Gy consolidative RT was used (therefore 20 Gy of RT total). RRs show good LC with doses >21 Gy. A recent study treated high-risk patients to 18 Gy and did not result in compromised LC or OS[40]; however, larger prospective studies are warranted.

Haas-Kogan, Secondary Analysis of CCG 3891/Matthay (*IJROBP*** 2003, PMID 12694821):** Secondary analysis of the Matthay CCG 3891 focusing on those who received 10 Gy to the primary (abdominal and mediastinal tumors with gross disease remaining postoperatively). For patients who received 10 Gy to the primary, the addition of 10 Gy of TBI and BMT decreased LR compared with those who received continuous CHT and no TBI (22% vs. 52%, *p* = .022). **Conclusion: There may be a dose–response relationship for EBRT (20 Gy better LC than 10 Gy).**

Wolden (*Pediatr Blood & Cancer*** 2018, PMID 29469198):** RR of 19 high-risk patients who received consolidation RT after STR of the primary to evaluate LC after 21 to 36 Gy. The 5-year cumulative LF was 17%; 30% LF in those receiving <30 Gy vs. 0% in those who received 30 to 36 Gy (*p* = .12). **Conclusion: A dose of 30 to 36 Gy is likely needed for optimal control of gross residual disease during consolidation in high-risk disease.**

Casey, MSKCC (*IJROBP*** 2019, PMID 30763661):** Prospective dose-reduction protocol at MSKCC for 25 high-risk NB patients after GTR; patients treated with 18 Gy BID over 6 days; primary objective to assess LC and patterns of failure. MFU 3.5 years. No failures within the RT field, three with marginal recurrence. The 3-year PFS and OS rates were 55% and 91% for patients in first CR (from induction CHT) and 43% and 76% for those not in metastatic CR. **Conclusion: Reduced-dose RT (18 Gy) with accelerated hyperfractionation did not compromise LC or survival in HR-NB patients after GTR.** *Comment: This was further investigated and presented at ASTRO 2024 (Jackson et al.), with 53 patients receiving dose reduction 15 Gy BID over 5 days, MFU 22 months, and 83% receiving protons. Four patients had LF at primary site at a median of 5.5 months. Estimated risk of LF at 2 years after RT was 8%. No acute toxicities above grade 2, and no late toxicities. More follow-up is needed.*

Is there a benefit with a boost to gross residual tumor after induction therapy?

Based on a retrospective comparative analysis of LRC among patients who underwent an incomplete resection on GOG A3973 and ANBL0532, there appears to be no benefit. The ongoing SIOPEN HR-NBL2 phase III trial will evaluate the role of a boost by randomizing patients who have undergone an incomplete resection to 21.6 Gy plus 14.4 Gy boost vs. no boost to residual gross disease.

Liu, COG ANBL0532 (*JCO*** 2020, PMID 32530765):** PRT of children with high-risk NB who received an increased local dose to residual primary tumor. Patients randomized to autologous SCT vs. tandem SCT after induction CHT. RT was then delivered to 21.6 Gy to preoperative tumor volume and an additional boost of 14.4 Gy to any gross residual disease for a total dose of 36 Gy. Primary endpoint of cumulative incidence of local progression (CILP). CILP, EFS, and OS were compared with the historical control COG A3973, where only 21.6 Gy was delivered without a boost. 323 patients received RT. The 5-year CILP, EFS, and OS rates of ANBL0532 and COG A3973 are shown in Table 63.8. **Conclusion: RT boost of gross residual disease after induction therapy does not significantly improve 5-year CILP.**

Table 63.8 Comparative 5-Yr Results of ANBL0532 vs. A3973						
Patients Receiving RT (*n* = 323 for ANBL0532 and *n* = 328 for A3973)				**RT After Incomplete Resection** (*n* = 74 for ANBL0532 and *n* = 47 for A3973)		
	CILP	**EFS**	**OS**	**CILP**	**EFS**	**OS**
COG ANBL0532	11%	56%	68%	16%	51%	68%
COG A3973	7%	47%	57%	11%	49%	57%
p value	.059	.009	.0088	.4126	.5084	.2835

Is there a benefit to tandem stem cell transplants?

Park, COG ANBL 0532 (*JAMA* 2019, PMID 31454045): PRT of 355 children with high-risk NB randomized to single autologous SCT vs. tandem SCT; median age 3 years. Tandem SCT improved 3-year EFS from 48% to 62% (*p* = .006). Only 70% were able to receive subsequent IO, and they had superior EFS than those not receiving IO. Improvement in EFS with tandem transplant persisted in the subgroup receiving IO. There was no OS benefit to tandem transplant (69% vs. 76%, *p* = .25); however, if patients ultimately received IO, a survival advantage was observed with tandem transplant (84% vs. 74%, *p* = .04). There was no significant difference in toxicity between the two regimens. **Conclusion: Tandem SCT improves EFS in patients with high-risk NB, even in the presence of IO.**

Is there a benefit to targeted immunotherapy in high-risk patients?

Dinutuximab (Ch14.18), a chimeric anti-GD2 antibody, improves OS but at the cost of high acute toxicity in the form of pain and capillary leak syndrome.

Yu, COG ANBL0032 (*NEJM* 2010, PMID 20879881; Update *Clin Cancer Res*, PMID 33504555): PRT of 226 patients randomized to IO vs. standard therapy after myeloablative therapy and stem cell rescue. The IO arm was ch14.18 (dinutuximab) with alternating GM-CSF and IL-2 (to stimulate Ab-dependent cell-mediated cytotoxicity) + isotretinoin vs. isotretinoin alone (standard arm). Ch14.18 is a chimeric anti-GD2 monoclonal Ab; GD2 is a surface protein on tissues of neuroectodermal origin.[46] IO improved 2-year EFS (66% vs. 46%, *p* = .01) and 2-year OS (86% vs. 75%, *p* = .02). Grade 3 to 4 pain was higher in the IO arm, with 52% of patients having grade 3 or 4 pain. Additionally, 23% and 25% of patients in that arm had capillary leak syndrome and hypersensitivity reaction, respectively. Early in the study, two patients were inadvertently given an overdose of IL-2 (>20 times the intended dose), with one of these patients consequently experiencing grade 5 toxicity in the form of capillary leak with pulmonary edema. **Conclusion: IO with anti-GD2 monoclonal antibodies shows improved outcomes compared with standard therapy.** *Comment: Closed early due to highly favorable results. The FDA approved ch14.18 (dinutuximab) in 2015 for use in combination with GM-CSF, IL-2, and isotretinoin for high-risk NB patients who achieve at least a partial response to standard multimodality therapy.[43] The update with 5-year EFS and OS demonstrates continued improvement in outcomes with the experimental arm: 5-year EFS 57% vs. 46%, p = .04; 5-year OS 73% vs. 57%, p = .045. Given the demonstrated OS benefit of adding dinutuximab in the maintenance setting, the ongoing COG ANBL 2131 phase III trial is assessing the role of adding dinutuximab to induction CHT.*

Is there a benefit to MIBG with I-131 or crizotinib in high-risk NB?

This is the question of the ongoing study COG ANBL1531. Iobenguane I-131 is essentially therapeutic MIBG including I-131 (diagnostic MIBG includes I-123) and has shown dramatic responses in relapsed/refractory cases. Crizotinib is active against ALK mutated tumors.[47]

INTERMEDIATE RISK

Is RT beneficial for intermediate-risk disease?

RT was shown to increase both EFS and OS when added to adjuvant CHT in the Castleberry study of POG C patients. However, in the modern era, additional genetic/biological risk stratification factors (such as N-myc status) are used to better risk-stratify patients. Thus, the current intermediate-risk patients (in whom RT is not a standard component of first-line therapy) are not the same group of patients as those in the Castleberry study. As in low-risk patients, RT is typically reserved for residual disease refractory to CHT, recurrent disease, or those who remain symptomatic.

Castleberry, POG (*JCO* 1991, PMID 2016621): PRT of 62 patients >1 year of age with POG stage C NB comparing surgery and CHT ± RT. All patients received AC CHT × 5 cycles. Patients randomized to RT received treatment to primary tumor and regional LNs. Age 12 to 24 months: total dose 18 to 24 Gy; age ≥24 months: total dose 24 to 30 Gy, with lower doses reserved for abdominal or thoracic paravertebral primary and SCV nodes. Second-look surgery was advised to evaluate response and to remove residual disease. Continuation CHT alternated AC with CDDP/teniposide for two courses each. Differences in CR, EFS, and OS rates were significant (see Table 63.9). **Conclusion: Children**

>1 year of age with POG stage C NB are a higher risk group in whom the addition of RT to CHT provides superior initial and long-term control compared with CHT alone. Metastatic failures in both treatment groups suggest a need for more aggressive CHT.

Table 63.9 Results of Castleberry Trial, RT for Intermediate-Risk Neuroblastoma			
	CR	**EFS**	**OS**
RT	76%	59%	73%
No RT	46%	32%	41%
p value	.013	.009	.008

Twist, COG ANBL0531 (*JCO* 2019, PMID 31386611): Phase III trial of 404 intermediate-risk patients with NB. Goal was to reduce therapy for subsets of patients using biology and a response-based algorithm, while maintaining 3-year OS of ≥95%. MYCN-amplified tumors were excluded. Stratification based on age, INSS stage, histology, N-myc status, LOH of 1p and/or 11q, and tumor ploidy. Treatment was CHT (± isotretinoin) × 2, 4, or 8 cycles and/or surgery based on prognostic markers. Prognostic markers included allelic status of 1p and 11q. The 3-year EFS and OS rates were 83% and 95%, respectively, for the entire cohort. OS for patients with localized disease was 100%. Infants with stage 4 tumors with favorable biology had a superior 3-year EFS compared with patients with ≥1 unfavorable biological features. **Conclusion: Favorable biological factors can tailor treatment strategies.**

LOW RISK

What is the treatment paradigm for low-risk disease?

Low-risk disease is the most common presentation of NB. Surgery is the mainstay of therapy if the tumor is deemed resectable. Residual disease may be observed if patient is ≤18 months old and has favorable risk factors (favorable histology and nondiploid tumors). CHT is reserved for unresectable, unfavorable, symptomatic, or progressive/recurrent disease. There is no role for routine adjuvant RT in low-risk patients, given the outcomes with salvage therapy.

Strother, COG P9641 (*JCO* 2012, PMID 22529259): 915 children with stage 2A and 2B disease underwent maximally safe resection with adjuvant CHT given if <50% resection at diagnosis, or with unresectable progressive disease after surgery. The 5-year EFS and OS rates were 89% and 97%, respectively. Patients with 2B disease who were >18 months old had significantly lower OS. Patients with unfavorable histology or diploid tumors had significantly lower EFS and OS. **Conclusion: Patients >18 months old with stage 2B disease or those with unfavorable histology or diploid tumors have higher rates of recurrence with observation after surgery, and adjuvant CHT may be warranted.**

Perez, CCG 3881 (*JCO* 2000, PMID 10623689): Prospective trial of 374 children with stage I to II NB. All children without N-myc amplification were treated with surgery alone, but laminotomy or RT was recommended if there was cord compression. Stage II patients <1 year with N-myc amplification received induction CHT, surgery, and RT to gross residual after surgery. Stage II patients >1 year with N-myc amplification were treated on CCG 3891 (see above). Results (Table 63.10): Recurrences among stage II patients were managed successfully in 38 of 43 children. Supplemental treatment necessary in only 10% of stage I and 20% of stage II. N-myc amplification, unfavorable histopathology, age >2, and LN+ predicted for a lower OS in stage II. **Conclusion: Stage I and II diseases represent a biologically favorable group with excellent prognosis. Surgery alone is sufficient initial treatment, regardless of other clinical or biological factors, with an OS of 99% for stage I and 98% for stage II.**

Table 63.10 Results of CCG 3881 Neuroblastoma			
	4-Yr EFS	**4-Yr OS**	**Deaths**
Stage I	93%	99%	1
Stage II	81%	98%	6
p value	.002	NS	

STAGE 4S

What are the outcomes for stage 4S disease?

Patients <1 year of age presenting with abdominal tumors can still have excellent outcomes (3-year EFS and OS >95%) if observed closely. Katzenstein et al. showed that patients who may require intervention are those who are symptomatic from their disease (hepatomegaly), very young (<2 months), or have unfavorable histology. The concern with very young patients is that they have a higher risk of rapid clinical decline without intervention. If CHT is given for symptomatic disease, it is generally given until cessation of symptoms. Early results of COG-ANBL0531 for patients with 4S disappointingly showed a lower 2-year OS of 81%, which was thought to be due to inclusion of patients who could not undergo biopsy due to poor clinical factors previously excluded from prior trials (see intermediate risk).

Katzenstein, POG Experience (*JCO* 1998, PMID 9626197): RR of 110 patients with stage D(S) NB registered on POG protocols. The 3-year OS was 85%. OS was 71% for patients ≤2 months of age, 68% for patients with diploid tumors, 44% for patients with N-myc amplification, and 33% for patients with unfavorable histology. No difference in OS between those who received CHT vs. no CHT (82% vs. 93%, *p* = .187), or between those who underwent GTR of primary tumor vs. STR/biopsy (90% vs. 78%, *p* = .083). **Conclusion: Survival of infants with stage D(S) NB is good. However, prognosis is poor in those of very young age and those with unfavorable biological factors.**

Nickerson, CCG 3881 (*JCO* 2000, PMID 10653863): Prospective study of 77 patients with stage 4S NB treated with supportive care only (*n* = 44), CHT (CYC 5 mg/kg/day × 5 days) + hepatic RT (4.5 Gy/3 fx; *n* = 22), CHT alone (*n* = 10), or RT alone (*n* = 1). The 5-year EFS was 86% and the 5-year OS was 92%. In 44 patients undergoing supportive care only, OS was 100%, compared with 81% for those requiring CHT for symptoms (*p* = .005). Five of six deaths occurred in patients <2 months of age. Patients aged ≤3 months at diagnosis had decreased EFS. The only factor predictive of improved OS was favorable Shimada histopathologic classification. **Conclusion: Minimal treatment is appropriate for infants with stage 4S NB disease except those <2 months with progressive abdominal disease.**

Nutchtern, COG-ANBL00P2 (*Ann Surg* 2012, PMID 22964741): Prospective trial of 87 patients with small adrenal masses and <6 months of age whose parents elected for observation or surgical resection. Followed by abdominal ultrasound and VMA/HMA measurements. Referred to surgery if >50% increase in mass volume OR >50% increase in urine catecholamine levels OR HMA:VMA ratio >2. Eighty-three patients were observed overall, with 16 (19%) ultimately requiring surgery. Of those, eight (50%) had stage I NB, one had stage 2B and one had 4S, two had low-grade adrenocortical neoplasm, and four were benign. MFU 3.2 years; 3-year EFS 98% and OS 100%. **Conclusion: Most infants <6 months with small adrenal masses can have excellent outcomes if closely observed without surgery.**

REFERENCES

1. Mahapatra S, CK. Neuroblastoma. *StatPearls*. https://www.ncbi.nlm.nih.gov/books/NBK448111
2. Heck JE, Ritz B, Hung RJ, Hashibe M, Boffetta P. The epidemiology of neuroblastoma: a review. *Paediatr Perinat Epidemiol*. 2009;23(2):125–143. doi:10.1111/j.1365-3016.2008.00983.x
3. Cook MN, Olshan AF, Guess HA, et al. Maternal medication use and neuroblastoma in offspring. *Am J Epidemiol*. 2004;159(8):721–731. doi:10.1093/aje/kwh108
4. Maris JM, Chatten J, Meadows AT, Biegel JA, Brodeur GM. Familial neuroblastoma: a three-generation pedigree and a further association with Hirschsprung disease. *Med Pediatr Oncol*. 1997;28(1):1–5. doi:10.1002/(SICI)1096-911X(199701)28:1<1::AID-MPO1>3.0.CO;2-P
5. Shimada H. Tumors of the neuroblastoma group. *Pathology (Phila)*. 1993;2(1):43–59. PMID: 9420930
6. Shimada H, Ambros IM, Dehner LP, et al. The international neuroblastoma pathology classification (the Shimada system). *Cancer*. 1999;86(2):364–372. PMID: 10421273
7. Hachitanda Y, Tsuneyoshi M, Enjoji M. Expression of pan-neuroendocrine proteins in 53 neuroblastic tumors: an immunohistochemical study with neuron-specific enolase, chromogranin, and synaptophysin. *Arch Pathol Lab Med*. 1989;113(4):381–384. PMID: 2495784
8. Sebire NJ, Gibson S, Rampling D, Williams S, Malone M, Ramsay AD. Immunohistochemical findings in embryonal small round cell tumors with molecular diagnostic confirmation. *Appl Immunohistochem Mol Morphol*. 2005;13(1):1–5. doi:10.1097/00129039-200503000-00001

9. Maris JM. Recent advances in neuroblastoma. *N Engl J Med*. 2010;362(23):2202–2211. doi:10.1056/NEJMra0804577

10. Hachitanda Y, Tsuneyoshi M, Enjoji M. An ultrastructural and immunohistochemical evaluation of cytodifferentiation in neuroblastic tumors. *Mod Pathol*. 1989;2(1):13–19. PMID: 2922387

11. Brodeur GM, Seeger RC, Schwab M, Varmus HE, Bishop JM. Amplification of N-myc in untreated human neuroblastomas correlates with advanced disease stage. *Science*. 1984;224(4653):1121–1124. doi:10.1126/science.6719137

12. Peifer M, Hertwig F, Roels F, et al. Telomerase activation by genomic rearrangements in high-risk neuroblastoma. *Nature*. 2015;526(7575):700–704. doi:10.1038/nature14980

13. Valentijn LJ, Koster J, Zwijnenburg DA, et al. TERT rearrangements are frequent in neuroblastoma and identify aggressive tumors. *Nat Genet*. 2015;47(12):1411–1414. doi:10.1038/ng.3438

14. Vik TA, Pfluger T, Kadota R, et al. (123)I-mIBG scintigraphy in patients with known or suspected neuroblastoma: results from a prospective multicenter trial. *Pediatr Blood Cancer*. 2009;52(7):784–790. doi:10.1002/pbc.21932

15. Shapiro B. Summary, conclusions, and future directions of [131I] metaiodobenzylguanidine therapy in the treatment of neural crest tumors. *J Nucl Biol Med*. 1991;35(4):357–363. PMID: 1823858

16. Brisse HJ, McCarville MB, Granata C, et al. Guidelines for imaging and staging of neuroblastic tumors: consensus report from the International Neuroblastoma Risk Group Project. *Radiology*. 2011;261(1):243–257. doi:10.1148/radiol.11101352

17. Yanik GA, Parisi MT, Naranjo A, et al. Validation of postinduction Curie scores in high-risk neuroblastoma: a Children's Oncology Group and SIOPEN Group report on SIOPEN/HR-NBL1. *J Nucl Med*. 2018;59(3):502–508. doi:10.2967/jnumed.117.195883

18. Matthay KK, Edeline V, Lumbroso J, et al. Correlation of early metastatic response by [123I] metaiodobenzylguanidine scintigraphy with overall response and event-free survival in stage IV neuroblastoma. *J Clin Oncol*. 2003;21(13):2486–2491. doi:10.1200/JCO.2003.09.122

19. Yanik GA, Parisi MT, Shulkin BL, et al. Semiquantitative mIBG scoring as a prognostic indicator in patients with stage 4 neuroblastoma: a report from the Children's Oncology Group. *J Nucl Med*. 2013;54(4):541–548. doi:10.2967/jnumed.112.112334

20. Barco S, Gennai I, Reggiardo G, et al. Urinary homovanillic and vanillylmandelic acid in the diagnosis of neuroblastoma: report from the Italian Cooperative Group for Neuroblastoma. *Clin Biochem*. 2014;47(9):848–852. doi:10.1016/j.clinbiochem.2014.04.015

21. Adams GA, Shochat SJ, Smith EI, et al. Thoracic neuroblastoma: a Pediatric Oncology Group study. *J Pediatr Surg*. 1993;28(3):372–378. doi:10.1016/0022-3468(93)90234-C

22. Evans AE, Albo V, D'Angio GJ, et al. Factors influencing survival of children with nonmetastatic neuroblastoma. *Cancer*. 1976;38(2):661–666. doi:10.1002/1097-0142(197608)38:2<661::AID-CNCR2820380206>3.0.CO;2-M

23. Hayes FA, Green A, Hustu HO, Kumar M. Surgicopathologic staging of neuroblastoma: prognostic significance of regional lymph node metastases. *J Pediatr*. 1983;102(1):59–62. doi:10.1016/S0022-3476(83)80287-X

24. Cotterill SJ, Ahrens S, Paulussen M, et al. Prognostic factors in Ewing's tumor of bone: analysis of 975 patients from the European intergroup cooperative ewing's sarcoma study group. *J Clin Oncol*. 2000;18(17):3108–3114. doi:10.1200/JCO.2000.18.17.3108

25. Castleberry RP, Shuster JJ, Altshuler G, et al. Infants with neuroblastoma and regional lymph node metastases have a favorable outlook after limited postoperative chemotherapy: a Pediatric Oncology Group study. *J Clin Oncol*. 1992;10(8):1299–1304. doi:10.1200/JCO.1992.10.8.1299

26. Peuchmaur M, d'Amore ES, Joshi VV, et al. Revision of the International Neuroblastoma Pathology Classification: confirmation of favorable and unfavorable prognostic subsets in ganglioneuroblastoma, nodular. *Cancer*. 2003;98(10):2274–2281. doi:10.1002/cncr.11773

27. Cohn SL, Pearson AD, London WB, et al. The International Neuroblastoma Risk Group (INRG) classification system: an INRG Task Force report. *J Clin Oncol*. 2009;27(2):289–297. doi:10.1200/JCO.2008.16.6785

28. Yoo SY, Kim JS, Sung KW, et al. The degree of tumor volume reduction during the early phase of induction chemotherapy is an independent prognostic factor in patients with high-risk neuroblastoma. *Cancer*. 2013;119(3):656–664. doi:10.1002/cncr.27775

29. Morris JA, Shcochat SJ, Smith EI, et al. Biological variables in thoracic neuroblastoma: a Pediatric Oncology Group study. *J Pediatr Surg*. 1995;30(2):296–303. doi:10.1016/0022-3468(95)90577-4

30. Nickerson HJ, Matthay KK, Seeger RC, et al. Favorable biology and outcome of stage IV-S neuroblastoma with supportive care or minimal therapy: a Children's Cancer Group study. *J Clin Oncol*. 2000;18(3):477–486. doi:10.1200/JCO.2000.18.3.477

31. Horner MJ, Ries LAG, Krapcho M, et al. SEER Cancer Statistics Review, 1975–2006. National Cancer Institute. http://seer.cancer.gov/csr/1975_2006

32. Monclair T, Brodeur GM, Ambros PF, et al. The international neuroblastoma risk group (INRG) staging system: an INRG Task Force report. *J Clin Oncol*. 2009;27(2):298–303. doi:10.1200/JCO.2008.16.6876

33. Brodeur GM, Pritchard J, Berthold F, et al. Revisions of the international criteria for neuroblastoma diagnosis, staging, and response to treatment. *J Clin Oncol.* 1993;11(8):1466–1477. doi:10.1200/JCO.1993.11.8.1466

34. Garaventa A, Poetschger U, Valteau-Couanet D, et al. Randomized trial of two induction therapy regimens for high-risk neuroblastoma: HR-NBL1.5 international society of pediatric oncology European neuroblastoma group study. *J Clin Oncol.* 2021;39(23):2552–2563. doi:10.1200/JCO.20.03144

35. Park JR, Kreissman SG, London WB, et al. Effect of tandem autologous stem cell transplant vs single transplant on event-free survival in patients with high-risk neuroblastoma: a randomized clinical trial. *JAMA.* 2019;322(8):746–755. doi:10.1001/jama.2019.11642

36. Zebrowska U, Balwierz W, Wechowski J, Wieczorek A. Survival benefit of myeloablative therapy with autologous stem cell transplantation in high-risk neuroblastoma: a systematic literature review. *Target Oncol.* 2024;19(2):143–159. doi:10.1007/s11523-024-01033-4

37. Sidell N, Altman A, Haussler MR, Seeger RC. Effects of retinoic acid (RA) on the growth and phenotypic expression of several human neuroblastoma cell lines. *Exp Cell Res.* 1983;148(1):21–30. doi:10.1016/0014-4827(83)90184-2

38. Larrosa C, Mora J, Cheung NK. Global impact of monoclonal antibodies (mAbs) in children: a focus on anti-GD2. *Cancers (Basel).* 2023;15(14):3729. doi:10.3390/cancers15143729

39. Liu KX, Naranjo A, Zhang FF, et al. Prospective evaluation of radiation dose escalation in patients with high-risk neuroblastoma and gross residual disease after surgery: a report from the Children's Oncology Group ANBL0532 study. *J Clin Oncol.* 2020;38(24):2741–2752. doi:10.1200/JCO.19.03316

40. Casey DL, Kushner BH, Cheung NV, et al. Reduced-dose radiation therapy to the primary site is effective for high-risk neuroblastoma: results from a prospective trial. *Int J Radiat Oncol Biol Phys.* 2019;104(2):409–414. doi:10.1016/j.ijrobp.2019.02.004

41. Ussowicz M, Wieczorek A, Dluzniewska A, et al. Factors modifying outcome after MIBG therapy in children with neuroblastoma—a national retrospective study. *Front Oncol.* 2021;11:647361. doi:10.3389/fonc.2021.647361

42. Strother DR, London WB, Schmidt ML, et al. Outcome after surgery alone or with restricted use of chemotherapy for patients with low-risk neuroblastoma: results of Children's Oncology Group study P9641. *J Clin Oncol.* 2012;30(15):1842–1848. doi:10.1200/JCO.2011.37.9990

43. Matthay KK, Villablanca JG, Seeger RC, et al. Treatment of high-risk neuroblastoma with intensive chemotherapy, radiotherapy, autologous bone marrow transplantation, and 13-cis-retinoic acid. *N Engl J Med.* 1999;341(16):1165–1173. doi:10.1056/NEJM199910143411601

44. Ladenstein R, Pötschger U, Gray J, et al. Toxicity and outcome of anti-GD2 antibody ch14.18/CHO in frontline, high-risk patients with neuroblastoma: final results of the phase III immunotherapy randomisation (HR-NBL1/SIOPEN trial). *J Clin Oncol.* 2016;34(15_suppl):10502.

45. Yu AL, Gilman AL, Ozkaynak MF, et al. Anti-GD2 antibody with GM-CSF, interleukin-2, and isotretinoin for neuroblastoma. *N Engl J Med.* 2010;363(14):1324–1334. doi:10.1056/NEJMoa0911123

46. Yang RK, Sondel PM. Anti-GD2 strategy in the treatment of neuroblastoma. *Drugs Future.* 2010;35(8):665. doi:10.1358/dof.2010.035.08.1513490

47. FDA approves first therapy for high-risk neuroblastoma. European Society for Medical Oncology. https://www.esmo.org/oncology-news/archive/fda-approves-first-therapy-for-high-risk-neuroblastoma

64 WILMS TUMOR

Salem Alfaifi, Praveen Pendyala, and Erin S. Murphy

QUICK HIT Wilms tumor (WT) is the most common abdominal tumor in children. It is managed with initial resection, followed by risk-adapted CHT ± RT. CHT is variable and usually consists of vincristine, actinomycin-D, and Adriamycin (with carboplatin/etoposide/cyclophosphamide added on protocol for higher risk patients). RT is delivered based on pathologic findings, as listed in Table 64.1, and should be delivered within 14 days postop. For stage IV, RT can be directed to the abdomen and whole lung separately, based on indications. Stage V is often approached with neoadjuvant CHT first to allow for nephron-sparing surgery.

Table 64.1 General Strategy of Postoperative RT for Wilms Tumor		
Indication	**Target**	**Dose**
Stage III, FH Stage IV, FH with hilar LNs Stage I–IV, UH Recurrent disease Residual flank disease	Flank	10.8 Gy/6 fx (+9 Gy/5 fx boost for diffuse anaplasia)
Surgical spillage Peritoneal seeding Malignant ascites Preoperative rupture	Whole abdomen	10.5 Gy/7 fx (+9 Gy/6 fx boost for diffuse anaplasia age >12 months or + 10.5 Gy/7 fx boost for diffuse unresectable implants)
Lung metastases	Whole lung irradiation	12 Gy/8 fx (10.5 Gy/7 fx if age <1)

EPIDEMIOLOGY: Most common abdominal tumor in children and accounts for 6% of all childhood cancers, with ~500 new cases per year in the United States. Median age at diagnosis: 3 to 4 years for unilateral tumors, 2 to 3 years for bilateral. Seventy-five percent of cases present before age 5. Bilateral cases occur in 4% to 8% of patients at presentation. Females are more commonly affected; F:M is 1.09:1 for unilateral tumors and 1.67:1 for bilateral tumors.[1,2]

RISK FACTORS: Paternal occupation as a machinist or a welder and maternal use of hair dye.[3] Also associated with congenital anomalies in 10% to 15% of cases:

- **WAGR: W**ilms tumor, **A**niridia, **G**U malformations, mental **R**etardation. Caused by alteration of 11p13 with deletion of *WT1* gene (Wilms tumor suppressor gene, important for normal kidney/gonadal development) and *PAX6* (aniridia gene); 30% risk of developing WT.
- **Beckwith–Wiedemann:** Macrosomia, hemihypertrophy, macroglossia, omphalocele, abdominal organomegaly, ear pits/creases. Caused by alteration of 11p15 locus, which causes loss of imprinting of genes; 5% risk of developing WT.
- **Denys–Drash syndrome**: Renal disease (proteinuria during infancy, nephrotic syndrome, renal failure), male pseudohermaphroditism, and Wilms. Caused by alteration of 11p13 locus, causing point mutation in zinc-finger regions of *WT1* gene; 50% to 90% risk of developing WT.[4]

ANATOMY: WT originates from the kidney parenchyma and drains to perinephric and para-aortic LNs.

PATHOLOGY: WT is an embryonic kidney tumor (Table 64.2), classically triphasic with blastemal, epithelial, and stromal elements. WT tends to be lobulated and solid, lacks calcifications, and may have soft and cystic areas. These tumors tend to be very large and often can compress adjacent structures, but only minority of cases show pathologic evidence of organ invasion.[1]

Table 64.2 Pathologic Types of Renal Tumors in Children		
Favorable histology (FH) Wilms tumor	Typical features (blastemal, epithelial, and stromal elements) without anaplastic or sarcomatous components.	
Unfavorable histology (UH) Wilms tumor; anaplastic Wilms tumor	Anaplasia refers to enlargement of nuclei, hyperchromatism of nuclei, and increased mitotic figures.	Focal anaplasia: sharply localized in the primary tumor. Diffuse anaplasia: nonlocalized or localized with significant nuclear unrest in the remainder of the tumor, outside tumor capsule, in metastases, or on random biopsy of the tumor.
Rhabdoid tumor of the kidney (RTK)	Typically diagnosed before 2 years of age with eosinophilic cytoplasm and hyaline globular inclusions (+ vimentin and cytokeratin), associated with primary CNS neoplasms (i.e., ATRT) and *INI1* mutations.	
Clear cell sarcoma of the kidney (CCSK)	4% of all childhood renal tumors.[5] About 5% present with metastases, most commonly in bone (40%–60%), compared with those with WT (2% incidence).[6] Tumor cells with abundant intracytoplasmic vesicles. No specific tumor markers but classically described as "chicken-wire" pattern with undifferentiated cells separated by fibrovascular septa.[7]	
Renal cell carcinoma	Approximately 6% of renal tumors in children, not included in classic studies; treatment is surgery alone, no clear role for adjuvant RT.	

All subtypes except FH are considered "high-risk" tumors.

GENETICS: WT is associated with genetic predisposing conditions in ~10% to 15% of cases.[8]

- Poor prognosis associated with LOH of 1p and/or 16q (worse if both).[9] Those with early-stage disease and loss of 1p16q are treated more aggressively with a three-drug regimen (as for stage III/IV).
- Gain of 1q is associated with inferior survival for unilateral FH WT.[10]
- Although Wilms is associated with inactivation of the *WT1* tumor suppressor gene in 5% to 10% of cases, about one-third of Wilms cases are associated with inactivation of a more recently described tumor suppressor gene *WTX* (unknown gene on X chromosome), which may be involved with normal kidney development. Tumors with *WTX* mutation lack *WT1* mutation. In contrast to *WT1*-associated Wilms, which required biallelic (two-hit) inactivation, *WTX* requires only one hit (i.e., the single X chromosome in males or the active X chromosome in females).[1,11]

SCREENING: If a predisposing condition is present, routine screening for WT is recommended with physical exam and renal US every 3 months until 7 years of age.[12]

CLINICAL PRESENTATION: Abdominal mass (83%), fever (23%), hematuria (21%), abdominal pain (37%). Can also have anemia (due to decreased EPO) and hypertension (from increased renin). See Table 64.3 for comparison between Wilms and neuroblastoma.

Table 64.3 Comparison Between Neuroblastoma and Wilms Tumor	
Neuroblastoma	**Wilms**
Younger children; typically, <2 years old	Slightly older; typically, 3–4 years old
Classic eggshell calcifications on x-ray in 85%	No tumor calcifications (but may have calcifications from hemorrhage)
Displaces kidney ("drooping lily" sign) but does not distort renal architecture	Disrupts renal architecture
Mets to LNs, bone marrow, liver, skin (rarely to lung or brain)	Mets to lung, liver, bone
Frequently crosses midline	Rarely crosses midline

WORKUP: H&P (including assessment for congenital anomalies).

Labs: Urinalysis including urinary catecholamines (to rule out neuroblastoma).

Imaging: Abdominal ultrasound including contralateral kidney and evaluation of thrombosis/extension into renal vein or IVC. MRI, CT chest, abdomen, pelvis, and CXR (studies have relied on whether pulmonary metastases are visible on CXR; positive CT with a negative CXR can present controversy).

Biopsy: In order to avoid local tumor spillage, *do not biopsy* unless unresectable or bilateral disease. If biopsy is necessary, use a posterior approach to avoid abdominal contamination and to contain bleeding or spillage if they occur. Once pathology is available, obtain further workup if CCSK (bone scan) or RTK (MRI brain).

PROGNOSTIC FACTORS: LOH 1p and/or 16q, gain of 1q, higher stage, unfavorable histology, and age >24 months portend a worse prognosis.[13]

STAGING: Two systems exist: National Wilms Tumor Study Group (NWTSG), often referred to as NWTS, and Société Internationale d'Oncologie Pédiatrique (SIOP) staging. The NWTS system is used in the United States and Canada and emphasizes postsurgical, pre-CHT staging to obtain the most "unadulterated" information (extent of primary, degree of anaplasia, presence of unusual histology, ± LNs). The SIOP system is used in Europe and utilizes neoadjuvant treatment with CHT and/or RT in an effort to reduce the extent of disease and increase en bloc resection, but at the expense of losing or obscuring some of the information listed earlier. NWTS staging is currently used by the COG and listed in Table 64.4.

Table 64.4 NWTS/COG Staging for Wilms Tumor		
I	Completely excised tumor with negative margins of resection. Tumor limited to kidney with renal capsule intact, no renal sinus vessel involvement, and no rupture or biopsy prior to removal.	
II	Tumor extends beyond kidney but is completely excised with negative margins. Extension includes penetration to renal capsule or soft tissue of the renal sinus, or tumor is present in blood vessels within the nephrectomy specimen but outside the renal parenchyma (including the renal sinus).	
III	Residual tumor following surgery, confined to abdomen. Any one of the following criteria may be present: • Abdominal or pelvic LNs involved by tumor • Tumor has penetrated through the peritoneal surface • Peritoneal implants are present • Gross or microscopic positive margins • Unresectable disease due to extension into vital structures • Tumor spillage either before or during surgery • Preoperative tumor biopsy (tru-cut, open, or fine needle aspiration) • Piecemeal resection of tumor (including tumor cells found in separately removed adrenal gland or tumor thrombus in separately removed vessel)	**Helpful mnemonic for stage III Wilms (SLURPPIB):** **S:** STR/+margin **L:** LN (abdominal) **U:** Unresectable **R:** Rupture/spillage **P:** Piecemeal resection (including thrombus not removed en bloc) **P:** Preoperative CHT required (unresectable) **I:** Implant (i.e., peritoneal involvement, including peritoneal penetration) **B:** Biopsy
IV	Distant metastases or LN metastases outside the abdomen or pelvis.	
V	Bilateral renal involvement present at diagnosis.	

Source: Data from Halperin EC, Constine LS, Tarbell NJ, Kun LE. *Pediatric radiation oncology.* Lippincott Williams & Wilkins; 2012.

TREATMENT PARADIGM

Surgery: Radical nephrectomy is the initial definitive treatment of choice for WT in the United States. Historically, nephrectomy alone (1930s) achieved cure in only 15% to 30% of patients, but it still may be appropriate in very low-risk patients (stage I FH, nephrectomy weight <550 g, and <2 years at time of diagnosis, 4-year EFS 90%).[14] About 90% to 95% of patients are resectable at diagnosis via wide transverse abdominal incision and radical nephrectomy with assessment of surgical margins and avoidance of spillage via a transperitoneal approach. Tumors that are marginally resectable or with large central necrosis, which may portend increased risk for spillage, may benefit from neoadjuvant therapy with CHT or RT. This is a complex surgery (10% of tumors involve renal vein; 15% involve IVC/atrium). Inspect/palpate abdominal cavity, liver, and LN for extent of tumor spread; examine and palpate opposite kidney; inspect and palpate renal vein to exclude tumor thrombus. Regional LN sampling for accurate staging. Tumor spillage incidence is 15% to 30% and is significantly associated with abdominal recurrence and mortality.[15,16] Incidence of surgical complications with nephrectomy (as per NWTS-4) is 11%. The most common complications are hemorrhage and SBO. Quality of surgery has prognostic importance (e.g., degree of LN sampling, spillage, unnecessary biopsies), and QA among COG surgeons is underway.

Chemotherapy: CHT has improved overall results for WT in the past two decades via NWTS and SIOP studies. In Europe, CHT is typically given preoperatively. In North America, it is given adjuvantly following initial nephrectomy. Preoperative CHT may be required if there is bulky, unresectable disease, bilateral WT, WT in a solitary kidney, or tumor thrombus in the IVC. The use of specific agents varies with risk stratification (Table 64.5). Stage I/II FH is typically treated with vincristine (VCR) and actinomycin-D. Stage III/IV and UH are typically treated with three or more agents, including Adriamycin. Adjuvant CHT should be started within 7 to 14 days of upfront nephrectomy and the timing should be coordinated with RT, if required, to avoid coadministration of full doses of actinomycin-D or Adriamycin with RT.[12]

Radiation: RT formerly played a much larger role in WT and was historically delivered postoperatively to the tumor bed at 2 Gy/day to 40 to 50 Gy. In the modern era, only ~25% of patients with WT are treated with RT (only 15% if metastatic disease is excluded). Traditional start for RT is by day 10 after surgery, no later than day 14, if surgery is designated day 0. A later RT start is linked to increased risk of abdominal recurrence in some studies. RT is given concurrently with VCR and actinomycin-D.

Indications: See Table 64.1. Typically, at least flank RT is indicated for stage III disease, unfavorable histology, or positive margins. Whole abdominal irradiation (WAI) indicated for mnemonic "**SPAR**" (**S**pillage during surgery, **P**eritoneal seeding, malignant **A**scites, or preoperative **R**upture).

Dose[12]: Flank RT dose is 10.8 Gy/6 fx with boost to a total dose of 21.6 Gy for gross residual disease. If ≥16 years old, stage III diffuse anaplasia, or I to III rhabdoid, flank RT dose is 19.8 Gy (+10.8 Gy boost to gross disease; total 30.6 Gy). WAI typically 10.5 Gy/7 fx or 21 Gy/14 fx for diffuse unresectable peritoneal implants. Whole lung irradiation (WLI) indicated for lung metastases at a dose of 12 Gy/8 fx (10.5 Gy if <1 year of age). WLI can be omitted if there is a CR to CHT and the tumor did not have 1q gain or combined LOH at 1p and 16q.[17,18] If WLI and flank are both indicated, can treat flank to 10.5 Gy simultaneous with WLI to 12 Gy or at separate times (do not feather or block to adjust for overlap).

Procedure: See *Handbook of Treatment Planning in Radiation Oncology*, Chapter 12.[19]

Toxicity:

Renal: Approximately 1% of patients with unilateral WT will have end-stage renal disease from chronic renal failure 20 years after diagnosis; 3% for patients with bilateral WT.[20]

Premature Mortality: Risk of death from all causes increased from 5% to 23% at 30 and 50 years of age, respectively, after WT diagnosis; 50% of excess deaths beyond 30 years from diagnosis were attributable to secondary neoplasms and 25% from cardiac diseases.[21]

Cardiac: The risk of CHF increases with increasing total dose of Adriamycin received, increasing amount of RT dose to the heart, and female gender; 1.7% of patients treated with Adriamycin on NWTS-1-4 developed CHF compared with 5.4% in patients treated with WLI.[1,22]

Pulmonary: About 10% of patients with pulmonary mets treated on NWTS-3 developed "diffuse interstitial pneumonitis of unknown etiology" (possibly radiation pneumonitis) after WLI (using 14 Gy). There were four additional cases of diffuse pneumonitis secondary to varicella and PJP. Give trimethoprim/sulfamethoxazole for PJP prophylaxis with WLI. The incidence of pneumonitis has subsequently decreased by reducing the dose of Adriamycin and actinomycin-D given concurrently with RT, as well as reducing WLI dose to 12 Gy.

Hepatic: In SIOP-9, 8% of children developed hepatotoxicity consistent with veno-occlusive disease with the combination of CHT and RT.[23]

Reproductive: Females who receive RT or CHT during childhood for unilateral WT have an increased risk for hypertension complicating pregnancy, fetal malpositioning, and premature labor.[24]

Musculoskeletal: RT is associated with the development of scoliosis and reduction in height, with severity increasing with younger age and increasing dose to the spine.[25]

Second Malignancies: GI, soft tissue sarcomas, and breast cancers are the most frequent secondary neoplasms to develop after treatment.[26] Cumulative incidence of invasive breast cancer for survivors who received lung RT is almost 15% by 40 years of age.[27]

Table 64.5 Summary of Wilms Tumor Treatment Paradigm per COG AREN 0532, AREN 0533, and AREN 0321 Studies[14,17,18,28–30]

Stage	Histology and Clinical Features	Adjuvant CHT	Adjuvant RT
I	Very low-risk tumors: stage I, age <2 years, FH, and tumor weight <550 grams	None	None
	FH but NOT meeting ALL very low risk criteria	EE4A, escalated to DD4A if LOH at 1p and 16q	
	Focal or diffuse anaplasia	DD4A	Flank RT
II	FH	EE4A, escalated to DD4A if LOH at 1p and 16q	None
	Focal anaplasia	DD4A	Flank RT
	Diffuse anaplasia	Regimen M + carboplatin	
III	FH	DD4A, escalated to Regimen M if LOH 1p and 16q	Flank/abdomen RT, boost gross disease
	Focal anaplasia	DD4A	
	Diffuse anaplasia	Regimen M + carboplatin (Regimen UH1)	
IV	FH, no LOH, lung nodules with CR at week 6	DD4A	Flank/abdomen for local stage III features + RT to other metastatic sites; no WLI (AREN 0533)
	FH, with LOH 1p and 16q OR lung nodules without CR at week 6	Regimen M	Flank/abdomen for local stage III features + RT to other metastatic sites + WLI
	Focal anaplasia	Regimen M + carboplatin (Regimen UH1)	
	Diffuse anaplasia	Regimen M + carboplatin + irinotecan (Regimen UH2)	

EVIDENCE-BASED Q&A

What are the findings from the most recent National Wilms Tumor Study (NWTS) 5?

The NWTS studies pooled patients with WT beginning in the 1970s with the goal of optimizing treatment outcomes. NWTS-5, along with AREN 0532, helped define the standard of care for very low-risk patients (stage I FH, <2 years old, and tumors <550 g); both studies showed surgery alone is sufficient treatment in this patient population with excellent survival and effective salvage options.[14,31] NWTS-5 also aimed to further identify and incorporate histologic and genetic markers in order to guide treatment intensification for certain subgroups of patients.

Dome, NWTS-5 (*JCO* 2006, PMID 16710034): Single-arm study of stage I anaplastic histology WT treated with VCR and dactinomycin and stage II to IV WT with anaplasia treated with VCR/Adriamycin/CYC/etoposide plus flank/abdominal RT (10.8 Gy + 10.8 Gy boost to bulky residual tumor). **Conclusion: 4-year EFS and OS for patients with diffuse anaplasia is worse than those with FH, and treatment intensification is warranted.**

Grundy, NWTS-5 (*JCO* 2005, PMID 16129848): Investigated prognostic significance of LOH 1p or 16q in patients with FH. For stages I to II FH, risk of relapse and death increased with LOH at 1p, 16q, or both. For stages III to IV FH, risk of relapse and death increased only with LOH for both 1p and 16q (relative risk = 2.4, p = .01 and relative risk = 2.7, p = .04). **Conclusion: LOH on chr 1p and 16q can be independent prognostic factors given the increased risk of relapse and death.**

What is the impact of RT in the setting of tumor spillage?

RT decreases abdominal tumor recurrence rates after tumor spillage.

Kalapurakal, NWTS 4 and 5 Pooled (*IJROBP* 2010, PMID 19395185): Analyzed influence of RT (flank and WAI) and CHT regimens on abdominal recurrence after intraoperative spillage of FH WT. Crude OR for risk of recurrence after 10 Gy RT vs. no RT was 0.35 (95% CI 0.15–0.78) and 0.08 (0.01–0.58) after 20 Gy. OR for CHT after adjusting for RT was not significant. For stage II patients (NWTS-4), 8-year RFS with and without spillage, respectively, was 79% vs. 87% (p = .07) and OS was 90% vs. 95% (p = .04). **Conclusion: RT (10 Gy or 20 Gy) reduced abdominal tumor recurrence rates after tumor spillage. Tumor spillage in stage II patients is associated with decreased RFS and significantly decreased OS.**

What study helps guide treatment in stage III FH WT?

The previous NWTS studies laid the foundation for the most recent AREN protocol, which incorporated previously identified prognostic factors. The results have helped define the standard of care for Wilms.

Fernandez, AREN 0532 (*JCO* 2018, PMID 29211618): 535 stage III FH WT treated with DD4A and RT. MFU 5.2 years; 4-year EFS and OS estimates 88% and 97%, respectively. Of 66 relapses, 58 occurred in the first 2 years, predominately pulmonary (n = 36). Improved EFS was associated with negative LNs and absence of LOH 1p or 16q (p < .01 for both); 4-year EFS 74% in those with both positive LNs and LOH 1p or 16q. **Conclusion: Overall favorable EFS and OS in stage III FH WT with DD4A and RT. Positive LNs and 1p or 16q LOH were highly predictive of worse EFS and should be considered a potential prognostic marker for future trials.**

What is the role of WLI in patients with FH Wilms who have pulmonary metastases detected by CT only? What is the role of Adriamycin in this setting?

In CT-detected lung metastases, there is no OS benefit with Adriamycin or WLI, though EFS is improved with Adriamycin.

Grundy, NWTS 4 and 5 Pooled (*Pediatr Blood Cancer* 2012, PMID 22422736): 417 patients with FH WT and isolated lung metastases. Compared outcomes by method of detection (CXR vs. CT only), use of WLI, and two- or three-drug CHT (dactinomycin and VCR ± Adriamycin). For patients with CT-only lung mets (negative CXR), 5-year EFS was greater with three drugs (including Adriamycin) with or without WLI vs. only two drugs (80% vs. 56%, p = .004); OS was not impacted (87% vs. 86%, p = .91). In this group, WLI did not improve 5-year EFS when adjusting for CHT regimen used (p = .52). There was no difference in OS with or without WLI. **Conclusion: Patients with CT-only lung mets have improved EFS but not OS with the addition of Adriamycin; they do not seem to benefit from WLI.**

For which patients with lung metastases can WLI be omitted?

WLI may not be necessary for patients with FH WT without 1p16q LOH who have a CR of lung nodules after 6 weeks of CHT.

Dix, AREN 0533 (*JCO* 2018, PMID 29659330): 292 patients with FH WT with isolated lung metastases who received DD4A × 6 weeks. If CR in the lungs, CHT continued without WLI. If PR in the lungs or 1p/16q LOH, they received WLI (12 Gy/8 fx) and four cycles of intensified CHT (Regimen M); 133 had CR and 159 had PR. Among the 133 patients with CR, 4-year EFS and OS estimates were 80% and 96%, respectively. Among the 159 patients with PR, 4-year EFS and OS estimates were 89% and 95%, respectively. **Conclusion: Excellent OS even with omission of WLI in patients with CR after CHT, although more events than anticipated. Patients with PR benefit from WLI and CHT intensification with improvement in EFS and OS.**

How is bilateral WT managed?

Bilateral WT accounts for 5% of cases and is associated with higher rates of ESRD compared with unilateral WT. The 20-year cumulative incidence of ESRD in bilateral WT is 3% (compared with <1% for unilateral

WT) and is even higher in patients with WAGR (50%) and Denys–Drash syndrome (75%).[20,32] AREN0534 utilized induction CHT, surgery, risk-adapted RT, and histology-directed CHT in an effort to maximally preserve renal parenchyma.

Dome, AREN0534 (*Ann Surg* 2017, PMID 28795993): 189 patients with bilateral WT treated with induction VCR, dactinomycin, and doxorubicin for 6 or 12 weeks based on radiographic response followed by surgery and further CHT. RT given for post-CHT stage III and IV disease. The 4-year EFS and OS rates were 82% and 95%, which compared favorably to the 4-year EFS and OS of 56% and 81% on NWTS-5. Twenty-three patients relapsed and seven had disease progression. After induction CHT, 84% underwent definitive surgical treatment in at least one kidney by 12 weeks and 39% retained parts of both kidneys. **Conclusions: Induction CHT followed by surgical resection, risk-adapted RT, and histology-directed postoperative CHT improves EFS, OS, and renal preservation compared with historical outcomes in stage V (bilateral) WT.**

REFERENCES

1. Halperin EC, Wazer DE, Perez CA, Brady LW. *Perez & Brady's Principles and Practice of Radiation Oncology.* 7th ed. Wolters Kluwer; 2019.
2. Siegel RL, Giaquinto AN, Jemal A. Cancer statistics, 2024. *CA Cancer J Clin.* 2024;74(1):12–49. doi:10.3322/caac.21820
3. Bunin GR, Nass CC, Kramer S, Meadows AT. Parental occupation and Wilms' tumor: results of a case-control study. *Cancer Res.* 1989;49(3):725–729. PMID: 2535965
4. Dome JS, Coppes MJ. Recent advances in Wilms tumor genetics. *Curr Opin Pediatr.* 2002;14(1):5–11. doi:10.1097/00008480-200202000-00002
5. Sebire NJ, Vujanic GM. Paediatric renal tumours: recent developments, new entities and pathological features. *Histopathology.* 2009;54(5):516–528. doi:10.1111/j.1365-2559.2008.03110.x
6. Miniati D, Gay AN, Parks KV, et al. Imaging accuracy and incidence of Wilms' and non-Wilms' renal tumors in children. *J Pediatr Surg.* 2008;43(7):1301–1307. doi:10.1016/j.jpedsurg.2008.02.077
7. Boo YJ, Fisher JC, Haley MJ, Cowles RA, Kandel JJ, Yamashiro DJ. Vascular characterization of clear cell sarcoma of the kidney in a child: a case report and review. *J Pediatr Surg.* 2009;44(10):2031–2036. doi:10.1016/j.jpedsurg.2009.06.023
8. Maciaszek JL, Oak N, Nichols KE. Recent advances in Wilms' tumor predisposition. *Hum Mol Genet.* 2020;29(R2):R138–R149. doi:10.1093/hmg/ddaa091
9. Phelps HM, Kaviany S, Borinstein SC, Lovvorn HN III. Biological drivers of Wilms tumor prognosis and treatment. *Children (Basel).* 2018;5(11):145. doi:10.3390/children5110145
10. Gratias EJ, Dome JS, Jennings LJ, et al. Association of chromosome 1q gain with inferior survival in favorable-histology Wilms tumor: a report from the Children's Oncology Group. *J Clin Oncol.* 2016;34(26):3189–3194. doi:10.1200/JCO.2015.66.1140
11. Rivera MN, Kim WJ, Wells J, et al. An X chromosome gene, WTX, is commonly inactivated in Wilms tumor. *Science.* 2007;315(5812):642–645. doi:10.1126/science.1137509
12. National Comprehensive Cancer Network. *NCCN Clinical Practice Guidelines in Oncology: Wilms Tumor (Nephroblastoma).* Version 2.2024; 2024.
13. Dome JS, Perlman EJ, Graf N. Risk stratification for Wilms tumor: current approach and future directions. *Am Soc Clin Oncol Educ Book.* 2014:215–223. doi:10.14694/EdBook_AM.2014.34.215
14. Fernandez CV, Perlman EJ, Mullen EA, et al. Clinical outcome and biological predictors of relapse after nephrectomy only for very low-risk Wilms tumor: a report from Children's Oncology Group AREN0532. *Ann Surg.* 2017;265(4):835–840. doi:10.1097/SLA.0000000000001716
15. Shamberger RC, Guthrie KA, Ritchey ML, et al. Surgery-related factors and local recurrence of Wilms tumor in National Wilms Tumor Study 4. *Ann Surg.* 1999;229(2):292–297. doi:10.1097/00000658-199902000-00019
16. Green DM, Breslow NE, D'Angio GJ, et al. Outcome of patients with stage II/favorable histology Wilms tumor with and without local tumor spill: a report from the National Wilms Tumor Study Group. *Pediatr Blood Cancer.* 2014;61(1):134–139. doi:10.1002/pbc.24658
17. Dix DB, Fernandez CV, Chi YY, et al. Augmentation of therapy for combined loss of heterozygosity 1p and 16q in favorable histology Wilms tumor: a Children's Oncology Group AREN0532 and AREN0533 study report. *J Clin Oncol.* 2019;37(30):2769–2777. doi:10.1200/JCO.18.01972
18. Dix DB, Seibel NL, Chi YY, et al. Treatment of stage IV favorable histology Wilms tumor with lung metastases: a report from the Children's Oncology Group AREN0533 study. *J Clin Oncol.* 2018;36(16):1564–1570. doi:10.1200/JCO.2017.77.1931
19. Videtic GMM, Woody NM, Vassil AD. *Handbook of Treatment Planning in Radiation Oncology.* 3rd ed. Springer Publishing Company; 2020.
20. Lange J, Peterson SM, Takashima JR, et al. Risk factors for end stage renal disease in non-WT1-syndromic Wilms tumor. *J Urol.* 2011;186(2):378–386. doi:10.1016/j.juro.2011.03.110

21. Wong KF, Reulen RC, Winter DL, et al. Risk of adverse health and social outcomes up to 50 years after Wilms tumor: the British Childhood Cancer Survivor Study. *J Clin Oncol.* 2016;34(15):1772–1779. doi:10.1200/JCO.2015.64.4344

22. Green DM, Grigoriev YA, Nan B, et al. Congestive heart failure after treatment for Wilms' tumor: a report from the National Wilms' Tumor Study group. *J Clin Oncol.* 2001;19(7):1926–1934. doi:10.1200/JCO.2001.19.7.1926

23. Bisogno G, de Kraker J, Weirich A, et al. Veno-occlusive disease of the liver in children treated for Wilms tumor. *Med Pediatr Oncol.* 1997;29(4):245–251. doi:10.1002/(SICI)1096-911X(199710)29:4<245::AID-MPO2>3.0.CO;2-M

24. Green DM, Lange JM, Peabody EM, et al. Pregnancy outcome after treatment for Wilms tumor: a report from the National Wilms tumor long-term follow-up study. *J Clin Oncol.* 2010;28(17):2824–2830. doi:10.1200/JCO.2009.27.2922

25. Hogeboom CJ, Grosser SC, Guthrie KA, Thomas PR, D'Angio GJ, Breslow NE. Stature loss following treatment for Wilms Tumor. *Med Pediatr Oncol.* 2001;36(2):295–304. doi:10.1002/1096-911X(20010201)36:2<295::AID-MPO1068>3.0.CO;2-Y

26. Termuhlen AM, Tersak JM, Liu Q, et al. Twenty-five year follow-up of childhood Wilms tumor: a report from the Childhood Cancer Survivor Study. *Pediatr Blood Cancer.* 2011;57(7):1210–1216. doi:10.1002/pbc.23090

27. Lange JM, Takashima JR, Peterson SM, Kalapurakal JA, Green DM, Breslow NE. Breast cancer in female survivors of Wilms tumor: a report from the National Wilms Tumor late effects study. *Cancer.* 2014;120(23):3722–3730. doi:10.1002/cncr.28908

28. Fernandez CV, Mullen EA, Chi YY, et al. Outcome and prognostic factors in stage III favorable-histology Wilms tumor: a report from the Children's Oncology Group Study AREN0532. *J Clin Oncol.* 2018;36(3):254–261. doi:10.1200/JCO.2017.73.7999

29. Daw NC, Chi YY, Kalapurakal JA, et al. Activity of vincristine and irinotecan in diffuse anaplastic Wilms tumor and therapy outcomes of stage II to IV disease: results of the Children's Oncology Group AREN0321 study. *J Clin Oncol.* 2020;38(14):1558–1568. doi:10.1200/JCO.19.01265

30. Daw NC, Chi YY, Kim Y, et al. Treatment of stage I anaplastic Wilms' tumour: a report from the Children's Oncology Group AREN0321 study. *Eur J Cancer.* 2019;118:58–66. doi:10.1016/j.ejca.2019.05.033

31. Shamberger RC, Anderson JR, Breslow NE, et al. Long-term outcomes for infants with very low risk Wilms tumor treated with surgery alone in National Wilms Tumor Study-5. *Ann Surg.* 2010;251(3):555–558. doi:10.1097/SLA.0b013e3181c0e5d7

32. Breslow NE, Collins AJ, Ritchey ML, Grigoriev YA, Peterson SM, Green DM. End stage renal disease in patients with Wilms tumor: results from the National Wilms Tumor Study Group and the United States Renal Data System. *J Urol.* 2005;174(5):1972–1975. doi:10.1097/01.ju.0000176800.00994.3a

65 EWING SARCOMA

Jenna E. Kocsis, Shauna R. Campbell, and Erin S. Murphy

QUICK HIT Ewing sarcoma (EWS) is the second most common primary bone tumor in children. Males are affected more than females, and peak age is 10 to 15 years of age. Important genetic mutations include t(11;22) and t(21;22). Workup includes evaluation of primary site with CT/MRI, PET/CT, bilateral bone marrow biopsies, and biopsy of the primary tumor. The overall treatment paradigm is shown in Table 65.1.

Table 65.1 General Treatment Paradigm for Ewing Sarcoma	
Induction (weeks 1–12)	VDC + IE × 6 cycles
Local control (week 13)	Surgery or RT or combined modality (see Table 65.2)
Consolidation	VDC + IE × 8–11 cycles ASAP after surgery; adjuvant RT (if indicated) starts cycle 1 of consolidation

EPIDEMIOLOGY: Described in 1921 by James Ewing as an undifferentiated tumor involving the diaphysis of long bones that is radiation-sensitive (in contrast to osteosarcoma).[1] Second most common primary bone tumor in children after osteosarcoma and the most lethal bone tumor. Approximately 200 cases per year (~3% of childhood cancers).[2,3] Peak incidence is between 10 and 15 years of age, with 30% of cases arising in children <10 years and another 30% in adults >20 years.[2] More common in Caucasian boys, and the M:F ratio is 1.5:1.[4]

RISK FACTORS: No known environmental or familial risk factors.[5] No convincing evidence of inheritance.

ANATOMY: Approximately 50% originate in an extremity (20%–30% proximal and 30%–40% distal) and ~50% central (45% pelvis, 35% chest wall, 10% spine, <10% remainder). Long bone tumors are usually present in the diaphysis, as opposed to osteosarcoma, which originates in the metaphysis.[6] Mnemonic for bone tumors "EG-MODE": **E**piphysis (**G**iant cell tumor), **M**etaphysis (**O**steosarcoma), **D**iaphysis (**E**wing sarcoma). A minority of EWS arise in soft tissue, and these patients with extraosseous Ewing sarcoma (EES) are more frequently older and female; the tumor often arises more within the axial rather than appendicular skeleton.[7–9] Ewing sarcoma family of tumors (ESFT) includes Ewing sarcoma of bone (ESB), EES, and primitive peripheral PNET (neuroepithelioma, adult neuroblastoma, Askin tumor, and paravertebral small cell tumor). EES has a more favorable prognosis, and localized EES is commonly managed with surgery alone.

PATHOLOGY: Generally, sarcomas are divided into two categories: (a) tumors displaying complex karyotypic abnormalities with no distinct pattern and (b) tumors associated with particular chromosomal translocations that result in specific fusion genes. ESFT belongs to the second category. Although controversial, ESFT is thought to originate from the postganglionic parasympathetic neural cells as opposed to neuroblastoma, which originates from the sympathetic system. An alternative theory is that ESFT originates from mesenchymal progenitor or mesenchymal stem cells.[10] Microscopically, ESFT appears as monomorphic sheets of small round blue cells usually with extensive necrosis, but morphology alone is insufficient for diagnosis. The cells have eosinophilic cytoplasm containing glycogen and stain for PAS. More than 90% of ESFT cells express the MIC2 glycoprotein (CD99). Depending on the degree of neuroectodermal differentiation (more common in PNETs), ESFT cells may also express neural cell markers such as NSE, S100, synaptophysin, CD57, anti-vimentin.[11] Histopathologic types: typical (i.e., classic) vs. atypical (lobular, alveolar, or organoid).[6]

GENETICS: Definitive diagnosis relies on identification of signature chromosomal translocations via FISH or PCR.[12] The defining genetic alteration is translation in the EWSR1 gene, with 85% to 90%

of cases displaying t(11;22)(q24;q12).[13,14] t(21;22)(q21;q12) is the second most common (~5%–10%), with a number of other less common translocations or structural aberrations in the remainder of cases (e.g., t[7;22], t[17;22], gain of chr 8 and 12, deletion of 1p, deletion of CDKN2A, mutations of STAG2 and TP53).[5,15–17] t(11;22)(q24;q12) results in fusion of the FLI-1 gene (DNA-binding transcription factor) on 11q24 with the EWS gene (RNA-binding protein) on 22q12.[18] EWS-FLI-1 is a transcription factor that impacts cell cycle regulation, apoptosis, and telomerase activity.[15] t(21;22)(q21;q12) results in EWS-ERG fusion product and phenotype is identical to EWS-FLI-1. Desmoplastic small round cell tumor, clear cell sarcoma, and malignant melanoma of soft parts also involve an EWSR1 translocation.[19–21] PNETs that are positive for EWSR translocation (CD99+) are classified and treated as peripheral PNET (pPNET), and if negative for the translocation they are a central PNET (cPNET) and treated like an embryonal tumor.

CLINICAL PRESENTATION: Patients often present with local symptoms of pain, stiffness, and/or swelling. Pain can be intermittent and worse at night. Bone or osseous metastatic lesions may present as pathologic fractures. Systemic symptoms include fever and weight loss.[22–24] Approximately 20% to 25% have overt metastases at presentation, most commonly in lung and bone (spine most common). Pelvis primary tumors are more likely to present with metastatic disease; ~25% in pelvic primaries vs. ~16% for other sites.[25] Micrometastases are assumed to be present at diagnosis in nearly all patients because of a high distant failure rate with local therapy alone. The risk of LN metastasis at diagnosis is low.[26] Askin tumor is a primary EWS of the rib that is more common in females. It is associated with direct pleural extension and a large extraosseous soft tissue mass.[6] The differential for EWS includes osteomyelitis, lymphoma of the bone, leukemia (chloroma), rhabdomyosarcoma, metastatic neuroblastoma, small cell osteosarcoma, eosinophilic granuloma, metastatic small cell lung cancer, or mesenchymal chondrosarcoma. Differential for small round blue cell tumors (mnemonic LEMONS): **L**ymphoma, **E**wing's, **M**edulloblastoma, **O**ther (rhabdomyosarcoma, pineoblastoma, ependymoblastoma, etc.), **N**euroblastoma, **S**mall cell carcinoma.

WORKUP: H&P.

Labs: CBC, BMP, LDH.

Imaging: Plain x-ray, CT and MRI of the involved primary site, CT chest, PET/CT preferred.[27] Plain x-ray findings range from lytic (75%) to sclerotic (25%), "moth-eaten," "onion skinning" (layers of reactive bone), "Codman's triangle" (displaced periosteum with cortical destruction; also present in osteosarcoma). It is often associated with a soft tissue mass. CT bone outlines bony destruction and soft tissue extent; enhances with contrast. MRI with contrast allows for better determination of the extent of disease, operability, edema, and involvement of adjacent organs. PET assesses tumor viability, evaluates for metastases (most helpful in LNs and bone), and is the most sensitive test for follow-up after treatment.[28] CT chest is more reliable for lung metastasis compared with PET.[27,29] SUV >5.8 is associated with worse survival.[30]

Procedures: Biopsy of the primary site should be performed by the surgeon who will be resecting the tumor to avoid compromising a subsequent surgery such as limb salvage. FNA provides inadequate diagnostic material, and CT-guided or ultrasound-guided core needle biopsy is instead utilized. Open biopsy should be done only if necrotic material on core. Always include biopsy site in the predicted operative site. If imaging or clinical symptoms demonstrate concern for metastatic disease or bone marrow involvement, consider bone marrow biopsy (at least unilateral).[28,31]

PROGNOSTIC FACTORS: Presence of metastases is the most important (bone or liver worse than lung, and multiple lung lesions worse than solitary).[25] Other poor factors can be remembered with the mnemonic "**MASSS**ive **LDH R**esponse": **M**ale gender, **A**ge >17, pelvic/axial **S**ite, **S**ize >8 cm, **S**tage (+mets), high **LDH**,[32] **R**esponse to CHT (>90% necrosis is a positive prognostic factor).[25,33] Fever, anemia, and elevated LDH correspond with a high volume of disease and worse prognosis.[32,34] Deletion of the short arm of chr 1p, homozygous deletions of CDKN2A and p16/p14ARF, and p53 mutations are associated with a poor response to CHT and worse prognosis.[35–37]

NATURAL HISTORY: Marked improvement in 5-year OS since 1975 (35%) to current 5-year OS (70%–80%) for nonmetastatic patients, principally due to the addition of intensive CHT. Metastases are not uniformly fatal, with average 5-year OS of ~30% in the modern era.[22] Distant failures remain the predominant pattern of failure for large tumors despite aggressive CHT.

STAGING: No formal staging. Stratification is by presence or absence of metastatic disease.

TREATMENT PARADIGM

Patients with localized EWS are treated with induction CHT, LC with surgery, RT, or combined modalities, followed by adjuvant CHT. Patients with metastatic EWS are also treated with multi-modality therapy using induction CHT followed by LC of the primary and limited metastatic sites with surgery and/or RT.

Chemotherapy: Induction CHT is given to all patients. Compressed VDC-IE (q14 days × 6 cycles) is the current standard. Agents: vincristine (VCR; neuropathy, constipation, myalgias, arthralgias, and cholestasis), doxorubicin (myocardial dysfunction and pancytopenia), cyclophosphamide (CYC; pancytopenia, dose-dependent hemorrhagic cystitis, infertility), ifosfamide (high incidence of hemorrhagic cystitis requiring use of Mesna and Fanconi syndrome of electrolyte wasting), etoposide (pancytopenia, anaphylactic reactions, and second malignancies such as AML). No role for further intensification with higher doses of CYC, ifosfamide, or doxorubicin due to increased toxicity and risk of second malignancy without an improvement in EFS and OS.[38] After local therapy, patients should resume systemic therapy as soon as possible given high rates of distant failures. A total of 14 to 17 cycles of CHT (including neoadjuvant cycles) are typically administered.[28]

Surgery: For LC, resection is preferred unless poor functional results are anticipated.[39,40] Resection provides pathologic information post-CHT and avoids second malignancy and late effects of RT. Resection without reconstruction can be done in small bones such as rib, clavicle, proximal fibula, distal scapula, metatarsals, metacarpals, and small iliac wing or pubic bone lesions. Results are typically very good for these "dispensable bones."[41,42] Large lesions may require allograft or endoprosthetic reconstructions. Unresectable disease may become resectable after neoadjuvant CHT, and RT can be considered preoperatively to facilitate the resection. Nodal dissection is not routinely indicated; however, if suggestion of nodal positivity on imaging, surgical pathology should be obtained since this would influence the RT target. In the metastatic setting, surgery may be helpful for limited pulmonary metastases or palliation at primary site.

Radiation: Potentially indicated preop, postop, or definitively for LC of the primary tumor and for treatment of metastases. Indications for postoperative RT (PORT) include close margins (<1 cm), poor histologic response (<90% necrosis), or tumor spill.[27,43] Adjuvant RT starts at the time of consolidation CHT (week 14) with VC-IE CHT given concurrently (doxorubicin held during RT). Preoperative RT is considered when close/positive margins are expected. Treat pre-CHT volume due to high rate of LF if post-CHT volumes are used.[44] Involved field rather than whole bone is sufficient.[45] Definitive RT is indicated for patients with tumors in locations unamenable to surgery with wider resection margins. Whole lung irradiation (WLI) is given as consolidation for patients with pulmonary metastases given an improvement in EFS.[28,46] Consider SRS/SBRT as consolidation for metastases as the EURO-EWING 99 trial showed improved 3-year EFS when LC is given to both the primary and metastatic disease.[47] Dose of RT as per AEWS 1031 in Table 65.2.

Table 65.2 Radiation Therapy Guidelines for Ewing Sarcoma Summary per AEWS 1031			
Situation	**Dose**	**Volumes**	**Concurrent CHT**
Preoperative	36 Gy	Pre-CHT GTV	VC-IE (no doxorubicin when given concurrently)
Definitive	45 Gy Cone down to 55.8 Gy	Pre-CHT GTV Gross residual/post-CHT GTV	VC-IE
Postoperative (i.e., microscopic)	50.4 Gy (>90% necrosis) 50.4 Gy (<90% necrosis)	Post-CHT GTV Pre-CHT GTV	VC-IE
Vertebral body	45 Gy Boost to 50.4 Gy	Pre-CHT GTV + 1 cm (entire VB + 0.5 cm) Post-CHT GTV + 0.5	VC-IE

(continued)

Table 65.2 Radiation Therapy Guidelines for Ewing Sarcoma Summary per AEWS 1031 (*continued*)

Situation	Dose	Volumes	Concurrent CHT
Involved nodal region	45 Gy with cone down to 55.8 Gy 50.4 Gy	LN unresected LN resected	
Lung metastases (per AEWS1221)	15 Gy at 1.5 Gy/fx 45 Gy at 1.8 Gy/fx or 30–40 Gy/5 fx with SBRT	Bilateral lungs (IMRT can be considered) Boost to primary/lung nodules	Hold CHT
Bone metastasis	45–56 Gy (consider SBRT, 40 Gy/5 fx)		

Notes:
– Do not treat across a joint or encompass an extremity circumferentially (spare strip of skin) unless absolutely necessary for tumor coverage.
– For intraoperative spill, boost pre-CHT volume.
– When using PORT, if there is microscopic residual, evaluate necrosis; if >90%, then 14.4 Gy boost to post-CHT GTV; if <90%, then 14.4 Gy boost to pre-CHT GTV.

Rib Primary or Askin Tumor: Do not attempt resection prior to CHT. Preoperative CHT improves negative margins (50% vs. 77%) and decreases need for PORT (5-year EFS 56%).[48] Some treat entire ipsilateral hemithorax (15–18 Gy, 1.5 Gy/fx) before reducing field to complete dose schedule as noted previously, especially if lung metastasis or positive pleural cytology present.[49] Some have used intrapleural colloidal P32 in addition to EBRT to spare lung while treating pleura. Include all areas of pleural involvement in the GTV regardless if RT is delivered pre- or postoperatively.

Metastatic Disease: Low-dose bilateral lung RT (15 Gy/10 fx) is used as a consolidative tool for lung metastases and is usually recommended after CHT, despite paucity of data. Bone metastases can be controlled with doses of 45 to 56 Gy, and SBRT can be considered for tumors initially ≤5 cm in max diameter per COG AEWS 1221. Treatment of metastatic disease is typically done after completion of CHT.

Toxicity: May potentiate bladder and cardiotoxicity from CHT. Acute toxicity is site-dependent. Late toxicity includes reduction of bone growth, soft tissue induration and fibrosis, lymphedema (try to spare skin strip), increased risk of pathologic fracture, and second malignancy. Older studies demonstrated loss of 25% remaining growth in limb for >50 Gy, particularly if including joint or epiphysis. May consider amputation and prosthesis in the very young as they recover function well. For pelvic tumors, remember to consider fertility preservation.

Second Malignancy: Rates reported from 7% to 9% at 20 years in recent studies. Risk is highest for doses >60 Gy and minimal for <48 Gy. The most common second tumor is osteosarcoma. In a recent review of RT-induced osteosarcoma, the most common primary was Ewing's (25%) and the median latency was 8 years.[50]

EVIDENCE-BASED Q&A

WHAT IS THE UTILITY OF CHT IN EWING SARCOMA?

CHT forms the cornerstone of therapy. Due to suboptimal outcomes with VDC-based CHT, efforts were made to add agents as well as to intensify the regimens (Table 65.3). VDCA was found to be superior to VAC (IESS-1), and subsequently high-dose intermittent VDCA was found to be superior to standard-dose VDCA (IESS-II).[51,52] Given the activity of IE in metastatic EWS, VDCA + IE was tested and found to be superior to high-dose intermittent VDCA for nonmetastatic patients (IESS-III).[53] Subsequently, dose intensification of 48 vs. 30 weeks of VDC + IE (IESS-IV) for local EWS demonstrated no benefit but showed that dropping actinomycin D was acceptable.[54] On AEWS0031, interval compression of q2 weeks of VDC + IE compared with q3 weeks was found to be superior and forms the current standard of care in the definitive setting.[54,55] AEWS1031 is the most recent trial providing up-to-date estimates on survival in nonmetastatic EWS as well as guidelines for RT volumes. It showed that the addition of VCR, topotecan, and CYC (VTC) to interval compressed CHT did not improve survival.[56]

Table 65.3 Summary of CHT Trials in EWS

Study Name	Randomization	Outcome Studied	Key Takeaway
IESS-I	VDCA vs. VAC	5-yr RFS (60% vs. 24%, SS), 5-yr OS (65% vs. 28%, SS)	VDCA is superior to VAC.
IESS-II[52]	High-dose intermittent VDCA vs. standard-dose VDCA	5-yr RFS (73% vs. 56%, SS), 5-yr OS (77% vs. 63%, SS)	High-dose intermittent VDCA is superior.
IESS-III[53]	VDCA + IE vs. high-dose intermittent VDCA	5-yr OS (72% vs. 61%, SS), 5-yr LR (9% vs. 28%, SS), 5-yr EFS (69% vs. 54%, SS)*	VDCA + IE is superior for nonmetastatic patients.
IESS-IV[54]	Dose intensification of 48 vs. 30 weeks of VDC + IE	5-yr EFS (70% vs. 72%, NS)	No benefit to dose intensification, but dropping actinomycin D is acceptable.
AEWS0031[55]	VDC-IE q3 weeks vs. VDC-IE q2 weeks	5-yr EFS (65% vs. 73%, SS), 5-yr OS (77% vs. 83%, SS)	Dose intense VDC-IE q2 weeks is standard of care.
AEWS1031[56]	VDC-IE vs. VDC-IE-VTC	5-yr EFS (78% vs. 79%, NS), 5-yr OS (86% vs. 88%, NS)	The addition of VTC did not improve OS. Study provides best survival estimates to date.

*Nonmetastatic population on IESS-III trial. There was no significant OS or EFS improvement in the metastatic arm.
VAC, VCR, actinomycin, CYC; VDCA: VCR, doxorubicin, CYC, actinomycin; VDC-IE, VCR, doxorubicin, CYC, ifosfamide, etoposide; VDC-IE-VTC: VCR, doxorubicin, CYC, ifosfamide, etoposide, VCR, topotecan, CYC.

What is the optimal local control modality: surgery or RT?

Classically, surgery has been performed for tumors that are surgically resectable, and definitive RT has been reserved for tumors that are unresectable. There are no prospective trials evaluating surgery vs. definitive RT. There are only RRs of either RCTs or institutional databases,[38,57,58] which suggest that surgery and definitive RT have similar outcomes (albeit with the inherent selection biases of institutional RRs). Furthermore, despite modern RT and surgical techniques, surgery + RT is associated with the lowest risk of LF for pelvic tumors.[58] Surgery is generally preferred if possible, but RT is preferred for patients who lack a function-preserving surgical option due to location (e.g., scapula, proximal humerus, skull, face, vertebrae) or extent of disease.

Schuck, Review of CESS 81, CESS 86, and EICESS 92 Trials (*IJROBP* 2003, PMID 12504050): Review of 1,058 patients who received varying LC modalities after induction CHT. Surgery as local therapy used when feasible, and adjuvant RT was given for poor histologic response or biopsy/ STR. Definitive RT for cases where surgical resection was not possible. Preoperative RT used for patients with expected close resection margins. See Table 65.4 for results. **Conclusion: Low rates of LF after induction CHT for resectable tumors. For intralesional resections, definitive RT was equivalent to surgery + PORT.** *Comment: RT patients were negatively selected with unfavorable tumor sites.*

Table 65.4 Combined Analysis of CESS 81 and 86 and EICESS 92 for Ewing Sarcoma

	5-Yr LF	5/10-Yr EFS
Surgery ± RT	8%	61%/55%
Preop RT	5%	59%/58%
RT alone	26%	47%/40%
p value	.001	.0001

Yock, INT 0091 (*JCO* 2006, PMID 16921035): PRT of 75 nonmetastatic pelvic EWS patients comparing VDCA vs. VDCA + IE to determine its influence on LC modality with respect to surgery, RT, or both (S + RT), which was chosen by the treating physicians. The effect of LC modality was assessed after adjusting for the size of tumor (<8 cm, ≥8 cm) and CHT type. Surgery was done in 12 patients, RT in 44, and S + RT in 19. The 5-year EFS and LF rates were 49% and 21% (16% LF only; 5% LF and distant failure). No significant difference in EFS or LF by tumor size (<8 cm, >8 cm), LC modality, or CHT. However, VDCA-IE seems to confer an LC benefit (11% vs. 30%, p = .06). **Conclusion: VDCA + IE is superior for pelvic tumors. Surgery and RT produce comparable outcomes as LC modalities.**

Ahmed, COG Trials (*IJROBP* 2017, PMID 28964585): Pooled analysis of 956 EWS patients treated on three COG protocols (INT-0091, INT-0154, and AEWS0031) identifying clinical and treatment variables associated with a higher risk of LF after treatment with IE-based CHT. LF rate for the entire cohort was 7% (4% for surgery, 15% for RT [p < .01] and 7% for S + RT [p = .12]). LF incidence was highest for pelvic tumors (5% extremity, 13% pelvis, 5% axial nonspine tumors, 9% extraskeletal tumors, and 4% spine tumors). Incidence of LF was higher for extremity and pelvis tumors treated with RT (SS). On MVA, age ≥18 years and treatment with RT were independent prognostic factors for higher LF rates. **Conclusion: Age ≥18 years and use of RT for LC especially for pelvis and extremity tumors are associated with higher risk of LF.**

Considering bone marrow is one contiguous space, should RT volumes include the entire involved bone?

Donaldson, POG-8346 (*IJROBP* 1998, PMID 9747829): A total of 178 patients with localized EWS. Adriamycin/CYC × 12 weeks, followed by VAC × 50 weeks. Local therapy was surgery when possible without functional loss, otherwise RT. RT alone (n = 94), randomized to whole bone (39.6 Gy, boost to pre-CHT + 2 cm to 55.8 Gy) vs. tailored port (pre-CHT + 2 cm to 55.8 Gy). Results: 5-year EFS differed by site, distal extremity 65%, central 63%, proximal extremity 46%, and pelvic/sacral 24%. LC for RT alone was 65%. No difference between whole bone and tailored port; 5-year LC differed by quality of RT, appropriate RT 80%, minor deviation 48%, and major deviation 15%. LF 62% in RT volume, 24% outside RT volume, and 14% indeterminate. **Conclusion: Involved field RT can be used over whole bone RT if appropriate volumes are defined by MRI.**

Does dose escalation lead to improved outcomes?

Laskar, Tata Memorial (*IJROBP* 2022, PMID 35568246): Single-institution phase III RCT of 95 patients with nonmetastatic unresectable EWS/PNET randomized between standard dose RT (SDRT 55.8 Gy/31 fx) vs. escalated dose RT (EDRT 70.2 Gy/39 fx). Median age was 17 years. The 5-year LC was significantly superior in EDRT (76% vs. 49%, p = .02). OS and DFS were higher in the EDRT arm but not statistically significant: 59% vs. 45% (p = .08) and 47% vs. 32% (p = .22), respectively. Incidence of grade ≥2 acute skin toxicity in EDRT vs. SDRT was 10% vs. 2% (p = .080), respectively, and no differences in late toxicity were seen. **Conclusion: EDRT results in improved LC with a trend toward improved OS without significant increase in toxicities.**

What is the role of SBRT for metastatic Ewing sarcoma?

Multiple RRs have shown excellent LC and minimal toxicity with the use of SBRT in metastatic EWS.[59–61] The EURO-E.W.I.N.G. 99 trial showed that 3-year EFS was improved in metastatic EWS patients when patients received local treatment to both primary and metastatic sites, and more recent data from Johns Hopkins suggest consolidative RT is independently associated with improved OS and PFS.[62] The COG study AEWS1221 established the new standard of care in metastatic patients, treating all sites of metastases with some form of local therapy.

Haeusler, EURO-E.W.I.N.G. 99 (*Cancer* 2009, PMID 19924786): Analysis of 120 patients with primary, disseminated, multifocal Ewing's evaluating the role of local treatment. Thirty-nine percent received local treatment to primary AND metastases, 34% to primary OR metastatic sites, and 27% received no local therapy. The 3-year EFS was 0.39 in those who received local treatment to both primary tumor and sites of metastases, compared with 0.17 in those with local treatment of either primary tumor OR metastases, and 0.14 in patients with no local therapy (p < .001). MVA showed absence of local treatment to be the major risk factor (HR = 2.21, p = .027). **Conclusion: Given the improvement in EFS, local therapy to all involved sites should be standard in the treatment of metastatic EWS.**

DuBois, AEWS1221 (*JCO* 2023, PMID 36669140): PRT of 298 patients with newly diagnosed metastatic EWS randomized to interval compressed VDC + IE (standard arm) vs. VDC + IE with ganitumab concurrent and adjuvant (experimental). Trial design included induction CHT, LC using surgery, RT, or surgery + RT, adjuvant CHT, and patients were recommended to receive RT to all metastatic sites (including use of WLI; RT could be conventional or SBRT). Primary endpoint EFS. The 3-year EFS and 3-year OS for standard vs. experimental arm were 37% vs. 39% and 60% vs. 57%, respectively. **Conclusion: Ganitumab did not improve EFS or OS when added to current standard of care VDC + IE in metastatic EWS. However, this study established the role of consolidative local therapy to all metastatic sites.**

REFERENCES

1. Angervall L, Enzinger FM. Extraskeletal neoplasm resembling Ewing's sarcoma. *Cancer.* 1975;36(1): 240–251. doi:10.1002/1097-0142(197507)36:1<240::AID-CNCR2820360128>3.0.CO;2-I

2. Glass AG, Fraumeni JF Jr. Epidemiology of bone cancer in children. *J Natl Cancer Inst.* 1970;44(1):187–199. PMID: 11515030

3. Esiashvili N, Goodman M, Marcus RB Jr. Changes in incidence and survival of Ewing sarcoma patients over the past 3 decades: Surveillance Epidemiology and End Results data. *J Pediatr Hematol Oncol.* 2008; 30(6):425–430. doi:10.1097/MPH.0b013e31816e22f3

4. Brown HK, Schiavone K, Gouin F, Heymann MF, Heymann D. Biology of bone sarcomas and new therapeutic developments. *Calcif Tissue Int.* 2018;102(2):174–195. doi:10.1007/s00223-017-0372-2

5. Buckley JD, Pendergrass TW, Buckley CM, et al. Epidemiology of osteosarcoma and Ewing's sarcoma in childhood: a study of 305 cases by the Children's Cancer Group. *Cancer.* 1998;83(7):1440–1448. doi:10.1002/ (SICI)1097-0142(19981001)83:7<1440::AID-CNCR23>3.0.CO;2-3

6. Halperin EC, Constine LS, Tarbell NJ, eds. *Pediatric Radiation Oncology.* 6th ed. Lippincott Williams & Wilkins; 2016.

7. Pradhan A, Grimer RJ, Spooner D, et al. Oncological outcomes of patients with Ewing's sarcoma: is there a difference between skeletal and extra-skeletal Ewing's sarcoma? *J Bone Joint Surg Br.* 2011;93(4):531–536. doi:10.1302/0301-620X.93B4.25510

8. Applebaum MA, Worch J, Matthay KK, et al. Clinical features and outcomes in patients with extraskeletal Ewing sarcoma. *Cancer.* 2011;117(13):3027–3032. doi:10.1002/cncr.25840

9. Raney RB, Asmar L, Newton WA Jr, et al. Ewing's sarcoma of soft tissues in childhood: a report from the Intergroup Rhabdomyosarcoma Study, 1972 to 1991. *J Clin Oncol.* 1997;15(2):574–582. doi:10.1200/ JCO.1997.15.2.574

10. Tirode F, Laud-Duval K, Prieur A, Delorme B, Charbord P, Delattre O. Mesenchymal stem cell features of Ewing tumors. *Cancer Cell.* 2007;11(5):421–429. doi:10.1016/j.ccr.2007.02.027

11. Riggi N, Stamenkovic I. The Biology of Ewing sarcoma. *Cancer Lett.* 2007;254(1):1–10. doi:10.1016/j .canlet.2006.12.009

12. Machado I, Noguera R, Pellin A, et al. Molecular diagnosis of Ewing sarcoma family of tumors: a comparative analysis of 560 cases with FISH and RT-PCR. *Diagn Mol Pathol.* 2009;18(4):189–199. doi:10.1097/ PDM.0b013e3181a06f66

13. Delattre O, Zucman J, Plougastel B, et al. Gene fusion with an ETS DNA-binding domain caused by chromosome translocation in human tumours. *Nature.* 1992;359(6391):162–165. doi:10.1038/359162a0

14. Zucman J, Delattre O, Desmaze C, et al. Cloning and characterization of the Ewing's sarcoma and peripheral neuroepithelioma t(11;22) translocation breakpoints. *Genes Chromosomes Cancer.* 1992;5(4):271–277. doi:10 .1002/gcc.2870050402

15. Riggi N, Suva ML, Stamenkovic I. Ewing's Sarcoma. *N Engl J Med.* 2021;384(2):154–164. doi:10.1056/ NEJMra2028910

16. de Alava E, Gerald WL. Molecular biology of the Ewing's sarcoma/primitive neuroectodermal tumor family. *J Clin Oncol.* 2000;18(1):204–213. doi:10.1200/JCO.2000.18.1.204

17. Urano F, Umezawa A, Yabe H, et al. Molecular analysis of Ewing's sarcoma: another fusion gene, EWS-E1AF, available for diagnosis. *Jpn J Cancer Res.* 1998;89(7):703–711. doi:10.1111/j.1349-7006.1998.tb03274.x

18. Hromas R, Klemsz M. The ETS oncogene family in development, proliferation and neoplasia. *Int J Hematol.* 1994;59(4):257–265. PMID: 8086619

19. Rabbitts TH, Forster A, Larson R, Nathan P. Fusion of the dominant negative transcription regulator CHOP with a novel gene FUS by translocation t(12;16) in malignant liposarcoma. *Nat Genet.* 1993;4(2):175–180. doi:10.1038/ng0693-175

20. Panagopoulos I, Hoglund M, Mertens F, Mandahl N, Mitelman F, Aman P. Fusion of the EWS and CHOP genes in myxoid liposarcoma. *Oncogene.* 1996;12(3):489–494. PMID: 8637704

21. Zucman J, Delattre O, Desmaze C, et al. EWS and ATF-1 gene fusion induced by t(12;22) translocation in malignant melanoma of soft parts. *Nat Genet.* 1993;4(4):341–345. doi:10.1038/ng0893-341

22. Durer S, Shaikh H, Durer C. *Ewing Sarcoma.* StatPearls Publishing; 2023. https://www.ncbi.nlm.nih.gov/ books/NBK559183

23. Widhe B, Widhe T. Initial symptoms and clinical features in osteosarcoma and Ewing sarcoma. *J Bone Joint Surg Am.* 2000;82(5):667–674. doi:10.2106/00004623-200005000-00007

24. Rud NP, Reiman HM, Pritchard DJ, Frassica FJ, Smithson WA. Extraosseous Ewing's sarcoma. A study of 42 cases. *Cancer.* 1989;64(7):1548–1553. doi:10.1002/1097-0142(19891001)64:7<1548::AID-CNCR2820640733>3 .0.CO;2-W

25. Cotterill SJ, Ahrens S, Paulussen M, et al. Prognostic factors in Ewing's tumor of bone: analysis of 975 patients from the European intergroup cooperative Ewing's Sarcoma study group. *J Clin Oncol.* 2000;18(17): 3108–3114. doi:10.1200/JCO.2000.18.17.3108

26. Cangir A, Vietti TJ, Gehan EA, et al. Ewing's sarcoma metastatic at diagnosis. Results and comparisons of two intergroup Ewing's sarcoma studies. *Cancer.* 1990;66(5):887–893. doi:10.1002/1097-0142(19900901)66: 5<887::AID-CNCR2820660513>3.0.CO;2-R

27. National Comprehensive Cancer Network. *NCCN Clinical Practice Guidelines in Oncology: Bone Cancer.* Version 1.2024. https://www.nccn.org/professionals/physician_gls/pdf/bone.pdf

28. Gupta A, Riedel RF, Shah C, et al. Consensus recommendations in the management of Ewing sarcoma from the National Ewing Sarcoma Tumor Board. *Cancer.* 2023;129(21):3363–3371. doi:10.1002/cncr.34942

29. Volker T, Denecke T, Steffen I, et al. Positron emission tomography for staging of pediatric sarcoma patients: results of a prospective multicenter trial. *J Clin Oncol.* 2007;25(34):5435–5441. doi:10.1200/JCO.2007.12.2473

30. Hwang JP, Lim I, Kong CB, et al. Prognostic value of SUVmax measured by pretreatment fluorine-18 fluorodeoxyglucose positron emission tomography/computed tomography in patients with Ewing Sarcoma. *PLoS One.* 2016;11(4):e0153281. doi:10.1371/journal.pone.0153281

31. Oberlin O, Bayle C, Hartmann O, Terrier-Lacombe MJ, Lemerle J. Incidence of bone marrow involvement in Ewing's sarcoma: value of extensive investigation of the bone marrow. *Med Pediatr Oncol.* 1995;24(6): 343–346. doi:10.1002/mpo.2950240602

32. Bacci G, Capanna R, Orlandi M, et al. Prognostic significance of serum lactic acid dehydrogenase in Ewing's tumor of bone. *Ric Clin Lab.* 1985;15(1):89–96. doi:10.1007/BF03029166

33. Marina N, Granowetter L, Grier HE, et al. Age, Tumor characteristics, and treatment regimen as event predictors in Ewing: a children's oncology group report. *Sarcoma.* 2015;2015:927123. doi:10.1155/2015/927123

34. Ferrari S, Bertoni F, Mercuri M, Sottili S, Versari M, Bacci G. Ewing's sarcoma of bone: relation between clinical characteristics and staging. *Oncol Rep.* 2001;8(3):553–556. doi:10.3892/or.8.3.553

35. Hattinger CM, Rumpler S, Strehl S, et al. Prognostic impact of deletions at 1p36 and numerical aberrations in Ewing tumors. *Genes Chromosomes Cancer.* 1999;24(3):243–254. doi:10.1002/(SICI)1098-2264(199903)24 :3<243::AID-GCC10>3.0.CO;2-A

36. de Alava E, Antonescu CR, Panizo A, et al. Prognostic impact of P53 status in Ewing sarcoma. *Cancer.* 2000;89(4):783–792. PMID: 10951341

37. Huang HY, Illei PB, Zhao Z, et al. Ewing sarcomas with p53 mutation or p16/p14ARF homozygous deletion: a highly lethal subset associated with poor chemoresponse. *J Clin Oncol.* 2005;23(3):548–558. doi:10.1200/JCO.2005.02.081

38. Miser JS, Goldsby RE, Chen Z, et al. Treatment of metastatic Ewing sarcoma/primitive neuroectodermal tumor of bone: evaluation of increasing the dose intensity of chemotherapy--a report from the Children's Oncology Group. *Pediatr Blood Cancer.* 2007;49(7):894–900. doi:10.1002/pbc.21233

39. DuBois SG, Krailo MD, Gebhardt MC, et al. Comparative evaluation of local control strategies in localized Ewing sarcoma of bone: a report from the Children's Oncology Group. *Cancer.* 2015;121(3):467–475. doi:10.1002/cncr.29065

40. Ahmed SK, Robinson SI, Arndt CAS, et al. Identification of patients with localized Ewing Sarcoma at higher risk for local failure: a report from the children's oncology group. *Int J Radiat Oncol Biol Phys.* 2017;99(5):1286–1294. doi:10.1016/j.ijrobp.2017.08.020

41. Sauer R, Jurgens H, Burgers JM, Dunst J, Hawlicek R, Michaelis J. Prognostic factors in the treatment of Ewing's sarcoma. The Ewing's Sarcoma Study Group of the German Society of Paediatric Oncology CESS 81. *Radiother Oncol.* 1987;10(2):101–110. doi:10.1016/S0167-8140(87)80052-X

42. Werier J, Yao X, Caudrelier JM, et al. A systematic review of optimal treatment strategies for localized Ewing's sarcoma of bone after neo-adjuvant chemotherapy. *Surg Oncol.* 2016;25(1):16–23. doi:10.1016/j .suronc.2015.11.002

43. Foulon S, Brennan B, Gaspar N, et al. Can postoperative radiotherapy be omitted in localised standard-risk Ewing sarcoma? An observational study of the Euro-E.W.I.N.G group. *Eur J Cancer.* 2016;61:128–136. doi:10.1016/j.ejca.2016.03.075

44. Donaldson SS. Ewing sarcoma: radiation dose and target volume. *Pediatr Blood Cancer.* 2004;42(5):471–476. doi:10.1002/pbc.10472

45. Donaldson SS, Torrey M, Link MP, et al. A multidisciplinary study investigating radiotherapy in Ewing's sarcoma: end results of POG #8346. Pediatric Oncology Group. *Int J Radiat Oncol Biol Phys.* 1998;42(1): 125–135. doi:10.1016/S0360-3016(98)00191-6

46. Paulussen M, Ahrens S, Craft AW, et al. Ewing's tumors with primary lung metastases: survival analysis of 114 (European Intergroup) Cooperative Ewing's Sarcoma Studies patients. *J Clin Oncol.* 1998;16(9): 3044–3052. doi:10.1200/JCO.1998.16.9.3044

47. Haeusler J, Ranft A, Boelling T, et al. The value of local treatment in patients with primary, disseminated, multifocal Ewing sarcoma (PDMES). *Cancer.* 2010;116(2):443–450. doi:10.1002/cncr.24740

48. Shamberger RC, LaQuaglia MP, Gebhardt MC, et al. Ewing sarcoma/primitive neuroectodermal tumor of the chest wall: impact of initial versus delayed resection on tumor margins, survival, and use of radiation therapy. *Ann Surg.* 2003;238(4):563–568. doi:10.1097/01.sla.0000089857.45191.52

49. Schuck A, Ahrens S, Konarzewska A, et al. Hemithorax irradiation for Ewing tumors of the chest wall. *Int J Radiat Oncol Biol Phys.* 2002;54(3):830–838. doi:10.1016/S0360-3016(02)02993-0

50. Koshy M, Paulino AC, Mai WY, Teh BS. Radiation-induced osteosarcomas in the pediatric population. *Int J Radiat Oncol Biol Phys.* 2005;63(4):1169–1174. doi:10.1016/j.ijrobp.2005.04.008

51. Nesbit ME Jr, Gehan EA, Burgert EO Jr, et al. Multimodal therapy for the management of primary, non-metastatic Ewing's sarcoma of bone: a long-term follow-up of the First Intergroup study. *J Clin Oncol.* 1990;8(10):1664–1674. doi:10.1200/JCO.1990.8.10.1664

52. Burgert EO Jr, Nesbit ME, Garnsey LA, et al. Multimodal therapy for the management of nonpelvic, localized Ewing's sarcoma of bone: intergroup study IESS-II. *J Clin Oncol.* 1990;8(9):1514–1524. doi:10.1200/JCO.1990.8.9.1514

53. Grier HE, Krailo MD, Tarbell NJ, et al. Addition of ifosfamide and etoposide to standard chemotherapy for Ewing's sarcoma and primitive neuroectodermal tumor of bone. *N Engl J Med.* 2003;348(8):694–701. doi:10.1056/NEJMoa020890

54. Granowetter L, Womer R, Devidas M, et al. Dose-intensified compared with standard chemotherapy for nonmetastatic Ewing sarcoma family of tumors: a Children's Oncology Group Study. *J Clin Oncol.* 2009;27(15):2536–2541. doi:10.1200/JCO.2008.19.1478

55. Womer RB, West DC, Krailo MD, et al. Randomized controlled trial of interval-compressed chemotherapy for the treatment of localized Ewing sarcoma: a report from the Children's Oncology Group. *J Clin Oncol.* 2012;30(33):4148–4154. doi:10.1200/JCO.2011.41.5703

56. Leavey PJ, Laack NN, Krailo MD, et al. Phase III trial adding vincristine-topotecan-cyclophosphamide to the initial treatment of patients with nonmetastatic Ewing Sarcoma: a children's oncology group report. *J Clin Oncol.* 2021;39(36):4029–4038. doi:10.1200/JCO.21.00358

57. Daw NC, Laack NN, McIlvaine EJ, et al. Local control modality and outcome for Ewing Sarcoma of the femur: a report from the children's oncology group. *Ann Surg Oncol.* 2016;23(11):3541–3547. doi:10.1245/s10434-016-5269-1

58. Ahmed SK, Robinson SI, Arndt CAS, et al. Pelvis Ewing sarcoma: Local control and survival in the modern era. *Pediatr Blood Cancer.* 2017;64(9). doi:10.1002/pbc.26504

59. Brown LC, Lester RA, Grams MP, et al. Stereotactic body radiotherapy for metastatic and recurrent ewing sarcoma and osteosarcoma. *Sarcoma.* 2014;2014:418270. doi:10.1155/2014/418270

60. Elledge CR, Krasin MJ, Ladra MM, et al. A multi-institutional phase 2 trial of stereotactic body radiotherapy in the treatment of bone metastases in pediatric and young adult patients with sarcoma. *Cancer.* 2021;127(5):739–747. doi:10.1002/cncr.33306

61. Parsai S, Sedor G, Smile TD, et al. Multiple site SBRT in pediatric, adolescent, and young adult patients with recurrent and/or metastatic Sarcoma. *Am J Clin Oncol.* 2021;44(3):126–130. doi:10.1097/COC.0000000000000794

62. Chang L, D'Amiano A, Bhatia R, et al. Impact of consolidative radiation on overall and progression-free survival in pediatric, adolescent, and young adult metastatic bone and soft tissue Sarcoma. *Int J Radiat Oncol Biol Phys.* 2024;118(2):474–484. doi:10.1016/j.ijrobp.2023.09.007

Katherine R. Amarell, Sarah M. C. Sittenfeld, and Erin S. Murphy

QUICK HIT Pediatric Hodgkin lymphoma (HL) accounts for ~7% of all childhood malignancies and is highly curable, with survival rates >90% across risk groups. Nodular sclerosis is the most common histology (similar to adult HL); however, mixed cellularity subtype is seen more frequently in pediatric HL compared with other age groups. Given the excellent cure rates, trials have been designed to evaluate de-escalation of CHT and RT based on risk stratification. Generally, RT is delivered per protocol based on the selection of systemic therapy and response criteria specified. Table 66.1 presents some general principles, but specifics are determined by paradigms set forth by the trials listed.

Table 66.1 General Treatment Paradigm for Pediatric Hodgkin Lymphoma	
Risk Group	**Suggested Treatment Options**
Low risk	1. Treatment per GPOH-2002, EuroNet-PHL-C1, AHOD0431 2. OEPA × 2C or AVPC × 3C ± ISRT (15–25.5 Gy) 3. Other possible CHT regimens: ABVD, VAMP, OPPA, COPP/ABV
Intermediate risk	1. Treatment per AHOD0031, EuroNet-PHL-C1 2. OEPA × 2C or ABVE-PC × 3C followed by response-adapted CHT (× 2C) ± ISRT (15–25.5 Gy) 3. Other possible CHT regimens: COPP/ABV, OPPA/COPP
High risk	1. Treatment per AHOD1331, EuroNet-PHL-C1 2. Bv-ABVE-PC × 2C or OEPA × 2C followed by response-adapted CHT (× 3–4C) ± ISRT (15–25.5 Gy) 3. Other possible CHT regimens: COPP/ABVD

EPIDEMIOLOGY: Of ~10,450 childhood cancer diagnoses per year, pediatric HL (age up to 21) represents ~7% (~1,180 cases).[1] Bimodal age distribution. Rarely diagnosed before age 5, has a male predominance (M:F ratio 2–3:1), and is more likely than adult HL to present as mixed cellularity (30%–35%) or nodular lymphocyte predominant (10%–20%) subtypes.[2] See Tables 66.2 and 66.3. The 5-year OS for all pediatric HL patients is 97%.[3]

RISK FACTORS

Pediatric HL: Increasing family size, lower SES status, and early EBV exposure.[4] EBV exposure is associated with mixed cellularity HL, and this disease tends to occur more in developing countries.

AYA HL: Higher SES, early birth order, small family size, and delayed EBV exposure.

Adults: Immunosuppression (HIV, organ/bone marrow transplant), autoimmune disorders, or immune dysfunction (there is evidence to suggest adult HL is biologically different and more aggressive compared with pediatric HL).

ANATOMY AND PATHOLOGY: See Chapter 52 for details.

Table 66.2 Histologic Classification and Relative Frequency of Pediatric HL				
	Histology	Pediatric Frequency	Adult Frequency	Markers
Classic Hodgkin	• **Lymphocyte rich (LR-HL)**	<5%	5%	CD15+, CD30+ Occasionally CD20+
	• **Nodular sclerosis (NS-HL)**	55%	≥70%	
	• **Mixed cellularity (MC-HL)**	30%–35%	~20%	
	• **Lymphocyte depletion (LD-HL)**	<5%	<5%	
Nodular lymphocyte predominance (NLP-HL)		5%–10%	5%	CD19+, CD20+, CD45+, CD15–, CD30–

Source: Data from Halperin EC, Constine LS, Tarbell NJ, Kun LE. *Pediatric Radiation Oncology.* 5th ed. Lippincott Williams and Wilkins; 2010.

CLINICAL PRESENTATION[4]: Painless adenopathy is the most common presentation. Approximately 80% have cervical LN involvement at presentation and >50% have mediastinal disease. Approximately one-third present with B symptoms: fevers (>38°C), drenching night sweats, and weight loss (>10% in the past 6 months). May see Pel–Ebstein fevers (cyclical spiking fevers up to 40°C, last ~1 week and remit for ~1 week; due to cytokine release), generalized pruritus, or alcohol-induced pain in tissues infiltrated by HL.

Table 66.3 Comparison of Pediatric and Adolescent/Young Adult Hodgkin Lymphoma

	Pediatric (Age <14 Yrs)	AYA (Age 15–35 Yrs)
Gender (M:F)	2–3:1	1.1–1.3:1
Site of disease	More commonly have cervical (80%) lymphadenopathy; many also have mediastinal disease; rare to have isolated mediastinal or subdiaphragmatic disease (<5%)	More commonly have mediastinal disease (75%)
Histology NS-HL MC-HL LD-HL NLP-HL	40%–45% 30%–45% 0%–3% 8%–20%	65%–80% 10%–25% 1%–5% 2%–8%
EBV-associated	27%–54%	20%–25%
Risk factors	Lower SES Increasing family size	Higher SES Smaller family size Early birth order
B symptoms at presentation	25%	30%–40%
Stage III/IV at presentation	30%–35%	40%
5-yr OS	>94%	90%

Source: Adapted from Halperin EC, Constine LS, Tarbell NJ. *Pediatric radiation oncology,* 6th ed. Lippincott Williams and Wilkins; 2016.

WORKUP AND STAGING: See Chapter 52.

PROGNOSTIC FACTORS: Poor prognostic factors include advanced stage, large mediastinal adenopathy, more than four subsites, B symptoms, poor histology, age (<10 years better than 11–16 years better than >20 years), male sex, slow response to CHT. Risk stratification per Table 66.4. CHIPS prognostic score for patients with COG Intermediate Risk (based on AHOD0031)[5]: stage IV disease, large mediastinal mass, albumin (<3.4), and fever were independent prognostic factors and were assigned 1 point each. EFS was 93% for patients with 0 points, 89% for patients with 1 point, 78% for patients with 2 points, and 69% for patients with 3 points.

Table 66.4 Risk Stratification Schemes for Pediatric HL[4]

Study Group	Low Risk	Intermediate Risk	High Risk
COG	IA/IIA, no bulk	Everyone else	IIIB/IVB
German	IA/B or IIA	IIB, IIIEA, IIIB	IIEB, IIIEA/B, IIIB, IVA/B
St. Jude/Stanford/Dana Farber	IA/IIA, no bulk, <3 sites	IB, IA–IIIA, ≥3 sites or bulk	Everyone else

Source: From Merchant TE, Kortmann RD. *Pediatric radiation oncology.* Springer International Publishing; 2018.

TREATMENT PARADIGM CLASSIC TYPE

In general, treatment paradigms are centered around protocols that have been established based on risk stratification (see Table 66.5).

Surgery: There is generally no role for surgery in HL beyond biopsy except for favorable stage IA NLP-HL, which can be treated with excision followed by observation (5-year OS ~100%).[6]

Chemotherapy: Historically, MOPP CHT was the backbone regimen used, but due to significant fertility impact, ABVD was introduced followed by derivatives of these regimens. with additional drugs to reduce the total dose of any single drug (see Table 66.6).

Radiation Therapy

Indications: Determined by the choice of CHT and should be followed per protocol. Involved-site RT (ISRT) is currently recommended for HL. Involved-field RT (IFRT) should only be used if it was used in the protocol being utilized for treatment. See ILROG guidelines on ISRT for details.[7,8]

Dose: Consolidative RT dose is determined by the paradigm chosen but typically ranges from 15 to 25.5 Gy. Acute effects at modern RT doses are minimal but may include fatigue, skin erythema, and esophagitis. Late effects drive protocol development and include secondary malignancy, heart disease, pulmonary fibrosis, skeletal hypoplasia, and infertility.

Table 66.5 Preferred Treatment Protocols Based on Risk Stratification			
Type/Stage	**Protocol Options**	**Initial Treatment**	**Indicated Therapies Based on Response**
Low risk	GPOH-2002/ EuroNet-PHL-C1	OEPA × 2C	*CR*: surveillance *PR*: IFRT with boost
Low risk	AHOD0431	AVPC × 3C	*RER*: surveillance *SER*: IFRT with boost
Intermediate risk	AHOD0031	ABVE-PC × 2C	*RER*: ABVE-PC × 2C → if CR then ± IFRT and if <CR then IFRT *SER*: ABVE-PC × 2C → if CR then IFRT, if < CR consider DECA followed by IFRT
Intermediate risk	EuroNet-PHL-C1	OEPA × 2C	*RER*: COPDAC × 2C then observe ± IFRT *SER*: COPDAC × 2C then IFRT to all sites and boost sites of inadequate disease
High risk	AHOD1331	Bv-ABVE-PC × 2C	*RER*: Bv-ABVE-PC × 3C + ISRT to sites of LMA *SER*: Bv-ABVE-PC × 3C + ISRT to sites of LMA with boost to sites of inadequate response
High risk	EuroNet-PHL-C1	OEPA × 2C	*RER*: COPDAC × 4C then observe ± IFRT *SER*: COPDAC × 4C then IFRT to all sites and boost sites of inadequate disease

LMA = large mediastinal adenopathy.
CR = complete response: >80% reduction in the product of the perpendicular diameters (PPD).
PR = partial response: >50% reduction in PPD.
RER = rapid early response: CR after 3C of AVPC (low risk) or CR after 2C of ABVE-PC (intermediate/high risk).
SER = slow early response: <CR after 3C of AVPC (low risk) or CR after 2C of ABVE-PC (intermediate/high risk).

Table 66.6 Common CHT Regimens in Pediatric Hodgkin Lymphoma	
MOPP	Nitrogen mustard, vincristine (VCR), procarbazine, prednisone *Toxicities include sterility, secondary leukemia (latent period 3–7 years with risk of 3%–5% at 7–10 years); historical regimen not used in the modern era*
ABVD	Adriamycin, bleomycin, vinblastine, dacarbazine *Toxicities include pulmonary and cardiovascular*
OEPA	VCR, etoposide, prednisone, adriamycin
OPPA	VCR, procarbazine, prednisone, adriamycin
AVPC	Doxorubicin, VCR, prednisone, cyclophosphamide (CYC)
ABVE-PC	Doxorubicin, bleomycin, VCR, etoposide, prednisone, CYC
Bv-ABVD-PC	Brentuximab vedotin, doxorubicin, VCR, etoposide, prednisone, CYC
CVbP	CYC, vinblastine, prednisolone *CVbP ± rituximab used for stages IA or IIA NLP-HL with incomplete resection*
COPDAC	CYC, VCR, prednisone, dacarbazine
COPP	CYC, VCR, procarbazine, prednisone
DECA	Dexamethasone, etoposide, cisplatin, cytarabine
VAMP	VCR, Adriamycin, methotrexate, prednisone

EVIDENCE-BASED Q&A

LOW-RISK/EARLY/FAVORABLE PEDIATRIC HODGKIN'S

Which early studies evaluated CHT deintensification in low-risk pediatric HL?

ABVD and MOPP led to excellent cure rates (>90%); however, they had significant associated toxicity. Initial trials focused on testing whether less-intensive CHT would lead to equivalent outcomes with improved toxicity. The German HD-90[9] and French MDH-90[10] trials demonstrated excellent outcomes with CHT deintensification + ISRT.

Is it possible to omit RT in patients who have a complete response (CR) to CHT?

This question was evaluated in HD-95, HD-2002, POG 8625, and CCG 5942. HD-95 and HD-2002 showed that in patients who achieve CR after 2C, RT can be omitted. However, POG 8625 showed that to omit RT, two additional cycles of CHT are required.[11] When CHT is further de-escalated from MOPP/ABVD, CCG 5942 showed that RT cannot be omitted (trial closed early).[12]

Dorffel, HD-95 (*JCO* 2013, PMID 23509321): Prospective, nonrandomized trial of 925 patients divided into early stage (TG1), intermediate stage (TG2), and advanced stage (TG3). RT was given as follows: if CR (on CT/MRI), no RT; if tumor reduction of >75%, IFRT to 25 Gy; and if residual tumors >50 cc (considered bulky), IFRT to 25 Gy with 10 to 15 Gy boost. IFRT was given to patients with poor CHT response; however, it was significantly associated with better EFS among intermediate- and high-risk patients but not among low-risk patients. No difference in OS. On QA, 2 of 17 relapses on the RT arm were due to poor-quality RT; 4 of 14 patients with stage IIA, who failed, had prolonged delay between CHT and RT. **Conclusion: The omission of RT after CR results in increased risk of treatment failures, most notably in advanced-stage patients (note: a nonrandomized observation). May omit RT after CR in early-stage (low-risk) patients because no EFS benefit was seen in this group.**

Mauz, Korholz, GPOH-HD-2002 study (*J Clin Oncol* 2010, PMID 20625128): 573 patients with classic HL <18 years old, stratified by early, intermediate, and high-risk disease, and received 2C of OEPA (girls received OPPA). If intermediate- or advanced-stage, patients received two to four more cycles of either COPP (females) or COPDAC (males). All patients received IFRT to 19.8 Gy except those in the early-stage group who had a CR. In the low-risk group, the 5-year EFS for those with and without RT was 93% and 92%, respectively. **Conclusion: RT can be omitted in early-stage HL patients with CR to CHT, confirming the results of the HD-95 study.**

Can RT be omitted in patients who have a rapid early response (RER)?

This question was evaluated on the AHOD0431 trial, which demonstrated that RER (defined as CR after 3C of AV-PC) does not adequately predict patients in which RT can be safely omitted (however, negative PET/CT after cycle 1 was prognostic). In contrast, the EuroNet-PHL-C1 study evaluated response-based management following OEPA CHT and found similar rates of 5-year EFS. Standard of care recommendations for omission of RT in low-risk disease are based on this trial.

Keller, AHOD 0431 (*Cancer 2018*, PMID 29738613): Phase II trial of 287 patients with low-risk HL examining AV-PC × 3C and no RT for CR (>80% reduction in PPD) after 3C. Patients with PR (>50% PPD) receive IFRT 21 Gy/14 fx. For those who failed after initial CR, if they failed as stage I/II, they received VI/DECA + IFRT 21 Gy. If they failed as advanced stage, they received high-dose CHT with autologous SCT. Study closed early due to higher risk for relapse in patients with CR who were PET+ after 1C. CR after 3C was achieved in 64%, PR in 35%, and stable disease in 2%. See Table 66.7 for additional results. Patients with MC-HL had significantly improved EFS compared with patients with NS-HL (95% vs. 76%, *p* = .008). **Conclusion: RER as defined in this trial does not adequately define a population in which RT can be avoided. PET response after one cycle of CHT is highly predictive of outcomes.**

Table 66.7 Results of AHOD 0431	
	4-Yr EFS (−PET vs. +PET After One Cycle of CHT)
Entire cohort	88% vs. 69% (p = .0007)
CR (no RT)	85% vs. 60% (*p* = .001)
PR (+RT)	96% vs. 70% (*p* = .015)

Muaz-Korholz, EuroNet-PHL-C1 Early Stage (*Lancet* 2023, PMID 36858722): Multi-institutional trial of children and adolescents with stage IA, IB, and IIA classic HL <18 years. Patients received 2C of OEPA followed by PET/CT. If <50% reduction in tumor volume and PET activity > mediastinal blood or background, then IFRT to 19.8 Gy/11 fx. Primary endpoint was EFS with goal of 5-year EFS of 90%. In those with adequate response (and thus no RT), 5-year EFS was 87% (95% CI 83%–90%), which was less than the target goal. For inadequate responders who received RT, 5-year EFS was 89% (95% CI 85–93%), which included the target goal in the 95% CI. **Conclusion: RT can be omitted for early-stage classic HL if adequate response to OEPA.** *Note: Although EFS target was not reached in the RT omission group, a post-hoc analysis showed that target was met for patients without bulky disease or elevated ESR. Therefore, in patients with additional risk factors, even in the setting of CR, the addition of IFRT may be beneficial*

INTERMEDIATE-HIGH RISK/ADVANCED/FAVORABLE PEDIATRIC HODGKIN'S

Can RT be avoided in patients with CR after CHT?

Several trials have evaluated whether RT can be eliminated for patients who have a CR to induction CHT. HD-95 and CCG 5942 studies showed that IFRT improved EFS but with no difference in OS.[12,13] TATA Memorial from India suggested that there was an OS benefit to IFRT after CR (caveat was that ~50% were AYA or adult HL).[14] However, POG 8725 trial (STNI) and CCG 521 (EFRT), both of which utilized large RT volumes, did not show an EFS or OS benefit to RT.[15,16] These trials together suggested that there may be patients in whom RT could be avoided without impacting oncologic outcome; however, selecting for this population remained unclear.

Is it possible to utilize CHT and/or RT response-based criteria to determine which intermediate-risk patients require escalation vs. de-escalation of treatment?

Early response has been shown in previous studies to be predictive of long-term outcomes. Therefore, the AHOD0031 trial was initiated and demonstrated that rapid early responders (defined as CR after 2C of ABVE-PC) have no benefit from IFRT. However, all others on the trial received IFRT.

Friedman, AHOD0031 (*JCO* 2014, PMID 25311218): PRT of 1,712 patients. All patients received 2C of ABVE-PC. CR defined as >80% PPD response, PR defined as >50% PPD response. Those with an RER (CR or PR) after 2C received two further cycles of ABVE-PC followed by repeat evaluation: if CR, then IFRT vs. no IFRT (randomized); if <CR, then IFRT. Those with SER randomized to ABVE-PC × 2C + IFRT or DECA × 2C + ABVE-PC × 2C + IFRT and all received IFRT. IFRT was 21 Gy/14 fx. The 4-year EFS was 85%; 87% for RER and 77% for SER (SS). The 4-year OS was 98%; 99% for RER and 95% for SER. For RERs with CR, 4-year EFS with IFRT was 88% vs. 84% without IFRT (NS). For RERs with PET-negative results at response assessment, 4-year EFS was 87% for patients who received IFRT vs. 87% for those who did not receive IFRT (NS). For SERs randomly assigned to DECA vs. no DECA, 4-year EFS was 79% vs. 75% (NS), respectively, and 71% vs. 55% (SS) for SERs with PET+ results at response assessment. **Conclusion: This trial was able to validate response-based therapeutic titration. For RERs with CR, IFRT could be safely omitted, and for SERs with PET+ disease, CHT augmentation is recommended.**

Dharmarajan, AHOD0031 Patterns of Failure (*IJROBP* 2015, PMID 25542311): A subset analysis of 198 patients (out of 244) enrolled on AHOD0031 who had developed relapse. Of these patients, 30% were RER/no CR, 26% were SER, 26% RER/CR/no IFRT, 16% were RER/CR/IFRT, and 2% remained uncategorized. Approximately three-fourths of relapses occurred at initially involved sites (bulky or nonbulky). First relapses rarely occurred at previously uninvolved or out-of-field sites. **Conclusion: Response-based therapy can help define treatment for selected RER patients, but it has not proven beneficial for patients with SER, nor has it facilitated refinement of IFRT treatment volumes. Therefore, IFRT remains standard of care.** *Comment: A second subset analysis evaluated which patients who achieved RER and CR benefitted from IFRT.[17] The results showed that most patients did not benefit from IFRT. However, those with anemia and bulky limited-stage disease had significantly improved 4-year EFS with the addition of IFRT (89% vs. 78%, p = .019).*

Muaz-Korholz, EuroNet-PHL-C1 Intermediate and Advanced Stage (*Lancet* 2022, PMID 34895479): Multi-institutional study of treatment groups 2 (intermediate-stage) and 3 (advanced-stage) consisting of patients with stage IIAE, IIB, IIBE, IIIA, IIIAE, IIIB, IIIBE, and all stage IV.

All patients underwent 2C of OEPA followed by randomization to 2C (Group 2) or 4C (Group 3) of COPP or COPDAC. If inadequate response on PET, patients underwent IFRT 19.8 Gy. Primary endpoint was EFS with goal of maintaining 90% EFS at 5 years. In adequate responders, EFS was 90%. The 5-year EFS in patients treated with COPP vs. COPDAC was 90% vs. 86%, respectively. **Conclusion: RT can be omitted in adequate responders who are treated with consolidation COPP or COPDAC. COPDAC may be less effective but is overall less toxic than COPP (gonadotoxic).**

Can response-adapted therapy be utilized in high-risk pediatric Hodgkin's?

High-risk patients were enrolled on AHOD0831 with the goal of treatment deintensification to limit alkylator exposure and reduce RT volumes based on initial CHT response while maintaining comparable OS (the first COG trial to use response-based RT volumes). AHOD1331 included the use of brentuximab vedotin as part of the CHT regimen and was shown to improve EFS and is now utilized in high-risk patients.

Kelly, AHOD0831 (*Br J Haematol* 2019, PMID 31180135): PRT of high-risk patients (stage IIIB/IVB) who received ABVE-PC × 2C. RER received two additional cycles of ABVE-PC, and SER received ifosfamide/vinorelbine × 2C + ABVE-PC × 2C. IFRT given to sites of initial bulk (>2.5 cm) and/or SER (21Gy/14fx). The 4-year second EFS (freedom from second relapse or malignancy) was 92%, which was below the projected baseline of 95% (*p* = .038). The 5-year first EFS and OS rates were 79% and 95%. Persistent PET+ disease at the end of CHT was especially high risk for relapse/early progression (8 out of 11 patients failed). **Conclusion: Despite not meeting prespecified target, EFS and OS rates were comparable to recent trials despite reduction in RT volumes.**

Castellino, AHOD1331 High Risk (*NEJM* 2022, PMID 36322844): Phase III trial of patients with stage IIB with bulk or stage IIIB, IVA, or IVB HL. Patients received 5C of Bv-ABVE-PC vs. ABVE-PC. Slow responding lesions (identified on PET/CT after 2C) and bulky mediastinal disease were given ISRT after the fifth cycle of CHT. Primary endpoint was 3-year EFS, which was 92% in the Bv-ABVE-PC arm vs. 88% in the ABVE-PC arm (SS). **Conclusion: The addition of brentuximab vedotin to standard of care therapy improves EFS with increased toxicity.**

How are patients with relapsed or refractory disease managed?

Refractory disease is marked by failure to achieve CR or good PR with initial CHT (~6% overall). Salvage therapy in this setting may include high-dose CHT ± RT with response rates of 50% to 70%, followed by autologous SCT. However, 5-year DFS is only ~20%. Relapsed disease is usually treated with high-dose CHT (HDC) and ASCT. The most common HDC is CBV or BEAM. In general, autologous SCT is preferred over allogeneic SCT due to toxicity and overall lack of graft vs. lymphoma effect. An RR of 1,200 patients with HL who underwent transplant showed that treatment-related mortality was 65% for allogeneic transplant vs. 12% for autologous transplant, and the 4-year OS was 25% vs. 37%, respectively (p = .005).[18] IFRT as part of salvage therapy has been shown to improve EFS and trended toward an improvement in OS (especially in RT-naïve patients) in several studies.[19]

*Whole lung irradiation: If treating lungs with RT, complete RT **after** the transplant. For RT to sites other than in the lung, consider RT **prior** to transplant (especially in the pelvis; RT prior to transplant prevents additional bone marrow toxicity to the new graft). Stem cells for transplant should be harvested prior to RT. Transplant has similar outcomes with or without TBI. If RT has been utilized prior to BMT, salvage RT may also be utilized to doses of 15 to 25 Gy.*

What is the risk for secondary malignancies in patients treated for Hodgkin lymphoma?

An observational study out of the Netherlands shows that the risk for secondary malignancies continues to increase even up to 40 years after treatment for HL.[20] The cumulative incidence of second cancers at 40 years was 48.5%. Compared with the general population, patients treated for HL had a standardized incidence ratio of 4.6 for the development of second cancers (equivalent to 121.8 excess cancer diagnoses per 10,000 person-years). The risk for secondary hematologic malignancies was lower in the more recent treatment years due to reduction in utilization of alkylating agents. However, reduction in solid tumors was not lower in more recent years (supradiaphragmatic RT was associated with lower second malignancies compared with mantle field RT). One study by O'Brien et al. showed that all patients who developed secondary leukemias (usually due to CHT) had a fatal course, whereas those who developed secondary solid tumors (usually due to RT) had a 5-year OS of 85%.[21]

REFERENCES

1. Ward E, DeSantis C, Robbins A, et al. Childhood and adolescent cancer statistics, 2014. *CA Cancer J Clin.* 2014;64(2):83–103. doi:10.3322/caac.21219
2. Punnett A, Tsang RW, Hodgson DC. Hodgkin lymphoma across the age spectrum: epidemiology, therapy, and late effects. *Semin Radiat Oncol.* 2010;20(1):30–44. doi:10.1016/j.semradonc.2009.09.006
3. CureSearch for Children's Cancer. *CureSearch for Children's Cancer Research—Home.* https://curesearch.org
4. Halperin EC, Constine LS, Tarbell NJ, Kun LE. *Pediatric Radiation Oncology.* 5th ed. Lippincott Williams & Wilkins; 2010.
5. Schwartz CL, Chen L, McCarten K, et al. Childhood hodgkin international prognostic score (CHIPS) predicts event-free survival in Hodgkin lymphoma: a report from the Children's Oncology Group. *Pediatr Blood Cancer.* 2017;64(4):e26278. doi:10.1002/pbc.26278
6. Appel BE, Chen L, Buxton AB, et al. Minimal treatment of low-risk, pediatric lymphocyte-predominant Hodgkin lymphoma: a report from the Children's Oncology Group. *J Clin Oncol.* 2016;34(20):2372–2379. doi:10.1200/JCO.2015.65.3469
7. Specht L, Yahalom J, Illidge T, et al. Modern radiation therapy for Hodgkin lymphoma: field and dose guidelines from the international lymphoma radiation oncology group (ILROG). *Int J Radiat Oncol Biol Phys.* 2014;89(4):854–862. doi:10.1016/j.ijrobp.2013.05.005
8. Hodgson DC, Dieckmann K, Terezakis S, et al. Implementation of contemporary radiation therapy planning concepts for pediatric Hodgkin lymphoma: guidelines from the international lymphoma radiation oncology group. *Pract Radiat Oncol.* 2015;5(2):85–92. doi:10.1016/j.prro.2014.05.003
9. Schellong G, Pötter R, Brämswig J, et al. High cure rates and reduced long-term toxicity in pediatric Hodgkin's disease: the German-Austrian multicenter trial DAL-HD-90. *J Clin Oncol.* 1999;17(12):3736–3744. doi:10.1200/JCO.1999.17.12.3736
10. Landman-Parker J, Pacquement H, Leblanc T, et al. Localized childhood Hodgkin's disease: response-adapted chemotherapy with etoposide, bleomycin, vinblastine, and prednisone before low-dose radiation therapy—results of the French society of pediatric oncology study MDH90. *J Clin Oncol.* 2000;18(7):1500–1507. doi:10.1200/JCO.2000.18.7.1500
11. Kung FH, Schwartz CL, Ferree CR, et al. POG 8625: a randomized trial comparing chemotherapy with chemoradiotherapy for children and adolescents with Stages I, IIA, IIIA1 Hodgkin Disease: a report from the Children's Oncology Group. *Pediatr Hematol Oncol.* 2006;23(5):362–368. doi:10.1097/00043426-200606000-00008
12. Wolden SL, Chen L, Kelly KM, et al. Long-term results of CCG 5942: a randomized comparison of chemotherapy with and without radiotherapy for children with Hodgkin's lymphoma—a report from the Children's Oncology Group. *J Clin Oncol.* 2012;30(26):3174–3180. doi:10.1200/JCO.2011.41.1819
13. Dörffel W, Rühl U, Lüders H, et al. Treatment of children and adolescents with Hodgkin lymphoma without radiotherapy for patients in complete remission after chemotherapy: final results of the multinational trial GPOH-HD95. *J Clin Oncol.* 2013;31(12):1562–1568. doi:10.1200/JCO.2012.45.3266
14. Laskar S, Gupta T, Vimal S, et al. Consolidation radiation after complete remission in Hodgkin's disease following six cycles of doxorubicin, bleomycin, vinblastine, and dacarbazine chemotherapy: is there a need? *J Clin Oncol.* 2004;22(1):62–68. doi:10.1200/JCO.2004.01.021
15. Weiner MA, Leventhal B, Brecher ML, et al. Randomized study of intensive MOPP-ABVD with or without low-dose total-nodal radiation therapy in the treatment of stages IIB, IIIA2, IIIB, and IV Hodgkin's disease in pediatric patients: a Pediatric Oncology Group study. *J Clin Oncol.* 1997;15(8):2769–2779. doi:10.1200/JCO.1997.15.8.2769
16. Hutchinson RJ, Fryer CJ, Davis PC, et al. MOPP or radiation in addition to ABVD in the treatment of pathologically staged advanced Hodgkin's disease in children: results of the Children's Cancer Group Phase III Trial. *J Clin Oncol.* 1998;16(3):897–906. doi:10.1200/JCO.1998.16.3.897
17. Charpentier A-M, Friedman DL, Wolden S, et al. Predictive factor analysis of response-adapted radiation therapy for chemotherapy-sensitive pediatric Hodgkin lymphoma: analysis of the Children's Oncology Group AHOD 0031 Trial. *Int J Radiat Oncol Biol Phys.* 2016;96(5):943–950. doi:10.1016/j.ijrobp.2016.07.015
18. Milpied N, Fielding AK, Pearce RM, et al. Allogeneic bone marrow transplant is not better than autologous transplant for patients with relapsed Hodgkin's disease. *J Clin Oncol.* 1996;14(4):1291–1296. doi:10.1200/JCO.1996.14.4.1291
19. Poen JC, Hoppe RT, Horning SJ. High-dose therapy and autologous bone marrow transplantation for relapsed/refractory Hodgkin's disease: the impact of involved field radiotherapy on patterns of failure and survival. *Int J Radiat Oncol Biol Phys.* 1996;36(1):3–12. doi:10.1016/S0360-3016(96)00277-5
20. Schaapveld M, Aleman BMP, van Eggermond AM, et al. Second cancer risk up to 40 years after treatment for Hodgkin's lymphoma. *N Engl J Med.* 2015;373(26):2499–2511. doi:10.1056/NEJMoa1505949
21. O'Brien MM, Donaldson SS, Balise RR, et al. Second malignant neoplasms in survivors of pediatric Hodgkin's lymphoma treated with low-dose radiation and chemotherapy. *J Clin Oncol.* 2010;28(7):1232–1239. doi:10.1200/JCO.2009.24.8062

Katherine R. Amarell, Praveen Pendyala, and Erin S. Murphy

QUICK HIT   There are a number of rare CNS tumors often presenting in childhood, which include ATRT, pineoblastoma, and intracranial GCT. Each composes <10% of childhood CNS malignancies and exhibits a wide variation in prognosis. Tumors that present in the very young tend to have a poor prognosis, and the patient's young age complicates treatment decisions, particularly the role of RT. One similarity between these tumors is the propensity for dissemination within the neuroaxis; therefore, CSF sampling and MRI of the brain and complete spine are essential components of staging. Tumors of the pineal region can be accessed via neuroendoscopy, at which time third ventriculostomy can be performed to relieve obstruction, sample CSF, and biopsy the tumor.

ATYPICAL TERATOID/RHABDOID TUMOR (ATRT)

Epidemiology: Rare and aggressive malignancy often found in infants <3 years old. ATRT can present in the supratentorial or infratentorial brain. Infratentorial tumors are more common in infants and patients >3 years of age and demonstrate more favorable survival. Disseminated disease, most commonly leptomeningeal involvement, is present in one-third of patients at diagnosis.[1,2]

Pathology/Genetics: ATRT is defined by loss of the SMARCB1 tumor suppressor gene on IHC. Germline mutations, rather than somatic, are associated with younger age at presentation and extracranial malignant rhabdoid tumors.[3]

Prognosis: The single prospective ATRT cooperative group trial ACNS0333 demonstrated a significant improvement over historical controls with 4-year OS of 43%.[1] This phase III trial set intense multimodality treatment as the standard of care.

Treatment Paradigm: Defined by ACNS0333.[1] Surgery is first recommended with a maximal safe resection. Postoperatively, two cycles of induction CHT include vincristine, methotrexate, etoposide, cyclophosphamide, and cisplatin. If after induction CHT there is persistent residual disease a second-look surgery is recommended. Consolidation CHT includes three cycles of carboplatin and thiotepa. RT follows consolidation CHT and consists of 50.4 Gy for patients <3 years of age and 54 Gy for those older. CSI to 23.4 to 36 Gy with a boost to gross disease can be considered for patients with metastatic disease. Historical reports found earlier RT was associated with improved outcomes,[4] but with the more recent addition of intensive multimodality therapy, the delay of RT to after CHT does not appear to be detrimental.[1]

PINEOBLASTOMA

Epidemiology: Pineoblastoma is the most aggressive (grade IV) primary pineal tumor. It is the second most common type of pineal gland tumor after germ cell tumor (GCT). It was previously categorized as a primary neuroectodermal tumor (PNET). Pineoblastoma is most common in children <5 years old and is associated with a poor prognosis, especially in younger children. Pineoblastoma commonly presents with elevated intracranial pressure (ICP) with hydrocephalus and has a significant risk of leptomeningeal and extracranial dissemination.

Imaging: On MRI, pineoblastomas are hyperdense and have no calcifications. The tumor often appears lobulated with poorly defined borders. Heterogeneously enhances with contrast.

Treatment Paradigm: Maximal safe resection is recommended; extent of resection is likely associated with improved outcomes.[5-7] RT, most commonly CSI, is associated with improved OS; however, infants and young children are often treated with intensive CHT alone as investigated on the Head Start I–III protocols.[8] For older children, CSI of 18 to 36 Gy with boost to 50.4 to 54 Gy for gross disease is standard, and these children are eligible for the high-risk medulloblastoma COG trials (see Chapter 58). CHT can be delivered prior to CSI for young children or those with less than GTR in which a second-look surgery after CHT could be beneficial.

INTRACRANIAL GERM CELL TUMOR (GCT)

Epidemiology: Intracranial GCT is a heterogeneous group of tumors that represent 3% of childhood CNS malignancies. GCTs are more commonly found in adolescents aged 10 to 20 years old. They spread through the subependymal lining and CSF, but rarely metastasize outside the CNS. Metastatic disease in the neuroaxis is present in 5% to 10% at diagnosis.

Pathology: GCTs are categorized by the WHO classification into pure germinoma and nongerminomatous germ cell tumors (NGGCTs), which represent two-thirds and one-third of cases, respectively. NGGCTs are further categorized as embryonal carcinoma, endodermal sinus/yolk sac tumor, choriocarcinoma, teratoma, and mixed tumors.

Tumor Markers: Elevation of beta-human chorionic gonadotropin (β-hCG) and alpha-fetoprotein (AFP) in the serum and/or CSF are tumor markers associated with subtypes of NGGCT (Table 67.1). Included is the most recent COG trial cutoff for pure germinoma categorization; syncytiotrophoblastic cells present in pure germinoma can cause a slight elevation of β-hCG.

Table 67.1 Tumor Markers		
	β-hCG (IU/L)	**AFP (µg/L)**
Pure germinoma	<50 to <100 (with pathologic confirmation)	<20 (or lab normal)
Immature teratoma **Pure endodermal sinus/yolk sac** **Choriocarcinoma**	100–1,000 >1,000 >1,000	20–50 >500 <20 or normal

Anatomy: Most commonly occur in the pineal gland, followed by the suprasellar region, which can be associated with diabetes insipidus. Due to subependymal spread, patients may have plaque-like spread along ventricular lining that is not visible on MRI but is an important factor guiding RT techniques. Pineal gland tumors can cause compression of the medial longitudinal fasciculus resulting in Parinaud syndrome, a constellation of upward gaze palsy, convergence nystagmus, and impaired pupillary constriction but preserved accommodation.

Workup: May be delayed due to nonspecific symptoms such as pituitary dysfunction or increased ICP due to obstruction of the cerebral aqueduct.[9,10]

Imaging: Includes contrast-enhanced MRI of the brain and entire spine. Occasionally, the primary tumor may be of subclinical size and not visible on imaging.[11] If GCT is found to involve both the suprasellar region and the pineal gland, the patient has bifocal disease, which is not metastatic. Bifocal disease is more commonly associated with pure germinoma.

Labs: Serum and CSF tumor markers as above (CSF via LP if safe).

Pathology: If safe, intracranial biopsy is necessary; complete resection is rare due to risks (occasionally done for teratoma). Occasionally, biopsy may obtain only a fraction of a mixed tumor and lead to inaccurate diagnosis.

Prognosis: Very favorable, with 5-year OS ~95% for pure germinomas, which are treatment-sensitive and require less intense therapy.[12] NGGCTs are more aggressive, but with multimodality treatment exhibit 5-year OS of 90%.[13] Given the excellent outcomes following therapy, decreasing treatment-associated morbidity has been a focus of most clinical trials, with specific attempts to move away from CSI for nonmetastatic disease and decrease RT dose.

Treatment Paradigm: Defined by subtype and utilizes multimodality therapy. The role of upfront surgery at diagnosis is often restricted to biopsy as the morbidity and mortality of upfront surgical resection can near 20%.[14] Second-look surgery is recommended for patients with inadequate radiographic tumor reduction following CHT but with normalization of serum and CSF tumor markers.[15]

Pure Germinoma: The current standard of care for nonmetastatic pure germinoma includes CHT with four cycles of carboplatin/etoposide, followed by RT to the whole ventricle plus a tumor bed boost. In prior studies of involved-field RT alone, over 80% of failures were located in the periventricular region, supporting whole ventricular irradiation (WVI) as standard.[16] If CHT is not given, full-dose CSI is an acceptable alternative. Metastatic patients should receive 21 to 24 Gy CSI with 9 to 12 Gy boost after CHT. The lower dose is often used for patients with a CR or PR to CHT. ACNS

1123 gave response-based RT after induction CHT, and patients with a CR received 18 Gy WVI plus 12 Gy tumor bed boost with excellent PFS of 94% and 100% OS.[17] Patients with a PR to induction CHT received 24 Gy WVI plus 12 Gy boost with PFS of 94% and OS of 93%. The now opened ACNS2321 germinoma trial includes patients with localized, bifocal, basal ganglia/thalamic, and metastatic disease and is evaluating response-based lower doses of RT. The SIOP-CNS-GCT-II prospective multicenter trial evaluated induction CHT followed by 24 Gy WVI without a boost to localized germinoma patients in CR after CHT, with 4-year EFS of 98%.

NGGCT: Nonmetastatic NGGCT is treated with six cycles of carboplatin/etoposide alternating with ifosfamide/etoposide prior to RT. CSI to 36 Gy with 18 Gy boost is the current RT standard; however, ACNS1123 investigated 30.6 Gy WVI with 23.4 Gy boost for patients with a CR or PR to CHT. The results demonstrated 3-year PFS of 88%; however, there was a unique pattern of failure in that all patients progressed in the spine.[18] The current NGGCT trial, ACNS 2021, includes WVI with full spine RT.

REFERENCES

1. Reddy AT, Strother DR, Judkins AR, et al. Efficacy of high-dose chemotherapy and three-dimensional conformal radiation for atypical teratoid/rhabdoid tumor: a report from the Children's Oncology Group Trial ACNS0333. *J Clin Oncol.* 2020;38(11):1175–1185. doi:10.1200/JCO.19.01776
2. Rorke LB, Packer R, Biegel J. Central nervous system atypical teratoid/rhabdoid tumors of infancy and childhood. *J Neurooncol.* 1995;24(1):21–28. doi:10.1007/BF01052653
3. Pawel BR. SMARCB1-deficient tumors of childhood: a practical guide. *Pediatr Dev Pathol.* 2018;21(1):6–28. doi:10.1177/1093526617749671
4. Pai Panandiker AS, Merchant TE, Beltran C, et al. Sequencing of local therapy affects the pattern of treatment failure and survival in children with atypical teratoid rhabdoid tumors of the central nervous system. *Int J Radiat Oncol Biol Phys.* 2012;82(5):1756–1763. doi:10.1016/j.ijrobp.2011.02.059
5. Hwang EI, Kool M, Burger PC, et al. Extensive molecular and clinical heterogeneity in patients with histologically diagnosed CNS-PNET treated as a single entity: a report from the Children's Oncology Group randomized ACNS0332 trial. *J Clin Oncol.* 2018;36(34):JCO2017764720. doi:10.1200/JCO.2017.76.4720
6. Jin MC, Prolo LM, Wu A, et al. Patterns of care and age-specific impact of extent of resection and adjuvant radiotherapy in pediatric pineoblastoma. *Neurosurgery.* 2020;86(5):E426–E435. doi:10.1093/neuros/nyaa023
7. Parikh KA, Venable GT, Orr BA, et al. Pineoblastoma—the experience at St. Jude Children's Research Hospital. *Neurosurgery.* 2017;81(1):120–128. doi:10.1093/neuros/nyx005
8. Abdelbaki MS, Abu-Arja MH, Davidson TB, et al. Pineoblastoma in children less than six years of age: the Head Start I, II, and III experience. *Pediatr Blood Cancer.* 2020;67(6):e28252. doi:10.1002/pbc.28252
9. Sethi RV, Marino R, Niemierko A, Tarbell NJ, Yock TI, MacDonald SM. Delayed diagnosis in children with intracranial germ cell tumors. *J Pediatr.* 2013;163(5):1448–1453. doi:10.1016/j.jpeds.2013.06.024
10. Mootha SL, Barkovich AJ, Grumbach MM, et al. Idiopathic hypothalamic diabetes insipidus, pituitary stalk thickening, and the occult intracranial germinoma in children and adolescents. *J Clin Endocrinol Metab.* 1997;82(5):1362–1367. doi:10.1210/jcem.82.5.3955
11. Liang L, Korogi Y, Sugahara T, et al. MRI of intracranial germ-cell tumours. *Neuroradiology.* 2002;44(5):382–388. doi:10.1007/s00234-001-0752-0
12. Calaminus G, Kortmann R, Worch J, et al. SIOP CNS GCT 96: final report of outcome of a prospective, multinational nonrandomized trial for children and adults with intracranial germinoma, comparing craniospinal irradiation alone with chemotherapy followed by focal primary site irradiation for patients with localized disease. *Neuro Oncol.* 2013;15(6):788–796. doi:10.1093/neuonc/not019
13. Goldman S, Bouffet E, Fisher PG, et al. Phase II trial assessing the ability of neoadjuvant chemotherapy with or without second-look surgery to eliminate measurable disease for nongerminomatous germ cell tumors: a Children's Oncology Group study. *J Clin Oncol.* 2015;33(22):2464–2471. doi:10.1200/JCO.2014.59.5132
14. Calaminus G, Bamberg M, Jurgens H, et al. Impact of surgery, chemotherapy and irradiation on long term outcome of intracranial malignant non-germinomatous germ cell tumors: results of the German Cooperative Trial MAKEI 89. *Klin Padiatr.* 2004;216(3):141–149. doi:10.1055/s-2004-822626
15. Calaminus G, Bamberg M, Harms D, et al. AFP/beta-HCG secreting CNS germ cell tumors: long-term outcome with respect to initial symptoms and primary tumor resection. Results of the cooperative trial MAKEI 89. *Neuropediatrics.* 2005;36(2):71–77. doi:10.1055/s-2005-837582
16. Alapetite C, Brisse H, Patte C, et al. Pattern of relapse and outcome of non-metastatic germinoma patients treated with chemotherapy and limited field radiation: the SFOP experience. *Neuro Oncol.* 2010;12(12):1318–1325. doi:10.1093/neuonc/noq093

17. Bartels U, Onar-Thomas A, Patel SK, et al. Phase II trial of response-based radiation therapy for patients with localized germinoma: a Children's Oncology Group study. *Neuro Oncol.* 2022;24(6):974–983. doi:10.1093/neuonc/noab270

18. Fangusaro J, Wu S, MacDonald S, et al. Phase II trial of response-based radiation therapy for patients with localized CNS nongerminomatous germ cell tumors: a Children's Oncology Group study. *J Clin Oncol.* 2019;37(34):3283–3290. doi:10.1200/JCO.19.00701

PART XII: Metastases and Palliative Radiation Therapy

68 BRAIN METASTASES

Winston Vuong, Martin C. Tom, and John H. Suh

QUICK HIT Brain metastases are the most common intracranial tumor. Surgery, WBRT, HA-WBRT, and SRS are all treatment options and can be performed in many combinations based on careful patient selection.[1] Key factors for patient selection include performance status, number and size of lesions, histology, systemic therapy options, and status of extracranial disease. Typically, surgery is reserved for large or symptomatic lesions or when a tissue sample is required. SRS is preferred over WBRT due to less neurocognitive side effects and QOL benefit for patients with limited- or intermediate-volume intracranial disease.

EPIDEMIOLOGY: Most common intracranial tumor, with ~200,000 cases per year. Brain metastases occur in up to 30% of patients with cancer and are the direct cause of death in 30% to 50% of those patients. Incidence has increased in the MRI era due to the detection of smaller lesions as well as advances in cancer treatment allowing for longer patient survival.[1,2] A solitary brain metastasis is defined as one intracranial lesion without evidence of extracranial disease; however, 80% of patients have multiple lesions. In contrast, a "single" brain metastases refers to one identifiable intracranial lesion with the presence of extracranial disease.

ANATOMY: Most commonly occur at the gray–white matter junction due to decrease in diameter of blood vessels. Typically spherical, well-demarcated lesions with edema: 80% supratentorial, 15% cerebellum, and 5% brainstem. The incidence of lesions in the hippocampal and perihippocampal region is 4.5%.[3]

PATHOLOGY: The most common histologies (overall prevalence) include the lung (50%), breast (20%), melanoma (10%), and colon (5%).[2] Histologies with the highest predilection for the development of brain metastases (neurotropism) include SCLC, melanoma, choriocarcinoma, and germ cell. Hemorrhagic lesions are typically melanoma, choriocarcinoma, testicular, thyroid, and renal cell. The most common pediatric histologies are sarcomas, Wilms tumor, and germ cell tumors.

CLINICAL PRESENTATION: Variable but most commonly include impaired cognitive function, motor weakness, sensory changes, headache, speech changes, nausea/vomiting, and seizures.[2]

WORKUP: H&P with detailed neurologic exam.

Imaging: Noncontrast head CT is often the first-line test performed to rule out intracranial hemorrhage. MRI with and without contrast is best to detect and characterize small metastases. A challenge in posttreatment surveillance is distinguishing radiation necrosis from tumor progression, and there are various advanced imaging modalities being explored. Advanced MRI sequences can include MR spectroscopy, diffusion-weighted imaging, and dynamic susceptibility contrast-enhanced MR perfusion. Novel amino acid PET radiotracers, such as fluciclovine, are under evaluation as well.[4]

Biopsy: May be necessary for solitary lesions (no extracranial disease) as up to 10% can be primary brain tumors,[5] although this is likely lower in the MRI era. For large solitary tumors with mass effect, resection can be therapeutic and diagnostic. For multiple lesions, >95% are metastatic rather than primary tumors and biopsy should be targeted to the most accessible lesion.

PROGNOSTIC FACTORS: Numerous prognostic systems have been developed and updated to reflect contemporary outcomes. The initial RPA (based on age, KPS, controlled primary, presence of extracranial metastases) was developed by the RTOG, followed by the GPA (based on age, KPS, number of brain metastases, and the presence or absence of extracranial metastases), then the diagnosis-specific GPA (Table 68.1), which was recently updated and is available at brainmetgpa. com.[6–8] Disease-specific factors vary in number of metastases that are prognostic, and other considerations include mutational status (NSCLC-adeno and melanoma), PD-L1 status (NSCLC-adeno), Hgb (RCC), and subtype (breast). Brain metastasis velocity (number of new brain metastases per year since initial SRS) ≥4 can help predict survival outcomes.[9] Prognostic factors for neurocognitive function are under development, with suggestion of ApoE-related genotypes and higher serum amyloid beta having worse neurocognitive decline with RT.[10,11]

Table 68.1 Diagnosis-Specific GPA[12]					
	0	0.5	1	1.5	2
Variable	NSCLC				
Age	≥70	<70			
KPS	≤70	80	90–100		
Number of brain mets	≥5	1–4			
Extracranial mets	Present	–	Absent		
EGFR and ALK (adenocarcinoma only)	Both negative or unknown	–	EGFR or ALK positive		
	Sum = MS (months) by GPA: Adenocarcinoma: 0–1 = 7; 1.5–2.0 = 13; 2.5–3.0 = 25; 3.5–4.0 = 46 Nonadenocarcinoma: 0–1 = 5; 1.5–2.0 = 10; 2.5–3.0 = 13; 3.5–4.0 = NA				
	Breast				
KPS	≤60	70–80	90–100		
Age	≥60	<60			
Number of brain mets	≥2	1			
Extracranial mets	Present	Absent			
Subtype	Triple negative	Luminal A (ER/PR+, HER2–)	–	HER2+ or Luminal B (triple +)	
	Sum = MS (months) by GPA: 0–1 = 6; 1.5–2.0 = 13; 2.5–3.0 = 24; 3.5–4.0 = 36				
	Renal				
KPS	≤70	–	80	–	90–100
Number of brain mets	≥5	1–4			
Extracranial mets	Present	Absent			
Hemoglobin	<11.1	11.1–12.5 or unknown	>12.5		
	Sum = MS (months) by GPA: 0–1 = 4; 1.5–2.0 = 12; 2.5–3.0 = 17; 3.5–4.0 = 35				
	Melanoma				
Age	≥70	<70			
KPS	≤70	80	90–100		
Number of brain mets	≥5	2–4	1		
Extracranial mets	Present	–	Absent		
BRAF	Negative or unknown	Positive			
	Sum = MS (months) by GPA: 0–1 = 5; 1.5–2.0 = 8; 2.5–3.0 = 16; 3.5–4.0 = 34				
	GI				
KPS	<70	–	80	–	90–100
Age	≥60	<60			
Number brain mets	≥4	2–3	1		
Extracranial mets	Present	Absent			
	Sum = MS (months) by GPA: 0–1 = 3; 1.5–2.0 = 7; 2.5–3.0 = 11; 3.5–4.0 = 17				

Source: Adapted from Sperduto PW, Mesko S, Li J, et al. Survival in patients with brain metastases: summary report on the updated diagnosis-specific graded prognostic assessment and definition of the eligibility quotient. *J Clin Oncol.* 2020;38(32):3773–3784. doi:10.1200/JCO.20.01255.

NATURAL HISTORY: Historically, the direct cause of death in 30% to 50% of patients who develop brain metastases, but estimates in the modern systemic therapy era suggest this has improved to 10% of deaths being attributable to CNS disease.[13] While all effective therapies are associated with varying levels of neurocognitive decline, uncontrolled brain metastases also drive worsening neurocognition. Postoperatively, there is an elevated risk of leptomeningeal disease (LMD), although this is often a focal/nodular type (i.e., nodular meningeal disease) that has a better prognosis than diffuse types. The types of LMD include diffuse vs. focal, nodular vs. classic, and pachymeningeal vs. leptomeningeal, and EANO-ESMO have formalized the diagnostic criteria for classifying the subtypes of LMD.[14–16]

TREATMENT PARADIGM

Medical: Glucocorticoids such as dexamethasone are first-line medical therapy to improve symptoms related to cerebral edema in up to 75% within 1 to 3 days. Acute side effects include insomnia, hyperglycemia, irritability, and weight gain. Effects from long-term use include Cushingoid appearance, gastric ulcers (require GI prophylaxis), osteopenia, and proximal muscle weakness. Radiosensitizers such as motexafin gadolinium[17] and efaproxiral[18] have been studied with no demonstrable benefit. Nitroglycerin is being explored as a radiosensitizer, although larger studies are needed.[19]

Neurocognitive Protectant: Memantine is an NMDA receptor antagonist used for dementia and can be given with WBRT (including HA-WBRT) to minimize neurocognitive decline as demonstrated on RTOG 0614 (see the following).

Surgery: Recommended for larger symptomatic lesions or when tissue diagnosis is necessary. A stereotactic approach with maximal safe resection is standard.

Systemic Therapy: Historically, there has been little role for CHT in the treatment of brain metastases due to the blood–brain barrier, with the exception of metastatic germ cell tumors (e.g., testicular); however, with new targeted agents, antibody–drug conjugates, and immunotherapies, there is evidence of improved intracranial efficacy.[10,11] Brain metastases from EGFR and ALK mutant NSCLC, PD-L1 expressing NSCLC, HER2+ breast cancer, and melanoma all have approved agents with intracranial efficacy; however, these have not yet been proven to replace local therapy.[20] Local therapy should not be deferred except for specific scenarios for asymptomatic patients as recommended by the ASCO-SNO-ASTRO 2022 guidelines.[21] Recent evidence suggests that SRS with concurrent targeted therapy can be safely performed based on the TURBO-NSCLC cohort, RTOG 1119, and T-DXd multi-institutional cohort.[22–24] The addition of SRS to EGFR or ALK-directed TKIs appears to improve CNS progression in EGFR/ALK-mutant NSCLC, but the addition of lapatinib to WBRT/SRS did not improve CR rates in HER2+ breast cancer brain metastases.

Radiation Therapy: RT is the cornerstone of treatment for brain metastases and is indicated in most patients except for those with exceptionally poor prognosis (see QUARTZ trial in the following). Options include SRS or WBRT (with or without hippocampal avoidance).

Dose: For WBRT, dose options include 30 Gy/10 fx (most common), 20 Gy/5 fx, and 8–10 Gy/1fx. Hippocampal avoidance whole-brain RT (HA-WBRT) is delivered with 30 Gy/10 fx. The use of HA-WBRT with SIB to metastases is under evaluation.[25–27]

SRS: Traditionally, SRS delivers a single high-dose treatment using multiple converging beams.[28] Metastases are often ideal targets for SRS considering they are small, spherical, well-demarcated, and located at the gray–white matter junction away from critical structures. Dosing is heterogenous and institutionally dependent, but can be performed per RTOG 9005 based on maximum diameter: 24 Gy for lesions ≤2 cm, 18 Gy for lesions 2.1 to 3.0 cm, and 15 Gy for 3.1 to 4 cm. Lesions ≥2 cm may have worse LC and may be treated with fractionated SRS (common doses include 27 Gy/3 fx or 30 Gy/5 fx)[29–32] or staged SRS delivered 2 to 4 weeks apart.[33,34]

Postoperative SRS to the cavity of a resected brain metastasis decreases the risk of LR. Dose varies by institution but can be defined by the N107C study: 20 Gy if cavity volume <4.2 mL, 18 Gy if 4.2 to 7.9 mL, 17 Gy if 8.0 to 14.3 mL, 15 Gy if 14.4 to 19.9 mL, 14 Gy if 20.0 to 29.9 mL, and 12 Gy if ≥30.0 mL, up to the maximal surgical cavity extent of 5 cm. Fractionated SRS can also be used (27 Gy/3 fx or 30 Gy/5 fx). Practice guidelines have been established by the ISRS as well.[35]

Preoperative SRS is currently being investigated on phase III trials, as it may address limitations of postoperative SRS including a higher incidence of LF, nodular meningeal disease, and radionecrosis compared with WBRT.[36] Dose escalation is also being explored.[37]

Of note, SCLC patients have historically been excluded from SRS studies, although recent retrospective data have shown potential for upfront SRS in this population[38] and phase II/III trials are currently ongoing.

Toxicity: Side effects of SRS include fatigue, headache, nausea, radionecrosis, damage to nearby critical structures (optic nerve, chiasm, brainstem), and neurocognitive decline (less than WBRT). Consensus guidelines on radionecrosis may inform post-SRS management.[39] Side effects of WBRT include fatigue, hair loss, skin erythema, headache, nausea, temporary muffled hearing, and neurocognitive decline.

Procedure: See *Handbook of Treatment Planning in Radiation Oncology*, Chapters 3 and 13.[40]

EVIDENCE-BASED Q&A

Is there a benefit to WBRT over best supportive care?

In poor-performance patients with NSCLC not eligible for SRS or resection, the benefit of WBRT is questionable based on the QUARTZ study.

Mulvenna, QUARTZ (*Lancet* 2016, PMID 27604504): PRT (noninferiority) of optimal supportive care (OSC) vs. 20 Gy/5 fx WBRT for NSCLC brain metastases in patients unsuitable for SRS or resection. Primary endpoint was QALY (calculated using EQ-5D) with a noninferiority margin of 7 QALY days. Enrolled 538 patients, 83% were GPA 0 to 2 and 38% had a KPS <70. Did not demonstrate a difference in OS (HR 1.06, $p = .81$) or QALY days (mean QALYs 46.4 days WBRT vs. 41.7 days OSC, 4.7 QALY-day difference with 90% CI −12.7 to 3.3). Dexamethasone use was not significantly different. There were nonsignificant suggestions that WBRT may offer a survival benefit in patients with better prognoses. **Conclusion: Although optimal supportive care noninferiority was not met, WBRT may be unnecessary in poor-performance patients.** *Note: Patients selected for this trial had poor performance at baseline; results may not apply to patients with more favorable performance status.*

What is the ideal dose of WBRT for patients with brain metastases?

RTOG 9104 compared standard 30 Gy/10 fx with 32/20 fx with boost to 54.4/34 fx BID and found no benefit to dose escalation with hyperfractionation. Shorter durations (10 Gy/1fx or 12 Gy/2 fx over 3 days) have worse time to neurologic deterioration, duration of improvement, and rate of complete disappearance of neurologic symptoms compared with 2- to 4-week regimens (20 Gy/5 fx, 30 Gy/10 fx, or 40 Gy/20 fx) based on the original RTOG data, although have similar response rates and can be considered in patients with poor prognosis.[40] 37.5 Gy/15 fx was common on older RTOG trials but has not demonstrated improved outcomes but did have increased toxicity.[21,41]

What is the role of surgery in patients with a single brain metastasis?

Surgery is beneficial for select patients and is typically reserved for patients with large and relatively few lesions in a resectable location. Three trials have looked at adding surgery to WBRT and two (Patchell I and Noordijk)[5,42] showed a survival benefit. The third did not show an OS benefit but enrolled poor-performance patients.[43] Contemporary trials have established surgery + SRS as the standard of care treatment option (see below Mahajan et al. and N107c) to maintain control rates while decreasing neurocognitive decline. Preoperative SRS is under evaluation.

Patchell I (*NEJM* 1990, PMID 2405271): PRT of 48 patients with single brain metastasis randomized to biopsy followed by WBRT vs. surgical resection with WBRT (36 Gy/12 fx). Of note, 6 of 54 patients (11%) were found to have a primary brain tumor or benign findings (pre-MRI era). The results are in Table 68.2. **Conclusion: Surgical resection + WBRT for a single brain metastasis improves OS compared with WBRT alone.**

Table 68.2 Patchell I Results

	LR	Time to LR	DM	MS	Time to Neurologic Death	Functional Independence
Biopsy + WBRT	52%	21 weeks	13%	15 weeks	26 weeks	8 weeks
Surgery + WBRT	20%	59 weeks	20%	40 weeks	62 weeks	38 weeks
p value	<.02	<.0001	.52	<.01	<.0009	<.005

Does WBRT improve outcomes after surgery?

Patchell II (JAMA 1998, PMID 9809728): PRT of 95 patients with one brain metastasis and KPS ≥70 randomized to surgery alone vs. surgery with postoperative WBRT (50.4 Gy/28 fx). Nearly all outcomes were improved except survival; however, the trial was not powered for survival. The results are in Table 68.3. **Conclusion: WBRT after surgical resection of a single brain met improves local and distant brain control.**

Table 68.3 Patchell II Results

	Any Recurrence	Distant Recurrence	LR	MS	Neurologic Death	Functional Independence
Surgery	70%	37%	46%	43 weeks	44%	35 weeks
Surgery + RT	18%	14%	10%	48 weeks	14%	37 weeks
p value	<.001	<.01	<.001	.39	.003	.61

Can SRS offer similar rates of control in the postoperative setting to WBRT but without the neurocognitive deficits?

In an attempt to maintain control rates while decreasing neurocognitive decline, SRS can be given to the resection cavity, with initial retrospective data favoring a 2-mm margin around the cavity.[35] Note that dosing to the resection cavity is often by volume rather than by diameter, but this varies by institution.

Brown, N107C (Lancet Oncol 2017, PMID 28687377): PRT of 194 patients with ≤4 metastases (all <3 cm) with resection of a single lesion (cavity <5 cm), then randomized to WBRT (with SRS to unresected metastases) vs. SRS alone to the cavity and unresected lesions. Co-primary endpoints were OS and cognitive deterioration-free survival (CDFS) at 6 months, defined as death or a drop by 1 standard deviation in one test (HVLT, COWA, Trailmaking A and B). Preferred sequencing was SRS to unresected metastases followed by WBRT within 14 days. Dosing to the surgical bed was 12 to 20 Gy depending on tumor volume (dosing to unresected lesions was 18–24 Gy depending on arm and diameter). No difference in OS (MS 12.2 months SRS vs. 11.6 months WBRT, *p* = .70). CDFS was improved in SRS arm: median 3.7 vs. 3.0 months (*p* < .0001). **Conclusion: Postoperative SRS provides comparable OS with less neurocognitive deterioration as compared with WBRT and is thus preferred.**

Mahajan, MDACC (Lancet Oncol 2017, PMID 28687375): PRT of 132 patients with one to three surgically resected metastases (surgical cavity ≤4 cm) were randomized to SRS (64 patients) vs. observation (68 patients). Primary endpoint was time to LR in the surgical cavity. Dose to surgical bed was based on resection bed volume. Results: MFU 11.1 months. Median OS was similar between the groups (5.4 months observation group vs. 7.5 months SRS, *p* = .24). The 12-month LRFS was inferior in the observation group (43%) vs. SRS (72%; *p* = .015). There were no adverse events or treatment-related deaths in either group. **Conclusion: Postop SRS lowers the risk of LR.** *Note: Neurocognitive outcomes not reported.*

Kayama, JCOG 0504 (JCO 2018, PMID 29924704): PRT (noninferiority) of 271 patients with ≤4 lesions surgically resected with only one lesion >3 cm randomized to SRS or WBRT after surgery. Primary endpoint was OS. MS 15.6 months on both arms, with HR of 1.05 (*p* = .027) meeting noninferiority criteria. Grades 2 to 4 cognitive dysfunction beyond 90 days was higher in the WBRT arm (16% vs. 8%, *p* = .048) but the proportion of patients whose MMSE did not worsen was similar in both arms. **Conclusion: With respect to OS, postoperative salvage SRS is noninferior to WBRT.**

What determines the dose of SRS?

Dosing is based on tumor diameter as established by RTOG 9005, but in practice varies significantly across institutions.[44] LC for larger metastases is suboptimal with single fx, and various attempts at improving outcomes for these patients are noted in the following.

Shaw, RTOG 9005 (*IJROBP* 2000, PMID 10802351): Phase I/II SRS dose escalation trial for patients with a recurrent primary brain tumor (36%) or metastases (64%) ≤4 cm after receiving previous brain RT ≥3 months prior. Treated to escalating dose levels. Maximum tolerated dose (MTD) was 15 Gy for tumors 3.1 to 4 cm and 18 Gy for tumors 2.1 to 3 cm. Investigators were unwilling to escalate above 24 Gy to tumors ≤2.0 cm even though MTD was not observed. A homogeneity index (ratio of max dose/prescription dose) of ≥2 was associated with increased toxicity. Incidence of radionecrosis was 11% at 2 years.

When added to standard WBRT, does an SRS boost improve survival?

SRS boost improves LC after WBRT, with no clear impact on OS.

Andrews, RTOG 9508 (*Lancet* 2004, PMID 15158627): Patients with one to three new brain metastases each ≤4 cm randomized to WBRT or WBRT + SRS boost. WBRT dose was 37.5 Gy/15 fx and boost was given 1 week after WBRT using RTOG 9005 SRS doses. While there was an improvement in LC, KPS, and steroid use in all patients in the WBRT + SRS arm, the primary endpoint of OS was not met (Table 68.4). Patients with a single metastasis did demonstrate a survival benefit with WBRT + SRS (preplanned stratification). On an unplanned subset analysis, patients in RPA class I, those with large metastases (>2 cm), squamous or NSCLC, or KPS 90 to 100 experienced a benefit that was not statistically significant after adjustment for unplanned subgroup analyses. **Conclusion: SRS boost improves LC after WBRT.**

Table 68.4 RTOG 9508 Results								
RTOG 9508	Mean Survival (Months)						1-Yr LC	Stable/Improved KPS at 6 Months
	Overall	Single Met	Tumor >2 cm*	RPA Class I*	Squamous/ NSCLC*	KPS 90–100*		
WBRT alone	6.5	4.9	5.3	9.6	3.9	7.4	71%	25%
WBRT + SRS	5.7	6.5	6.5	11.6	5.9	10.2	82%	42%
p value	.136	.039	.045	.045	.051	.071	.013	.033

*Subset analysis: p value for significance = .0056.

If SRS boost does not improve survival compared with WBRT alone, does WBRT improve survival when added to SRS?

Aoyama (*JAMA* 2006, PMID 16757720): Randomized 132 patients with one to four brain metastases all ≤3 cm to WBRT (30 Gy/10 fx) with SRS vs. SRS alone. SRS doses alone were 22 to 25 Gy for tumors ≤2 cm and 18 to 20 Gy for tumors >2 cm and reduced by 30% if given after WBRT. Fortynine percent had a single metastasis; 83% were RPA class II. Primary endpoint OS. Closed early on interim analysis because of the higher than anticipated sample size needed to show a difference in OS. Complete results in Table 68.5. Rates of LR and any recurrence were decreased significantly by WBRT. **Conclusion: The addition of WBRT does not confer a survival benefit when added to SRS, although not sufficiently powered for this endpoint.**

Table 68.5 Aoyama Trial Results						
	MS (Months)	Neurologic Death	1-Yr Any Recurrence	1-Yr LR	1-Yr Distant Recurrence	Neurologic Preservation
SRS alone	8.0	19%	76%	27.5%	64%	70%
WBRT + SRS	7.5	23%	47%	11%	42%	72%
p value	.42	.64	<.001	.002	.003	.99

If survival is not improved by adding SRS to WBRT, do the neurocognitive risks of adding WBRT to SRS outweigh the benefits?

The addition of WBRT to SRS leads to increased neurocognitive decline without a survival benefit compared with SRS alone in patients with limited brain metastases (Table 68.6).[45,46]

Table 68.6 SRS vs. SRS + WBRT in Patients With 1–3 Brain Metastases		
Study	Primary Endpoint	Results
Chang, MD Anderson (2009)[45]	Deterioration of HVLT-R-TR by 5 pts at 4 months	• HVLT-R-TR decline in 23% of SRS arm vs. 49% WBRT + SRS arm • LC and distant control improved with SRS + WBRT
Kocher, EORTC (2011)[46]	Time to WHO performance status >2	• No difference in time to PS >2 • No difference in OS (~11 months) • WBRT improved LF and in-brain failure
Sahgal meta-analysis (2015)[47]		• SRS + WBRT with better LC • Age ≤50: lower hazard of mortality with SRS alone (MS: 13.6 vs. 8.2 months) • Age >50 benefit from WBRT in terms of distant brain failure
Brown, NCCTG N0574 (2016)[48]	Decline in any of six cognitive tests at 3 months	• Cognitive decline higher after WBRT + SRS • QOL improved with SRS, no difference in functional independence • In-brain control was better in WBRT arm; no difference in OS

If WBRT is associated with a decline in neurocognitive function, what are some possible strategies to avoid this?

Adding memantine and hippocampus-sparing are two strategies to decrease the neurocognitive detriment associated with WBRT. RTOG 0933 limited the hippocampus to 16 Gy max dose and D100% ≤9 Gy and found that HA-WBRT preserved memory and QOL more than WBRT in a historical control.[49] Secondary analyses of NRG CC001 have suggested the primary benefit of hippocampal avoidance in patients living at least 4 months.[50]

Brown, RTOG 0614 (*Neuro-Oncol* 2013, PMID 23956241): PRT of patients with KPS ≥70 and stable systemic disease randomized to receive 20 mg of memantine vs. placebo during and after WBRT for a total of 24 weeks. Dose was uptitrated by 5 mg weekly, starting at 5 mg daily up to 10 mg BID for weeks 4 to 24. Primary endpoint was decline in HVLT-R-DR at 24 weeks compared with baseline, which trended toward improvement ($p = .059$), but statistical power was limited due to patient loss. The memantine arm did have statistically significant longer time to cognitive decline, lower probability of cognitive failure, and superior results for executive function, processing speed, and delayed recognition at 24 weeks. **Conclusion: Memantine is a well-tolerated medication and patients who received memantine compared with placebo had better cognitive function over time, although patient loss to follow-up limited the statistical significance of the primary endpoint.**

Brown, NRG CC001 (*JCO* 2020, PMID 32058845): Randomized phase III trial of 518 patients with brain metastases, stratified by RPA and prior SRS/surgery, randomized to WBRT (30 Gy/10 fx) + memantine vs. HA-WBRT + memantine. Primary endpoint was time to neurocognitive failure, defined as an established decline in one of the neurocognitive tests (HVLT, Trailmaking, or COWA). No difference in OS, intracranial PFS, or toxicity between arms. Cognitive failure risk significantly lower in the HA-WBRT arm compared with the WBRT arm (HR 0.76, 95% CI 0.60–0.98). The lower cognitive failure was secondary to statistically significantly less deterioration in executive functioning at 4 months and learning and memory at 6 months. On MVA, age >61 years was also significant for time-to-cognitive failure (HR 0.635, $p = .0016$). HA-WBRT was also associated with less fatigue, difficulty remembering things, speaking, interference of neurologic symptoms with daily activities, and fewer cognitive symptoms (all $p < .05$). **Conclusion: HA-WBRT has comparable efficacy to standard WBRT, but better preserves neurocognitive function with the benefit first appreciated at 4 months posttreatment.**

How many metastases are necessary to warrant WBRT rather than SRS?

The standard of care for patients with limited-volume brain metastases is SRS alone to avoid WBRT, but the specific number or volume remains unclear. Observational data have suggested no detriment in survival for SRS up to 10 lesions, and emerging studies are suggesting feasibility and safety of treating >10 lesions without compromising OS, neurologic death-free survival, or neurologic deterioration.[51,52] Some studies support intracranial tumor volume over number as a better indicator of when SRS is appropriate and have recommended using a threshold of <15 to 30 cc.

Yamamato, Japan (*Lancet Oncol* 2014, PMID 24621620): Prospective observational study of patients with 1 to 10 new metastases (maximum <3 cm) treated with SRS alone. Patients with 5 to 10 lesions were compared with patients with one tumor and patients with two to four tumors. Primary endpoint OS. No OS difference between the 5–10 cohorts when compared to the 2–4 cohorts (noninferior). The rate of adverse events was also similar. **Conclusion: SRS may be suitable in patients with up to 10 brain metastases.**

Li, MDACC (ASTRO Abstract 2020): Phase III RCT of 72 patients with 4 to 15 untreated nonmelanoma brain metastases randomized to SRS (*n* = 36) or WBRT (*n* = 36). Prior SRS to one to three brain metastases with at least 3 months interval was permitted. Median number of brain metastases was 8, and 31 patients were evaluable for primary endpoint of neurocognition using HVLT-R-TR at 4 months. WBRT-treated patients had greater decline in HVLT-R-TR compared with SRS patients (*p* = .041). MS 10.4 months for SRS and 8.4 months for WBRT (*p* = .45). **Conclusion: Nonmelanoma patients with 4–15 brain metastases can be treated with SRS to better preserve neurocognition without a detriment in OS based on abstract results.** *Note: Trial was closed early as HA-WBRT became standard.*

What treatment options are there for large metastases that are not amenable to surgical resection?

Larger tumors treated with SRS have suboptimal LC using RTOG 9005 dosing.[44,53] Strategies to improve LC include fractionated[29–32,53] and staged SRS[33,34,54] with the goal of dose escalation while limiting toxicity such as radionecrosis.[18] Data from prospective studies investigating these SRS techniques to determine the optimal dose, fractionation, and timing for large brain metastases will be important to guide future standards.

What doses can be safely given in the preoperative setting for those with large brain metastases?

Murphy, CCF (*Neuro Oncol* 2024, PMID 38656347): Phase I dose escalation in 35 patients/36 lesions measuring at least 2 cm in cohorts of >2 to 3 cm, >3 to 4 cm, and >4 to 6 cm. The MTD of the >2–3 cm cohort was not reached and was 18 Gy for the other two cohorts. At MFU of 64 months, 6-month LC was 86% and 12-month LC was 77%. One out of 35 patients developed grade 3 radiation necrosis and the 2-year rate of LMD was 0%. **Conclusion: The MTD for preop SRS in large lesions was not reached in tumors up to 3 cm but was 18 Gy for tumors >3 cm.**

Can SRS be considered for patients with brain metastases from small cell lung cancer?

Historically, SCLC patients have been excluded from SRS studies due to concern that omission of WBRT would decrease OS, as these patients have a high risk of short-interval CNS progression compared with other histologies. However, FIRE-SCLC reports that, although WBRT is associated with superior time to CNS progression, there was no OS advantage, as is seen with other histologies.

Rusthoven, FIRE-SCLC (*JAMA Oncol* 2020, PMID 32496550): Multicenter cohort study that analyzed the outcomes of 710 patients treated with SRS for SCLC brain mets (no prior PCI or WBRT) and used propensity score-matched analysis to compare with the outcomes from a WBRT cohort. After propensity score matching, 187 patients in each SRS and WBRT cohort were analyzed for OS. Median OS favored SRS vs. WBRT (6.5 vs. 5.2 months, *p* = .003), and median time to CNS progression was improved with WBRT (9.0 months for SRS vs. not reached for WBRT, *p* < .003). **Conclusion: Upfront SRS does not appear to have a detriment to OS in this matched cohort, so the role of WBRT should be reconsidered given the neurocognitive detriment; however, this analysis should not be used to conclude SRS is associated with superior OS.**

Gaebe, SRS vs. WBRT Meta-Analysis (*Lancet Oncol* 2022, PMID 35644163): Meta-analysis including seven studies evaluating OS following WBRT ± SRS boost vs. SRS alone for SCLC brain mets. The SRS-alone cohort was only 8.5% of patients. OS following SRS alone was longer than following WBRT (HR 0.77, 95% CI 0.72–0.83; 7 studies, n = 18,130) but not WBRT + SRS boost (HR 1.17, 95% CI 0.78–1.75; 4 studies, n = 1,167). **Conclusion: Survival outcomes are similar with SRS compared with WBRT in patients with brain metastases from SCLC.**

Given the distant intracranial failure of SRS and neurocognitive decline associated with WBRT, what alternative modality can be considered for whole brain consolidation after SRS?

In patients with NSCLC with ≤10 brain mets without driver mutations, tumor-treating fields (TTF) are an emerging therapy based on the METIS (EF-25) trial for consolidation after SRS with improved time to intracranial progression and deterioration free-survival compared with best supportive care, with no negative impact on cognition. Final publication is pending.[55]

What is the role of craniospinal irradiation (CSI) in patients with LMD over involved-field RT (IFRT)?

IFRT has been the standard of care, although there are promising randomized phase II data suggesting that CSI may be superior (CNS PFS and OS), pending further validation.

Yang, MSKCC (*JCO* 2022, PMID 35802849): Phase II RCT of 63 patients with LMD from NSCLC or breast cancer randomized 2:1 to proton CSI (pCSI) vs. photon IFRT. At planned interim analysis, pCSI demonstrated superior CNS PFS (7.5 vs. 2.3 months, p < .001) and OS (9.9 vs. 6.0 months, p = .029), without difference in G3/4 AE. Thirty-five patients with other solid tumors were enrolled in a nonrandomized exploratory group, resulting in a median CNS PFS of 5.8 months and OS of 6.6 months. **Conclusion: pCSI appears to have superior CNS PFS and OS compared with IFRT without compromise in toxicity.** Limitation: It remains unclear if pCSI is superior to or significantly less toxic than modern photon CSI. For now, it appears that safe delivery of higher volumes of CNS RT for LMD may be beneficial and proton therapy may facilitate this. NRG BN014 is an ongoing randomized phase III study of IFRT vs. pCSI for LMD from breast or NSCLC.

REFERENCES

1. Suh JH, Kotecha R, Chao ST, Ahluwalia MS, Sahgal A, Chang EL. Current approaches to the management of brain metastases. *Nat Rev Clin Oncol.* 2020;17(5):279–299. doi:10.1038/s41571-019-0320-3
2. Nichols EM, Patchell RA, Regine WF, et al. Palliation of brain and spinal cord metastases. In: *Perez and Brady's Principles and Practice of Radiation Oncology.* 7th ed. Lippincott Williams & Wilkins; 2018.
3. Wiegreffe S, Sarria GR, Layer JP, et al. Incidence of hippocampal and perihippocampal brain metastases and impact on hippocampal-avoiding radiotherapy: a systematic review and meta-analysis. *Radiother Oncol.* 2024;197:110331. doi:10.1016/j.radonc.2024.110331
4. Tom MC, DiFilippo FP, Jones SE, et al. 18F-fluciclovine PET/CT to distinguish radiation necrosis from tumor progression for brain metastases treated with radiosurgery: results of a prospective pilot study. *J Neurooncol.* 2023;163(3):647–655. doi:10.1007/s11060-023-04377-5
5. Patchell RA, Tibbs PA, Walsh JW, et al. A randomized trial of surgery in the treatment of single metastases to the brain. *N Engl J Med.* 1990;322(8):494–500. doi:10.1056/NEJM199002223220802
6. Gaspar L, Scott C, Rotman M, et al. Recursive partitioning analysis (RPA) of prognostic factors in three Radiation Therapy Oncology Group (RTOG) brain metastases trials. *Int J Radiat Oncol Biol Phys.* 1997;37(4):745–751. doi:10.1016/S0360-3016(96)00619-0
7. Sperduto PW, Berkey B, Gaspar LE, Mehta M, Curran W. A new prognostic index and comparison to three other indices for patients with brain metastases: an analysis of 1,960 patients in the RTOG database. *Int J Radiat Oncol Biol Phys.* 2008;70(2):510–514. doi:10.1016/j.ijrobp.2007.06.074
8. Sperduto PW, Mesko S, Li J, et al. Survival in patients with brain metastases: summary report on the updated diagnosis-specific graded prognostic assessment and definition of the eligibility quotient. *J Clin Oncol.* 2020;38(32):3773–3784. doi:10.1200/JCO.20.01255
9. Farris M, McTyre ER, Cramer CK, et al. Brain metastasis velocity: a novel prognostic metric predictive of overall survival and freedom from whole-brain radiation therapy after distant brain failure following upfront radiosurgery alone. *Int J Radiat Oncol Biol Phys.* 2017;98(1):131–141. doi:10.1016/j.ijrobp.2017.01.201
10. Huntoon K, Anderson SK, Ballman KV, et al. Association of circulating markers with cognitive decline after radiation therapy for brain metastasis. *Neuro Oncol.* 2023;25(6):1123–1131. doi:10.1093/neuonc/noac262
11. Wefel JS, Deshmukh S, Brown PD, et al. Impact of apolipoprotein E genotype on neurocognitive function in patients with brain metastases: an analysis of NRG Oncology's RTOG 0614. *Int J Radiat Oncol Biol Phys.* 2024;119(3):846–857. doi:10.1016/j.ijrobp.2023.12.004

12. Sperduto PW, Mesko S, Li J, et al. Survival in patients with brain metastases: summary report on the updated diagnosis-specific graded prognostic assessment and definition of the eligibility quotient. *J Clin Oncol.* 2020;38(32):3773–3784. doi:10.1200/JCO.20.01255

13. Schnurman Z, Mashiach E, Link KE, et al. Causes of death in patients with brain metastases. *Neurosurgery.* 2023;93(5):986–993. doi: 10.1227/neu.0000000000002542

14. Kirkpatrick JP. Classifying leptomeningeal disease: an essential element in managing advanced metastatic disease in the central nervous system. *Int J Radiat Oncol Biol Phys.* 2020;106(3):587–588. doi:10.1016/j.ijrobp.2019.12.016

15. Gutiérrez-Valencia E, Sánchez I, Valles A, et al. Pachymeningeal disease: a systematic review and metanalysis. *J Neurooncol.* 2023;165(1):29–39. doi:10.1007/s11060-023-04476-3

16. Le Rhun E, Weller M, van den Bent M, et al. Leptomeningeal metastasis from solid tumours: EANO–ESMO Clinical Practice Guideline for diagnosis, treatment and follow-up. *ESMO Open.* 2023;8(5):101624. doi:10.1016/j.esmoop.2023.101624

17. Mehta MP, Rodrigus P, Terhaard CHJ, et al. Survival and neurologic outcomes in a randomized trial of motexafin gadolinium and whole-brain radiation therapy in brain metastases. *J Clin Oncol.* 2003;21(13):2529–2536. doi:10.1200/JCO.2003.12.122

18. Suh JH, Stea B, Nabid A, et al. Phase III study of efaproxiral as an adjunct to whole-brain radiation therapy for brain metastases. *J Clin Oncol.* 2006;24(1):106–114. doi:10.1200/JCO.2004.00.1768

19. Arrieta O, Hernández-Pedro N, Maldonado F, et al. Nitroglycerin plus whole intracranial radiation therapy for brain metastases in patients with non-small cell lung cancer: a randomized, open-label, phase 2 clinical trial. *Int J Radiat Oncol Biol Phys.* 2023;115(3):592–607. doi:10.1016/j.ijrobp.2022.02.010

20. Di Lorenzo R, Ahluwalia MS. Targeted therapy of brain metastases: latest evidence and clinical implications. *Ther Adv Med Oncol.* 2017;9(12):781–796. doi:10.1177/1758834017736252

21. Gondi V, Bauman G, Bradfield L, et al. Radiation therapy for brain metastases: an ASTRO clinical practice guideline. *Pract Radiat Oncol.* 2022;12(4):265–282. doi:10.1016/j.prro.2022.02.003

22. Pike LRG, Miao E, Boe LA, et al. Tyrosine kinase inhibitors with and without up-front stereotactic radiosurgery for brain metastases from EGFR and ALK oncogene–driven non–small cell lung cancer (TURBO-NSCLC). *J Clin Oncol.* 2024;42(30):3606–3617. doi:10.1200/JCO.23.02668

23. Kim IA, Winter KA, Sperduto PW, et al. Concurrent lapatinib with brain radiation therapy in patients with HER2+ breast cancer with brain metastases: NRG Oncology–KROG/RTOG 1119 phase 2 randomized trial. *Int J Radiat Oncol Biol Phys.* 2024;118(5):1391–1401. doi:10.1016/j.ijrobp.2023.07.019

24. Khatri VM, Mestres-Villanueva MA, Yarlagadda S, et al. Multi-institutional report of trastuzumab deruxtecan and stereotactic radiosurgery for HER2 positive and HER2-low breast cancer brain metastases. *NPJ Breast Cancer.* 2024;10(1):100. doi:10.1038/s41523-024-00711-w

25. Westover KD, Mendel JT, Dan T, et al. Phase II trial of hippocampal-sparing whole brain irradiation with simultaneous integrated boost for metastatic cancer. *Neuro Oncol.* 2020;22(12):1831–1839. doi:10.1093/neuonc/noaa092

26. Lebow ES, Hwang WL, Zieminski S, et al. Early experience with hippocampal avoidance whole brain radiation therapy and simultaneous integrated boost for brain metastases. *J Neurooncol.* 2020;148(1):81–88. doi:10.1007/s11060-020-03491-y

27. Chia BSH, Leong JY, Ong ALK, et al. Randomised prospective phase II trial in multiple brain metastases comparing outcomes between hippocampal avoidance whole brain radiotherapy with or without simultaneous integrated boost: HA-SIB-WBRT study protocol. *BMC Cancer.* 2020;20(1):1045. doi:10.1186/s12885-020-07565-y

28. Suh JH. Stereotactic radiosurgery for the management of brain metastases. *N Engl J Med.* 2010;362(12):1119–1127. doi:10.1056/NEJMct0806951

29. Minniti G, D'Angelillo RM, Scaringi C, et al. Fractionated stereotactic radiosurgery for patients with brain metastases. *J Neurooncol.* 2014;117(2):295–301. doi:10.1007/s11060-014-1388-3

30. Kim YJ, Cho KH, Kim JY, et al. Single-dose versus fractionated stereotactic radiotherapy for brain metastases. *Int J Radiat Oncol Biol Phys.* 2011;81(2):483–489. doi:10.1016/j.ijrobp.2010.05.033

31. Remick JS, Kowalski E, Khairnar R, et al. A multi-center analysis of single-fraction versus hypofractionated stereotactic radiosurgery for the treatment of brain metastasis. *Radiat Oncol.* 2020;15(1):128. doi:10.1186/s13014-020-01522-6

32. Ernst-Stecken A, Ganslandt O, Lambrecht U, Sauer R, Grabenbauer G. Phase II trial of hypofractionated stereotactic radiotherapy for brain metastases: results and toxicity. *Radiother Oncol.* 2006;81(1):18–24. doi:10.1016/j.radonc.2006.08.024

33. Dohm A, McTyre ER, Okoukoni C, et al. Staged stereotactic radiosurgery for large brain metastases: local control and clinical outcomes of a one-two punch technique. *Neurosurgery.* 2018;83(1):114–121. doi:10.1093/neuros/nyx355

34. Angelov L, Mohammadi AM, Bennett EE, et al. Impact of 2-staged stereotactic radiosurgery for treatment of brain metastases ≥ 2 cm. *J Neurosurg.* 2018;129(2):366–382. doi:10.3171/2017.3.JNS162532

35. Redmond KJ, De Salles AAF, Fariselli L, et al. Stereotactic radiosurgery for postoperative metastatic surgical cavities: a critical review and International Stereotactic Radiosurgery Society (ISRS) practice guidelines. *Int J Radiat Oncol Biol Phys.* 2021;111(1):68–80. doi:10.1016/j.ijrobp.2021.04.016

36. Routman DM, Yan E, Vora S, et al. Preoperative stereotactic radiosurgery for brain metastases. *Front Neurol.* 2018;9:959. doi: 10.3389/fneur.2018.00959

37. Murphy ES, Yang K, Suh JH, et al. Phase I trial of dose escalation for preoperative stereotactic radiosurgery for patients with large brain metastases. *Neuro Oncol.* 2024;26(9):1651–1659. doi:10.1093/neuonc/noae076

38. Rusthoven CG, Yamamoto M, Bernhardt D, et al. Evaluation of first-line radiosurgery vs whole-brain radiotherapy for small cell lung cancer brain metastases: the FIRE-SCLC cohort study. *JAMA Oncol.* 2020;6(7):1028–1037. doi:10.1001/jamaoncol.2020.1271

39. Vellayappan B, Lim-Fat MJ, Kotecha R, et al. A systematic review informing the management of symptomatic brain radiation necrosis after stereotactic radiosurgery and International Stereotactic Radiosurgery Society recommendations. *Int J Radiat Oncol Biol Phys.* 2024;118(1):14–28. doi:10.1016/j.ijrobp.2023.07.015

40. Videtic GMM, Vassil AD, Woody NM. *Handbook of Treatment Planning in Radiation Oncology.* Springer Publishing Company; 2020.

41. Trifiletti DM, Ballman KV, Brown PD, et al. Optimizing whole brain radiation therapy dose and fractionation: results from a prospective phase 3 trial (NCCTG N107C [Alliance]/CEC.3). *Int J Radiat Oncol Biol Phys.* 2020;106(2):255–260. doi:10.1016/j.ijrobp.2019.10.024

42. Noordijk EM, Vecht CJ, Haaxma-Reiche H, et al. The choice of treatment of single brain metastasis should be based on extracranial tumor activity and age. *Int J Radiat Oncol Biol Phys.* 1994;29(4):711–717. doi:10.1016/0360-3016(94)90558-4

43. Mintz AH, Kestle J, Rathbone MP, et al. A randomized trial to assess the efficacy of surgery in addition to radiotherapy in patients with a single cerebral metastasis. *Cancer.* 1996;78(7):1470–1476. doi:10.1002/(SICI)1097-0142(19961001)78:7<1470::AID-CNCR14>3.0.CO;2-X

44. Shaw E, Scott C, Souhami L, et al. Single dose radiosurgical treatment of recurrent previously irradiated primary brain tumors and brain metastases: final report of RTOG protocol 90-05. *Int J Radiat Oncol Biol Phys.* 2000;47(2):291–298. doi:10.1016/S0360-3016(99)00507-6

45. Chang EL, Wefel JS, Hess KR, et al. Neurocognition in patients with brain metastases treated with radiosurgery or radiosurgery plus whole-brain irradiation: a randomised controlled trial. *Lancet Oncol.* 2009;10(11):1037–1044. doi:10.1016/S1470-2045(09)70263-3

46. Kocher M, Soffietti R, Abacioglu U, et al. Adjuvant whole-brain radiotherapy versus observation after radiosurgery or surgical resection of one to three cerebral metastases: results of the EORTC 22952-26001 study. *J Clin Oncol.* 2011;29(2):134–141. doi:10.1200/JCO.2010.30.1655

47. Sahgal A, Aoyama H, Kocher M, et al. Phase 3 trials of stereotactic radiosurgery with or without whole-brain radiation therapy for 1 to 4 brain metastases: individual patient data meta-analysis. *Int J Radiat Oncol Biol Phys.* 2015;91(4):710–717. doi:10.1016/j.ijrobp.2014.10.024

48. Brown PD, Jaeckle K, Ballman KV, et al. Effect of radiosurgery alone vs radiosurgery with whole brain radiation therapy on cognitive function in patients with 1 to 3 brain metastases: a randomized clinical trial. *JAMA.* 2016;316(4):401–409. doi:10.1001/jama.2016.9839

49. Gondi V, Pugh SL, Tome WA, et al. Preservation of memory with conformal avoidance of the hippocampal neural stem-cell compartment during whole-brain radiotherapy for brain metastases (RTOG 0933): a phase II multi-institutional trial. *J Clin Oncol.* 2014;32(34):3810–3816. doi:10.1200/JCO.2014.57.2909

50. Cherng HR, Sun K, Bentzen S, et al. Evaluating the heterogeneity of hippocampal avoidant whole brain radiotherapy treatment effect: a secondary analysis of NRG CC001. *Neuro Oncol.* 2024;26(5):911–921. doi:10.1093/neuonc/noad226

51. Yamamoto M, Kawabe T, Sato Y, et al. Stereotactic radiosurgery for patients with multiple brain metastases: a case-matched study comparing treatment results for patients with 2–9 versus 10 or more tumors. *J Neurosurg.* 2014;121(suppl 2):16–25. doi:10.3171/2014.8.GKS141421

52. Nagai N, Koide Y, Shindo Y, et al. Retrospective non-inferiority study of stereotactic radiosurgery for more than ten brain metastases. *J Neurooncol.* 2023;163(2):385–395. doi:10.1007/s11060-023-04358-8

53. Minniti G, Scaringi C, Paolini S, et al. Single-fraction versus multifraction (3 × 9 Gy) stereotactic radiosurgery for large (>2 cm) brain metastases: a comparative analysis of local control and risk of radiation-induced brain necrosis. *Int J Radiat Oncol Biol Phys.* 2016;95(4):1142–1148. doi:10.1016/j.ijrobp.2016.03.013

54. Yomo S, Hayashi M, Nicholson C. A prospective pilot study of two-session Gamma Knife surgery for large metastatic brain tumors. *J Neurooncol.* 2012;109(1):159–165. doi:10.1007/s11060-012-0882-8

55. Mehta MP, Gondi V, Ahluwalia MS, et al. Results from METIS (EF-25), an international, multicenter phase III randomized study evaluating the efficacy and safety of tumor treating fields (TTFields) therapy in NSCLC patients with brain metastases. *J Clin Oncol.* 2024;42(16_suppl):2008–2008. doi:10.1200/JCO.2024.42.16_suppl.2008

Sean M. Parker, Ehsan H. Balagamwala, Samuel T. Chao, and Andrew D. Vassil

QUICK HIT Up to 80% of advanced cancer patients develop bone metastases. The most common primary sites include the breast, lung, and prostate. A variety of fractionation regimens are used, with 8 Gy/1 fx, 20 Gy/5 fx, and 30 Gy/10 fx being the most common. Factors that influence treatment technique and dose/fractionation include performance status, logistics, tumor size and location, histology, prior surgery or RT, neurologic deficits, impending fracture, soft tissue component, physician preference, and patient's goals. Pain relief is expected in approximately two-thirds of patients, and median time to pain response is ~3 weeks. Multiple studies have demonstrated no difference in pain control between single- and multifraction regimens; however, single fraction may entail a higher retreatment rate (perhaps due to physician bias). Pain flare may occur in up to one-third of patients and is treated with a short steroid course. SBRT is increasingly utilized in the upfront setting for oligometastatic disease, high KPS patients, or radioresistant histology. The role of radiopharmaceuticals (e.g., Ra-223, Lu-177-617-PSMA) is evolving and increasingly considered for multifocal bone metastases. Prophylactic RT to high-risk bone metastases has demonstrated efficacy in reducing skeletal-related events (SREs).

EPIDEMIOLOGY: Up to 80% of patients with advanced solid tumors develop bone metastasis to the spine, pelvis, or extremities, and over half of people who die of cancer are thought to have bone involvement.[1,2] The most common primary tumor sites are the breast, prostate, lung, thyroid, and kidney. Metastases to bone most often occur in the red marrow distribution: spine (lumbar > thoracic) > pelvis > ribs > femur > skull.

ANATOMY: Axial skeleton includes the skull, spine, sternum, and ribs. Appendicular skeleton includes long bones and appendixes. Long bones consist of epiphysis (end), metaphysis, and diaphysis (shaft). Two types of bone: cortical and trabecular. Cortical bone, found in the diaphysis of long bones, is dense, making up 80% of skeletal mass and providing strength/protection; ~3% replaced per year. Trabecular bone is spongy, contains red marrow, and is found inside long bones (concentrated at ends), vertebral bodies, inner pelvic bones, and other large flat bones; ~25% replaced per year.

PATHOLOGY: Bone metastases primarily occur via hematogenous spread and less commonly from direct extension (e.g., oral cavity cancer invading the mandible). A combination of tumor factors (cell adhesion molecules that bind to receptors on the cells of the marrow and bone matrix) and the bony microenvironment (growth factors released and activated during bone resorption) contribute to preferential metastasis to bone.[3] Normal bone is constantly remodeled via bone-building osteoblasts and bone-reabsorbing osteoclasts. Bony metastasis causes a dysregulation of normal bone remodeling that can manifest as osteoblastic, osteolytic, or mixed lesions. Bone destruction by osteolytic metastasis is mediated by osteoclasts, which are activated by factors produced by tumor cells, such as TGF-β, PTH-rP, IL-1, and IL-6. Although classically certain cancers are thought to be primarily osteoblastic or osteolytic, the vast majority have components of both processes. *Osteoblastic:* prostate, SCLC, Hodgkin lymphoma, and carcinoid. *Osteolytic:* renal cell, melanoma, multiple myeloma (MM), NSCLC, thyroid, and NHL. *Mixed:* breast, GI, and squamous cell cancers.

CLINICAL PRESENTATION: The most common presenting symptom is pain, followed by reduced mobility (70%), pathologic fractures (10%–20%), hypercalcemia (10%–15%), spinal cord/nerve compression (5%), and reduced marrow function.

WORKUP: H&P to assess for pain onset/severity, sensory or motor dysfunction, ambulation, urinary/bowel retention or incontinence. Physical exam to evaluate the symptomatic site for soft tissue extension, relationship to nearby neurovascular structures, limb edema, muscle strength, and range of motion.

Imaging: X-ray of the entire involved bone for appendicular skeletal metastases (most specific) to evaluate bone structure, extent of involvement, pathologic fracture, or any risk of impending fracture. Small lesions are difficult to assess on x-ray as nearly half of bone mineral content must be lost to be visible. Bone scan (Tc-99m), which detects osteoblastic activity (less effective when osteolysis dominates), is often first line. Skeletal survey XR can be helpful in cases where osteolysis predominates, such as MM. CT is more sensitive than XR and may be useful in assessing pathologic fracture risk or guiding biopsies. MRI is most sensitive (91%–100%) and better assesses neurovascular compression and marrow involvement, especially for spine metastases. PET/CT is very sensitive in detecting osteolytic metastases (~98%) but less specific (~56%).[4] Neoplasms with lower metabolic rates (like prostate cancer) are not typically evident on FDG-PET, but histology-specific PET scans (e.g., fluciclovine, PSMA-PET) have improved detection.[5,6]

Biopsy: Tissue diagnosis should be strongly considered in patients with solitary bone lesions without a history of cancer or as a first metastatic relapse. CT-guided FNA or core biopsy is preferred. In cases of pathologic fracture, biopsy can be performed as component of the surgical revision.

PROGNOSTIC FACTORS: Dependent on underlying histology and extent of metastatic disease.

TREATMENT PARADIGM

Surgery: Surgery is considered to prevent or treat pathologic fractures. Both lytic and blastic lesions reduce bone strength. Historically, 2- to 3-cm cortical involvement or lytic destruction of ≥50% of the width of bone was concerning for impending fracture. Mirels 12-point scoring system is commonly utilized to predict risk for fracture (Table 69.1).[7] Prophylactic fixation is considered for lesions with functionally limiting pain exacerbated by weight bearing or in patients with persistent pain after RT.

Table 69.1 Mirels Nomogram for Pathologic Fracture Risk of Bone Metastases[7]			
Points	**1**	**2**	**3**
Site	Upper limb	Lower limb	Peritrochanteric
Degree of pain	Mild	Moderate	Severe
Radiographic nature	Blastic	Mixed	Lytic
Size of cortex	<1/3	1/3–2/3	>2/3
Some add 1 point for femoral lesions proximal to lesser trochanter, proximal humeral lesions, breast cancer, no bisphosphonates, and osteoporosis.			
≤7 points = <10% fracture risk → observe. 8 points = 15% fracture risk → consider fixation. 9 points = 33% fracture risk → prophylactic fixation. ≥10 points = >50% fracture risk → prophylactic fixation.			

Source: Adapted from Mirels H. The Classic: metastatic disease in long bones—a proposed scoring system for diagnosing impending pathologic fractures. *Clin Orthop Relat Res.* 2003;415(suppl):S4–S13. doi:10.1097/01.blo.0000093045.56370.dd.

Femoral metastases account for two-thirds of pathologic fractures requiring intervention. Femoral neck fractures undergo total hip arthroplasty (replacing the femoral head and acetabulum) or proximal femoral endoprosthesis. Intertrochanteric region fractures are managed with open reduction and internal fixation without prosthesis (better gait). Lytic disease below intertrochanteric area is treated with an intramedullary rod. Postoperative fractionated RT of the entire bone metastasis and surgical hardware reduces the risk of disease progression, compromising hardware integrity.[8]

Medical Management

Bisphosphonates: Decrease SREs by inhibiting osteoclast-mediated bone resorption and promoting repair by stimulating osteoblast differentiation and bone formation.[9,10] Zoledronate and pamidronate are the most common and are administered as monthly IV infusions. Zoledronate also induces apoptosis and inhibits tumor cell adhesion to the extracellular matrix. Bisphosphonates may prolong time to first SRE and reduce rates of fracture, RT, surgery, and hypercalcemia.[9,10] Toxicities include osteonecrosis (1%–2%), hypocalcemia, and renal insufficiency.

RANK-L Inhibitors: RANK/RANK-ligand/osteoprotegerin (RANK/RANK-L/OPG) pathway regulates osteoclast maturation, differentiation, and survival. This pathway is disrupted in the metastatic setting due to increased RANK expression.[11] Denosumab, a monoclonal antibody that inhibits RANK-L, is approved for prevention of SREs in patients with bone metastasis from solid tumors. A meta-analysis of three phase III trials suggests denosumab for solid tumor bone metastases is superior to zoledronic acid in reducing first SRE or hypercalcemia of malignancy.[12] Bone-modifying agents are recommended by ASCO for all patients with MM and those with bone metastases from solid tumors.[13–15]

Radiation

RT is the cornerstone of bone metastasis treatment in the palliative and postoperative settings. Conventional EBRT is most frequently utilized, although SBRT/SRS and radiopharmaceuticals now play an increasingly important role. Recent prospective data support an emerging paradigm of prophylactic RT for asymptomatic high-risk bone metastases to reduce SREs.[16]

EBRT: For conventional fractionation, the 2024 ASTRO guidelines suggest the following as recommended doses: 8 Gy/1 fx, 20 Gy/5 fx, 24 Gy/6 fx, 20 Gy/10 fx (for MM), or 30 Gy/10 fx.[17] Equivalent pain relief but higher retreatment rates is reported with single-fraction RT, although this may be secondary to physician bias.[18–20] The use of other modalities (e.g., surgery, RFA, cryoablation, bisphosphonates, radiopharmaceuticals) does not obviate the role of EBRT for painful bone metastases.

SBRT/SRS: SBRT to nonspine metastases may improve pain control and can be considered for select patients with good KPS without neurologic symptoms.[17,21] For nonspine osseous metastases, the most common SBRT doses include 12 Gy/1 fx (size ≥4 cm), 16 Gy/1 fx (size <4 cm), 30 Gy/3 fx, or 35 Gy/5 fx.[21–23] The clearest indication for spine SRS is in the retreatment setting (20 Gy/10 fx is also a common retreatment regimen). For spine SRS, the most common fractionation schemes include 16–18 Gy/1 fx or 24 Gy/1–2 fx. Doses of ≥20 Gy per fraction are associated with increased risk of VCF.[24] Guidelines are published for contouring of definitive spine SRS, postoperative spine SRS, and for response assessment (SPINO).[25–27] Use of SBRT for oligometastatic disease is detailed in Chapter 73.

Radiopharmaceuticals: Radioactive agents are administered intravenously and localize to the site of osteoblastic activity, thereby delivering dose simultaneously to all sites of bony disease. Myelosuppression is the major toxicity. The most used isotopes are beta emitters and alpha emitters. Early trials evaluating beta emitters (Sr-89, Sm-153, P-53) demonstrated modest improvements in pain response at the cost of increased hematologic toxicity. Ra-223 offers the advantage of an alpha emitter with high LET and short range (10 µm in bone and soft tissue), thus reducing toxicity. More recently, the PSMA-tagged beta emitter Lu-177-PSMA-617 has emerged as an effective treatment option for metastatic CRPC.

Procedure: See *Handbook of Treatment Planning in Radiation Oncology*, Chapter 14.[28]

EVIDENCE-BASED Q&A

Is there a benefit to longer fractionation schemes for uncomplicated bone metastases?

Several large prospective trials as well as a meta-analysis showed no difference in pain relief (~2/3) between single-fraction and multifraction regimens. Retreatment rates are higher after single-fraction RT, perhaps due to physician bias.[29] Complicated bone metastases (fractures, cord compression, previous RT) were excluded from these trials.

Steenland, Dutch Bone Metastasis Study (*Radiother Oncol* 1999, PMID 10577695): PRT of 1,171 patients randomized to 8 Gy/1 fx vs. 24 Gy/6 fx. Weekly questionnaires used for self-assessment after treatment, and primary endpoint was pain score (0–10). Response in 71% (median time to response 3 weeks in both groups), with no differences in pain medication usage, QOL, or side effects between regimens. More patients were retreated in the single-fx group (25% vs. 7%). However, among single-fx patients, time to retreat and pain score at retreat were lower, suggesting physicians may offer retreatment more readily to single-fx patients. Axial cortical involvement >30 mm (p = .01) and circumferential cortical involvement >50% (p = .03) were predictive of fracture. **Conclusion: Single fraction provides similar pain response compared with multifraction, but patients may be at a higher risk for retreatment.**

Hartsell, RTOG 9714 (*JNCI* 2005, PMID 15928300): PRT of 898 patients with breast or prostate cancer with one to three painful bone metastases randomized to 8 Gy/1 fx vs. 30 Gy/10 fx. No difference in overall response rate (66%), CR (~15%), and PR (~50%). More frequent grades 2 to 4 acute toxicities (mostly GI-related) in the 30 Gy arm (17% vs. 10%, $p = .002$). No difference in late toxicity (4%), fracture rates (4%–5%), or narcotic use at 3 months. Higher rate of retreatment with single fx (18% vs. 9%, $p < .001$). **Conclusion: A single fraction of 8 Gy provides similar efficacy in pain relief, with less acute toxicity but higher rates of retreatment than 30 Gy/10 fx.**

Chow, Toronto Meta-Analysis (*JCO* 2007, PMID 17416863; Update *Clin Oncol* 2012, PMID 22130630): Meta-analysis of 25 PRT with over 5,600 patients comparing single- with multi-fx schedules. No difference in overall response rate (60% vs. 61%), CR (23% vs. 24%), acute toxicity, or pathologic fracture risk (3.3% vs. 3.0%). Retreatment was more likely in the single-fx group (20% vs. 8%, $p < .001$). **Conclusion: Single- and multifraction regimens provide equal pain relief.**

What is the best dose for single-fraction palliative RT?

The Toronto Meta-Analysis on Dose included 24 trials (3,233 patients) randomizing patients to single-fraction arms (4–15 Gy) and noted a dose–response relationship. The optimal single-fraction dose was found to be 8 Gy/1 fx.[30]

What is the expected time to pain response with EBRT?

Median time to pain response is ~3 weeks with either single-fraction or multifraction EBRT regimens.[20,31] *Palliative RT may be effective in patients with limited life spans as 40% will have pain reduction by 10 days.*[32]

Does SBRT relieve pain from nonspine bone metastases more effectively than EBRT?

Five trials have compared pain response between SBRT and conventionally fractionated EBRT, with a majority focusing on spine metastases.[33,34] *Among nonspine metastases, two randomized trials demonstrate conflicting data. The Nguyen MDACC trial demonstrated noninferiority of SBRT with improved pain response. A phase II trial by Ito et al. did not demonstrate improved pain response but was underpowered due to a high dropout rate.*[23] *A meta-analysis including seven spine- and nonspine-focused trials found SBRT improved complete pain response but not overall pain response.*[35]

Nguyen, MDACC (*JAMA Oncol* 2019, PMID 31021390): Phase II noninferiority (10% margin) RCT of 160 patients with painful bone metastases randomized to SBRT (12 Gy for ≥4 cm lesions, 16 Gy for <4 cm; prophylactic dexamethasone recommended) vs. EBRT 30 Gy/10 fx (no prophylactic dexamethasone). The SBRT group had more pain response (CR or PR; primary endpoint) at 2 weeks (62% vs. 36%, $p = .01$), 3 months (72% vs. 49%, $p = .03$), and 9 months (77% vs. 46%, $p = .03$). No difference in treatment toxicity; 1-year local PFS 100% with SBRT vs. 91% with EBRT ($p = .01$). Subset analysis suggested the 16 Gy group had the highest rate of/most durable pain response. **Conclusions: SBRT is noninferior to EBRT for pain control and time to local progression. SBRT had significantly higher pain response at 2 weeks, 3 months, and 9 months.** *Note: High attrition rate due to cancer deaths. Not all time points were significantly different (i.e., 1 and 6 months).*

What are pain flares and what is the incidence?

A pain flare is a temporary worsening of bone pain in the irradiated site that usually occurs in the first few days after RT (80% occur in the first 5 days). Up to 40% of patients treated with RT may develop a pain flare in the first 10 days after RT, and the flare often lasts 1 to 2 days.[36] *Prophylactic dexamethasone 4 mg BID for 5 days has been prospectively demonstrated to treat (and possibly prevent) pain flares.*[37]

What is the role of RT after orthopedic stabilization?

RT promotes remineralization/bone healing, alleviates pain, improves functional status, reduces the risk for subsequent fracture or loss of fixation, and is associated with prolonged survival.[38,39] *Disadvantages include the potential effects on uninvolved bone and postoperative wound healing. RT is generally started within 2 to 4 weeks after surgery, although wound healing is prioritized. Covering the entire implant reduces the risk of LR.*[8] *The optimal dose/fractionation is unclear as there are limited data regarding single-fraction treatments, so 30 Gy/10 fx is typically recommended.*

Can prophylactic RT reduce SREs?

SREs occur in approximately two-thirds of patients with bone metastases and can significantly impact patient mobility, hospitalizations, and QOL. Retrospective data and the below prospective trial suggest prophylactic RT to high-risk bone metastases reduces the risk of developing SREs and hospitalizations.[16,40]

Gillespie, MSKCC (*JCO* 2023, PMID 37748124): Phase II RCT of 78 patients (≥5 metastases) and 122 asymptomatic high-risk bone metastases (bulky ≥2 cm, hip/shoulder/SI joint disease, long bone occupying one-third to two-thirds cortical thickness, or junctional spine) randomized to SOC vs. prophylactic RT. MFU 2.5 years. Primary endpoint of SRE (pathologic fracture, cord compression, surgical intervention, palliative RT for pain) was reduced in prophylactic RT group (HR 0.08, 95% CI 0.01–0.66). Although not powered to detect OS, median OS was improved with RT (1.7 vs. 1.0 years, *p* = .018). No difference in QOL or opioid-free survival. **Conclusion: Prophylactic RT to high-risk bone metastases reduces SREs and may improve OS.**

What is the evidence for retreatment of bone metastasis?

About 20% of patients will require retreatment of bone metastasis and the frequency is expected to increase as systemic therapies improve. Retreatment is feasible and provides pain relief in 50% to 60%.[41,42] It is recommended to wait at least 4 weeks after initial RT before considering re-RT to allow for full response from initial course. Patients with good response to prior RT are more likely to respond. Single fraction appears to have similar efficacy as multifraction regimens for uncomplicated metastases. It is important to carefully evaluate OARs, and more conformal planning may be considered to safely meet constraints.

Chow, NCIC SC 20 (*Lancet Oncol* 2014, PMID 24369114): RCT of 425 patients with painful (≥2 using Brief Pain Inventory) bone metastases previously treated with RT randomized to 8 Gy/1 fx vs. 20 Gy in multiple fractions. Primary endpoint of overall pain response at 2 months was 28% in the 8 Gy arm vs. 32% in the 20 Gy arm. Toxicity, including lack of appetite and diarrhea, was worse in the 20 Gy arm. **Conclusion: 8 Gy was noninferior and less toxic than 20 Gy for re-RT of painful bone metastases.**

What is the role of hemibody irradiation?

Hemibody RT, either with single- or multi-fraction regimens, may be indicated in those with extensive bony disease, especially in cases when radiopharmaceuticals are not available or contraindicated. An extended SSD technique is utilized, and fields are matched at the umbilicus or L4/5. Lung blocks may be necessary to limit lung dose to 6 to 7 Gy. Typically, 6 Gy/1 fx is given for the upper body and 8 Gy/1 fx to the lower body. Alternate doses include 15 Gy/5 fx or 20–30 Gy/8–10 fx delivered three fractions weekly. Typically, the other half of the body is treated 6 to 8 weeks later.

What is the role of radiopharmaceuticals for the treatment of extensive bony metastases?

Radiopharmaceuticals are radioactive agents that are administered intravenously and localize to the site of osteoblastic activity, thereby delivering dose simultaneously at sites of disease. The most common isotopes used are beta emitters (Sr-89, Sm-153, P-53, Lu-177) and alpha emitters (Ra-223). In the ALSYMPCA trial, Ra-223 (compared with placebo for bony metastatic prostate cancer) demonstrated improved OS and time to first SRE[43,44]; however, these findings were not reproduced on ERA-223 when Ra-223 was given in combination with abiraterone.[45] More recently, the targeted radiopharmaceutical Lu-177-PSMA-617 has demonstrated improved OS when added to SOC for mCRPC.[46]

Sartor, VISION (*NEJM* 2021, PMID 34161051): Phase III RCT of 831 men with metastatic CRPC treated with at least one AR inhibitor and one to two taxane regimens who had PSMA positive PET scans. Randomized to SOC (excluded Ra-223, CHT, immunotherapy) +/− Lu-177-PSMA-617. Lu-177-PSMA-617 + SOC significantly prolonged both imaging-based PFS (median 8.7 vs. 3.4 months, *p* < .001) and OS (median 15.3 vs. 11.3 months, *p* < .001). Grade 3 adverse events were higher (53% vs. 38%), but QOL was not adversely affected. **Conclusion: In patients with metastatic CRPC who have received SOC treatment with AR inhibitors and taxanes, the addition of Lu-177-PSMA-617 improves OS.**

Is there a role for spine SRS as compared with fractionated RT?

With true cord compression, the role of SRS is limited, given the duration of planning required for SRS and the need for ≥3 mm separation for the cord/thecal sac. The literature currently suggests an LC benefit, although this is primarily retrospective. RTOG 0631 compared patient-reported pain outcomes between the two modalities; it excluded patients with <3 mm of separation from the cord/thecal sac. It showed no significant difference in pain score between SRS and EBRT. More recently, CCTG SC.24 showed that 24 Gy in 2 fx provided higher pain CR rates compared with 20 Gy in 5 fx. The risk of pain flare after spine SBRT is ~15% and is adequately treated with a short course of steroids. The risk of new or progressive vertebral compression fractures is also ~15% and increases with dose/fraction ≥20 Gy.[17]

Ryu, RTOG 0631 (*JAMA Oncol* 2023, PMID 37079324): Randomized multi-institution phase II/III study of 339 patients with one to three sites of spinal metastatic disease randomized 2:1 to SBRT 16 or 18 Gy in 1 fx vs. EBRT 8 Gy in 1 fx to involved vertebral level plus one level above and below. Epidural extension permitted as long as ≥3 mm of separation from cord. Primary endpoint: pain control (3-point improvement on Numerical Rating Pain Scale [NRPS] at treated site 3 months posttreatment). No significant difference in pain score between the SRS group (–3.00 points) and the EBRT group (–3.83 points), nor in the proportion of patients with pain response (SBRT 40% vs. EBRT 58%, one-sided $p = .99$). **Conclusion: SBRT is not superior to EBRT for pain palliation in spine metastases.**

Sahgal, CCTG SC.24 (*Lancet Oncol* 2021, PMID 34126044): Randomized multi-institution phase II/III study of 229 patients with ≤3 consecutive involved spinal segments randomized 1:1 to SBRT 24 Gy/2 fx vs. EBRT 20 Gy/5 fx. Primary endpoint: complete pain response at 3 months posttreatment. MFU 6.7 months. At 3 months, pain CR rate was higher in the SRS group compared with the EBRT group (36% vs. 16%, $p < .001$). This difference was maintained at 6 months (33% vs. 16%, $p = .004$) and on MVA (OR 3.47, 95% CI 1.77–6.80). **Conclusion: SRS offers higher pain CR rates compared with EBRT.** *Note: On separate secondary analysis, SRS with improved LC (94% vs. 76%) and lower retreatment rates (2% vs. 16%) at 12 months.*

REFERENCES

1. Mundy GR. Metastasis to bone: causes, consequences and therapeutic opportunities. *Nat Rev Cancer.* 2002;2(8):584–593. doi:10.1038/nrc867
2. Nielsen OS. Palliative radiotherapy of bone metastases: there is now evidence for the use of single fractions. *Radiother Oncol.* 1999;52(2):95–96. doi:10.1016/s0167-8140(99)00109-7
3. Barghash RF, Abdou WM. Pathophysiology of metastatic bone disease and the role of the second generation of bisphosphonates: from basic science to medicine. *Curr Pharm Des.* 2016;22(11):1546–1557. doi:10.2174/1381612822666160122093810
4. Sullivan GJ, Carty FL, Cronin CG. Imaging of bone metastasis: an update. *World J Radiol.* 2015;7(8):202–211. doi:10.4329/wjr.v7.i8.202
5. Turpin A, Girard E, Baillet C, et al. Imaging for metastasis in prostate cancer: a review of the literature. *Front Oncol.* 2020;10:55. doi:10.3389/fonc.2020.00055
6. Kao CH, Hsieh JF, Tsai SC, Ho YJ, Yen RF. Comparison and discrepancy of 18F-2-deoxyglucose positron emission tomography and Tc-99m MDP bone scan to detect bone metastases. *Anticancer Res.* 2000;20(3B):2189–2192. PMID: 10928175
7. Mirels H. The Classic: metastatic disease in long bones—a proposed scoring system for diagnosing impending pathologic fractures. *Clin Orthop Relat Res.* 2003;415(suppl):S4–S13. doi:10.1097/01.blo.0000093045.56370.dd
8. Rosen DB, Haseltine JM, Bartelstein M, et al. Should postoperative radiation for long bone metastases cover part or all of the orthopedic hardware? Results of a large retrospective analysis. *Adv Radiat Oncol.* 2021;6(6):100756. doi:10.1016/j.adro.2021.100756
9. Berenson JR, Lichtenstein A, Porter L, et al. Long-term pamidronate treatment of advanced multiple myeloma patients reduces skeletal events. *J Clin Oncol.* 1998;16(2):593–602. doi:10.1200/JCO.1998.16.2.593
10. Ross JR, Saunders Y, Edmonds PM, Patel S, Broadley KE, Johnston SRD. Systematic review of role of bisphosphonates on skeletal morbidity in metastatic cancer. *BMJ.* 2003;327(7413):469. doi:10.1136/bmj.327.7413.469
11. Boyce BF, Xing L. Functions of RANKL/RANK/OPG in bone modeling and remodeling. *Arch Biochem Biophys.* 2008;473(2):139–146. doi:10.1016/j.abb.2008.03.018

12. Lipton A, Fizazi K, Stopeck AT, et al. Superiority of denosumab to zoledronic acid for prevention of skeletal-related events: a combined analysis of 3 pivotal, randomised, phase 3 trials. *Eur J Cancer.* 2012;48(16): 3082–3092. doi:10.1016/j.ejca.2012.08.002

13. Anderson K, Ismaila N, Flynn PJ, et al. Role of bone-modifying agents in multiple myeloma: American Society of Clinical Oncology clinical practice guideline update. *J Clin Oncol.* 2018;36(8):813–818. doi:10.1200/JCO.2017.76.6402

14. Poznak CV, Somerfield MR, Barlow WE, et al. Role of bone-modifying agents in metastatic breast cancer: an American Society of Clinical Oncology–Cancer Care Ontario focused guideline update. *J Clin Oncol.* 2017;35(35):3978–3985. doi:10.1200/JCO.2017.75.4614

15. Saylor PJ, Rumble RB, Tagawa S, et al. Bone health and bone-targeted therapies for prostate cancer: ASCO endorsement of a Cancer Care Ontario guideline. *J Clin Oncol.* 2020;38(15):1736–1743. doi:10.1200/JCO.19.03148

16. Gillespie EF, Yang JC, Mathis NJ, et al. Prophylactic radiation therapy versus standard of care for patients with high-risk asymptomatic bone metastases: a multicenter, randomized phase II clinical trial. *J Clin Oncol.* 2023;41(36):5564–5572. doi:10.1200/JCO.23.00753

17. Alcorn S, Cortés ÁA, Bradfield L, et al. External beam radiation therapy for palliation of symptomatic bone metastases: an ASTRO clinical practice guideline. *Pract Radiat Oncol.* 2024;14(4):e213–e225. doi:10.1016/j.prro.2024.04.018

18. Chow E, Zeng L, Salvo N, Dennis K, Tsao M, Lutz S. Update on the systematic review of palliative radiotherapy trials for bone metastases. *Clin Oncol.* 2012;24(2):112–124. doi:10.1016/j.clon.2011.11.004

19. Hartsell WF, Scott CB, Bruner DW, et al. Randomized trial of short- versus long-course radiotherapy for palliation of painful bone metastases. *J Natl Cancer Inst.* 2005;97(11):798–804. doi:10.1093/jnci/dji139

20. Steenland E, Leer JW, van Houwelingen H, et al. The effect of a single fraction compared to multiple fractions on painful bone metastases: a global analysis of the Dutch Bone Metastasis Study. *Radiother Oncol.* 1999;52(2):101–109. doi:10.1016/s0167-8140(99)00110-3

21. Nguyen QN, Chun SG, Chow E, et al. Single-fraction stereotactic vs conventional multifraction radiotherapy for pain relief in patients with predominantly nonspine bone metastases. *JAMA Oncol.* 2019;5(6): 872–878. doi:10.1001/jamaoncol.2019.0192

22. Chmura S, Winter KA, Robinson C, et al. Evaluation of safety of stereotactic body radiotherapy for the treatment of patients with multiple metastases. *JAMA Oncol.* 2021;7(6):845–852. doi:10.1001/jamaoncol.2021.0687

23. Ito K, Nakajima Y, Onoe T, et al. Phase 2 clinical trial of stereotactic body radiation therapy for painful nonspine bone metastases. *Pract Radiat Oncol.* 2021;11(2):e139–e145. doi:10.1016/j.prro.2020.10.003

24. Sahgal A, Atenafu EG, Chao S, et al. Vertebral compression fracture after spine stereotactic body radiotherapy: a multi-institutional analysis with a focus on radiation dose and the spinal instability neoplastic score. *J Clin Oncol.* 2013;31(27):3426–3431. doi:10.1200/JCO.2013.50.1411

25. Thibault I, Chang EL, Sheehan J, et al. Response assessment after stereotactic body radiotherapy for spinal metastasis: a report from the SPIne response assessment in Neuro-Oncology (SPINO) group. *Lancet Oncol.* 2015;16(16):e595–e603. doi:10.1016/S1470-2045(15)00166-7

26. Cox BW, Spratt DE, Lovelock M, et al. International Spine Radiosurgery Consortium consensus guidelines for target volume definition in spinal stereotactic radiosurgery. *Int J Radiat Oncol Biol Phys.* 2012;83(5): e597–e605. doi:10.1016/j.ijrobp.2012.03.009

27. Redmond KJ, Robertson S, Lo SS, et al. Consensus contouring guidelines for postoperative stereotactic body radiation therapy for metastatic solid tumor malignancies to the spine. *Int J Radiat Oncol Biol Phys.* 2017;97(1):64–74. doi:10.1016/j.ijrobp.2016.09.014

28. Videtic GM, Woody NW, Vassil AD. Palliative treatment. In: *Handbook of Treatment Planning in Radiation Oncology.* 3rd ed. Demos Medical; 2020.

29. Nieder C. Repeat palliative radiotherapy for painful bone metastases. *Lancet Oncol.* 2014;15(2):126–128. doi:10.1016/S1470-2045(13)70581-3

30. Dennis K, Makhani L, Zeng L, Lam H, Chow E. Single fraction conventional external beam radiation therapy for bone metastases: a systematic review of randomised controlled trials. *Radiother Oncol.* 2013;106(1): 5–14. doi:10.1016/j.radonc.2012.12.009

31. Yarnold JR. 8 Gy single fraction radiotherapy for the treatment of metastatic skeletal pain: randomised comparison with a multifraction schedule over 12 months of patient follow-up. *Radiother Oncol.* 1999;52(2): 111–121. doi:10.1016/S0167-8140(99)00097-3

32. McDonald R, Ding K, Brundage M, et al. Effect of radiotherapy on painful bone metastases: a secondary analysis of the NCIC Clinical Trials Group Symptom Control Trial SC.23. *JAMA Oncol.* 2017;3(7):953–959. doi:10.1001/jamaoncol.2016.6770

33. Ryu S, Deshmukh S, Timmerman RD, et al. Stereotactic radiosurgery vs conventional radiotherapy for localized vertebral metastases of the spine. *JAMA Oncol.* 2023;9(6):800–807. doi:10.1001/jamaoncol.2023.0356

34. Sahgal A, Myrehaug SD, Siva S, et al. Stereotactic body radiotherapy versus conventional external beam radiotherapy in patients with painful spinal metastases: an open-label, multicentre, randomised, controlled, phase 2/3 trial. *Lancet Oncol.* 2021;22(7):1023–1033. doi:10.1016/S1470-2045(21)00196-0

35. Ito K, Saito T, Nakamura N, Imano N, Hoskin P. Stereotactic body radiotherapy versus conventional radiotherapy for painful bone metastases: a systematic review and meta-analysis of randomised controlled trials. *Radiat Oncol.* 2022;17(1):156. doi:10.1186/s13014-022-02128-w

36. Hird A, Chow E, Zhang L, et al. Determining the incidence of pain flare following palliative radiotherapy for symptomatic bone metastases: results from three Canadian cancer centers. *Int J Radiat Oncol Biol Phys.* 2009;75(1):193–197. doi:10.1016/j.ijrobp.2008.10.044

37. Chow E, Meyer RM, Ding K, et al. Dexamethasone in the prophylaxis of radiation-induced pain flare after palliative radiotherapy for bone metastases: a double-blind, randomised placebo-controlled, phase 3 trial. *Lancet Oncol.* 2015;16(15):1463–1472. doi:10.1016/S1470-2045(15)00199-0

38. Townsend PW, Rosenthal HG, Smalley SR, Cozad SC, Hassanein RE. Impact of postoperative radiation therapy and other perioperative factors on outcome after orthopedic stabilization of impending or pathologic fractures due to metastatic disease. *J Clin Oncol.* 1994;12(11):2345–2350. doi:10.1200/JCO.1994.12.11.2345

39. Townsend PW, Smalley SR, Cozad SC, Rosenthal HG, Hassanein RE. Role of postoperative radiation therapy after stabilization of fractures caused by metastatic disease. *Int J Radiat Oncol Biol Phys.* 1995;31(1): 43–49. doi:10.1016/0360-3016(94)E0310-G

40. Shulman RM, Meyer JE, Li T, Howell KJ. External beam radiation therapy (EBRT) for asymptomatic bone metastases in patients with solid tumors reduces the risk of skeletal-related events (SREs). *Ann Palliat Med.* 2018;7(4):1004–1011. doi:10.21037/apm.2018.10.04

41. Chow E, van der Linden YM, Roos D, et al. Single versus multiple fractions of repeat radiation for painful bone metastases: a randomised, controlled, non-inferiority trial. *Lancet Oncol.* 2014;15(2):164–171. doi:10.1016/S1470-2045(13)70556-4

42. Huisman M, van der Bosch MAAJ, Wijlemans JW, van Vulpen M, van der Linden YM, Verkooijen HM. Effectiveness of reirradiation for painful bone metastases: a systematic review and meta-analysis. *Int J Radiat Oncol Biol Phys.* 2012;84(1):8–14. doi:10.1016/j.ijrobp.2011.10.080

43. Parker C, Nilsson S, Heinrich D, et al. Alpha emitter radium-223 and survival in metastatic prostate cancer. *N Engl J Med.* 2013;369(3):213–223. doi:10.1056/NEJMoa1213755

44. Hoskin P, Sartor O, O'Sullivan JM, et al. Efficacy and safety of radium-223 dichloride in patients with castration-resistant prostate cancer and symptomatic bone metastases, with or without previous docetaxel use: a prespecified subgroup analysis from the randomised, double-blind, phase 3 ALSYMPCA trial. *Lancet Oncol.* 2014;15(12):1397–1406. doi:10.1016/S1470-2045(14)70474-7

45. Smith M, Parker C, Saad F, et al. Addition of radium-223 to abiraterone acetate and prednisone or prednisolone in patients with castration-resistant prostate cancer and bone metastases (ERA 223): a randomised, double-blind, placebo-controlled, phase 3 trial. *Lancet Oncol.* 2019;20(3):408–419. doi:10.1016/S1470-2045(18)30860-X

46. Sartor O, de Bono J, Chi KN, et al. Lutetium-177-PSMA-617 for metastatic castration-resistant prostate cancer. *N Engl J Med.* 2021;385(12):1091–1103. doi:10.1056/NEJMoa2107322

Cole Billena and Samuel T. Chao

QUICK HIT   Malignant spinal cord compression (mSCC) is considered an oncologic emergency and defined as any radiographic compression of the spinal cord or cauda equina secondary to an extradural or intramedullary malignancy. The most common presenting symptom is pain. Severity of symptoms can vary depending on the degree of compression, from asymptomatic to frank paraplegia, which may be reversible or irreversible. Initial treatment usually involves steroids (dexamethasone 10 mg loading dose, followed by 4 mg every 6 hours). Surgical evaluation should be obtained, and if surgical intervention is indicated, postoperative RT should follow, typically 30 Gy/10 fx about 2 to 4 weeks after surgery. If no surgical intervention is indicated, standard conventional fractionation is typically 30 Gy/10 fx or 20 Gy/5 fx. The use of SRS is established for re-RT and an evolving area for nonurgent treatment of spinal metastases in the absence of cord compression.

EPIDEMIOLOGY: Among patients with cancer, the annual incidence of mSCC is 2.5% to 3.4%, ranging from 0.2% in pancreatic cancer to 8% in multiple myeloma (MM). Most cases are due to lung, breast, and prostate cancer. The highest proportional incidence is observed in MM, lymphoma, and prostate cancer.[1,2] In pediatrics, mSCC is observed in 5% of cancer patients and is most commonly caused by Ewing sarcoma and neuroblastoma.[3]

ANATOMY: The *spinal cord* extends from the foramen magnum to L1–L2 in adults. In children, the spinal cord extends more inferiorly (L2–L4). The *dural sac* surrounds the spinal cord and 31 nerve roots, which are cervical (8), thoracic (12), lumbar (5), sacral (5), and coccygeal (1). The sacral nerve roots S3 to S5 originate from the terminal segment of the spinal cord, called the *conus medullaris*. The *filum terminale* is a thin connective tissue filament that originates from the conus medullaris and is fused to the periosteum of the coccygeal bone. The *cauda equina* is defined as the lumbar and sacral spinal nerves located in the lumbar cistern from L1–L2 to S2.[4,5] The *spinal meninges*, from deep to superficial, are composed of the pia mater, arachnoid mater, and the dura mater. The *epidural space* is superficial to the dura mater and contains fat and a venous plexus. The *gray matter* of the spinal cord is composed of lower motor nuclei anteriorly and sensory nuclei posteriorly. The *white matter* of the spinal cord is composed of the dorsal columns (proprioception), lateral spinothalamic tract (pain, temperature), ventral spinothalamic tract (touch sensation), anterior corticospinal tract (axial musculature), and lateral corticospinal tract (extremities).

PATHOLOGY: mSCC occurs through two main mechanisms—external compression typically arising from the vertebral body (more common; hematogenous spread) and internal compression due to intramedullary metastasis. Obstruction of the epidural venous plexus leads to the development of vasogenic edema of the white matter and then the gray matter. Untreated, spinal cord infarction can ultimately develop.

CLINICAL PRESENTATION: Back pain is the most common presenting symptom, occurring in 83% to 95% of cases, typically most pronounced at night or early in the morning when adrenal steroid secretion is at its lowest.[6,7] Back pain often precedes neurologic symptoms by several weeks. An estimated 60% to 85% of patients present with weakness, with 48% to 77% nonambulatory. Sensory symptoms present in ~50% and can be described as "band-like," ascending, or "saddle" anesthesia/paresthesias, depending on location.[8] Physical exam findings may include upper motor neuron signs of spasticity, hyperactive reflexes, Babinski sign, and lower motor neuron signs of atrophy, flaccidity, and loss of reflexes.

Spinal Cord Syndromes

Transection of the Cord: Loss of all sensory modalities (proprioception, vibration, touch), weakness below the level of transection, bowel/bladder dysfunction.

Ventral Cord Syndrome: Weakness, loss of pain and temperature sensation.

Dorsal Cord Syndrome: Loss of proprioception and vibration, weakness, ataxia.

Cauda Equina: Radiculopathy, leg weakness and sensory loss, saddle anesthesia, bowel/bladder incontinence/retention. Bowel/bladder dysfunction is a late finding that can present in up to 50% of patients.[7]

WORKUP: Full H&P, focused on neurologic exam.

Imaging: MRI of the entire spine with and without gadolinium. If MRI cannot be obtained, CT myelography is similar in terms of sensitivity and specificity for cord compression.[9]

Biopsy: Indicated for patients who are not surgical candidates and have an undiagnosed primary cancer, new oligometastasis, or if there is a discordance between the primary lesion and spinal lesion.

PROGNOSTIC FACTORS: Pretreatment neurologic function is the strongest predictor of post-treatment neurologic function.[6,10] Ambulatory function after treatment is more likely in those whose motor deficits develop more slowly (>2 weeks).[11] If nonambulatory at presentation, outcomes are improved if treatment is begun <12 hours after loss of ambulation.[12] Underlying tumor type and disease extent also influence outcomes.

TREATMENT PARADIGM

The epidural spinal cord compression scale is based on a 6-point grading system to quantify the degree of spinal cord or thecal sac compression to help determine management: grade 0: bone only disease; grade 1a: epidural impingement, no deformation of thecal sac; grade 1b: deformation of thecal sac, no spinal cord abutment; grade 1c: deformation of thecal sac and spinal cord abutment, but no cord compression; grade 2: spinal cord compression but visible CSF around cord; grade 3: spinal cord compression with no visible CSF around cord.[13]

Medical Treatment: Early initiation of high-dose corticosteroids is standard management of mSCC. Typically, patients are started on 10-mg dexamethasone, followed by 4 mg q6 hours. Several studies have evaluated the benefit of steroid dose escalation with doses of 96 to 100 mg compared with 10 to 16 mg and have demonstrated no benefit with respect to pain control, ambulation rates, or neurologic outcomes, but have noted higher incidence of serious adverse effects, such as perforated gastric ulcer, psychosis, and death from infection.[14-16] Duration of steroid taper should be initiated based on severity of symptoms, clinical response, and definitive management. Initiation of CHT should be considered with CHT-sensitive disease (SCLC, lymphoma, Ewing sarcoma, germ cell tumors, neuroblastoma).

Surgical Treatment: Assessing spinal stability is important in surgical decision-making. In the event of spinal instability, the degree of spinal instability, neurologic symptoms, and location of disease dictate management. Percutaneous vertebroplasty and kyphoplasty are minimally invasive procedures for patients without anterior extension of disease. The Spine Instability Neoplastic Score (SINS) takes into account six different factors of clinical and radiographic findings, and a score of >7 warrants surgical consultation.[17] Surgery provides immediate relief of compression and is beneficial when a histologic diagnosis is unknown, in a previously irradiated site of compression, or when a patient has progressive neurologic deterioration with poor response to steroids. Postsurgical ambulatory rates range between 70% and 90%. Surgical morbidity and mortality rates range from 5% to 10%.[18,19] Various surgical options are outlined in Table 70.1.

Table 70.1 Surgical Options in mSCC					
	Corpectomy	**Laminectomy**	**Separation Surgery**	**Vertebroplasty**	**Kyphoplasty**
Procedure	Removal of vertebral body via thoracotomy or retroperitoneal approach; delays RT for 6 weeks to allow for fusion.	Removal of posterior arch of vertebrae (unclear if it adds benefit compared with RT alone and may destabilize spine)[20]	Debulking and instrumentation to increase margin between tumor and spinal cord/thecal sac.	Percutaneous injection of bone cement (PMMA) under fluoroscopy into a collapsed vertebral body	Inflatable bone tamps introduced into the vertebral body; once inflated, the bone tamps variably restore the height of the vertebral body, while creating a cavity to fill with viscous bone cement
Candidates	Good life expectancy and good-performing patients (see Patchell trial)[19]	Anterior extension of posterior disease	Most commonly used to create adequate margin for adjuvant SRS	Patients with spinal instability but without anterior extension	

Radiation

EBRT: Indications: postoperatively (typically 2–4 weeks after surgery, except after corpectomy, which requires 6 weeks for fusion) or in nonsurgical candidates. The goal of RT is palliation of pain and LC for prevention or reduction of neurologic deficits. Studies have demonstrated a 70% improvement in pain and LC rates >75%.[21] Typical doses include 30 Gy/10 fx, 20 Gy/5 fx, and 8 Gy/1 fx. For radiosensitive histologies, such as MM, 20 Gy/10 fx may be appropriate.[22] Several series demonstrated between 67% and 82% retention of ambulation following RT and about one-third of patients who were nonambulatory regained the ability to walk following RT.[10,21] In the retreatment setting, consider lower doses of 20 Gy/10 fx or consider SRS in patients with extended life expectancy. Side effects are dependent on location and length of spine being treated and can include mucositis, dysphagia, nausea, diarrhea, or cytopenia.

SRS: Generally, not indicated for mSCC given tumor proximity to the cord and the time required to initiate therapy. The clearest indication for SRS is re-RT, but patients with radioresistant histologies with asymptomatic/minimally symptomatic disease or following separation surgery with gross residual disease may also benefit. Contraindications include significant epidural extension (a gap of >3 mm between the spinal cord and the edge of the lesion is ideal). A rate of >85% long-term pain control even in radioresistant patients has been observed.[23] Common SRS doses include 16–18 Gy/1 fx, 24 Gy/1–2 fx, and 30 Gy/5 fx.[24,25] Side effects include acute pain flare (15%), fatigue, nausea, diarrhea, vertebral fracture, myelopathy (<1%).[26]

Procedure: See *Handbook of Treatment Planning in Radiation Oncology*, Chapter 13.[27]

EVIDENCE-BASED Q&A

What is the value of surgical decompression in addition to RT?

The addition of surgery (corpectomy) to RT in patients with a single site of mSCC with paraplegia present <48 hours improves median survival, ambulation rate, length of ambulation retention, and ability to regain walking, with no change in hospitalization time.

Patchell (*Lancet* 2005, PMID 16112300): PRT of 101 patients with confirmed cancer, life expectancy >3 months, single site of MRI-confirmed displaced cord, with at least one neurologic sign or symptom, and who were paraplegic <48 hours randomized to surgery with postop RT (30 Gy/10 fx) vs. RT alone. Surgery was primarily corpectomy. Lymphoma, MM, leukemia, and germ cell tumors were excluded. Primary endpoint was the ability to walk (at least four steps unassisted with or without a cane/walker). Secondary endpoints were urinary continence, muscle strength, functional status, need for steroids/opioids, and OS. Of note, 20% in the RT group clinically deteriorated and required surgery. See Table 70.2 for results. **Conclusion: Decompressive surgery + RT is superior to RT alone for patients with mSCC.**

Table 70.2 Results of Patchell Trial for mSCC					
	Ambulation Rate at the End of Treatment (Primary Endpoint)	Ambulation Retention Time (Primary Endpoint)	Median Survival (Secondary Endpoint)	Regained Ability to Walk	Length of Hospitalization
Surgery + RT	84%	122 days	126 days	62%	10 days
RT alone	57%	13 days	100 days	19%	10 days
p value	.001	.003	.03	.01	

Is there an ideal dose/fractionation regimen to use for mSCC?

Typical dose and fractionations include 20 Gy/5 fx and 30 Gy/10 fx; however, a superior dosing and fractionation schedule with regard to efficacy and toxicity has not been identified in prospective randomized trials, and several trials support single-fx EBRT. Therefore, clinical decision-making should incorporate patient prognosis, functional status, disease burden, histology, future treatment plans, and patient convenience.

Thirion, ICORG 05-03 (*BJC* 2020, PMID 32157242): Phase III noninferiority RCT of 73 patients comparing 10 Gy/1 fx vs. 20 Gy/5 fx for mSCC with no surgical intervention. Hematologic/germ cell malignancies and prior treatment not eligible. Primary endpoint: change in mobility at 5 weeks by modified Tomita score (a mobility scale that had three possible scores: 1 = "Unaided," 2 = "With walking aid," and 3 = "Bed-bound"). Median age 69, KPS 70, 60% male; 34% prostate, 26% breast, 10% lung; 71% T-spine, 20% L-spine. MFU 5.6 months. Average change in mobility score was −0.06 in single-fx group and −0.3 in multi-fx group, which met the predefined noninferiority criterion. No difference in posttreatment bladder control or MS (6.6 months single-fx vs. 6.0 months multi-fx). No difference in grades 2 to 3 acute or late AEs in multi-fx (26%) vs. single-fx (11%) group (p = .069). **Conclusion: With respect to mobility preservation, 10 Gy/1 fx is noninferior to 20 Gy/5 fx.**

Hoskin, SCORAD III (*JAMA* 2019, PMID 31794625): RCT of 686 patients comparing EBRT 8 Gy/1 fx vs. 20 Gy/5 fx. Spinal cord or cauda equina (C1–S2) compression confirmed by MRI/CT scan, treatable within a single RT field, life expectancy >8 weeks, and no previous RT to the same area required. Primary endpoint was ambulatory status at 8 weeks graded from 1 to 4 (grades 1–2 defined as ambulatory); 73% male; median age 70 years; 44% prostate, 19% lung, 12% breast. Grades 1 to 2 at week 8: 69% of patients in the single-fx group vs. 73% in the multi-fx group (p = .06). The 12-week OS was 50% in the single-fx group vs. 55% in the multi-fx group. **Conclusion: 8 Gy in 1 fx did not meet noninferiority criterion for primary endpoint of ambulatory status at 8 weeks, with the caveat that the lower bound of confidence interval overlapped with the noninferiority margin, making the clinical relevance of this finding unclear.**

Rades, SCORE-2 (*JCO* 2016, PMID 26729431; Update *IJROBP* 2019, PMID 31415797): PRT noninferiority study of 203 patients with mSCC and intermediate to poor life expectancy randomized to 20 Gy/5 fx vs. 30 Gy/10 fx. Primary endpoint was 1-month overall response, defined as improvement or no further progression of motor deficits. See Table 70.3 for results. On secondary analysis of patient-reported outcomes, there was no difference in complete pain relief (24% vs. 20%, NS) or overall pain relief (53% vs. 57%, NS) at 1 month. **Conclusion: 20 Gy/5 fx is noninferior to 30 Gy/10 fx in patients with intermediate to poor life expectancy.**

Table 70.3 Results of Rades Randomized Trial				
	Overall Motor Function Response Rate	Ambulatory Rate (at 1 Month)	Local PFS (at 6 Months)	OS (at 6 Months)
20 Gy/5 fx	87%	72%	75%	42%
30 Gy/10 fx	90%	74%	82%	38%
p value	.73	.86	.51	.68

Maranzano (*JCO* 2005, PMID 15738534): PRT of 300 patients with mSCC randomized to 16 Gy/2 fx (given with a 6-day break in between fractions) vs. split-course RT (15 Gy/3 fx → 4-day rest → 15 Gy/5 fx; total of 30 Gy/8 fx over 2 weeks). Approximately 60% of patients in each arm had pain relief, 70% in each arm were able to walk, and 90% had good bladder function. OS and toxicity were equivalent. **Conclusion: Both hypofractionated RT schedules are effective with acceptable toxicity.**

Is there a role for spine SRS as compared with fractionated RT?

With true cord compression, the role of SRS is limited given the duration of planning required for SRS and the need for ≥3 mm separation for the cord/thecal sac. See Chapter 68 for more information on spine SRS.

REFERENCES

1. Mak KS, Lee LK, Mak RH, et al. Incidence and treatment patterns in hospitalizations for malignant spinal cord compression in the United States, 1998–2006. *Int J Radiat Oncol Biol Phys*. 2011;80(3):824–831. doi:10.1016/j.ijrobp.2010.03.022

2. Loblaw DA, Laperriere NJ, Mackillop WJ. A population-based study of malignant spinal cord compression in Ontario. *Clin Oncol (R Coll Radiol)*. 2003;15(4):211–217. doi:10.1016/s0936-6555(02)00400-4

3. Klein SL, Sanford RA, Muhlbauer MS. Pediatric spinal epidural metastases. *J Neurosurg*. 1991;74(1):70–75. doi:10.3171/jns.1991.74.1.0070

4. Binokay F, Akgul E, Bicakci K, Soyupak S, Aksungur E, Sertdemir Y. Determining the level of the dural sac tip: magnetic resonance imaging in an adult population. *Acta Radiol*. 2006;47(4):397–400. doi:10.1080/02841850600580323

5. Scharf CB, Paulino AC, Goldberg KN. Determination of the inferior border of the thecal sac using magnetic resonance imaging: implications on radiation therapy treatment planning. *Int J Radiat Oncol Biol Phys*. 1998;41(3):621–624. doi:10.1016/s0360-3016(98)00094-3

6. Bach F, Larsen BH, Rohde K, et al. Metastatic spinal cord compression. Occurrence, symptoms, clinical presentations and prognosis in 398 patients with spinal cord compression. *Acta Neurochir (Wien)*. 1990;107(1-2):37–43. doi:10.1007/BF01402610

7. Helweg-Larsen S, Sørensen PS. Symptoms and signs in metastatic spinal cord compression: a study of progression from first symptom until diagnosis in 153 patients. *Eur J Cancer*. 1994;30A(3):396–398. doi:10.1016/0959-8049(94)90263-1

8. Bilsky MH. New therapeutics in spine metastases. *Expert Rev Neurother*. 2005;5(6):831–840. doi:10.1586/14737175.5.6.831

9. Loblaw DA, Perry J, Chambers A, Laperriere NJ. Systematic review of the diagnosis and management of malignant extradural spinal cord compression: the Cancer Care Ontario Practice Guidelines Initiative's Neuro-Oncology Disease Site Group. *J Clin Oncol*. 2005;23(9):2028–2037. doi:10.1200/JCO.2005.00.067

10. Maranzano E, Latini P. Effectiveness of radiation therapy without surgery in metastatic spinal cord compression: final results from a prospective trial. *Int J Radiat Oncol Biol Phys*. 1995;32(4):959–967. doi:10.1016/0360-3016(95)00572-G

11. Rades D, Heidenreich F, Karstens JH. Final results of a prospective study of the prognostic value of the time to develop motor deficits before irradiation in metastatic spinal cord compression. *Int J Radiat Oncol Biol Phys*. 2002;53(4):975–979. doi:10.1016/S0360-3016(02)02819-5

12. Zaidat OO, Ruff RL. Treatment of spinal epidural metastasis improves patient survival and functional state. *Neurology*. 2002;58(9):1360–1366. doi:10.1212/WNL.58.9.1360

13. Bilsky MH, Laufer I, Fourney DR, et al. Reliability analysis of the epidural spinal cord compression scale. *J Neurosurg Spine*. 2010;13(3):324–328. doi:10.3171/2010.3.SPINE09459

14. George R, Jeba J, Ramkumar G, Chacko AG, Tharyan P. Interventions for the treatment of metastatic extradural spinal cord compression in adults. *Cochrane Database Syst Rev*. 2015;2015(9):CD006716. doi:10.1002/14651858.CD006716.pub3

15. Graham PH, Capp A, Delaney G, et al. A pilot randomised comparison of dexamethasone 96 mg vs 16 mg per day for malignant spinal-cord compression treated by radiotherapy: TROG 01.05 Superdex study. *Clin Oncol (R Coll Radiol)*. 2006;18(1):70–76. doi:10.1016/j.clon.2005.08.015

16. Vecht CJ, Haaxma-Reiche H, van Putten WL, de Visser M, Vries EP, Twijnstra A. Initial bolus of conventional versus high-dose dexamethasone in metastatic spinal cord compression. *Neurology*. 1989;39(9):1255–1257. doi:10.1212/WNL.39.9.1255

17. Mendel E, Bourekas E, Gerszten P, Golan JD. Percutaneous techniques in the treatment of spine tumors: what are the diagnostic and therapeutic indications and outcomes? *Spine (Phila Pa 1976)*. 2009;34(22Suppl):S93–S100. doi:10.1097/BRS.0b013e3181b77895

18. Rades D, Huttenlocher S, Dunst J, et al. Matched pair analysis comparing surgery followed by radiotherapy and radiotherapy alone for metastatic spinal cord compression. *J Clin Oncol.* 2010;28(22):3597–3604. doi:10.1200/JCO.2010.28.5635

19. Patchell RA, Tibbs PA, Regine WF, et al. Direct decompressive surgical resection in the treatment of spinal cord compression caused by metastatic cancer: a randomised trial. *Lancet.* 2005;366(9486):643–648. doi:10.1016/S0140-6736(05)66954-1

20. Young RF, Post EM, King GA. Treatment of spinal epidural metastases. Randomized prospective comparison of laminectomy and radiotherapy. *J Neurosurg.* 1980;53(6):741–748. doi:10.3171/jns.1980.53.6.0741

21. Maranzano E, Bellavita R, Rossi R, et al. Short-course versus split-course radiotherapy in metastatic spinal cord compression: results of a phase III, randomized, multicenter trial. *J Clin Oncol.* 2005;23(15):3358–3365. doi:10.1200/JCO.2005.08.193

22. Terpos E, Morgan G, Dimopoulos MA, et al. International Myeloma Working Group recommendations for the treatment of multiple myeloma-related bone disease. *J Clin Oncol.* 2013;31(18):2347–2357. doi:10.1200/JCO.2012.47.7901

23. Jin R, Rock J, Jin JY, et al. Single fraction spine radiosurgery for myeloma epidural spinal cord compression. *J Exp Ther Oncol.* 2009;8(1):35–41. PMID: 19827269

24. Yamada Y, Bilsky MH, Lovelock DM, et al. High-dose, single-fraction image-guided intensity-modulated radiotherapy for metastatic spinal lesions. *Int J Radiat Oncol Biol Phys.* 2008;71(2):484–490. doi:10.1016/j.ijrobp.2007.11.046

25. Yamada Y, Katsoulakis E, Laufer I, et al. The impact of histology and delivered dose on local control of spinal metastases treated with stereotactic radiosurgery. *Neurosurg Focus.* 2017;42(1):E6. doi:10.3171/2016.9.FOCUS16369

26. Sahgal A, Atenafu EG, Chao S, et al. Vertebral compression fracture after spine stereotactic body radiotherapy: a multi-institutional analysis with a focus on radiation dose and the spinal instability neoplastic score. *J Clin Oncol.* 2013;31(27):3426–3431. doi:10.1200/JCO.2013.50.1411

27. Videtic GMM, Vassil AD, Woody NM. *Handbook of Treatment Planning in Radiation Oncology.* Springer Publishing Company; 2020.

71 SUPERIOR VENA CAVA SYNDROME

Anirudh Bommireddy and Gregory M. M. Videtic

QUICK HIT SVC syndrome is an urgent clinical scenario but not an emergency unless presenting with clinically severe airway, neurologic, or hemodynamic compromise. Treatment decision-making is best directed by patient performance, underlying tumor histology, and overall stage. Patients with SVC syndrome do not have worse prognosis than patients without it (for the same stage and histologic diagnosis). In stable patients, pursue completion of staging and workup prior to initiating treatment. When emergent intervention is required, intravascular stenting may provide the most rapid relief. In the United States, the most common malignancies associated with SVC syndrome are NSCLC, SCLC, and lymphoma. Overall, 60% to 80% respond to CHT or RT within 2 weeks (common treatment approaches are listed in Table 71.1).

Table 71.1 General Treatment Approaches for SVC Syndrome	
Supportive care	Head elevation with high-flow oxygen. Data are unclear for use of steroids as it may obscure diagnosis. Diuretics used to reduce intravascular pressure.
CHT	Consider as initial treatment for SCLC, lymphoma, and germ cell tumors.
RT	Consider hypofractionated RT for urgent relief with initiation of definitive course if clinically appropriate. Consider palliative RT as initial treatment in advanced/emergent patients for histologies other than SCLC, lymphoma, and germ cell tumors.
Intravascular stenting	Consider if rapid relief is necessary, patient unable to tolerate tumor-directed therapy, or if symptoms are refractory to prior previous modalities.

EPIDEMIOLOGY: There are ~15,000 cases per year in the United States, with survival dependent on the underlying etiology.[1]

ANATOMY: The SVC carries about one-third of total venous return including drainage from the head, arms, and upper torso including the mediastinum (Table 71.2). It contains low-pressure blood flow and is thin-walled and easily compressible. The brachiocephalic (innominate) veins join to form the SVC beginning at the sternal angle. The SVC then extends inferiorly along the right lateral side of the ascending aorta and inserts into the right atrium. The azygos vein enters the SVC posteriorly just above the pericardial reflection. When obstructed, blood flow is diverted through collateral vessels including the internal mammary, intercostal, esophageal, lateral thoracic, paraspinal, and azygos veins, ultimately to the IVC.

Table 71.2 Anatomy of Mediastinum			
	Boundaries	Contents	Etiology of Malignant SVC Syndrome
Superior mediastinum	Below thoracic inlet at T1 to above the plane between sternal angle and T4/T5	Thymus, trachea, SVC, aortic arch, esophagus, lymph nodes, vagus/phrenic/recurrent laryngeal nerve	NHL, lung, thymoma, thymic carcinoma, thyroid cancer, germ cell tumors
Anterior mediastinum	Between pericardium and sternum	Thymus, fat, lymph nodes	NHL, Hodgkin's, thyroid cancer, thymoma, germ cell tumors, metastasis
Middle mediastinum	Pericardium and its contents, from T5 to T8	Heart, great vessels (including distal SVC), mainstem bronchi, lymph nodes, phrenic nerve	NHL, lung cancer, sarcoma, thymoma, teratoma, mesothelioma
Posterior mediastinum	Between pericardium and vertebral column, from T8 to T12	Esophagus, descending aorta, thoracic duct, azygos vein, lymph nodes, vagus nerve	NHL, nerve sheath tumors, pheochromocytoma, ganglioma/neuroblastoma

PATHOLOGY: SVC syndrome was previously associated with untreated infections such as tuberculosis, syphilis, or aortic aneurysms. Due to more advanced antibiotics, malignancy now accounts for 70% to 90% of cases.[1-3] Common malignant etiologies include NSCLC (50%) > SCLC (25%) > NHL (12%) > metastasis (9%) > germ cell tumors > thymoma > others. SVC syndrome is more common in SCLC at 10% compared with 2% of NSCLC patients. Overall, 2% to 4% of patients with primary lung malignancy will develop SVC syndrome during the course of their disease.[1,4,5] Other benign causes include thrombosis (related to intravascular devices), thyroid goiter, postradiation fibrosis, CHF, and aortic aneurysm. Fibrosing mediastinitis, often associated with granulomatous disease, requires biopsy for confirmation.

CLINICAL PRESENTATION: The severity of symptoms is related to the degree and time frame of SVC obstruction with subsequent collateralization (Table 71.3). Dyspnea and facial/neck swelling are the most common presenting symptoms. Medical emergencies are characterized by clinical symptoms including airway obstruction, neurologic compromise, or hemodynamic instability.[6] Symptoms are commonly exacerbated by leaning forward or lying supine. One-third of patients develop symptoms over 2 weeks.[1] In most cases, symptoms gradually progress over several weeks and then get better over time due to the development of collateral vessels.

Table 71.3 Proposed Grading System for SVC Syndrome[6]

Grade	Category	Incidence	Definition
0	Asymptomatic	10%	Asymptomatic radiographic SVC obstruction
1	Mild	25%	Edema/vascular distention in head or neck, cyanosis, plethora
2	Moderate	50%	Edema in head or neck with associated symptoms (dysphagia; cough; mild or moderate movement impairment of head, jaw, or eyelid; visual disruption)
3	Severe	10%	Mild/moderate cerebral edema (headache, dizziness), laryngeal edema, or diminished cardiac reserve (syncope after bending)
4	Life-threatening	5%	Cerebral edema with associated confusion or obtundation, laryngeal edema with stridor, or significant hemodynamic compromise leading to syncope due to SVC obstruction
5	Life-threatening	<1%	Death

Note: Some argue this grading system can be used to delineate which patients need urgent treatment: patients having grades 1–3 amenable to diagnostic and staging procedures first and those with grade 4+ necessitating emergent stenting.[7]
Source: Adapted from Yu JB, Wilson LD, Detterbeck FC. Superior vena cava syndrome - a proposed classification system and algorithm for management. *J Thorac Oncol.* 2008;3(8):811–814. doi:10.1097/JTO.0b013e3181804791.

WORKUP: H&P with focus on previous malignancies and intravascular procedures, risk factors for coagulopathy and granulomatous disease.

Imaging: CXR, CT chest with contrast with attention to collateral vessels.[8,9] Ultrasound to assess for thrombus.

Procedures: Biopsy (bronchoscopic, CT-guided, mediastinoscopy/mediastinotomy, or via thoracentesis).[10,11] Further workup per histologic diagnosis.

PROGNOSTIC FACTORS: Prognosis is determined by underlying histology. Negative factors specific to SVC syndrome include cerebral edema, laryngeal edema, hypotension, syncope, and headache. SVC obstruction does not predict for worse outcomes in patients with treatment-responsive tumors compared with those without SVC.[12-17]

NATURAL HISTORY: After SVC obstruction, increased central venous pressure (may be increased from 2 to 8 mmHg to between 20 and 30 mmHg) diverts venous return through collateral circulation.[8,18,19] Obstruction above the junction of azygos vein causes venous congestion of the head, neck, and arms. Obstruction below the azygos vein leads to distention of veins in the thorax and abdomen. Laryngeal edema may lead to dyspnea, stridor, cough, and dysphagia.[6] Symptoms are related to time of onset, with protracted onset allowing time for collaterals to develop and therefore reduced symptoms. Disruption of cardiac output is usually temporary due to collateral development.

TREATMENT PARADIGM

Supportive: Head elevation and supplemental oxygen. Dexamethasone may be helpful to reduce cerebral edema or for treatment of steroid-responsive malignancies (lymphoma). The role of diuretics is unclear based on a single retrospective study of 107 patients with similar symptomatic improvement (84%) regardless of use of steroids, diuretics, or neither.[20]

Surgery: There is no standard role for surgery in SVC syndrome, but it can be considered in definitive management of the underlying malignancy. Resection or bypass grafting is generally reserved for surgically managed tumors (e.g., thymoma) and those with progressive or persistent symptoms (>6 months). A common approach is sternotomy/thoracotomy with resection and/or reconstruction of the SVC.[21-23]

Chemotherapy: For CHT-responsive histologies such as SCLC, germ cell tumors, or lymphoma, CHT is often the initial treatment of choice in order to allow time for staging and RT planning. CHT should be dosed according to the underlying histology. In one systematic review of 46 studies, ~77% of SCLC patients had resolution of symptoms with an average time of 7 to 14 days.[5]

Radiation: For palliation, RT doses ranging from 8–10 Gy/1 fx to 30 Gy/10 fx may be reasonable depending on function of the patient and disease status.[24] Patients with curable disease but in need of urgent palliation may benefit from a higher dose per fraction upfront (3–4 Gy/fx) to alleviate symptoms, with dose-adapted definitive RT at standard 1.8–2 Gy/fx after 2 to 3 days with total doses based on histology for curative intent. Symptomatic relief can be apparent in 72 hours but can take up to 4 weeks.[5] Up to 20% of patients do not obtain symptomatic relief from RT. Among those who do respond, ~20% will have recurrent obstruction.[17] Symptomatic relief may occur without complete SVC patency after treatment.[25] As per review of 24 CHT/RT studies, there were no reports of worsening symptoms with RT.[5,26]

Intravascular Stent: Intravascular stenting is the most rapid treatment for SVC syndrome.[5] Stent placement should be considered in those with severe symptoms (e.g., airway compromise or cerebral edema), an inability to tolerate tumor-directed therapy, or a low probability of response to CHT/RT (e.g., mesothelioma). Symptomatic improvement occurs in 75 to 100% of patients and typically occurs within 48 to 72 hours. Complication rate is 3% to 7%.[1,27,28] A small phase III study from Japan (32 patients) demonstrated significant superiority of stent placement compared with other management.[29] Early complications include infection, pulmonary embolism, stent migration, hematoma, bleeding, and perforation/rupture of SVC (rare). Late complications include bleeding (1%–14%) or death (1%–2%) from anticoagulation and stent failure with reocclusion.[30] Relative contraindications include asymptomatic patients and those with an inability to lie flat.

EVIDENCE-BASED Q&A

Is it safe to delay intervention to pursue workup?

Yes, except when symptoms concerning for urgent treatment are present (e.g., airway compromise, cerebral edema). There have been three separate RRs of 107, 63, and 249 patients with SVC syndrome, and there was no evidence of serious complications resulting from delay in treatment of SVC obstruction while diagnostic workup was completed.[2,10,31]

Should histology play a role when considering initial treatment for SVC syndrome?

For patients with SCLC, NHL, or germ cell tumor, CHT is recommended as the initial treatment of choice. Symptomatic improvement usually occurs within 1 to 2 weeks from treatment initiation. The degree and timing of response to CHT are less in NSCLC, and symptomatic relief can be more rapidly achieved with an intravascular stent or RT.

REFERENCES

1.   Wilson LD, Detterbeck FC, Yahalom J. Clinical practice. Superior vena cava syndrome with malignant causes. *N Engl J Med.* 2007;356(18):1862–1869. doi:10.1056/NEJMcp067190

2.   Yellin A, Rosen A, Reichert N, Lieberman Y. Superior vena cava syndrome. The myth - the facts. *Am Rev Respir Dis.* 1990;141(5 Pt 1):1114–1118. doi:10.1164/ajrccm/141.5_Pt_1.1114

3. Martins SJ, Pereira JR. Clinical factors and prognosis in non-small cell lung cancer. *Am J Clin Oncol.* 1999;22(5):453–457. doi:10.1097/00000421-199910000-00006

4. Houman M, Ksontini I, Ben Ghorbel I, et al. Association of right heart thrombosis, endomyocardial fibrosis, and pulmonary artery aneurysm in Behcet's disease. *Eur J Intern Med.* 2002;13(7):455. doi:10.1016/s0953-6205(02)00134-6

5. Rowell NP, Gleeson FV. Steroids, radiotherapy, chemotherapy and stents for superior vena caval obstruction in carcinoma of the bronchus: a systematic review. *Clin Oncol (R Coll Radiol).* 2002;14(5):338–351. doi:10.1053/clon.2002.0095

6. Yu JB, Wilson LD, Detterbeck FC. Superior vena cava syndrome - a proposed classification system and algorithm for management. *J Thorac Oncol.* 2008;3(8):811–814. doi:10.1097/JTO.0b013e3181804791

7. Talapatra K, Panda S, Goyle S, Bhadra K, Mistry R. Superior vena cava syndrome: A radiation oncologist's perspective. *J Cancer Res Ther.* 2016;12(2):515–519. doi:10.4103/0973-1482.177503

8. Kim HJ, Kim HS, Chung SH. CT diagnosis of superior vena cava syndrome: importance of collateral vessels. *AJR Am J Roentgenol.* 1993;161(3):539–542. doi:10.2214/ajr.161.3.8352099

9. Parish JM, Marschke RF Jr, Dines DE, Lee RE. Etiologic considerations in superior vena cava syndrome. *Mayo Clin Proc.* 1981;56(7):407–413. PMID: 7253702

10. Mineo TC, Ambrogi V, Nofroni I, Pistolese C. Mediastinoscopy in superior vena cava obstruction: analysis of 80 consecutive patients. *Ann Thorac Surg.* 1999;68(1):223–226. doi:10.1016/s0003-4975(99)00455-5

11. Dosios T, Theakos N, Chatziantoniou C. Cervical mediastinoscopy and anterior mediastinotomy in superior vena cava obstruction. *Chest.* 2005;128(3):1551–1556. doi:10.1378/chest.128.3.1551

12. Urban T, Lebeau B, Chastang C, Leclerc P, Botto MJ, Sauvaget J. Superior vena cava syndrome in small-cell lung cancer. *Arch Intern Med.* 1993;153(3):384–387. PMID: 8381263

13. Sculier JP, Evans WK, Feld R, et al. Superior vena caval obstruction syndrome in small cell lung cancer. *Cancer.* 1986;57(4):847–851. doi:10.1002/1097-0142(19860215)57:4<847::aid-cncr2820570427>3.0.co;2-h

14. Dombernowsky P, Hansen HH. Combination chemotherapy in the management of superior vena caval obstruction in small-cell anaplastic carcinoma of the lung. *Acta Med Scand.* 1978;204(6):513–516. doi:10.1111/j.0954-6820.1978.tb08482.x

15. Warde P, Payne D. Does thoracic irradiation improve survival and local control in limited-stage small-cell carcinoma of the lung? A meta-analysis. *J Clin Oncol.* 1992;10(6):890–895. doi:10.1200/JCO.1992.10.6.890

16. Wurschmidt F, Bunemann H, Heilmann HP. Small cell lung cancer with and without superior vena cava syndrome: a multivariate analysis of prognostic factors in 408 cases. *Int J Radiat Oncol Biol Phys.* 1995;33(1):77–82. doi:10.1016/0360-3016(95)00094-F

17. Spiro SG, Shah S, Harper PG, Tobias JS, Geddes DM, Souhami RL. Treatment of obstruction of the superior vena cava by combination chemotherapy with and without irradiation in small-cell carcinoma of the bronchus. *Thorax.* 1983;38(7):501–505. doi:10.1136/thx.38.7.501

18. Trigaux JP, Van Beers B. Thoracic collateral venous channels: normal and pathologic CT findings. *J Comput Assist Tomogr.* 1990;14(5):769–773. doi:10.1097/00004728-199009000-00017

19. Gonzalez-Fajardo JA, Garcia-Yuste M, Florez S, Ramos G, Alvarez T, Coca JM. Hemodynamic and cerebral repercussions arising from surgical interruption of the superior vena cava. Experimental model. *J Thorac Cardiovasc Surg.* 1994;107(4):1044–1049. PMID: 8159025

20. Schraufnagel DE, Hill R, Leech JA, Pare JA. Superior vena caval obstruction. Is it a medical emergency? *Am J Med.* 1981;70(6):1169–1174. doi:10.1016/0002-9343(81)90823-8

21. Magnan PE, Thomas P, Giudicelli R, Fuentes P, Branchereau A. Surgical reconstruction of the superior vena cava. *Cardiovasc Surg.* 1994;2(5):598–604. PMID: 7820520

22. Bacha EA, Chapelier AR, Macchiarini P, Fadel E, Dartevelle PG. Surgery for invasive primary mediastinal tumors. *Ann Thorac Surg.* 1998;66(1):234–239. doi:10.1016/s0003-4975(98)00350-6

23. Chen KN, Xu SF, Gu ZD, et al. Surgical treatment of complex malignant anterior mediastinal tumors invading the superior vena cava. *World J Surg.* 2006;30(2):162–170. doi:10.1007/s00268-005-0009-x

24. Straka C, Ying J, Kong FM, Willey CD, Kaminski J, Kim DW. Review of evolving etiologies, implications and treatment strategies for the superior vena cava syndrome. *Springerplus.* 2016;5:229. doi:10.1186/s40064-016-1900-7

25. Ahmann FR. A reassessment of the clinical implications of the superior vena caval syndrome. *J Clin Oncol.* 1984;2(8):961–969. doi:10.1200/JCO.1984.2.8.961

26. Egelmeers A, Goor C, van Meerbeeck J, van den Weyngaert D, Scalliet P. Palliative effectiveness of radiation therapy in the treatment of superior vena cava syndrome. *Bull Cancer Radiother.* 1996;83(3):153–157. doi:10.1016/0924-4212(96)81747-6

27. Fagedet D, Thony F, Timsit JF, et al. Endovascular treatment of malignant superior vena cava syndrome: results and predictive factors of clinical efficacy. *Cardiovasc Intervent Radiol.* 2013;36(1):140–149. doi:10.1007/s00270-011-0310-z

28. Sobrinho G, Aguiar P. Stent placement for the treatment of malignant superior vena cava syndrome - a single-center series of 56 patients. *Arch Bronconeumol.* 2014;50(4):135–140. doi:10.1016/j.arbres.2013.10.009

29. Takeuchi Y, Arai Y, Sone M, et al. Evaluation of stent placement for vena cava syndrome: phase II trial and phase III randomized controlled trial. *Support Care Cancer.* 2019;27(3):1081–1088. doi:10.1007/s00520-018-4397-5

30. Watkinson AF, Yeow TN, Fraser C. Endovascular stenting to treat obstruction of the superior vena cava. *BMJ.* 2008;336(7658):1434–1437. doi:10.1136/bmj.39562.512789.80

31. Gauden SJ. Superior vena cava syndrome induced by bronchogenic carcinoma: is this an oncological emergency? *Australas Radiol.* 1993;37(4):363–366. doi:10.1111/j.1440-1673.1993.tb00096.x

David S. Buchberger, Matthew C. Ward, and Andrew D. Vassil

The goal of palliative RT is to increase quality of life and is most often applied when quantity of life cannot be reasonably improved. Palliative RT should be focused on the near term, be completed in a short time, in a convenient manner, without undue risks, and at minimal expense.[1] Deviation from these priorities risks an unnecessary burden on patients during a difficult time.

PALLIATION OF INCURABLE HEAD AND NECK CANCER

Locoregional disease can be distressing for patients especially with poor performance status, advanced medical comorbidities, and/or metastatic disease, which preclude aggressive management. Symptoms of progressive disease warranting consideration of palliative RT include pain, odynophagia, otalgia, dysphagia, airway obstruction (cough, dyspnea), and ulceration/bleeding/ necrosis. Short courses of RT are available to minimize side effects and reduce such symptoms (Table 72.1). Concurrent systemic therapy is typically avoided given the known increase in sequalae without a known benefit to quality of life.

Table 72.1 Selected Palliative Regimens for H&N Cancer		
Regimen	Dose	Notes
Quad Shot[2–5]	14 Gy/4 fx BID over 2 days with ≥6-hour interval; repeat at 4-week intervals for up to three to four total cycles (42 Gy/12 fx)	Phase I–II trials did not enroll patients with previous RT or give concurrent CHT, but both appear safe
Hypo[6]	30 Gy/5 fx at least 3 days apart; additional 6 Gy boost to tumors ≤3 cm	No previous RT
Christie[7]	50 Gy/16 fx, 4–5 fx per week	
Italy[8]	50 Gy/20 fx with 2-week midtreatment break	
SCAHRT[9]	30 Gy/10 fx, 3- to 5-week break, if tolerated, then followed by additional 30–36 Gy/10–12 fx	
IHF2SQ[10]	6 Gy/2 fx, days 1 and 3 during the first, third, and fifth weeks of platinum CHT	Concurrent CHT, no previous RT

SALVAGE OF LOCOREGIONALLY RECURRENT HEAD AND NECK CANCER

For patients with carcinoma of the H&N arising within or adjacent to a previous RT field, more aggressive options may be reasonable through the use of re-RT (loosely defined here as ≥100 Gy cumulative doses). Data for a survival benefit to re-RT over systemic therapy are lacking and limited primarily to retrospective outcomes. Absolute contraindications to aggressive re-RT include tumor adjacent to critical structures in which damage would be catastrophic such as the brainstem or spinal cord. Relative contraindications include poor performance status, distant metastatic disease, and short time interval since previous RT (≤6 months). Salvage surgery is optimal when possible.

Classic techniques for re-RT include hyperfractionated RT to doses of ~60 Gy with variable schedules including treatment breaks.[11,12] More modern techniques treat to 60 to 72 Gy without a break. Retrospective outcomes do not support elective nodal radiation.[13] Hyperfractionation may allow for dose escalation, but outcomes appear similar.[13] SBRT is an evolving option with doses of 35 to 44 Gy given in 5 fx every other day.[14] SBRT carries the advantage of convenience with more durable LC than other palliative regimens and late effects seem comparable.[15]

Our preference is to utilize an RPA model for patient selection.[16] In the postsurgical adjuvant re-RT setting, for RPA class I patients with risk factors according to the GORTEC trial,[17] we often recommend 60–66 Gy/30–33 fx to the tumor bed alone. For nonoperable class II patients, we often recommend 66 Gy/33 fx with CHT to the gross tumor plus margin. For RPA class III patients regardless of resection status, we consider short-course palliative retreatment or SBRT, as long-term survival is not thought to be possible even with protracted regimens. This approach closely mirrors the recently published American Radium Society Appropriate Use Criteria for H&N re-RT.[18]

ADRENAL METASTASES PALLIATION

The adrenal gland is a common site of metastasis from other primary tumors (lung being the most common), but with <5% of patients symptomatic at detection.[19] When symptomatic, pain (lower chest, abdomen, back, or flank) is most often reported. Other signs and symptoms include adrenal insufficiency, peritoneal hemorrhage, and IVC thrombosis. For symptomatic/palliative intent, RT is effective and standard regimens such as 20 Gy/5 fx, 30 Gy/10 fx, 36 Gy/20 fx, or 45 Gy/20 fx have been used.[20]

With increasing imaging surveillance of cancer patients, incidence of asymptomatic adrenal metastases is rising.[21] For patients with limited metastatic disease, adrenalectomy is the preferred treatment.[22] Other interventions include percutaneous ablation, conventional RT, and SBRT. While rare (and should be considered in the context of bilateral adrenal metastases), adrenal insufficiency may be associated with weakness, weight loss, hypotension, hypoglycemia, hyponatremia, and hyperkalemia. Treatment is with glucocorticoids and mineralocorticoids. There are limited data for SBRT but ideally BED >100 Gy can be achieved while respecting normal tissue tolerance. See Table 72.2 for example regimens.

Table 72.2 Selected Series of SBRT for Adrenal Metastases			
Series	N (patients)	Dose (Median/Mode)	Dose (Range)
Rochester[23]	30	40 Gy/10 fx	16 Gy/4 fx to 50 Gy/10 fx
Florence[24]	48	36 Gy/3 fx	30–54 Gy
Milan[25]	34	32 Gy/4 fx	20 Gy/4 fx to 45 Gy/18 fx
MDACC[26]	43	60 Gy/10 fx	50 Gy/4 fx to 63 Gy/9 fx

RENAL PALLIATION

Metastatic deposits in the kidneys from cancers originating in extrarenal sites are relatively rare.[27–30] When they occur, limited series utilizing SBRT report encouraging control with acceptable toxicity.[31] With the landmark publication of FASTRAK II[32] (see Chapter 47) demonstrating the safety and efficacy of primary SBRT in the treatment of localized RCC, there has been a renewed interest in the use of SBRT for palliation of the primary tumor in metastatic RCC.[33] As the primary lesion can be associated with significant bleeding and pain, SBRT offers a noninvasive means of symptom management with additional immune-modulatory and cytoreductive effects that could potentially improve oncologic outcomes.[33] Two ongoing RCTs are currently assessing the use of SBRT in this setting. CYTOSHRINK (NCT04090710) is a phase II study randomizing patients with de novo metastatic RCC to SBRT + immunotherapy (IO) or IO alone with a primary endpoint of PFS. SBRT doses range from 30 to 40 Gy/5 fx. NRG-GU012 or SAMURAI (NCT05327686) is another phase II study in which patients with metastatic RCC are randomized to SBRT + IO vs. IO alone (VEGF inhibitors can also be used) with primary endpoints of nephrectomy and radiographic PFS.

LIVER PALLIATION

The liver represents a common source of visceral metastatic disease. Patients with low volume and solitary metastatic disease may be considered for curative resection or SBRT (see Chapter 73). In colorectal cancer, 5- and 10-year OS of 40% and 25% are reported in such cases, respectively.[34]

Optimal candidates for ablative RT have preserved performance status, adequate liver function, solitary liver metastasis, and uninvolved liver volume >700 cc.[35] KRAS mutations carry a higher rate of LF.[36] Both 3 and 5 fx regimens of SBRT have been used. For 3 fx regimens, prescription dose of ≥48 Gy (48–54 Gy) is recommended when safe.[37]

Other modalities such as RFA, cryotherapy, laser-induced thermotherapy, HIFU, TACE chemoembolization, or Y90 embolization have been employed as well.

In cases of advanced or refractory symptomatic hepatic metastases, RT to the whole liver can afford effective palliation of symptoms/signs such as pain (from capsule distention), nausea/anorexia, jaundice, and constitutional symptoms such as weight loss, fevers, or night sweats. Premedication with antinausea medication with or without dexamethasone is recommended when treating large volumes of liver. A number of regimens have safely been employed, including 8 Gy/1 fx,[38] 10 Gy/2 fx,[39] 21 Gy/7 fx,[40] and 30 Gy/15 fx.[35] In 2024, a phase III RCT assessed the effectiveness of whole-liver palliative RT in 66 patients with HCC (35%) or liver metastases (65%) and worsening liver pain (with disease involving >50% of the liver, >10 lesions, >10 cm lesion or multiple lesions with at least one >6 cm, or vascular invasion).[41] Patients were randomized to best supportive care or palliative single-fx whole-liver RT (8 Gy); prior radioembolization was not permitted. An improvement in hepatic pain of at least two points on the Brief Pain Inventory was observed in 16 out of 24 patients in the RT group at 1 month vs. 4 out of 18 patients in the supportive care group (67% vs. 22%, p = .0042). G3–4 adverse events included abdominal pain (three patients in the RT arm vs. one in the supportive care arm) and ascites (two patients in the RT arm vs. one in the supportive care arm).[41]

LUNG PALLIATION

Patients with primary lung cancer or progressive pulmonary metastases can present with symptoms including hemoptysis, cough, dyspnea, and chest pain. A definitive approach should be considered for those patients deemed nonmetastatic. For those in whom poor performance status and/or advanced medical comorbidities preclude aggressive management, a palliative approach is appropriate.

Treatment must be triaged according to urgency. In otherwise stable patients, locoregional control, relief of symptoms, limiting toxicity, maintaining quality of life, patient convenience, and cost of care are all important considerations. Early referral to a palliative care specialist is encouraged. Endoscopic interventions such as bronchoscopy with laser ablation ± endobronchial stenting may be helpful for rapid relief of central airway obstruction. Thoracentesis with drainage catheter placement can aid for pleural effusions. Endovascular stenting can aid for SVC syndrome (see Chapter 71).

Various RT fractionation schemes have been employed. ASTRO guidelines suggest protracted regimens (30 Gy/10 fx) for patients with a good performance status.[42] While survival and symptom scores are improved with higher dose schedules, the latter comes with the cost of higher treatment-related toxicity. Shorter courses are appropriate for patients with compromised performance status. Regimens to consider: 10 Gy/1 fx, 16–17 Gy/2 fx, 20 Gy/5 fx, 30 Gy/10 fx, 36 Gy/12 fx, 39 Gy/13 fx.[42,43]

PELVIC PALLIATION

RT is effective for palliation of pelvic progression of urogenital and anorectal malignancies. The most common symptoms include pain, bleeding, and obstruction (urinary or bowel). In addition to presenting symptoms, consideration should be given to the tumor burden (both at local level as well as systemic), prognosis, performance status, ongoing treatments, and personal preferences.

Palliative pelvic exenteration may be considered for select patients who are medically fit, are amenable to gross resection (no major peripheral nerve involvement, no direct invasion of common iliac vessels, or bony invasion at pelvic sidewall or sacrum), and have minimal extrapelvic disease.[44] Exenteration often requires both urinary and fecal diversion through ostomies.

For recurrent rectal cancer, experience exists for both definitive and perioperative re-RT (see Chapter 37 for details). More limited experience exists for re-RT (e.g., 50 Gy/20–25 fx) of other malignancies.[45]

For those with metastatic, unresectable, or medically inoperable disease, RT is the standard option for palliation. A wide variety of clinical scenarios mandate careful application of RT. Accepted regimens beyond standard doses of 20 Gy/5 fx or 30 Gy/10 fx are noted in Table 72.3. Other palliative modalities such as transarterial embolization (TAE) and nerve blocks can be considered for bleeding and pain, respectively.

Table 72.3 Selected Palliative Regimens for Miscellaneous Pelvic Malignancies

Regimen	Dose	Notes
Quad Shot/RTOG 8502[46,47]	14.8 Gy/4 fx BID over 2 days with ≥6-hour interval; repeat at 4-week intervals for up to three total cycles (44.4 Gy/12 fx)	Break of 2 weeks no different than 4-week break (NS increase in acute effects)[48]
RTOG 7905[49]	10 Gy/1 fx once every 4 weeks for up to 3 treatments	Abandoned due to grades 3–4 late effects of 45%
MRC BA09 (UK)[50]	PRT 35 Gy/10 fx vs. 21 Gy/3 fx	Tested in bladder cancer only; no differences in efficacy or toxicity

SIMULATION-FREE DELIVERY

Simulation-free RT has emerged as an effective means for expediting palliative treatments without compromising effectiveness. Institutional experiences reporting on the use of recent diagnostic CT scans for palliative treatment planning in lieu of simulation scans have shown an encouraging benefit in treatment planning time reduction (~50% shorter time interval from consult to plan generation) without significant deviation in RT delivery.[51] In 2024, the results of the phase II DART trial (Diagnostic CT-Enabled Planning: Results of a Randomized Trial in Palliative Radiation Therapy) comparing the delivery of palliative RT planned with diagnostic CT scans vs. simulation CT scans were published.[52] Patients ($n = 33$) were randomized to have CT simulation-based (all patients were undergoing same-day simulation and treatment) planning or diagnostic CT-based planning for their palliative RT. The most used fractionation regimens were 20 Gy/5 fx and 8 Gy/1 fx (30 Gy/10 fx and 4 Gy/2 fx also used). The use of diagnostic CTs for planning was found to notably reduce the time patients spent at the cancer center (5 hours vs. 30 minutes) with no major deviations in plan quality or delivery.[52] Simulation-free RT is an attractive option for safely and effectively expediting palliative RT, especially at busy centers where the simulation schedule may be consistently full.

REFERENCES

1. Lutz ST, Jones J, Chow E. Role of radiation therapy in palliative care of the patient with cancer. *J Clin Oncol.* 2014;32(26):2913–2919. doi:10.1200/JCO.2014.55.1143
2. Corry J, Peters LJ, Costa ID, et al. The "QUAD SHOT" - a phase II study of palliative radiotherapy for incurable head and neck cancer. *Radiother Oncol.* 2005;77(2):137–142. doi:10.1016/j.radonc.2005.10.008
3. Paris KJ, Spanos WJ Jr, Lindberg RD, Jose B, Albrink F. Phase I–II study of multiple daily fractions for palliation of advanced head and neck malignancies. *Int J Radiat Oncol Biol Phys.* 1993;25(4):657–660. doi:10.1016/0360-3016(93)90012-K
4. Lok BH, Jiang G, Gutiontov S, et al. Palliative head and neck radiotherapy with the RTOG 8502 regimen for incurable primary or metastatic cancers. *Oral Oncol.* 2015;51(10):957–962. doi:10.1016/j.oraloncology.2015.07.011
5. Gamez ME, Agarwal M, Hu KS, Lukens JN, Harrison LB. Hypofractionated palliative radiotherapy with concurrent radiosensitizing chemotherapy for advanced head and neck cancer using the "QUAD-SHOT regimen". *Anticancer Res.* 2017;37(2):685–691. doi:10.21873/anticanres.11364
6. Porceddu SV, Rosser B, Burmeister BH, et al. Hypofractionated radiotherapy for the palliation of advanced head and neck cancer in patients unsuitable for curative treatment - "Hypo Trial". *Radiother Oncol.* 2007;85(3):456–462. doi:10.1016/j.radonc.2007.10.020
7. Al-Mamgani A, Tans L, van Rooij PH, Noever I, Baatenburg de Jong RJ, Levendag PC. Hypofractionated radiotherapy denoted as the "Christie scheme": an effective means of palliating patients with head and neck cancers not suitable for curative treatment. *Acta Oncol.* 2009;48(4):562–570. doi:10.1080/02841860902740899
8. Minatel E, Gigante M, Franchin G, et al. Combined radiotherapy and bleomycin in patients with inoperable head and neck cancer with unfavourable prognostic factors and severe symptoms. *Oral Oncol.* 1998;34(2):119–122. doi:10.1016/S1368-8375(97)00073-0
9. Bledsoe TJ, Noble AR, Reddy CA, et al. Split-course accelerated hypofractionated radiotherapy (SCAHRT): a safe and effective option for head and neck cancer in the elderly or infirm. *Anticancer Res.* 2016;36(3): 933–939. PMID: 26976981
10. Monnier L, Touboul E, Durdux C, Lang P, St Guily JL, Huguet F. Hypofractionated palliative radiotherapy for advanced head and neck cancer: the IHF2SQ regimen. *Head Neck.* 2013;35(12):1683–1688. doi:10.1002/hed.23219

11. Spencer SA, Harris J, Wheeler RH, et al. Final report of RTOG 9610, a multi-institutional trial of reirradiation and chemotherapy for unresectable recurrent squamous cell carcinoma of the head and neck. *Head Neck.* 2008;30(3):281–288. doi:10.1002/hed.20697

12. Langer CJ, Harris J, Horwitz EM, et al. Phase II study of low-dose paclitaxel and cisplatin in combination with split-course concomitant twice-daily reirradiation in recurrent squamous cell carcinoma of the head and neck: results of radiation therapy oncology group protocol 9911. *J Clin Oncol.* 2007;25(30):4800–4805. doi:10.1200/JCO.2006.07.9194

13. Caudell JJ, Ward MC, Riaz N, et al. Volume, dose, and fractionation considerations for IMRT-based reirradiation in head and neck cancer: a multi-institution analysis. *Int J Radiat Oncol Biol Phys.* 2018;100(3): 606–617. doi:10.1016/j.ijrobp.2017.11.036

14. Vargo JA, Ferris RL, Ohr J, et al. A prospective phase 2 trial of reirradiation with stereotactic body radiation therapy plus cetuximab in patients with previously irradiated recurrent squamous cell carcinoma of the head and neck. *Int J Radiat Oncol Biol Phys.* 2015;91(3):480–488. doi:10.1016/j.ijrobp.2014.11.023

15. Vargo JA, Ward MC, Caudell JJ, et al. A multi-institutional comparison of SBRT and IMRT for definitive reirradiation of recurrent or second primary head and neck cancer. *Int J Radiat Oncol Biol Phys.* 2018;100(3): 595–605. doi:10.1016/j.ijrobp.2017.04.017

16. Ward MC, Riaz N, Caudell JJ, et al. Refining patient selection for reirradiation of head and neck squamous carcinoma in the IMRT era: a multi-institution cohort study by the MIRI Collaborative. *Int J Radiat Oncol Biol Phys.* 2018;100(3):586–594. doi:10.1016/j.ijrobp.2017.06.012

17. Janot F, de Raucourt D, Benhamou E, et al. Randomized trial of postoperative reirradiation combined with chemotherapy after salvage surgery compared with salvage surgery alone in head and neck carcinoma. *J Clin Oncol.* 2008;26(34):5518–5523. doi:10.1200/JCO.2007.15.0102

18. Ward MC, Koyfman SA, Bakst RL, et al. Retreatment of recurrent or second primary head and neck cancer after prior radiation: executive summary of the American Radium Society Appropriate Use Criteria. *Int J Radiat Oncol Biol Phys.* 2022;113(4):759–786. doi:10.1016/j.ijrobp.2022.03.034

19. Shiue K, Song A, Teh BS, et al. Stereotactic body radiation therapy for metastasis to the adrenal glands. *Expert Rev Anticancer Ther.* 2012;12(12):1613–1620. doi:10.1586/era.12.125

20. Short S, Chaturvedi A, Leslie MD. Palliation of symptomatic adrenal gland metastases by radiotherapy. *Clin Oncol (R Coll Radiol).* 1996;8(6):387–389. doi:10.1016/S0936-6555(96)80087-2

21. Mitchell IC, Nwariaku FE. Adrenal masses in the cancer patient: surveillance or excision. *Oncologist.* 2007;12(2):168–174. doi:10.1634/theoncologist.12-2-168

22. Sastry P, Tocock A, Coonar AS. Adrenalectomy for isolated metastasis from operable non-small-cell lung cancer. *Interact Cardiovasc Thorac Surg.* 2014;18(4):495–497. doi:10.1093/icvts/ivt526

23. Chawla S, Chen Y, Katz AW, et al. Stereotactic body radiotherapy for treatment of adrenal metastases. *Int J Radiat Oncol Biol Phys.* 2009;75(1):71–75. doi:10.1016/j.ijrobp.2008.10.079

24. Casamassima F, Livi L, Masciullo S, et al. Stereotactic radiotherapy for adrenal gland metastases: university of Florence experience. *Int J Radiat Oncol Biol Phys.* 2012;82(2):919–923. doi:10.1016/j.ijrobp.2010.11.060

25. Scorsetti M, Alongi F, Filippi AR, et al. Long-term local control achieved after hypofractionated stereotactic body radiotherapy for adrenal gland metastases: a retrospective analysis of 34 patients. *Acta Oncol.* 2012;51(5):618–623. doi:10.3109/0284186X.2011.652738

26. Chance WW, Nguyen QN, Mehran R, et al. Stereotactic ablative radiotherapy for adrenal gland metastases: factors influencing outcomes, patterns of failure, and dosimetric thresholds for toxicity. *Pract Radiat Oncol.* 2017;7(3):e195–e203. doi:10.1016/j.prro.2016.09.005

27. Derweesh IH, Ismail HR, Magi-Galluzzi C, Hale J, Goldfarb DA. Non-small cell lung carcinoma metastatic to the kidney. *Can J Urol.* 2006;13(5):3281–3282. PMID: 17076953

28. Finke NM, Aubry MC, Tazelaar HD, et al. Autopsy results after surgery for non-small cell lung cancer. *Mayo Clin Proc.* 2004;79(11):1409–1414. doi:10.4065/79.11.1409

29. Barry-Brooks M, Yoo DC, Chaump M, Noto RB. Non-small cell lung cancer with unsuspected distant metastasis to the kidney seen on PET/CT. *Med Health R I.* 2012;95(5):144–146. PMID: 22808631

30. Cai J, Liang G, Cai Z, Yang T, Li S, Yang J. Isolated renal metastasis from squamous cell lung cancer. *Multidiscip Respir Med.* 2013;8(1):2. doi:10.1186/2049-6958-8-2

31. Verma V, Simone CB 2nd. Stereotactic body radiation therapy for metastases to the kidney in patients with non-small cell lung cancer: a new treatment paradigm for durable palliation. *Ann Palliat Med.* 2017;6(2): 96–103. doi:10.21037/apm.2017.03.06

32. Siva S, Bressel M, Sidhom M, et al. Stereotactic ablative body radiotherapy for primary kidney cancer (TROG 15.03 FASTRACK II): a non-randomised phase 2 trial. *Lancet Oncol.* 2024;25(3):308–316. doi:10.1016/S1470-2045(24)00020-2

33. Ali M, Mooi J, Lawrentschuk N, et al. The role of stereotactic ablative body radiotherapy in renal cell carcinoma. *Eur Urol.* 2022;82(6):613–622. doi:10.1016/j.eururo.2022.06.017

34. Abdalla EK, Vauthey JN, Ellis LM, et al. Recurrence and outcomes following hepatic resection, radiofrequency ablation, and combined resection/ablation for colorectal liver metastases. *Ann Surg.* 2004;239(6): 818–825. doi:10.1097/01.sla.0000128305.90650.71

35. Hoyer M, Swaminath A, Bydder S, et al. Radiotherapy for liver metastases: a review of evidence. *Int J Radiat Oncol Biol Phys.* 2012;82(3):1047–1057. doi:10.1016/j.ijrobp.2011.07.020

36. Hong TS, Wo JY, Borger DR, et al. Phase II study of proton-based stereotactic body radiation therapy for liver metastases: importance of tumor genotype. *J Natl Cancer Inst.* 2017;109(9). doi:10.1093/jnci/djx031

37. Chang DT, Swaminath A, Kozak M, et al. Stereotactic body radiotherapy for colorectal liver metastases: a pooled analysis. *Cancer.* 2011;117(17):4060–4069. doi:10.1002/cncr.25997

38. Soliman H, Ringash J, Jiang H, et al. Phase II trial of palliative radiotherapy for hepatocellular carcinoma and liver metastases. *J Clin Oncol.* 2013;31(31):3980–3986. doi:10.1200/JCO.2013.49.9202

39. Bydder S, Spry NA, Christie DR, et al. A prospective trial of short-fractionation radiotherapy for the palliation of liver metastases. *Australas Radiol.* 2003;47(3):284–288. doi:10.1046/j.1440-1673.2003.01177.x

40. Leibel SA, Pajak TF, Massullo V, et al. A comparison of misonidazole sensitized radiation therapy to radiation therapy alone for the palliation of hepatic metastases: results of a Radiation Therapy Oncology Group randomized prospective trial. *Int J Radiat Oncol Biol Phys.* 1987;13(7):1057–1064. doi:10.1016/0360-3016(87)90045-9

41. Dawson LA, Ringash J, Fairchild A, et al. Palliative radiotherapy versus best supportive care in patients with painful hepatic cancer (CCTG HE1): a multicentre, open-label, randomised, controlled, phase 3 study. *Lancet Oncol.* 2024;25(10):1337–1346. doi:10.1016/S1470-2045(24)00438-8

42. Rodrigues G, Videtic GM, Sur R, et al. Palliative thoracic radiotherapy in lung cancer: an American Society for Radiation Oncology evidence-based clinical practice guideline. *Pract Radiat Oncol.* 2011;1(2):60–71. doi:10.1016/j.prro.2011.01.005

43. Macbeth FR, Bolger JJ, Hopwood P, et al. Randomized trial of palliative two-fraction versus more intensive 13-fraction radiotherapy for patients with inoperable non-small cell lung cancer and good performance status. *Clin Oncol (R Coll Radiol).* 1996;8(3):167–175. doi:10.1016/S0936-6555(96)80041-0

44. Finlayson CA, Eisenberg BL. Palliative pelvic exenteration: patient selection and results. *Oncology (Williston Park).* 1996;10(4):479–484.

45. Kamran SC, Harshman LC, Bhagwat MS, et al. Characterization of efficacy and toxicity after high-dose pelvic reirradiation with palliative intent for genitourinary second malignant neoplasms or local recurrences after full-dose radiation therapy in the pelvis: a high-volume cancer center experience. *Adv Radiat Oncol.* 2017;2(2):140–147. doi:10.1016/j.adro.2017.01.001

46. Spanos WJ Jr, Clery M, Perez CA, et al. Late effect of multiple daily fraction palliation schedule for advanced pelvic malignancies (RTOG 8502). *Int J Radiat Oncol Biol Phys.* 1994;29(5):961–967. doi:10.1016/0360-3016(94)90389-1

47. Spanos W Jr, Guse C, Perez C, Grigsby P, Doggett RL, Poulter C. Phase II study of multiple daily fractionations in the palliation of advanced pelvic malignancies: preliminary report of RTOG 8502. *Int J Radiat Oncol Biol Phys.* 1989;17(3):659–661. doi:10.1016/0360-3016(89)90120-X

48. Spanos WJ Jr, Perez CA, Marcus S, et al. Effect of rest interval on tumor and normal tissue response - a report of phase III study of accelerated split course palliative radiation for advanced pelvic malignancies (RTOG-8502). *Int J Radiat Oncol Biol Phys.* 1993;25(3):399–403. doi:10.1016/0360-3016(93)90059-5

49. Spanos WJ Jr, Wasserman T, Meoz R, Sala J, Kong J, Stetz J. Palliation of advanced pelvic malignant disease with large fraction pelvic radiation and misonidazole: final report of RTOG phase I/II study. *Int J Radiat Oncol Biol Phys.* 1987;13(10):1479–1482. doi:10.1016/0360-3016(87)90314-2

50. Duchesne GM, Bolger JJ, Griffiths GO, et al. A randomized trial of hypofractionated schedules of palliative radiotherapy in the management of bladder carcinoma: results of medical research council trial BA09. *Int J Radiat Oncol Biol Phys.* 2000;47(2):379–388. doi:10.1016/S0360-3016(00)00430-2

51. Schiff JP, Zhao T, Huang Y, et al. Simulation-free radiation therapy: an emerging form of treatment planning to expedite plan generation for patients receiving palliative radiation therapy. *Adv Radiat Oncol.* 2023;8(1):101091. doi:10.1016/j.adro.2022.101091

52. O'Neil M, Laba JM, Nguyen TK, et al. Diagnostic CT-enabled planning (DART): results of a randomized trial in palliative radiation therapy. *Int J Radiat Oncol Biol Phys.* 2024;120(1):69–76. doi:10.1016/j.ijrobp.2024.03.005

Salem Alfaifi, Ian W. Winter, Martin C. Tom, Rahul D. Tendulkar, and Ehsan H. Balagamwala

QUICK HIT   Oligometastatic disease (OMD) refers to a state between localized and widely metastatic cancer, wherein some patients may benefit from metastasis-directed therapy (MDT). OMD has been generally defined in several prospective trials as ≤3 to 5 lesions. Subgroups include synchronous, metachronous, oligoprogressive, and oligopersistent disease. Rationales for aggressive local treatment include a potential PFS benefit, to spare patients from prolonged systemic therapy, or to avoid a change in systemic therapy that is otherwise effective. Prospective trials have demonstrated favorable oncologic outcomes with MDT across various cancer histologies, particularly in oligometastatic prostate cancer. Furthermore, prostate-directed RT in low-volume metastatic prostate cancer improved OS in a randomized trial subset and is now included as an option in NCCN guidelines.

BACKGROUND: In 1995, Hellman and Weichselbaum defined the term oligometastases as limited-volume metastatic disease with a favorable prognosis where treatment of the oligometastatic site(s) may impact survival.[1] They described cancer as existing on a biological spectrum extending from localized to systemic disease, but with many intermediate states. They hypothesized that some patients with OMD may benefit from local therapy and achieve a durable response or, in some cases, cure. Modern improvements in imaging, systemic therapy, and less invasive local therapies (SBRT and minimally invasive surgery) have allowed further study of MDT to manage OMD.[2]

DEFINITIONS: Numerous definitions and subsets of OMD have emerged, with significant heterogeneity and differing prognoses. OMD is most commonly defined as ≤3 to 5 (or up to 10) metastatic lesions[3]; however, some have argued that there is no biologically defined upper limit and that OMD should apply to any state where all sites of disease can be safely treated with MDT.[4] General terminology includes the following: (a) synchronous: OMD at the time of initial diagnosis, with the primary tumor and limited number of metastases detected simultaneously; (b) metachronous: oligometastatic recurrence following primary therapy at least 3 to 6 months after the initial diagnosis, also referred to as oligorecurrence; (c) oligoprogression: few lesions progress on a background of otherwise controlled metastatic disease; (d) oligopersistence: few lesions persist after systemic therapy.[4] A more comprehensive classification scheme has been proposed (Table 73.1).

Table 73.1 EORTC and ESTRO Proposed OMD Classification[5]

DE NOVO OMD No history of OMD or polymetastatic disease	REPEAT OMD History of OMD, no polymetastatic disease	INDUCED OMD History of polymetastatic disease treated with systemic therapy
Synchronous OMD OMD present at diagnosis or within ~6 months	**Repeat Oligorecurrence** OMD at diagnosis treated with local or systemic therapy → systemic therapy-free interval → new/ growing OMD	**Induced Oligorecurrence** Polymetastatic disease treated with systemic therapy → systemic therapy-free interval → growing or regrowing OMD
Metachronous Oligorecurrence Primary treated in nonmetastatic state → systemic therapy-free interval → OMD at recurrence (>6 months after first diagnosis)	**Repeat Oligoprogression** OMD at diagnosis treated with local or systemic therapy → on systemic therapy → growing or regrowing OMD	**Induced Oligoprogression** Polymetastatic disease treated with systemic therapy → on systemic therapy → growing or regrowing OMD
Metachronous Oligoprogression Primary treated in nonmetastatic state → on systemic therapy → OMD (>6 months after first diagnosis)	**Repeat Oligopersistence** OMD at diagnosis treated with local or systemic therapy → on systemic therapy → persistent nonprogressive OMD	**Induced Oligopersistence** Polymetastatic disease treated with systemic therapy → on systemic therapy → persistent nonprogressive OMD

Source: Adapted from Guckenberger M, Lievens Y, Bouma AB, et al. Characterisation and classification of oligometastatic disease: a European Society for Radiotherapy and Oncology and European Organisation for Research and Treatment of Cancer consensus recommendation. *Lancet Oncol.* 2020;21(1):e18–e28. doi:10.1016/S1470-2045(19)30718-1.

EPIDEMIOLOGY: Oligometastatic states are not uncommon, but owing to the lack of a uniform definition the incidence/prevalence is difficult to quantify. In a series of patients at MSKCC with sarcoma, 19% presented with isolated pulmonary metastasis as the first site of failure.[6] In a series of patients with CRC at British Columbia Cancer Agency, 46% of those with metastatic disease presented with isolated hepatic metastases, 38% of these had one to three sites of disease.[7] In a patterns of failure analysis of patients with recurrent locally advanced or metastatic lung cancer treated with first-line systemic CHT, 53% of patients were considered eligible for consolidative SBRT at the time of first failure, with a median of three lesions.[8]

EVIDENCE-BASED Q&A

Are there any prospective studies assessing the role of MDT in oligometastatic NSCLC?

Two randomized phase II trials in patients with oligometastatic NSCLC after first-line systemic therapy were closed early due to a PFS benefit with MDT to all sites, one of which also demonstrated an OS benefit. These formed the basis of phase II/III NRG LU002. Additionally, NROGC-002 and SINDAS studies have highlighted the role of RT in EGFR+ oligometastatic NSCLC receiving EGFR-TKI, which was shown to improve PFS and OS. Furthermore, the CURB trial has shown improved PFS when oligoprogressive lesions are treated with SBRT in addition to receiving the standard of care systemic agent, while STOP trial, which included lung cancer (44%) and other solid cancers, showed only a lesional control benefit but not PFS nor OS. See Table 73.2 for a review of studies evaluating the role of RT in oligometastatic/oligoprogressive NSCLC.

Gomez, "Oligomez" (*Lancet Oncol* 2016, PMID 27789196; Update *JCO* 2019, PMID 31067138): Phase II randomized multicenter study of 49 patients with ≤3 NSCLC oligometastases (not including primary lesion) after first-line therapy without progressive disease (PD) randomized to local consolidative therapy (LCT; via RT [no standard dose] or surgery ± maintenance therapy) vs. maintenance therapy alone (or surveillance). Primary endpoint: PFS. Study was terminated early (49 of 74 patients accrued) because at 12.4 months MFU the LCT arm had significantly improved PFS (median 12 vs. 4 months, p = .0054). With updated 38.8-month MFU, PFS benefit persisted (median 14 vs. 4 months, p = .022). Despite crossover to LCT arm, OS was improved in the LCT arm (median 41 vs. 17 months, p = .017). Grade 3 adverse events were similar in both arms, with no grade 4+ toxicity. Exploratory analysis suggested that late LCT (after progression) may still improve OS. **Conclusion: In patients with oligometastatic NSCLC after first-line systemic therapy, LCT prolongs PFS and OS.** *Note: Study performed prior to immunotherapy era.*

Iyengar, UTSW NSCLC Oligomets (*JAMA Oncol* 2018, PMID 28973074): Phase II study of 29 patients with oligometastatic NSCLC (primary lesion and ≤5 metastases) without EGFR/ALK mutation following induction CHT without PD randomized to maintenance CHT vs. SBRT (various doses) to all sites and primary followed by maintenance CHT. Primary endpoint: PFS. Trial stopped early due to interim analysis showing significant improvement in PFS with SBRT + maintenance CHT (9.7 vs. 3.5 months, p = .01). Similar toxicity. **Conclusion: In patients with oligometastatic NSCLC that did not progress after induction CHT, consolidative SBRT prior to maintenance CHT nearly triples PFS.**

Iyengar, NRG LU002 (2024 ASCO Annual Meeting Abstract): Phase II study of 215 patients with oligometastatic NSCLC with ≤3 metastatic sites (excluding primary) exhibiting at least stable disease after four cycles of first-line systemic therapy. Patients were randomized 1:2 to maintenance systemic therapy or LCT (RT and/or surgery) to all lesions followed by maintenance systemic therapy. Primary endpoint: PFS. Ninety percent of patients received IO-based systemic therapy. MFU was 22 months. Estimated 1- and 2-year PFS rates were 48% and 36% in the maintenance systemic therapy arm and 52% and 40% in the LCT + maintenance systemic therapy arm, respectively (p = .66; HR 0.93, 95% CI 0.66–1.31). OS HR between the two arms was 1.05 (0.70–1.56). Grade 3+ pneumonitis was higher in the LCT group (10% vs. 1%). **Conclusion: In patients with oligometastatic NSCLC that did not progress after first-line systemic therapy, local consolidative therapy prior to maintenance therapy did not improve PFS or OS.** *Note: Study closed to accrual early due to failure to meet primary endpoint of PFS and will not move to phase III portion of the study.*

Table 73.2 Further Studies Evaluating the Role of RT in Oligometastatic/Oligoprogressive NSCLC				
Trial	Population	Intervention	Outcome	Conclusion
NROGC-002 (phase III)[9]	EGFR mut NSCLC with oligo-organ metastases*	EGFR-TKI + concurrent thoracic RT (60 Gy to primary tumor and +ve regional LNs) ± RT to oligomets (clinician-determined)	*PFS:* 17.1 vs. 10.6 months ($p = .004$) *OS:* 34.4 vs. 26.2 months ($p = .029$) *Tx-related AE:* 12% vs. 5%	OS and PFS improved with adding concurrent thoracic RT to EGFR-TKI.
SINDAS (phase III)[10]	EGFR mut NSCLC with synchronous oligomets (1–5), ≤2 lesions in any one organ	First-gen EGFR-TKI ± RT 25–40 Gy/5 fx to primary tumor, involved regional LNs, and all mets	*PFS:* 20.2 vs. 12.5 months ($p < .001$) *OS:* 25.5 vs. 17.4 months ($p < .001$) *G3–4 pneumonitis:* 6% vs. 1%	OS and PFS improved with adding concurrent thoracic RT to EGFR-TKI.
CURB (phase II)[11]	NSCLC or breast cancer with extracranial oligoprogressive after first-line therapy (1–5 lesions)	SOC[†] ± SBRT to all oligoprogressive lesions 27–30 Gy/3 fx or 30–50/5 fx	*PFS:* (NSCLC subgroup) 10 vs. 2.2 months ($p = .0039$)	PFS improved with SBRT to oligoprogressive lesions.
STOP (phase II)[12]	NSCLC (44%) + other[‡] with ≤5 sites of oligoprogression on systemic therapy	SOC ± SBRT to oligoprogressive lesions Conventional palliative doses allowed in SOC arm	*PFS:* 8.4 vs. 4.3 months ($p = .91$) *OS:* 31.2 vs. 27.4 months ($p = .22$) *Lesional control:* 70% vs. 38% ($p = .0015$)	Improved lesional control with SBRT, but no difference in OS or PFS.

*Oligo-organ metastases: only one to three organs are involved by metastatic lesions (i.e., there can be more than five met lesions as long as no more than three organs are involved).

[†]SOC: standard of care systemic therapy.

[‡]STOP trial initially included NSCLC only but later expanded the inclusion criteria to include all nonhematologic malignancies for accrual purposes. While subablative doses were recommended in the SOC arm, 35% of patients had protocol deviation and received high-dose or ablative SBRT or withdrew from the study.

Are there any prospective studies assessing the role of MDT in oligometastatic breast cancer?

On recent phase II trials, no PFS or OS improvement was observed when adding MDT to oligometastatic/oligoprogressive breast cancer. See Table 73.3.

Table 73.3 Metastasis-Directed Therapy in Oligometastatic Breast Cancer				
Trial	Population	Intervention	Outcome	Conclusion
CURB (phase II)[11]	NSCLC or breast cancer with extracranial oligoprogressive after first-line therapy (1–5 lesions)	SOC* ± SBRT to all oligoprogressive lesions 27–30 Gy/3 fx or 30–50/5 fx	*PFS* (breast subgroup): 4.4 vs. 4.2 months ($p = .43$)	No PFS benefit with SBRT to oligoprogressive lesions
BR002[†] (phase II)[13]	Breast with ≤5 oligomets on first-line systemic therapy for ≤12 months without progression	SOC ± MDT (SBRT or resection) SBRT in 93% and SR in 2%	*PFS:* 19.5 vs. 23 months ($p = .36$) *3-yr OS:* ~70% in both	No signal for PFS or OS improvement; did not proceed to phase III
EXTEND (phase II)[14]	Breast ($n = 43$) with ≤5 oligomets	SOC ± MDT (local treatment to all sites of disease)	*PFS:* 15.6 vs. 24.9 months ($p = .86$) *2-yr OS:* 81% vs. 100% ($p = .52$) *LC* for treated lesions: 100%	No PFS or OS improvement

*SOC: standard of care systemic therapy.

[†]ASCO Abstract.

Are there any prospective studies assessing the role of MDT in OMD in diseases other than NSCLC and breast cancer?

SABR-COMET was a randomized phase II trial that included various histologies and found SABR to all OMD sites was associated with improved OS compared with standard therapy. Given the screening design of the study, results are to be confirmed in phase III studies. Other studies have demonstrated benefit in prostate cancer, CRC, pancreatic cancer, RCC, and sarcomas.[15–21]

Palma, SABR-COMET (*Lancet* 2019, PMID 30982687; Update *JCO* 2020, PMID 32484754): Phase II randomized screening trial ($p < .2$ considered significant) of 99 patients with OMD of various types (controlled primary and 1–5 lesions) randomized (1:2) to standard palliative treatment vs. SABR to all metastatic sites. Primary endpoint OS. SABR arm improved 5-year OS (42% vs. 18%, stratified log-rank $p = .006$). Three (4.5%) grade 5 toxicities in the SABR arm. **Conclusion: SABR to all sites is associated with improved OS but with 4.5% treatment-related deaths. A phase III trial is needed to confirm the results (SABR-COMET-3 and SABR-COMET-10 are ongoing).** *Comment: 93% of patients had one to three lesions, limiting extrapolation to four to five lesions. Higher proportion of patients in the SABR arm had prostate cancer (21% vs. 6% in the control arm); however, sensitivity analysis included in the update suggests the benefit of SABR persisted even in patients without prostate cancer.*

Ruers, EORTC 40004 Colorectal Liver Metastases (*Ann Oncol* 2012, PMID 22431703; Update *JNCI* 2017, PMID 28376151): Randomized phase II study of 119 patients with unresectable CRC liver metastases (<10, no extrahepatic disease) randomized to systemic therapy alone vs. systemic therapy with RFA (± resection). Primary endpoint of 30-month OS was no different between arms, 62% for combined treatment vs. 58% for systemic treatment alone ($p = .22$), but mPFS was improved 17 vs. 10 months ($p = .025$). Long-term outcomes at MFU of 9.7 years showed improved MS of 46 months in combined therapy vs. 41 months with systemic treatment alone (HR 0.58, $p = .01$). **Conclusion: Aggressive local treatment can prolong OS in patients with unresectable liver metastases from CRC. However, the study did not meet its primary endpoint of 30-month OS as the control arm had a higher than anticipated survival.**

Treasure, PulMiCC Colorectal Lung Metastases (*Trials* 2019, PMID 31831062): Phase III study of 65 patients with CRC and OMD to lungs (amenable to resection) randomized to active monitoring ± metastasectomy. Primary endpoint OS. No benefit to metastectomy, with an HR for death within 5 years of 0.82 (95% CI 0.43–1.56). No treatment-related deaths or major AEs. **Conclusion: Metastectomy for lung-only colorectal oligometastasis does not improve OS.** *Note: Study limited by poor recruitment and low sample size.*

Gore, RTOG 0937 SCLC (*JTO* 2017, PMID 28648948): Phase II trial of 86 oligometastatic ES-SCLC (1–4 extracranial mets) patients with PR/CR to CHT randomized to PCI ± consolidative RT (c-RT) to both chest and metastases. PCI 25 Gy/10 fx, consolidative RT 45 Gy/15 fx. MFU 9 months. No difference in 1-year OS (60% PCI vs. 51% PCI + c-RT). Time to progression favored PCI + c-RT (HR 0.53, $p = .01$). One patient in each arm had grade 4 toxicity and one had grade 5 pneumonitis with PCI + c-RT. Trial closed at interim analysis for futility. **Conclusion: After PCI, consolidative RT to the chest and oligometastases (1–4) did not improve 1-year OS, but did delay progression.**

Ludmir, EXTEND Pancreatic Adenocarcinoma (*JCO* 2024, PMID 39102622): Phase II randomized trial of 41 patients with ≤5 OMD sites from pancreatic adenocarcinoma (ACA), randomized 1:1 to MDT + systemic therapy vs. systemic therapy alone. Primary endpoint: PFS. MFU 17 months; mPFS 10.3 vs. 2.5 months (HR 0.34, $p = .03$). No MDT-related grade ≥3 toxicity. **Conclusion: MDT addition to systemic therapy significantly improved PFS in patients with oligometastatic pancreatic ACA.**

OLIGOMETASTATIC PROSTATE CANCER

Does RT to the prostate improve outcomes in men with oligometastatic prostate cancer?

Across all disease sites, treatment of the primary tumor (surgery or RT) in the setting of oligometastatic cancer is controversial, with a large meta-analysis of 11 prospective trials demonstrating no improvement in PFS or OS.[22] However, among patients receiving RT for "low burden" metastatic disease, risk of death was reduced for those with prostate cancer. ADT ± prostate-directed RT for metastatic prostate cancer has been tested in two RCTs (HORRAD and STAMPEDE Arm H), with both trials ultimately demonstrating no survival benefit among an unselected cohort. However, subset analysis of HORRAD suggested a benefit for those with low volume metastatic disease. Subsequently, Arm H of the STAMPEDE trial was amended to test the hypothesis that prostate-directed RT would benefit low burden patients (using the CHAARTED definition below). Results of the prespecified analysis showed an OS benefit with prostate RT (compared with ADT alone) for low-volume patients, which was confirmed in the STOPCAP meta-analysis of both trials.[23] A secondary analysis of STAMPEDE Arm H showed that the survival benefit decreased continuously as the number of bone metastases increased.[24] NCCN has since added prostate-directed RT as an option for low-volume de novo metastatic prostate cancer, defined as either nonregional LN-only disease OR less than four bone metastases without visceral/other metastases. Note that neither HORRAD or STAMPEDE included PET scans, elective nodal RT, abiraterone/enzalutamide/apalutamide, surgery, or MDT.

Boevé, HORRAD (*Eur Urol* **2019, PMID 30266309):** Phase III RCT of 432 men with de novo prostate metastatic to bone (any amount detected on bone scan) and PSA ≥20 randomized to ADT ± prostate RT (70 Gy/35 fx daily or 57.76 Gy/19 fx 3 days/week). MFU 47 months. The primary endpoint of OS was no different with RT (45 vs. 43 months in the control arm, $p = .4$). Time to PSA progression improved with RT (15 vs. 12 months, $p = .02$). Exploratory subgroup analysis suggested men with ≤4 bone metastases may benefit, although this did not reach significance (HR 0.68, 95% CI 0.42–1.1). **Conclusion: In an unselected group of men with metastatic prostate cancer, prostate-directed RT did not improve OS compared with ADT alone. However, due to small sample size, cannot exclude benefit for ≤4 bone metastases.**

Parker, STAMPEDE Arm H (*Lancet* **2018, PMID 30355464;** *PlosMed* **2022, PMID 35671327):** Phase III RCT of 2,061 men with de novo metastatic prostate cancer (assessed by bone scan and CT or MRI) randomized to lifelong ADT (later allowed docetaxel) ± prostate RT (either 55 Gy/20 fx daily in 4 weeks or 36 Gy/6 fx weekly over 6 weeks). MFU 37 months. Primary endpoint of OS was no different for the entire cohort with RT (median 48 vs. 46 months; 3-year OS 65% vs. 62%, $p = .266$), but prostate-directed RT improved FFS (median 17 vs. 13 months, $p < .0001$). Prespecified subgroup analysis was stratified by metastatic burden (per CHAARTED definition): high burden: (a) ≥4 bone metastases with ≥1 outside the vertebral bodies or pelvis, or (b) visceral metastases. In those with low metastatic burden, prostate-directed RT improved OS (3-year OS 81% vs. 73% in control, $p = .007$). No difference in high metastatic burden group. 2022 update: At MFU of 61 months, prostate RT continued to demonstrate an OS benefit in low-volume (median OS: 86 vs. 64 months; 5-year OS: 65% vs. 53%, $p < .001$) but not high-volume disease (5-year OS: 35% vs. 30%, $p < .164$). There was no evidence of interaction in the treatment effect by RT schedule. **Conclusion: Prostate-directed RT improved OS over ADT alone in those with low-volume de novo metastatic prostate cancer.**

Burdett, STOPCAP Meta-Analysis (*Eur Urol* **2019, PMID 30826218):** Meta-analysis of HORRAD and STAMPEDE trials above. Overall, the addition of prostate RT to ADT showed no improvement in OS or PFS, but did improve bPFS and FFS by ~10% at 3 years. Among those with low volume (defined as ≤4 bone metastases), prostate RT improved OS by ~7% at 3 years (77% vs. 70%, $p = .007$). **Conclusion: Prostate-directed RT should be considered for men with ≤4 bone metastases at presentation.** *Comment: Unable to use STAMPEDE/CHAARTED metastatic burden definition because HORRAD did not collect data on visceral metastases.*

Fizazi, PEACE-1 (*Lancet* **2022, PMID 35405085; Update Bossi,** *Lancet* **2024, PMID 39580202):** Phase III PRT of 1,173 patients with de novo metastatic prostate cancer randomized in a 2 × 2 design to standard of care (SOC; initially ADT with or without docetaxel, then required docetaxel), SOC + abiraterone, SOC + prostate RT, or SOC + abiraterone + prostate RT. RT was 74 Gy/37 fx. Addition of abiraterone resulted in a median rPFS (4.5 vs. 2.2 years, $p < .0001$) and OS benefit (5.7 vs. 4.7 years, $p = .03$). A predefined subset of 505 patients had low-volume disease (0–3 bone metastases ± LNs), 252 in RT arms and 253 in non-RT arms. Adding prostate RT to SOC improved rPFS in patients with low-volume disease treated with abiraterone (7.5 years in the SOC + abiraterone + prostate RT group vs. 4.4 years in the SOC + abiraterone group, $p = .019$), but not in patients not treated with abiraterone (2.6 years in the SOC + prostate RT group vs. 3 years in the SOC group, $p = .61$). For OS, the two groups receiving prostate RT were pooled together. In patients with low-volume disease, OS was not influenced by prostate RT (7.5 years for SOC + prostate RT ± abiraterone vs. 6.7 years for SOC ± abiraterone, $p = .86$). RT reduced the risk of serious GU events, regardless of metastatic burden, without increasing overall toxicity. **Conclusion: Addition of abiraterone improved PFS and OS among de novo metastatic patients. The addition of prostate RT in low volume de novo OMD did not improve OS, but the best outcomes for rPFS and OS were seen in the combination**

group of SOC + abiraterone + prostate RT. **Prostate-directed RT reduced the risk of serious GU events, regardless of metastatic burden.**

What is the role of MDT to oligorecurrent hormone-sensitive prostate cancer?

The phase II SABR-COMET trial included various-histology oligometastatic cancer (16% prostate) and demonstrated SABR to all sites was associated with improved OS compared with standard therapy.[25] Long-term pooled analysis of the ORIOLE and STOMP trials detailed below demonstrated improved PFS with MDT for prostate cancer.[26] EXTEND further evaluated the role of MDT in the setting of intermittent ADT for oligometastatic disease.

Ost, STOMP (*JCO* 2018, PMID 29240541): Phase II study of 62 patients with metachronous asymptomatic oligorecurrent (≤3 extracranial lesions by choline PET) prostate cancer with bF randomized to surveillance vs. MDT via SBRT (30 Gy/3 fx) or surgery. Indication to start ADT was symptomatic progression, progression to >3 metastases, or progression of known lesions; asymptomatic progression in ≤3 could receive further MDT. Primary endpoint was ADT-free survival. At MFU of 3 years, MDT improved the median ADT-free survival (21 vs. 13 months, $p = .11$; trial designed where $p < .2$ is significant). QOL was similar. No grades 2 to 5 toxicities were was observed. **Conclusion: ADT-free survival was longer with MDT than with surveillance alone for oligorecurrent prostate cancer.**

Phillips, ORIOLE (*JAMA Oncol* 2020, PMID 32215577): Phase II multicenter study of 54 men with oligorecurrent hormone-sensitive prostate cancer (previously treated with curative surgery or RT and who had not received ADT within 6 months) and ≤3 metastases detected by conventional imaging randomized to observation vs. SABR (19.5–48 Gy/3–5 fx) to all sites. Primary endpoint was 6-month rate of progression (by PSA, imaging, symptom progression, ADT initiation, or death), which was improved with SABR (19% vs. 61%, $p = .005$). PFS also improved with SABR (NR vs. 5.8 months, $p = .002$). Patients had baseline PSMA PET (blinded to treatment team), and of the SABR group those that had all PET-avid sites treated (20 of 36 patients) had significant improvement in 6-month progression (5% vs. 38%), PFS, and DMFS. No grade ≥3 AEs with SABR. **Conclusion: Compared with observation, SABR improves outcomes for oligometastatic prostate cancer, which is enhanced by total consolidation of all PET-avid sites.**

Tang, EXTEND (*JAMA Oncol* 2023, PMID 37022702): Phase II randomized trial of 87 patients investigating MDT for patients with oligometastatic prostate cancer treated with intermittent ADT. Patients with ≤5 metastases treated with ADT for >2 months were randomized to ADT ± MDT, with planned break in ADT at 6 months after enrollment until disease progression. MFU 22 months. Seventy-two percent had received prior definitive treatment to the prostate. Seventy-four percent had one to two metastatic lesions. The addition of MDT improved mPFS (16 months vs. not reached, $p < .001$) and median eugonadal testosterone PFS (not reached vs. 6.1 months, $p = .03$). The incidence of failure at new sites was also reduced with MDT (33% vs. 41%). **Conclusion: In men receiving intermittent ADT for oligometastatic prostate cancer, the addition of MDT prolongs PFS and facilitates a prolonged period of eugonadal testosterone levels.**

What is the role of MDT to oligometastases in patients with castrate-resistant prostate cancer (CRPC)?

Francolini, ARTO (*JCO* 2023, PMID 37733977): Multicenter phase II RCT of 157 patients with oligometastatic CRPC (<3 nonvisceral metastatic lesions) randomized to abiraterone alone vs. abiraterone with SBRT to all sites of disease. Primary endpoint was biochemical response (≥50% drop from baseline within 6 months of treatment). Biochemical response significantly favored the addition of MDT (OR 5.34, 2.05–13.88). Complete biochemical response was more likely with MDT (OR 4.22, 2.12–8.38). PFS was also improved with SBRT (OR 0.35, 0.21–0.57). **Conclusion: Addition of SBRT to abiraterone in men with oligometastatic CRPC improves biochemical response and PFS.**

Rans, MEDCARE (*Eur Urol Oncol* 2024, PMID 38664137): Phase II single-arm, nonrandomized trial of 20 patients with mCRPC who underwent MDT to 38 oligoprogressive lesions. Primary endpoint was time to next-line systemic treatment (NEST-FS). MFU 28 months. Median NEST-FS was 17 months and 2-year NEST-FS was 35%. MDT was well-tolerated with no early or late grade 3+ toxicity. **Conclusion: MDT to oligoprogressive lesions in patients with mCRPC appears feasible with prolonged time to initiation of next-line systemic therapy.**

What is the management of patients with oligorecurrent lymph node-positive prostate cancer?

Treatment options can include ADT alone, SBRT ± ADT, EBRT ± ADT, and PLND ± EBRT ± ADT. Salvage PLND was initially suggested to have a potential benefit; however, more recent analyses suggest poor oncologic outcomes (89% having biochemical recurrence [BCR], 69% with clinical recurrence within 10 years, and 57% with PSA persistence after surgery). Even with PSMA-PET guidance, salvage PLND results in a 2-year BCR-free survival of 38%. The De Bleser retrospective study[27] suggested decreased LN recurrence with pelvic nodal RT vs. SBRT at the cost of increased toxicity. The OLIGOPELVIS GETUG P07 trial suggests a benefit to high-dose salvage pelvic EBRT (54 Gy/30 fx with SIB to 66.6 Gy for PET+ LN) combined with 6 months of ADT. The ongoing PEACE V STORM trial is examining the role of MDT + 6 months ADT vs. elective nodal RT (ENRT), with early acute toxicity results reported.

Supiot, OLIGOPELVIS GETUG P07 (*Eur Urol* 2021, PMID 34247896; Update Vaugier, *Eur Urol* 2025, PMID 38490854): Phase II trial of 67 patients with nodal oligorecurrence with ≤5 LNs detected by F18-fluorocholine PET. Patients underwent salvage pelvic EBRT to 54 Gy/30 fx with an SIB to 66.6 Gy for PET+ LN combined with 6 months of ADT. At MFU of 49 months, the 2- and 3-year PFS rates were 81% and 58%, respectively, with an mPFS of 45.3 months. BRFS was 58% and 46% at 2- and 3-year, respectively, with a median BRFS of 25.9 months. G2+ GI/GU AEs were 2% and 10%, respectively. Update: 5-year PFS, BRFS, and ADT-free survival rates were 39%, 31%, and 64%, respectively. **Conclusion: Aggressive salvage EBRT + ADT for pelvic nodal oligorecurrences shows promising activity; however, interpretation is limited in the absence of randomized data.**

Ost, PEACE V STORM (*Eur Urol Oncol* 2023, PMID 37821242): Phase II trial of 196 patients with pelvic nodal oligorecurrence (≤5 LNs) on PET following prior primary treatment with RP or RT randomized to MDT + 6 months ADT vs. ENRT + 6 months ADT. Primary endpoint was MFS. MDT included SBRT (30 Gy/3 fx with 3-mm PTV) or salvage LN dissection. ENRT included 45 Gy/25 fx to the pelvis with SIB to 65 Gy to PET+ nodes. Patients without prior RT to the prostate were suggested salvage bed RT as well. Fifty-eight percent of patients had a single node, 26% had two nodes, and 16% had three to five nodes. Ninety-two percent of patients in the MDT group received SBRT, while 8% had salvage LND. Grade 2+ GU (8% for MDT, 13% for ENRT, *p* = .42) and GI (3% vs. 4%, *p* = .95) toxicity did not differ significantly between the two groups. There were no differences in clinically significant QOL from baseline. Grade ≥2 GU and GI toxicities were higher in patients receiving prostate bed RT. **Conclusion: In patients with oligorecurrent pelvic LNs, there were no clinically meaningful differences in acute toxicity for MDT vs. ENRT.** *Note: Results for the primary endpoint of MFS are not yet published.*

REFERENCES

1. Hellman S, Weichselbaum RR. Oligometastases. *J Clin Oncol.* 1995;13(1):8–10. doi:10.1200/JCO.1995.13.1.8
2. Palma DA, Bauman GS, Rodrigues GB. Beyond oligometastases. *Int J Radiat Oncol Biol Phys.* 2020;107(2): 253–256. doi:10.1016/j.ijrobp.2019.12.023
3. Palma DA, Olson R, Harrow S, et al. Stereotactic ablative radiotherapy for the comprehensive treatment of 4-10 oligometastatic tumors (SABR-COMET-10): study protocol for a randomized phase III trial. *BMC Cancer.* 2019;19(1):816. doi:10.1186/s12885-019-5977-6
4. Lievens Y, Guckenberger M, Gomez D, et al. Defining oligometastatic disease from a radiation oncology perspective: an ESTRO-ASTRO consensus document. *Radiother Oncol.* 2020;148:157–166. doi:10.1016/j.radonc.2020.04.003
5. Guckenberger M, Lievens Y, Bouma AB, et al. Characterisation and classification of oligometastatic disease: a European Society for Radiotherapy and Oncology and European Organisation for Research and Treatment of Cancer consensus recommendation. *Lancet Oncol.* 2020;21(1):e18–e28. doi:10.1016/S1470-2045(19)30718-1
6. Gadd MA, Casper ES, Woodruff JM, McCormack PM, Brennan MF. Development and treatment of pulmonary metastases in adult patients with extremity soft tissue sarcoma. *Ann Surg.* 1993;218(6):705–712. doi:10.1097/00000658-199312000-00002
7. Ksienski D, Woods R, Speers C, Kennecke H. Patterns of referral and resection among patients with liver-only metastatic colorectal cancer (MCRC). *Ann Surg Oncol.* 2010;17(12):3085–3093. doi:10.1245/s10434-010-1304-9
8. Rusthoven KE, Hammerman SF, Kavanagh BD, Birtwhistle MJ, Stares M, Camidge DR. Is there a role for consolidative stereotactic body radiation therapy following first-line systemic therapy for metastatic lung cancer? A patterns-of-failure analysis. *Acta Oncol.* 2009;48(4):578–583. doi:10.1080/02841860802662722

9. Sun H, Li M, Huang W, et al. Thoracic radiotherapy improves the survival in patients with EGFR-mutated oligo-organ metastatic non-small cell lung cancer treated with epidermal growth factor receptor-tyrosine kinase inhibitors: a multicenter, randomized, controlled, phase III trial. *J Clin Oncol.* 2024;42(28):JCO2302075. doi:10.1200/JCO.23.02075

10. Wang XS, Bai YF, Verma V, et al. Randomized trial of first-line tyrosine kinase inhibitor with or without radiotherapy for synchronous oligometastatic EGFR-mutated non-small cell lung cancer. *J Natl Cancer Inst.* 2023;115(6):742–748. doi:10.1093/jnci/djac015

11. Tsai CJ, Yang JT, Shaverdian N, et al. Standard-of-care systemic therapy with or without stereotactic body radiotherapy in patients with oligoprogressive breast cancer or non-small-cell lung cancer (Consolidative Use of Radiotherapy to Block [CURB] oligoprogression): an open-label, randomised, controlled, phase 2 study. *Lancet.* 2024;403(10422):171–182. doi:10.1016/S0140-6736(23)01857-3

12. Schellenberg D, Gabos Z, Duimering A, et al. Stereotactic ablative radiation for oligoprogressive cancers: results of the randomized phase 2 STOP trial. *Int J Radiat Oncol Biol Phys.* 2024. doi:10.1016/j.ijrobp.2024.08.031

13. Chmura SJ, Winter KA, Woodward WA, et al. NRG-BR002: a phase IIR/III trial of standard of care systemic therapy with or without stereotactic body radiotherapy (SBRT) and/or surgical resection (SR) for newly oligometastatic breast cancer (NCT02364557). *J Clin Oncol.* 2022;40(16_suppl):1007. doi:10.1200/JCO.2022.40.16_suppl.1007

14. Reddy JP, Sherry AD, Fellman B, et al. Adding metastasis-directed therapy to standard-of-care systemic therapy for oligometastatic breast cancer (EXTEND): a multicenter, randomized phase 2 trial. *Int J Radiat Oncol Biol Phys.* 2024. doi:10.1016/j.ijrobp.2024.10.030

15. Ruers T, Punt C, Van Coevorden F, et al. Radiofrequency ablation combined with systemic treatment versus systemic treatment alone in patients with non-resectable colorectal liver metastases: a randomized EORTC Intergroup phase II study (EORTC 40004). *Ann Oncol.* 2012;23(10):2619–2626. doi:10.1093/annonc/mds053

16. Ruers T, Van Coevorden F, Punt CJ, et al. Local treatment of unresectable colorectal liver metastases: results of a randomized phase II trial. *J Natl Cancer Inst.* 2017;109(9). doi:10.1093/jnci/djx015

17. Treasure T, Farewell V, Macbeth F, et al. Pulmonary metastasectomy versus continued active monitoring in colorectal cancer (PulMiCC): a multicentre randomised clinical trial. *Trials.* 2019;20(1):718. doi:10.1186/s13063-019-3837-y

18. Gore EM, Hu C, Sun AY, et al. Randomized phase II study comparing prophylactic cranial irradiation alone to prophylactic cranial irradiation and consolidative extracranial irradiation for extensive-disease small cell lung cancer (ED SCLC): NRG Oncology RTOG 0937. *J Thorac Oncol.* 2017;12(10):1561–1570. doi:10.1016/j.jtho.2017.06.015

19. Tang C, Msaouel P, Hara K, et al. Definitive radiotherapy in lieu of systemic therapy for oligometastatic renal cell carcinoma: a single-arm, single-centre, feasibility, phase 2 trial. *Lancet Oncol.* 2021;22(12):1732–1739. doi:10.1016/S1470-2045(21)00528-3

20. Navarria P, Baldaccini D, Clerici E, et al. Stereotactic body radiation therapy for lung metastases from sarcoma in oligometastatic patients: a phase 2 study. *Int J Radiat Oncol Biol Phys.* 2022;114(4):762–770. doi:10.1016/j.ijrobp.2022.08.028

21. Ludmir EB, Sherry AD, Fellman BM, et al. Addition of metastasis-directed therapy to systemic therapy for oligometastatic pancreatic ductal adenocarcinoma (EXTEND): a multicenter, randomized phase II trial. *J Clin Oncol.* 2024;42(32):3795–3805. doi:10.1200/JCO.24.00081

22. Ryckman JM, Thomas TV, Wang M, et al. Local treatment of the primary tumor for patients with metastatic cancer (PRIME-TX): a meta-analysis. *Int J Radiat Oncol Biol Phys.* 2022;114(5):919–935. doi:10.1016/j.ijrobp.2022.06.095

23. Burdett S, Boevé LM, Ingleby FC, et al. Prostate radiotherapy for metastatic hormone-sensitive prostate cancer: a STOPCAP systematic review and meta-analysis. *Eur Urol.* 2019;76(1):115–124. doi:10.1016/j.eururo.2019.02.003

24. Ali A, Hoyle A, Haran ÁM, et al. Association of bone metastatic burden with survival benefit from prostate radiotherapy in patients with newly diagnosed metastatic prostate cancer. *JAMA Oncol.* 2021;7(4):555–563. doi:10.1001/jamaoncol.2020.7857

25. Harrow S, Palma DA, Olson R, et al. Stereotactic radiation for the comprehensive treatment of oligometastases (SABR-COMET): extended long-term outcomes. *Int J Radiat Oncol Biol Phys.* 2022;114(4):611–616. doi:10.1016/j.ijrobp.2022.05.004

26. Deek MP, van der Eecken K, Sutera P, et al. Long-term outcomes and genetic predictors of response to metastasis-directed therapy versus observation in oligometastatic prostate cancer: analysis of STOMP and ORIOLE trials. *J Clin Oncol.* 2022;40(29):3377–3382. doi:10.1200/JCO.22.00644

27. De Bleser E, Jereczek-Fossa BA, Pasquier D, et al. Metastasis-directed therapy in treating nodal oligorecurrent prostate cancer: a multi-institutional analysis comparing the outcome and toxicity of stereotactic body radiotherapy and elective nodal radiotherapy. *Eur Urol.* 2019;76(6):732–739. doi:10.1016/j.eururo.2019.07.009

PART XIII: Benign Diseases

Ahmed Halima, Rahul D. Tendulkar, and Chirag Shah

QUICK HIT   Radiation therapy is used for a number of benign conditions (see Table 74.1).

Table 74.1 Quick Hit Radiation Treatment for Benign Diseases	
Disease	**Radiation Treatment**
Heterotopic ossification	7 Gy/1 fx AP/PA <24 hours before surgery or within 72–96 hours after surgery.
Osteoarthritis	3 Gy/6 fx twice weekly on nonconsecutive days is most commonly used. In patients who do not respond after 6–12 weeks, a second course can be delivered.
Hidradenitis suppurativa	7.5 Gy/5 fx daily. Can consider 4–15 Gy/1–10 fx. Wait at least 3 months since previous course before considering retreatment.
Keloids	21 Gy/3 fx for most locations and 18 Gy/3 fx for earlobe 24–72 hours after surgical excision. 37.5 Gy/5 fx if RT is used definitively.
Graves ophthalmopathy	Treat underlying thyroid disease first. 20 Gy/10 fx.
Desmoid tumors	50 Gy for microscopic disease and 55–58 Gy to gross disease.
Pterygium	Use Sr-90 or Y-90 (β emitter), giving 8–10 Gy on days 0 (<8 hours postop), 7, and 14 after surgery. EBRT dose 24–60 Gy/3–6 fx.
AVM	SRS, usually 15–30 Gy. Dose can be estimated according to volume using $27/\sqrt[3]{Volume}$.[1]
Coronary restenosis	15–20 Gy/1 fx using intravascular brachytherapy, typically with Sr-90 source, at 2 mm depth, 5 cm active length.
Glomus tumor	Embolization and surgery ± postop RT (PORT), or RT alone: 45–50 Gy; or SRS 14–16 Gy.
Juvenile nasopharyngeal angiofibroma	30–36 Gy/10–12 fx, up to 50 Gy/25 fx if inoperable.
Langerhans cell histiocytosis	6–8 Gy as prophylaxis against bone fracture.
Gynecomastia	Prophylactic RT effective if given before ADT, using 9 Gy/1 fx or 12–15 Gy/3 fx with 9–12 MeV electrons. 20 Gy/5 fx has 90% pain relief for mammalgia after DES.
Orbital pseudotumor	20 Gy/10 fx.
Pigmented villonodular synovitis	30–50 Gy, LC >80%.
Peyronie disease	8–36 Gy at 2–3 Gy/fx. Penis positioned upright in tube, using 4–8 MeV electrons or 4–6 MV photons.
Splenomegaly	Variety of RT doses can be used for palliation, most commonly 10 Gy/10 fx over 2 weeks but lower doses can be used (5 Gy/5 fx). Monitor blood counts on treatment.
Plantar warts	10 Gy/1 fx may be considered for refractory cases.
Dupuytren disease/plantar fibromas	RT can be used for palmar/plantar nodules without significant contractures, 30 Gy/10 fx split course with an 8- to 12-week break, or 21 Gy/7 fx.
Refractory ventricular tachycardia	SBRT 25 Gy/1 fx delivered to the arrhythmogenic ventricular scar identified with cardiac MRI/SPECT/CT and electrophysiologic mapping for target delineation.
Choroidal hemangioma	20 Gy/10 fx or brachytherapy with I-125 plaques. Higher dose (30 Gy) can be used for diffuse type.

HETEROTOPIC OSSIFICATION (HO): Formation of mature bone in periarticular soft tissue occurs in 30% to 40% of patients beginning 3 to 6 weeks after total hip arthroplasty (60%–80% incidence if high risk).[2] Graded per Brooker classification (Table 74.2).[3] Risk factors: prior HO, trauma, burns, acetabular fracture, ankylosing spondylitis, Paget disease, skeletal hyperostosis, hypertrophic osteoarthritis. RT dose is 7 Gy/1 fx AP/PA, given within 24 hours preop or within 72 to 96 hours postop (before mesenchymal cell differentiation).[4,5] Preop RT effectiveness equivalent to PORT[6]; 10% rate of HO recurrence following RT.[4–6] Other treatment options include indomethacin, although a randomized trial showed that RT with 7 Gy/1fx was more effective.[7,8]

Table 74.2 Brooker's Classification for Heterotopic Ossification[3]	
I	Isolated bone islands in the soft tissue
II	Bone spurs originating from two adjacent articulating bones at least 1 cm apart
III	Bone spurs originating from two adjacent articulating bones decreasing the space between the two bones to <1 cm
IV	Bony ankylosis between proximal femur and pelvis

Source: Data from Hug KT, Alton TB, Gee AO. Classifications in brief: Brooker classification of heterotopic ossification after total hip arthroplasty. *Clin Orthop Relat Res.* 2015;473(6):2154–2157. doi:10.1007/s11999-014-4076-x.

OSTEOARTHRITIS (OA): Most common form of arthritis. OA is among the fastest increasing health condition and a major cause of disability.[9] Pathophysiology includes a complex interaction of "wear and tear" and a proinflammatory response that leads to damage of joint tissues, including ligaments, articular cartilage, and bone.[10] This alters joint mechanics and leads to pain. Multiple treatment options exist including NSAIDs, weight loss/physical activity, physical therapy, and surgical interventions. Low-dose radiation therapy (LDRT) has been used for decades in the management of OA, with the hypothesized mechanism of action being an anti-inflammatory response associated with LDRT.[11] Response rates to RT are typically estimated at 60% to 70%.[11] Of note, some smaller studies have failed to demonstrate a benefit as compared with sham RT, although there were limitations to these studies.[11] The most common prescription is 3 Gy/6 fractions, delivered twice weekly on nonconsecutive days.[12] Lower doses of RT have been evaluated as well (as low as 0.3 Gy/6 fx twice weekly). In case of persisting pain or insufficient relief 6 to 12 weeks after RT, a second RT course may be considered. Currently, DEGRO guidelines provide level 2 to 4 recommendations for the treatment of OA with RT for patients older than 40 who do not respond to non-RT treatments to limit risk of second malignancy.[13] Limited side effects have been noted with current dosing regimens. Guidelines exist on treatment planning.[14]

HIDRADENITIS SUPPURATIVA: Chronic autoinflammatory condition characterized by painful boils of the sweat glands with associated abscesses and fistulas. Commonly affects intertriginous sites: axilla, breasts, perineum, and perianal region. Staging via Hurley system (Table 74.3).[15] Management includes antibiotics (tetracycline or clindamycin), antiandrogens, and/or retinoids for mild disease. Flares can be treated with intralesional triamcinolone injection and antibiotics. Moderate to severe disease is treated with an immunomodulating agent, immunosuppressants, and/or surgery. No completed PRTs, but RT can be used in those with stage 2 to 3 disease who fail maximal medical therapy or are ineligible for standard therapy. A terminated prospective study from Montefiore used 7.5 Gy/5 fx over 1 week (NCT03040804). The largest RR of 231 patients used 3 to 10 Gy in 0.5 to 1.5 Gy per fraction; CR in 38% and PR in 40% with no adverse effects reported.[16]

Table 74.3 Hurley System for Hidradenitis Suppurativa	
I	Abscess formation (single or multiple), no sinus tracts or cicatrization/scarring
II	Limited disease with recurrent abscesses with sinus tracts and scarring, single or multiple separated lesions
III	Diffuse or almost diffuse involvement, or multiple interconnected sinus tracts and abscesses across the entire area

Source: Data from Alikhan A, Sayed C, Alavi A, et al. North American clinical management guidelines for hidradenitis suppurativa: a publication from the United States and Canadian Hidradenitis Suppurativa Foundations: Part I: Diagnosis, evaluation, and the use of complementary and procedural management. *J Am Acad Dermatol.* 2019;81(1):76–90. doi:10.1016/j.jaad.2019.02.067.

KELOIDS: Excess scar tissue after stressors including skin incision, piercing, burn, acne, skin tension, or infection. LR >50% after surgery alone. RT given within 24 to 72 hours after surgical excision: 21 Gy/3 fx for most locations and 18 Gy/3 fx if on the earlobe.[17] LC 75%.[17-19] Definitive RT dose is 37.5 Gy/5 fx.[18] Other options include steroid injection, cryotherapy, pulsed-dye laser, interferon, or topical agents.[20]

GRAVES OPHTHALMOPATHY: Presents with proptosis, altered vision, periorbital edema, and extraocular muscle dysfunction. Pathology shows lymphocytic infiltration of retro-orbital fat due to T-cell invasion and glycosaminoglycan production by fibroblasts.[21] The underlying thyroid disease should be treated first if possible. RT dose is 20 Gy/10 fx with 5 × 5 cm lateral fields using 6 MV photons and 5° posterior tilt or half-beam block.[22-24] RT is usually given after a failed trial of steroids. Response rate to RT is 50% to 70%.[22-27] More recently, teprotumumab, an insulin-like growth factor I receptor (IGF-1R) inhibitor, was recently approved for use in patients with Grave ophthalmopathy.[28] Other options include surgical decompression.

DESMOID TUMORS (I.E., FIBROMATOSIS): Nonencapsulated, locally invasive tumor that rarely metastasizes. Associated with familial adenomatous polyposis, Gardner syndrome (mutation *CTNNB1* gene, B-catenin), and prior trauma. Extra-abdominal types are less destructive and occur in the shoulder, chest, back, thigh, and H&N. Abdominal type arises from the rectus muscle, often in young peri- or postpartum women; may regress with antiestrogen therapy. Intra-abdominal type arises in iliac fossa, pelvis, or mesentery (associated with Gardner syndrome, may be >10 cm), in young women unrelated to gestation. Treatment is surgery with wide margins. RT indicated for unresectable, close margins or gross disease not amenable to re-resection.[29,30] Treat microscopic disease to 50 Gy, gross disease to 55 to 58 Gy, with large margins.[31] LC is 70% to 85% for RT of either gross or microscopic disease. Regression is slow. Alternative options include sulindac, tamoxifen, and systemic therapy with Nirogacestat, a gamma secretase inhibitor, recently approved.[31-35] Sorafenib, an oral multikinase inhibitor, is associated with increased PFS and can be used for progressive, refractory, or symptomatic tumors.[36]

PTERYGIUM: Pterygium is a relatively common ocular surface disease characterized by a wing-shaped, benign fibrovascular growth at the cornea/conjunctiva junction, located nasally.[37] Risk factors include fair skin, UV light, or dust exposure. Surgery alone has a 30% to 70% recurrence rate. Adjuvant RT decreases recurrence to 15%. Use Sr-90 or Y-90 (β emitter), giving 8 to 10 Gy on days 0 (<8 hours postop), 7, and 14 after surgery.[38,39]

ARTERIOVENOUS MALFORMATION: Untreated, the annual risk of spontaneous hemorrhage is 1% to 4% and mortality 1%. Grading system is Spetzler–Martin on a scale of 1 to 5 (size: 0–3 vs. 3–6 vs. >6 cm; eloquent brain region: yes vs. no; venous drainage: deep vs. superficial), which predicts for operative mortality (not risk of hemorrhage).[40] Low risk: treat with observation or surgery. High-risk lesions can be treated with SRS, dose ~16 to 30 Gy to margin of nidus.[41-43] Dose can be estimated according to AVM volume using $27/\sqrt[3]{\text{Volume}}$.[44] Control rate 45% at 1 year and 80% at 2 years, depending on size. Risk of bleeding (5%–10%) persists after SRS during latency period of ~2 years until obliteration. Risk of permanent injury is 3% to 4%.[45]

CORONARY RESTENOSIS: Intravascular brachytherapy (IVBT) is an option to prevent coronary restenosis.[46] Typically, source is Sr-90, although Ir-192, P-32, or I-125 has been used. RT dose 15–20 Gy/1 fx at 2 mm depth, 5 cm active length. RT improves restenosis rates compared with placebo, 15% to 20% vs. 50%. Drug-eluting stents (paclitaxel, sirolimus) were found to have better outcomes compared with IVBT, but intravascular brachytherapy may be an option for select patients after failure of drug-eluting stents.[47]

GLOMUS TUMOR: Also known as chemodectoma/nonchromaffin paraganglioma/carotid body tumor (chromaffin-producing). Generally benign (only 1%–5% malignant). Usually presents as a painless mass; may also present with ear pain, pulsation, tinnitus, bone destruction, or CN palsies. Rare LN or DM (<5%). Origin is neural crest (chief cells of paraganglia in adventitia of dome in jugular bulb). Occurs in carotid body (60%–70%), temporal bone (along internal jugular vein = glomus jugulare; along tympanic branch of CN IX = glomus tympanicum). Can present with bluish mass behind tympanic membrane. Staged by Glasscock–Jackson or McCabe–Fletcher classifications.[48] Contrast-enhancing (hypervascular) with areas of low attenuation (necrosis and hemorrhage).

Treatment options include (a) embolization and surgery ± PORT (surgery plus PORT leads to tumor control of >90%)[49]; (b) RT alone 45 to 50 Gy; or (c) SRS 14 to 16 Gy. LC >90% at 10 years.[50]

JUVENILE NASOPHARYNGEAL ANGIOFIBROMA: Red vascular mass in nasopharynx (NPX) of young boys ~12 to 15 years of age, presenting with epistaxis or nasal obstruction. Can have bone destruction, spreading into the paranasal sinuses, infratemporal fossa, orbit, or middle cranial fossa. May have androgynous hormone receptors (rarely spontaneously regresses after puberty). Often associated with hemorrhage, so biopsy is contraindicated. Treatment is embolization and surgery if limited to NPX or nasal cavity. RT 30–36 Gy/10–12 fx, up to 50 Gy/25 fx if inoperable with intracranial spread. LC 80% to 90%, but tumors regress slowly.[51,52]

LANGERHANS CELL HISTIOCYTOSIS: Previously known as histiocytosis X. Common sites of single eosinophilic granulomas are bone, skin, and LNs; multiple sites include liver, spleen, marrow, GI, and CNS. It can involve single organ (older children/adults) or diffuse multisystem disease (young children). Heterogeneous prognosis. Electron microscopy shows Birbeck granules. Associated diseases include solitary eosinophilic granuloma (<2 years, excellent prognosis), Hans–Schuller–Christian (>2 years, good prognosis, triad of exophthalmos, diabetes insipidus, and skull lesions), and Letterer–Siwe (<2 years, wasting, rash, otitis, lymphadenopathy, bleeding, fulminant, acute, fatal). Treatment options include steroids, etoposide, and vinblastine. RT is used for prophylaxis against bone fracture with doses of 6 to 8 Gy.[53]

GYNECOMASTIA: Incidence of up to 90% of patients on antiandrogens or estrogens. Prophylactic RT effective if given before ADT, using 9 Gy/1 fx or 12–15 Gy/3 fx with 9 to 12 MeV electrons, or tangential Co-60 or 4 MV photons; 20 Gy/5 fx has 90% pain relief for mammalgia after DES. Tamoxifen represents another alternative with increasing use.[54]

ORBITAL PSEUDOTUMOR (A.K.A. ORBITAL PSEUDOLYMPHOMA): Typically, unilateral inflammation, but may be bilateral. Diagnosis of exclusion: differential includes Graves', lymphoma, and lymphoid hyperplasia. Up to 30% progress to lymphoma. About 50% respond to steroids. Consider surgery or immunosuppression. RT dose 20 Gy/10 fx (technique as per Graves').[55]

PEYRONIE DISEASE: Inflammation of tunica albuginea in the corpus cavernosa that progresses to hard plaques or bands on the dorsum of penis, causing painful upward angulation. Up to 50% spontaneously resolve in 12 to 18 months. Treatment includes surgery, steroid injections, verapamil, and RT (if early). RT dose 8 to 36 Gy at 2–3 Gy/fx. Penis positioned upright in tube, using 4 to 8 MeV electrons or 4 to 6 MV photons.[56]

PIGMENTED VILLONODULAR SYNOVITIS: Proliferation in synovial cells of tendon sheaths and joint capsules. LR after synovectomy in 45%. RT dose 30 to 50 Gy; LC >80%.[57,58]

SPLENOMEGALY: Associated with myeloproliferative disorders or CLL. Variety of RT doses can be used for palliation, most common 10 Gy/10 fx over 2 weeks but lower doses can be used (5 Gy/5 fx). Monitor blood counts on treatment; 85% to 90% response rate.[59]

PLANTAR WARTS: Treatment options include surgery, salicylic ointment, liquid nitrogen cryotherapy, or bleomycin injection. Superficial RT can be used in refractory cases; dose is 10 Gy/1 fx.[60]

DUPUYTREN DISEASE: Relatively common condition caused by progressive fibrosis of the palmar fascia resulting in fascial thickening and nodule formation. Staged using the Tubiana staging (Table 74.4).[61] Some lesions regress spontaneously. Glucocorticoid injection may be helpful in patients with nodules.[62] Fasciotomy or fasciectomy for severe functional impairment. RT can be used to prevent progression and provide symptomatic relief in mild to moderate disease (nodules only, or with mild contractures up to 10°). Regression of nodules occurs in ~60% of patients, and only rarely is surgery needed within 1 year after RT. Typical dose regimens include 30 Gy/10 fx split course, with an 8- to 12-week break, or 21 Gy/7 fx.[63]

Table 74.4 Tubiana Staging of Dupuytren Contracture[61]	
0	No deficit in the joint extension
N	Nodule but without contracture
1	Contracture 0–45°
2	Contracture 45–90°
3	Contracture 90–135°
4	Contracture >135°

Source: Hindocha S, Stanley JK, Watson JS, Bayat A. Revised Tubiana's staging system for assessment of disease severity in Dupuytren's disease—preliminary clinical findings. *Hand.* 2008;3(2):80–86. doi:10.1007/s11552-007-9071-1.

PLANTAR FIBROMAS: Also known as Ledderhose disease. Plantar fibromatosis is similar to Dupuytren disease but with nodules arising in the arch of the foot, with RT used in a similar fashion. In one series, after treatment with 30 Gy/10 fx split course, 71% of patients experienced regression and the rest had stable disease in 1 to 4 years.[64] A randomized phase III trial showed improved pain relief and quality of life with RT compared with sham RT.[65]

VENTRICULAR TACHYCARDIA: Refractory ventricular tachycardia can be treated with electrophysiology-guided radioablation with SBRT (20–25 Gy/1 fx) to the arrhythmogenic scar identified by cardiac MRI, SPECT, or Cardiac CT. Electrophysiologic planning is incorporated for delineation of PTV.[66-71] A prospective phase III trial (RADIATE-VT) is currently recruiting patients to catheter-based ablation or SBRT for patients with recurrent ventricular tachycardia.

CHOROIDAL HEMANGIOMA: Two types: diffuse and circumscribed. If progressive, can lead to visual loss depending on the location. Diffuse type occurs in children and is almost always associated with Sturge–Weber syndrome. Circumscribed type occurs in adults. Localized disease is treated with EBRT with 18 to 20 Gy with 2 Gy/fx, with 64% rate of reattachment of the retina.[72] Brachytherapy is also an option in localized hemangiomas using I-125 plaques, with an average dose of 30 Gy, with excellent outcomes.[25,73] Diffuse type can be treated with 30 Gy/15 fx with photons or protons.

REFERENCES

1. Missios S, Bekelis K, Al-Shyal G, Rasmussen PA, Barnett GH. Stereotactic radiosurgery of intracranial arteriovenous malformations and the use of the K index in determining treatment dose. *Neurosurg Focus.* 2014;37(3):E15. doi:10.3171/2014.7.Focus14157
2. Neal B, Gray H, MacMahon S, Dunn L. Incidence of heterotopic bone formation after major hip surgery. *ANZ J Surg.* 2002;72(11):808–821. doi:10.1046/j.1445-2197.2002.02549.x
3. Hug KT, Alton TB, Gee AO. Classifications in brief: Brooker classification of heterotopic ossification after total hip arthroplasty. *Clin Orthop Relat Res.* 2015;473(6):2154–2157. doi:10.1007/s11999-014-4076-x
4. Gregoritch SJ, Chadha M, Pelligrini VD, Rubin P, Kantorowitz DA. Randomized trial comparing preoperative versus postoperative irradiation for prevention of heterotopic ossification following prosthetic total hip replacement: preliminary results. *Int J Radiat Oncol Biol Phys.* 1994;30(1):55–62. doi:10.1016/0360-3016(94)90519-3
5. Seegenschmiedt MH, Makoski HB, Micke O. Radiation prophylaxis for heterotopic ossification about the hip joint—a multicenter study. *Int J Radiat Oncol Biol Phys.* 2001;51(3):756–765. doi:10.1016/S0360-3016(01)01640-6
6. Konski A, Pellegrini V, Poulter C, et al. Randomized trial comparing single dose versus fractionated irradiation for prevention of heterotopic bone: a preliminary report. *Int J Radiat Oncol Biol Phys.* 1990;18(5):1139–1142. doi:10.1016/0360-3016(90)90450-X
7. Kölbl O, Knelles D, Barthel T, Kraus U, Flentje M, Eulert J. Randomized trial comparing early postoperative irradiation vs. the use of nonsteroidal antiinflammatory drugs for prevention of heterotopic ossification following prosthetic total hip replacement. *Int J Radiat Oncol Biol Phys.* 1997;39(5):961–966. doi:10.1016/S0360-3016(97)00496-3
8. Pakos EE, Ioannidis JP. Radiotherapy vs. nonsteroidal anti-inflammatory drugs for the prevention of heterotopic ossification after major hip procedures: a meta-analysis of randomized trials. *Int J Radiat Oncol Biol Phys.* 2004;60(3):888–895. doi:10.1016/j.ijrobp.2003.11.015

9.   Global, regional, and national burden of osteoarthritis, 1990-2020 and projections to 2050: a systematic analysis for the Global Burden of Disease Study 2021. *Lancet Rheumatol.* 2023;5(9):e508–e522. doi:10.1016/S2665-9913(23)00163-7

10. Yunus MHM, Nordin A, Kamal H. Pathophysiological perspective of osteoarthritis. *Medicina (Kaunas).* 2020;56(11):614. doi:10.3390/medicina56110614

11. Dove APH, Cmelak A, Darrow K, et al. The use of low-dose radiation therapy in osteoarthritis: a review. *Int J Radiat Oncol Biol Phys.* 2022;114(2):203–220. doi:10.1016/j.ijrobp.2022.04.029

12. Niewald M, Müller LN, Hautmann MG, et al. ArthroRad trial: multicentric prospective and randomized single-blinded trial on the effect of low-dose radiotherapy for painful osteoarthritis depending on the dose—results after 3 months' follow-up. *Strahlenther Onkol.* 2022;198(4):370–377. doi:10.1007/s00066-021-01866-2

13. Ott OJ, Niewald M, Weitmann HD, et al. DEGRO guidelines for the radiotherapy of non-malignant disorders. Part II: Painful degenerative skeletal disorders. *Strahlenther Onkol.* 2015;191(1):1–6. doi:10.1007/s00066-014-0757-3

14. Alvarez B, Montero A, Hernando O, et al. Radiotherapy CT-based contouring atlas for non-malignant skeletal and soft tissue disorders: a practical proposal from Spanish experience. *Br J Radiol.* 2021;94(1124):20200809. doi:10.1259/bjr.20200809

15. Alikhan A, Sayed C, Alavi A, et al. North American clinical management guidelines for hidradenitis suppurativa: a publication from the United States and Canadian Hidradenitis Suppurativa Foundations: Part I: Diagnosis, evaluation, and the use of complementary and procedural management. *J Am Acad Dermatol.* 2019;81(1):76–90. doi:10.1016/j.jaad.2019.02.067

16. Frohlich D, Baaske D, Glatzel M. Radiotherapy of hidradenitis suppurativa—still valid today? *Strahlenther Onkol.* 2000;176(6):286–289. PMID: 10897256

17. Renz P, Hasan S, Gresswell S, Hajjar RT, Trombetta M, Fontanesi J. Dose effect in adjuvant radiation therapy for the treatment of resected keloids. *Int J Radiat Oncol Biol Phys.* 2018;102(1):149–154. doi:10.1016/j.ijrobp.2018.05.027

18. Mankowski P, Kanevsky J, Tomlinson J, Dyachenko A, Luc M. Optimizing radiotherapy for keloids: a meta-analysis systematic review comparing recurrence rates between different radiation modalities. *Ann Plast Surg.* 2017;78(4):403–411. doi:10.1097/SAP.0000000000000989

19. Ogawa R, Miyashita T, Hyakusoku H, Akaishi S, Kuribayashi S, Tateno A. Postoperative radiation protocol for keloids and hypertrophic scars: statistical analysis of 370 sites followed for over 18 months. *Ann Plast Surg.* 2007;59(6):688–691. doi:10.1097/SAP.0b013e3180423b32

20. Limmer EE, Glass DA. A review of current keloid management: mainstay monotherapies and emerging approaches. *Dermatol Ther.* 2020;10(5):931–948. doi:10.1007/s13555-020-00427-2

21. Bahn RS. Pathophysiology of Graves' ophthalmopathy: the cycle of disease. *J Clin Endocrinol Metab.* 2003;88(5):1939–1946. doi:10.1210/jc.2002-030010

22. Prummel MF, Terwee CB, Gerding MN, et al. A randomized controlled trial of orbital radiotherapy versus sham irradiation in patients with mild Graves' ophthalmopathy. *J Clin Endocrinol Metab.* 2004;89(1):15–20. doi:10.1210/jc.2003-030809

23. Mourits MP, van Kempen-Harteveld ML, García MB, Koppeschaar HP, Tick L, Terwee CB. Radiotherapy for Graves' orbitopathy: randomised placebo-controlled study. *Lancet.* 2000;355(9214):1505–1509. doi:10.1016/S0140-6736(00)02165-6

24. Petersen IA, Kriss JP, McDougall IR, Donaldson SS. Prognostic factors in the radiotherapy of Graves' ophthalmopathy. *Int J Radiat Oncol Biol Phys.* 1990;19(2):259–264. doi:10.1016/0360-3016(90)90532-O

25. Augsburger JJ, Freire J, Brady LW. Radiation therapy for choroidal and retinal hemangiomas. *Front Radiat Ther Oncol.* 1997;30:265–280. doi:10.1159/000425713

26. Bradley EA, Gower EW, Bradley DJ, et al. Orbital radiation for Graves ophthalmopathy: a report by the American Academy of Ophthalmology. *Ophthalmology.* 2008;115(2):398–409. doi:10.1016/j.ophtha.2007.10.028

27. Prummel MF, Mourits MP, Blank L, Berghout A, Koornneef L, Wiersinga WM. Randomized double-blind trial of prednisone versus radiotherapy in Graves' ophthalmopathy. *Lancet.* 1993;342(8877):949–954. doi:10.1016/0140-6736(93)92001-A

28. Douglas RS, Kahaly GJ, Patel A, et al. Teprotumumab for the treatment of active thyroid eye disease. *N Engl J Med.* 2020;382(4):341–352. doi:10.1056/NEJMoa1910434

29. Cates JM, Stricker TP. Surgical resection margins in desmoid-type fibromatosis: a critical reassessment. *Am J Surg Pathol.* 2014;38(12):1707–1714. doi:10.1097/PAS.0000000000000276

30. Janssen ML, van Broekhoven DL, Cates JM, et al. Meta-analysis of the influence of surgical margin and adjuvant radiotherapy on local recurrence after resection of sporadic desmoid-type fibromatosis. *Br J Surg.* 2017;104(4):347–357. doi:10.1002/bjs.10477

31. Ballo MT, Zagars GK, Pollack A. Radiation therapy in the management of desmoid tumors. *Int J Radiat Oncol Biol Phys.* 1998;42(5):1007–1014. doi:10.1016/S0360-3016(98)00285-5

32. Tsukada K, Church JM, Jagelman DG, et al. Noncytotoxic drug therapy for intra-abdominal desmoid tumor in patients with familial adenomatous polyposis. *Dis Colon Rectum.* 1992;35(1):29–33. doi:10.1007/BF02053335

33. Quast DR, Schneider R, Burdzik E, Hoppe S, Möslein G. Long-term outcome of sporadic and FAP-associated desmoid tumors treated with high-dose selective estrogen receptor modulators and sulindac: a single-center long-term observational study in 134 patients. *Fam Cancer.* 2016;15(1):31–40. doi:10.1007/s10689-015-9830-z

34. Desurmont T, Lefèvre JH, Shields C, Colas C, Tiret E, Parc Y. Desmoid tumour in familial adenomatous polyposis patients: responses to treatments. *Fam Cancer.* 2015;14(1):31–39. doi:10.1007/s10689-014-9760-1

35. Hansmann A, Adolph C, Vogel T, Unger A, Moeslein G. High-dose tamoxifen and sulindac as first-line treatment for desmoid tumors. *Cancer.* 2004;100(3):612–620. doi:10.1002/cncr.11937

36. Gounder MM, Mahoney MR, Van Tine BA, et al. Sorafenib for advanced and refractory desmoid tumors. *N Engl J Med.* 2018;379(25):2417–2428. doi:10.1056/NEJMoa1805052

37. Shahraki T, Arabi A, Feizi S. Pterygium: an update on pathophysiology, clinical features, and management. *Ther Adv Ophthalmol.* 2021;13:25158414211020152. doi:10.1177/25158414211020152

38. Ali AM, Thariat J, Bensadoun RJ, et al. The role of radiotherapy in the treatment of pterygium: a review of the literature including more than 6000 treated lesions. *Cancer Radiother.* 2011;15(2):140–147. doi:10.1016/j.canrad.2010.03.020

39. Nishimura Y, Nakai A, Yoshimasu T, et al. Long-term results of fractionated strontium-90 radiation therapy for pterygia. *Int J Radiat Oncol Biol Phys.* 2000;46(1):137–141. doi:10.1016/S0360-3016(99)00419-8

40. Spetzler RF, Martin NA. A proposed grading system for arteriovenous malformations. *J Neurosurg.* 1986;65(4):476–483. doi:10.3171/jns.1986.65.4.0476

41. Flickinger JC, Kondziolka D, Maitz AH, Lunsford LD. An analysis of the dose–response for arteriovenous malformation radiosurgery and other factors affecting obliteration. *Radiother Oncol.* 2002;63(3):347–354. doi:10.1016/S0167-8140(02)00103-2

42. Byun J, Kwon DH, Lee DH, Park W, Park JC, Ahn JS. Radiosurgery for cerebral arteriovenous malformation (AVM): current treatment strategy and radiosurgical technique for large cerebral AVM. *J Korean Neurosurg Soc.* 2020;63(4):415–426. doi:10.3340/jkns.2020.0008

43. Sethi A, Chee K, Chatain GP, et al. Time-dosed stereotactic radiosurgery for the treatment of cerebral arteriovenous malformations: an early institution experience and case series. *Neurosurg Pract.* 2023;4(4):e00060. doi:10.1227/neuprac.0000000000000060

44. Karlsson B, Lindquist C, Steiner L. Prediction of obliteration after gamma knife surgery for cerebral arteriovenous malformations. *Neurosurgery.* 1997;40(3):425–431. doi:10.1097/00006123-199703000-00001

45. Joshi NP, Shah C, Kotecha R, et al. Contemporary management of large-volume arteriovenous malformations: a clinician's review. *J Radiat Oncol.* 2016;5:239–248. doi:10.1007/s13566-016-0261-8

46. Detloff LR, Ho EC, Ellis SG, Ciezki JP, Cherian S, Smile TD. Coronary intravascular brachytherapy for in-stent restenosis: a review of the contemporary literature. *Brachytherapy.* 2022;21(5):692–702. doi:10.1016/j.brachy.2022.05.004

47. Benjo A, Cardoso RN, Collins T, et al. Vascular brachytherapy versus drug-eluting stents in the treatment of in-stent restenosis: a meta-analysis of long-term outcomes. *Catheter Cardiovasc Interv.* 2016;87(2):200–208. doi:10.1002/ccd.25998

48. Brady LW, Yaeger TE. *Encyclopedia of Radiation Oncology.* Springer; 2013.

49. Manzoor NF, Yancey KL, Aulino JM, et al. Contemporary management of jugular paragangliomas with neural preservation. *Otolaryngol Head Neck Surg.* 2021;164(2):391–398. doi:10.1177/0194599820938660

50. Jacob JT, Pollock BE, Carlson ML, Driscoll CL, Link MJ. Stereotactic radiosurgery in the management of vestibular schwannoma and glomus jugulare: indications, techniques, and results. *Otolaryngol Clin North Am.* 2015;48(3):515–526. doi:10.1016/j.otc.2015.02.010

51. Lee JT, Chen P, Safa A, Juillard G, Calcaterra TC. The role of radiation in the treatment of advanced juvenile angiofibroma. *Laryngoscope.* 2002;112(7):1213–1220. doi:10.1097/00005537-200207000-00014

52. López F, Triantafyllou A, Snyderman CH, et al. Nasal juvenile angiofibroma: current perspectives with emphasis on management. *Head Neck.* 2017;39(5):1033–1045. doi:10.1002/hed.24696

53. Lian C, Lu Y, Shen S. Langerhans cell histiocytosis in adults: a case report and review of the literature. *Oncotarget.* 2016;7(14):18678–18683. doi:10.18632/oncotarget.7892

54. Viani GA, Bernardes da Silva LG, Stefano EJ. Prevention of gynecomastia and breast pain caused by androgen deprivation therapy in prostate cancer: tamoxifen or radiotherapy? *Int J Radiat Oncol Biol Phys.* 2012;83(4):e519–e524. doi:10.1016/j.ijrobp.2012.01.036

55. Mendenhall WM, Lessner AM. Orbital pseudotumor. *Am J Clin Oncol.* 2010;33(3):304–306. doi:10.1097/COC.0b013e3181a07567

56. Seegenschmiedt MH, Micke O, Niewald M, et al. DEGRO guidelines for the radiotherapy of non-malignant disorders. *Strahlenther Onkol.* 2015;191(7):541–548. doi:10.1007/s00066-015-0818-2

57. Heyd R, Micke O, Berger B, Eich HT, Ackermann H, Seegenschmiedt MH. Radiation therapy for treatment of pigmented villonodular synovitis: results of a national patterns of care study. *Int J Radiat Oncol Biol Phys.* 2010;78(1):199–204. doi:10.1016/j.ijrobp.2009.07.1747

58. Heyd R, Seegenschmiedt M, Micke O. The role of external beam radiation therapy in the adjuvant treatment of pigmented villonodular synovitis. *Z Orthop Unfall.* 2011;149(6):677–682. doi:10.1055/s-0030-1250687

59. Zaorsky NG, Williams GR, Barta SK, et al. Splenic irradiation for splenomegaly: a systematic review. *Cancer Treat Rev.* 2017;53:47–52. doi:10.1016/j.ctrv.2016.11.016

60. Perez CA, Lockett MA, Young G. Radiation therapy for keloids and plantar warts. In: *The Radiation Therapy of Benign Diseases.* Karger Publishers; 2001:135–146.

61. Hindocha S, Stanley JK, Watson JS, Bayat A. Revised Tubiana's staging system for assessment of disease severity in Dupuytren's disease—preliminary clinical findings. *Hand.* 2008;3(2):80–86. doi:10.1007/s11552-007-9071-1

62. Ketchum LD, Donahue TK. The injection of nodules of Dupuytren's disease with triamcinolone acetonide. *J Hand Surg Am.* 2000;25(6):1157–1162. doi:10.1053/jhsu.2000.18493

63. Seegenschmiedt MH, Olschewski T, Guntrum F. Radiotherapy optimization in early-stage Dupuytren's contracture: first results of a randomized clinical study. *Int J Radiat Oncol Biol Phys.* 2001;49(3):785–798. doi:10.1016/s0360-3016(00)00745-8

64. Attassi M, Seegenschmiedt H. Radiotherapy is effective in the treatment of progressive plantar fibromatosis (Morbus Ledderhose). *Int J Radiat Oncol Biol Phys.* 2001;51(3):47.

65. de Haan A, van Nes JGH, Kolff MW, et al. Radiotherapy for Ledderhose disease: results of the LedRad-study, a prospective multicentre randomised double-blind phase 3 trial. *Radiother Oncol.* 2023;185:109718. doi:10.1016/j.radonc.2023.109718

66. Cuculich PS, Schill MR, Kashani R, et al. Noninvasive cardiac radiation for ablation of ventricular tachycardia. *N Engl J Med.* 2017;377(24):2325–2336. doi:10.1056/NEJMoa1613773

67. Gerard IJ, Bernier ML, Hijal T, et al. Stereotactic arrhythmia radioablation for ventricular tachycardia (StAR-VT): a single institution, dose de-escalation, phase II trial. *Int J Radiat Oncol Biol Phys.* 2022;114(3):e416–e417. doi:10.1016/j.ijrobp.2022.07.1605

68. Gupta A, Sattar Z, Chaaban N, et al. Stereotactic cardiac radiotherapy for refractory ventricular tachycardia in structural heart disease patients: a systematic review. *Europace.* 2024:euae305. doi:10.1093/europace/euae305

69. Miszczyk M, Sajdok M, Bednarek J, et al. Stereotactic management of arrhythmia - radiosurgery in treatment of ventricular tachycardia (SMART-VT). Results of a prospective safety trial. *Radiother Oncol.* 2023;188:109857. doi:10.1016/j.radonc.2023.109857

70. Ninni S, Gallot-Lavallée T, Klein C, et al. Stereotactic radioablation for ventricular tachycardia in the setting of electrical storm. *Circ Arrhythm Electrophysiol.* 2022;15(9):e010955. doi:10.1161/CIRCEP.122.010955

71. Wight J, Bigham T, Schwartz A, et al. Long term follow-up of stereotactic body radiation therapy for refractory ventricular tachycardia in advanced heart failure patients. *Front Cardiovasc Med.* 2022;9:849113. doi:10.3389/fcvm.2022.849113

72. Schilling H, Sauerwein W, Lommatzsch A, et al. Long-term results after low dose ocular irradiation for choroidal haemangiomas. *Br J Ophthalmol.* 1997;81(4):267–273. doi:10.1136/bjo.81.4.267

73. Lewis GD, Li HK, Quan EM, Scarboro SB, Teh BS. The role of eye plaque brachytherapy and MR imaging in the management of diffuse choroidal hemangioma: an illustrative case report and literature review. *Pract Radiat Oncol.* 2019;9(5):e452–e456. doi:10.1016/j.prro.2019.05.007

ABBREVIATIONS

2D	two-dimensional
3D-CRT	3D-conformal radiation therapy
5-ARI	5α-reductase inhibitors
5-FU	5-fluorouracil
AA	anaplastic astrocytoma
AA/P	abiraterone acetate/prednisolone
AAD	American Academy of Dermatology
AASLD	American Association for the Study of Liver Diseases
ABR	auditory brainstem response
ABS	American Brachytherapy Society
ABV	Adriamycin, bleomycin, vinblastine
ABVD	Adriamycin, bleomycin, vinblastine, dacarbazine
ABVE	doxorubicin, bleomycin, vincristine, etoposide
ABVE-PC	doxorubicin, bleomycin, vincristine, etoposide, prednisone, cyclophosphamide
AC	Adriamycin, cyclophosphamide
ACA	adenocarcinoma
ACC	adenoid cystic carcinoma
ACCP	American College of Chest Physicians
ACM	all-cause mortality
ACOG	American College of Obstetricians and Gynecologists
ACR	American College of Radiology
ACS	American College of Surgeons
AC-T	doxorubicin, cyclophosphamide, paclitaxel
ACTH	adrenocorticotropic hormone
AD	autosomal dominant
ADH	antidiuretic hormone
ADL	activities of daily living
ADT	androgen deprivation therapy
AE	adverse event
AF	altered fractionation
AFP	alpha-fetoprotein
AGC	atypical glandular cells
AHT	adjuvant hormonal therapy
AI	aromatase inhibitors
AIDS	acquired immunodeficiency syndrome

AJCC	American Joint Committee on Cancer
AK	actinic keratosis
ALBI	albumin-bilirubin
ALK	anaplastic lymphoma kinase
ALL	acute lymphoblastic lymphoma/leukemia
ALN	axillary lymph node
ALND	axillary lymph node dissection
ALP	alkaline phosphatase
AMA	American Medical Association
AML	acute myeloid leukemia
AO	anaplastic oligodendroglioma
AOA	anaplastic oligoastrocytoma
AP/PA	anterior–posterior/posterior–anterior
APC	argon plasma coagulation
APL	acute promyelocytic leukemia
APR	abdominoperineal resection
AR	androgen receptor
Ara-C	cytarabine
ARR	absolute risk reduction
AS	active surveillance
ASBS	American Society of Breast Surgeons
ASCCP	American Society for Colposcopy and Cervical Pathology
ASC-H	atypical squamous cells, cannot exclude high-grade squamous intraepithelial lesion
ASCO	American Society of Clinical Oncology
ASCT	autologous stem cell transplant
ASCUS	atypical squamous cells of undetermined significance
ASTRO	American Society for Radiation Oncology
ATA	American Thyroid Association
ATC	anaplastic thyroid cancer
ATRA	all-trans-retinoic acid
ATRT	atypical teratoid/rhabdoid tumor
ATRX	alpha thalassemia/mental retardation syndrome X-linked
AUA	American Urological Association
AUC	area under the curve
AVM	arteriovenous malformation
AVPC	doxorubicin, vincristine, prednisone, cyclophosphamide
AYA	adolescent and young adults

B2M	beta-2 microglobulin
BAER	brainstem auditory evoked response
BC	breast cancer
BCC	basal cell carcinoma
BCG	bacillus Calmette–Guerin
BCL	B-cell lymphoma
BCLC	Barcelona clinic liver cancer
BCM	breast cancer mortality
BCNU	1,3-bis(2-chloroethyl)-1-nitrosourea
BCS	breast-conserving surgery
BCSM	breast cancer-specific mortality
BCT	breast-conserving therapy
bDFS	biochemical disease-free survival
BEACOPP	bleomycin, etoposide, Adriamycin, cyclophosphamide, vincristine, procarbazine, prednisone
BEAM	carmustine, etoposide, cytarabine, melphalan
BED	biologically effective dose
BED10	biological equivalent dose assuming alpha-beta ratio of 10
BEP	bleomycin, etoposide, cisplatin
bF	biochemical failure
BFFS	biochemical failure-free survival
B-HCG	beta-human chorionic gonadotropin
BID	twice daily
BM	bone marrow
BMI	body mass index
BMP	basic metabolic panel
BMT	bone marrow transplant
bNED	biochemical no evidence of disease
BNI	Barrow Neurological Institute
BOS	base of skull
BOT	base of tongue
bPFS	biochemical progression-free survival
BPH	benign prostatic hyperplasia
BReCADD	brentuximab vedotin, etoposide, cyclophosphamide, doxorubicin, dacarbazine, and dexamethasone
bRFS	biochemical recurrence-free survival
BSC	best supportive care
BSG	brainstem glioma

BSO	bilateral salpingo-oophorectomy
BUN	blood urea nitrogen
BV	brentuximab vedotin
Bv-ABVE-PC	brentuximab vedotin, doxorubicin, vincristine, etoposide, prednisone, cyclophosphamide
C	cycles
CALGB	cancer and leukemia group B
CAP	chest, abdomen, pelvis
CAPOX	capecitabine and oxaliplatin
CAR	chimeric antigen receptor
CAR-T	chimeric antigen receptor T-cell
CBC	complete blood count
CBE	contralateral breast event
CBV	carmustine, cyclophosphamide, etoposide
CC	cholangiocarcinoma
CCNU	lomustine
cCR	clinical complete response
cCRT	concurrent chemotherapy and radiation therapy
CCSK	clear cell sarcoma of the kidney
CD	cluster of differentiation
CDC	Centers for Disease Control and Prevention
CDDP	cisplatin
CDKN2A/B	cyclin-dependent kinase inhibitor 2A/B
CEA	carcinoembryonic antigen
CECT	contrast-enhanced computed tomography
CEM43	cumulative equivalent minutes at 43°C
CExP	carcinoma ex pleomorphic adenoma
CF	conventional fractionation
CFS	colostomy-free survival
CHF	congestive heart failure
CHOP	cyclophosphamide, doxorubicin, vincristine, prednisone
Chr	chromosome
CHT	chemotherapy
CI	confidence interval
CIR	cumulative incidence of recurrence
CIS	carcinoma in situ
CISS	constructive interference in steady-state sequence
CKC	cold-knife conization

CLL	chronic lymphocytic leukemia
CMF	cyclophosphamide, methotrexate, 5-FU
CML	chronic myeloid leukemia
CMP	comprehensive metabolic panel
CMT	combined-modality therapy
CN	cranial nerve
CNS	central nervous system
CODOX-M	cyclophosphamide, cytarabine, vincristine, doxorubicin, methotrexate
COG	Children's Oncology Group
COMS	Collaborative Ocular Melanoma Study
COPDAC	cyclophosphamide, vincristine, prednisone, dacarbazine
COPP	cyclophosphamide, vincristine, procarbazine, prednisone
COWA	controlled oral word association
CP	craniopharyngioma
CPA	cerebellopontine angle
CPI	checkpoint inhibitor
cPNI	clinical perineural invasion
CPT	charged particle therapy
CR	complete response
CRC	colorectal cancer
CRM	circumferential resection margin
CRPC	castrate-resistant prostate cancer
CRT	chemoradiotherapy
CS	Curie Score
cSCC	cutaneous squamous cell carcinoma
CSF	cerebrospinal fluid
CSI	craniospinal irradiation
CSS	cancer-specific survival
CT	computed tomography
CTV	clinical target volume
CV	cardiovascular
CVA	cerebrovascular accident
CVAD	cyclophosphamide, vincristine, doxorubicin, dexamethasone
CVP	cyclophosphamide, vincristine, prednisolone
CW	chest wall
CXR	chest x-ray
CYC	cyclophosphamide
D&C	dilatation and curettage

DC	distant control
DCE MRI	dynamic contrast-enhanced magnetic resonance imaging
DCIS	ductal carcinoma in situ
DD4A	vincristine, doxorubicin, dactinomycin
ddMVAC	dose-dense methotrexate, vinblastine, doxorubicin, cisplatin
DECA	dexamethasone, etoposide, cisplatin, cytarabine
DES	diethylstilbestrol
DeVIC	dexamethasone, etoposide, ifosfamide, carboplatin
DFR	delayed free recall
DFS	disease-free survival
DIBH	deep inspiration breath hold
DIC	disseminated intravascular coagulation
DIL	dominant intraprostatic lesion
DIPG	diffuse intrinsic pontine glioma
DL	dogleg
DLBCL	diffuse large B-cell lymphoma
DLCO	diffusion capacity for carbon monoxide
DLT	dose-limiting toxicity
DM	distant metastasis
DMFS	distant metastasis-free survival
DMFSP	dermatofibrosarcoma protuberans
DMG	diffuse midline glioma
dMMR	deficient mismatch repair
DNA	deoxyribonucleic acid
DOI	depth of invasion
DRE	digital rectal exam
DRTF	disease-related treatment failures
DS	double strength
DSS	disease-specific survival
DTI	direct to implant
DVH	dose volume histogram
DVT	deep vein thrombosis
DWI	diffusion-weighted imaging
EASL	European Association for the Study of the Liver
EAU	European Association of Urology
EBER	Epstein–Barr encoding region
EBRT	external beam radiation therapy
EBUS	endobronchial ultrasound

EBV	Epstein–Barr virus
EC	etoposide, carboplatin
ECE	extracapsular extension
ECF	epirubicin, cisplatin, fluorouracil
ECOG	Eastern Cooperative Oncology Group
ED	erectile dysfunction
EE4A	dactinomycin, vincristine
EES	extraosseous Ewing sarcoma
EFRT	extended-field radiation therapy
EFS	event-free survival
EGFR	epidermal growth factor receptor
EIC	extensive intraductal component
EMR	endoscopic mucosal resection
EMVI	extramural venous invasion
ENE	extranodal extension
ENI	elective nodal irradiation
ENRT	elective nodal radiation therapy
EORTC	European Organisation for Research and Treatment of Cancer
EP	etoposide, cisplatin
EPE	extraprostatic extension
EPO	erythropoietin
EPOCH	etoposide, vincristine, doxorubicin, cyclophosphamide, prednisolone
EPP	extrapleural pneumonectomy
EQ-5D	EuroQol 5 Dimension
EQD2	equivalent dose in 2 Gy per fraction
ER	estrogen receptor
ERCP	endoscopic retrograde cholangiopancreatography
ESB	Ewing sarcoma of bone
ESD	endoscopic submucosal dissection
ESFT	Ewing sarcoma family of tumors
ESMO	European Society for Medical Oncology
ESR	erythrocyte sedimentation rate
ESRD	end-stage renal disease
ESS	endometrial stromal sarcoma
ES-SCLC	extensive stage small cell lung cancer
ESTRO	European Society for Radiotherapy and Oncology
ETE	extrathyroidal extension
ETP	early thymocyte precursor

EUA	exam under anesthesia
EUS	endoscopic ultrasound
EWS	Ewing sarcoma
FAP	familial adenomatous polyposis
FDA	Food and Drug Administration
FDG	fluorodeoxyglucose
FEV1	forced expiratory volume in 1 second
FFBF	freedom from biochemical failure
FFDM	freedom from distant metastases
FFDP	freedom from disease progression
FFLP	freedom from local progression
FFLR	freedom from locoregional recurrence
FFP	freedom from progression
FFS	failure-free survival
FFTF	freedom from treatment failure
FH	favorable histology
FIGC	familial intestinal gastric cancer
FIGO	International Federation of Gynecology and Obstetrics
FIR	favorable intermediate risk
FISH	fluorescence in situ hybridization
FL	follicular lymphoma
FLAIR	fluid attenuated inversion recovery
FLIPI	Follicular Lymphoma International Prognostic Index
FLOT	5-FU, leucovorin, oxaliplatin, docetaxel
F-MISO	18F-fluoromisonidazole
FNA	fine needle aspiration
FOLFIRINOX	fluorouracil, irinotecan, oxaliplatin, leucovorin
FOLFOX	fluorouracil, oxaliplatin, leucovorin
FS	fibrosarcoma
FSH	follicle stimulating hormone
FSRT	fractionated stereotactic radiation therapy
FTC	follicular thyroid cancer
FU	follow-up
fx	fractions
G3/4	grade 3/4
GAPPs	gastric adenocarcinoma and proximal polyposis
GBM	glioblastoma
GC	genomic classifier

GCT	germ cell tumors
GEJ	gastroesophageal junction
GELA	Groupe d'Etude des Lymphomes de l'Adulte
GELOX	gemcitabine, oxaliplatin, L-asparaginase
GEP	gene expression profile
GERD	gastroesophageal reflux disease
GFAP	glial fibrillary acidic protein
GH	growth hormone
GHSG	German Hodgkin Study Group
GI	gastrointestinal
GIST	gastrointestinal stromal tumor
GKRS	Gamma Knife radiosurgery
GLUT-1	glucose transporter 1
GnRH	gonadotropin-releasing hormone
GPA	Graded Prognostic Assessment
GS	Gleason score
GTR	gross total resection
GTV	gross tumor volume
GU	genitourinary
Gy	Gray
GyE	Gray-equivalents
GYN	gynecologic
H&N	head and neck
H&P	history and physical examination
HA	headache
HAART	highly active antiretroviral therapy
HA-PCI	hippocampal avoidance prophylactic cranial irradiation
HA-WBRT	hippocampal avoidance whole brain radiation therapy
HBV	hepatitis B virus
HCC	hepatocellular carcinoma
HCRC	hereditary clear cell renal carcinoma
HCT	hematopoietic cell transplant
HCV	hepatitis C virus
HD	Hodgkin disease
HDGC	hereditary diffuse gastric cancer
HD-MTX	high-dose methotrexate
HDR	high-dose rate
HDR-BT	high-dose rate brachytherapy

HDT	high-dose chemotherapy
HER2	human epidermal growth factor receptor 2
HFSRT	hypofractionated stereotactic radiation therapy
HFX	hyperfractionated radiation therapy
Hgb	hemoglobin
HHV8	human herpesvirus-8
HIF-1α	hypoxia-inducible factor 1-alpha
HIFU	high-intensity focused ultrasound
HIR	high intermediate risk
HIV	human immunodeficiency virus
HL	Hodgkin lymphoma
HNCUP	head and neck cancer of unknown primary
HNPCC	hereditary nonpolyposis colorectal cancer
HNSCC	head and neck squamous cell carcinoma
HO	heterotopic ossification
HPF	high-powered field
HPRC	hereditary papillary cell renal carcinoma
HPV	human papillomavirus
HR	hazard ratio
HR-QoL	health-related quality of life
HSC	hematopoietic stem cell
HSCT	hematopoietic stem cell transplant
HSIL	high-grade squamous intraepithelial lesion
HTLV	human T-cell lymphotropic virus
HVLT	Hopkins Verbal Learning Test
HYP	hyperthermia
Hypofx	hypofractionation
IBC	inflammatory breast cancer
IBD	inflammatory bowel disease
IBE	ipsilateral breast events
IBTR	ipsilateral breast tumor recurrence
ICHD-3	International Classification of Headache Disorders
ICI	immune checkpoint inhibitor
ICP	intracranial pressure
ICR	intracranial recurrence
IDC	invasive ductal carcinoma
IDH	isocitrate dehydrogenase
IDL	isodose line

IDRF	imaging-defined risk factors
IE	ifosfamide, etoposide
IELSG	International Extranodal Lymphoma Study Group
IF	involved-field
IFL	inguinofemoral lymphadenectomy
IFN-α	interferon alfa
IFRT	involved-field radiation therapy
IGF-IR	insulin-like growth factor I receptor
IGRT	image-guided radiation therapy
IGSRT	image-guided superficial radiation therapy
IHC	immunohistochemistry
IJ	internal jugular
ILC	invasive lobular carcinoma
ILD	interstitial lung disease
ILROG	International Lymphoma Radiation Oncology Group
IM	internal mammary
ImmTAC	immune-mobilizing monoclonal T-cell receptor against cancer
IMN	internal mammary node
IMRT	intensity-modulated radiation therapy
INI	involved nodal irradiation
INR	international normalized ratio
INRGSS	International Neuroblastoma Risk Group Staging System
INRT	involved-node radiation therapy
INSS	International Neuroblastoma Staging System
IO	immunotherapy
IORT	intraoperative radiation therapy
IPI	International Prognostic Index
IPS	International Prognostic Score
IPSS	International Prostate Symptom Score
IR	intermediate risk
IRS	Intergroup Rhabdomyosarcoma Study
IRSG	Intergroup Rhabdomyosarcoma Study Group
ISCL	International Society for Cutaneous Lymphomas
ISH	in-situ hybridization
ISRT	involved-site radiation therapy
IT-ADT	intermediate-term androgen deprivation therapy
ITC	isolated tumor cells
ITGCNU	intratubular germ cell neoplasia of unclassified type

ITM	in-transit metastasis
ITT	intention to treat
IV	Intravenous
IVBT	intravascular brachytherapy
IVC	inferior vena cava
JPA	juvenile pilocytic astrocytoma
JRSGC	Japanese Research Society for Gastric Cancer
KPS	Karnofsky Performance Status
LABC	locally advanced breast cancer
LAR	low anterior resection
LC	local control
LC-CRT	long-course chemotherapy and radiation therapy
LCIS	lobular carcinoma in situ
LCNEC	large-cell neuroendocrine carcinoma
LCV	leucovorin
LDH	lactate dehydrogenase
LD-HL	lymphocyte depleted Hodgkin lymphoma
LDR	low-dose rate
LDRT	low-dose radiation therapy
LD-WBRT	low-dose whole brain radiation therapy
LE	local excision
LET	linear energy transfer
LF	local failure
LFS	laryngectomy-free survival
LFT	liver function test
LGG	low-grade gliomas
LH	luteinizing hormone
LHRH	luteinizing hormone-releasing hormone
LINAC	linear accelerator
LIQ	lower inner quadrant
LIR	low intermediate risk
LI-RADS	Liver Imaging Reporting and Data System
LMA	large mediastinal adenopathy
LMD	leptomeningeal disease
LMS	leiomyosarcoma
LN	lymph node
LND	lymph node dissection
LOH	loss of heterozygosity

LOQ	lower outer quadrant
LP	lumbar puncture
LPFS	local progression-free survival
LR	local recurrence
LRC	locoregional control
LRF	locoregional failure
LRFS	local recurrence-free survival
LR-HL	lymphocyte-rich Hodgkin lymphoma
LRR	locoregional recurrence
LS	liposarcoma
LSIL	low-grade squamous intraepithelial lesion
LSRT	local superficial radiation therapy
LSS	limb salvage surgery
LS-SCLC	limited-stage small-cell lung cancer
LT-ADT	long-term androgen deprivation therapy
LUTS	lower urinary tract symptoms
LVI	lymphovascular invasion
LVSI	lymphovascular space invasion
M:F	male-to-female ratio
MAID	mesna, doxorubicin, ifosfamide, dacarbazine
MALT	mucosa-associated lymphoid tissue
MB	medulloblastoma
MCB	multicatheter brachytherapy
MCC	Merkel cell carcinoma
MC-HL	mixed cellularity Hodgkin lymphoma
MDACC	MD Anderson Cancer Center
MDADI	MD Anderson Dysphagia Index
MDH	mean heart dose
MDT	metastasis-directed therapy
MELD	model for end-stage liver disease
MEN1	multiple endocrine neoplasia 1
MEN2	multiple endocrine neoplasia 2
MeV	mega electron volt
MF	mycosis fungoides
MFH	malignant fibrous histiocytoma
mFOLFIRINOX	modified FOLFIRINOX
MFS	metastasis-free survival
MFU	median follow-up

MG	myasthenia gravis
MGMT	methylguanine methyltransferase
MGUS	monoclonal gammopathy of undetermined significance
MI	myometrial invasion
MIBC	muscle-invasive bladder cancer
MIBG	metaiodobenzylguanidine
MIPI	Mantle Cell Lymphoma International Prognostic Index
MKI	Mitosis-Karyorrhexis Index
MLD	mean liver dose
MLO	mediolateral oblique
MM	multiple myeloma
MMC	mitomycin C
MMR	mismatch repair
MMRd	mismatch repair deficient tumors
MMSE	Mini-Mental State Exam
MOPP	nitrogen mustard, vincristine, procarbazine, prednisone
mOS	median overall survival
Mp	multiparametric
MPE	myxopapillary ependymoma
MPEC	multipolar electrocoagulation
mPFS	median progression-free survival
MPM	malignant pleural mesothelioma
MPNST	malignant peripheral nerve sheath tumor
MPV	methotrexate, procarbazine, vincristine
MRCP	magnetic resonance cholangiopancreatography
MRF	mesorectal fascia
MRI	magnetic resonance imaging
MRM	modified radical mastectomy
MS	median survival
mSCC	malignant spinal cord compression
MSI	microsatellite instability
MSKCC	Memorial Sloan Kettering Cancer Center
MSS	melanoma-specific survival
MTC	medullary thyroid cancer
MTD	maximally tolerated dose
MTIC	3-methyl-(triazen-1-yl)imidazole-4-carboximide
MTOL	more than one line
MTX	methotrexate

MUGA	multigated acquisition scan
MUM	multiple myeloma oncogene
MVA	multivariate analysis
MVD	microvascular decompression
MVI	macrovascular invasion
MYC	myelocytomatosis oncogene
MZL	marginal zone lymphoma
NACT	neoadjuvant chemotherapy
NALIRINOX	liposomal irinotecan, oxaliplatin, leucovorin, 5-FU
NASH	nonalcoholic steatohepatitis
NB	neuroblastoma
NCCN	National Comprehensive Cancer Network
NCDB	National Cancer Database
NCF	neurocognitive test failure
NEC	not elsewhere classified
NED	no evidence of disease
NF	neurofibromatosis
NF1	neurofibromatosis type 1
NF2	neurofibromatosis type 2
NFS	neurological functional score
NGGCT	nongerminomatous germ cell tumor
NHL	Non-Hodgkin lymphoma
NHT	neoadjuvant hormonal therapy
NK	natural killer
NK-T-cell	natural killer T-cell
NLP-HL	nodular lymphocyte predominate Hodgkin lymphoma
NMIBC	non–muscle-invasive bladder cancer
NMSC	nonmelanoma skin cancer
NNT	number needed to treat
NOM	nonoperative management
NOS	not otherwise specified
NPC	nasopharyngeal cancer
NPV	negative predictive value
NPVM	nonpulmonary visceral metastases
NPX	nasopharynx
NR	not reached
NS	not statistically significant
NSCLC	non–small-cell lung cancer

NSE	neuron-specific enolase
NSGCT	nonseminomatous germ cell tumor
NS-HL	nodular sclerosis Hodgkin lymphoma
NSMP	no specific molecular profile tumor
nsRPLND	nerve-sparing retroperitoneal lymph node dissection
NTE	normal tissue effects
NTR	near total resection
OA	osteoarthritis
OAR	organs at risk
OCP	oral contraceptive pill
OC-SCC	oral cavity squamous cell carcinoma
OEPA	vincristine, etoposide, prednisone, Adriamycin
OLT	orthotopic liver transplant
OM	overall mortality
OMD	oligometastatic disease
OPC	oropharynx cancer
OPG	osteoprotegerin
OPPA	vincristine, procarbazine, prednisone, Adriamycin
OPTN	Organ Procurement and Transplantation Network
OR	odds ratio
ORR	objective response rate
OS	overall survival
OSHA	Occupational Safety and Health Administration
OTT	overall treatment time
P/D	pleurectomy and decortication
PA	para-aortic
PAB	posterior axillary boost
PAC	cisplatin, doxorubicin, cyclophosphamide
PA-LND	para-aortic lymphadenectomy
PAS	para-aortic strip
PBI	partial breast irradiation
PBrI	partial breast re-irradiation
PBT	proton beam therapy
PCA3	prostate cancer antigen 3
PCI	prophylactic cranial irradiation
PCLBCL	primary cutaneous B-cell lymphoma
PCM	prostate cancer mortality
PCNSL	primary central nervous system lymphoma

pCO2	partial pressure of carbon dioxide
pCR	pathologic complete response
PCR	polymerase chain reaction
PCSM	prostate cancer-specific mortality
PCSS	prostate cancer-specific survival
PCV	procarbazine, lomustine (CCNU), vincristine
PD	progressive disease
PDGF	platelet-derived growth factor
PDR	pulsed dose rate
PDT	photodynamic therapy
PET	positron emission tomography
PET/CT	positron emission tomography/computed tomography
PF	posterior fossa
PFS	progression-free survival
PFT	pulmonary function test
PHQ-9	Patient Health Questionnaire-9
PitNET	pituitary neuroendocrine tumor
PJP	*Pneumocystis jirovecii* pneumonia
PLND	pelvic lymph node dissection
PLNRT	pelvic lymph node radiation therapy
PM	parameningeal
PMMA	polymethyl methacrylate
PMRT	postmastectomy radiation therapy
PN	partial nephrectomy
PNET	primitive neuroectodermal tumors
PNI	perineural invasion
pO2	partial pressure of oxygen
Pola-R-CHP	polatuzumab vedotin-piiq, rituximab, cyclophosphamide, doxorubicin, prednisone
POLE	DNA polymerase-epsilon mutated tumors
PORT	postoperative radiation therapy
PORT	prostate-only radiation therapy
PPD	product of the perpendicular diameters
PPV	positive predictive value
PR	partial response
PRDR	pulsed reduced dose rate
PRL	prolactin
PRT	prospective randomized trial

PRV	planning risk volume
PS	performance status
PSA	prostate-specific antigen
PSADT	prostate-specific antigen doubling time
PSC	primary sclerosing cholangitis
PSMA	prostate-specific membrane antigen
PTC	papillary thyroid cancer
PTCL	peripheral T-cell lymphoma
PTHC	percutaneous transhepatic cholangiography
PTHrP	parathyroid hormone-related protein
PTV	planning target volume
PUVA	psoralen plus ultraviolet A
PVI	protracted venous infusion
Q	quadrantectomy
QALY	quality-adjusted life-years
QD	once daily
QOD	every other day
QOL	quality of life
R0	negative margin resection
R1	microscopically positive margin
R2	macroscopically positive margin
R-ACVBP	rituximab, doxorubicin, cyclophosphamide, vindesine, bleomycin, prednisone
RADS	reporting and data system
RAI	radioactive iodine
RANO	Response Assessment in Neuro-Oncology
Rb	retinoblastoma
RBC	red blood cell
RCC	renal cell carcinoma
R-CHOP	rituximab, cyclophosphamide, doxorubicin, vincristine, prednisone
RCT	randomized controlled trial
R-CVP	rituximab, cyclophosphamide, vincristine, prednisone
Rd	lenalidomide, dexamethasone
RECIST	Response Evaluation Criteria in Solid Tumors
R-EPOCH	rituximab, etoposide, cyclophosphamide, doxorubicin, vincristine, prednisone
RER	rapid early response
re-RT	re-irradiation
REZ	root entry zone
RF	regional failure

RFA	radiofrequency ablation
RFI	recurrence-free interval
RFR	recurrence-free rates
RFS	recurrence-free survival
R-Hyper-CVAD	rituximab, cyclophosphamide, vincristine, doxorubicin, dexamethasone
RILD	radiation-induced liver disease
RM	radical mastectomy
R-MPV	rituximab, methotrexate, procarbazine, vincristine
R-MPV-A	rituximab, methotrexate, procarbazine, vincristine, cytarabine
RMS	rhabdomyosarcoma
RN	radical nephrectomy
RNI	regional nodal irradiation
RP	radical prostatectomy
RPA	recursive partitioning analysis
rPFS	radiographic progression-free survival
RPLND	retroperitoneal lymph node dissection
RPN	retropharyngeal lymph node
RPS	retroperitoneal sarcoma
RR	retrospective review
RRFS	regional relapse-free survival
RS	Reed–Sternberg
RT	radiation therapy
RTK	rhabdoid tumor of the kidney
RTOG	Radiation Therapy Oncology Group
RT-PCR	reverse transcriptase polymerase chain reaction
RUQ	right-upper quadrant
SBO	small bowel obstruction
SBP	selective bladder preservation
SBRT	stereotactic body radiation therapy
SCC	squamous cell carcinoma
SCCUP	squamous cell carcinoma of unknown primary
SCLC	small-cell lung cancer
SCM	sternocleidomastoid
SCPL-CHEP	supracricoid partial laryngectomy with cricohyoidopexy
SC-RT	short-course radiation therapy
SCT	stem cell transplantation
SCV	supraclavicular
SEER	Surveillance, Epidemiology, and End Results

SEP	solitary extramedullary plasmacytoma
SER	slow early response
SES	socioeconomic status
SFRT	spatially fractionated radiation therapy
SGL	supraglottic laryngectomy
SGO	Society of Gynecologic Oncology
SHH	sonic hedgehog
SIB	simultaneous integrated boost
SINS	Spine Instability Neoplastic Score
S-ITM	satellitosis or in-transit metastasis
SLL	small lymphocytic lymphoma
SLN	sentinel lymph node
SLNB	sentinel lymph node biopsy
SMA	superior mesenteric artery
SMAC	Sarcoma Meta-Analysis Collaboration
SMILE	dexamethasone, methotrexate, ifosfamide, L-asparaginase, etoposide
SMT	single modality therapy
SMV	superior mesenteric vein
SND	selective nodal dissection
SNI	selective nodal irradiation
SNUC	sinonasal undifferentiated carcinoma
SOC	standard of care
SOT	solid organ transplant
SPECT	single-photon emission computed tomography
SPEP	serum protein electrophoresis
SP-EPN	spinal ependymoma
SRE	skeletal-related events
SRF	subretinal fluid
SRS	stereotactic radiosurgery
SS	statistically significant
ST	supratentorial
ST-ADT	short-term androgen deprivation therapy
STD	sexually transmitted diseases
STR	subtotal resection
STS	soft tissue sarcoma
SUV	standardized uptake value
SV	seminal vesicles
SVC	superior vena cava

SVI	seminal vesical invasion
SWOG	Southwest Oncology Group
TACE	transcatheter arterial chemoembolization
TACE-DEB	transarterial chemoembolization with drug-eluting beads
TAE	transarterial embolization
TAH/BSO	total abdominal hysterectomy/bilateral salpingo-oophorectomy
TARE	transarterial radioembolization
TBI	total body irradiation
TC	docetaxel, cyclophosphamide
Tc-99m	technetium-99m
TCC	transitional cell carcinoma
TCHP	docetaxel, carboplatin, trastuzumab, pertuzumab
T-DM1	trastuzumab emtansine
TE/I	tissue expander/implant
TERT	telomerase reverse transcriptase
Tg	thyroglobulin
TGF-β	transforming growth factor beta
TGN	trigeminal neuralgia
TIP	paclitaxel, ifosfamide, cisplatin
TKI	tyrosine kinase inhibitor
TL	total laryngectomy
TLM	transoral laser microsurgery
TLM/TOLM	transoral laser microsurgery
TM	total mastectomy
TMB	tumor mutational burden
TME	total mesorectal excision
TMT	Trailmaking Test
TMZ	temozolomide
TNBC	triple-negative breast cancer
TNMB	tumor-node-metastasis-blood
TNT	total neoadjuvant therapy
TORS	transoral robotic surgery
TPCV	thioguanine, procarbazine, lomustine/CCNU, vincristine
TPF	docetaxel, cisplatin, 5-FU
TROG	Trans-Tasman Radiation Oncology Group
TRUS	transrectal ultrasound
TSEBT	total skin electron beam therapy
TSET	total skin electron therapy

TSH	thyroid-stimulating hormone
TSS	transsphenoidal surgery
TTF	tumor treating fields
TUR	transurethral resection
TURBT	transurethral resection of bladder tumor
TURP	transurethral resection of the prostate
TVUS	transvaginal ultrasound
UC	ulcerative colitis
UDES	undifferentiated endometrial sarcoma
UES	upper esophageal sphincter
UH	unfavorable histology
UIQ	upper inner quadrant
UIR	unfavorable intermediate risk
ULN	upper limit of normal
UM	uveal melanoma
UOQ	upper outer quadrant
UPEP	urine protein electrophoresis
UPS	undifferentiated pleomorphic sarcoma
US	ultrasound
USPSTF	U.S. Preventive Services Task Force
UTI	urinary tract infection
UV	ultraviolet
UVA	univariate analysis
UVA1	ultraviolet A1
UVB	ultraviolet B
VA	vincristine and actinomycin D
VAC	vincristine, actinomycin D, cyclophosphamide
VAC/VI	vincristine, actinomycin D, and cyclophosphamide/vincristine and irinotecan
VAI	vincristine, actinomycin D, ifosfamide
VAIN	vaginal intraepithelial neoplasia
VAMP	vincristine, Adriamycin, methotrexate, prednisone
VATS	video-assisted thoracoscopic surgery
VBT	vaginal brachytherapy
VCR	vincristine
VDC	vincristine, doxorubicin, cyclophosphamide
VDCA	vincristine, doxorubicin, cyclophosphamide, actinomycin
VEGF	vascular endothelial growth factor
VHL	von Hippel–Lindau

VI	vincristine, ifosfamide
VI/DECA	vinorelbine, ifosfamide, dexamethasone, etoposide, cisplatin, cytarabine
VIE	vincristine, ifosfamide, etoposide
VIN	vulvar intraepithelial neoplasia
VIP	vasoactive intestinal peptide
VMA/HVA	vanillylmandelic acid/homovanillic acid
VNPI	Van Nuys Prognostic Index
VP Shunt	ventriculoperitoneal shunt
VRd	bortezomib, lenalidomide, dexamethasone
VS	vestibular schwannoma
VTC	vincristine, topotecan, cyclophosphamide
VTE	venous thromboembolism
W&W	watch and wait
WAI	whole abdominal irradiation
WBI	whole breast irradiation
WBRT	whole brain radiation therapy
WE	wide excision
WHO	World Health Organization
WLE	wide local excision
WLI	whole lung irradiation
WPOI	worst pattern of invasion
WPRT	whole pelvic radiation therapy
WT	Wilms tumor
WVI	whole ventricular irradiation
XP	xeroderma pigmentosum
XR	x-ray
yr	year

INDEX